PeriAnesthesia Nursing Core Curriculum

Preprocedure, Phase I and Phase II PACU Nursing

American Society of PeriAnesthesia Nurses

PeriAnesthesia Nursing Core Curriculum

- Preprocedure,
- Phase I and Phase II
- PACU Nursing

SECOND EDITION

Lois Schick, MN, MBA, RN, CPAN, CAPA
PeriAnesthesia Nurse Consultant
Per Diem Staff Nurse
Exempla Lutheran Medical Center
Wheatridge, Colorado

Pamela E. Windle, MS, RN, NE-BC, CPAN, CAPA, FAAN
Nurse Manager
St. Luke's Episcopal Hospital
Houston, Texas

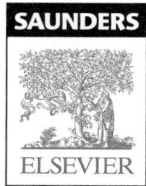

SAUNDERS

ELSEVIER

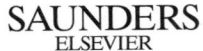

SAUNDERS
ELSEVIER

3251 Riverport Lane
St. Louis, Missouri 63043

PERIANESTHESIA NURSING CORE CURRICULUM:
PREOPERATIVE, PHASE I AND PHASE II PACU NURSING   978–1–4160–5193–0
Copyright © 2010 by Saunders, an imprint of Elsevier Inc.

Notice

Knowledge and best practice in this field are constantly changing. As new research and experience broaden our knowledge, changes in practice, treatment and drug therapy may become necessary or appropriate. Readers are advised to check the most current information provided (i) on procedures featured or (ii) by the manufacturer of each product to be administered, to verify the recommended dose or formula, the method and duration of administration, and contraindications. It is the responsibility of the practitioner, relying on their own experience and knowledge of the patient, to make diagnoses, to determine dosages and the best treatment for each individual patient, and to take all appropriate safety precautions. To the fullest extent of the law, neither the Publisher nor the Authors assumes any liability for any injury and/or damage to persons or property arising out of or related to any use of the material contained in this book.

The Publisher

Previous edition copyrighted 2004

Library of Congress Cataloging-in-Publication Data
American Society of PeriAnesthesia Nurses.
    Perianesthesia nursing core curriculum : preprocedure, phase I, and phase II PACU nursing/ American Society of PeriAnesthesia Nurses ; Lois Schick, Pamela E. Windle. – 2nd ed.
       p. ; cm.
    Includes bibliographical references and index.
    ISBN 978–1–4160–5193–0 (pbk. : alk. paper) 1. Post anesthesia nursing. 2. Clinical competence. 3. Postoperative care. I. Schick, Lois. II. Windle, Pamela E. III. Title.
    [DNLM: 1. Postanesthesia Nursing–education–Outlines. 2. Clinical Competence–standards–Outlines. 3. Postoperative Care–education–Outlines. 4. Postoperative Care–nursing–Outlines. WY 18.2 A5128p 2010]
    RD51.3A43 2010
    617′.919–dc22   2009033174

Acquisitions Editor: Tamara A. Myers
Publishing Services Manager: Deborah Vogel
Project Manager: Brandilyn Tidwell
Designer: Karen Pauls

Printed in the United States
Last digit is the print number: 9 8 7 6 5 4 3 2 1

To my parents and 11 older siblings, who have always encouraged me to just be "me." I thank them for their support, love, guidance, and for being there throughout the years. A special thank you to all nurses I have worked with and have had the opportunity to share nursing stories with over the years.

Lois Schick

To all perianesthesia nurses, especially my staff in the Post Anesthesia Care Unit (PACU) and Surgical Observation Unit (SOU) at St. Luke's Episcopal Hospital, Houston, Texas, who for the past 25 years have consistently shown commitment in their daily practices, shared their knowledge, and provided me with their expertise and insights. Working with them to provide the best postoperative care management for all types of patients has been a great privilege and an honor.

To David, my husband, and my two children, Cynthia and Michael, for their understanding of my dedication and love of my career, and for their support and patience throughout this endeavor; as well as to my brothers Junior, Alan, Peter, and Philip, and sisters Elsie, Jane, and Tina, and especially to my loving parents, Mary and Lorenzo, who believed in me! Thank you all!

Pamela E. Yang Windle

CONTRIBUTORS

JENNIFER ALLEN, MSQSM, RN, CPAN
Department Head
Post Anesthesia Care Unit
National Naval Medical Center
Bethesda, Maryland

SUSAN M. ANDREWS, MA, BAN, RN, CAPA
Perioperative Manager
Medical College of Georgia Health System
Augusta, Georgia

MEG BETURNE, MSN, RN, CPAN, CAPA
Perianesthesia Coordinator
Baystate Orthopedic Surgery Center
Springfield, Massachusetts

COURTNEY BROWN, MSN, CCRN, CRNA
Clinical Education Coordinator
Nurse Anesthesia Program
Wake Forest University Baptist Medical
    Center
Winston Salem, North Carolina

NANCY BURDEN, MS, RN, CPAN, CAPA
Director of Ambulatory Surgery
Bay Care Health System
Trinity, Florida

THERESA L. CLIFFORD, MSN, RN, CPAN
Perianesthesia Staff Nurse/Educator
Post Anesthesia Care Unit
Mercy Hospital
Portland, Maine

LAURA CURRIE, MS, RN
Clinical Specialist
Baystate Medical Center
Springfield, Massachusetts

JANE C. DIERENFIELD, BSN, RN, CPAN, CAPA
Kona Community Hospital
Kealakekua, Hawaii

KATHLEEN P. DONOHUE, BSN, RN, CAPA
Nurse Manager
Baltimore Washington Medical Center
Glen Burnie, Maryland

KATHLEEN FALKENSTEIN, PhD, RN, CCTC, PNP-BC
Assistant Professor
Drexel University
College of Nursing and Health Professions
Philadelphia, Pennsylvania

ROSE FERRARA-LOVE, MSN, RN-BC, CNE
Nursing Faculty
AKMC – Citizens School of Nursing
New Kensington, Pennsylvania

SUSAN JANE FETZER, PhD, MBA, RN
Associate Professor
College of Health and Human Services
University of New Hampshire
Durham, New Hampshire

SUSAN FOSSUM, BSN, RN, CPAN
CNIV, Staff Developer
Post Anesthesia Care Unit /Operating Room
University of California, Davis Medical Center
Sacramento, California

BARBARA A. GODDEN, MHS, RN, CPAN, CAPA
PACU Clinical Nurse Coordinator
Sky Ridge Medical Center
Lone Tree, Colorado

SUSAN GOODWIN, MS, RN, CNS, CPAN
Clinical Nurse Specialist
OU Medical Center
Oklahoma City, Oklahoma

GARY M. GUSICK, PhD, RN, CCNS
Clinical Nurse Specialist
St. Luke's Episcopal Hospital
Houston, Texas

VALLIRE D. HOOPER, PhD, RN, CPAN, FAAN
Assistant Professor
PhD Program Assistant
School of Nursing, Medical College of Georgia
Augusta, Georgia

BECKI L. HOYLE, RN, CPAN, CAPA
Patient Care Coordinator/Clinical Nurse
    Educator
Post Anesthesia Care Unit
Medical Center of the Rockies
Loveland, Colorado

SEEMA S. HUSSAIN, BSN, RN, CAPA
Staff Nurse
National Naval Medical Center
Bethesda, Maryland

H. LYNN KANE, MSN, MBA, RN, CCRN
Clinical Nurse Specialist
Thomas Jefferson University Hospital
Philadelphia, Pennsylvania

DINA A. KRENZISCHEK, PhD, MAS, RN, CPAN
Nurse Manager
Johns Hopkins Hospital
Baltimore, Maryland

LAURA S. KRIEGER, BS, RN, CCRN
Education Consultant
Med Ed Consulting Corporation
Littleton, Colorado

MAUREEN E. LISBERGER, BS, RN, CCRN, CPAN
PACU Nurse
Presbyterian St. Luke's Medical Center
Denver, Colorado

MYRNA E. MAMARIL, MS, RN, CPAN, CAPA, FAAN
Nurse Manager
Johns Hopkins Hospital
Baltimore, Maryland

LYNDA MARKS, RN, CAPA
Nurse Informatics
Littleton Adventist Hospital
Littleton, Colorado

REX A. MARLEY, MS, CRNA, RRT
Chief Nurse Anesthetist
Northern Colorado Anesthesia Professional
    Consultants
Fort Collins, Colorado

DONNA R. McEWEN, BSN, RN, CNOR
Senior Instructional Designer
Independent Perioperative Nursing
    Consultant
Optum Health, United Health Care
San Antonio, Texas

MAUREEN F. McLAUGHLIN, MS, RN, CPAN, CAPA
Clinical Educator
Post Anesthesia Care Unit
Lahey Clinics
Burlington, Massachusetts

BONNIE NIEBUHR, MS, RN, CAE
Chief Executive Officer, ABPANC
New York, New York

KIM A. NOBLE, PhD, RN, CPAN
Temple University, Department of Nursing
College of Health Professions
Philadelphia, Pennsylvania

DENISE O'BRIEN, MSN, RN, ACNS-BC, CPAN, CAPA, FAAN
Clinical Nurse Specialist
Post Anesthesia Care Unit
Department of Operating Rooms
Ypsilanti, Michigan

JAN ODOM-FORREN, PhD, RN, CPAN, FAAN
Instructor
University of Kentucky
Lexington, Kentucky;
Perianesthesia Consultant
Staff RN, Phase II Recovery
Baptist Hospital East
Louisville, Kentucky

NANCY O'MALLEY, MA, RN, CPAN, CAPA
Perioperative Clinical Educator
Perioperative Services
Parker Adventist Hospital
Parker, Colorado

JUDITH H. POOLE, MBA/MHA, RNC-OB, EFM
Nurse Manager
Birthing Care/Special Maternity Care
Presbyterian Hospital
Matthews, North Carolina

DONNA M. DEFAZIO QUINN, MBA, BSN, RN, CPAN, CAPA
Director Orthopaedic Surgery Center
Concord, New Hampshire

MARY (CONNIE) REDMOND, MSN, RN, CAPA
Former Staff Nurse
Alegent Health Bergan Mercy Medical Center
Omaha, Nebraska

WANDA RODRIGUEZ, MA, RN, CCRN, CPAN
Clinical Nurse Specialist
Post Anesthesia Care Unit
Memorial Sloan-Kettering Cancer Center
New York, New York

JACQUELINE M. ROSS, MSN, RN, CPAN
Patient Safety Analyst
Perianesthesia Consultant
Ohio IDTC
Columbus, Ohio

NANCY M. SAUFL, MS, RN, CPAN, CAPA
Coordinator Preadmission Testing
    Department
Florida Hospital Memorial System
Ormond Beach, Florida

MAUREEN SCHNUR, MS, RN, CPAN
Nurse Manager, Perioperative Programs
Children's Hospital Boston
Boston, Massachusetts

JUDY STEVENSON, BSN, RN, CCRN, CEN
Clinical Instructor
St. John Medical Center
Tulsa, Oklahoma

KERRIE K. TALBOT, BSN, RN
Clinical Education Specialist
Day Surgery/Post Anesthesia Care Unit
Connecticut Children's Medical Center
Hartford, Connecticut

JOANNE E. THOMPSON, MSN, RNC-OB, CNS
Perinatal Clinical Nurse Specialist
Presbyterian Hospital
Matthews, North Carolina

SARA N. WALDRON, BSN, RN, CPAN
Clinical Staff Registered Nurse
Post Anesthesia Care Unit
Unit Education Coordinator
Carondelet St. Joseph's Hospital
Tucson, Arizona

VALERIE S. WATKINS, BSN, RN, CAPA
Clinical Nurse IV
PreProcedure Services
University of Colorado Hospital
Aurora, Colorado

LINDA WILSON, PhD, RN, CPAN, CAPA, BC, CNE
Assistant Professor
College of Nursing and Health Professions
Drexel University
Philadelphia, Pennsylvania

KENNETH D. WITCHER, ASN, RN
Clinical Nurse Specialist
National Naval Medical Center
Bethesda, Maryland

REVIEWERS

JENNIFER ALLEN, MSQSM, RN, CPAN
Department Head
Post Anesthesia Care Unit
National Naval Medical Center
Bethesda, Maryland

SUSAN M. ANDREWS, MA, BAN, RN, CAPA
Perioperative Manager
Medical College of Georgia Health System
Augusta, Georgia

SANDRA BARNES, MS, RN, CPAN
Associate Director of Clinical Operations
Westchester Medical Group
White Plains, New York

MARCIA BIXBY, MS, RN, CS, CCRN
Critical Care Clinical Nurse Specialist
Randolph, Massachusetts

AIDA P. CADORNA, BA, BSE, RN, CCRN, CPAN
Nurse Clinician IV
Post Anesthesia Care Unit
St. Luke's Episcopal Hospital
Houston, Texas

KAREN CANNON, MN, RN, CAPA
Retired Nurse
Bozeman, Montana

SHELLY L. CANNON, BSN, RN, CPAN
Staff Nurse Pre-surgery/Post Anesthesia
    Care Unit
Exempla Lutheran Medical Center
Wheat Ridge, Colorado

MARTHA L. CLARK, MSN, RN, CPAN
University Pointe Surgical Hospital
West Chester, Ohio

THERESA L. CLIFFORD, MSN, RN, CPAN
Perianesthesia Staff Nurse/Educator
Post Anesthesia Care Unit
Mercy Hospital
Portland, Maine

MARCIA CORY, RN, CPAN
Patient Care Services Manager
Kaiser Permanente Sacramento Medical Center
Sacramento, California

KATHY DALEY, MSN, RN, CNS, CCRN, CMC-CSC, CPAN
Cardiovascular Clinical Specialist
Mission Hospitals
Clinical Support and Development
Ashville, North Carolina

JoANN DESELMS, RN, CAPA
Staff Nurse Ambulatory Surgery Post
    Anesthesia Care Unit
Exempla Lutheran Medical Center
Wheat Ridge, Colorado

SUSAN JANE FETZER, PhD, MBA, RN
Associate Professor
College of Health and Human Services
University of New Hampshire
Durham, New Hampshire

MARJORIE A. GEISZ-EVERSON, PhD, CRNA
Instructor, School of Nursing
Louisiana State University Health Sciences
    Center
New Orleans, Louisiana

JUDY GRAHAM-GARCIA, MN, CRNA
Chief, Anaesthesia Association of
    Massachusetts
CRNA Northshore Medical Center
Salem, Massachusetts;
Part-time Faculty
Boston College
Chestnut Hill, Massachusetts

BARBARA A. HANNAH, EdD, MS, RN, CPAN
Nursing Education Program Manager
Department of Nursing Education
Jane Phillips Medical Center
Bartlesville, Oklahoma

BECKI HOYLE, RN, CPAN, CAPA
Patient Care Coordinator/Clinical Nurse
    Educator
Post Anesthesia Care Unit
Medical Center of the Rockies
Loveland, Colorado

MAUREEN V. IACONO, BSN, RN, CPAN
Nurse Manager
Post Anesthesia Care Unit
St. Joseph's Hospital
Syracuse, New York

DOLLY IRELAND, MSN, RN, CAPA, CPN
Clinical Nursing Educator
Perianesthesia Surgical Services
Ambulatory Service
Mount Clemens Regional Medical Center
Mount Clemens, Michigan

SUSAN M. IRVIN, DNP, ACNS-BC, CAPA
Retired Nurse
Bartlett, Tennessee

KIM KRAFT, BSN, RN, CPAN
Perianesthesia Nurse Clinician
Surgical Services
St. John's Mercy Medical Center
St. Louis, Missouri

DIANA M. LIND, DO
Ophthalmologist
Lind Eye Care
Kearney, Nebraska

JAN LOPEZ, BSN, RN, CPAN, CAPA
Clinical Resource Nurse
Post Anesthesia Care Unit
St. Luke's Hospital
Kansas City, Missouri

KANDACE K. MAIER, BSN, RN, NP, CPAN
Staff Nurse Post Anesthesia Care Unit
Sky Ridge Medical Center
Lone Tree, Colorado

MYRNA MAMARIL, MS, RN, CPAN, CAPA, FAAN
Nurse Manager
Johns Hopkins Hospital
Baltimore, Maryland

KATHLEEN J. MENARD, MS, RN, CPAN, CAPA
Clinical Nurse III
Interventional Radiology
UMass Memorial Medical Center –
   Memorial Campus
Worcester, Massachusetts

DANIEL D. MOOS, MS, CRNA
Nurse Anesthetist
Kearney Anesthesia Associates PC
Kearney, Nebraska;
Adjunct Faculty/Clinical Instructor
School of Nurse Anesthesia
Bryan LGH College of Health Sciences
Lincoln, Nebraska

DEBBY NIEHAUS, BSN, RN, CPAN
Clinical Nurse III
TriHealth – North Perioperative Services
Bethesda North Ambulatory Surgery Center
Cincinnati, Ohio

ERNESTINE NUNES, RN, CPAN, CNOR
Surgical Services Educator
Post Anesthesia Care Unit/Operating
   Room/Short Stay Surgery
Hanford Community Medical Center
Hanford, California

NANCY O'MALLEY, MA, RN, CPAN, CAPA
Perioperative Clinical Educator
Perioperative Services
Parker Adventist Hospital
Denver, Colorado

AMELIA PACARDO, BSN, RN, CCRN, CPAN
Nurse Clinician IV
Post Anesthesia Care Unit
St. Luke's Episcopal Hospital
Houston, Texas

ELLEN L. POOLE, PhD, RN, CCRN, CPAN
Professor of Nursing
Chamberlain College of Nursing
Phoenix, Arizona

EMILIE A. RAMOS, BSN, RN, CCRN, CPAN
Nurse Clinician IV
Post Anesthesia Care Unit
St. Luke's Episcopal Hospital
Houston, Texas

MARY (CONNIE) REDMOND, MSN, RN, CAPA
Former Staff Nurse
Alegent Health Bergan Mercy
   Medical Center
Omaha, Nebraska

WANDA RODRIGUEZ, MA, RN, CCRN, CPAN
Clinical Nurse Specialist
Post Anesthesia Care Unit
Memorial Sloan-Kettering Cancer Center
New York, New York

JACQUELINE M. ROSS, MSN, RN, CPAN
Patient Safety Analyst
Perianesthesia Consultant
Ohio IDTC
Columbus, Ohio

NANCY M. SAUFL, MS, RN, CPAN, CAPA
Coordinator Preadmission Testing
   Department
Florida Hospital Memorial System
Ormond Beach, Florida

ALLAN SCHWARTZ, DDS, CRNA
Dentist/Nurse Anesthetist
Heartland Dental Care ProDental
Columbia, Missouri

MARY SEITENBACH, BSN, RN, CPAN
Chest Pain Center Coordinator
Exempla Good Samaritan Medical Center
Lafayette, Colorado

LYNN SEKERES, MSN, RN, CCRN, CPAN
Staff Nurse Phase I Post Anesthesia Care
    Unit
University of Pittsburgh Medical
    Center – Montefiore
Pittsburgh, Pennsylvania

CHERIE A. SLOAN, BSN, RN, CPAN
Staff Nurse
Kaiser Permanente
Anaheim, California

DAPHNE STANNARD, PhD, RN, CCRN, CCNS, FCCM
PeriAnesthesia Clinical Nurse Specialist
Perioperative Division
University of California San Francisco
    Medical Center
San Francisco, California

VALERIE S. WATKINS, BSN, RN, CAPA
Clinical Nurse IV
PreProcedure Services
University of Colorado Hospital
Aurora, Colorado

ANNETTE S. WILLIAMS, BSN, RN, CPAN
Staff Nurse/Phase I Post Anesthesia Care
    Unit
Memorial Hospital at Gulfport
Gulfport, Mississippi

LINDA WILSON, PhD, RN, CPAN, CAPA, CNE, BC
Assistant Professor
College of Nursing and Health Professions
Drexel University
Philadelphia, Pennsylvania

FOREWORD

The American Society of PeriAnesthesia Nurses (ASPAN) is pleased to offer this second edition of the *PeriAnesthesia Nursing Core Curriculum*. While the roots of nursing knowledge are embedded in day-to-day practice, seeds of change in care delivery models and constant transformations in medicine have driven the need to update this essential text. This edition provides updated subject matter for the wide range of perianesthesia practices and has been created by clinical experts in perianesthesia nursing.

The core tenets in this curriculum are intended to provide guidance to cover the spectrum of perianesthesia nursing, from preoperative or preprocedural assessments and planning to day-of-surgery or procedure care, through phase I and phase II levels of care. In addition, these concepts of practice are intended to offer guidance regardless of the location of that care. This includes the acute care setting, ambulatory or free-standing facilities, and office based practices, to name a few. New topics are integrated throughout the text to reflect a growing body of evidence and to address emerging trends in care. Improvements in this edition include the grouping of the physiology and assessment of related body systems with the respective surgical or procedural principles to make these chapters complete, self-contained references. Two new chapters include coverage of the latest information on "Postoperative and Postdischarge Nausea and Vomiting" and "Bariatric Care."

ASPAN's most strategic goal is to be recognized as the leading association for perianesthesia education, nursing practice, standards, and research. The depth and value this edition will bring towards that goal is immense. As a core curriculum, it will provide guidance for nurses seeking certification, a map for creating unit based competencies, reference for clinical orientation of new staff and new perianesthesia nurses, as well as a resource for the fundamentals and standards of practice.

ASPAN offers this text as a comprehensive review for the assessment and care of patients of all ages presenting with a wide variety of medical findings, surgeries, and procedures in all phases and settings of perianesthesia care.

Theresa Clifford, MSN, RN, CPAN
ASPAN President 2009-2010

PREFACE

The specialty of perianesthesia nursing is performed in a variety of settings. Once practiced only in the "recovery room," nurses now care for perioperative and postprocedure patients in an array of surroundings—hospital-based and freestanding. Perianesthesia nursing encompasses caring for patients during the preanesthesia phase (preadmission and day of procedure), in PACUs (phase I and II), ambulatory care settings, extended observation settings, and special procedure areas (endoscopy, radiology, cardiovascular, oncology, etc.), labor and delivery suites, pain management services, and physician and dental offices. Nurses caring for perianesthesia patients need to possess a variety of skills and expertise. Patients undergoing operative and invasive procedures come to the facility either as a planned event or an emergency. Being able to assess the patient, develop an individualized plan of care, implement the plan, and evaluate the results requires proficiency in perianesthesia nursing.

This review text is designed to be a resource for nurses working in the perianesthesia setting. It is intended to cover perianesthesia knowledge essential to practice in both the hospital-based or freestanding settings. Regardless of individual practice settings, there is a group of core competencies essential to providing good nursing care. This text is divided into seven sections to address those competencies:
- Professional Competencies
- Environment of Care
- Life Span Considerations
- Competency of Preoperative Assessment
- Core Competencies of PACU Nursing
- Surgical Specialties
- Ambulatory Surgical Nursing Competencies

This text is also a resource for nurses preparing to take either the CPAN or CAPA certification examination. Certification in one's specialty is a way to promote quality of care to the general public, the nursing profession, and the individual nurse. When a nurse achieves certification in his or her specialty, this demonstrates commitment to his or her nursing career, provides tremendous personal satisfaction, and provides opportunities for career advancement.

The text uses an outline format to delineate areas of perianesthesia nursing practice. The text is not designed to be a complete study guide. The nurse must identify his or her own areas of strengths and weaknesses, seek out additional resources, and develop an individualized study plan that will meet his or her needs.

Although designed to assist nurses in preparation of the CPAN or CAPA examination, this book can be used for other purposes such as:
- A study guide for nurses new to the perianesthesia setting
- Development of an orientation plan for the PACU
- Development of perianesthesia nursing competencies
- A reference guide for student nurses rotating through the PACU

The chapter authors are experts in their fields of practice, and many of them are certified in their specialties. The information presented in this text is as accurate and current as possible. Each chapter has been reviewed to ensure accuracy. The development of this core curriculum was sponsored by and supported by the American Society of PeriAnesthesia Nurses (ASPAN).

Lois Schick and Pam Windle

ACKNOWLEDGMENTS

This second edition of the *Core Curriculum* has been updated with two new chapters to reflect evidence based practice. These chapters, "Postoperative Nausea and Vomiting," and "Bariatric Care," provide updated current practice concepts. Evidence-based practices were added to the Research chapter. Revisions were made to the surgical specialties chapters to combine care concepts. In this edition, inception to its final reality, we encountered numerous challenges but none so monumental that they could not be overcome. We wish to thank the previous authors and our current authors who contributed chapters, as well as to the reviewers who provided insightful suggestions and recommendations for updating each chapter in this second edition. The time, energy, and dedication that each author and reviewer exhibited is a reflection of their devotion to our nursing specialty.

We wish to thank Tamara A. Myers, Acquisition Editor at Elsevier, for her expertise in coordinating this project. Words cannot describe our gratitude for her continued assistance and support. She was always there with encouragement and words of kindness, keeping us on track to get the project done.

Our sincere appreciation goes to Brandi Tidwell, Project Manager at Elsevier, for her dedication in assisting each chapter author with any desired changes in their manuscript and getting the final proofs ready in a timely manner. Her assistance in getting the final product to print on time is greatly appreciated. We extend our gratitude to the numerous other members of Elsevier's team and thank them for bringing this project to fruition.

We could not have accomplished the re-write of this book without the opportunity provided by the American Society of PeriAnesthesia Nurses (ASPAN) to recognize the continued need for an updated evidenced based core curriculum. This text will assist the perianesthesia nurse in enhancing his or her knowledge and skills in preparation for taking their certification examination(s) and for providing comprehensive care to patients and families.

A special thank you goes to my two sisters Jean Newton and Lavonne Hougen who were there over the past 2 years to encourage and support me while editing this book. Thank you to the ASPAN 2008-2009 Board of Directors for their understanding and support during my presidency year. Without their support and encouragement, this would have been an impossible task for me. I cannot thank Donna Quinn, the first Core Curriculum co-editor, and our new co-editor Pam Windle, as well as Tamara Myers at Elsevier, enough for their expertise and support during this time of writing.

Lois Schick

A special thank you to my husband David Windle for his patience, support, and understanding of the dedicated weekends spent editing this book. Thank you also to my mentor and teacher Lois Schick for her assistance as co-editor, and Tamara Myers for her continual support and encouragement.

Pam Windle

CONTENTS

PROFESSIONAL COMPETENCIES

1 Evolution of Perianesthesia Care

JAN ODOM-FORREN
THERESA L. CLIFFORD

OBJECTIVES

At the conclusion of this chapter, the reader will be able to:

1. Describe three of the earliest recovery rooms.
2. Name the decade when recovery rooms became commonplace.
3. Name the one historical event that contributed most to the advent of recovery rooms.
4. Name three advances in medical technology that led to an increase in ambulatory surgeries.
5. List three reasons for consumer acceptance of ambulatory surgery.
6. Describe the development of the American Society of PeriAnesthesia Nurses (ASPAN).
7. Describe three benefits brought to perianesthesia nursing by ASPAN.

I. EARLY BEGINNINGS
  A. Early beginnings of recovery room and ambulatory surgery
    1. Trephining of the skull and amputations identified in the year 3500 B.C. as evidenced by cave drawings
    2. New Castle Infirmary, New Castle, England (1751): rooms reserved for dangerously ill or major surgery patients
    3. Florence Nightingale, London, England (1863): separate rooms for patients to recover from immediate effects of anesthesia
    4. Ambulatory surgeries performed at Glasgow Royal Hospital for Sick Children in Scotland from 1898 to 1908
      a. Surgeries were performed on 8988 children.
      b. Surgeries included orthopedic problems, cleft lip and cleft palate, spina bifida, skull fracture, hernias, and others.
      c. None of the children required hospital admission.
    5. Information from Glasgow Hospital presented at a meeting of the British Medical Association in 1909
    6. Twentieth century
      a. First general anesthesia in ambulatory surgery reported in Sioux City, Iowa, in 1918
      b. 1920s and 1930s: complexity of surgeries increased
      c. 1923: Johns Hopkins Hospital, Baltimore, Maryland, three-bed neurosurgical recovery unit opened by Dandy and Firor
      d. World War II: recovery units created to provide adequate level of nursing care during nursing shortage
      e. 1942: Mayo Clinic, Rochester, Minnesota
      f. 1944: New York Hospital
      g. 1945: Ochsner Clinic, New Orleans, Louisiana
      h. 1940s and 1950s: early ambulation after surgery came into acceptance

    B. Value of recovery room demonstrated in improving surgical care
      1. Anesthesia Study Commission of the Philadelphia County Medical Society report (1947): one third of preventable postsurgical deaths during an 11-year period could have been eliminated by improved postoperative nursing care.
      2. Operating Room Committee for New York Hospital (1949) stated that adequate recovery room service was necessary for any hospital that provided surgical services.
II. ACCEPTANCE AND DECLINE OF RECOVERY ROOMS
    A. Impact of changing technology on patient care
      1. 1950s: more knowledge of common postanesthesia complications
      2. 1950s and 1960s: growth of surgical intensive care and postoperative respiratory support
      3. Expanding complex surgical procedures
      4. Expanding technology led to outpatient complex surgeries.
        a. Microscopic surgeries abounded
        b. New lasers were developed (yttrium argon gas, argon, carbon dioxide).
        c. New laparoscopic instruments facilitated shorter, less invasive laparoscopic procedures.
        d. More endoscopic procedures were being performed as outpatient procedures.
        e. Video equipment and computer-assisted surgeries were now being performed.
        f. Fiberoptics led to advances in ophthalmic surgeries, most of which are performed in outpatient settings.
      5. Change in anesthesia techniques and medications
      6. 1970s: recovery rooms managed routine postanesthesia patients, including ambulatory, routine, and critically ill patients receiving respiratory and circulatory support.
      7. Many diagnostic procedures done in ambulatory settings
        a. X-ray procedures
        b. Laboratory tests
        c. Physical therapy
        d. Cardiopulmonary tests
        e. Pain blocks
    B. Recovery rooms lose viability and identity.
      1. Staffing: shortage of skilled personnel
      2. No organized body of knowledge pertinent to postanesthesia
        a. Staff performance evaluated on the basis of trial and error
        b. No territorial restrictions: in some places considered to be extension of operating room
        c. No established standards of care
III. AMBULATORY SURGERY FOCUS
    A. Ambulatory surgery programs established
      1. The nation's first ambulatory surgery program opened at Butterworth Hospital in Grand Rapids, Michigan, in 1961, and staff performed 879 ambulatory surgeries between 1963 and 1964.
      2. A formal ambulatory surgery program began at the University of California–Los Angeles in 1962.
      3. In 1968, the Dudley Street Ambulatory Surgery Center opened in Providence, Rhode Island.
      4. The nation's first freestanding surgery facility was opened in 1970 by Dr. Wallace Reed and Dr. John Ford in Phoenix, Arizona.
        a. In 1971, the American Medical Association endorsed the use of surgicenters.
        b. In 1974, the Society for the Advancement of Freestanding Ambulatory Surgery was formed, which was the precursor for the current Federated Ambulatory Surgery Association (FASA).
      5. The American Society for Outpatient Surgeons (now known as American Association of Ambulatory Surgery Centers) was formed in 1978, paving the way for surgery being performed in doctors' offices.

      a. The 1980s brought a shortage of inpatient hospital beds.

      b. In 1980, the Omnibus Budget Reconciliation Act authorized reimbursement for outpatient surgery.

      c. In 1981, the American College of Surgeons (ACS) approved the concept of ambulatory surgery units (ASUs) as preadmission units for scheduled inpatients.

      d. In 1983, Porterfield and Franklin advocated for office outpatient surgery.

      e. The Society for Ambulatory Anesthesia was formed in 1984.

B. The ambulatory surgery concept proliferated in the 1980s.

    1. Hospital-affiliated ambulatory surgery accounted for 9.8 million operations (45%) performed within hospital settings by 1987.

    2. By 1988, 984 freestanding outpatient surgery centers performed more than 1.5 million surgical operations.

    3. By 1989, there were 984 Medicare-participating freestanding ambulatory surgery centers in the United States.

    4. The list of approved procedures that can be conducted in surgery centers was expanded in 1987 by the Health Care Financing Administration (HCFA), now known as the Centers for Medicare and Medicaid Services.

    5. In 1989, HCFA revised the payment schedule for outpatient surgeries performed on Medicare patients.

C. Freestanding recovery sites

    1. In 1979, the first freestanding recovery care center opened in Phoenix, Arizona.

      a. Patients were transported directly to the recovery care center from hospital post anesthesia care units (PACUs), from the ASU, and from physicians' offices.

      b. Some patients were transferred there from hospitals on their second or third postoperative day.

    2. The limits of stay for recovery care centers are defined by state regulation.

    3. In the 1980s, the concept of 23-hour units led to guest services being developed for patients living more than 1 hour away from the site where the surgery was to be performed (hospital hotels; medical motels).

      a. Freestanding medical motels are considered a comfortable, affordable, convenient place to recuperate.

      b. Patients are cared for by family members.

      c. Home health nurses make visits, or a nurse is stationed onsite.

    4. In 1996, data from the National Center for Health Statistics Data Center

      a. An estimated 31.5 million surgical and nonsurgical procedures were performed during 20.8 million ambulatory visits in 1996.

      b. An estimated 17.5 million (84%) of the ambulatory surgery visits were in hospitals and 3.3 million (16%) were in freestanding centers in 1996.

      c. In 2000, 63% of all surgeries were performed in outpatient settings.

    5. In 2005, there were more than 4200 ambulatory surgery centers that provided over 12 million surgeries annually.

D. Economics of ambulatory surgery

    1. Cost control, a primary force in the development of ambulatory surgery

      a. In 1988, 58% of surgery centers contracted with health maintenance organizations and 52% with preferred provider organizations.

      b. In 1990, the American Hospital Association reported that more than 50% of all hospital-based surgical procedures were done on an outpatient basis.

      c. In the 1990s, 23 home observation units (recovery centers) were established in the United States.

      d. The percentage of outpatient procedures approved for payment under Medicare increased.

        (1) In 1982, 450 procedures approved

        (2) By the early 1990s, 2500 approved procedures

        (3) On July 1, 2003, 282 additional procedures added

e. Third-party payers require many surgeries to be performed in an ambulatory setting to avoid the cost of hospitalization.

f. Many freestanding centers have contractual arrangements with managed care plans, rehabilitation centers, and nursing homes.

g. Outpatient facilities eliminate the costs of cafeteria, laundry, and the need for 24-hour staffing.

h. Outpatient procedures eliminate unnecessary lab, x-ray, and electrocardiogram services.

i. Patients recovering in 23-hour units are considered nonhospitalized for purposes of reimbursement by Medicare and third-party payers.

E. Legislation encouraged growth of ambulatory centers.

  1. Relaxation of legislation began to occur in the 1980s.

  2. By 1987, the Omnibus Budget Reconciliation Act provided for less reimbursement to hospitals, providing rates equal to those for ambulatory surgery centers.

  3. The Omnibus Budget Reconciliation Act of 1989 again increased the reimbursement rates for assigned surgical procedures in ambulatory centers.

  4. Ambulatory centers became certified by accepted certifying agencies.

F. Consumer acceptance of ambulatory surgery

  1. Awareness

    a. Increased marketing led to increased consumer awareness.

    b. Greater awareness led to greater demand for surgery in ambulatory settings.

    c. Consumers saw more physician involvement in ambulatory settings.

    d. Patient consumers felt more involved and took part in decisions.

    e. Few problems were seen with quality of care.

  2. Convenience

    a. Flexible hours

    b. Early admission and same-day discharge

    c. Less time lost from work

    d. Units easily accessible

  3. Wellness philosophy well accepted

    a. Patients could walk to the operating room.

    b. Patients could recover on stretchers or in recliners.

    c. Parents could remain with children during induction; parents and sometimes families could be present postoperatively.

    d. Patients were able to keep dentures, eyeglasses, and hearing aids with them.

    e. Patients felt more involved in decision-making for their care.

    f. Family visitation encouraged in phase I PACUs

  4. Reimbursement

    a. Reimbursement provided by Medicare for outpatient procedures for the elderly made ambulatory surgery a viable alternative.

    b. Employers were paying less, and consumers found ambulatory settings less expensive, making outpatient surgery an attractive option.

IV. EMERGENCE OF ORGANIZED RECOVERY ROOM GROUPS

A. Need to identify a special body of knowledge and skills required for practice

  1. Groups form to develop educational opportunities.

    a. Nineteen groups organized in United States

    b. Florida Society of Anesthesiologists initiated yearly seminar in 1969.

      (1) Attended by nurses from United States and Canada

      (2) Dr. Frank McKechnie: very supportive of recovery room nurses

  2. Series of seminars sponsored by American Society of Anesthesiologists (ASA)—1970s

    a. Supported by solid attendance and strong interest from nurses in the specialty

    b. Interest shown in development of recovery room nursing organization

   B. Local and state organizations form national group.
      1. Regional nursing representatives met with ASA Care Team to organize national postanesthesia nurses' association.
      2. Goals established
         a. Education for postanesthesia nurses
         b. Recognition of postanesthesia nursing as a specialty
      3. 1979: steering committee formed
         a. Selection of name: American Society of Post Anesthesia Nurses (ASPAN)
         b. Preparation of bylaws
         c. Incorporation
         d. First ASPAN president: Ina Pipkin, RN, from Seattle, Washington
      4. First meeting of board of directors held October 1980, in Orlando, Florida
      5. April 1982: charter for component status granted to Alabama and Florida
 V. FIRST YEARS (October 1980 to April 1982)
   A. Financial development
      1. ASA grant for legal expenses
      2. Membership dues
   B. Internal organization developed.
      1. Committees appointed.
      2. Newsletter, *Breathline*, begun in 1981.
      3. Membership increased.
         a. First national conference planned.
         b. Regional educational meetings held.
VI. ASPAN DEVELOPMENTS
   A. Publications
      1. 1981: *Breathline* (ASPAN's newsletter)
      2. 1983: *Guidelines for Standards of Care*
      3. 1984: *Post Anesthesia Nursing Review for Certification*
      4. 1986: *Standards of Nursing Practice*
      5. 1986: *Journal of Post Anesthesia Nursing (JoPAN)*
      6. 1986: *Redi-Ref*, ed 1
      7. 1990: *Fifty Years of Progress in Post Anesthesia Nursing 1940-1990*
      8. 1991: *Standards of Post Anesthesia Nursing Practice*
      9. 1991: *Core Curriculum for Post Anesthesia Nursing Practice*, ed 2
     10. 1992: *Standards of Post Anesthesia Nursing Practice*
     11. 1992: *ASPAN Resource Manual*
     12. 1993: *Postanesthesia and Ambulatory Surgery Nursing Update* (WB Saunders, publisher)
     13. 1994: Pediatrics added to *Redi-Ref*
     14. 1994: *ASPAN Resource Manual* published in collaboration with American Board of Post Anesthesia Nursing
     15. 1994: *Ambulatory Post Anesthesia Nursing Outline: Content for Certification*
     16. 1995: *Core Curriculum for Post Anesthesia Nursing Practice*, ed 3
     17. 1995: *Standards of Perianesthesia Nursing Practice*
     18. 1996: *Certification Review for Perianesthesia Nursing*
     19. 1996: *Research Primer*
     20. 1997: *Competency Based Orientation and Credentialing program*, ed 1
     21. 1998: *Redi-Ref*, ed 2
     22. 1998: *Standards of Perianesthesia Nursing Practice*. New additions include:
         a. Guidelines for preadmission phase
            (1) Preadmission
            (2) Day of surgery/procedure
         b. Guidelines for phase III (addresses ongoing care for those patients requiring extended observations/interventions after transfer/discharge from phase I or phase II)
         c. New position statements

      (1) "Minimum Staffing in Phase I PACU"
      (2) "Registered Nurse Use of Unlicensed Assistive Personnel"
      (3) "Intensive Care Unit (ICU) Overflow Patients"

23. 1999: Core Curriculum for Ambulatory Perianesthesia Nursing Practice
24. 1999: Core Curriculum for Perianesthesia Nursing Practice, ed 4
25. 1999 Position statements
    a. "Fast Tracking"
    b. "Pain Management"
    c. "On Call/Work Schedule"
26. 2000 *Standards* included a "Joint Position Statement on ICU Overflow Patients," developed by ASPAN, American Association of Critical Care Nurses (AACN), and ASA's Anesthesia Care Team Committee and Committee on Critical Care Medicine and Trauma Medicine.
27. 2001: *Competency Based Orientation and Credentialing Program for the Unlicensed Assistive Personnel in the Perianesthesia Setting*, ed 1
28. 2002: *Standards* included position statement on the "Nursing Shortage."
29. 2003: *Competency Based Orientation and Credentialing Program*, ed 2
30. 2003: *Prevention of Unplanned Perioperative Hypothermia Guidelines*
31. 2003: *Pain and Comfort Clinical Practice Guidelines* and *Resource Manual*
32. 2003 Position Statements approved included:
    a. "Medical/Surgical Overflow Patients in the PACU and Ambulatory Care Unit"
    b. "Visitation in Phase I Level of Care"
    c. "Smallpox Vaccination Programs"
33. 2003: *Breathline* approved for online access
34. 2004: *Redi-Ref*, ed 3
35. 2004: *PeriAnesthesia Nursing Core Curriculum: Preoperative, Phase I and Phase II PACU Nursing*, ed 1
36. August 2005: *ASPAN'S Evidence-Based Practice Model* introduced
37. 2006: *Evidence-Based Clinical Practice Guideline for the Prevention and/or Management of PONV/PDNV*
38. *2006-2008 Standards of PeriAnesthesia Nursing Practice.* Additions include:
    a. "The Joint Commission Universal Protocol for Preventing Wrong Site, Wrong Procedure, Wrong Person Surgery"
    b. New position statements:
      (1) "Safe Medication Administration"
      (2) "Cultural Diversity and Sensitivity in Perianesthesia Nursing Practice"
      (3) "Perianesthesia Safety"
39. December 2007: ASPAN's Safety Model introduced, "Perianesthesia Nursing's Essential Role in Safe Practice," published in *JoPAN*
40. 2007: *Competency Based Orientation and Credentialing Program for the Unlicensed Assistive Personnel in the Perianesthesia Setting*, ed 2
41. February 2008: *ASPAN's Perianesthesia Data Elements Model* introduced
42. *2008-2010 Standards of PeriAnesthesia Nursing Practice*
    a. "Smallpox Vaccination Program" position statement retired
    b. New position statements:
      (1) "The Geriatric Patient"
      (2) "Advocacy"
43. 2009: *A Competency Based Orientation and Credentialing Program for the Registered Nurse in the PeriAnesthesia Setting*, ed 2
44. 2009: *ASPAN PeriAnesthesia Data Elements (PDE)*
45. 2009: *ASPAN Safety Toolkit*
46. 2009: *Evidence Based Clinical Practice Guideline for the Promotion of Perioperative Normothermia*
47. 2009: *New additional position statements*
    a. "The Pediatric Patient"
    b. "The Workplace Violence"
48. 2009: *"Go Green" initiatives*
    a. *Breathline* – only available online
    b. ASPAN Educational syllabus – only available online

B. Certification
   1. 1985: American Board of Post Anesthesia Nursing Certification (ABPANC) established (see Appendix A)
   2. Certification examination developed to recognize knowledge and skill of practitioners
   3. November 1986: certification examination first administered, 172 nurses certified
   4. Annual certified postanesthesia nurse recognition day at national conference
   5. 1991: certification examination expanded to include ambulatory surgery nurses who work in preoperative and phase II areas
   6. 1993-1994: separate certification examinations under development for phase I PACU nurses and ambulatory postanesthesia nurses: Certified postanesthesia nurse (CPAN) and certified ambulatory postanesthesia nurse (CAPA) designations
   7. November 1994: CAPA examination first administered
   8. 1996: name changed to American Board of PeriAnesthesia Nursing Certification (ABPANC)
   9. 1998: 4191 CPANs, 1183 CAPAs, and 100 with dual certification
   10. 2003: 3921 CPANs, 1730 CAPAs, and 202 with dual certification
   11. 2008: 5371 CPANs, 3210 CAPAs, and 297 with dual certification
   12. 2009: Computer Based Testing for CPAN and CAPA started
C. Education
   1. 1982: national conference and annual educational program started
   2. Regional core curriculum workshops (2-day program available)
   3. Regional ambulatory surgery workshops
   4. Regional interpersonal and leadership skills workshops
   5. ASPAN videotapes: overviews of postanesthesia nursing
   6. 1993: national ASPAN Lecture Series established
   7. 1993: joint ASPAN/Association of periOperative Registered Nurses (AORN) Ambulatory Surgery Symposium
   8. 1994: cosponsored Governmental Affairs Workshop with American Association of Nurse Anesthetists (AANA), AORN, and the American Veterans Association of Nurse Anesthetists
   9. September 1994: sponsored first Volunteer Leadership Institute in Richmond, Virginia
   10. 1997: patient education videos on general anesthesia, conscious sedation, and regional anesthesia developed
   11. Continuing education articles available in *JoPAN*
   12. 1998: Consensus Conference for Perioperative Normothermia held in Bethesda, Maryland
   13. 2001: Consensus Conference for Pain and Comfort held in Nashville, Tennessee
   14. 2008: second consensus meeting for Normothermia guideline held in St. Louis, Missouri
D. Specialty representation
   1. Member of National Federation for Specialty Nursing Organizations (NFSNO) since June 1983
      a. 1990: Federation presidents invited for Nurses Day Luncheon given by Barbara Bush at the White House with ASPAN President attending
   2. Member of National Organization Liaison Forum (NOLF)
   3. Established official liaison with ASA
   4. Official liaisons with following organizations
      a. Society of Gastroenterology Nurses and Associates
      b. Society of Critical Care Medicine
      c. FASA
   5. Increased networking with the following
      a. AANA
      b. AORN
      c. AACN

6. 1992: organizational affiliate of American Nurses Association (ANA)
7. 1994-1996: ASPAN elected to NFSNO Executive Board
8. 1994: ASPAN elected to NOLF Board
9. 1994: ASPAN represented at AORN Perioperative World Conference in Adelaide, Australia
10. Nursing Summit held in Chicago—a coalition of all nursing leadership to discuss Nursing's Agenda for Healthcare Reform
11. September 2000: ASPAN started the first Component Development Institute, focusing on leadership, education, research, clinical practice, and advocacy
12. 2003: NOLF and NFSNO combine to form new organization of the Alliance: Nurses Organizations Alliance.
13. Fall 2002: ASPAN president represented at the 10th Congress of the Cuban Nursing Society and the first Colloquium on Natural and Traditional Medicine in Havana, Cuba.
14. 2004: ASPAN partners with the AANA, American Association of Surgical Physician Assistants, ACS, ASA, AORN, and the Association of Surgical Technologists to form the Council on Surgical and Perioperative Safety (CSPS), dedicated to promote a culture of patient safety and a caring perioperative workplace environment.
15. 2003: ASPAN begins partnership with the British Anaesthetic and Recovery Nurses Association (BARNA), and seven ASPAN delegates attended the BARNA Conference
16. July 2006: ASPAN represented at the Nursing Terminology Summit, Nashville, Tennessee
17. September 2006: ASPAN represented at the first summit of the newly formed Society for Perioperative Assessment and Quality Improvement
18. October 2006: ASPAN president invited for the first time to attend the ACS in Chicago
19. October 2007: ASPAN president participated in the Irish Anaesthetic and Recovery Nurses Association Conference and began a partnership in Waterford, Ireland.
20. November 2007: two ASPAN past presidents were co-leaders for the 2007 People to People delegation to China
21. May 2008: ASPAN president participated in Canadian conference.

E. Other highlights
1. 1983: members encouraged to change name of workplace from recovery room to PACU
2. 1989: postanesthesia nurse awareness week established
3. 1989: definition of immediate postanesthesia nursing expanded to include preoperative and phase II areas to incorporate ambulatory nurses working only in those areas
4. 1989: presidential award established
5. 1989: AACN formally recognized postanesthesia nursing as a critical care specialty.
6. 1991: clinical excellence and outstanding achievement awards established
7. 1991: ASPAN becomes an ANA approver and provider of continuing education.
8. 1992-1993: research committee offers grants and conducted the first Delphi study to establish postanesthesia and ambulatory surgery nursing priorities.
9. 1993: ASPAN Foundation established with first board of trustees
10. 1993: organizational task force appointed to look at size and structure of ASPAN Board, dues structure, and membership voting
11. 1994: approved concept of specialty practice groups
12. 1994: Ontario, Canada, becomes ASPAN's first affiliate member.
13. 1994: online communication by means of Internet between officers and national office

14. 1995: change of ASPAN's name to American Society of PeriAnesthesia Nurses approved, effective July 1, 1996
15. 1995: funds for first scholarship awards donated by the ASPAN Foundation
16. 1996: one dues structure initiated (one payment includes national and component membership)
17. 1996: ASPAN website created (www.aspan.org)
18. 1996: *Journal of Post Anesthesia Nursing* name changed to *Journal of PeriAnesthesia Nursing*
19. April 10, 1997: newly structured board of directors met for first time in Denver, Colorado, after the ASPAN Conference.
20. 1997: ASPAN Foundation receives seat, and ASPAN member attends AANA Foundation Research Scholars Program.
21. April 21, 1998: first meeting of the ASPAN Representative Assembly at National Conference in Philadelphia
22. 2006-2007: ASPAN Safe Staffing Group conducted a multidisciplinary meeting and developed an ASPAN Fatigue Checklist as a guide for members.
23. 2007: ASPAN Research Committee conducted the second Delphi study for ASPAN members' research priorities.
24. 1998: ASPAN membership is more than 10,000 with 40 components.
25. 2008: ASPAN membership is 13,403.

F. Specialty interest groups
  1. Preoperative Assessment, chartered 1996-1997
  2. Management, chartered 1998-1999
  3. Pain Management, chartered 1999-2000
  4. Publications, chartered 2002-2003
  5. Pediatric, chartered 2003-2004
  6. Geriatric, chartered 2004-2005
  7. Advanced Degree, chartered 2004-2005
  8. Perianesthesia Nurse Educator, chartered 2007-2008

G. Past presidents of ASPAN and national conference themes
  1. Ina Pipkin, 1982; First National Conference
  2. Hallie Ennis, 1983; Nurses in Action
  3. Jeanne Maher, 1984; New Horizons
  4. Marilyn Glaser, 1985; Caring, Sharing, and All That Jazz
  5. Clara Conn, 1986; Spirit of 86
  6. Meg Danielson Alexander, 1987; ASPAN Directions for Change
  7. Jane Sutton, 1988; Challenge of Excellence
  8. Anne Allen, 1989; Magic of Caring
  9. Deborah Johnson, 1990; Sailing into the Future
  10. Debby Niehaus, 1991; Bridging Knowledge and Growth
  11. Cindy Smith, 1992; In Session
  12. Jan Odom-Forren, 1993; Goldmine of Knowledge
  13. Dolly Ireland, 1994; Reaching for Excellence
  14. Denise O'Brien, 1995; Champions of Caring
  15. Lois Roberts, 1996; Proud Past, Bright Future
  16. Terry McLean, 1997; Attaining New Heights, Change and Transition
  17. Lisa Jeran, 1998; Professional Growth through Knowledge and Fitness
  18. Maureen Iacono, 1999; New Milestones in a New Millennium
  19. Myrna Mamaril, 2000; Creating Visions for the Future
  20. Nancy Saufl, 2001; Making the Connection Through Teaching, Touch, and Technology
  21. Susan Shelander, 2002; Transforming Vision into Reality, Our Journey, Our Legacy
  22. Linda Wilson, 2003; Reach Beyond the Horizon—Make Dreams a Reality
  23. Sandra Barnes, 2004; Circles of Influence—Shaping Tomorrow's Definition of Perianesthesia Nursing

24. Dina Krenzischek, 2005; Vision in Action—Values, Power, Unity, Passion
25. Meg Beturne, 2006; Perianesthesia Nursing Diversity—Touch the World That Touches You
26. Pamela Windle, 2007; Soaring on the Magical Journey to Excellence
27. Susan Fossum, 2008; Be the Voice—Advocacy Through Education, Practice, Research, and Legislative Involvement
28. Lois Schick, 2009; Dreams Create Lasting Legacies
29. Theresa Clifford, 2010; Roots of Knowledge, Seeds of Transformation

BIBLIOGRAPHY

1. American Society of Post Anesthesia Nurses: *Fifty years of progress in post anesthesia nursing 1940–1990*, Richmond, VA, 1990, The Society.
2. American Society of Post Anesthesia Nurses: *ASPAN resource manual*, Richmond, VA, 1992, The Society.
3. Aquavella JV: Ambulatory surgery in the 1990s. *J Ambul Care Manage* 13(1):21–24, 1990.
4. Barone CP, Pablo CS, Barone GW: A history of the PACU. *J Perianesth Nurs* 19(4):237–241, 2003.
5. Bendixen H, Kinney J: History of intensive care: American College of Surgeons. In Kinney JM, Bendixen HH, Powers SR Jr, eds: *Manual of surgical intensive care*, Philadelphia, 1977, WB Saunders.
6. Burden N: Outpatient surgery: A view through history. *J Perianesth Nurs* 20(6):435–437, 2005.
7. Burden N: PACU nursing: Our today, our tomorrows. *J Post Anesth Nurs* 3(4):222–228, 1988.
8. Burden N, Quinn D, O'Brien D, et al: *Ambulatory surgical nursing*, ed 2, Philadelphia, 2000, WB Saunders.
9. Clifford TL, Windle PE, Wilson L: ASPAN perianesthesia data elements: The model. *J Perianesth Nurs* 23(1):49–52, 2008.
10. DeFazio-Quinn D, editor: *Ambulatory surgical nursing core curriculum*, Philadelphia, 1999, WB Saunders.
11. Drain CB, Odom-Forren J: *Perianesthesia nursing: A critical care approach*, ed 5, St Louis, 2008, WB Saunders.
12. Dunn F, Shupp M: The recovery room: A wartime economy. *Am J Nurs* 43(3):279–281, 1943.
13. Feeley TW, Macario A: The postanesthesia care unit. In Miller R, ed: *Anesthesia*, ed 6, New York, 2004, Churchill Livingstone.
14. Fetzer SJ: Practice characteristics of the dual certificant: CPAN/CAPA, *J Perianesth Nurs* 12(4):240–244, 1997.
15. Frost E, editor: *Post anesthesia care unit: Current practices*, ed 2, St Louis, 1990, Mosby.
16. Kozak LJ, Hall RP, Lawrence L: Ambulatory surgery in the United States, 1994. In *Centers for Disease Control and Prevention: Advance data*, Hyattsville, MD, 1997, National Center of Health Care Statistics.
17. Krenzischek D, Clifford TL, Windle PE, et al: Patient safety: Perianesthesia nursing's essential role in safe practice. *J Perianesth Nurs* 22(6):385–392, 2007.
18. Litwack K: *Post anesthesia care nursing*, ed 2, St Louis, 1995, Mosby.
19. Luczun ME: Postanesthesia nursing: Past, present, and future. *J Post Anesth Nurs* 5(4):282–285, 1990.
20. Mamaril ME, Ross JM, Krenzischek D, et al: The ASPAN's EBP conceptual model: Framework for perianesthesia practice and research. *J Perianesth Nurs* 21(3):157–167, 2006.
21. Niebuhr BH, Muenzen P: Foundation for newly revised CPAN and CAPA certification examinations. *J Perianesth Nurs* 16(3):163–173, 2001.
22. Ruth H, Haugen F, Grove DD: Anesthesia study commission. *JAMA* 135(14):881–884, 1947.
23. Schneider M: Trends in postanesthesia nursing. *J Post Anesth Nurs* 2(3):183–188, 1987.
24. Surgical Center Association: *Meeting America's surgical needs*. Available at: www.ascassociation.org/openhouse/Surgicalneeds.pdf. Accessed July 12, 2008.
25. Wetchler BV: *Anesthesia for ambulatory surgery*, ed 2, Philadelphia, 1990, Lippincott.
26. White PF: *Outpatient anesthesia*, New York, 1990, Churchill Livingstone.

2 Standards for Ethical Practice

BARBARA A. GODDEN

OBJECTIVES
At the conclusion of this chapter, the reader will be able to:

1. Describe the importance of standards as they relate to perianesthesia nursing practice.
2. Describe the contents of the American Society of PeriAnesthesia Nurses (ASPAN) Standards of Perianesthesia Nursing Practice.
3. Define competency-based practice.
4. Identify important ethical principles.
5. List the steps for ethical decision-making.

I. DEFINITION OF STANDARD
   A. Established by authority, custom, or general consent
   B. Model for quality or quantity
   C. Standardized for everyone
   D. Determined by what a reasonably prudent nurse acting under the same circumstance would do
   E. Describes the responsibilities for which the nursing profession is accountable
   F. Provides direction for professional nursing practice
   G. Framework for the evaluation of care
II. EVOLUTION OF NURSING STANDARDS
   A. Before 1950
      1. Florence Nightingale
      2. Reports of court cases
   B. *Code of Ethics* published by the American Nurses Association (ANA) in 1950
      1. Nursing care without prejudice
      2. Confidential care
      3. Safe care
   C. Standards of professional nursing practice
      1. Pertain to general or specialty practice
      2. First generic nursing standards in 1973 by the ANA Congress for Nursing Practice
      3. Specialty standards followed beginning in 1974.
III. SOURCES OF STANDARDS
   A. Accrediting organizations
      1. The Joint Commission (TJC)
      2. Accreditation Association for Ambulatory Healthcare
      3. American Association for the Accreditation of Ambulatory Surgical Facilities
   B. ANA
   C. Hospital policies and procedures
   D. Specialty organizations
   E. Nursing texts and articles
   F. Common practice

IV. STANDARD CRITERIA
  A. Standard: authoritative statement articulated and disseminated by the profession by which the quality of practice, service, or education can be judged
  B. Rationale: delineates the importance to perianesthesia practice
  C. Outcome: measures the results of activity (per The Joint Commission, care should meet the same standards of practice wherever the care is provided)
  D. Criteria: describes principles and actual activities used in implementing practices to meet the standard
V. ANA STANDARDS—*NURSING: SCOPE AND STANDARDS OF PRACTICE*
  A. Original standards published in 1973
  B. Apply to all registered nurses in clinical practice
  C. Standards of care: describe a competent level of nursing care
    1. Assessment: collect pertinent patient health information
    2. Diagnosis: analyze assessment data to determine nursing diagnosis
    3. Outcome identification: identify individualized expected patient outcomes
    4. Planning: develop a plan of care specific for the patient
    5. Implementation: implement nursing interventions identified in the plan of care
    6. Evaluation: evaluate patient's outcomes on an ongoing basis
  D. Standards of professional performance: describe a competent level of behavior in the professional role
    1. Quality of care: systematic evaluation of the quality and effectiveness of the nursing practice
    2. Performance appraisal: evaluate own nursing practice with professional practice standards and any relevant regulations
    3. Education: maintain current knowledge and competency in nursing practice
    4. Collegiality: interact and contribute to the professional development of peers and other health care providers
    5. Ethics: decision-making and advocating ethical actions on behalf of the patient
    6. Collaboration: work together with other heath care providers, the patient, and family for patient care
    7. Research/evidence-based practice (EBP): review and incorporate research and EBP findings into daily nursing care
    8. Resource utilization: utilize research findings for individualized patient care
VI. AGENCY FOR HEALTHCARE RESEARCH AND QUALITY, FORMERLY THE AGENCY FOR HEALTHCARE POLICY AND RESEARCH
  A. Established in 1989
  B. Goal to enhance quality, appropriateness, effectiveness of health care
  C. Standard of practice: patients will receive care according to the standard
  D. Guideline: to guide practitioners, patients, and consumers in health care decisions
  E. First guidelines in 1992: *Acute Pain Management* goals:
    1. Reduce the incidence and severity of patients' acute postoperative or posttraumatic pain.
    2. Educate patients about the need to communicate unrelieved pain.
    3. Enhance patient comfort and satisfaction.
    4. Contribute to fewer postoperative complications and shorter lengths of stay.
VII. *STANDARDS OF PERIANESTHESIA NURSING PRACTICE 2008–2010*
  A. ASPAN history of standards
    1. 1983: *Guidelines for Standards of Care* published
    2. 1986: *Standards of Nursing Practice* published
    3. 1989: definition expanded to include preoperative and phase II areas
    4. 1991: *Standards of Post Anesthesia Nursing Practice* published; included data for initial, ongoing, and discharge assessment for phase I and phase II
    5. 1992: *Standards of Post Anesthesia Nursing Practice* published
    6. 1995: *Standards of Perianesthesia Nursing Practice* published; included preanesthesia, preprocedural, phase I and phase II postanesthesia information

  7. 1998: *Standards of Perianesthesia Nursing Practice,* revised; included the addition of postanesthesia phase III for patients requiring extended observation

  8. 2000: *Standards of Perianesthesia Nursing Practice,* revised

  9. 2002: *Standards of Perianesthesia Nursing Practice,* revised

  10. 2004: *Standards of Perianesthesia Nursing Practice,* revised

  11. 2006: *Standards of Perianesthesia Nursing Practice,* revised

  12. 2008: *Standards of Perianesthesia Nursing Practice,* revised

B. Perianesthesia nursing scope of practice

 1. Assessment, diagnosis, intervention, evaluation of physical and psychosocial problems, and risk for problems resulting from the administration of sedation, analgesia, and/or anesthetic agents and techniques

 2. Nursing practice is systematic in nature and includes:

  a. Nursing process

  b. Decision-making

  c. Analytical and scientific thinking

  d. Inquiry

 3. The scope of practice includes, but is not limited to:

  a. Preanesthesia level of care

   (1) Preadmission

   (2) Day of surgery/procedure

  b. Postanesthesia levels of care

   (1) Phase I

   (2) Phase II

   (3) Extended observation

 4. The environment of care includes, but is not limited to:

  a. Hospitals

  b. Ambulatory surgery units (ASUs)/centers

  c. Procedure areas (i.e., cardiology, electroconvulsive therapy, GI/endoscopy, interventional and diagnostic radiology, oncology, pain management, etc)

  d. Labor and delivery

  e. Office-based settings

C. Perianesthesia nursing encompasses the following continuum of care:

 1. Preanesthesia phase

  a. Preadmission: preparation, interviewing, assessment, identification of potential or actual problems

  b. Day of surgery/procedure: validation of existing information; completion of preparation

 2. Postanesthesia phase I: immediate postanesthesia period; basic life-sustaining needs, constant vigilance

 3. Postanesthesia phase II: prepare the patient/significant other for home or extended care environment

 4. Extended observation (formerly phase III): provide ongoing care for patients requiring extended observation/intervention after discharge from phase I or phase II

D. The scope of perianesthesia nursing practice is regulated by:

 1. Hospital or facility policies and procedures

 2. State and federal regulatory agencies

 3. National accreditation bodies

 4. Professional nursing organizations

E. Perianesthesia nursing interacts with other professional groups to advance the delivery of quality care. These groups include but may not be limited to:

 1. American Association of Colleges of Nursing (AACN)

 2. American Association of Critical Care Nurses (AACN)

 3. American Association of Nurse Anesthetists (AANA)

 4. American Association of Surgical Physician Assistants (AASPA)

 5. American Board of Perianesthesia Nursing Certification (ABPANC)

 6. American College of Surgeons (ACS)

      7. ANA
      8. American Radiologic and Interventional Nurses (ARIN)
      9. American Society of Anesthesiologists (ASA)
    10. American Society of Pain Management Nurses (ASPMN)
    11. American Society of Plastic Surgery Nurses (ASPSN)
    12. Anesthesia Patient Safety Foundation (APSF)
    13. Association of Surgical Technologists (AST)
    14. Association of Women's Health, Obstetric and Neonatal Nurses (AWHONN)
    15. Association of periOperative Registered Nurses (AORN)
    16. British Anaesthetic & Recovery Nurses Association (BARNA)
    17. Council on Surgical and Perioperative Safety (CSPS)
    18. Foundation for Ambulatory Surgery Association (FASA)
    19. Irish Anaesthetic & Recovery Nurses Association (IARNA)
    20. National Association of Perianesthesia Nurses of Canada (NAPNC)
    21. National League for Nursing (NLN)
    22. National Student Nurses Association (NSNA)
    23. Nursing Organizations Alliance (NOA)
    24. Society for Ambulatory Anesthesia (SAA)
    25. Society of Gastroenterology Nurses and Associates (SGNA)
    26. Society for Perioperative Assessment and Quality Improvement (SPAQI)
    27. Society of Office-Based Anesthesia (SOBA)

F. Perianesthesia standards for ethical practice
    1. Specific context in which to apply the ANA *Code of Ethics*
    2. Moral commitment to uphold values and ethical obligations related to perianesthesia nursing
    3. Strive to ensure:
      a. Competency
        (1) Maintains personal accountability
        (2) Participates in professional continuing education
        (3) Adheres to ASPAN's standards
        (4) Complies with institutional policies and procedures
        (5) Accepts responsibility/accountability
        (6) Participates in performance improvement
        (7) Uses competency-based orientation
        (8) Remains current on new products/procedures
        (9) Practices with compassion and respect
       (10) Incorporates research and evidence into practice
      b. Responsibilities to patients
        (1) Provides quality care
        (2) Adheres to safe patient practices
        (3) Explains procedures
        (4) Maintains patient confidentiality
        (5) Participates in patient teaching
        (6) Answers questions accurately
        (7) Communicates pertinent information
        (8) Respects advance directives
        (9) Provides communication aids
       (10) Advocates for spiritual comfort
       (11) Respects patient's decisions
       (12) Protects patients from harm
       (13) Advocates for patients
       (14) Delegates tasks appropriately
       (15) Aggressively provides pain control/comfort measures
       (16) Includes the patient's family and/or support system
       (17) Evaluates the patient's environment for safety
       (18) Ensures that all patients are cared for by a registered nurse

      c. Professional responsibilities
        (1) Adheres to national regulations, standards, facility policies, procedures
        (2) Provides comparable level of care regardless of physical setting
        (3) Discusses patient information appropriately
        (4) Maintains accurate patient records
        (5) Safeguards patient confidentiality/information
        (6) Participates in activities that contribute to development of the nursing profession
        (7) Promotes certification
        (8) Acts as a mentor/preceptor
        (9) Demonstrates responsible management of resources
        (10) Maintains an awareness of changing practice issues
        (11) Recognizes a need to care for one's self
        (12) Follows policies, procedures, and laws to protect patients
        (13) Identifies/reports unethical practice
      d. Collegiality
        (1) Collaborates with peers, colleagues, and other health care providers
        (2) Promotes respectful relationships with colleagues
      e. Research
        (1) Identifies problems to be considered for research
        (2) Obtains appropriate institutional review board approvals
        (3) Protects the rights of research participants
        (4) Protects patient confidentiality
        (5) Uses evidence and findings to support clinical practice
G. Standards
    1. Standard I: Patient rights
    2. Standard II: Environment of care
    3. Standard III: Staffing and personnel management
    4. Standard IV: Performance improvement
    5. Standard V: Research
    6. Standard VI: Assessment
    7. Standard VII: Planning and implementation
    8. Standard VIII: Evaluation
H. ASPAN Clinical Practice Guidelines
    1. ASPAN *Clinical Guideline for the Prevention of Unplanned Perioperative Hypothermia*
    2. ASPAN *Clinical Guideline for Pain and Comfort*
    3. ASPAN *Clinical Guideline for Postoperative Nausea and Vomiting/Postdischarge Nausea and Vomiting*
I. Resources in the ASPAN 2008-2010 *Standards of Perianesthesia Nursing Practice*
    1. Nine provisions of the ANA *Code of Ethics for Nurses With Interpretive Statements*
    2. Patient classification and recommended staffing guidelines
      a. Preanesthesia phase
        (1) Preadmission
        (2) Day of surgery/procedure
      b. Postanesthesia phase
        (1) Phase I level of care
        (2) Phase II level of care
      c. Extended observation level of care
      d. Blended levels of care
    3. Components of initial, ongoing, and discharge assessment and management
      a. Preadmission
      b. Day of surgery/procedure
      c. Initial assessment: phase I
      d. Ongoing assessment and management: phase I
      e. Discharge assessment: phase I

       f. Initial assessment: phase II

       g. Ongoing assessment and management: phase II

       h. Discharge assessment: phase II

       i. Initial/ongoing/discharge assessment and management: extended observation

    4. Recommended equipment for preanesthesia phase, post anesthesia care unit (PACU) phase I, phase II, and extended observation

    5. ASA standards

       a. "Statement on Routine Preoperative Laboratory and Diagnostic Screening"

       b. ASA "Basic Standards for Preanesthesia Care"

       c. ASA "Standards for Postanesthesia Care"

    6. Competent support staff

    7. ANA position statement: "Role of the Registered Nurse in the Management of Analgesia by Catheter Techniques (Epidural, Intrathecal, Intrapleural, or Peripheral Nerve Catheters)"

       a. AWHONN Position Statement: "Role of the Registered Nurse in the Care of the Pregnant Woman Receiving Analgesia/Anesthesia by Catheter Techniques (Epidural, Intrathecal, Spinal, PCEA Catheters)"

    8. "The Role of the Registered Nurse in the Management of Patients Undergoing Sedation for Short-Term Therapeutic, Diagnostic or Surgical Procedures"

    9. Safe transfer of care

    10. ASPAN 2006 Internet resources

    11. TJC *Universal Protocol for Preventing Wrong Site, Wrong Procedure, Wrong Person Surgery*

    12. Recommended Competencies for the Perianesthesia Nurse

    13. Resource for Infection Control

  J. ASPAN position statements in the *2008-2010 ASPAN Standards*

    1. "A Position Statement on Entry into Nursing Practice"

    2. "A Position Statement on the Perianesthesia Patient with a Do-Not-Resuscitate Advance Directive"

    3. "A Position Statement on Perianesthesia Advanced Practice Nursing"

    4. "A Position Statement on Minimum Staffing in Phase I PACU"

    5. "A Position Statement on Registered Nurse Utilization of Unlicensed Assistive Personnel (UAP)"

    6. "A Position Statement on Fast Tracking"

    7. "A Position Statement on On Call/Work Schedule"

       a. "ASPAN Fatigue Evaluation Checklist"

    8. "A Joint Position Statement on Intensive Care Unit Overflow Patients" developed by ASPAN, AACN, and ASA's Anesthesia Care Team Committee and Committee on Critical Care Medicine and Trauma Medicine

    9. "A Position Statement on the Nursing Shortage"

    10. "A Position Statement for Medical-Surgical Overflow Patients in the PACU and ASU"

    11. "A Position Statement on Visitation in Phase I Level of Care"

    12. "A Position Statement on Safe Medication Administration"

    13. "A Position Statement on Cultural Diversity and Sensitivity in Perianesthesia Nursing Practice"

    14. "A Position Statement on Perianesthesia Safety"

    15. "A Position Statement on the Geriatric Patient"

    16. "A Position Statement on Advocacy"

VIII. COMPETENCY-BASED PRACTICE

  A. Comprehensive guide to competency and skill development for the perianesthesia nurse

  B. May be used to orient the new perianesthesia nurse

  C. May be used for annual skills renewal and annual updates for the perianesthesia nurse

D. Provides the perianesthesia nurse a framework of essential performance criteria, thus establishing basic competencies needed to practice in diverse perianesthesia settings

E. Guidelines for using UAP in the perianesthesia setting
   1. Value of using competent UAP in perianesthesia settings
   2. Foremost concern is to promote a safe environment for the perianesthesia patient.
   3. Perianesthesia nursing profession defines and supervises the education, training, and utilization of UAPs involved in direct patient care.
   4. Perianesthesia RN is responsible for and accountable for the provision of nursing practice.
   5. Perianesthesia RN supervises and determines appropriate utilization of any UAP involved in direct patient care.
   6. Purpose of the UAP is to enable the professional perianesthesia nurse to provide nursing care for the patient.

F. Competencies for the RN
   1. Mentoring
   2. Critical thinking
   3. Preanesthesia care
      a. Preanesthesia testing
      b. Preprocedural teaching
      c. Preanesthesia history and assessment
      d. Day of surgery preparation
   4. Airway management
   5. Circulation
   6. Neurological
   7. Renal
   8. Moderate sedation and analgesia
   9. Anesthesia agents and adjuncts
      a. General inhalation agents
      b. Muscle relaxants
      c. Regional anesthesia
      d. Intravenous agents
   10. Perianesthesia fluid management and resuscitation
   11. Pain and comfort management
   12. Nausea and vomiting
   13. Malignant hyperthermia
   14. Thermoregulation
   15. Age-specific competencies
   16. Postoperative education and teaching
   17. Medical imaging/interventional radiology
   18. Documentation/legal
   19. Transcultural nursing
   20. EBP in the perianesthesia setting

G. Competency-based orientation for the UAP
   1. Introduction
   2. Patient rights, confidentiality, and communication skills
   3. Basic infection, prevention, and control practices
   4. Preoperative testing
   5. Basic life support
   6. Airway management
   7. Care of the patient requiring monitoring
   8. Care of the patient receiving intravenous fluids
   9. Pain assessment and management
   10. Care of the patient requiring comfort measures
   11. Care of the patient with nausea and vomiting
   12. Care of the patient requiring oral or nasal suctioning
   13. Care of the patient requiring oral intake

14. Care of the patient with catheters and drains
15. Care of the patient with hypothermia
16. Care of the patient with malignant hyperthermia
17. Care of the patient with seizure disorder
18. Care of the patient requiring antiembolism devices
19. Assisting with ambulation
20. Safe transport of the perianesthesia patient

To obtain a copy of the *2008-2010 Standards of Perianesthesia Nursing Practice; A Competency Based Orientation and Credentialing Program for the Registered Nurse in the Perianesthesia Setting 2009*; and/or *A Competency Based Orientation and Credentialing Program for the Unlicensed Assistive Personnel in the Perianesthesia Setting 2007*; contact ASPAN at 10 Melrose Avenue, Suite 110, Cherry Hill, NJ 08003; at 1-877-737-9696 (toll-free); or at www.aspan.org.

IX. ETHICAL ISSUES
   A. Ethics
      1. The science relating to moral action and moral values
      2. Concerned with motives and attitudes and their relation to the good of the individual
   B. Professional responsibilities and duties
      1. Duty of veracity: a duty to tell the truth
      2. Rule of confidentiality: a duty to control disclosure of personal information about patients to others
      3. Health Insurance Portability and Accountability Act
         a. Requires health care organizations to comply with federal regulations for privacy and electronic transactions
         b. Portability standards
         c. Accountability standards
         d. Privacy standards
      4. Duty of advocacy: nurse supports the best interests of the individual patient
      5. Accountability: answerable to others for one's actions
      6. Duty of fidelity: obligation to be faithful to commitments to self and others
   C. Ethical theories
      1. Utilitarianism: defines "good" as happiness or pleasure
         a. Greatest good for the greatest number of people
         b. The end justifies the means
      2. Deontology: system of ethical decision-making based on moral obligation or commitment to others
         a. Emphasis on the dignity of human beings
      3. Principalism: incorporates various existing ethical principles and attempts to resolve conflicts by applying one or more of them
   D. Ethical principles
      1. Beneficence: views the primary goal of health care as doing good for patients
      2. Nonmaleficence: requirement that health care providers prevent or do no harm to their patients
      3. Autonomy: freedom of action as chosen by an individual
      4. Justice: duty to be fair to all people
   E. Ethical decision-making: goal is to determine right from wrong in certain situations in which the lines are unclear.
      1. Decision-making process
         a. Obtain as much information as possible.
         b. State the problem or dilemma as clearly as possible.
         c. List all possible choices of action.
         d. Evaluate the consequences of each choice.
         e. Make a decision.
      2. Moral model
         a. Massage the dilemma.
         b. Outline the options.
         c. Resolve the dilemma.

    d. Act by applying chosen option.

    e. Look back and evaluate entire process.

  F. Relationship of law and ethics

    1. Legal system is founded on rules and regulations that are formal and binding; ethical values are subject to philosophical, moral, and individual interpretation.

    2. Legal right may or may not be ethical.

    3. Moral right may or may not be a legal right.

    4. Law influences ethical decision-making, and ethics can influence legal decision-making.

  G. "Perianesthesia Standards for Ethical Practice," included in ASPAN's *2008-2010 Standards of Perianesthesia Nursing Practice*

  H. ANA: *Code of Ethics for Nurses With Interpretive Statements* (nine provisions approved June 30, 2001)

    1. The nurse practices with compassion and respect.

    2. The nurse's primary commitment is to the patient.

    3. The nurse advocates for the health, safety, and rights of the patient.

    4. The nurse is accountable for individual nursing practice.

    5. The nurse owes the same duties to self as to others.

    6. The nurse participates in maintaining and improving health care environments and conditions.

    7. The nurse participates in the advancement of the profession.

    8. The nurse collaborates with other health professionals.

    9. The profession of nursing is responsible for articulating nursing values, for maintaining the integrity of the profession, and for shaping social policy.

  I. The nursing shortage

    1. The ANA, the National Council of State Boards of Nursing, and the National Federation of Licensed Practical Nursing, Inc: "Joint Statement on Maintaining Professional and Legal Standards During a Shortage of Nursing Personnel"

    2. ASPAN: "A Position Statement on the Nursing Shortage"

BIBLIOGRAPHY

1. Agency for Healthcare Research and Quality: *Clinical practice guideline: Acute pain management: Operative or medical procedures and trauma*, AHCPR Publication No 92–00322, Rockville, MD, 1992, US Dept of Health and Human Services.

2. Agency for Healthcare Research and Quality: *The patient care partnership.* Available at: www.ahrq.org. Accessed November 20, 2008.

3. American Hospital Association: *The patient care partnership.* Available at: www.aha.org/aha/issues/communicating-with-patients/pt-carepartnership. Accessed February 10, 2008.

4. American Nurses Association: *Code for nurses with interpretive statements*, Washington, DC, 2001, American Nurses Publishing.

5. American Nurses Association: *Nursing: Scope and standards of practice*, Washington, DC, 2004, American Nurses Publishing.

6. American Nurses Association: *ANA position statements.* Available at: www.nursingworld.org/mainmenucategories/healthcareand policyissues/anapositionstatements. Accessed February 10, 2008.

7. American Society of PeriAnesthesia Nurses: *2008–2010 Standards of perianesthesia nursing practice*, Cherry Hill, NJ, 2008, American Society of PeriAnesthesia Nurses.

8. American Society of PeriAnesthesia Nurses: *A competency based orientation and credentialing program for unlicensed assistive personnel in the perianesthesia setting*, Cherry Hill, NJ, 2007, American Society of PeriAnesthesia Nurses.

9. American Society of PeriAnesthesia Nurses: *A competency based orientation and credentialing program for the registered nurse in the perianesthesia setting*, Cherry Hill, NJ, 2009, American Society of PeriAnesthesia Nurses.

10. American Society of PeriAnesthesia Nurses: Position statements. Available at: www.aspan.org. Accessed February 10, 2008.

11. Association of periOperative Registered Nurses: *Standards, recommended practices, and guidelines*, Denver, CO, 2007, Association of periOperative Registered Nurses.

12. Brent NJ: *Nurses and the law: A guide to principles and applications*, Philadelphia, 1997, WB Saunders.

13. Brunsen CD, Eichhorn JH: Risk management: Avoiding complications and litigation. In White PF, editor: *Ambulatory anesthesia and surgery*, Philadelphia, 1997, WB Saunders.

14. Burden N, Quinn D, O'Brien D, et al: *Ambulatory surgical nursing*, ed 2, Philadelphia, 2000, WB Saunders.

15. Connelly J: Emotions, ethics and decision making in primary care. *J Clin Ethics* 9(3):225–234, 1998.

16. D'Arcy Y: Practice guidelines, standards, consensus statements, position papers: What they are, how they differ. *American Nurse Today* 2(10):23–24, 2007.

17. Follin SA, editor: *Nurse's legal handbook*, ed. 5, Philadelphia, 2004, Lippincott Williams & Wilkins.

18. Gastmans C: Challenges to nursing values in a changing nursing environment. *Nurs Ethics* 5(3):236–245, 1998.

19. Gray C: Understanding and complying with HIPAA. *J Perianesth Nurs* 18(3):182–185, 2003.

20. Green C: Ethical issues in perianesthesia nursing. *J Perianesth Nurs* 15(4):229–236, 2000.

21. Gue DG, Fox S: *Guide to medical privacy and HIPAA*, Washington, DC, 2002, Thompson Publications Group.

22. Guido GW: *Legal issues in nursing*, ed 2, Stamford, CT, 1997, Appleton & Lange.

23. National Guideline Clearinghouse. Available at: www.guideline.gov/. Accessed November 20, 2008.

24. Odom J: Implementation of nursing standards. In Quinn D, editor: *Ambulatory surgical nursing core curriculum*, Philadelphia, 1999, WB Saunders.

25. Odom J: Legal and ethical issues. In Quinn D, editor: *Ambulatory surgical nursing core curriculum*, Philadelphia, 1999, WB Saunders.

26. Redman BK, Fry ST: Nurses' ethical conflicts: What is really known about them? *Nurs Ethics* 7(4):360–366, 2000.

27. Saufl NM: Standards for ethical practice. In DeFazio Quinn D, Schick L, editors: *Perianesthesia nursing core curriculum: Preoperative, phase I and phase II PACU nursing*, St Louis, 2004, WB Saunders.

28. *The HIPAA privacy, security, transaction, and code sets, and national resources, 1996.* Available at: www.hipaadvisory.com. Accessed February 10, 2008.

29. The Joint Commission: *2008 Hospital accreditation standards*, Oakbrook Terrace, IL, 2008, The Joint Commission.

30. United States Congress: *Health Insurance Portability and Accountability Act of 1996*, 104th Congress, Public Record, 104–191.

31. White G: The code of ethics for nurses. *Am J Nurs* 101(10):73–75, 2001.

32. Wood J: Ethical decision-making. *J Perianesth Nurs* 16(1):6–10, 2001.

33. Zickuhr MT: Nursing practice, nursing standards, and nursing practice. In Litwack K, editor: *Core curriculum for perianesthesia nursing practice*, ed 4, Philadelphia, 1999, WB Saunders.

Patient and Family Education

VALERIE S. WATKINS

OBJECTIVES

At the conclusion of this chapter, the reader will be able to:

1. Define the education process and use the nursing process to provide patient and family education (assessment, nursing diagnosis, planning, implementation, and evaluation).
2. Define The Joint Commission (TJC) standards for patient and family education.
3. Identify the developmental stages of learner.
4. List patient education that addresses the five teaching domains.
5. List components of patient teaching using the three domains of learning.
6. Describe teaching strategies that meet the needs of patients with different learning styles.
7. Describe methods for evaluation of patient education.
8. Identify documentation and information obtained from evaluations to improve the education process.

I. TJC STANDARDS FOR PATIENT AND FAMILY EDUCATION
   A. TJC's rationale for patient and family education is to provide patients sufficient information to make decisions and take responsibility for self-management and activities related to their needs.
   B. Expectations (Box 3-1)
   C. TJC is not looking for evidence of what is taught but what the patient knows.
II. ASSESSMENT
   A. Assessing learning needs
      1. Defined as gaps in knowledge that exist between desired level of performance and actual level of performance
         a. Gaps exist because of a lack of knowledge, attitude, or skills.
         b. Identify the learner.
         c. Choose the right setting.
         d. Collect data about the learner.
         e. Collect data from the learner.
         f. Involve members of the health care team.
         g. Prioritize needs.
         h. Determine the availability of educational resources.
         i. Access demands of the organization.
         j. Take time-management issues into account.
   B. Readiness to learn: willingness or ability to accept information
      1. Assessment of readiness to learn
         a. Physical readiness
            (1) Measures of ability
            (2) Complexity of task

▪ BOX 3-1
▪ **THE JOINT COMMISSION 2009 STANDARD**

Provision of Care
The hospital provides patient education and training based on each patient's needs and abilities.

Elements of Performance
- The hospital performs a learning needs assessment for each patient, which includes the patient's cultural and religious beliefs, emotional barriers, desire and motivation to learn, physical or cognitive limitations, and barriers to communication.
- The hospital provides education and training to the patient based on his or her assessed needs.
- The hospital coordinates the patient education and training provided by all disciplines involved in the patient's care, treatment, and services.
- Based on the patient's condition and assessed needs, the education and training provided to the patient by the hospital include any of the following:
  - An explanation of the plan for care, treatment, and services
  - Basic health practices and safety
  - Information on the safe and effective use of medications
  - Nutrition interventions (for example, supplements) and modified diets
  - Discussion of pain, the risk for pain, the importance of effective pain management, the pain assessment process, and methods for pain management
  - Information on oral health
  - Information on the safe and effective use of medical equipment or supplies provided by the hospital
  - Habilitation or rehabilitation techniques to help the patient reach maximum independence
- The hospital evaluates the patient's understanding of the education and training it provided

From The Joint Commission: *Comprehensive accreditation manual for ambulatory care (CAMAC)*, Oakbrook Terrace, IL, 2009, The Joint Commission.

          (3) Environmental effects
          (4) Health status
          (5) Gender
          (6) Primary language
     b. Emotional readiness
          (1) Anxiety level
          (2) Support system
          (3) Motivation
          (4) Risk-taking behavior
          (5) Frame of mind
          (6) Developmental stage
     c. Experimental readiness
          (1) Level of aspiration
          (2) Past coping mechanism
          (3) Cultural background
          (4) Locus of control
          (5) Orientation
     d. Knowledge readiness
          (1) Present knowledge base
          (2) Cognitive ability
          (3) Learning disabilities
          (4) Learning styles
  C. Assessing learning styles
     1. Visual: learn through seeing.
       a. Like to see the big picture or diagrams
       b. To coincide with the verbal instructions, prefer

        (1) Demonstrations
        (2) Watching videos
        (3) Written material
  2. Auditory: Learn through hearing.
    a. Like to listen to
        (1) Audio tapes
        (2) Lectures
        (3) Debates
        (4) Discussion
        (5) Verbal instructions
  3. Kinesthetic: learn through physical activities and through direct involvement.
    a. Like to be "hands-on," moving, touching, experiencing
    b. Will respond well to hands-on learning with equipment and return demonstration of skills
  4. Determine learning style (way that individual processes information).
    a. Adults
        (1) Use more than one method of learning
        (2) Have a primary learning preference
    b. Children have a more defined preference for one of the learning styles.
    c. May need to use more than one method to provide information
D. Developmental stages of learner: specific patient population requirements will have bearing on ability to learn and interact
  1. Age-specific—infant, child, adolescent, adult, and geriatric
    a. Emotional, cognitive, communication, educational
    b. Developmental age—not just age of patient
  2. Are there any developmental delays or injuries that may have impacted the ability to learn?
    a. Family's, significant other's, or guardian's expectations for and involvement in care
    b. Emotional or behavioral disorders
    c. Alcoholism or drug dependency
    d. Possible victims of abuse or neglect
    e. Patients with history of posttraumatic stress disorder or previous unpleasant experiences
    f. Cultural preferences
    g. Past and present health care practices
    h. Language barriers
        (1) Legislation requires the use of qualified interpreters for limited English proficiency patients representing the largest minority group in the area.
        (2) The patient has the option of declining the interpreter and using a family member or friend, but this must be documented on the patient record.
        (3) Qualified interpreters must be used for all "life-threatening" information (unless declined by the patient) such as
            (a) Diagnosis
            (b) Patient histories
            (c) Surgical procedures
            (d) Medical procedure
            (e) Procedural consents
            (f) Discharge instructions
        (4) Information can be taken and given over the phone via an authorized interpreter if the interpreter is not available to come to the hospital or facility site.

E. Stress
  1. Can be physiological, psychological, or emotional
  2. Some individuals are more vulnerable than others.
  3. Responses can be behavioral, psychological, or physiological.
  4. Children are more vulnerable when a number of stressors are present.
  5. Identify behaviors indicative of stress.
  6. Must listen to children—be aware of fears and concerns.
  7. Physical comforting and reassuring are beneficial to children.
F. Coping: individual reactions to stressors
  1. Strategies are specific to the person.
  2. Styles are relatively unchanging personality characteristics or outcomes of coping.
  3. Children have a more internal center of control.
  4. Strategies that use relaxation are effective in reducing stress.
G. Pediatric concerns when addressing educational needs (see Chapter 10)
  1. Pediatric stages of growth and development
  2. Psychosocial development (Erikson)
    a. Experiences can be favorable or unfavorable.
    b. Birth to 1 year (trust vs mistrust)
      (1) Establishment of trust dominates.
      (2) Trust exists in relationship to someone or something.
    c. One to 3 years (autonomy vs shame and doubt)
      (1) Autonomy is centered on the children's increased ability to control their bodies, themselves, and their environments.
      (2) Children want to do things for themselves by using newly acquired motor skills.
        (a) Walking
        (b) Climbing
        (c) Mental powers of selection and decision-making
      (3) Much of learning is acquired through imitation of activities and behavior.
      (4) Negative feelings arise when
        (a) Made to feel small and self-conscious
        (b) Consequences of behavior and choices are negative
        (c) Shamed by others
        (d) Forced to be dependent in areas where independence has been demonstrated
    d. Three to 6 years (initiative vs guilt)
      (1) Characterized by energetic and intrusive behavior and a strong imagination; explore the world with all of their senses and abilities.
      (2) No longer guided by outsiders; develop a conscience that warns and protects or threatens them.
      (3) A sense of guilt occurs when in conflict with others or made to feel that their behaviors are bad.
      (4) Must learn to maintain initiative without encroaching on the rights of others.
    e. Six to 12 years (industry vs inferiority)
      (1) Want to engage in activities and behaviors that they can complete. They need a sense of achievement.
      (2) They learn to compete and cooperate with others, and learn the rules.
      (3) Important for learning to develop relationships with others.
      (4) May feel inadequate and inferior if too much is expected of them or they believe they cannot measure up to standards set for them by others.
    f. Twelve to 18 years (identity vs role confusion)
      (1) Adolescent-development is characterized by rapid and marked physical changes.

       (2) Adolescents' perception of their bodies changes and diminishes.

       (3) They become overly preoccupied with others' perceptions of themselves.

       (4) Adolescents face difficulty in dealing with concepts that others expect of them and the values of society.

3. Cognitive development (Piaget)

  a. Consists of age-related changes that occur in mental activities.

  b. Intelligence enables individuals to make adaptations to the environment that increase the probability of survival.

  c. Three stages of reasoning

       (1) Intuitive

       (2) Concrete operational

       (3) Formal operational

  d. Concrete reasoning for children begins at about 7 years of age.

  e. Birth to 2 years (sensorimotor)

       (1) Six substages that are governed by sensations

       (2) Progress from simple reflex activity to simple repetitive behaviors to imitative behavior

       (3) Develop a sense of cause and effect

       (4) Display a high level of curiosity, experimentation, and enjoyment of new things

       (5) Begin to develop a sense of self; become aware of a sense of permanence

       (6) Begin to use language and thought

  f. Two to 7 years (preoperational)

       (1) Interpret objects in sense of relationships or the use to themselves. Unable to see things from any perspective but their own

       (2) See things in sense of concrete and tangible; lack the ability to use deductive reasoning

       (3) Use imaginative play, questioning, and other interactions to develop the ability to make associations between ideas

       (4) Thought is dominated by what children see, hear, or experience. Have increasing use of language and symbols to represent objects in their environment

  g. Seven to 11 years (concrete operations)

       (1) Become increasingly logical and articulate

       (2) Able to sort, classify, order, and organize information to use in problem solving

       (3) Develop a new concept of permanence

       (4) Able to deal with multiple aspects of a situation simultaneously

       (5) Do not have the ability to deal with abstract concepts

       (6) Problems are solved in concrete systematic methods based on what children recognize.

       (7) Become less self-centered through interactions with others; thinking becomes socialized

       (8) Can consider points of view outside their own

  h. Eleven to 15 years (formal operations)

       (1) Able to be adaptable and flexible

       (2) Can think in abstract terms and symbols, and are able to draw logical conclusions from observations

       (3) Can make hypotheses and test them

       (4) Consider abstract, theoretical, and philosophical matters

       (5) May confuse the ideal with the practical, but in most cases can deal with the contradictions and resolve issues

       (6) Nonsocial stimulating experience that starts outside the child

       (7) Attention attracted by objects in the environment

      (a) Light
      (b) Color
      (c) Taste
      (d) Odors
      (e) Textures
      (f) Consistencies
    (8) Use of body senses to experience

H. Fears
    1. Vary with age
      a. Infants
        (1) Birth to 6 months: loss of support, loud noise, bright lights, sudden movement
        (2) Seven to 12 months: strangers, sudden appearance of unexpected and looming objects, animals, or heights
      b. Toddlers (1–3 years): separation from parents, the dark, loud or sudden noise, injury, strangers, certain persons (e.g., the physician), certain situations (e.g., trip to the dentist), animals, large objects or machines, change in environment
      c. Preschoolers (3–5 years): separation from parent, supernatural beings (e.g., monsters or ghosts), animals, the dark, noises, "bad" people, injury, death
      d. School-age children (6–12 years): supernatural beings, injury, storms, the dark, staying alone, separation from parent, things seen on television or in movies, injury, tests and failure in school, consequences related to unattractive physical appearance, death
      e. Adolescents: inept social performance, social isolation, sexuality, drugs, war, divorce, crowds, gossip, public speaking, plane and car crashes, death

I. Adult concerns when addressing educational needs
    1. Early adulthood: 20 to 40 years (intimacy vs isolation)
      a. Have a commitment to work and relationships
        (1) Have they planned appropriately for the impact that surgery may have on their work, social, and personal life?
      b. Concerned with emancipation from parents and in building an independent lifestyle
      c. Concerned with forming an intimate bond with another and choosing a mate
        (1) The adult seeks love, commitment, and industry of an intense, lasting relationship.
        (2) Relationships include mutual trust, cooperation, acceptance, sharing of feelings and goals.
        (3) Without secure personal identity, the adult cannot form a love relationship; may result in a lonely, isolated, withdrawn person.
      d. Has reached maximum potential for growth and development
      e. All body systems operate at peak efficiency.
      f. Nutritional needs depend on maintenance and repair requirements and on activity levels.
      g. Sensible nutrition is a major problem for many adults.
      h. Cognitive function has reached a new level of formal operations and the capacity for abstract thinking.
      i. Less egocentric, operates in a more realistic and objective manner
      j. Is close to the maximum ability to acquire and use knowledge
      k. Work is an important factor in the young adult and is tied closely with ego identity.
      l. Begins to self-reflect in the late 20s to early 30s:
        (1) "Where am I going?"
        (2) "Why am I doing these things in my life?"
      m. The 30s are characterized by settling down.

   n. Strives to establish a niche in society and to build a better life
   o. Risk for stress is increased since there are many situations that require choices to be made.
   p. Single parents often have additional stress of decreased financial resources for themselves and/or children.
2. Middle adulthood: 40 to 64 years (generativity vs stagnation)
   a. Realization that life is half over
   b. Accepting and adjusting to the physical changes of middle age
      (1) Effects of aging are becoming more apparent—wrinkles, graying or thinning hair, changes in body function, redistribution of fat deposits, decreased physical stamina and abilities.
      (2) Decreased respiratory capacity and cardiac function, visual changes
      (3) Sensory function remains intact except for some visual changes (e.g., decreased accommodation for near vision or presbyopia)
      (4) Women—menopause:
         (a) Decrease in estrogen and progesterone
         (b) Attendant symptoms of
            (i)   Atrophy of reproductive organs
            (ii) Hot flashes
            (iii) Mood swings
      (5) Men: decrease in testosterone, which causes
         (a) Decreased sperm and semen production
         (b) Less intense orgasms
   c. Adjusting to aging parents
   d. Reviewing and redirecting career goals
   e. Helping adolescent children in their search for identity
      (1) Often feel caught in a "squeeze" between simultaneously changing needs of adolescent children and aging parents
   f. Accepting and relating to the spouse as a person
   g. Coping with an empty nest at home
   h. Aware of occasional death of peers—reminder of own mortality
   i. Leading causes of death: cardiovascular disease, cancer, and stroke
   j. Morbidity increased
      (1) Often related to increase in obesity
      (2) Resulting hypertension, cardiovascular disease, diabetes, mobility dysfunction, and arthritis
      (3) Chronic smoking leads to health problems.
   k. Intelligence levels remain generally constant.
      (1) Is further enhanced by knowledge that comes with
         (a) Life experiences
         (b) Self-confidence
         (c) A sense of humor
         (d) Flexibility
      (2) Interested in how new knowledge is applied, not just in learning for learning's sake
   l. Adults have an urge to contribute to the next generation.
      (1) Wants to be needed, to leave something behind
      (2) If fulfillment does not occur, stagnation is experienced—boredom, a sense of emptiness in life, which leads to being inactive, self-absorbed, self-indulgent, a chronic complainer.
   m. Role realignment occurs in relationships with aging parents.
      (1) Once parents die, middle-aged adults are more vulnerable and realize limited quantities of time are left.
   n. Be alert for
      (1) Depressive symptoms
      (2) Suicide risk factors
      (3) Abnormal bereavement
      (4) Signs of physical abuse or neglect

      (5) Malignant skin lesions

      (6) Peripheral arterial disease

      (7) Other body dysfunction

      (8) Signs and symptoms apply to young and late adulthood.

3. Maturity—65 years to death (integrity vs despair)

   a. Fastest growing segment of the population

   b. Developmental tasks include:

      (1) Adjusting to changes in physical strength and health

      (2) Forming a new family role as an in-law and/or a grandparent

      (3) Adjusting to retirement and reduced incomes

      (4) Developing postretirement activities that enhance self-worth and usefulness

      (5) Arranging satisfactory physical living quarters

      (6) Adjusting to the death of spouse, family members, and friends

      (7) Conducting a life review

      (8) Preparing for the inevitability of one's own death

   c. Illness affects aging people more than those in other age groups.

      (1) Incidence of chronic disease increases.

      (2) Resistance to illness decreases.

      (3) Recuperative power decreases.

      (4) Body aches and pains increase.

      (5) Increasingly dependent on the health care system for advice, health teaching, and physical care

   d. Widely diverse response to disease and health concerns is dependent on

      (1) Subjective attitude

      (2) Physical activity

      (3) Nutrition

      (4) Personal habits

      (5) Occurrence of physical illness

   e. Intellectual function depends on factors such as

      (1) Motivation

      (2) Interest

      (3) Sensory impairment

      (4) Educational level

      (5) Deliberate caution

      (6) Tendency to conserve time and emotional energy rather than acting assertively

   f. Decreased ability for complex decision-making

      (1) Do not provide information for more than one task at a time.

      (2) Giving a list of directions produces confusion and inability to follow-through.

   g. Decreased speed of performance—requires more time to process and to complete tasks

   h. Memory may be affected.

      (1) If so, short-term memory more so than long-term memory

   i. Retirement often involves financial adjustment.

      (1) May impact ability to manage disease processes if money is not available for medications or food

   j. Options to live alone may change as ability to care for self decreases.

   k. Reminded of limited time remaining as aging continues

      (1) Life review occurs.

   l. Feels content with life or has feelings of futility, despair, resentment, hopelessness, and a fear of death

   m. Decreased ability to read materials in normal or small font size

   n. Loses ability to read materials printed in or on backgrounds of green and blue

J. Consider options for obtaining information.
  1. Informal conversations
  2. Questionnaires
  3. Observations
  4. Structured interviews
    a. Telephone
    b. Face to face
  5. Focus groups
  6. Patient charts
  7. Risk management reports
  8. Committee requests
  9. Professional society standards or requirements
  10. Changes in patient populations
  11. Patterns of care delivery
  12. Regulatory requirements
K. Consider barriers in assessment.
  1. Cultural
  2. Religious
  3. Physical limitations
  4. Cognitive limitations
  5. Language
  6. Financial barriers
  7. Consider your own biases.
    a. Ethnicity
    b. Religion
    c. Elderly
    d. Alcohol use
    e. Obesity
    f. Children
    g. Female/male hang-ups
    h. The key to developing education to meet the needs of the patient requires nurses to understand their own biases and how they affect their views and the care they provide.
L. Start with what the learner knows.
  1. Determine what the patient, family, or significant other feels that they need to know.
    a. Collect data from the patient, family, or significant other.
  2. Educational background and primary language
  3. Cultural factors
    a. "Do you seek the advice of another health practitioner?"
    b. "Do you use herbs or other medications or treatments?"
    c. "What language do you use most often when speaking and writing?"
  4. What knowledge, skills, values, and attitudes does the patient have?
III. NURSING DIAGNOSIS
  A. Analyze assessment. Identify potential problems.
    1. Preoperative
      a. Knowledge deficits, absence or deficiency of cognitive information
        (1) Process issues
        (2) Safety issues
        (3) Risks for injury, infection
        (4) Anxiety
        (5) Hypothermia or hyperthermia
        (6) Potential coping inability, ineffective coping
        (7) Ineffective or absent support system
        (8) Body image disturbance
        (9) Caregiver role strain
        (10) Risk for altered development

         (11) Fears

         (12) Fluid volume deficits

         (13) Latex allergy risk or problem

         (14) Impaired mobility

         (15) Pain management concerns (acute and chronic)

         (16) Nutritional deficits and concerns

    2. Postoperative

       a. Knowledge deficits and risks for developing problems

         (1) Airway management problems

         (2) Safety concerns

         (3) Hypothermia or hyperthermia

         (4) Nutritional concerns and needs

         (5) Altered mental status

         (6) Activity intolerance or inability

         (7) Aspiration risk

         (8) Body image disturbance

         (9) Caregiver role strain

         (10) Communication impaired

         (11) Risk for altered, delayed, or regressed development

         (12) Altered family processes

         (13) Fear

         (14) Fluid volume deficit or excess

         (15) Grieving

         (16) Latex allergy risk or problem

         (17) Impaired mobility

         (18) Nausea and vomiting

         (19) Impaired memory

         (20) Ineffective pain management (acute and chronic)

         (21) Nutritional concerns and deficits

         (22) Impaired skin integrity

         (23) Altered sleep patterns and inadequate sleep

         (24) Impaired tissue integrity

         (25) Urinary elimination concerns

         (26) Altered sexuality

         (27) Risk for development of constipation

   3. Determine specific problems of patient and family or significant other.

   4. Nursing diagnosis may be formal or informal.

      a. May be incorporated into a care process model or map

   5. Diagnosis may be related to altered health responses or dysfunction.

      a. May be anticipated or actual problems

  B. May use the teaching-learning process

   1. Similar to nursing process

      a. Assessing learning needs and learning readiness

      b. Developing learning objective. Objectives must be specific, attainable, measurable, and short-term statements.

      c. Planning and implementing patient teaching

      d. Evaluating patient learning

   2. Documenting patient teaching and learning

   3. Both processes repeat with ongoing assessment and evaluation, redirecting the planning and teaching.

IV. PLANNING

  A. Develop a teaching plan based on learning outcomes/objectives to meet the patient's needs.

   1. Address immediate and emerging needs—explain rationale for what will be occurring.

      a. Physical

      b. Psychological

      c. Social

      d. Nutritional status

      e. Functional status

      f. Pain

      g. Necessary diagnostic tests based on patient's diagnosis and condition—not routine testing

      h. Discharge planning

  2. Starts at first contact with patient and progresses through each additional contact

  3. Develop learning objectives.

      a. Desired outcomes

        (1) State the desired patient behavior or performance.

        (2) Reflect an observable, measurable activity.

        (3) May add conditions or modifiers as required to clarify what, where, when, or how the behavior will be performed.

        (4) Include criteria specifying the time by which learning should have occurred.

      b. Learning objectives can reflect the learner's command of simple to complex concepts.

      c. Must be specific about what behaviors and knowledge (cognitive, psychomotor, affective) the learner must have to accomplish the desired outcome. Examples:

        (1) Describe signs and symptoms of wound infection.

        (2) Identify equipment needed for wound care.

        (3) Describe appropriate actions if questions or complications arise.

  4. Select specific content to be addressed.

  5. Motivation for learning. Set realistic goals as a motivating factor.

      a. Internal is more lasting and more self-directive.

      b. Need for learning is recognized.

        (1) Five learning principles

          (a) Principle 1: learning is influenced by personal factors, such as past experiences, culture, age, ability to learn, and beliefs about health.

          (b) Principle 2: students learn more when they perceive a need to learn and when they have a clear overview of the plan.

          (c) Principle 3: learning is facilitated when the learner is accepted and respected as a person of worth in a mutually trusting relationship without fear of criticism or ridicule.

          (d) Principle 4: people learn through their five senses: seeing, hearing, feeling, smelling, and tasting.

          (e) Principle 5: learning is facilitated when students have knowledge of how well they are performing in a learning experience.

        (2) Patients who are ill do not absorb information well—this improves as health returns.

      c. Encourage motivation.

        (1) Provide nonthreatening environment.

        (2) Encourage self-direction and independence.

        (3) Demonstrate a positive attitude about patient's ability to learn.

        (4) Offer continuing support and encouragement as attempts are made to learn.

        (5) Create learning situations in which the patient is likely to succeed.

B. Consider the patient as an individual with specific needs, abilities, values, knowledge, and skills.

  1. Prioritize needs.

      a. Maslow's hierarchy of needs provides a guideline for determining patient needs.

        (1) Physiological needs (basic needs)

        (2) Safety and security needs (freedom from fear)

(3) Belonging and love needs (give and receive affection)

(4) Esteem needs (need to be perceived as competent)

(5) Self-actualization needs (need to fill one's potential)

b. Involve patient and family in determining what they consider important to learn.

2. Determine availability of resources.

a. Focus on what is available and what information can be provided to patient and family for present and/or future use.

b. Internet

(1) Expect that patients have already searched for information.

(2) Be aware of the information available.

(3) Be prepared to teach your patients how to access information and what sites are most reliable.

(4) Use as a teaching tool through your health care organization.

(5) Be aware that most patient information is written at a 10th grade level.

3. Consider time-management issues.

a. What can be provided in the time frame available?

b. Minimize distractions.

4. Teach basics before progressing to more difficult concepts.

5. Allow time for questions and review of contents for clarification.

C. Develop patient education that addresses the five teaching domains.

1. Situational and procedural information

a. Provide description of what to expect of the perioperative experience.

b. Examples:

(1) Explain process—preoperatively, intraoperatively, postoperatively.

(2) Who will patient come into contact with?

(3) Timing of events

(4) Family's or significant other's role in process

(5) Children—what parental or guardian role is, when parent or guardian will leave child and when will return

2. Sensation and discomfort information

a. What the patient may feel, see, and hear

b. Examples:

(1) "What will occur?" "How will you feel?"

(2) Environmental description, uniforms, masks

(3) Pain management

(4) Anxiety

(5) "What will you hear?"

(a) Hearing is last sense to leave.

(b) Hearing is first sense to return.

(c) May hear things even if not completely awake

3. Patient role information

a. Behavior expectation

b. Examples

(1) Explain procedures and follow-up.

(2) "Nothing by mouth" (NPO) guidelines, including medications to take and to hold

(3) Home preparations and care needs after discharge for self and/or family

(4) Appropriate clothing for discharge

(5) Need for safe transportation home after discharge

4. Skills training

a. Explanation of specific skills needed postoperatively

b. Examples:

(1) Teach skills (e.g., how to do a dressing change, empty drains, management of pain).

      5. Psychosocial support

         a. Interaction between patient and the care providers

         b. Examples:

            (1) Assist in decision-making.

            (2) Reinforce what may already be known.

            (3) Change: provide alternative behaviors or thoughts.

            (4) Maximize current level of functioning.

D. Develop components of patient teaching using the three domains of learning.

    1. Affective and attitude learning (feeling domain)

       a. Addresses attitudes, behaviors, and feelings

       b. Most difficult domain in which to affect learning

    2. Psychomotor learning (skills/doing domain)

       a. Motor skills

       b. Best taught by demonstration and hands-on experiences

       c. Provide the opportunity to practice.

       d. Return demonstration (e.g., use of incentive spirometer, crutch walking demonstration and practice)

    3. Cognitive learning (thinking domain)

       a. Addresses the patient's understanding

       b. Incorporates use of facts, details, and information basic to intellectual learning

       c. Multiple methods best address this learning need.

       d. People remember:

          (1) 10% of what they read

          (2) 20% of what they hear

          (3) 30% of what they see

          (4) 50% of what they see and hear

          (5) 90% of what they say and do

    4. Select teaching strategies to be used based on information obtained in needs assessment.

       a. Explanation (cognitive)

       b. One-to-one discussion (affective, cognitive)

       c. Answering questions (cognitive)

       d. Demonstration (psychomotor)

       e. Discovery (cognitive, affective)

       f. Group discussions (affective, cognitive)

       g. Practice (psychomotor)

       h. Printed and audiovisual materials (cognitive)

       i. Role playing (affective, cognitive)

       j. Modeling (affective, psychomotor)

       k. Computer-assisted learning programs (all types of learning)

E. Suitability of education materials used for patients

    1. Use of printed material is an economical one

    2. Allows the patient to proceed at own pace

    3. Use of a variety of media is more successful

    4. Disadvantages

       a. One in five adults is functionally illiterate, reading at or below the fifth grade level.

          (1) Because of shame and embarrassment, patients rarely admit they are functionally illiterate.

       b. Research shows that low literacy and poor health care are closely related.

       c. Five percent of the population cannot read English.

       d. Many individuals who are illiterate have normal or above-average intelligence.

    5. Many computer programs have built-in features that will calculate the readability of your document.

    6. Tell the patients what they need to know, not what is nice to know.

F. Strategies for improving readability

    1. Writing

        a. Reading materials should be at a fifth grade or lower reading level.

        b. Vocabulary—use short words.

            (1) Use simple, smaller words.

            (2) Use words of less than three syllables.

        c. Define words that are difficult to understand.

        d. Do not use abbreviations or acronyms.

        e. Sentence construction—use short sentences, no more than 10 to 20 words.

            (1) Avoid the use of medical terminology; use lay terminology—explain in terms the patient and family can understand.

            (2) Active voices (present tense)—avoid passive voice.

            (3) It is more easily understood.

            (4) Conversational style, use you and your.

            (5) Put most important information first.

            (6) If possible, make the first word the topic of the sentence and the first sentence of the paragraph the topic sentence.

    2. Design

        a. Typography

            (1) Type size and font make text easy or difficult to read at all levels.

            (2) Select simple type style (serif or sans serif).

            (3) Type size is at least 12 point.

            (4) Use typographic cues (boldface, size, color) to emphasize key points.

            (5) Avoid ALL CAPS, *italics,* or fancy lettering.

            (6) Justify text to left, leave right side jagged.

        b. Headers, subheadings, or captions

            (1) Helps the reader to focus attention on the message

            (2) Use both lowercase and uppercase letters.

            (3) Less than seven independent items—more easily remembered

            (4) Three to five items for lower literacy levels

        c. Layout

            (1) Layout and sequence of information are consistent, easy to predict flow.

            (2) Visual cuing devices (shading, boxes, arrows) are used to direct attention to specific points or key content.

            (3) Allow for plenty of white space.

            (4) Use of color supports and is not distracting from the message. Do not use pastels.

            (5) Line length is 30 to 50 characters and spaces.

            (6) High contrast between paper and type

            (7) Paper has nongloss or low-gloss surface.

            (8) Use of bullets helps, especially when summarizing

        d. Graphics (illustrations, lists, tables, charts, graphs)

            (1) Material is judged by first impression.

            (2) Friendly, attractive, and clearly portrays intent of material

        e. Type of illustration

            (1) Illustrations are on the same page adjacent to the text.

            (2) Use design layouts that allow eye movement from left to right, as in reading.

            (3) Simple line drawings promote realism without distracting details.

            (4) Avoid medical textbook drawings or abstract art or symbols.

        f. Relevance of illustrations

            (1) Use to illustrate concepts or procedures

               (a) Keep simple

        (2) Avoid nonessential details such as room background, elaborate borders, and unneeded color.
    g. Graphics
        (1) If used, must have clear explanations (step by step, or how-to instructions)
        (2) Easily misunderstood
    h. Captions
        (1) Can quickly tell a reader what the graphic is about and where to focus
        (2) Brief and simple

V. IMPLEMENTATION

  A. Teaching is performed using specific methods of instruction and tools.
    1. Optimal time for learning depends primarily on the learner.
    2. Pace of the teaching session affects learning.
    3. Environment selected must be conducive to learning.
      a. Avoid distractions (i.e., noise and interruptions).
    4. Teaching aids can foster learning and help focus learner's attention.
    5. Learning is more effective when learners discover the content for themselves.
      a. Provide stimulating motivation and stimulating self-direction.
      b. Provide feedback.
    6. Repetition reinforces learning.
    7. Organize information ahead of time.
    8. Use lay person's vocabulary.
    9. Teaching strategies
  B. Use specific teaching strategies.
    1. Group teaching
    2. Computer-assisted instruction
    3. Discovery and problem solving
    4. Behavior modification
  C. Develop teaching strategies that meet the needs of patients with different learning styles.
  D. Role of play in development
    1. Play has therapeutic and moral value and assists in development of
      a. Sensorimotor skills
      b. Intellectual development
      c. Socialization
      d. Creativity
      e. Self-awareness
    2. Content of play
      a. Social-affective play
        (1) Takes pleasure in relationships with people
        (2) Starts with smiling and cooing, progresses to initiating games and activities
        (3) Varies among cultures
      b. Sense-pleasure play
      c. Skill play
        (1) Repeat actions over and over
        (2) Determination to accomplish and develop new skills may produce a sense of frustration and pain.
      d. Unoccupied behavior
        (1) Not playful, but focus attention on anything that strikes the children's interest
        (2) Daydream, fiddle with clothes or other objects, or walk aimlessly
      e. Dramatic or pretend play
        (1) Dramatic or symbolic play begins in late infancy (11–13 months).
        (2) Predominant form of play in preschool child

          (3) As interactions with others increase, children attribute meaning to activities.

          (4) Acting out daily events provides modeling of behaviors of family and members of society.

          (5) Interacting with the environment develops a greater understanding of the world.

      f. Games

          (1) Found in all cultures

          (2) Repetitive activities allow progression to more complicated games and activities.

          (3) Challenge development of independent skills: puzzle solving, playing solitaire, computer or video games

          (4) Different ages participate in different games—simple to more complex.

          (5) Preschoolers hate to lose and will try to cheat or change the rules, or demand exceptions.

          (6) School-age children and adolescents enjoy competitive games—mental and physical.

  E. Transcultural teaching

    1. Obtain teaching materials, pamphlets, and instructions in various languages used by patients in the health care setting.

      a. Use a translator to evaluate materials.

    2. Use visual aids, such as pictures, charts, or diagrams, to communicate meaning.

      a. Audiovisual material may help portray the intent of simple information.

    3. Use concrete rather than abstract words.

      a. Use simple language—short sentences, short words.

      b. Present only one idea at a time.

    4. Allow time for questions.

    5. Avoid the use of medical terminology.

    6. If understanding another's pronunciation is a problem, validate a brief meaning in writing.

    7. Use humor cautiously.

    8. Do not use slang words or colloquialisms.

    9. Do not assume that a patient who nods, uses eye contact, or smiles is indicating an understanding of what is being taught.

    10. Invite and encourage questions during teaching.

    11. When explaining procedures or functioning related to personal areas of the body, it might be appropriate to have a nurse of the same sex do the teaching.

    12. Include the family in the planning and teaching.

    13. Consider the patient's time orientation.

    14. Identify cultural health practices and beliefs.

      a. Provide education to patient in preferred language.

      b. Provide written materials in preferred language.

    15. Provide documentation of education to patient and family.

      a. Verbally

      b. Written form

    16. Provide patients with information about available resources that will facilitate habilitation or rehabilitation.

    17. Promote the patient education process among appropriate staff and disciplines that are providing care or services.

    18. Care is planned for and coordinated by the facility providing the patient services.

VI. EVALUATION

  A. Develop methods of evaluation for patient education materials and processes.

    1. Both an ongoing and final process

    2. Evaluate achievement of desired outcomes.

    a. Established by patient, family, significant other, and nursing collaboration

    b. Learning objectives and goals of education directed by nursing diagnosis

       (1) Cognitive learning demonstrated by acquisition of knowledge that directly impacts behavior changes

       (2) Psychomotor learning is best evaluated by observing how well the client carries out a procedure.

       (3) Affective learning is more difficult to observe. May be evaluated by determining

          (a) Whether patient has made changes to behaviors that will improve long-term health status

          (b) Patient obtaining health education that impacts long-term health

3. Evaluation of content

    a. Purpose

       (1) Is it clearly stated?

       (2) Is it clearly understood?

    b. Content topics

       (1) That which is of greatest interest will become focus of patient efforts.

    c. Scope

       (1) Limited to purpose or objectives

    d. Summary and review

       (1) Reinforces and reiterates information addressed

4. Learning stimulation and motivation

    a. Interaction included in text and/or graphic

       (1) Chemical changes occur when the patient responds to the questions.

       (2) Memory is enhanced and retention occurs.

       (3) Moves to long-term memory

       (4) Ask to solve problems, to make choices, or to demonstrate.

    b. Desired behavior patterns are modeled, shown in specific terms.

       (1) People learn more readily by observation and by doing it themselves, rather than by being told.

    c. Motivation

       (1) More motivated to learn when the tasks or behaviors are doable

       (2) Divide complex tasks into small parts—will experience small successes in understanding or problem solving.

5. Cultural appropriateness

    a. Cultural match: logic, language, experience (LLE)

       (1) Does the LLE match the intended audience?

    b. Cultural image and examples

       (1) Present cultural images and examples in a realistic and positive way.

6. Evaluate the effectiveness of the teaching that was provided by the nurse.

    a. Consider all factors of the teaching experience.

       (1) Timing

       (2) Teaching strategies

       (3) Amount of information provided

       (4) Was the teaching helpful?

       (5) Was the patient, family, or significant other overwhelmed by the amount or type of information?

       (6) Request feedback from the patient, family, and significant other.

       (7) Were the needs of the patient considered when providing the education?

       (8) Were the patient's preferences for learning considered in providing the education?

7. Use information obtained from evaluations to improve the education process.

8. Effectiveness of education is evaluated by changes in behavior, knowledge attained, attitudes, and skills development.

   9. Methods of evaluation
      a. Concurrent and retrospective
         (1) Self-report of patient, family, or significant other
         (2) Direct observation
         (3) Retain copy of materials provided to patient.
   10. Methods of measurement
      a. Defined quality indicators that determine patient outcomes
      b. Observation
      c. Interview
      d. Checklist
      e. Written or oral testing
      f. Patient demonstrates comprehension of information provided in postprocedural behaviors.
      g. Patient satisfaction surveys
      h. Postprocedure contacts
         (1) Surveys
         (2) Telephone contact
         (3) Other contacts
   11. Use feedback to improve the process for the future.
VII. DOCUMENTATION OF TEACHING PROCESS
   A. Provides a legal record that the teaching occurred
      1. Include actual information and skills taught.
      2. Teaching strategies used
      3. Time framework and content for each class
      4. Teaching outcomes and methods of evaluation
   B. Provides a record for referral and review with the patient at a later date (e.g., follow-up phone contact)
   C. Did the patient respond to the education?
   D. Documentation components
      1. Patient and family learning needs
      2. Readiness to learn and learning style
      3. Learning objectives
      4. Information taught
      5. Teaching methods (e.g., brochures, models, video, demonstration)
      6. Patient and family response to teaching
      7. How learning outcomes were determined
      8. Need for additional teaching
      9. Resources provided
   E. Were the tools and methods used appropriate?
   F. Were there any barriers to assessing, planning, and delivering the education?
   G. Were the evaluation and analysis objective?

BIBLIOGRAPHY

1. Aldridge MD: Writing and designing readable patient education materials. *Nephrol Nurs J* 31(4):373–377, 2004.
2. Bastable SB: *Nurse as educator: Principles of teaching and learning*, ed 3, Sudbury, MA, 2008, Jones and Bartlett.
3. Berman AJ, Burke K, Erb G, et al: *Fundamentals of nursing: Concepts, process, and practice*, ed 6, Upper Saddle River, NJ, 2000, Prentice Hall Health.
4. Bernier MJ: Preoperative teaching received and valued in day surgery setting. *AORN J* 77(3):563–572, 575–578, 581–582, 2003.
5. Brownson K: Education handouts. Are we wasting our time? *J Nurses Staff Dev* 14(4):176–182, 1998.
6. Burden N: *Ambulatory surgical nursing*, ed 2, Philadelphia, 2000, WB Saunders.
7. Canobbio MM: *Mosby's handbook of patient teaching*, ed 2, St Louis, 2006, Mosby.
8. Cutilli C: Do your patients understand? Providing culturally congruent patient education. *Orthop Nurs* 25(3):218–226, 2006.
9. DeFazio-Quinn D, editor: *Ambulatory surgical nursing core curriculum*, Philadelphia, 1999, WB Saunders.

10. Doak CC, Doak LG, Root JH: *Teaching patients with low literacy skills*, ed 2, Philadelphia, 1996, Lippincott Williams and Wilkins.

11. Engel JK: *Mosby's pocket guide to pediatric assessment*, ed 5, St Louis, 2006, Mosby.

12. Habel M: Getting your message across patient teaching, part 3. *Nurs Spectr 2005*. Available at: www.patienteducationupdate.com/2006–04–01/article3.asp. Accessed March 9, 2009.

13. Jarvis C: *Physical examination and health assessment*, ed 5, Philadelphia, 2008, WB Saunders.

14. The Joint Commission: *2009 Comprehensive accreditation manual for hospitals: The official handbook*, Oak Brook, IL, 2007, Joint Commission Resources.

15. The Joint Commission: *Comprehensive accreditation manual for ambulatory care (CAMAC)*, Oakbrook Terrace, IL, 2009, The Joint Commission.

16. Kutner M, Greenberg E, Jin Y, et al: *Literacy in everyday life: Results from the 2003 National Assessment of Adult Literacy*, Washington D.C., 2007, U.S Department of Education. National Center for Education Statistics. Available at: www.nces.ed.gov/pubs2007/2007480.pdf. Accessed: April 30, 2008.

17. Litwack K: *Core curriculum for perianesthesia nursing practice*, ed 4, Philadelphia, 1999, WB Saunders.

18. London F: Moving beyond teaching check-lists. *Patient Education Update Newsletter* (3): Fall 2005.

19. Redman BK: *The practice of patient education*, ed 10, St Louis, 2007, Mosby.

20. White S: *Assessing the nation's health literacy: Key concepts and findings of the National Assessment of Adult Literacy (NAAL)*, Chicago, 2008, American Medical Association Foundation.

21. Winslow EH: Patient education materials. *Am J Nurs* 101(10):33–39, 2001.

22. Wong DL, Whaley LF, Wilson D, et al: *Whaley & Wong's nursing care of infants and children*, ed 6, St Louis, 1999, Mosby.

Evidence-Based Practice and Nursing Research

SUSAN JANE FETZER

OBJECTIVES

At the conclusion of this chapter, the reader will be able to:

1. Define evidence-based practice, nursing research, and research utilization.
2. Rank the strength of their contribution and list the major sources of evidence used to develop clinical practice guidelines.
3. Describe the link between research and the development of evidence-based practice.
4. Describe the nurse's role in protection of patients from unethical or harmful research.
5. Identify the components of a research proposal.
6. Differentiate the research process from the quality assurance process.
7. Identify three areas of perianesthesia nursing practice that are in need of research.
8. Identify three methods of applying ambulatory perianesthesia research in practice.

I. DEFINITION OF EVIDENCE-BASED PRACTICE (EBP)
  A. Problem-solving approach to clinical decision-making
  B. Research utilization
     1. Is one part of EBP
     2. Assessment of single research report
     3. Research study results will suggest change or support existing practice.
  C. Requires search for best and latest evidence
     1. Scientific evidence
     2. Experiential evidence of patient and provider
  D. Four components
     1. Analysis of best research
     2. Integrating clinical expertise
     3. Integrating patient values and cultural needs
     4. Integrating preferences of patient, family, and community
  E. Approach is systematic and rigorous.
  F. Requires synthesis of quality of evidence
  G. Conscientious integration of evidence in practice
II. GOAL OF EBP
  A. Implement effective nursing interventions
  B. Provide quality cost-effective care
  C. Reduce variations in practice
  D. Improve patient outcomes
III. STIMULI FOR EBP INITIATIVES
  A. Unusual or low-frequency clinical practice
  B. Indicated when outcome of care differs between similar patient situations
  C. Reference for developing nursing policies and procedures

IV. STEPS OF EBP
   A. Assess need for practice change; formulate a clinical question.
      1. Develop a problem-focused clinical question.
         a. Derived from recurrent clinical problem
         b. Encouraged by a quality improvement (QI) recommendation
         c. Stimulated by a benchmarking report
      2. Develop a knowledge-focused clinical question.
         a. New practice is identified.
            (1) Recently published research
            (2) Scientific paper at conference
            (3) Published clinical practice guideline
         b. Unit is interested in maintaining competency.
      3. Clinical question developed using PICO question format
         a. P—population of interest
         b. I—intervention of interest
         c. C—comparison intervention
         d. O—outcome
         e. Example: in patients undergoing bowel resection [P], does prewarming to 38° C [I], compared with no prewarming [C], result in less postoperative hypothermia [O]?
   B. Collect evidence.
      1. Sources of evidence
         a. Meta-analysis
            (1) Collection of multiple quantitative studies on the research question
            (2) Sample for analysis composed of the research studies identified
            (3) Application of statistical techniques to combine results into one data set
            (4) Determines strength of relationship between variables
            (5) Highest level of evidence to determine practice effectiveness
            (6) Example: a meta-analysis of studies of nurses' job satisfaction
         b. Systematic reviews
            (1) Collection of evidence related to specific clinical issue
            (2) Quantitative studies with similar methodology
            (3) Rigorous search designed to ensure complete database
            (4) Summary of findings provided
            (5) Highest level of evidence to determine practice effectiveness
            (6) Examples:
               (a) *Cochrane Database of Systematic Reviews*
               (b) Joanna Briggs Institute
         c. Integrative literature reviews
            (1) Similar to systematic review
            (2) Includes qualitative and quantitative studies
            (3) Draws narrative conclusions from summary of findings
            (4) Provides understanding of state of the science
            (5) Example: the relationship between nurse educational level and patient safety
         d. Metasummary
            (1) Synthesis of multiple qualitative studies
            (2) Provides narrative understanding of selected phenomenon
         e. Metasynthesis
            (1) Similar to metasummary
            (2) Develops a new theory or framework for topic
         f. EBP guidelines
            (1) General outline for specific course of action
            (2) Systematically developed
            (3) Recommendations supported by evidence
            (4) Developed by experts who have evaluated evidence
            (5) Goal is to translate evidence from research evaluations into practice

          (6) Formats of guidelines
            (a) Decision trees
            (b) Algorithms
            (c) Protocols
            (d) Clinical pathways
          (7) Sources of guidelines
            (a) National Guideline Clearinghouse
            (b) Agency for Healthcare Research and Quality
            (c) PeriAnesthesia guidelines
               (i) Normothermia
               (ii) Postoperative nausea and vomiting
               (iii) Pain and comfort
      g. Original clinical studies
         (1) Located through databases or indexes
            (a) *Cumulative Index to Nursing and Allied Health Literature*
            (b) *PubMed*
         (2) Types of clinical studies
            (a) Randomized controlled clinical trial (RCT)
            (b) Quantitative studies
               (i) Quasi-experimental
               (ii) Correlational
               (iii) Descriptive
            (c) Qualitative studies

C. Evidence appraisal
  1. Evidence appraised (critiqued) based on criteria
    a. Merit
    b. Feasibility
    c. Utility
  2. Evidence rated based on strength and quality
  3. Strength of evidence
    a. Level I—meta-analysis of multiple controlled studies; systematic review, evidence-based clinical guideline
    b. Level II—single, well-designed RCT
    c. Level III—quasi-experimental study, not randomized, single group
    d. Level IV—well-designed, nonexperimental study: correlation, descriptive, qualitative
    e. Level V—case report, program evaluation data
    f. Level VI—expert opinion, nationally known authorities
  4. Quality of evidence
    a. A—well-designed study
    b. B—observational study or controlled trials with less consistent results
    c. C—dramatic results but lacks controlled trial, evidence not consistent
    d. D—study has major flaw, findings suspect
  5. Evidence summarized
    a. Narrative summary
    b. Table of evidence

D. Integrate evidence into practice recommendations.
  1. Practice guidelines
    a. General outline for specific course of action
  2. Practice protocols
    a. Specific actions for direct application of an intervention

E. Implement practice change.
  1. Pilot study or demonstration project
  2. Evaluate need for change.
    a. Adopt a practice change based on evidence.
    b. Adapt a practice change based on evidence and setting characteristics.
    c. Reject a practice change for nonapplicability to the situation.

   3. Rogers' Theory of Diffusion of Innovation
      a. Guide for implementing changes in practice based on research
      b. Five-stage process
         (1) Knowledge—first awareness of innovation
         (2) Persuasion—attitude formation toward innovation
         (3) Decision—determination to adopt or reject innovation
         (4) Implementation—using innovation in practice
         (5) Confirmation—reconsider adoption or rejection of innovation
   F. Evaluate and monitor practice change.
      1. QI monitoring
      2. Conduct an original research study.
V. DEVELOPING AN EVIDENCE-BASED CULTURE
   A. Creation of environment that allows questions of current practices and actions
   B. Policies and procedures supported by literature citations
   C. Research committee is active.
      1. Inservice staff
         a. Promote positive attitude toward EBP.
         b. Methods of critical appraisal
         c. Accessing databases
         d. Steps of the research process
         e. Grading evidence
      2. Facilitate journal clubs.
      3. Change agents for EBP
         a. Champion a positive attitude toward research.
         b. Identify clinical practice questions.
   D. Resources needed to support EBP culture
      1. Time to reflect on practice
      2. Time to access and review evidence
      3. Consultants with research expertise
      4. Access to databases
      5. Authority to implement change
VI. DEFINITION OF NURSING RESEARCH
   A. Research: process of applying the scientific method designed to develop or contribute to generalizable knowledge
   B. Scientific method: controlled, systematic process for conducting studies in which data are collected under constant conditions to decrease error so that all data are collected in the same manner
   C. Nursing research: process of applying the scientific method to answer questions about nursing education, nursing practice, and nursing administration
VII. GOALS OF PERIANESTHESIA NURSING RESEARCH
   A. Maximize perianesthesia patient outcomes from nursing interventions.
   B. Validate a unique body of perianesthesia knowledge that impacts perianesthesia nursing.
   C. Maximize the effectiveness and efficiency of perianesthesia nursing care delivery.
VIII. OBJECTIVES OF PERIANESTHESIA NURSING RESEARCH
   A. Validate interventions used by perianesthesia nurses.
   B. Uncover perianesthesia phenomena not previously realized.
   C. Develop and test theories able to explain, predict, and control perianesthesia nursing practice and patient outcomes.
   D. Substantiate the unique contribution of perianesthesia nurses as health care providers.
IX. DEVELOPING AND PLANNING A RESEARCH STUDY
   A. Phases of a research study
      1. Proposal development
      2. Institutional review board (IRB) approval
      3. Data collection

        4. Analysis

        5. Communication of findings

    B. Proposal development

        1. A proposal is the plan the researcher intends to implement to solve the research problem by answering the research question or supporting the research hypothesis.

        2. Proposal precedes the implementation of a research study

           a. Assists the researcher to think through all steps in a study so nothing is missed

           b. Allows the researcher to make changes before investing time and money in procedures that may not be appropriate

           c. Encourages researcher to plan study with such clarity that it can be replicated (e.g., reproduced with another group)

           d. Provides an opportunity for peer review that allows constructive criticism from others who are knowledgeable about topic and research process for purpose of improving the study

           e. Proposal reviewed by the human subjects committee or IRB before data collection

X. COMPONENTS OF A RESEARCH PROPOSAL

    A. Introduction and problem statement (Box 4-1)

        1. Introduction: defines problem and provides background information so reader can understand why study needs to be conducted

        2. One to two paragraphs at the beginning of a research proposal that introduces the topic to the reader

        3. Problem statement: description of a dilemma or situation

           a. Dilemma or situation requires resolution by scientific inquiry and the development of new knowledge.

           b. Situation has not been satisfactorily resolved by past research studies.

           c. Dilemma exists because of a knowledge gap in the nursing literature.

           d. Example of perianesthesia nursing introduction and problem statement:

■ BOX 4-1

■ **EXAMPLE OF A PERIANESTHESIA NURSING INTRODUCTION AND PROBLEM STATEMENT**

> Pain is a common problem in the post anesthesia care unit (PACU) resulting in negative consequences for the patient. Length of stay in the PACU contributes to total cost of the surgical experience. Unrelieved pain is one of the most common causes of delayed stay in the PACU, therefore, contributing to higher cost.
>
>   Traditionally medications have been used to provide pain relief in the PACU. The effect of medications differs from person to person because of great variability in personal responses to pain. Experts have suggested that a combination of pharmaceutical and nonpharmaceutical therapies have the greatest potential for providing optimal pain relief. Music and quiet conversation by staff have the potential to provide pain relief and improve patient satisfaction with the PACU experience. The effect of music with noise control in the PACU on pain reports is not known.

        4. Perianesthesia topics that can be developed into research problems

           a. Preoperative examples:

               (1) Effectiveness of take-home preoperative video on patient compliance with preoperative regimen

               (2) Completeness of data provided by patient for preoperative database

               (3) Appropriate scheduling of preadmission visits

           b. Phase I examples:

               (1) Role of registered nurse during conscious sedation

               (2) Speed of patient rewarming on pain management

               (3) Role of PACU visitation on patient, family, and staff

           c. Phase II examples:

               (1) Validity of discharge criteria for regional anesthesia patients

               (2) Effectiveness of postoperative telephone calls in measuring patient outcomes

               (3) Use of bladder scanner to determine postoperative voiding necessity

B. Purpose statement
1. Provides a direction the researcher will take to solve the research problem
2. Includes the extent of the research project and the clinical context in which the researcher is interested
3. Presents one sentence that clarifies and provides the specific reason for the research
4. Example of perianesthesia nursing purpose statement:
   a. The purpose of the study was to investigate the effect of soothing music and control of noise on patients' perceived pain in PACU.
5. Perianesthesia purpose statements related to research problems
   a. Preoperative examples:
      (1) The purpose of the study is to determine the effectiveness of a take-home preoperative video on patient compliance with the preoperative regimen.
      (2) The purpose of the study is to describe the completeness of the data provided by the patient for the preoperative database.
      (3) The purpose of the study is to determine the most appropriate scheduling of preadmission visits.
   b. Phase I examples:
      (1) The purpose of the study is to describe the role of the registered nurse during moderate sedation and analgesia.
      (2) The purpose of the study is to determine the relationship between the speed of patient rewarming and perceived pain.
      (3) The purpose of the study is to determine the difference between scheduled and open PACU visitation on patient satisfaction.
   c. Phase II examples:
      (1) The purpose of the study is to determine the validity of temperature as a discharge criterion for regional anesthesia patients.
      (2) The purpose of the study is to determine the effectiveness of postoperative telephone calls in measuring patient satisfaction.
      (3) The purpose of the study is to determine the relationship between bladder scan volume and postoperative voiding urgency after spinal anesthesia.
C. Review of literature
1. Presents and clarifies what has been previously written or studied on the proposed topic
2. The researcher seeks out available solutions to the research problem in the existing literature before planning the study.
3. Includes a written summary of previous research related to the study problem and purpose
4. Provides the reader with a comprehensive background on the research topic
5. Types of literature
   a. Research-based literature—qualitative or quantitative research studies that follow steps of the scientific method found in nursing and nonnursing journals
   b. Theoretical—opinions or empirical experience articles found in nursing and non-nursing journals
   c. Research-based literature preferred
6. Literature review breadth and depth
   a. Breadth—wide variety of topics because area of research not well defined
   b. Depth—focused review on single concept when area of research is extensively documented in existing literature
D. Research question
1. Study purpose narrowed down further to focus on one or two research questions and/or hypotheses
2. Research question
   a. Definition: an interrogative statement posed by the researcher when little is known about the topic

      b. Used when there is insufficient current research to predict a relationship between two characteristics (variables) or an effect of one variable on another

      c. Components include the group to be studied and the characteristics (variables) under investigation.

  3. Perianesthesia nursing research questions

      a. Preoperative examples:

        (1) What preoperative information do cataract patients retain?

        (2) How do parents describe the effect of pediatric preoperative tours on the child's behavior?

        (3) What are the characteristics of patients who do not comply with fasting limits (e.g., nothing by mouth [NPO]) preoperatively?

      b. Phase I examples:

        (1) What are the educational characteristics of RNs administering conscious sedation?

        (2) What is the older nurse's experience of being on-call?

        (3) How long does it take an elderly patient to regain movement after spinal anesthesia?

      c. Phase II examples:

        (1) What is the effect of ketorolac on discharge temperature of elderly patients?

        (2) What is the most frequent reason for inability to contact patients by phone for discharge follow-up?

        (3) What are the factors associated with the ambulatory perianesthesia nurse's proficiency with cardiopulmonary resuscitation?

  E. Research hypothesis

    1. Definition: a formal declaration of an expected relationship or cause and effect between two characteristics (variables) made by the researcher based on established theory and/or past research

    2. Statement that offers a potential solution to the research problem that can be supported by the existing literature and the researcher's experience

    3. Always determined before the study and offers a framework for the research methodology

    4. Components of a hypothesis

      a. Group being studied

      b. Characteristics (variables) being studied

      c. The direction of the expected relationship (e.g., positive, negative, increased, decreased)

    5. Perianesthesia nursing research hypotheses

      a. Preoperative examples:

        (1) Cataract patients who are provided with face-to-face preoperative education will remember more information than cataract patients who are given an audiovisual preoperative video.

        (2) Patients scheduled for breast biopsy will report more anxiety if the time between preadmission interview and day of surgery is longer than 3 days.

        (3) There is a positive relationship between patient educational level and compliance with NPO guidelines.

      b. Phase I examples:

        (1) There will be a positive relationship between the PACU nurse's years of experience and comfort with administering moderate sedation and analgesia.

        (2) Patients who receive intravenous ketorolac preoperatively will report less postoperative pain than patients who receive intravenous ketorolac intraoperatively.

        (3) Patients who receive supplemental oxygen during postoperative transport to PACU will report less nausea than patients who do not receive supplemental oxygen.

    c. Phase II examples:
       (1) Discharge assessment phone calls placed after 5 PM will be more successful than phone calls placed before 5 PM.
       (2) There is a negative relationship between duration of preoperative NPO status and ability to void before discharge in cystoscopy patients.
       (3) Pediatric patients who participate in preoperative pediatric tours will recover faster than patients who do not participate.

F. Research variables
  1. Definition: any quality or characteristic that is likely to change and/or is observed or measured by the researcher
  2. Independent variable (IV): a characteristic selected by the researcher and believed to affect another characteristic (i.e., dependent variable [DV])
  3. DV: the characteristic believed by the researcher to change when the IV is changed
  4. IV is the cause or antecedent; DV is the effect or outcome.
  5. Demographic variables are characteristics of the group (e.g., patients, providers, units) being measured (i.e., gender, age, type of anesthesia, type of surgery, education, phase).
  6. IV, DV, and demographic variables require definition and measurement by the researcher; other characteristics, which may impact the research study, should be controlled.
  7. IV and DV are found in the purpose statement and the research question or the hypothesis.
  8. Perianesthesia nursing variables of interest
    a. Preoperative examples:
       (1) Type of preoperative teaching strategy (e.g., face to face, video)
       (2) Timing of preadmission visits (e.g., 2 days before surgery, day of surgery)
       (3) Preoperative temperature
    b. Phase I examples:
       (1) Postoperative temperature
       (2) Report of nausea
       (3) Oxygen saturation
    c. Phase II examples:
       (1) Duration of time to discharge
       (2) Bladder volume
       (3) Report of pain
    d. Examples of demographic variables—patients:
       (1) Age
       (2) Gender
       (3) Surgical procedure
    e. Examples of demographic variables—providers:
       (1) Years of experience
       (2) Certification status
       (3) Educational background
    f. Examples of demographic variables—units:
       (1) Phase of recovery provided
       (2) Number of beds
       (3) Types of patients (e.g., specialty unit, general unit)
  9. Examples linking IV and DV of interest:
    a. Type of teaching strategy (IV) and preoperative knowledge using a posttest score (DV)
    b. Time of preadmission visit (IV) and anxiety behavior (DV)
    b. Type of health care provider (IV) and patient satisfaction (DV)
    c. Warming device (IV) and postoperative temperature (DV)
    d. Intravenous fluid administration volume (IV) and time to postoperative void (DV)
    e. Certification of RN provider (IV) and amount of conscious sedation administered (DV)

      f. Use of ketorolac (IV) and postoperative pain (DV)

      g. Postoperative phone call (IV) and patient satisfaction (DV)

      h. Use of pediatric tours (IV) and child anxiety behavior upon discharge (DV)

G. Methodology

   1. Definition: the blueprint or plan taken by the researcher to collect the data required to answer the research question or support the research hypothesis

   2. Includes all procedures required to collect the research data: design, sample, setting, instrument, procedure, data analysis

   3. Includes rationales for decisions on how, when, and where data are collected, as these decisions may affect the research results

   4. Researcher designs the methodology so that the findings will have implications for nursing in general, not just the group being studied (e.g., generalizability).

   5. Research design

      a. Definition: the approach the researcher will use to collect the data

        (1) Qualitative

        (2) Quantitative

      b. Depends on the purpose of the study and the research question or hypothesis

      c. Qualitative research design

        (1) Focuses on the experience from the perspective of the patient

        (2) Emphasizes the holistic approach to the patient

        (3) Seeks to examine meaning of and insight into a patient's experience

        (4) Used when previous research on the topic is limited or absent

        (5) Data collected using words and narratives of patients

        (6) Topics using qualitative research designs in perianesthesia nursing

          (a) Preoperative examples:

            (i)   Experience of waiting for surgery

            (ii) Patient's account of preadmission screening

            (iii) Narrative response to advanced directive questions before surgery

          (b) Phase I examples:

            (i)   Patient's account of the experience of postanesthetic shivering

            (ii) One patient's account of midazolam-induced amnesia

            (iii) Experience of parents during the child's surgery

          (c) Phase II examples:

            (i)   A narrative response to inquiry about satisfaction with caregivers

            (ii) Patients' experience with postdischarge nausea

            (iii) Parental satisfaction with discharge instructions

      d. Quantitative research design

        (1) Focuses on understanding one part of the patient's experience

        (2) Emphasis placed on one or two selected variables of interest to the researcher

        (3) Used when a variable is in need of description (e.g., descriptive research), a relationship is being examined (e.g., correlational research), or cause and effect is being tested (e.g., experimental research)

        (4) Data collected for quantitative research can be reduced to numbers for statistical analysis.

        (5) Topics using quantitative research designs in perianesthesia nursing

          (a) Preoperative examples:

            (i)   Characteristics of patients who fail to follow preoperative instructions (descriptive research)

            (ii) Effect of pediatric tours on parental anxiety (experimental research)

            (iii) Relationship between NPO duration and preoperative blood pressure (correlational research)

(b) Phase I examples:
    (i)   Relationship between fluid volume replacement intraoperatively and incidence of postoperative nausea (correlational research)
    (ii) Incidence of hypothermia among elderly patients (descriptive study)
    (iii) Effect of Reiki therapy on report of postoperative pain (experimental study)
(c) Phase II examples:
    (i)   Effect of ketorolac on discharge temperature (experimental research)
    (ii) Incidence of postdischarge nausea (descriptive research)
    (iii) Relationship between admission temperature and discharge temperature (correlational research)

6. Research sample
  a. Definition: the individuals (i.e., patients, nurses, and family members) who agree to participate and provide data for the research study
  b. Individuals who provide data referred to as participants (qualitative design) or subjects (quantitative design)
  c. Sample selected from the population of all individuals with the characteristic of interest
  d. Sample selected so that the individuals are representative of all the individuals who are known to have the variable(s) of interest to the researcher
  e. Sample size
    (1) Qualitative design: data collected from participants until data saturation is obtained
    (2) Quantitative design considerations
      (a) Number of variables being studied
      (b) Type of variables being studied
      (c) Statistical analysis selected
      (d) Ability of the instrument measuring outcome variable to detect differences
    (3) Power analysis (statistical calculation) used to determine number of subjects
  f. Types of sampling methods
    (1) Simple random sample
      (a) Random selection of study subjects from population of interest using flip of a coin or random numbers table
      (b) Example: sample randomly selected from the population of thyroidectomy patients because it would be difficult and costly to study all patients in this category
    (2) Stratified random samples
      (a) Dividing subjects into layers or strata on the basis of specific attributes
      (b) Example: PACU nurse wishes to study implementation of PACU standards of practice; hospitals are stratified by geographic location (east, west, north, south) and bed size (<100, 100–300, >300).
    (3) Systematic random sampling
      (a) Random selection of sample from a list or membership roster
      (b) Example: American Society of PeriAnesthesia Nurses (ASPAN) membership roster (population of PACU nurses) used to obtain a sample of PACU nurses for a study on attitudes toward research
    (4) Cluster sample
      (a) Selection of a cluster of institutions in a geographic area
      (b) Example: sample of patients selected from several PACUs from several hospitals in a metropolitan area

        (5) Convenience or accidental sample
- (a) Obtaining subjects within readily available location or handy population
- (b) Example: PACU nurse studies effect of music therapy on pain in first 50 adult perianesthesia patients having orthopedic surgery who agree to participate.
- (c) Problem with convenience samples: Patients studied may not be representative of all patients admitted to all PACUs in all states.

        (6) Purposive sample
- (a) Selected intentionally on the basis of a particular attribute and frequently used in instrument development
- (b) Example: PACU nurse testing the ability of a new questionnaire to measure attitudes of ambulatory surgical patients' families regarding family visits in PACU would purposefully ask surgical patients' family members to participate in study. (Note: Families studied may not be representative of all types of ambulatory surgical patients' families.)

  g. Sample criteria
- (1) Researcher makes decision on demographic characteristics of participants or subjects for the study.
- (2) Inclusion criteria—demographic characteristics the researcher desires
- (3) Exclusion criteria—demographic characteristics that will make the participant or subject ineligible for the study
- (4) Examples of selection criteria for perianesthesia nursing research sample:
  - (a) Fifty male patients having regional anesthesia for herniorrhaphy
  - (b) All cataract patients requiring conscious sedation during the month of June
  - (c) Every other adult patient requiring general anesthesia who is not allergic to aspirin
  - (d) Children from 3 to 7 years of age who are accompanied by a parent
  - (e) Registered nurses who have been members of ASPAN for at least 10 years

7. Research setting
- **a.** Definition: location or environmental condition under which the study data are collected
- **b.** A description of the setting allows the reader to determine whether the research environment is similar to the reader's environment and whether the findings are applicable to the reader's practice.
- **c.** Examples of a perianesthesia nursing research setting:
  - (1) Waiting area of preadmission testing department
  - (2) Phase I PACU of a rural acute care facility with four operating suites and six postanesthesia bays
  - (3) Hospital-based surgery center caring for 30 pediatric surgical cases per week
  - (4) Operating room with temperature controlled at 60° F and humidity of 75%
  - (5) Waiting area of the surgeon's office
  - (6) Patient's home

8. Research instrument
- **a.** Definition: any device (e.g., monitor, questionnaire, interview) that produces or records data required by the research project
- **b.** Selection of the instrument depends on the variable being studied, the availability of the instrument, the expertise of the researcher, and the subject's capabilities.
- **c.** The instrument should be able to actually measure what the researcher intends (i.e., be a valid representation of the variable).
- **d.** The instrument should be able to collect consistent measurements of the variable being studied (i.e., be a reliable representation of the variable).

      e. The researcher describes the instrument clearly before the data are collected.
        (1) Reports or establishes the instrument's reliability
        (2) Reports or establishes the instrument's validity
        (3) Describes the nature of the instrument (e.g., number of questions, type of questions, type of device)
        (4) Provides rationale for selection of the instrument
        (5) Provides reference for instrument and any previous study using the instrument
      f. Examples of perianesthesia nursing research instruments:
        (1) Visual Analog Pain Scale
        (2) Tympanic thermometer in core mode
        (3) Speilberger's State–Trait Anxiety Questionnaire
        (4) Postanesthesia discharge criteria modified by Aldrete
        (5) Written posttest on care of surgical dressing
    9. Research procedure
      a. Definition: description of the steps taken to implement research data collection, including the selection of the sample, the identification of the setting, the administration of the research instrument, and any protocols for the IV
      b. Procedure provided with sufficient detail to allow the study to be replicated (repeated with a different group of participants) by other researchers.
      c. Procedure described in chronological order of implementation
   10. Data analysis methods
      a. Definition: procedures used to analyze the data
      b. Qualitative analysis will include ways in which the researcher will determine themes.
      c. Quantitative analysis
        (1) Descriptive procedures, correlational procedures, or tests of hypotheses
        (2) Based on the type of data collected and the format of hypothesis
        (3) Statistical experts consulted to determine appropriate statistical procedures

XI. ETHICAL ISSUES IN NURSING RESEARCH
  A. The researcher is required to protect the vulnerable patient from harmful effects and to ensure that benefits to participants outweigh risks of participating in the research.
  B. Ethical research behaviors include objectivity, cooperation with institutional guidelines, integrity, and honesty.
  C. Any research on human subjects requires review and approval by an IRB or human subjects committee *before* collecting data.
    1. Composition of the IRB includes nurses, physicians, and other health care professionals; clergy, community members, attorneys, and ethicists also participate on the IRB.
    2. IRB independently determines the ethical implications of the research methodology.
    3. IRB determines the requirements for participant's informed consent either in writing or verbally.

XII. COMMUNICATING THE RESULTS OF A RESEARCH PROJECT
  A. Upon completion of data collection, the researcher includes in the report findings, discussion of findings, conclusions, implications, and recommendations.
  B. Findings
    1. A demographic summary of the sample is provided.
    2. Results of the data analysis are provided in the order of the research questions or hypotheses.
    3. Tables are used to illustrate findings.
    4. Statistical notations are used to describe findings (e.g., $P = .001$).

C. Discussion of findings
  1. An interpretation of the findings
  2. Related research that supports or refutes the study findings is discussed from the perspective of the researcher's findings.
  3. Examples of perianesthesia nursing research findings:
     a. Findings from this study indicated that face-to-face preoperative instructions improve posttest scores significantly more than video teaching did.
     b. Findings of this study revealed that 2 days before surgical intervention is the appropriate time for a preadmission interview.
     c. Findings from this study did not identify a difference in patient satisfaction between care delivered by unlicensed providers and licensed providers.
     d. Findings from this study indicated no difference in postoperative temperature between patients who received ketorolac and patients who received acetaminophen.
     e. Findings from this study showed that postoperative follow-up phone calls made in the afternoon were more successful than those made in the morning.
D. Conclusions
  1. Definition: one or two specific statements of new knowledge that have been revealed by the research findings
  2. The conclusion attempts to answer the research problem presented at the beginning of the study.
  3. Examples of perianesthesia nursing research conclusions:
     a. The findings of the study support the conclusion that patients who receive face-to-face preoperative teaching learn better.
     b. The conclusion of this study is that the timing of preoperative visits can impact patient anxiety related to their surgical experience.
     c. The conclusion of this study is that level of patient education is a predictor of compliance with NPO guidelines.
     d. The research findings support the conclusion that pediatric preoperative tours reduce parental anxiety but have no effect on the child's anxiety before discharge.
     e. The findings of the study support the conclusion that patients who receive preoperative analgesics have less postoperative nausea.
E. Implications and recommendations
  1. Definition: suggestions offered by the researcher as to ways the research conclusions could be used in nursing practice, nursing education, nursing administration, or by future researchers
  2. Implications for practice translate the research findings into usable interventions to improve patient outcomes.
  3. At least one implication is reported for each research conclusion.
  4. Examples of perianesthesia nursing research implications:
     a. The study suggests that preoperative teaching be conducted by trained perianesthesia nurses during individualized face-to-face sessions.
     b. The study findings suggest that preadmission visits should be scheduled a maximum of 2 days before the day of surgery.
     c. The study findings recommend that NPO guidelines be explained based on the patient's educational level.
     d. The study findings suggest that parental tours may be just as effective as pediatric tours in reducing postoperative anxiety behaviors of children.
     e. The researcher recommends that the study be repeated using male and female patients of a wide range of ages.
XIII. QI AND THE RESEARCH PROCESS
  A. QI (e.g., quality assurance, total QI, and total quality management) projects are designed to measure performance against preestablished criteria (see Chapter 9).
  B. Purpose of QI project is to solve an institutional problem or improve or evaluate current practice.

■ TABLE 4-1
■ ■ **Comparison Between Research and Quality Improvement Using Key Characteristics**

Characteristic	Research	Quality Improvement
Seeks to solve a problem	Yes	Yes
Seeks to develop new knowledge	Yes	No
Requires defining the problem	Yes	Yes, but problem may be to examine current practice for improvement areas
Requires a purpose statement	Yes	No
Requires a question or hypothesis to be answered	Yes	No
Project supported by outside literature	Yes	No
Sample representative of population	May be, if using quantitative methods	No, sample of convenience
Sample size important	Yes	No
Setting described for replication	Yes, important for future researchers	No, setting is institution specific
Instrument has preestablished validity and reliability	Yes, validity and reliability strengthen study	Not needed, frequently an institution-created tool is used
Procedure clearly described	Yes, permits replication	Not necessary because one person is collecting data
Multiple methods used for data analysis depending on type of question or hypothesis	Yes, use of themes, descriptive, correlational, and effect statistics	No, data analyzed using descriptive statistics (mean, percentage)
Institutional review board approval required	Yes, mandatory	No, permission to survey granted by institution's administration
Findings, discussion, conclusion, recommendations follow from question or hypothesis	Yes, findings presented as generalizable results	No, findings discussed in light of improvement of quality and lessons learned
Publication in peer-reviewed journal	Yes, results disseminated to encourage knowledge development	No, results shared with internal stakeholders

    C. Goal of QI
       1. Improve systems and processes
       2. Improve outcome
    D. QI projects do not follow all the steps of the research process (Table 4-1).
    E. Framework of QI
       1. Plan
       2. Do
       3. Study
       4. Act
 XIV. DISSEMINATING RESEARCH FINDINGS
    A. Research findings can be disseminated in a variety of venues.
       1. Poster displays at national and local conferences and meetings of professional organizations
       2. Oral presentations at national and local conferences
       3. Local and national publications
          a. Specialty journals: *Journal of PeriAnesthesia Nursing, Breathline*
          b. Clinical journals: *Association of periOperative Registered Nurses Journal, American Journal of Critical Care, American Association of Nurse Anesthetists Journal*

      c. Research journals: *Nursing Research, Applied Nursing Research, Western Journal of Nursing Research*

XV. PROFESSIONAL RESPONSIBILITY FOR EBP AND RESEARCH

    A. Nurses have a professional responsibility to practice in accordance with the most current evidence.

    B. Nurses have a professional responsibility to maintain current practice by reading, discussing, and participating in nursing research.

    C. Research utilization should be included in all professional job descriptions.

    D. Perianesthesia nurses participating in nursing research are responsible for:

        1. Being aware of the research purpose and methodology

        2. Validating that the research project has undergone IRB review

        3. Advocating for the participant's informed consent

        4. Supporting the research data collection procedure where possible

BIBLIOGRAPHY

1. Agency for Healthcare Research and Quality: Available at: www.ahrq.gov. Accessed November 19, 2008.
2. American Society of PeriAnesthesia Nurses: Available at: www.aspan.org. Accessed November 19, 2008.
3. Brown SJ: *Evidence-based nursing: The research-practice connection*, Philadelphia, 2008, Jones & Bartlett.
4. Burns N, Grove SK: *Understanding nursing research: Building an evidence-based practice*, ed 4, Philadelphia, 2006, Saunders.
5. Fetzer SJ, Vogelsang J: *Research primer for perianesthesia nurses*, Thorofare, NJ, 2001, American Society of PeriAnesthesia Nurses.
6. Macnee CL, McCabe S: *Understanding nursing research*, ed 2, Philadelphia, 2008, Lippincott.
7. McSherry R, Artley A, Holioran J: Research awareness: An important factor for evidence-based practice? *Worldviews Evid Based Nurs* 3(3):103–115, 2006.
8. National Guideline Clearinghouse. Available at: www.guideline.gov. Accessed November 19, 2008.
9. Ridley RT: The relationship between nurse educational level and patient safety: An integrative review. *J Nurs Educ* 47(4):149–156, 2008.
10. Shertzer KE, Keck JF: Music in the PACU environment. *J Perianesth Nurs* 16(2):90–102, 2001.
11. The Cochrane Collaboration: *Cochrane collection*. Available at: www.cochrane.org/reviews/. Accessed November 19, 2008.
12. The Joanna Briggs Institute. Available at: www.joannabriggs.edu.au/about/home.php. Accessed November 19, 2008.
13. Zangra GA, Soeken KL: A meta-analysis of studies of nurses' job satisfaction. *Res Nurs Health* 30(4):445–458, 2007.

5 Legal Issues

JAN ODOM-FORREN

OBJECTIVES

At the conclusion of this chapter, the reader will be able to:

1. Identify five common causes of nursing liability.
2. Discuss methods for prevention of a malpractice suit.
3. Describe the four elements of negligence.
4. Discuss phases of litigation that can occur with a malpractice suit.

I. LEGAL CONCEPTS
   A. Sources of law
     1. Constitutional—system of laws for governance of a nation; may be federal or state
     2. Statutory—made by the legislative branch of the government
     3. Administrative—laws enacted by administrative agencies charged with implementing particular legislation
     4. Judicial—laws made by the courts that interpret legal issues that are in dispute
   B. Types of law
     1. Common law—derived from principles rather than rules and regulations
     2. Civil law—based on rules and regulations
       a. Administered through courts as damages or money compensation
       b. Most important area is tort law, which involves compensation to those wrongfully injured
     3. Criminal law—conduct that is offensive or harmful to society as a whole
     4. Substantive law—concerns the wrong, harm, or duty that caused the lawsuit
     5. Procedural law—concerns the process and rights of the individual charged with violating substantive law
   C. Legal definitions (Box 5-1)
   D. Negligence law
     1. Tort law—a civil wrong that allows the injured party to seek reparation; concerns any action or omission that harms someone
       a. Negligence
       b. Malpractice
       c. Assault and battery
       d. Invasion of privacy
       e. False imprisonment
       f. Defamation
     2. Essential elements of professional negligence (malpractice)
       a. Duty—once you, as a nurse, undertake the care of a patient, you are under a duty to act in accordance with the standard of care (e.g., you establish a duty to the patient when you take report on a patient in the post anesthesia care unit and accept that patient into your care).

■ BOX 5-1
■ **LEGAL TERMINOLOGY**

Assault
An attempt or threat that causes a person to fear physical touch or injury

Battery
The unauthorized touching of an individual's body, any extension of it, or anything attached to it in an offensive or injurious manner

Defendant
Person or entity against whom plaintiff's allegations are made

Expert Witness
A person who serves to educate the court and jury about the subject under consideration, including the appropriate standard of care

Malpractice (Professional Negligence)
A type of negligence that involves a standard of care that can be reasonably expected from professionals (e.g., attorneys, nurses, physicians, accountants); failure to act as a reasonably prudent nurse would act under similar circumstances

Negligence
Deviation from the standard of care that a reasonable person would use in a certain set of circumstances

Plaintiff
The person or party who brings the lawsuit and alleges harm

Standard of Care
The care and judgment exercised by a reasonable, prudent person (nurse) under the same or similar circumstances

   b. Breach of duty—failure to act in accordance with the standard of care
      (1) May be an act of omission (e.g., a failure to administer a medication that was ordered)
      (2) May be an act of commission (e.g., administration of a medication to which the patient had an allergy)
   c. Causation—plaintiff must prove that the breach of duty was the cause of damages (e.g., the administration of the medication to which the patient had an allergy caused an anaphylactic shock, resulting in the patient's death).
      (1) Most difficult element to prove
   d. Damages—actual loss or damages must be established (e.g., death, nerve damage, fracture).
   e. Plaintiff must prove all four elements of negligence for the cause of action to succeed.
3. Employer liability
   a. Respondent superior—"let the master speak"—employer is vicariously liable for negligent acts of employee if the act occurred during an employment relationship and within part of the employee's job responsibilities.
   b. Corporate liability—health care delivery system can be sued when it breaches any direct duty to the patient.
4. *Res ipsa loquitur*—"the thing speaks for itself"; a rule of evidence that allows a supposition of negligence on the part of the defendant (e.g., permanent loss of neuromuscular control of arm after routine hysterectomy)
   a. Defendant must be solely in control at the time injury occurred, and injury would not have occurred if defendant had exercised due care.
   b. Plaintiff must have done nothing to contribute to negligence (e.g., foreign object left inside patient after surgery).

5. Intentional torts—intent is necessary, and there must be a willful action against the injured person.
   a. Assault—an action that causes apprehension or unwarranted touching (e.g., threatening a patient)
   b. Battery—unauthorized touching of one person by another (e.g., lack of consent for treatment)
   c. False imprisonment—unjustifiable detention of a person without a legal warrant (e.g., not allowing a patient to go who wants to leave against medical advice)
6. Quasi-intentional torts
   a. Invasion of privacy—patient's right to privacy is recognized.
      (1) Using a person's likeness or name without consent for commercial advantage
      (2) Unreasonable intrusion into person's private affairs
      (3) Public disclosure of private facts about a person
      (4) Placing a person in a false light in the public's eye
   b. Defamation—wrongful injury to another's reputation
      (1) libel (written form)
      (2) slander (spoken form)
7. Standards of care—minimal requirements that define an acceptable level of care
   a. May be established by:
      (1) State Nurse Practice Act
      (2) Federal agency guidelines and regulations
      (3) American Nurses Association
      (4) American Society of PeriAnesthesia Nurses or other national specialty organization
      (5) The Joint Commission or other accrediting bodies, such as Accreditation Association for Ambulatory Health Care
      (6) Hospital or ambulatory surgery facility rules and procedures
      (7) State Board of Nursing
      (8) Common practice
      (9) Nursing texts and articles
   b. Determined by expert witnesses for judicial system
      (1) Essential in professional negligence cases
II. LIABILITY ISSUES
   A. Possible causes of nursing liability for the perianesthesia nurse
      1. Failure to adequately assess or monitor a patient
         a. Nurse must possess competency to assess and/or monitor patient.
         b. Assessment and monitoring of patient are actually performed.
         c. If assessment and monitoring reveal reportable condition, nurse must notify physician.
         d. Nurse must continue to assess and monitor to evaluate effectiveness of intervention.
      2. Errors in the use of equipment
      3. Errors in medication or treatment
         a. Failure to follow seven rights:
            (1) Right drug
            (2) Right dose
            (3) Right patient (two identifiers)
            (4) Right route
            (5) Right time
            (6) Right reason
            (7) Right documentation
      4. Failure to communicate
         a. To another nurse
         b. Confirmation of physician orders
         c. Changes in patient condition to a physician

5. Patient falls
6. Operating room errors (e.g., sponges/instruments left inside patient)
7. Mix-ups during patient transfers and/or before surgery (e.g., wrong surgery on patient)
8. Failure to report or act on deviations from accepted practice
   a. Nurses expected to exercise independent judgment and object when physician's orders are inappropriate
   b. Report facts to manager or otherwise follow chain of command.
9. Failure to follow a physician's order promptly and accurately
10. Failure to follow institutional or facility procedures
11. Failure to properly teach patient or caregiver accurate and appropriate discharge instructions
    a. Should receive discharge instructions before admission or surgery
    b. Use preprinted discharge instructions.
    c. Give verbal and written instructions.
12. Premature discharge for the ambulatory surgery patient
13. Failure to ensure the presence of an informed caregiver (responsible adult)
14. Failure to assess the ambulatory surgery patient on admission (e.g., nothing by mouth status, any signs or symptoms that might affect reaction to anesthesia or surgery, medication use that day)

B. Prevention of liability
   1. Documentation
      a. Accurate and comprehensive documentation
      b. Purposes of documentation
         (1) To communicate the patient's condition to other health professionals
         (2) To assess for improvements that might be needed by risk management and quality management
         (3) To obtain data for research
         (4) To obtain reimbursement—from the government and insurance
         (5) As a legal record
         (6) To use as data for quality-of-care review
      c. Nurses' notes first place an attorney will look
         (1) Written with time and date and in chronological order
         (2) Contains most detailed information regarding the patient
      d. Documentation guidelines
         (1) Chart accurately.
            (a) It is very difficult to prove that something was done if it is not charted.
            (b) On the other hand, deliberate inaccuracies can totally destroy defense and expose nurse to criminal charges of fraud.
         (2) Chart objectively.
            (a) Describe only what you observe.
            (b) Do not use words such as "seems," "apparently," or "appears."
         (3) Write legibly, and use standard abbreviations adopted by the health care facility.
         (4) Do not use the chart to criticize or complain.
            (a) Use other appropriate avenues if there is criticism of another nurse.
         (5) Do not destroy or obliterate documentation.
            (a) Do not use correction fluid or any other kind of eradicator.
            (b) Draw one line through the error, initial, and date the line.
         (6) Do not leave vacant lines; sign every entry.
         (7) Chart as promptly as possible after the care is given.
         (8) Correct grammar, spelling, and punctuation make a difference.
         (9) Do not chart for someone else or allow someone else to chart for you.
        (10) Use appropriate procedure for documenting a late entry.
        (11) Document patient and/or family teaching.

(12) Document disposition of any personal belongings.

(13) Document any nursing interventions and patient responses to those interventions.

(14) Document any communication with a physician or supervisor concerning a patient's condition.

2. Electronic documentation guidelines
   a. Protect the user identification code or password given for personal use.
      (1) No one else should be given access to that password or document for the user.
   b. Only access information and document in chart as authorized to do so.
      (1) An attempt to access an electronic chart on a patient without authorization is a breach of confidentiality and privacy.
   c. Never ignore electronic reminders that information is coded incorrectly, important data overlooked, or flags for critical information about the patient (e.g., lab work).
      (1) Systems alert nurses if a portion of the nursing process is absent.
   d. Know the facility procedure for how to handle late entries.
   e. Stay updated when changes in documentation format occur.
3. Incident reports
   a. Use has changed from punitive measure to a documentation of unusual events.
      (1) Should be no fear of reprisal or other negative consequences
      (2) Atmosphere of trust and cooperation essential for system to be of best value
   b. All actual and potential injuries must be reported.
      (1) Should be initiated by the person who observed the event or the first to become aware of the incident
      (2) Incorporate patient's description into the report by use of direct quotes.
   c. Documentation should be factual and objective.
      (1) Include information regarding patient, description of the incident, any injuries sustained, and outcome of event.
   d. Allows risk manager to assess situation and decide on best corrective action
   e. Record fact about event in nurses' notes, but not fact that incident report filed.
4. Telephone calls
   a. Document any telephone calls made to report changes in patient condition.
   b. Important information to include
      (1) Specific time call was made
      (2) Who made the call?
      (3) Who was called?
      (4) To whom information was given
      (5) All information given
      (6) All information received
   c. When obtaining consents (and any other time appropriate), have another witness listen in (total of two witnesses).
5. Personal accountability
   a. Know your state Nurse Practice Act.
   b. Know the national standards for perianesthesia nursing practice.
   c. Continuing education is essential.
      (1) Read professional journals and books.
      (2) Attend pertinent seminars.
      (3) Maintain membership in professional organization pertinent to specialty.
   d. Policies and procedures

      (1) Will be held accountable for knowing and following hospital or ambulatory facility's policies and procedures

      (2) Should not conflict with one another

      (3) Should reflect actual practice

  e. Patient relations

      (1) Important aspect of prevention of liability

      (2) Old adage is true: "Happy patient rarely sues."

      (3) Do not criticize other health care providers in the presence of the family or patient.

      (4) Maintain good communication and rapport with the patient and family.

III. LEGAL PROCESS

  A. Phases of litigation

    1. Evaluation for suit—review of medical record

    2. Pleadings

      a. Complaint—outlines alleged negligence, states the injury, and may indicate an amount of compensation demanded

        (1) Notify insurer and hospital after complaint received.

      b. Answer—defendant is allowed a certain period to respond to allegations.

        (1) Attorney prepares the answer.

    3. Prelitigation panels—required by some states

      a. Medical review panel

      b. Medical tribunal

      c. Arbitration panel

    4. If you've been sued

      a. Do not discuss the case with anyone other than the risk manager or your attorney.

      b. Do not talk to the plaintiff, the plaintiff's attorney, or anyone testifying for the plaintiff.

      c. Do not discuss with reporters.

      d. Do not alter patient's chart or hide any information from your attorney.

    5. Discovery (pretrial phase)—attempts to narrow issues for trial by gathering and clarifying facts

      a. Interrogatories—list of written questions that seeks information to support or refute the complaint

      b. Production of documents—may be requested (e.g., ambulatory surgery facility records, incident reports, anesthesia records, policies and procedures, discharge teaching forms)

      c. Deposition—oral testimony of any person thought to have information pertaining to the case

        (1) Testimony given under oath

        (2) Recorded by court reporter

    6. Settlement negotiations—may continue throughout process and occur at any time in the process.

    7. Trial of lawsuit—may be a judge or jury trial.

      a. Jury selection

      b. Opening statements by plaintiff and defendant

      c. Plaintiff presents case—uses expert witnesses.

      d. Defendant presents case—uses expert witnesses.

      e. Defense may make motion for directed verdict against plaintiff—argues that the plaintiff has not met the burden of proof.

      f. Closing statements by plaintiff and defendant

      g. Jury instructions by the judge

      h. Jury deliberations

      i. Verdict

      j. Appeal (optional)

IV. ISSUES OF CONSENT
   A. Informed consent
      1. Consent obtained after the patient has been fully informed by the physician or dentist about the risks and benefits of the treatment, alternatives, and consequences of no treatment
      2. Types of consent
         a. Express—given by direct words, either written or oral
         b. Implied—inferred by the patient's conduct or may be legally presumed in emergency situations
      3. Treatment without consent
         a. Assault and/or battery
         b. Negligent failure to obtain consent
      4. Exceptions to duty to disclose
         a. Some emergency situations—life or well-being of the individual is threatened, and consent cannot be obtained or would result in a delay of treatment.
         b. Therapeutic privilege—physician believes information would be harmful to the patient; very restricted.
         c. Patient has waived right to consent—does not want to be informed.
         d. Lack of decision-making capacity—information must be shared with proxy decision-maker or guardian.
      5. Documentation of consents
         a. Nurses who sign as witnesses are only witnessing signature of person signing consent form.
         b. If patient has additional questions, nurse should refer questions to physician.
         c. If physician fails to discuss questions further with the patient, nurse must report that information through the appropriate chain of command.
         d. If English is not primary language of patient, an interpreter must be used.
   B. Advanced directives
      1. Living will—directive from competent individual to medical personnel and family members regarding treatment he or she wishes to receive when he or she can no longer make the decisions himself or herself
      2. Natural Death Act
         a. State-legislated legally recognized living wills with statutory enforcement
         b. Protects practitioner and ensures patient's wishes are followed
      3. Durable power of attorney for health care—allows competent patients to appoint an individual to make health care decisions if they become incompetent to do so
      4. Patient Self-Determination Act
         a. Passed in 1990 as part of federal Omnibus Budget Reconciliation Act
         b. Requires hospitals and other facilities on admission to advise all patients of their rights to refuse treatments and of any relevant state laws dealing with advanced directives
      5. Do-not-resuscitate directives—require documentation that the patient's decision was made after consultation with physician and understanding of options
      6. Health Insurance Portability and Accountability Act of 1996
         a. Major goal is to ensure proper protection of individuals' health information.
         b. Major purpose is to limit the circumstances in which an individual's protected health information may be disclosed.

BIBLIOGRAPHY

1. Aiken TD, Catalano JT: *Legal, ethical, and political issues in nursing*, ed 2, Philadelphia, 2004, Davis.

2. American Society of PeriAnesthesia Nurses: *Standards of perianesthesia nursing practice 2008-2010*, Cherry Hill, NJ, 2009, American Society of PeriAnesthesia Nurses.

3. Ashley RC: How do I know if I have been sued as a nurse and what do I do? *Crit Care Nurse* 22(3):82–83, 2002.

4. Ashley RC: The anatomy of a lawsuit: Part 1. *Crit Care Nurse* 22(4):68–69, 2002.

5. Ashley RC: The anatomy of a lawsuit: Part 2. *Crit Care Nurse* 22(5):82–83, 2002.

6. Berry FA: What to do when sued. *Curr Rev Post Anesth Care Nurs* 14(19):153–160, 2002.

7. Brent NJ: *Nurses and the law: A guide to principles and applications*, ed 2, Philadelphia, 2001, WB Saunders.

8. De Kornfeld TJ: Medico-legal considerations in the recovery room. *Curr Rev Post Anesth Care Nurs* 14(3):17–24, 1992.

9. Dynamic Nursing Education: *Safe medication administration*. Available at: http://dynamicnursingeducation.com/class.php?class_id=38&pid=15. Accessed November 20, 2008.

10. Feutz-Harter S: Nursing case law update. *J Nurs Law* 1(2):57–61, 1994.

11. Fiesta J: Failure to assess. *Nurs Manage* 24(9):16–17, 1993.

12. Flores JA: What if you're named in a lawsuit? *RN* 65(12):65–68, 2002.

13. Guido GW: *Legal issues in nursing*, ed 2, Stamford, CT, 1997, Appleton & Lange.

14. Hall JK: *Nursing: Ethics and law*, Philadelphia, 1996, WB Saunders.

15. Joel LA: *The nursing experience: Trends, challenges, and transitions*, ed 5, New York, 2005, McGraw Hill.

16. Kemmy JA: OR nursing law: Legal implications of perioperative documentation. *AORN J* 57(4):954, 956, 968, 1993.

17. Kowalski K, Yoder-Wise P: *Rapid reference for nurses*, Sudbury, MA, 2006, Jones & Bartlett.

18. Litwack K: *Post anesthesia care nursing*, ed 2, St Louis, 1995, Mosby.

19. Odom J: Legal issues in perianesthesia nursing. *Dissector J Perioper Nurs Coll N Z Nurse Organ* 30(4):9–11, 2003.

20. O'Keefe JE: *Nursing practice and the law: Avoiding malpractice and other legal risks*, Philadelphia, 2001, Davis.

21. Springhouse Corporation: *Nurse's handbook of law and ethics*, Springhouse, PA, 1992, Springhouse.

22. Tammelleo AD: Patient sues nurse for failure to obtain consent. *Regan Rep Nurs Law* 33(10):4, 1993.

23. United States Department of Health and Human Services: *Summary of the HIPAA privacy rule, 2003*. Available at: www.hhs.gov/ocr/privacysummary.pdf. Accessed November 20, 2008.

24. White PF, editor: *Ambulatory anesthesia and surgery*, Philadelphia, 1997, WB Saunders.

25. Zuffoletto JM: OR nursing law: Anatomy of a lawsuit. *AORN J* 56(5):933–936, 1992.

26. Zuffoletto JM: OR nursing law: Proving causation, damages in malpractice cases. *AORN J* 58(3):589–592, 1993.

ENVIRONMENT OF CARE

6 Practice Settings, Policies, and Procedures

SARA N. WALDRON

OBJECTIVES
At the conclusion of this chapter, the reader will be able to:

1. Define the scope of practice for perianesthesia nursing.
2. Describe the preanesthesia phase of care.
3. Explain the three phases of postanesthesia care.
4. List three inpatient and three outpatient settings where perianesthesia nursing care is delivered.
5. Differentiate between a policy and a procedure.
6. Describe how a procedure is used to implement a policy.
7. Name three agencies or organizations that influence perianesthesia policies and procedures.
8. Identify policies and procedures that define practice in perianesthesia nursing settings.

I. SCOPE OF PRACTICE
   A. Perianesthesia scope of nursing practice involves:
      1. Assessment and intervention for, and diagnosis and evaluation of physical or psychosocial problems or risks for problems that may result from the administration of sedation/analgesia or anesthetic agents and techniques
      2. Care of the patient and family/significant other along the perianesthesia continuum
         a. Physical
         b. Psychological
         c. Educational
         d. Cultural
         e. Spiritual
   B. Perianesthesia nursing practice is based on knowledge of:
      1. Physiological and psychological responses
      2. Vulnerability of patients subjected to:
         a. Sedation/analgesia
         b. Anesthetic agents and techniques
         c. Specific surgical or procedural interventions
      3. Principles of age-specific medical-surgical nursing and critical care nursing
      4. Evidence-based practice
   C. Perianesthesia nursing roles encompass:
      1. Clinical practice
      2. Education
      3. Research
      4. Management

     5. Administration

     6. Consultation

     7. Advocacy

 D. Perianesthesia nursing practice occurs in, but may not be limited to:

     1. Hospital settings (inpatients and outpatients)

         a. Preadmission assessment/testing unit

         b. Preoperative/preprocedural holding area

         c. Post anesthesia care unit

         d. Same-day surgery units

         e. Extended observation

         f. Labor and delivery

         g. Emergency department

         h. Special procedure areas

            (1) Interventional radiology

            (2) Endoscopy

            (3) Cardiac catheterization lab

            (4) Electroconvulsive therapy (ECT)

            (5) Pain management clinic

     2. Outpatient settings

         a. Ambulatory surgery unit

            (1) Hospital based

            (2) Free-standing center

         b. Special procedure clinics

            (1) Interventional radiology

            (2) Endoscopy

            (3) Cardiac catheterization

            (4) ECT

            (5) Pain management clinic

         c. Office-based practice

            (1) Dental

            (2) Dermatology

            (3) Ophthalmology

            (4) Plastic surgery

 E. Perianesthesia nursing during all levels of care includes the patient's family/ significant other and other supports whenever possible.

     1. Preanesthesia phase

         a. Preadmission: preparation for surgery/procedure

            (1) Identify potential and/or actual problems

               (a) Interview

               (b) Physical assessment

               (c) Diagnostic testing

            (2) Develop plan of care

            (3) Education/teaching

          b. Day of surgery/procedure: final preparation for surgery/procedure

            (1) Review/confirm collected data

            (2) Physical assessment

            (3) Implement plan of care

            (4) Education/teaching

         c. Preanesthesia patients separated from patients undergoing procedure and/ or recovering from sedation/anesthesia

     2. Postanesthesia

         a. Phase I: acute care in the immediate postanesthesia period

            (1) Focus on safety and comfort during recovery from:

               (a) Sedation/analgesia

               (b) Anesthetic agents and techniques

               (c) Specific surgical or procedural interventions

            (2) Utilize and amend plan of care.

      (3) Prepare patient for transition to:
        (a) Critical care inpatient unit
        (b) General inpatient unit
        (c) Phase II
        (d) Extended observation
      (4) Phase I care provided in close proximity to where sedation/anesthesia is administered

b. Phase II: care after the acute phase of recovery from sedation, analgesia, and anesthetic agents

      (1) Patient and/family/significant other readied for discharge to self or assisted care
        (a) Resolve elements in plan of care.
        (b) Conclude education/teaching.
        (c) Facilitate discharge arrangements.
      (2) Patient is discharged to:
        (a) Home
        (b) Presurgical/preprocedural care setting/facility
        (c) Extended observation
      (3) Phase II care is provided in:
        (a) Phase I unit
        (b) Proximity to phase I unit
        (c) Another area of the facility

c. Extended observation—ongoing patient observation after discharge from:

      (1) Phase I level of care
        (a) Patient meets discharge criteria but is waiting for transfer to inpatient unit.
        (b) Patient meets discharge criteria but is waiting for transition to phase II level of care.
      (2) Phase II level of care
        (a) Patient requires prolonged observation until final outpatient discharge.
        (b) Patient is waiting discharge to family/caregiver or facility.
      (3) Extended observation is provided in:
        (a) Phase I unit
        (b) Phase II unit
        (c) Another area of the facility
      (4) Extended observation may include overnight stay.

II. POLICIES AND PROCEDURES

  A. Policy

    1. Definition

      a. Set of principles used as a guide for action

      b. Organizational rules to define desired outcomes

        (1) Define the means to achieve organizational goals.
        (2) Reflect and support organization's vision and mission.
        (3) Consistent with all applicable legal and regulatory requirements

    2. The purpose of a policy is to:

      a. Give direction: the action to take in a particular situation

      b. Define responsibility and accountability: who is expected to take action

      c. Define boundaries: specific actions included or excluded

      d. Provide consistency: same action in each circumstance

      e. Support objective decision-making: reference for deciding course of action and clarifying misunderstandings

      f. Promote compliance: how to meet professional standards or external regulatory requirements

      g. Assign authority: who oversees defined actions

      h. Establish benchmarks: assess performance related to expectations of policy

    B. Procedure
- **1.** Definition
  - **a.** Instructions with detailed steps how to accomplish a task
  - **b.** Specific directions how to implement a policy
- **2.** The purpose of a procedure is to:
  - **a.** Provide all information necessary to complete the task/action
  - **b.** Explain concisely how to do a task
  - **c.** Establish organization's approved method of achieving the goal(s) of a policy
  - **d.** Serve as a:
    - (1) Guide for learning new tasks
    - (2) Resource for teaching new personnel
    - (3) Standard to assess performance related to compliance with accepted procedure

C. Policy and procedure format
- **1.** Defined by organization and consistently applied. Includes:
  - **a.** Authorizing signatures
  - **b.** Approving body
  - **c.** Dates of implementation, review, and revision
  - **d.** Item, page and section numbering
- **2.** Policy commonly followed by procedure in same document
  - **a.** Policy includes:
    - (1) Reason the policy exists
    - (2) Definition of terms
    - (3) Assignment of responsibilities
  - **b.** Procedure includes:
    - (1) Necessary resources/equipment
    - (2) Sequential steps
    - (3) Time frame requirements
    - (4) Documentation guidelines
    - (5) References
- **3.** Policies and procedures require a process for review and revision.
- **4.** Policies and procedures are readily accessible to staff.
  - **a.** Written
  - **b.** Electronic format

D. Perianesthesia policies and procedures
- **1.** Guide and define the delivery of care in the perianesthesia setting
  - **a.** Congruent with:
    - (1) American Nurses Association *Code of Ethics for Nurses With Interpretive Statements*
    - (2) American Hospital Association *Patient Care Partnership*
    - (3) American Society of PeriAnesthesia Nurses *Perianesthesia Standards for Ethical Practice*
  - **b.** Comply with standards of accrediting bodies
    - (1) Joint Commission
    - (2) Centers for Medicare and Medicaid Services
    - (3) Accreditation Association for Ambulatory Health Care
    - (4) American Association for the Accreditation of Ambulatory Surgical Facilities
  - **c.** Consistent with state regulatory and licensing agencies
    - (1) Board of Nursing
    - (2) Health department/services
- **2.** Benefit from collaboration among administrators, managers, and direct care perianesthesia nursing providers.
- **3.** Incorporate research findings and evidence-based practices.
- **4.** Require systematic review and timely revision in response to changes in:
  - **a.** Standards of practice
  - **b.** Regulatory requirements
  - **c.** Technology

E. The number and scope of policies and procedures in any practice setting is determined by the:
   1. Nature of the perianesthesia unit or care area
   2. Type of health care facility
   3. Procedures performed
   4. Services provided
   5. Characteristics of the patient population
F. Examples of perianesthesia policies and procedures.
   1. Administrative
      a. Unit description, hours of operation
      b. Job descriptions, hiring prerequisites, required certifications
      c. Staffing patterns, availability, call back
      d. Attire, professional conduct, personal communication devices
      e. Employee health, annual testing or screening
   2. Patient rights
      a. Health Insurance Portability and Accountability Act (HIPAA)
      b. Consents
         (1) Surgical, procedural, anesthesia, blood products
         (2) Emergency, minors, incompetency
      c. Advance directives
      d. Power of attorney
      e. Ethical treatment
   3. Environment of care
      a. Supplies: inventory, procurement, storage
      b. Equipment operation and maintenance
      c. Fire and safety plans
      d. Emergency preparedness and disaster response
      e. Infection control, personal protective equipment
      f. Hazardous material management: medical waste, anesthetic gases
      g. Security: patients, staff, visitors, volunteers
      h. Access to unit, restricted areas, visitation
   4. Patient care (specific to each level of perianesthesia care)
      a. Patient care management
         (1) Anesthesia provider responsibilities and availability
         (2) Physician orders: procurement and implementation
         (3) Chain of command: nursing, medical, surgical, administrative
      b. Admission and discharge criteria
      c. Standards of care: diagnosis and age-specific patient care plans, or treatment protocols
      d. Nurse-patient ratios
      e. Assessment and monitoring guidelines
      f. Medications: storage, access, administration, controlled substances, wastage, documentation
      g. Patient education, discharge planning
      h. Patient transportation, transfers
      i. Translation services
   5. Quality management/performance improvement
      a. Staff orientation
      b. Continuing education
      c. Individual performance evaluation, competency assessment
      d. Unit-specific and organizational performance improvement program
   6. Information management
      a. Medical record access, storage
      b. Confidentiality and security
      c. Release of information

BIBLIOGRAPHY

1. American Society of Anesthesiologists: *Standards for post anesthesia care, 2004*. Available at: www.asahq.org/publicationsandservices/standards/36.pdf. Accessed June 20, 2008.
2. American Society of PeriAnesthesia Nurses: *Standards of perianesthesia nursing practice 2008–2010*, Cherry Hill, NJ, 2009, American Society of PeriAnesthesia Nurses.
3. Drain CF, Odom-Forren J, editors: *Perianesthesia nursing: A critical care approach*, ed 5, St Louis, 2009, Saunders.
4. Page SB: *Establishing a system of policies and procedures*, ed 6, Westerville, OH, 2002, Process Improvement.
5. The Joint Commission: *Comprehensive accreditation manual for hospitals*, Oakbrook Terrace, IL, 2008, The Joint Commission.

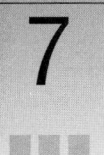

7 Regulatory Agencies and Accreditation

NANCY BURDEN

OBJECTIVES

At the conclusion of this chapter, the reader will be able to:

1. List three activities of the Office of the Inspector General.

2. Give three examples of activities addressed by state nurse practice acts.

3. Name at least three agencies within the U.S. Department of Health and Human Services (HHS).

4. Describe the major components of Health Insurance Portability and Accountability Act (HIPAA) regulations.

5. Give five examples of issues administered or regulated by state or local agencies.

I. REGULATORY AND ACCREDITATION ISSUES OVERVIEW
  A. Standards are the foundation from which the nurse develops and expands an individual and collective level of service.
    1. Standards related to the care of the patient are created and promulgated primarily by professional societies and educational institutions.
    2. Professional nursing and medical standards, however, must function within a larger collection of regulations, laws, and requirements.
  B. Most laws and regulations exist to protect the
    1. Public
    2. Patients
    3. Health care workers
    4. Financial and economic issues
  C. All levels of government—federal, state, and local—exert control over various areas of practice.
    1. Participation in Medicare, Medicaid, and other federally funded programs is dependent on meeting numerous requirements.
    2. Examples include the requirement to:
      a. Provide translation service for non–English-speaking patients (Civil Rights Act)
      b. Provide advance notice of financial responsibility to people covered by Medicare who may be accessing services that are not covered by the federal insurance plan (Centers for Medicare & Medicaid Services [CMS])
    3. Accreditation is a voluntary decision.
    4. Federal and private payers expect providers will be accredited by a national accrediting body.
II. PROFESSIONAL REGULATIONS
  A. National Council of State Boards of Nursing
    1. National Council of Licensure Examination for RN
    2. National standard examination with single passing standard

    B. Nursing boards and state nurse practice acts
       1. Regulate professional nursing practice and licensing.
       2. Identify scope of practice (e.g., administration of anesthetic agents for sedation/analgesia).
       3. Protect autonomy of the professional nurse.
       4. Protect public health.
          a. Standards for safe nursing care
          b. Issuing licenses
          c. Monitoring licensed nurses' compliance to state laws
          d. Disciplinary actions for unsafe practice
       5. Require that ethical and professional conduct standards be met, such as American Nurses Association's *Code for Nurses.*
       6. Regulations vary by state.
       7. Some reciprocity of requirements from state to state but separate licensing
    C. Certification boards—voluntary
       1. Specialty specific
          a. Certified Post Anesthesia Nurse
          b. Certified Ambulatory PeriAnesthesia Nurse
          c. Certified Nurse Operating Room
          d. Certified Gastroenterology Registered Nurse
          e. Registered Nurse—Board Certified in Pain Management
          f. Certified Administrator Surgery Center
       2. Testing function separate from educational entity of professional organization
       3. Promotes high level of education, experience, and application
       4. Demonstrates to public and peers commitment to professional excellence
    D. Other health care providers with professional regulation
       1. Physicians
       2. Nurse anesthetists
       3. Advanced registered nurse practitioners
       4. Physician assistants
       5. Radiology technologists
       6. Pharmacists
III. FACILITY-SPECIFIC REGULATIONS
    A. Policies and procedures (e.g., human resources, clinical, administrative)
       1. Identify methods and reasons to perform in a specific manner.
       2. Apply consistently and fairly.
       3. Ensure that practice conforms to policies.
    B. Emergency management plans and policies
    C. Employment requirements and job descriptions
    D. Patient and employee rights and responsibilities
    E. Drug-free/smoke-free workplace regulations
IV. COUNTY AND LOCAL REGULATIONS
    A. Business licensing
    B. Fire and disaster plans
    C. Emergency management plans
    D. Building codes and permits
    E. Impact fees
    F. Environmental regulations
V. STATE REGULATIONS
    A. Laws and statutes vary by state.
    B. Often define and/or enforce federal mandates
    C. Examples
       1. Facility licensing: hospitals, ambulatory surgery centers, pharmacies
       2. Professional licensing
       3. Risk management laws
       4. Insurance coverage requirements
       5. Biohazardous waste handling

      6. Pharmacy licensing and regulation

      7. Public health laws

      8. Radiation control

      9. Health statistics reporting

     10. Child, adult, elder abuse reporting

VI. FEDERAL REGULATIONS, STANDARDS, AND GUIDELINES

  A. U.S. Department of HHS

      1. Far-reaching regulatory control, umbrella department for many agencies

      2. CMS

      3. Fraud prevention and reporting

      4. Freedom of Information Act

      5. Biologicals (blood, organs, tissues)

      6. Poverty guidelines

      7. National Practitioner Data Bank (NPDB)

      8. Agency for Healthcare Research and Quality (AHRQ)

      9. Food and Drug Administration (FDA)

     10. Centers for Disease Control and Prevention (CDC)

  B. Americans With Disabilities Act, 1990

      1. Administered by Department of Justice, Civil Rights Division

      2. Protects against discrimination based on disabilities

      3. Applies to prospective and current employees and workplace issues, as well as to the public's access to facilities and services

      4. Removes barriers to access—physical, process, and attitudinal

      5. Reasonable modification of policies, practices, and procedures to accommodate

      6. Auxiliary aids such as qualified interpreters, telecommunications devices for the deaf, large print materials

        a. Interpreters should have medical terminology skills.

        b. Do not use family members.

        c. Cannot pass along cost of interpreter to patients

      7. Sets hiring and interviewing guidelines

      8. Expects reasonable accommodation for otherwise qualified candidates

  C. CDC

      1. Component of the Department of HHS

      2. Mission: to promote health and quality of life by preventing and controlling disease, injury, and disability

        a. Monitors health

        b. Detects and investigates health problems

        c. Conducts research to enhance prevention

        d. Develops and advocates sound public health policies

        e. Implements prevention strategies

        f. Promotes healthy behaviors

        g. Fosters safe and healthful environments

        h. Provides leadership and training

      3. Recommends disease prevention strategies affecting health care workers

        a. Hand washing standards

        b. Tuberculosis screening for health care workers

        c. Immunization against hepatitis

      4. Guideline for hand hygiene in health care settings

      5. Provides accurate health care information

      6. Investigates disease outbreaks

  D. Civil Rights Acts of 1957, 1960, 1964, 1968, 1973, 1980

      1. Administered by Department of Justice, Civil Rights Division

      2. Ten program-related sections

      3. Antidiscrimination statutes, broader than only health care

      4. Prohibit discrimination on basis of national origin, race, age, gender, and other factors

     5. Develop comprehensive language assistance program
       a. Assess facility's language needs
       b. Develop formal written policy
       c. Train staff
       d. Monitor program continually
  E. Clinical Laboratory Improvement Amendments (CLIA) Program
     1. CMS regulates all laboratory testing to ensure quality.
     2. Labs must be certified to receive Medicare or Medicaid reimbursement.
     3. CLIA waivers for specific point-of-care testing apparatus
       a. Competency requirements
       b. Required controls for test equipment
  F. CMS (formerly Health Care Financing Administration)
     1. Medicare and Medicaid
       a. Payment and coordination of health care benefits
       b. Fraud and abuse prevention and reporting
       c. False Claims Act (protects and rewards whistleblowers who report fraudulent claims against federal government)
       d. Anti-kickback statutes
     2. State Children's Health Insurance Program
     3. Health Insurance Portability and Accountability Act of 1996 (HIPAA of 1996)
     4. CLIA
  G. Consolidated Omnibus Budget Reconciliation Act (COBRA) of 1986
     1. Applies to certain former employees, spouses, dependent children, retirees
     2. Right to temporary continuation of health insurance coverage at group rates upon loss of employment
  H. U.S. Drug Enforcement Administration
     1. Controlled Substances Act, Title II of the Comprehensive Drug Abuse Prevention and Control Act of 1970
       a. Categorizes drugs regulated under federal laws into five schedules based upon the substance's medicinal value, harmfulness, and potential for abuse or addiction
         (1) Schedule I: highest (heroin, lysergic acid diethylamide [LSD], hashish
         (2) Schedule II: high (morphine, phencyclidine (PCP), codeine, cocaine, methadone, meperidine, Benzedrine, etc.)
         (3) Schedule III: medium (codeine with aspirin or Tylenol, anabolic steroids, etc.)
         (4) Low (Darvon, Talwin, phenobarbital, Equanil, Librium, diazepam, etc.)
         (5) Lowest (over-the-counter or prescription compounds with codeine, Lomotil, Robitussin-AC, etc.)
       b. System of distribution for those authorized to handle controlled substances
       c. Registration of those authorized to handle controlled substances
       d. Documentation and inventory control requirements
       e. Storage security regulations
       f. Periodic inspections
     2. Works in conjunction with U.S. Department of HHS
  I. Emergency Medical Treatment and Active Labor Act
     1. Part of COBRA of 1986
     2. Regulations passed in 1998
     3. Part of code that governs Medicare (Section 1867[a] of the Social Security Act)
     4. Applies only to "participating hospitals," those that are providers for CMS beneficiaries
     5. Primary purpose: to prevent hospitals from rejecting, refusing to treat, or transferring patients to "charity hospitals" or "county hospitals" because they are unable to pay or are covered under the Medicare or Medicaid programs
     6. Hospitals must provide stabilizing treatment for emergency medical conditions.
  J. Employee Retirement Income Security Act
     1. To ensure pension and other promised benefits
     2. Connected to Internal Revenue Code

     K. Fair Labor Standards Act
       1. Also known as Wage and Hour Regulations
       2. Defines exempt and nonexempt requirements for overtime
       3. Clarifies how pay issues are to be communicated
       4. Sets guidelines for age-appropriate work and hours
     L. HIPAA of 1996
       1. Title I: protects health insurance for workers who change or lose their jobs
       2. Title II: Administrative Simplification Standards
         a. Electronic health transactions
         b. Unique identifiers
         c. Security and electronic signature
         d. Privacy and confidentiality
       3. Congress added Administrative Simplification Standards section to standardize code sets, formats, and identifiers to save money.
       4. Protected health information (PHI)
       5. Privacy Rule: empowers patients and gives them more control over their PHI, how it is used, where it is shared
       6. Three areas where PHI can be shared freely, albeit confidentially
         a. T—Treatment
         b. P—Payment
         c. O—Operations
       7. Provides for civil and criminal penalties for noncompliance
    M. Patient Self-Determination Act
       1. Advance directives
         a. Living will
         b. Durable power of attorney
       2. Facility must have written policies and procedures that meet requirements for advance directives.
       3. Written information for patients—requirements vary by type of medical facility
       4. Educate staff on advance directive policies and requirements.
     N. NPDB
       1. Under HHS, Bureau of Health Professionals
       2. Created to improve quality of health care by:
         a. Encouraging agencies and state licensing boards to identify and discipline those engaging in unprofessional behavior
         b. Restricting ability for those practitioners to move from state to state
       3. Requiring reporting by health care facilities
       4. Using databank for credentialing and recredentialing licensed independent practitioners
       5. Access to information restricted to entities that meet eligibility requirements
 VII. OFFICE OF THE INSPECTOR GENERAL (OIG)
     A. Work authorized by the Inspector General Act of 1978
     B. Independent units within federal departments to:
       1. Conduct audits and investigate programs and operations
       2. Coordinate and recommend policies to promote economy, efficiency, and effectiveness
       3. Prevent and detect fraud and abuse
       4. Keep authorities informed about need for corrective action
     C. Work Plan: developed annually to identify areas most worthy of attention by the OIG
VIII. FEDERAL AGENCIES AND OTHER ORGANIZATIONS ADDRESSING QUALITY AND SAFETY
     A. AHRQ
       1. Arm of Department of HHS
       2. Federal agency for research on health care quality, costs, outcomes, and patient safety
       3. Research goals

        a. Identify most effective ways to organize, manage, finance, and deliver high-quality care.
        b. Reduce medical errors.
        c. Improve patient safety.
    4. Supports improvements in health outcomes
    5. Develops strategies to strengthen quality measurement and improvement
    6. Identifies strategies to improve health care access, fosters appropriate use, and reduces unnecessary expenditures
  B. Medical device reporting
    1. U.S. FDA
    2. Safe Medical Devices Act of 1990, 1997, 2000
    3. Objective: provide mechanism to identify and monitor significant adverse events related to medical devices
    4. Responsibilities by manufacturers and device users (medical facilities)
    5. MedWatch Program is mandatory reporting mechanism.
    6. Deaths or serious injuries must be reported within 10 workdays.
    7. Center for Devices and Radiological Health
  C. National Fire Protection Association
    1. International nonprofit organization
    2. Mission: to reduce the worldwide burden of fire and other hazards on the quality of life by providing and advocating consensus codes and standards, research, training, and education
    3. Develops, publishes, and disseminates timely consensus codes and standards intended to minimize the possibility and effects of fire and other risks
    4. Standards referenced by agencies and regulator bodies for compliance
  D. Occupational Safety and Health Administration
    1. Division of the U.S. Department of Labor
    2. Williams-Steiger Occupational Safety and Health Act of 1970
    3. Protection of workers. Examples:
        a. Environmental safety standards (e.g., fire safety, escape routes)
        b. Ergonomic controls
        c. Hazard communication standard (e.g., material safety data sheets)
        d. Materials handling and storage hazards and controls
        e. Needlestick Safety and Prevention Act
    4. Exposure control plan
        a. Occupational exposure to bloodborne pathogens—Standard 29 CFR 1910.1030
        b. Determine employee exposure risk.
        c. Outline methods to control exposure.
        d. Use engineering controls and work safety practices to improve safety (e.g., needleless systems, one-hand techniques).
        e. Provide personal protective equipment.
        f. Housekeeping, laundry practices
        g. Hepatitis B vaccination program
        h. Evaluate exposures.
        i. Documentation
    5. Workplace inspection priorities
        a. Imminent danger
        b. Fatal accidents
        c. Employee complaint
        d. Referral by other government agency
        e. Employer with high accident rate
        f. Follow-up
  E. Surgical Care Improvement Project (SCIP)
    1. National quality partnership of 36 organizations, companies, and agencies
    2. Seeking continued hospital involvement

       3. Goal to reduce the incidence of surgical complications nationally by 25% by the year 2010

       4. Focus areas

         a. Cardiac

         b. Infections

         c. Respiratory

         d. Venous thromboembolism

         e. End-stage renal disease

       5. Surgical site infections

         a. Responsible for 14% to 16% of all hospital-acquired infections

         b. Cost for each patient developing an infection: $3152 and up to 7 days of hospitalization

         c. Manage glucose levels.

         d. Avoid shaving skin preoperatively.

         e. Proper type and timing of preoperative antibiotics

         f. Proper perioperative thermoregulation

    F. Institute for Healthcare Improvement

       1. Protecting 5 Million Lives From Harm campaign

       2. Some is not a number. Soon is not a time.

       3. Voluntary initiative to protect 5 million people from medical harm between December 2006 and December 2008

       4. Carried over from 100,000 Lives campaign

         a. Deploy rapid response teams.

         b. Deliver reliable, evidence-based care for acute myocardial infarction.

         c. Prevent adverse drug events by implementing medication reconciliation.

         d. Prevent central line infections.

         e. Prevent surgical site infections by reliably delivering the correct perioperative antibiotics at the proper time.

         f. Prevent ventilator-associated pneumonia.

       5. Additional interventions

         a. Prevent harm from high alert medications … starting with a focus on anticoagulants, sedatives, narcotics, and insulin.

         b. Reduce surgical complications by reliably implementing all the changes in care recommended by SCIP.

         c. Prevent pressure ulcers.

         d. Reduce methicillin-resistant *Staphylococcus aureus* infection.

         e. Deliver reliable, evidence-based care for congestive heart failure.

         f. Get boards on board.

IX. WORLD HEALTH ORGANIZATION (WHO)

    A. World Alliance for Patient Safety

    B. WHO Guidelines on Hand Hygiene in Health Care (Advanced Draft): A Summary

       1. Indications for hand washing

       2. Hand hygiene technique

       3. Surgical hand preparation

       4. Selection of agents

       5. Skin care

       6. Glove use

       7. Other aspects of hand hygiene

       8. Health care worker training

       9. Government and institutional responsibilities

    C. Benefits of improved hand hygiene

X. ACCREDITING AGENCIES: VOLUNTARY OPTIONS

    A. Joint Commission

       1. Acute care, ambulatory, long-term care and other types of health care programs

       2. Recognized by third-party payers and government agencies

      3. Surveys are unannounced
      4. Strong emphasis on safety initiatives
      5. Publishes National Patient Safety Goals and Sentinel Event Alerts
   B. Accreditation Association for Ambulatory Health Care, Inc.
      1. Surveys many types of ambulatory health care providers
      2. Emphasizes constructive consultation and education
      3. Recognized by third-party payers and government agencies
   C. American Association for Accreditation of Ambulatory Surgery Facilities
      1. To ensure high standards in office-based surgery
      2. Single specialty and multispecialty facilities owned and operated by surgeons who are certified by a board recognized by the American Board of Medical Specialties
      3. Requires peer review and quality and process improvement programs to be in place

BIBLIOGRAPHY

1. Accreditation Association for Ambulatory Health Care, Inc. Available at: www.aaahc. org. Accessed November 21, 2008.
2. Agency for Healthcare Research and Quality. Available at: www.ahrq.org. Accessed November 20, 2008.
3. American Association for Accreditation of Ambulatory Surgery Facilities. Available at: www.aaaasf.org. Accessed November 21, 2008.
4. Boyce J, Pittet D: Guideline for hand hygiene in health-care settings. Recommendations of the Healthcare Infection Control Practices Advisory Committee and the HICPA/ SHEA/APIC/IDSA Hand Hygiene Task Force. *Infect Control Hosp Epidemiol* 23(suppl 12):S3-S40, 2002.
5. Cuming R, Rocco T, McEachern A: Improving compliance with occupational safety and health administration standards. *AORN J* 87(2):347–360, 2008.
6. Fosmire MS: *Frequently asked questions about the Emergency Medical Treatment and Active Labor Act (EMTALA).* Available at: www. emtala.com/faq.htm. Accessed February 16, 2008.
7. Gaberson K: Not your mother's nursing school. *AORN J* 87(2):287–292, 2008.
8. Institute for Healthcare Improvement: *Protecting 5 million lives from harm.* Available at: www.ihi.org/IHI/Programs/ Campaign/. Accessed November 21, 2008.
9. Medscape Today: *Surgical Care Improvement Project (SCIP).* Available at: www.medscape. com/viewarticle/557689. Accessed November 21, 2008.
10. National Council of State Boards of Nursing: *What boards do.* Available at: www.ncsbn. org/126.htm. Accessed February 13, 2008.
11. National Fire Protection Association. Available at: www.nfpa.org. Accessed November 21, 2008.
12. National Practitioner Data Bank Healthcare Integrity and Protection Data Bank. Available at: www.npdb-hipdb.com/. Accessed November 21, 2008.
13. The Joint Commission. Available at: www. jointcommission.org. Accessed November 21, 2008.
14. United States Centers for Disease Control and Prevention. Available at: www.cdc. gov/about/organization/cio.htm. Accessed February 12, 2008.
15. United States Department of Health & Human Services: *Office of the Inspector General work plan fiscal year 2008.* Available at: oig.hhs.gov/publications/docs/workplan/ 2008/Work_Plan_FY_2008.pdf. Accessed February 13, 2008.
16. United States Department of Health & Human Services: *Office for Civil Rights— HIPAA.* Available at: www.hhs.gov/ocr/ hipaa. Accessed February 16, 2008.
17. United States Department of Health & Human Services, Center for Devices and Radiological Health: *Medical device reporting: An overview.* Available at: www.fda. gov/cdrh/. Accessed February 13, 2008.
18. United States Department of Justice, Civil Rights Division: *Civil Rights Division activities and programs.* Available at: www.usdoj.gov/ crt/activity.html. Accessed February 16, 2008.
19. United States Department of Justice: *Americans With Disabilities Act.* Available at: www.ada. gov. Accessed November 21, 2008.
20. United States Department of Labor Occupational Safety and Health Administration: *Frequently asked questions,* August

2007. Available at: www.osha.gov/as/opa/osha-faq.html. Accessed February 13, 2008.

21. United States Drug Enforcement Administration: Available at: www.dea.gov. Accessed February 13, 2008.

22. United States Equal Employment Opportunity Commission: *Americans With Disabilities Act questions and answers.* Available at: www.usdoj.gov/crt/ada/q%26aeng02.htm. Accessed February 16, 2008.

23. World Health Organization: *WHO guidelines on hand hygiene in health care (advanced draft): A summary.* Available at: www.who.int/patientsafety/events/05/HH_en.pdf. Accessed February 16, 2008.

DINA A. KRENZISCHEK

OBJECTIVES

At the conclusion of this chapter, the reader will be able to:

1. Define patient safety.
2. Describe the American Society of PeriAnesthesia Nurses (ASPAN) position statement on perianesthesia safety.
3. List 2009 The Joint Commission (TJC) National Patient Safety Goals, patient safety resources, and Council on Surgical and Perioperative Safety (CSPS) safety goals.
4. List perianesthesia safety net, harm levels, and methods of reporting/analysis.
5. Identify key elements of safety culture, including workplace civility.

I. OVERVIEW
  A. Patient safety
    1. The core of standard practice of perianesthesia nurses
    2. Considered the highest priority
    3. The freedom from accidental injury caused by medical care or medical error
    4. The achievement of intended outcomes
  B. Safety is defined as
    1. A condition of being safe from undergoing or causing hurt or loss
    2. Protection against failure, breakage, or accident
  C. ASPAN position statement on perianesthesia safety
    1. Responsible in defining the principles of safe quality nursing practice in the perianesthesia setting
    2. Highly committed to the culture of safety
    3. A collective of shared knowledge and beliefs regarding safe health care practice settings and the provision of safe practice
    4. Prevention of any incidence or risk of injury, danger, or harm
    5. Goal is to promote a safe perianesthesia care setting and provide guidelines for best practices.
II. CORE VALUES AND TENETS OF A SAFETY CULTURE
  A. Communication
    1. Reporting errors/safe practices
    2. Ensuring a complete and systematic approach to hand-off processes and transfer of care
    3. Developing and using effective listening skills
  B. Advocacy
    1. Protecting patient from harm
    2. Upholding ethics of care
    3. Maintaining patients' rights
    4. Seeking and implementing best practices
  C. Competency
    1. Achieving and supporting professional competence in clinical practice
    2. Initiating, supporting, and providing education for staff and patients
    3. Demonstrating appropriate clinical judgment and critical thinking
    4. Measuring and monitoring quality measures and nurse-sensitive indicators

   D. Efficiency/timeliness
   1. Maintaining a healthy environment of care
   2. Providing timely interventions and reports
   3. Appreciating cues and initiating appropriate interventions
   E. Teamwork
   1. Collaborating with health care providers
   2. Building mutual trust between all health care providers
   3. Supporting an organizational culture of safety
III. 2009 TJC SAFETY GOALS AND KEY POINTS
   A. Goal 1: Improve the accuracy of patient identification.
   1. Use two identifiers for:
      a. Medication administration/IV fluids
      b. Blood products
      c. Blood samples and specimens
      d. Blood transfusion
      e. Treatment procedures
      f. Charts and forms
   2. Final verification process before surgery or procedure
   B. Goal 2: Improve the effectiveness of communication among caregivers.
   1. Hand-off communication: verbalize accurate, clear, complete, interactive
   2. Read back including critical results and provider's orders
   3. List of abbreviations, acronyms, symbols, and dose—not used
   4. Timeliness of reporting, receipt of critical test results and values
   5. Standardized approach to hand-off communications
   C. Goal 3: Improve the safety of using medications.
   1. Review and verify allergies.
   2. Be alert and take action on look-alike/sound-alike medications.
   3. Label medications, containers, and solutions.
   4. Attention to anticoagulant therapy, insulin, cardiac medications, etc.
   5. Verify unclear orders.
   6. Avoid distraction and interruptions during medication administration.
   D. Goal 7: Reduce the risk of health care–associated infection.
   1. Wash hands (15 seconds) before and after patient contact.
   2. Assess and report any signs of infection.
   3. Implement evidence-based practices to prevent health care–associated infections.
   4. Implement best practices or evidence-based guidelines to prevent central line–associated bloodstream infections.
   5. Implement best practices for preventing surgical site infections.
   6. Implement and encourage others to follow isolation protective techniques.
   E. Goal 8: Accurately and completely reconcile medications across the continuum of care.
   1. Obtain and verify medication list from patient (name, unit dose, dose amount, frequency, last dose).
   2. Reconcile medication list to provider's order.
   3. Document any changes noted.
   4. Communicate the completed reconciled list to the next receiving unit nurse, including other assessments.
   5. Communicate and educate patient directly and family as needed when patient is going home, using the completed reconciled list.
   6. Report any inconsistency or problems to the provider.
   F. Goal 9: Reduce the risk of patient harm resulting from falls.
   1. Follow institutional fall precaution protocol.
   2. Follow institutional restraint protocol including any competency training
   3. Stay with patient or delegate someone to assist patient when dressing to go home.
   4. Adjust patient assignment depending upon the needs of high- risk patients.
   G. Goal 10: Reduce the risk of influenza and pneumococcal disease in institutionalized older adults.
   1. Follow institutional flu vaccine protocol.

        2. Follow administration protocol of pneumococcus vaccine.

        3. Report any known cases of influenza.

   H. Goal 11: Reduce the risk of surgical fires.

        1. Assess and report any equipment with damaged electrical parts.

        2. Manage patient's injuries as a result of fire that occurred intraoperatively.

   I. Goal 13: Encourage patients' active involvement in their own care as a patient safety strategy.

        1. Encourage patients and families to report safety concerns.

        2. Identify ways of reporting and communicate to patient and family members.

        3. Identify process of correcting patient and family concerns in a timely manner.

   J. Goal 14: Prevent health care–associated pressure ulcers (decubitus ulcers).

        1. Assess areas of potential pressure ulcer.

        2. Follow institutional protocol for management of high-risk patients, including documentation.

   K. Goal 15: The organization identifies safety risks inherent in its patient population.

        1. Identify patients with risk for suicide.

        2. Assess and document potential signs of suicidal behaviors.

        3. Report any problem to the provider and facilitate psychiatric consult as ordered.

        4. Provide resource to watch patient and determine type of resource when transferring patient to a receiving unit.

   L. Goal 16: Improve recognition and response to changes in a patient's condition.

        1. Provide competency training to staff to meet the needs of the population to be served, including critically ill patients.

  M. Implement universal protocol.

        1. Conduct a preprocedure/surgical verification process.

        2. Facilitate the marking of the procedure site.

        3. Time out before starting a procedure.

IV. PATIENT SAFETY RESOURCES

   A. Agency for Healthcare Research and Quality

        1. Clinical practice guidelines

        2. Evidence-based practice

        3. Patient safety

        4. Funding opportunities

        5. *Be Involved in Your Healthcare Tips*

           a. 20 tips to help prevent medical errors

        6. *Healthcare 411*

           a. Latest findings, news, and consumer information

   B. Institute for Safe Medication Practices

        1. Alerts for patients

           a. Cancer treatment, safe medication, medication samples, and medicine reviews

   C. National Committee for Quality Assurance

        1. Strategies to improve care

        2. Indicators

        3. Protocols

        4. Cost reduction

        5. Disease management

        6. Measurement

   D. National Guideline Clearinghouse

        1. Evidence-based practice guidelines

   E. National Patient Safety Foundation

        1. Patient safety resources

        2. Safety organizations

        3. Safety definitions

        4. Safety advisories

           a. Tips for improving patient safety

    F. TJC
        1. *Sentinel Event Alerts*
            a. Medical error prevention guideline for safe treatment
    G. World Health Organization
            a. Protection against failure or accident

V. CSPS
    A. All members of the multidisciplinary perioperative care team participate to achieve optimal patient outcomes.
    B. Members include:
        1. American Association of Nurse Anesthetists (AANA)
        2. American Association of Surgical Physician Assistants (AASPA)
        3. American College of Surgeons (ACS)
        4. American Society of Anesthesiologists (ASA)
        5. American Society of PeriAnesthesia Nurses (ASPAN)
        6. Association of PeriOperative Registered Nurses (AORN)
        7. Association of Surgical Technologists (AST)
    C. Core principles endorsed
        1. Correct site surgery
        2. Sharps safety in the OR
        3. Prevention of retained foreign objects
        4. Fire safety
        5. Prevention of venous thromboembolism
        6. Prevention of health care–associated infections
        7. Audible physiological alarms
        8. Transfer-of-care principles
        9. Universal nomenclature
        10. Standardized glossary of times
        11. Consideration for other core principles
            a. Practitioner competency and credentialing
            b. Systems-based issues
            c. Communication issues
            d. Violence in the workplace

VI. ASPAN PERIANESTHESIA SAFETY NET, HARM LEVEL, REPORTING, AND ANALYSIS
    A. Perianesthesia safety net
        1. Improve the accuracy of patient identification and final verification before procedures to prevent identification errors.
        2. Improve the effectiveness of communication among caregivers.
        3. Improve the safety of using medications, and monitor medication errors.
        4. Eliminate wrong-site, wrong-patient, wrong-procedure surgery.
        5. Improve the safety of using infusion pumps, equipment, or both.
        6. Improve the effectiveness of clinical alarm systems.
        7. Reduce the risk of health care–associated infections.
        8. Reduce the risk of patient harm resulting from falls.
        9. Reduce the risk of influenza and pneumococcal disease in institutionalized older adults.
        10. Reduce the risk of surgical fires.
        11. Implement applicable *National Patient Safety Goals* and associated requirements by components and practitioner sites.
        12. Encourage the active involvement of patients and their families in the patient's care.
        13. Prevent health care–associated pressure ulcers.
        14. Identify safety risks inherent in the patient population (including suicide risk).
        15. Other
            a. Laboratory test problems
            b. Radiology/imaging test problems
            c. Transfusion

      d. Behavioral

      e. Care coordination

      f. Staffing-related problems

        (1) Cause of harm to patient

        (2) Contributory causes to adverse outcomes

      g. Physician order entry–related problems

      h. Other adverse events

  B. Harm levels

    1. National Coordinating Council for Medication Error Reporting and Prevention Index

      a. Category A: circumstances or events that have the capacity to cause error

      b. Category B: an error that occurred but did not reach the patient

      c. Category C: an error that occurred and did reach the patient but did not cause harm

      d. Category D: an error that occurred, reached the patient, and required monitoring to confirm that it resulted in no harm to the patient and/or required intervention to preclude harm

      e. Category E: an error that occurred that may have contributed to, or resulted in, temporary harm to the patient and required intervention

      f. Category F: an error that occurred that may have contributed to, or resulted in, temporary harm to the patient and required initial or prolonged hospitalization

      g. Category G: an error that occurred that may have contributed to, or resulted in, permanent patient harm

      h. Category H: an error that occurred that required intervention necessary to sustain life

      i. Category I: an error that occurred that may have contributed to, or resulted in, the patient's death

  C. Methods of reporting and analysis

    1. Reporting

      a. Situation-Background-Assessment-Recommendation (SBAR) method introduced by TJC (Box 8-1)

      b. SBAR used in reporting of events at the institutional, department, and unit-based levels and during performance improvement and unit-based staff meetings to reduce unsafe practices

    2. Analysis

      a. Risk management review

        (1) Process in building defense by collecting data related to exposure

        (2) Documents circumstances

        (3) Establishes probable cause, liability, and losses

        (4) Identifies risk leading to future events

      b. Peer review

        (1) An organized effort whereby practicing professionals review quality and appropriateness of service ordered or performed by their professional peers

        (2) Determines whether standard of care has been violated

        (3) Determines whether additional action is warranted

        (4) Ensures adequate training and competency

      c. Failure mode error analysis

        (1) Procedure for analysis of potential failure modes within a system for the classification by severity or determination of the failure's effect upon the system

        (2) Risk analysis technique/systematic thinking

        (3) Failure mode: effects, severity, causes, and action

        (4) Examines functions and process

      d. Root cause analysis

        (1) A problem-solving method for identifying the root causes of problem or event

■ BOX 8-1
■ **SBAR** REPORTING METHOD

Situation (S): What is the problem or main issue?
- Patient (Mr. Smith) was admitted to the post anesthesia care unit (PACU) with an oxygen saturation of 89%, and the oxygen tank was found to be empty. Patient was sleepy and not easily arousable.

Background (B): What are the circumstances of the situation?
- Mr. Smith is a 55-year-old patient who has had a bilateral knee replacement.
- Anesthesia technique: received epidural anesthesia but failed and general anesthesia.
- Analgesia: intraoperatively, received a total of 3000 micrograms fentanyl and 4 mg Hydromorphone. At the end of the case, received an additional 100 mcg fentanyl and 2 mg Hydromorphone for severe pain.

Assessment (A): What do you think is the problem?
- Preoperatively, patient reported that he has low pain threshold and would like his pain controlled.
- Portable oxygen tank was sent to the OR with the stretcher as part of routine, but PSI (pounds per square inch), the amount of oxygen in the tank was not checked and recorded.
- Oxygen tank was used during transport, but PSI was not checked.
- Upon PACU admission, oxygen tank was found to be empty, and patient was sleepy with shallow breathing and low oxygen saturation.

Recommendations (R): What needs to be done to correct the problem?
- Review practice standard regarding portable oxygen check. If no standard, develop a practice standard including PSI check before use, documentation and reporting of problem upon patient transfer.
- Disseminate, educate, and implement new standard.
- Follow-up audit for compliance and report findings.

        (2) Scientific method
        (3) Multidisciplinary approach
        (4) Focuses on obtaining information about lost system control
        (5) Getting at root of the problem, seeking real cause
VII. SAFETY CULTURE AND WORKPLACE CIVILITY
   A. Safety culture
     1. Framework for consideration:
       a. Developing a system-wide approach to patient safety
         (1) Vision statement
         (2) Leadership visibility and commitment to patient safety
         (3) Understanding different models of errors
       b. Create a safety culture in the unit-based environment
         (1) Level of compassion and concern for patient safety
         (2) Competency and training
         (3) Recognition and security for reporting errors
         (4) Recognition and security for identifying improvement opportunities
         (5) Learning environment where errors are valued
         (6) Opportunities for improvements
         (7) Open to interactions with patients, family, and health care team
         (8) Removal of culture of blame
         (9) Safe environment built from the bottom
         (10) Culture of safety supported from the top
         (11) Use of safety checklist/safety standards
   B. Workplace civility
     1. Rapidly changing, stressful environment
     2. Civility is an ethical role, implemented to maintain teamwork in a safe environment.
     3. Constant awareness of others based on restraint, respect, and consideration
     4. Rules of considerate conduct (Table 8-1)

■ TABLE 8-1
■ ■ **Rules of Considerate Conduct**

Rule	Key Points
1. Pay attention	Makes meaningful interaction possible
2. Acknowledge others	Gives honor to a person
3. Think the best	Decent thing to do and source of healthful innocence in our lives
4. Listen	Plan, show, and be a cooperative listener
5. Be inclusive	Feeling of welcome and acceptance
6. Speak kindly	Speaking with consideration and kindness is the heart of civil behavior
7. Don't speak ill	Nice but needs to be built
8. Accept and give praises	Deepest principle in human nature
9. Respect even a subtle "no"	Most elementary and significant rule of respect
10. Respect others' opinions	Respect for the whole person
11. Mind your body	Validate who we are
12. Be agreeable	Cultivate ability to consider that you might be wrong and ability to admit that you do not know
13. Keep it down and rediscover silence	Silence is the ability to hear others
14. Respect other people's timeliness	Punctuality is nonnegotiable
15. Respect other people's space	Most elementary way of consideration
16. Apologize earnestly and thoughtfully	A decent thing to do
17. Assert yourself	Stand up for own right in a diplomatic manner
18. Avoid personal questions	Respect privacy of others
19. Care for your guests	Guests should not feel that they must earn your hospitality
20. Be a considerate guest	Respect time of arrival and departure and do not bring a surprise guest
21. Think twice before asking favors	Solve your own problem and only turn to others as a last resort
22. Refrain from idle complaints	Speak up to bring good change but not unwanted misery
23. Give constructive criticism	You speak with the intention to help with a problem but not to humiliate
24. Respect the environment and be gentle to animals	Nature is in danger, and we must defend it from ourselves
25. Don't shift responsibility and blame	Rude and unfair by blaming someone

Adapted from Forni PM: *Choosing civility: The twenty-five rules of considerate conduct,* New York, 2002, St. Martin's Press.

BIBLIOGRAPHY

1. American Society of PeriAnesthesia Nurses: *Standards of perianesthesia nursing practice 2008–2010.* Cherry Hill, NJ, 2009, American Society of PeriAnesthesia Nurses.
2. Cohen MR, ed: *Defining medication errors,* ed 2, Washington, DC, 2007, American Pharmacists Association.
3. Forni PM: *Choosing civility: The twenty-five rules of considerate conduct,* New York, 2003, St. Martin's Press.
4. Frankel A: *Strategies for building a hospital wide culture of safety,* JCR, 2006, Oak Brook, IL.
5. Institute of Medicine: *Patient safety: Achieving a new standard of care,* Washington, DC, 2004, National Academic Press.
6. Iowa Department of Public Health: Promoting and Protecting the Health of Oawans. Available at: www.idph.state.ia.us/patient_safety/resources. Accessed November 24, 2008.
7. Kim H, Hathen-Vaires N, Capuano T, Morgan G, Bende-Kovitz R: Peer case review sharpens event analysis. *J Nurs Care Qual* 23(4):296–304, 2008.

8. Kohn LT, Corrigan JM, Donaldson MS, eds: *To err is human: Building a safer health system*, Washington, DC, 1999, National Academy Press.

9. Leape LL: A systems analysis approach to medical error. *J Eval Clin Pract* 3(3):213–222, 1997.

10. Lin L, Liang BA: Addressing the nursing work environment to promote patient safety. *Nurs Forum* 42(1):20–30, 2007.

11. Merriam-Webster Dictionary: *Safety*. Available at: www.merriam-webster.com/dictionary/safety. Accessed November 24, 2008.

12. Nieva VF, Sorra J: Safety culture assessment: A tool for improving patient safety in healthcare organizations. *Qual Saf Health Care* 12(suppl 2):ii17-ii23, 2003.

13. Spath PL, ed: *Investigating sentinel events: How to find and resolve root causes*, Forest Groove, OR, 1998, Brown-Spath & Associates.

14. Spath PL, ed: *Error reduction in health care*, San Francisco, 2000, AHA Press/Jossey-Bass.

15. The Joint Commission: *2009 National patient safety goals*. Available at: www.jointcommission.org/PatientSafety/NationalPatientSafetyGoals/. Accessed November 24, 2008.

Continuous Quality Improvement

MEG BETURNE

OBJECTIVES

At the conclusion of this chapter, the reader will be able to:

1. Define quality in health care.
2. Describe the process of continuous quality improvement (CQI).
3. Describe the concept of total quality management (TQM).
4. Recognize major changes in health care that have had an impact on quality improvement (QI).
5. Identify aspects and key dimensions of quality.
6. List useful sources of data collection.
7. List useful tools for identifying patterns or trends.
8. Recognize issues in perianesthesia settings that affect quality.

I. QUALITY IN HEALTH CARE
   A. Doing the right things right the first time
   B. According to Donadbedian, quality depends on:
      1. Practitioner assessment and/or patient and health system contributions
      2. How health and responsibility for health are defined
      3. Whether maximally or optimally effective care is sought
      4. Whether the optimum is defined according to individual or social preference
   C. Juran Institute defines quality as:
      1. Freedom from deficiencies: any avoidable intervention required to achieve an equivalent patient outcome
      2. Product features: both services and goods that attract and satisfy patients, meet customer expectations, and distinguish one practitioner or organization from others
   D. Institute of Medicine (IOM): quality of care is the degree to which health services for individuals and populations increase the likelihood of desired health outcomes and are consistent with current professional knowledge.
   E. Agency for Healthcare Research and Quality: quality in health care means:
      1. Providers deliver the right care to right patient at the right time in the right way.
      2. Patients can access timely care, have understandable and accurate information about benefits and risks, are protected from unsafe care services and products, and have understandable and reliable information on their care.
      3. Clinicians and patients have their rights respected.
   F. Concept of value

$$\text{Value} = \frac{\text{Quality of Care or Service} + \text{Outcome}}{\text{Cost}}$$

   1. Require proof (positive outcomes) that the quality of care received is the best possible for dollars spent and minimize adverse patient outcomes
   2. Value-added is key—it includes issues related to access, convenience, service, relationships with physicians, safety, and innovation.

  G. Incremental stages of quality
    1. Technical quality relies on quality tools, processes, and technology with customer perspective of "persuade them."
    2. Functional quality relies on people and judgment with customer perspective of "satisfy them."
    3. Competitive quality relies on time and flexibility with a customer perspective of "attract them."
    4. Forward quality relies on long-term planning and intuition with customer perspective of "building trust."
II. CQI
  A. Systematic approaches/models to the continuous study and improvement of the processes of providing health care services to meet the needs of individuals and others
  B. Shewhart cycle: statistical quality control and cycle for continuous improvement PDCA (plan, do, check, act)

$$\text{Improvement} = \text{Plan} \rightarrow \text{Do} \rightarrow \text{Check} \rightarrow \text{Act}$$

  C. FOCUS PDCA model
    1. Find
    2. Organize
    3. Clarify
    4. Understand
    5. Select
  D. Feiggenbaum

$$\text{Total Quality Control} = \text{Quality Development} + \text{Quality Maintenance} + \text{Quality Improvement}$$

  E. Organizational Dynamics FADE approach
    1. Focus on problem.
    2. Analyze problem.
    3. Develop a plan for improvement.
    4. Execute the plan.
  F. Ernst and Young IMPROVE model
    1. Identify problem.
    2. Measure impact.
    3. Prioritize causes.
    4. Research root causes.
    5. Outline alternatives.
    6. Validate solutions.
    7. Execute solutions and standardize.
  G. QI process
    1. Use of team collaborative efforts to study and improve specific existing processes at all levels
    2. Prioritizing and analyzing causes of existing process failure, dysfunction, or inefficiency
    3. Systematically instituting optimal solutions to chronic problems
    4. Analyzing and disseminating best-practice information to staff, patients, and families
    5. Using scientific problem-solving method to improve process performance and achieve stated goals
    6. Holding the gains through monitoring system
  H. Six Sigma strategy
    1. Disciplined approach to process improvement
    2. Define costs and benefits.
    3. Measure input and output.
    4. Analyze causes of current or anticipated defects.
  I. Lean-thinking approach
    1. Use of thought process based on lean principles of:
      a. Understanding value

       b. Identifying value stream

       c. Making service flow

       d. Pulling flow from demand (flexibility)

       e. Setting targets for perfection

J. The Joint Commission (TJC)

  1. Continuous improvement of patient care outcomes

  2. Identification of functions and processes with the most significant impact on outcomes

  3. Emphasis on integrated system rather than independent units

  4. Emphasis on consistent performance standards

  5. Use of national performance measurement system for patient outcomes and care processes

  6. Continual data collection, risk adjustment, and analysis

  7. Use of comparative data for performance improvement

K. Traditional ways of monitoring, evaluating, and measuring quality

  1. Retrospective: chart audit

     a. Peer review process used in hospitals until 1970s

     b. Small sample of patient records reviewed by medical staff with judgment made as to the quality of care provided

     c. Problems confirmed and solutions identified

     d. Increased emphasis on appropriateness of care in 1980s

  2. Prospective, concurrent, and focused monitoring and analysis processes in place

     a. On-line clinical data

     b. Observation of actual process of care

     c. Referrals

     d. Special study, case mix, or other data summaries

     e. Incident/occurrence reports

  3. Evaluation process

     a. In-depth assessment of quality of care when

       (1) A threshold (trigger point) is reached

       (2) A compliance level is/is not met

       (3) Control limits are exceeded

  4. Indicators

     a. Monitor the quality of all aspects of care.

     b. Gauge actual performance and compare with targeted objective or standard.

     c. Include

       (1) Clinical criteria

       (2) Clinical standards

       (3) Practice guidelines

       (4) Protocols

       (5) Performance database

     d. Stated in objective terms

     e. Condition or procedure specific

     f. Focus on discrete populations.

     g. Accuracy, risk adjustment, and cost are measured through control of information technology.

     h. Identify opportunities to improve care.

     i. Based on current knowledge or structure and projected needs, standards, or industry changes

     j. Classified as outcome or process

     k. Address issues of structure.

  5. Structure standards

     a. Qualifications of the providers

     b. Physical facility, equipment, and other resources

     c. Characteristics of the organization and its financing

6. Outcomes
  a. Things that do (or do not) happen as a result of medical interventions
    (1) Complication rates
    (2) Functional capacity and performance
    (3) Cost-effectiveness
    (4) Patient satisfaction
  b. Serve as red flags
  c. Objective measurements of outcomes
    (1) Patient satisfaction
    (2) Efficiency
    (3) Cost reduction
    (4) Results of service
  d. Most important concerns
    (1) Positive patient outcomes
    (2) Cost-effective delivery of care
    (3) Provide return on investment
  e. Number one competitive factor next to cost in health care
  f. Integrative: include contributions of providers and patients
  g. Survey target areas for The Joint Commission and Accreditation Association for Ambulatory Health care
  h. One of most crucial expectations of managed care and third-party payers
  i. Endpoint of outcomes research—clinical practice guidelines, which are intended to assist practitioners and patients in choosing appropriate health care for specific conditions
7. Nursing-sensitive quality indicators
  a. Performance measures that capture patient care or its outcomes most affected by nursing care
  b. Can be used to create a nursing report card for the organization
  c. Examples: pressure ulcers, patient falls, nosocomial infection rate for central lines, staffing mix, patient satisfaction, and staff satisfaction
L. Common steps in QI process
  1. Identify/focus on priority areas.
  2. Collect data/measure performance.
  3. Assess performance.
  4. Take action for improvement.
  5. Effective team development and interaction
  6. Use of statistical, analytical, and consensus tools
  7. Failure mode and effects analysis
    a. Improvement projects with significant impact
    b. Wise to conduct proactive team
    c. Identify risks of any process step failure.
    d. Analyze the potential severity if any process step fails.
    e. Select appropriate responses to minimize impact.
M. CQI key processes relative to data
  1. Identify current available data sources.
  2. Identify critical information needs.
  3. Define data elements.
  4. Determine data collection plan.
  5. Acquire/collect data.
  6. Aggregate and display data.
  7. Analyze data.
  8. Interpret data/information.
  9. Act on information/knowledge.
  10. Report data/information/knowledge/decision.
  11. Collect more data to monitor/analyze the decision.
N. QI team approach
  1. An ongoing interdisciplinary/cross-functional team selected from those who collect or use data and are trained in group process

      2. Each site, discipline, department, team, and committee collecting data identified
      3. Data to be collected determined by indicators/performance measures
      4. Resources provided for the team to hit targets and meet objectives
      5. Mechanisms in place for information management education
      6. Reviews/monitors internal report from teams
      7. Establishes improvement priorities
      8. Determines how data defined

O. CQI demands
      1. Corporate and organizational commitment to mission, money, management, material
      2. Organization-wide culture that talks and acts like quality
      3. Identification and understanding of customers, their needs and expectations
      4. Ongoing pursuit of customer satisfaction
      5. Team emphasis on perfecting systems in delivery of patient care to affect good outcomes
      6. Constant learning and improving
      7. Interdisciplinary and cross-functional collaboration
      8. A planned, systematic approach organized around flow of patient care

P. Responsibility of health care professionals with process and report to administrative and governing bodies
      1. Understand principles.
      2. Articulate process of
         a. Data measurement
         b. Analysis
         c. Improvement
         d. Development of effective strategies
      3. Recognize and be sensitive to the differences in quality services as opposed to products.
      4. Move quality to the top through the commitment to excellence.
      5. Validate current practice or identify opportunities for improvement using these criteria:
         a. Total cost
         b. Impact
         c. Benefit/cost relationship
         d. Cultural impact
         e. Resistance to change
         f. Risk
         g. Health, safety, and the environment

III. TQM
    A. Evolved from Japanese industry after World War II
      1. Edward Deming
         a. Developed sampling and data QI strategies and assisted the Japanese in developing high-quality merchandise
         b. Expanded statistical methodologies beyond manufacturing to sales and service
         c. Created a constancy of purpose toward improvement with the aim of becoming competitive
         d. Advocated for leadership perpetuating continuous improvement
         e. Promoted the attainment of profound knowledge
         f. Demonstrated an understanding of harnessing sources of variation
         g. Believed QI means all employees trying every day to do their jobs better to accomplish the transformation
         h. Philosophy for QI adapted by American automakers in the 1980s
      2. Joseph Juran
         a. Expert in quality control who assisted Japanese to apply this method in business functions such as design, marketing, distribution, sales, and service delivery

       b. Quality control handbook considered the bible for the QI movement

       c. Identified the elements of a system to measure, improve, and lead to optimal outcomes

       d. Efficiency (resource use) and quality (performance) viewed as aspects of the whole

       e. Developed the Juran Quality Trilogy: simple, logical model for understanding quality management

$$\text{Quality Trilogy} = \begin{cases} \text{Quality = Fitness for use} \\ \text{Quality control (i.e., finances)} \\ \text{Quality planning (i.e., budgeting)} \\ \text{Quality improvement (i.e., cost reduction)} \end{cases}$$

       f. Principles adopted by health care organizations in the late 1980s

  3. Kaoru Ishikawa

       a. Use of total quality control for open communication

       b. Changed product design in accordance with customer tastes and attitudes

       c. Encouraged gaining knowledge

       d. Promoted company-wide quality assurance emphasizing the importance of customer

       e. Believed in quality first, respect for humanity, full participatory and cross functional management to solve problems

  4. Philip B. Crosby

       a. Known for "zero defects" as performance standard

       b. Focused on prevention

B. TQM philosophy

  1. Broad management philosophy promoting quality and leadership commitment; provides the energy and rationale for implementation of the process of CQI

  2. Creates an environment of continuous improvement of people skills and processes and builds excellence into every aspect of organization

  3. Processes continuously improve quality resulting in:

       a. Increased customer satisfaction

       b. Increased productivity

       c. Increased profits

       d. Increased market share

       e. Decreased costs

  4. Key concepts

       a. Top management leadership

       b. Creating corporate framework for quality

       c. Transformation of corporate culture

       d. Customer and process focus

       e. Collaborative approach to process improvement

       f. Employee education and training

       g. Learning by practice and teaching

       h. Benchmarking

       i. Quality measures and statistics

       j. Recognition and reward

       k. Management integration

  5. Fosters a belief in the value of customers, employees/staff, management, and teamwork

  6. Views quality as an entity subject to measurement, scientific method, and data-driven problem solving

  7. Offers something new to health care

       a. New way of looking at delivery of care

       b. New paradigm for management (flattens organizational chart)

       c. New way of identifying and responding to those who benefit from provision of services (customers)

8. Customer concept in TQM
   a. Identify needs, expectations, and preferences.
   b. Rely on health care providers for services and products.
   c. External customers: those outside the organization receiving services from the organization or vendors
      (1) Patient and family
      (2) Physician
      (3) Purchasers (insurance companies, health plans, government agencies)
      (4) Regulators and accrediting agencies
      (5) Vendors/suppliers (goods and services, including registries)
      (6) Educational institutions
      (7) Attorneys
      (8) Community businesses, agencies, and residents
   d. Internal customers: those performing work, but dependent on others performing work, within the organization
      (1) Admitting/front office staff
      (2) Administrative staff
      (3) Ancillary staff
      (4) Care coordination/social services staff
      (5) Human resource staff
      (6) Physicians
      (7) Nurses, technical associates, medical assistants
      (8) Pharmacists
      (9) Performance improvement/quality management staff
      (10) Volunteers
   e. Health care customer focus
      (1) Truly committed to delivering value
      (2) Seeking insight for QI activities
      (3) Addressing true needs and value-based expectations
      (4) Optimizing outcomes
      (5) Enhancing performance of internal processes
      (6) Building trust, respect, and loyalty in relationships

IV. ASPECTS OF QUALITY: THE MAP
   A. Measurable quality
      1. Compliance with or adherence to standards that are guidelines for excellence
      2. May take the form of protocols or practice guidelines
      3. Establishment of acceptable expectations for processes of care and patient outcomes
      4. Acceptable compliance basis for
         a. Licensure
         b. Accreditation
         c. Certification
         d. Awards
         e. Reimbursement
   B. Appreciative quality
      1. Comprehension and appraisal of excellence beyond minimal standards and criteria
      2. Peer review bodies rely on professionals' judgments in determining quality of patient-practitioner interactions.
      3. Use of expert witnesses to determine reasonable or negligent professional behavior
   C. Perceptive quality
      1. Degree of excellence perceived and judged by recipient or observer of care
      2. Quality based more on degree of caring than technical competence and physical environment

V. KEY DIMENSIONS OF QUALITY PERFORMANCE
  A. Appropriateness: relevance
   1. Degree to which health care satisfies patients
     a. Sensitivity to timing issues
     b. Logical flow of activities
     c. Tactful, clear communication, including patient feedback
   2. Correct, suitable resource utilization as judged by peers
   3. Doing the right things in accordance with the purpose
  B. Availability
   1. Degree to which appropriate care and services are accessible and obtainable
   2. Ease and convenience with which health care can be reached in the face of financial, organizational, cultural, and emotional barriers (access)
  C. Competency
   1. Practitioner's ability (technical and interpersonal skills) to use the best available knowledge and judgment
     a. Ability to convey trust and confidence
     b. Ability to perform the promised service dependably and accurately
     c. Ability for tactful problem solving
     d. Willingness to help patients and provide prompt service
     e. Empathetic caring and individualized attention to patients and families
   2. Degree to which practitioner adheres to professional and organizational standards of practice and care
  D. Continuity
   1. Coordination of needed health care services for patient or specified population among all practitioners and across all involved organizations over time
   2. Delivery of needed health care as coherent, unbroken succession of services
  E. Effectiveness
   1. Power of particular procedure or treatment to improve health status and positive results of care delivery
   2. Degree to which care is provided in correct manner, given the current state of knowledge to achieve desired or projected outcome(s)
   3. Performance that is equivalent to stated requirements (doing the right things right)
  F. Efficacy
   1. Potential, capacity, or capability of care to produce the desired effect or outcome as already shown through scientific research (evidence-based) findings
  G. Efficiency
   1. Delivery of a maximum number of comparable units of health care for a given unit of health resources used
   2. Relationship between outcomes and resources used to deliver care
   3. Combination of skill and economy of energy in producing a desired result
   4. Organization and supervision to combat variation in patient care
  H. Prevention/early detection
   1. Degree to which interventions, including identification of risk factors, promote health and prevent disease
  I. Respect and caring
   1. Degree to which those providing services recognize
     a. Sensitivity for patient's needs
     b. Expectations
     c. Individual differences
   2. Degree to which individual or designee is involved in his/her own care and decisions
  J. Safety
   1. Degree to which health care intervention minimizes risks of adverse outcome for both provider and patient
   2. Degree to which organizational environment is free from hazard or danger

        3. Degree to which the risk of an intervention and care environment is reduced for patients and others, including practitioners

   K. Timeliness

        1. Degree to which care is provided to individuals at the most beneficial or necessary time

        2. Degree to which services are provided to customers in accordance with their perception of promptness

   L. Tangibles

        1. Appearance of physical facilities, equipment, personnel, and communication materials (brochures, educational handouts)

        2. Clear directions—easily readable signage

VI. CHANGES IN HEALTH CARE AFFECTING QUALITY

   A. 1970-1980: start of Medicare reform with Diagnosis Related Groups (DRG) and Medicare Prospective Payment systems appeared.

   B. 1980-1990: the following services began:

        1. Health maintenance organizations (HMOs) and preferred provider organizations (PPOs)

        2. Bundling of fees with high competition

        3. Delivery system redesign, downsizing, mergers, and reengineering

   C. 1990-2000: the following services began:

        1. Prenegotiated payment for sets of services

        2. Point of service plans

        3. Capitation payment

        4. Integrated delivery systems (horizontal and vertical)

        5. Preferred providers within networks

        6. Provider sponsored organizations with direct Medicare contract

   D. 2000-2009: the following started:

        1. Closure of facilities due to lack of reimbursement

        2. Pay for performance

        3. Consumer directed health plans

   E. Continued reduced length of stay in inpatient settings and use of hospitalists to manage inpatient care

   F. Specialists taking on more primary care responsibility for certain chronic conditions, such as congestive heart failure, chronic obstructive pulmonary disease, or catastrophic injuries

   G. Implementation of health promotion programs for members and disease management programs for specific populations of patients

   H. Risk reality

        1. Exorbitant increases in medical malpractice in many states, resulting in movement or closure of some practitioner specialist practices and attempts to get malpractice tort reform through Congress

        2. Litigious atmosphere based on increased patient/consumer awareness, greater expectation from medical technology, increased injury, and claims and awards for errors of omission and commission

        3. Depersonalization of doctor-patient relationship

   I. Increased tension between physicians and managed care due to perceived interference in their practice, administrative burden, and impact on income

   J. Academic health centers that provide graduate medical education, formerly financed through higher fee-for-service billing and Medicare reimbursement, need to be adequately funded now.

   K. IOM reports

        1. *Leading Health Indicators for Healthy People 2010: First Interim Report* (1998)

        2. *Statement on Quality of Care: National Roundtable on Health Care Quality—The Urgent Need to Improve Health Care Quality* (1998)

        3. *To Err is Human: Building a Safer Health System* (1999): discussed the thousands of Americans who die each year from medical errors and the importance on patient safety

4. *Crossing the Quality Chasm: A New Health System for the 21st Century* (2001) described
   a. Broader quality issues
   b. Defined six aims of care
      (1) Safe
      (2) Effective
      (3) Patient-centered
      (4) Timely
      (5) Efficient
      (6) Equitable
   c. Presented 10 rules for care delivery redesign
5. *Healthcare Quality Report* (2002) established:
   a. Standardized performance measures
   b. Uniform set of guidelines
   c. Strategies that encourage adoption of best practices by providers
   d. Comparative quality reports
   e. National health information infrastructure and a centralized data repository
   f. Support for development of computerized clinical records
6. *Leadership by Example: Coordinating Government Roles in Improving Health Care Quality* (2002)
7. *Keeping Patients Safe: Transforming the Work Environment of Nurses* (2003): Identifies solutions to problems in health care organization work environments. This includes:
   a. Blueprint of actions for all organizations that rely on nursing care addressing issues of
      (1) Management practices
      (2) Work design
      (3) Workforce capability
      (4) Organizational culture of safety
   b. Presented evidence to address public policy questions:
      (1) Nurse work hours
      (2) Nurse staffing levels
      (3) Mandatory overtime
8. *Health Professionals Education: A Bridge to Quality* (2003):
   a. Presents a vision for institutions and programs involved in clinical education
   b. Recommends the implementation of a core set of competencies in five areas to include:
      (1) Delivering of patient-centered care
      (2) Working as part of interdisciplinary teams
      (3) Focusing on QI
      (4) Practicing evidence-based medicine
      (5) Using information technology
   c. Targets various approaches to use including:
      (1) Fostering enhanced training environments
      (2) Leveraging oversight organizations
      (3) Initiating public reporting
9. *Medicare's Quality Improvement Organization Program: Maximizing Potential* (2006):
   a. Proposed a major restructuring of a quality improvement organization so that it can become a vital natural resource integral to strategies of
      (1) Performance measurement
      (2) Payment incentives
      (3) Public reporting
   b. Focus is on offering technical assistance to practitioners and providers aimed at building for QI.
10. *America's Healthcare Safety Net: Revisiting the 2000 IOM Report* (2007):
    a. Reflected on the rising numbers of

(1) Underinsured and uninsured people
(2) High immigration levels
(3) The aftermath of Hurricane Katrina
(4) New policy and fiscal pressures on care for vulnerable populations
b. Safety net providers find it difficult to meet growing needs for prescription drugs and specialty services (mental health care).
11. *Knowing What Works in Health Care: A Roadmap for the Nation* (2008):
a. Provides a blueprint for a national program to provide unbiased information about what really works in health care and to assess the effectiveness of clinical services
b. This national program would develop and promote rigorous standards for creating clinical practice guidelines that might minimize utilization of questionable services and target services to patients most likely to benefit.
L. Institute for Healthcare Improvement programs/campaigns
1. 100,000 Lives Campaign (December 2004-June 2006)
a. Included six interventions
(1) Deploy rapid response teams at the first sign of patient decline.
(2) Deliver reliable, evidence-based care for acute myocardial infarction.
(3) Prevent central line infections.
(4) Prevent surgical site infections.
(5) Prevent adverse drug events by implementing medication reconciliation.
(6) Prevent ventilator-associated pneumonia.
b. Total of 3100 hospitals participated
c. Estimated 122,000 lives saved in 18 months
2. 5 Million Lives Campaign (December 2006-December 2008)
a. Accelerating efforts to reduce nonfatal harm, while continuing to fight needless deaths
b. 4000 U.S. hospitals enlisted in this initiative to improve patient safety and to adopt six interventions that reduce patient injuries and save lives
c. Example interventions include:
(1) Preventing harm from high-alert medications
(2) Reducing surgical complications
(3) Preventing pressure ulcers
(4) Reducing methicillin-resistant *Staphylococcus aureus* (MRSA) infection
(5) Delivering reliable, evidence-based care for congestive heart failure
(6) Defining and spreading best-known leveraged processes so that hospital boards of directors can become far more effective in accelerating organizational progress toward safe care
d. Participating hospital boards provided useful resources
(1) Campaign materials
(2) Getting started kit
(3) Campaign mentor hospitals that will provide support, advice, clinical expertise, and tips on implementation efforts
e. Advice given on how to set powerful aims, build foundation, build will, and drive execution of the campaign at individual interested hospitals.
f. Tools
(1) Safety dashboards and data PowerPoint
(2) Guidelines for using patients' stories in the campaign
(3) Whole system measures kit
(4) Detailed information on the process
(5) Outcome measures
(6) Recordings of campaign calls for boards of directors
(7) Companion slide set

3. Strategic initiatives that will power future programs include:
   a. New health partnerships
   b. Pursuing perfection
   c. Creating models of excellence
   d. Safer patient initiative
   e. Transforming care at the bedside
   f. Improving staff satisfaction
   g. Improving care on medical-surgical units
   h. Understanding models that can improve patient experiences and positively impact the entire health communities at a reasonable per capita cost
M. Leapfrog Group: offers hospital rewards program for improvement in clinical areas based on performance measures

VII. SOURCES OF DATA COLLECTION—INTERNAL
  A. Objective questionnaires, surveys, and interviews
    1. Should be consumer oriented
    2. Solicit both consumer complaints and opinions.
    3. Mail-back questionnaires tend to generate low response (20%-40%).
  B. Postoperative phone call
    1. Vital for evaluating patient's postoperative condition, reinforcing teaching, and obtaining performance feedback
  C. Direct observation
  D. Patient focus groups
  E. Open-ended interviews, either structured or informal
  F. Computer-based patient input through available websites or dedicated computer terminals in hospitals
  G. Input from family and friends
  H. Satisfaction gap analysis
  I. Patient/client records (demographic, treatment data, and perception of care)
  J. Indexes: permanent topical collections of medical record data required by state laws; to locate cases for statistics and research
  K. Registers: permanent chronological listings for maintaining certain statistics (e.g., births, deaths)
  L. Reports on:
    1. Clinical research
    2. Case mix
    3. Risk management/claims
    4. Patient and environmental safety
    5. Utilization management
    6. Infection control
  M. Clinical review findings:
    1. Blood use
    2. Pharmacy and therapeutics function
    3. Functional outcome status
  N. Medication records
  O. Variance reports (clinical paths)
  P. Department/service quality measurement reports and minutes (physicians, nursing, ancillary staff)
  Q. Occurrence/other generic screening reports, including sentinel events and root cause analysis
  R. Reviews and audits
    1. Data on cost of poor quality—identifies forces that oppose or support options selected
    2. Records of quality department
    3. Internal audit with all financial reports
    4. Management engineering
    5. Aggregate performance measure data (process and outcome)
  S. Employee satisfaction surveys and staff input questionnaires
  T. Long-term strategic goals
  U. Issues uncovered during TJC visit

VIII. SOURCES OF DATA—EXTERNAL
  A. Reference databases/performance measure report systems (Maryland Quality Indicator Project), download offers automated retrieval from the computerized source
  B. Accreditation reports
  C. State inspection/licensure reports
  D. Third-party payer and employer reports
  E. Centers for Disease Control and Prevention reports
  F. Recent scientific, clinical, and management literature (e.g., MEDLINE)
  G. Sentinel event alerts from TJC
  H. Evidence-based practice guidelines and clinical algorithms/protocols (e.g., National Guideline Clearinghouse)
  I. Well-formulated/updated performance measures (e.g., National Quality Measures Clearinghouse)
  J. Validated clinical pathways
  K. Identified best practices
  L. State/regional/national rates and thresholds
  M. Comparative report cards
IX. USEFUL TOOLS FOR IDENTIFYING PATTERNS OR TRENDS
  A. Checklist: identifies how often certain events are happening; simple tool to assist in data collection
  B. Flowchart: pictorial representation showing the steps of a process (a graphic sequence of events)
  C. Histogram: data-gathering tool used to show frequency of events, distribution showing patterns
  D. Control chart: a "run chart" with statistically determined upper control limits and lower control limits (determines how much variation can be expected)
  E. Pareto chart: a special form of vertical bar graph to help determine which problems to solve in what order (highest to lowest)
  F. Cause-and-effect diagram (Fishbone diagram): represents relationship between some effect and all possible causes; organizes potential causes of a problem to help find the root cause
  G. Scatter diagram: a display of possible relationship between one variable and another in order to test for possible cause and effect
  H. Benefit/cost analysis
  I. Control spreadsheet
  J. Run chart: a tool for displaying the variation in data over time
  K. Useful process tools
    1. Brainstorming: group process used to create as many ideas, concerns, or problems in as short a time as possible
    2. Affinity diagram: used to organize large volumes of ideas or issues into major categories
    3. Delphi technique: tool used to reach team consensus concerning a particular goal or task
    4. Multivoting: a technique used to prioritize a long list of possibilities and to move the team toward consensus
    5. Prioritizing matrix: used to select one option from a group of alternatives and promotes objective decision-making
    6. Events and causal factors chart: combines flowchart and affinity diagram to identify and document both the sequence of events leading up to an occurrence and the relevant conditions affecting each event or step in the sequence
    7. Force field analysis: a technique that displays the driving (positive) and restraining (negative) forces surrounding any change
    8. Task list: a listing of things to do or obtain in order to keep the team on schedule or to inventory information; it can be converted to a detailed action plan if appropriate

      9. Gantt chart: project-planning tool for developing schedules; a graphic display, a type of bar chart (i.e., bars on a horizontal time scale)

     10. Storyboard: visual display of the team and pertinent data/information, analyses, and decisions made during the improvement process

X. UNIQUE ISSUES FOR AMBULATORY CARE

  A. Sources of care are sometimes scattered in place and time, with no common medical record and inadequate communication systems.

  B. Primary care and specialist providers' roles and obligations to the patient are ill-defined, and there may be conflict between the expectations of the patient and the public and those self-defined by the practitioners.

  C. In managed care, actual authorization of treatment may be controlled by medical group, independent practice association, or health plan rather than the primary care physician or specialist.

  D. Expected outcomes of ambulatory care are difficult to predict because of the lack of studies of the natural history of ambulatory conditions; adverse outcomes that are to be prevented may not occur anywhere close to time of health care interaction, so they cannot be easily monitored or tracked back to care episode.

  E. Patients are in control of their own diet, medications, personal habits and lifestyle, and care encounters; poor health outcomes result from patients' failure to seek care early, comply with recommended treatment, or return for follow-up care.

  F. Percentage of cost may come from the patient or be under a managed care contract; there is a constant delicate balance in decision-making between cost, benefit, and risk of non-treatment.

  G. Payment structure: fixed or packaged fees for standard surgical procedures (PPO/HMO); complications or unplanned admissions to the hospital may incur more expenses.

  H. Overnight observation and pain control at a 23-hour extended observation unit in the ambulatory surgery or designated hospital unit is less costly than at the acute care hospital setting; allows more complicated and extensive list of procedures to be done at a lower-cost outpatient setting.

  I. Free-standing center must have predetermined plan and agreement with hospital for emergency admission of patients to ensure continuity of quality care.

  J. Transient but disturbing side effects such as postoperative pain, nausea and vomiting, dysphagia, and extended somnolence may influence a patient-based assessment for quality of care; delayed recovery may prevent discharge home and require need for continued care and observation overnight.

  K. Short length of stay; brief window to obtain desired outcomes

  L. Families and significant others share responsibility for postoperative care at home.

  M. Emphasize on active patient involvement with wellness as the focus.

  N. Cross-training of nurses and support personnel reduces the number of different persons treating a patient and enhances continuity of care.

  O. Simplified paperwork and documentation leaves more time for direct care.

  P. Age no longer a barrier; well-controlled systemic disease does not disqualify patient from receiving care in an ambulatory setting.

    1. Elderly patient: minimizes separation from family and environment but must consider risks of anesthetic, surgery, and home care

    2. Younger patient: premature infant or ex-preemies that need postoperative apnea monitoring not appropriate candidates

  Q. Teaching

    1. Encompasses all ages of patients

    2. Thorough postoperative instructions to patient and family member or significant other

    3. Use of collaborative approach with patient, including patient empowerment

4. Nurses must consider:
   a. Educational background of patient, family member, or significant other
   b. Literacy: knowledge, skills, values, and attitudes of patient
   c. Determine readiness to learn, learning style, and timeliness of instructions
   d. Language barriers
   e. Physical impairments (deaf patient requiring signer to interpret verbal instructions) and mental or physical handicaps
   f. When and where to obtain follow-up care documented
   g. What to do in case of emergency documented
   h. Patient and family compliance
   i. Patient safety
R. Traditional outcomes: have historically been assessed in terms of surgical and anesthesia-related complications
   1. Unplanned hospital admissions
   2. Prolonged recovery time after anesthesia
   3. Unscheduled postoperative physician or emergency department visit
   4. Mortality
   5. Major morbidity
S. More recent outcomes focus on patient experience.
   1. Incidence of postoperative nausea and vomiting
   2. Pain or surgical discomfort
   3. Dizziness
   4. Sore throat
   5. Shivering
   6. Return to usual activities
   7. Patient satisfaction
XI. ISSUES IN POST ANESTHESIA CARE UNIT (PACU), PHASE I
A. Severe adverse events
   1. Return of patient to the operating room because of
      a. Loss of peripheral pulses
      b. Large blood loss
      c. Hematoma formation
      d. Wound dehiscence
   2. Patient reintubation
   3. Inability to extubate patient (delayed awakening and/or return of muscular strength and function)
   4. Issues of respiratory compromise:
      a. Laryngospasm/bronchospasm
      b. Croup
      c. Stridor
      d. Wheezing
      e. Retractions
   5. Spontaneous pneumothorax
   6. Emergence delirium
   7. Malignant hyperthermia
   8. New onset of ST depression or elevation
   9. New onset of life-threatening dysrhythmia
   10. Patient with chest pain, changes in electrocardiogram, rise in level of cardiac enzymes, nausea and sweating (rule out myocardial infarction)
   11. Marked hypotension, hypertension, tachycardia, or bradycardia
   12. Pulmonary embolism, pulmonary edema
   13. Inability to maintain adequate oxygen saturation, greater than 90%, in patients with a baseline saturation of 90% or greater preoperatively
   14. Marked fluid imbalance noted from assessing output, skin turgor, and blood pressure
   15. Tissue injury, burn, and skin breakdown
   16. Severe hypothermia

B. Disturbing events that may influence patient assessment
   1. Surgical pain and referred pain
   2. Nausea and vomiting
   3. Shivering
   4. Mild hypothermia
   5. Full bladder
   6. Pruritis
   7. Delay in moving extremities after regional and local anesthesia
   8. Headache, muscle aches
   9. Pins and needles sensation, numbness in extremities
   10. Drug reaction (nonanaphylactic)
   11. Somnolence
C. Other patient care issues
   1. High level of noise and increased use of lights may cause overstimulation.
   2. Lack of privacy with only curtains separating patients
   3. Delay in reaching PACU from the operating room
   4. Prolonged stay in PACU because of unavailability of nursing unit beds
   5. Inadequate supply of beds for morbidly obese patients
   6. Close proximity of preoperative and postoperative patients
   7. Close proximity of adult and pediatric patient populations
   8. Close proximity of PACU patients and intensive care unit overflow patients
   9. Less chance for visitation because of overcrowded conditions
   10. Lack of appropriate isolation rooms for the increased number of MRSA and vancomycin-resistant enterococci (VRE) cases
   11. Acute pain issues in a chronic pain patient
   12. Presence of phase I and phase II patients in the same recovery area, requiring a different focus and approach to care
D. Staff satisfaction issues
   1. Presence of automated medication/supply dispensing devices reduces time spent in ordering and stocking; keeps adequate supply in close proximity to patient care areas.
   2. Proper use of unlicensed assistive personnel enables the PACU nurse to provide nursing care for the patient.
   3. Simplified nursing flow sheets, checklists, and computer documentation allows more time for direct care.
   4. Practice guidelines, established protocols, policies, and standards guide the PACU nurse from admission to discharge of patients.

BIBLIOGRAPHY

1. Agency for Healthcare Research and Quality: *ARHQ quality indicators*. Available at: www.qualityindicators.ahrq.gov. Accessed October 31, 2008.
2. American Nurses Association: *National database of nursing quality indicators*. Available at: www.nursingquality.org. Accessed October 29, 2008.
3. Caldwell C, Brexler J, Gillem T: *Lean six-sigma for healthcare*, Milwaukee, WI, 2005, American Society for Quality.
4. Donadbedian A: The quality of care. How can it be assessed? *JAMA* 260(12):23–30, 1743–1748, 1988.
5. Elwood PM: Shattuck lecture–outcomes management: A technology of patient experience. *N Engl J Med* 318(23):1549–1556, 1988.
6. Feigenbaum AV, Fiegenbaum DS: The future of quality. *Quality Progress* 11:24–29, 2004.
7. Goonan KJ: *The Juran prescription*, San Francisco, 1995, Jossey-Bass.
8. Harry M, Schroeder R: *Six sigma: The breakthrough strategy revolutionizing the world's top corporations*, New York, 2000, Currency/Doubleday.
9. Institute for Healthcare Improvement: *Improving quality and achieving quality: A guide for hospital leaders*. Available at www.ihi.org/ihi. Accessed September 15, 2008.
10. Institute of Medicine of the National Academics: *Crossing the quality chasm: A new health system for the 21st century*. Available at: www.iom.edu/?id=22346. Accessed November 24, 2008.

11. Juran JM, Godfrey AB: *Juran's quality handbook*, ed 5, New York, 1999, McGraw-Hill.

12. Kelley D: *How to use control charts for healthcare*, Milwaukee, WI, 1999, Quality Press.

13. Leap Frog Group Hospital Rewards Program. Available at: www.leapfroggroup.org. Accessed October 29, 2008.

14. Leape LL, Berwick DM: Five years after *To Err Is Human*: What have we learned? *JAMA* 293(19):2384–2390, 2005.

15. Lucas JM: The essential six sigma. *Quality Progress* 35(1):27–31, 2002.

16. National Quality Forum: *Safe practices for better healthcare. A consensus report summary.* Available at: www.ahrq.gov/qual/nqfpract. htm. Accessed November 24, 2008.

17. Poppendieck M: *Principles of lean thinking*. Available at: www.poppendieck.com. Accessed October 29, 2008.

18. Shared visions-new pathways. *Jt Comm Perspect* 22(10):1, 3, 2002.

19. Shortell SM, Anderson DA, Gilles, R, et al: Building integrated systems: The holographic organization. *Healthc Forum J* 36(2):20–26, 1993.

20. Sloan FA, Morrisey MA, Valvona J: Case shifting and the Medicare prospective payment. *Am J Public Health* 78(5):553–556, 1988.

21. Spath P: Uncover root causes with E&CF charts. *Hosp Peer Rev* 25(7):96–98, 2000.

22. The Joint Commission: *2009 National Patient Safety Goals: Joint Commission on Accreditation of Healthcare Organizations.* Available at: www.jointcommission.org/ PatientSafety/National PatientSafetyGoals. Accessed September 8, 2008.

23. The Joint Commission: *2009 National patient safety goals*, Oakbrook Terrace, IL, 2009, The Joint Commission.

24. *Tools for performance measurement in health care*, Oakbrook Terrace, IL, 2002, The Joint Commission.

25. United States National Library of Medicine: *US sets hospital infection control goals.* Available at www.nlm.nih.gov. Accessed October 29, 2008.

26. Womack JP: *Lean thinking: A look back and a look forward*. Available at: www.lean.org/ Lean/Community/Registered/Articles. cfm. Accessed November 24, 2008.

LIFE SPAN
CONSIDERATIONS

10 Human Growth and Development

DONNA M. DEFAZIO QUINN

OBJECTIVES

At the conclusion of this chapter, the reader should be able to:

1. Define growth and development.

2. Identify the stages of growth and development.

3. Compare Freud's theory of psychosocial development with Erikson's psychosocial stages.

4. List Piaget's four stages of cognitive development.

5. Explain the five stages of language development.

6. Describe the effects of positive influence on the development of self-esteem.

7. Identify eight factors that could influence growth and development.

I. OVERVIEW OF GROWTH AND DEVELOPMENT
  A. Definition
    1. Growth and development
      a. Often used interchangeably
      b. Each has distinct definition
    2. Growth
      a. Implies a change in quantity (quantitative change)
        (1) An increase in physical size of a whole or any of its parts
        (2) Can be measured in:
          (a) Inches, centimeters (height)
          (b) Kilograms, pounds (increased organ mass, weight)
          (c) Numbers (increased vocabulary, increased number of relationships with others, increased number of physical skills that can be performed)
      b. Increase in number and size of cells
        (1) Reflected in an increase in the size and weight of the whole or any of its parts
    3. Development
      a. A complex concept not easily measured or studied
      b. Gradual growth and expansion; viewed as a qualitative change
        (1) Increased function (skill) and complexity (capacity)
        (2) Occurs through growth, maturation, and learning
      c. Move from lower case to a more advanced stage of complexity
        (1) Continuous, orderly series of conditions
        (2) Leads to activities, new motives for activities, and eventual patterns of behavior
        (3) Expansion of capabilities to provide greater facility in functioning
      d. Developmental process
        (1) Continuous, complex, and irreversible
        (2) Involves aging

    (a) Most rapid during fetal stage

    (b) Is a lifelong process

  e. Progression of development

   (1) Simple to complex

    (a) Infant's vocalizations before speech refinement

   (2) Sequence of changes leading to particular attainments

   (3) General to specific

    (a) Infant's palmar grasp before acquiring finer control of pincer grasp

   (4) From head to toe (cephalocaudally)

    (a) Infant gains head and neck control before gaining control of trunk and limbs.

   (5) From inner to outer (proximodistally)

    (a) Control of near structures before control of structures farther away from the body center

    (b) Infant coordinates arms to reach before gaining hand and finger coordination.

  f. Predictability of development

   (1) Sequence of development is invariable.

   (2) Precise age will vary.

   (3) Wide normal range allows for individual variances.

  g. Uniqueness of development

   (1) Each child has own genetic potential for growth and development.

   (2) May be deterred or modified at any stage

II. FACTORS INFLUENCING GROWTH AND DEVELOPMENT

 A. Genetics (heredity)

  1. Inherent characteristics influence development.

   a. Sex of child directs pattern of growth and behavior of others toward child.

   b. Physical characteristics are inherited.

    (1) Can influence how child grows and interacts with environment

 B. Gender

  1. Sex differences that influence behaviors in childhood

   a. Boys

    (1) More aggressive physically

    (2) Engage in rough and tumble play

    (3) Aggressive fantasies

    (4) Competitive behavior more common

    (5) Difficulty sitting still

    (6) Engage in more exploratory behavior

    (7) High activity level in presence of other boys

    (8) Greater impulsiveness

    (9) Subject to distraction

    (10) More extensive sphere of relationships

    (11) Highly oriented toward peer groups

    (12) Congregate in large groups

    (13) View themselves as more powerful and with more control over events

    (14) Respond to a challenge, especially when it appeals to their ego or competitive feelings

   b. Girls

    (1) More aggressive verbally

    (2) More likely to associate in pairs or small groups

    (3) Involved in more intense relationships with a few close friends

    (4) More concerned with the welfare of the group

    (5) More apt to compromise in situations involving conflict

    (6) May be superior regarding motivation to achieve

    (7) More likely to comply to adult commands

    (8) More nurturing or helping behavior

   C. Environment
      1. Before birth
         a. Prenatal factors
            (1) Maternal disease (diabetes)
            (2) Alcohol intake
               (a) Exhibit prenatal and postnatal growth deficiencies in height and weight
               (b) May produce significant central nervous system alterations that may not be evident until the child is older
            (3) Fetal exposure to drugs such as marijuana, cocaine, and heroin
               (a) Associated with intrauterine growth retardation and prematurity
            (4) Smoking may produce smaller infant.
         b. Socioeconomic status
   D. Culture
      1. Includes habits, beliefs, language, values, ethnicity, demographic setting, socioeconomic class, parental occupation, and family structure
         a. Attitude and expectations differ with respect to the sex of the child.
   E. Lifestyle
      1. Different family structures
         a. Two parents
         b. One parent
         c. Extended family
         d. Other variations
      2. Family relationships a major determinant of how children grow and progress
   F. Nutrition
      1. Single most important influence on growth
      2. Satisfactory nutrition closely related to good health throughout lifetime
      3. Malnutrition
         a. Defined as undernutrition, primarily resulting from insufficient calorie intake
         b. Need a continuous supply of nutrients
         c. Poor nutrition may have negative influence on development from time of implantation of ovum until birth
         d. Severe maternal malnutrition associated with permanent reduction in total number of fetal brain cells
            (1) Has critical effect on child's intellectual functioning
         e. Malnutrition may result from:
            (1) Inadequate dietary intake
               (a) Quality
               (b) Quantity
            (2) Disease that interferes with:
               (a) Appetite
               (b) Digestion
               (c) Absorption
            (3) Excessive physical activity
            (4) Inadequate rest
            (5) Disturbed interpersonal relationships
            (6) Other environmental or psychological factors
   G. Health status
      1. Diseases that affect growth and development
         a. Skeletal (dwarfism)
         b. Chromosome anomalies (Turner syndrome)
         c. Disorders of metabolism
            (1) Vitamin D–resistant rickets
            (2) Mucopolysaccharidoses
            (3) Endocrine disorders

        d. Klinefelter syndrome and Marfan syndrome

        e. Chronic illness

        f. Congenital cardiac anomalies

        g. Respiratory disorders

           (1) Cystic fibrosis

        h. Digestive malabsorptive syndromes

        i. Defects in digestive enzyme systems

        j. Metabolic diseases

H. Neuroendocrine

    1. Possible relationship exists between hypothalamus and endocrine system that influences growth.

    2. Peripheral nervous system may influence growth.

        a. Muscles deprived of nerve supply degenerate.

    3. All hormones affect growth in some manner.

        a. Growth hormone, thyroid hormone, and androgens given to a person deficient in these hormones

           (1) Stimulates protein anabolism

           (2) Produces retention of elements essential for building protoplasm and bony tissue

I. Play

    1. Activity with meaning and purpose

    2. May be directly related to expanding:

        a. Social development

        b. Intellectual development

        c. Motor development

        d. Language development

    3. Play used to accomplish developmental tasks and master the environment

J. School

    1. Contributes to development in the form of:

        a. Skill training

        b. Cultural transmission

        c. Self-actualization

K. Neighborhood

    1. Offers child opportunity to experience world outside the home

        a. Accepting

        b. Supportive of child's physical and psychosocial needs

        c. Reinforcing of child's self-confidence and safety

L. Season, climate, and oxygen concentration

    1. Some evidence that:

        a. Growth in height faster in spring and summer months

        b. Growth in weight more rapid in autumn and winter

    2. Effects of hypoxia on growth

        a. Children with disorders that produce chronic hypoxia characteristically smaller than same children of chronological age

        b. Children native to high altitudes smaller than children of lower altitudes

M. Stress

    1. Abnormal conditions that tend to disrupt normal functions of the body or mind

    2. Imbalance between environmental demands and coping resources

    3. Some children more vulnerable than others

        a. Affected by age, temperament, life situation, and state of health

        b. Response can be behavioral, physiological, or psychological

    4. Methods of coping

        a. Respond by trying to change the circumstance (primary control coping)

           (1) Tantrums

           (2) Aggressive behavior

        b. Trying to adjust to circumstances (secondary control coping)

           (1) Withdrawal

           (2) Submission

     5. Fear
       a. Emotional reaction to a specific real or unreal threat or danger
          (1) Child perceives threat
             (a) Person
             (b) Animal
             (c) Situation
          (2) Perceives threat to be stronger than himself or herself and capable of harm
       b. Alleviate fear by:
          (1) Presence of adult who will offer protection
          (2) Becoming familiar with source of threat (animal)
  N. Media
     1. Television
       a. Pervasive force
       b. Primary source of socialization in children
       c. Major source of information
          (1) Unhealthy messages regarding sex and violence
          (2) Alcohol consumption synonymous with having a good time
          (3) Food products promoting unhealthy nutritional practices
     2. Internet
       a. Instantaneous access to unlimited material; informative and detrimental
       b. Potential exposure to illegal activities
          (1) Parental controls need to be in place to limit Internet access to age-appropriate sites.
     3. Reading materials
       a. Books, newspapers, magazines
          (1) Provide enjoyment
          (2) Increase child's knowledge
     4. Movies
       a. Not closely associated with reality
       b. Usually provide opportunity for desirable social learning
       c. Child may be unable to distinguish between reality and fantasy.
          (1) Results in fears
     5. Cell phone
       a. Continuous contact with others
          (1) Parents
          (2) Friends
  O. Responsible adults
     1. Can influence positive choices (life decisions, media, social, etc.)
     2. Interact with child to identify right from wrong
III. STAGES OF GROWTH AND DEVELOPMENT (Box 10-1)
  A. Prenatal
     1. Period of life from conception to birth
       a. Crucial period in developmental process
       b. Health and well-being of the infant directly related to adequate prenatal care
       c. Direct relationship between maternal health and certain manifestations in the newborn
  B. Newborn or neonatal
     1. From birth through the first month of life
     2. Major physical adjustment to extrauterine existence
  C. Infancy
     1. Begins at end of first month of life and ends at 1 year of age
     2. Period of rapid motor, cognitive, and social development
     3. Establishes basic trust
       a. Foundation for future relationships
  D. Early childhood (Box 10-2)
     1. Toddler
       a. From 1 to 3 years

■ BOX 10-1
■ **DEVELOPMENTAL AGE PERIODS**

Prenatal Period: Conception to Birth
Germinal: Conception to approximately 2 weeks
Embryonic: 2 to 8 weeks
Fetal: 8 to 40 weeks (birth)
　A rapid growth rate and total dependency make this one of the most crucial periods in the developmental process. The relationship between maternal health and certain manifestations in the newborn emphasizes the importance of adequate prenatal care to the health and well-being of the infant.

Infancy Period: Birth to 12 Months
Neonatal: Birth to 27 to 28 days
Infancy: 1 to approximately 12 months
　The infancy period is one of rapid motor, cognitive, and social development. Through mutuality with the caregiver (parent), the infant establishes a basic trust in the world and the foundation for future interpersonal relationships. The critical first month of life, although part of the infancy period, is often differentiated from the remainder because of the major physical adjustments to extrauterine existence and the psychological adjustment of the parent.

Early Childhood: 1 to 6 Years
Toddler: 1 to 3 years
Preschool: 3 to 6 years
　This period, which extends from the time the children attain upright locomotion until they enter school, is characterized by intense activity and discovery. It is a time of marked physical and personality development. Motor development advances steadily. Children at this age acquire language and wider social relationships, learn role standards, gain self-control and mastery, develop increasing awareness of dependence and independence, and begin to develop a self-concept.

Middle Childhood: 6 to 11 or 12 Years
Frequently referred to as the "school age," this period of development is one in which the child is directed away from the family group and centered around the wider world of peer relationships. There is steady advancement in physical, mental, and social development, with emphasis on developing skill competencies. Social cooperation and early moral development take on more importance with relevance for later life stages. This is a critical period in the development of the self-concept.

Later Childhood: 11 to 19 Years
Prepubertal: 10 to 13 years
Adolescence: 13 to approximately 18 years
　The tumultuous period of rapid maturation and change known as adolescence is considered to be a transitional period that begins at the onset of puberty and extends to the point of entry into the adult world—usually high school graduation. Biological and personality maturation are accompanied by physical and emotional turmoil, and there is redefining of the self-concept. In the late adolescent period, the young person begins to internalize all previously learned values to focus on an individual, rather than a group, identity.

From Hockenberry MJ: *Wong's essentials of pediatric nursing,* ed 8, St Louis, 2009, Mosby.

　　2. Preschool
　　　　a. From 3 to 6 years
　　3. Characteristics of early childhood
　　　　a. Intense activity and discovery
　　　　b. Marked physical and personality development
　　　　c. Motor development advances steadily.
　　　　d. Acquire language skills.
　　　　e. Expand social relationships.
　　　　f. Learn role standards.
　　　　g. Gain self-control and mastery.

■ BOX 10-2
■ EMERGING PATTERNS OF BEHAVIOR FROM 1 TO 5 YEARS OF AGE*

15 Months
Motor: Walks alone; crawls up stairs
Adaptive: Makes a tower of three cubes; makes a line with crayon; inserts raisin in bottle
Language: Jargon; follows simple commands; may name a familiar object (e.g., ball)
Social: Indicates some desire or needs by pointing; hugs parents

18 Months
Motor: Runs stiffly; sits on small chair; walks up stairs with one hand held; explores drawers and wastebaskets
Adaptive: Makes a tower of four cubes; imitates scribbling; imitates vertical stroke; dumps raisin from bottle
Language: Ten words (average); names pictures; identifies one or more parts of body
Social: Feeds self, seeks help when in trouble; may complain when wet or soiled; kisses parents with pucker

24 Months
Motor: Runs well; walks up and down stairs, one step at a time; opens doors; climbs on furniture; jumps
Adaptive: Tower of seven cubes (6 at 21 months); scribbles in circular pattern; imitates horizontal stroke; folds paper once imitatively
Language: Puts three words together (subject, verb, object)
Social: Handles spoon well; often tells immediate experiences; helps to undress; listens to stories when shown pictures

30 Months
Motor: Goes up stairs alternating feet
Adaptive: Tower of nine cubes; makes vertical and horizontal strokes, but generally will not join them to make a cross; imitates circular stroke, forming closed figure
Language: Refers to self by pronoun "I"; knows full name
Social: Helps put things away; pretends in play

36 Months
Motor: Rides tricycle; stands momentarily on one foot
Adaptive: Tower of ten cubes; imitates construction of "bridge" of three cubes; copies circle; imitates cross
Language: Knows age and sex; counts three objects correctly; repeats three numbers or a sentence of six syllables
Social: Plays simple games (in "parallel" with other children); helps in dressing (unbuttons clothing and puts on shoes); washes hands

48 Months
Motor: Hops on one foot; throws ball overhand; uses scissors to cut out pictures; climbs well
Adaptive: Copies bridge from model; imitates construction of "gate" of five cubes; copies cross and square; draws man with two to four parts besides head; identifies longer of two lines
Language: Counts four pennies accurately; tells a story
Social: Plays with several children with beginning of social interaction and role-playing; goes to toilet alone

60 Months
Motor: Skips
Adaptive: Draws triangle from copy; names heavier of two weights
Language: Names four colors; repeats sentence of ten syllables; counts ten pennies correctly
Social: Dresses and undresses; asks questions about meaning of words; engages in domestic role-playing

*Data are derived from those of Gesell (as revised by Knobloch), Shirley, Provence, Wolf, Bailey, and others. After 5 years of age, the Stanford-Binet, Wechsler-Bellevue, and other scales offer the most precise estimates of developmental level. To have their greatest value, they should be administered only by an experienced and qualified person.
From Kliegman RM, Behrman RE, Jenson HB, et al: *Nelson textbook of pediatrics,* ed 18, Philadelphia, 2007, Saunders.

       h. Develop increasing awareness of dependence and independence.

       i. Begin to develop self-concept.

  E. Middle childhood or school-age years

    1. From age 6 to 11 or 12 years

    2. Child is directed away from family group and centered around peer relationships.

    3. Steady advancement in physical, mental, and social development

    4. Emphasis on developing skill competencies

    5. Social cooperation and moral development take on importance.

       a. Relevant for later life stages

    6. Critical period in the development of self-concept

  F. Later childhood or adolescence and young adulthood

    1. From the beginning of the 12th year to the end of the 21st year

    2. Period of rapid maturation and change

    3. Considered to be a transition that begins with the onset of puberty and extends to the point of entry into the adult world

    4. Biological and personality maturation accompanied by physical and emotional turmoil

    5. Self-concept redefined

    6. In late adolescence, the child begins to internalize all previously learned values and focus on an individual rather than a group identity.

IV. ASSESSMENT OF GROWTH AND DEVELOPMENT

  A. Assessment of growth

    1. Obtain accurate assessments at regular intervals.

    2. Record and plot data on growth charts.

       a. Allows for comparison with statistical norms

    3. Assessments include:

       a. Height

       b. Weight

       c. Head circumference

       d. Body mass index

  B. Assessment of development

    1. Complex process

    2. Gather data from many sources.

       a. Observations

         (1) Activities of daily living (eating, playing, dressing)

         (2) Communication patterns

         (3) Interaction skills

         (4) Emotional responses

       b. Interviews

       c. Physical exams

       d. Interactions with child and parents

V. THEORIES OF DEVELOPMENT—OVERVIEW (Table 10-1)

  A. Freudian

    1. Psychosocial

    2. Emphasis on development of personality

  B. Erikson

    1. Psychosocial development

  C. Piaget

    1. Cognitive development

  D. Kohlberg

    1. Moral development

  E. Sullivan

    1. Interpersonal development

  F. Skinner, Watson

    1. Learning theory; behaviorism.

    2. Focus entirely on behavior.

    3. Internalize processes such as thoughts and feelings.

■ TABLE 10-1
■ ■ **Summary of Personality, Cognitive, and Moral Development Theories**

Stage/ Age	Psychosexual Stages (Freud)	Psychosocial Stages (Erikson)	Cognitive Stages (Piaget)	Moral Judgment Stages (Kohlberg)
I. Infancy (Birth–1 year)	Oral-sensory	Trust vs mistrust	Sensorimotor (birth–2 years)	
II. Toddlerhood (1–3 years)	Anal-urethral	Autonomy vs shame and doubt	Preoperational thought, preconcep- tual phase (transductive reasoning, [e.g., specific to specific]) (2-4 years)	Preconventional (premoral) level Punishment and obedience orientation
III. Early childhood (3–6 years)	Phallic- locomotion	Initiative vs guilt	Preoperational thought, intuitive phase (transductive reasoning) (4-7 years)	Preconventional (premoral) level Naïve instrumental orientation
IV. Middle childhood (6–12 years)	Latency	Industry vs inferiority	Concrete operations (inductive reasoning and beginning logic) (7-11 years)	Conventional level Good-boy, nice-girl orientation Law-and-order orientation
V. Adolescence (12–18 years)	Genitality	Identity and repudiation vs identity confusion	Formal operations (deductive and abstract reasoning) (11-15 years)	Postconventional or principled level Social-contract orientation Universal ethical principle orientation (no longer included in revised theory)

From Hockenberry MJ: *Wong's essentials of pediatric nursing,* ed 8, St Louis, 2009, Mosby.

    G. Maslow
        1. Humanistic
        2. Focus on characteristics that contribute to healthy personality development.
VI. FREUDIAN (Table 10-2)
    A. Three components of personality
        1. Id
            a. Develops during birth
            b. The unconscious mind
            c. Inborn component that drives instincts
            d. Obeys pleasure principle of immediate gratification of needs
                (1) Raw libido seeking pleasure
        2. Ego
            a. Develops during toddler years
            b. Represents the conscious mind
                 (1) Reality component
                (2) Mediates conflict
            c. Functions as conscious or controlling self
            d. Finds realistic means of gratifying instincts
            e. Blocks irrational thinking of the Id

■ TABLE 10-2
■ **Theories of Growth and Development**

	Piaget's Periods of Cognitive Development	Freud's Stages of Psychosexual Development	Erikson's Stages of Psychosocial Development	Kohlberg's Stages of Moral Development
Infancy	Period 1 (birth–2 yr): Sensorimotor period Reflexive behavior is used to adapt to environment; egocentric view of the world; development of object permanence	Oral stage Mouth is a sensory organ; infant takes in and explores during oral passive substage (first half of infancy); infant strikes out with teeth during oral aggressive substage (latter half of infancy).	Trust vs mistrust Development of a sense that the self is good when consistent, predictable, reliable care is received; characterized by hope.	Premorality or preconventional morality, stage 0 (0–2 yr): Naiveté and egocentrism No moral sensitivity; decisions are made on the basis of what pleases the child; infants like or love what helps them and dislike what hurts them; no awareness of the effect of their actions on others. "Good is what I like and want."
Toddlerhood	Period 2 (2–7 yr): Preoperational thought Thinking remains egocentric, becomes magical, and is dominated by perception.	Anal stage Major focus of sexual interest is anus; control of body functions is major feature.	Autonomy vs shame and doubt Development of sense of control over the self and body functions; exerts self; characterized by will	Premorality or preconventional morality, stage 1 (2–3 yr): Punishment-obedience orientation Right or wrong is determined by physical consequences: "If I get caught and punished for doing it, it is wrong. If I am not caught or punished, then it must be right."
Preschool age		Phallic or Oedipal/Electra stage Genitals become focus of sexual curiosity; superego (conscience) develops; feelings of guilt emerge.	Initiative vs guilt Development of a can-do attitude about the self; behavior becomes goal-directed, competitive, and imaginative; initiation into gender role; characterized by purpose	Premorality or preconventional morality, stage 2 (4–7 yr): Instrumental hedonism and concrete reciprocity Child conforms to rules out of self-interest: "I'll do this for you if you do this for me"; behavior is guided by an "eye for an eye" orientation. "If you do something bad to me, then it's OK if I do something bad to you."

	Cognitive development (Piaget)	Psychosexual development (Freud)	Psychosocial development (Erikson)	Moral development (Kohlberg)
School age	Period 3 (7-11 yr): Concrete operations. Thinking becomes more systematic and logical, but concrete objects and activities are needed.	Latency stage. Sexual feelings are firmly repressed by the superego; period of relative calm	Industry vs inferiority. Mastering of useful skills and tools of the culture; learning how to play and work with peers; characterized by competence	Morality of conventional role conformity, stage 3 (7-10 yr): Good-boy or good-girl orientation. Morality is based on avoiding disapproval or disturbing the conscience; child is becoming socially sensitive. Kohlberg's stages of moral development. Morality of conventional role conformity, stage 4 (begins at about 10-12 yr): Law and order orientation. Right takes on a religious or metaphysical quality. Child wants to show respect for authority, and maintain social order; obeys rules for their own sake.
Adolescence	Period 4 (11 yr to adulthood): Formal operations. New ideas can be created; situations can be analyzed; use of abstract and futuristic thinking; understands logical sequences of behavior	Puberty or genital stage. Stimulated by increasing hormone levels; sexual energy wells up in full force, resulting in personal and family turmoil	Identity vs role confusion. Begins to develop a sense of "I"; this process is lifelong; peers become of paramount importance; child gains independence from parents; characterized by faith in self	Morality of self-accepted moral principles, stage 5: Social contract orientation. Right is determined by what is best for the majority; exceptions to rules can be made if person's welfare is violated; the end no longer justifies the means; laws are for mutual good and mutual cooperation.
Adulthood			Intimacy vs isolation. Development of the ability to lose the self in genuine mutuality with another. Characterized by love	

Continued

■ TABLE 10-2
■ ■ Theories of Growth and Development—cont'd

Piaget's Periods of Cognitive Development	Freud's Stages of Psychosexual Development	Erikson's Stages of Psychosocial Development	Kohlberg's Stages of Moral Development
Adulthood—cont'd		Generativity vs stagnation Production of ideas and materials through work; creation of children; characterized by care	Morality of self-accepted moral principles Stage 6: Personal principle orientation Achieved only by the morally mature individual; few people reach this level; these people do what they think is right, regardless of others' opinions, legal sanctions, or personal sacrifice; actions are guided by internal standards; integrity is of utmost importance; may be willing to die for their beliefs
		Ego integrity vs despair Realization that there is order and purpose to life; characterized by wisdom	Morality of self-accepted moral principles Stage 7: Universal principle orientation This stage is achieved by only a rare few; Mother Theresa, Gandhi, and Socrates are examples; these individuals transcend the teachings of organized religion and perceive themselves as part of the cosmic order, understand the reason for their existence, and live for their beliefs.

From James SR, Ashwill JW: *Nursing care of children*, Philadelphia, 2007, Saunders.

3. Superego
    a. Develops during preschool years
    b. Conscience
    c. Functions as moral arbitrator
        (1) Puts good or bad labels on behavior
    d. Represents the ideal
    e. Prevents individual from expressing undesirable instincts that could threaten social order
B. Psychosexual development (Table 10-3)
    1. Stages of development
        a. Oral
        b. Anal
        c. Phallic
        d. Latency
        e. Genital
    2. Sexual instincts significant in development of personality
    3. Psychosexual used to describe any sensual pleasure
    4. Theory focuses on desire to satisfy biological needs.
        a. Theory difficult to verify
        b. Of little value when attempting to predict future behaviors
        c. Psychosexual development usually complete by 6 years of age
C. Oral stage
    1. Birth to 1 year of age
    2. Sources of pleasure
        a. Sucking
        b. Biting
        c. Chewing
        d. Vocalizing

■ TABLE 10-3
■ ■ **Personality Traits Associated with Freud's First Three Stages of Psychosexual Development**

Stage	Age	Source of Pleasure	Personality Traits
Oral	Birth to 1 year	Oral activities Sucking Biting Chewing Vocalizing	Pessimism or optimism Determination or submission Gullibility or suspiciousness Admiration or envy Cockiness or self-belittlement
Anal	1 to 3 years	Anal region Withhold or expel feces	Stinginess or overgenerosity Constrictedness or expansiveness Rigid punctuality or tardiness Stubbornness or acquiescence Orderliness or messiness
Phallic	3 to 6 years	Genitals	Brashness or bashfulness Stylishness or plainness Gaiety or sadness Blind courage or timidness Gregariousness or isolationism

From Quinn DMD: *Ambulatory surgical nursing core curriculum,* Philadelphia, 1999, Saunders.

      3. Oral personality traits
        a. If met, child develops positive personality traits; if need is not met, child develops negative personality traits.
          (1) Pessimism or optimism
          (2) Determination or submission
          (3) Gullibility or suspiciousness
          (4) Admiration or envy
          (5) Cockiness or self-belittlement

D. Anal stage
  1. One to 3 years of age
  2. Focus on anal region
  3. Child develops ability to withhold or expel feces at will.
  4. Toilet training can have lasting effects on personality development.
  5. Anal personality traits
    a. Stinginess or overgenerosity
    b. Constrictedness or expansiveness
    c. Rigid punctuality or tardiness
    d. Stubbornness or acquiescence
    e. Orderliness or messiness

E. Phallic stage
  1. Three to 6 years of age
  2. Focus on genitals
  3. Recognition of difference between sexes
  4. Phallic personality traits
    a. Brashness or bashfulness
    b. Stylishness or plainness
    c. Gaiety or sadness
    d. Blind courage or timidity
    e. Gregariousness or isolationism

F. Latency period
  1. Six to 12 years of age
  2. Elaboration of previous learned traits and skills
  3. Physical and psychic energies funneled into acquiring knowledge of vigorous play

G. Genital stage
  1. Twelve years and over
  2. Begins at puberty
  3. Genital organs a major source of sexual tensions and pleasures
  4. Energy used to form friendships and prepare for marriage

H. Nursing implications of Freud's theory
  1. Children and parents may have many questions concerning:
    a. Normal sexual development
    b. Sex education
  2. Nurses must understand normal sexual growth and development.
    a. Assist children and parents to form healthy attitudes about sex.

VII. ERIKSON (see Table 10-2)
  A. Theory of psychosocial development most widely used
    1. Outlines a sequence of phases of psychosocial development
    2. Provides a theoretic basis for much of the emotional care that is given to children
  B. Emphasis on healthy personality rather than pathological approach
    1. Stresses rational and adaptive natures of individual
    2. Explains child's behaviors in mastering developmental tasks
  C. Eight stages of development
    1. Each stage has two components—favorable and unfavorable aspect of conflict.
    2. Progression to next stage depends on resolution of conflict.
    3. Conflict never mastered completely—remains a recurrent problem throughout life.

    D. Trust versus mistrust stage (stage I)
        1. Birth to 1 year of age
        2. "Getting" and "taking in" from all the senses
        3. Exists only in relation to something or someone
        4. Consistent, loving care by mother essential to development of trust
        5. Mistrust develops when:
            a. Trust-promoting activities absent
            b. Basic needs inconsistently or inadequately met
        6. Individual develops quality of hope and belief that one can attain deep and essential wishes.
            a. Results in faith and optimism
    E. Autonomy versus shame and doubt (stage II)
        1. One to 3 years of age
        2. Development centered on child's ability to control his or her body, himself or herself, and the environment
        3. Uses his or her power to do things independently
            a. Walking
            b. Climbing
            c. Selection and decision-making
        4. Learns to conform to social rules
        5. Doubt and shame arise when:
            a. Child made to feel unimportant or self-conscious
            b. Choices are disastrous
            c. Shamed by others
            d. Forced to be independent when he or she is capable of assuming control
        6. Achieves autonomy through imitation
            a. Parents are key socializing intermediaries.
            b. Results in self-control and willpower
    F. Initiative versus guilt stage (stage III)
        1. Three to 6 years of age
        2. Characterized by vigorous, intrusive behavior and a strong imagination
        3. Explores physical world with all senses
        4. Develops a conscience
        5. Responds to an inner voice that warns and threatens
        6. Guilt arises when:
            a. Child undertakes goals or activities that are in conflict with those of parent
            b. Made to feel activities are bad
        7. Achieves initiative through identification
            a. Family is key socializing agent.
            b. Results in direction and purpose; ability to imagine and pursue
    G. Industry versus inferiority stage (stage IV)
        1. Six to 12 years of age
        2. Carries tasks and activities through to completion
        3. Learns to compete and cooperate with others
        4. Learns rules
        5. Successful child develops a sense of mastery and self-assurance.
        6. Inferiority develops when:
            a. Too much is expected of child
            b. Child believes he or she cannot meet standards set for him or her by others.
        7. Achieves industry through education
            a. Teachers and peers are socializing agents.
            b. Develops competence, skill, and intelligence to complete task
    H. Identity versus role confusion stage (stage V)
        1. Twelve to 18 years of age
        2. Characterized by marked physical changes

3. Engrossed in how he or she appears to others as compared with his or her own self-concept
4. Struggle with:
    a. Ability to maintain current role and future role as defined by peers
    b. Integrating concepts and values with those of society
    c. Decision for an occupation
5. Role confusion develops when unable to resolve core conflicts.
6. Mastering identity results in devotion and fidelity.
7. Achieves identity through peer pressure and role experimentation

I. Intimacy versus isolation stage (stage VI)
    1. Occurs in early adulthood
    2. Intimacy established on a sense of identity
    3. Capacity to develop:
        a. An intimate love relationship
        b. Intimate interpersonal relationships with friends, partners, and significant others
    4. Isolation develops when intimacy not present.
    5. Intimacy develops when there is mutuality among peers.
    6. Key socializing agents
        a. Lovers
        b. Spouses
        c. Close friends
    7. Develops affiliation and love

J. Generativity versus stagnation stage (stage VII)
    1. Young and middle adulthood
    2. Creation and care of next generation
    3. Essential element is to nourish and nurture.
    4. Failure results in self-absorption and stagnation.
    5. Key socializing agents are spouse, children, and cultural norms.
        a. Results in production and care; commitment and concern for what has been generated

K. Ego integrity versus despair stage (stage VIII)
    1. Old age
    2. Results from satisfaction with life and acceptance of what has been
    3. Despair is a result of remorse for what might have been.
    4. Ego integrity results in renunciation and wisdom and concern with life in the face of death.
    5. Process achieved through introspection.

VIII. PIAGET: COGNITIVE DEVELOPMENT (see Table 10-2)
    A. Provides a basis for learning about and understanding cognitive development
        1. Believes learning should be geared to the child's level of understanding and that the child should be an active participant in the learning process
        2. Cognitive development is a process by which developing individuals become acquainted with the world and objects it contains.
            a. Allows child ability to:
                (1) Reason abstractly
                (2) Think in a logical manner
                (3) Organize intellectual functions into higher structures
    B. Sequence of four stages of intellectual development (sensorimotor, preparational, concrete operational, formal operational)
        1. Prior practice or teaching has little effect on development of new cognitive skills.
        2. Suitable cognitive maturity or readiness necessary to progress to next stage
    C. Sensorimotor (stage I)
        1. Birth to 2 years of age
        2. Consists of substages that are governed by sensations through which simple learning takes place
        3. Progresses from simple reflex activities to simple repetitive behaviors that imitate behaviors

    4. Develops sense of cause and effect
      a. Directs behavior toward object
      b. Solves problems through trial and error
      c. High level of curiosity
      d. Develops sense of self through interactions with environment
        (1) Able to differentiate self from environment
    5. Awareness that object has permanence
      a. Important prerequisite for all other mental activity
  D. Preoperational (stage II)
    1. Two to 7 years of age
    2. Egocentricity is predominant characteristic.
      a. Defined as inability to put oneself in place of another
    3. Interprets objects and events in terms of their relationship or use of them
    4. Sees only his or her perspective
      a. Cannot see another's point of view
    5. Preoperational thinking is concrete and tangible.
    6. Lacks ability to make deductions or generalizations
    7. Thoughts dominated by what he or she sees, hears, and experiences
    8. Increasing ability to use language to represent objects in his or her environment
    9. Increasing ability to elaborate on concepts and make simple associations between ideas
   10. Cannot understand that for every action or operation, there is an action or operation that cancels it
   11. Develops intuitive reasoning later in stage
   12. Begins to understand weight, length, size, and time
  E. Concrete operational (stage III)
    1. Seven to 11 years of age
    2. Thoughts become more logical and coherent.
    3. Able to problem solve
    4. Classifies, sorts, orders, and organizes facts
    5. Able to deal with a number of different aspects of a situation simultaneously
    6. Unable to deal with abstract
    7. Problem solves in concrete, systematic fashion, based on what he or she can perceive
    8. Thoughts become less self-centered
    9. Can consider points of view other than his or her own
   10. Develops socialized thinking
  F. Formal operational (stage IV)
    1. Twelve to 15 years of age
    2. Characterized by adaptability and flexibility
    3. Can think in terms of the abstract
    4. Able to draw conclusions from a set of observations
    5. Can make and test hypotheses
    6. May confuse the ideal with the practice
IX. KOHLBERG: MORAL DEVELOPMENT (see Table 10-2)
  A. Based on cognitive development theory
    1. Provides anticipatory guidance to parents about expectations and discipline of children
  B. Proceeds in an invariant sequence of six stages
  C. Cannot acquire higher levels of moral reasoning until appropriate cognitive development has occurred
  D. Preconventional level of morality
    1. Morality is external.
      a. Children conform to rules imposed by adults.
    2. Stage 1—the punishment and obedience orientation (age 2-3 years)
      a. Child determines whether action good or bad based on consequences
      b. Obeys those in power
      c. Avoids punishment
      d. Possesses no concept of the underlying moral order

      3. Stage 2—the instrumental relativist orientation (age 4-7 years)
        a. The right behavior is that which satisfies the child's own needs.
        b. Possesses elements of fairness, reciprocity, and equal sharing
        c. Do not possess elements of loyalty, gratitude, or justice
   E. Conventional level
     1. Child concerned with:
       a. Conformity and loyalty
       b. Maintaining, supporting, and justifying the social order
       c. Personal expectations of those significant to him or her
     2. Child values maintenance of family regardless of consequences.
     3. Stage 3—the interpersonal concordance or "good boy–nice girl" orientation (age 7-10 years)
       a. Behavior that meets approval of others viewed as good
       b. Conformity to the norm is the "natural" behavior.
       c. Earn approval by being "nice"
     4. Stage 4—the "law and order" orientation (age 10-12 years)
       a. Correct behavior is:
         (1) Obeying rules
         (2) Doing one's duty
         (3) Showing respect for authority
         (4) Maintaining social order
       b. Rules and authority can be social or religious.
   F. Postconventional, autonomous, or principled level
     1. Child reaches cognitive formal operational stage.
     2. Attempts to define moral values and principles
     3. Stage 5—the social contract, legalistic orientation (adolescence)
       a. Correct behavior defined in terms of general individual rights and standards agreed to by society
       b. Emphasis on:
         (1) Legal point of view
         (2) Possibility of changing law in terms of societal needs and rational considerations
     4. Stage 6—universal ethical principles (principles conscience)
       a. Moral reasoning based on abstract reasoning
       b. Uses universal ethical principles
         (1) Action is never a means, but always an end in itself.
       c. People rarely if ever reach stage 6.
X. SULLIVAN
   A. Interpersonal development
     1. Recognizes importance of environment in development
     2. Has some predictive value
     3. Does not recognize biological maturation process
   B. Emphasis on interpersonal relationships and importance of social approval or disapproval in developing a self-concept
     1. Unfavorable reactions result in tension and anxiety.
     2. Favorable reactions result in comfort and security.
   C. Infants
     1. Mother gratifies and comforts child.
     2. Relationship gradually extends to other family members.
   D. Toddler
     1. Becomes more outgoing
     2. Directs social gestures to wider audience
       a. Relatives
       b. Neighborhood children
     3. Engages in aspects of social learning
       a. Peer play
       b. Family events

    E. School age

      1. Wider range of relationships

        a. Authority figures at school and in community

      2. Develops peer relationships

      3. Shares intimacy and common interests with peers

    F. Adolescent

      1. Personal identity

        a. Friends of same sex

        b. Friends of opposite sex

XI. SKINNER, WATSON: LEARNING THEORY

    A. Learning occurs when behavior changes as a result of experience.

    B. Conditioning

      1. Learning through association

        a. Establishing a connection between a stimulus and a response

      2. Operant or instrumental conditioning

        a. Involves rewards or reinforcements to encourage specific behaviors

        b. Applicable to toddler and preschooler learning

      3. Avoidance conditioning

        a. Discourages undesirable behaviors through punishment

        b. Success depends on child's subjective assessment of reward or punishment.

    C. Child

      1. Acquires new behaviors

      2. Produces alterations in existing behavior through:

        a. Forming associations through conditioning

        b. Observing models

      3. Behavior is determined (conditioned) by:

        a. Environmental events

        b. Experiences

        c. Consequences

      4. Rewarded behaviors are repeated.

      5. Punished behaviors are not repeated.

XII. MASLOW: HUMANISTIC THEORY

    A. Focuses on attributes or characteristics that contribute to healthy personality development

    B. Concerned with uniqueness and potential of individuals

      1. Humans motivated by two need systems

        a. Basic

          (1) Food, water, and shelter

        b. Growth needs—internally motivated and reinforced

          (1) Beauty

          (2) Self-fulfillment

      2. Needs arranged in a hierarchy

        a. Lower-level needs assume dominance.

        b. When one level need is satisfied, the next becomes predominant.

    C. Theory does not address developmental stages or shaping of human behaviors.

XIII. BIOLOGICAL GROWTH

    A. Age categories

      1. Birth to 6 months

      2. Six to 12 months

      3. Toddlers

      4. Preschoolers

      5. School-age children

      6. Adolescent

      7. Adult

    B. During childhood, variations in growth of tissues and organs produce changes in body proportions.

   C. First year
      1. Period of rapid growth
      2. Lengthening of trunk
      3. Accumulation of subcutaneous fat
   D. First year to puberty
      1. Legs grow more rapidly.
      2. Body becomes slender and elongated.
   E. Puberty
      1. Feet and hand sizes increase.
         a. Appear large in relation to rest of body
         b. Source of embarrassment
      2. Trunk growth increases.
      3. Onset of puberty approximately 2½ years earlier for girls than boys
      4. Rapid linear growth followed by lateral growth
      5. Child "fills out" during later stages of adolescent growth.
   F. Height
      1. Occurs as a result of skeletal growth
      2. Considered a stable measurement of general growth
      3. When maturation of skeleton is complete, linear growth ceases.
   G. Weight
      1. Weight gain considered indication of satisfactory growth progress in child
      2. Variable
      3. Subject to numerous intrinsic and extrinsic factors
   H. Neurologic growth
      1. Rapid brain cell growth from 30 weeks to 1 year of age
      2. Growth consists of:
         a. Increase in cytoplasm around nuclei of existing cells
         b. Increase in number and intricacy of communication with other cells
         c. Advancing peripheral axons in relation to expanding body dimensions
      3. Brain growth
         a. Measured by head circumference
         b. Increases six times during first year
      4. Lymph tissue
         a. Lymph nodes, thymus, spleen, tonsils, adenoids, blood lymphocytes
            (1) Increase rapidly
            (2) Reach adult dimensions by age 6
            (3) Tissue reaches size approximately twice that of adult by age 12.
               (a) Rapid decline to stable adult dimension by adolescence
XIV. LANGUAGE DEVELOPMENT
   A. Child born with mechanism and capacity to develop speech and language skills
      1. Requires intact physiological function of:
         a. Respiratory system
         b. Speech control center in cerebral cortex
         c. Articulation and resonance structures of the mouth and nasal cavity
      2. Child also requires:
         a. Intact and discriminating auditory apparatus
         b. Intelligence
         c. A need to communicate
         d. Stimulation
   B. Components of language
      1. Phonology—learned first
         a. Basic units of sound that are combined to produce words
      2. Semantics of language—learned next
         a. Words and sentences convey an expressed meaning.
      3. Gain knowledge of syntax
         a. The form or structure of language (rules)
      4. Pragmatics
         a. Principles specifying how language is used in different contexts and situations

C. Stages of language development
  1. Prelinguistic stage
    a. Period before child speaks first meaningful word
    b. Develops systematically over first 10 to 12 months
    c. Involves crying, cooing, and babbling
  2. Holophrastic stage
    a. Speech consists of one- or two-word statements.
    b. Includes holophrases
      (1) Single words with meaning of entire sentence
  3. Telegraphic stage
    a. Speech includes content words only.
    b. From 18 to 24 months
  4. Preschool period
    a. Produce lengthy sentences
    b. Speech increases in complexity.
    c. From 30 months to 5 years
  5. Middle childhood period
    a. Refines language skill
    b. Increases linguistic competence
    c. From 6 to 14 years
    d. Uses bigger words
    e. Understands complex syntactic structures of language
D. Theories of language development
  1. Learning theory
    a. Language acquired as child hears and responds to speech.
    b. How child learns to speak (two theories)
      (1) Operant conditioning—adults reinforce child's attempt to produce grammatical speech
      (2) Acquires language by listening to and imitating speech of adults
  2. Nativists theory
    a. Inborn linguistic processor specialized for language learning
    b. Critical period for language development exists.
    c. Most proficient at learning language between 2 years of age and puberty
  3. Interactional proponents
    a. Child biologically prepared to acquire language
    b. Recognizes crucial role of environment in language learning
E. Factors affecting language development
  1. Delayed, lack of, or impaired speech can result from:
    a. Congenital structural defects of mouth and nasopharynx
    b. Hearing deficit
    c. Neurological dysfunction
    d. Maternal deprivation
    e. Emotional factors
F. Guidelines for communicating with children (Box 10-3)
  1. Do not exclude child in interactions.
  2. Nonverbal communication conveys the most significant message.
G. Communicating with families (Box 10-4)
XV. SELF-CONCEPT AND SELF-ESTEEM
  A. Self-concept
    1. Perception of whole self
    2. Not present at birth
      a. Develops gradually as a result of unique experiences
      b. Learned during childhood
      c. A product of socialization
    3. Subjective; may not reflect reality
    4. Answers the question "Who am I?" and "What am I?"

■ BOX 10-3
■ **GUIDELINES FOR COMMUNICATING WITH CHILDREN**

- Allow children time to feel comfortable.
- Avoid sudden or rapid advances, broad smiles, extended eye contact, or other gestures that may be seen as threatening.
- Talk to the parent if the child is initially shy.
- Communicate through transition objects such as dolls, puppets, stuffed animals before questioning a young child directly.
- Give older children the opportunity to talk without the parents present.
- Assume a position that is at eye level with child.
- Speak in a quiet, unhurried, and confident voice.
- Speak clearly, be specific, and use simple words and short sentences.
- State directions and suggestions positively.
- Offer a choice only when one exists.
- Be honest with children.
- Allow them to express their concerns and fears.
- Use a variety of communication techniques.

From Hockenberry MJ: *Wong's essentials of pediatric nursing,* ed 7, St Louis, 2005, Mosby.

■ BOX 10-4
■ **COMMUNICATING WITH FAMILIES**

- Include all involved family members. One essential step toward achieving a family-centered care environment is to develop open lines of communication with the family.
- Encourage families to write down their questions.
- Remain nonjudgmental.
- Give families both verbal and nonverbal signals that send a message of availability and openness.
- Respect and encourage feedback from families.
- Families come in various shapes, sizes, colors, and generations.
- Avoid assumptions about core family beliefs and values.
- Respect family diversity.

From James SR, Ashwill JW: *Nursing care of children,* Philadelphia, 2007, Saunders.

5. Formed by:
   a. Self-selected mental images
   b. Attitudes
   c. How he or she thinks others see him or her
B. Self-esteem (Box 10-5)
   1. Personal, subjective judgment of one's worthiness
   2. The value an individual places on self
      a. Derived from and influenced by social groups
      b. Individual's perception of how he or she is valued by others
   3. Factors affecting child's development of self-esteem
      a. Temperament
      b. Personality
      c. Ability and opportunity to accomplish age-appropriate developmental tasks
      d. Significant others
      e. Social roles undertaken
      f. Expectations of social roles

■ BOX 10-5
■ **SELF-ESTEEM IN CHILDREN: COMMUNICATION PRACTICES**

Techniques to Enhance Self-Esteem	Practices That Harm Self-Esteem
▪ Praise efforts and accomplishments.	▪ Criticize efforts and accomplishments.
▪ Use active listening skills.	▪ Be too busy to listen.
▪ Encourage expression of feelings.	▪ Tell children how they should feel.
▪ Acknowledge feelings.	▪ Give no support for dealing with feelings.
▪ Use developmentally based discipline.	▪ Use physical punishment.
▪ Use "I" statements.	▪ Use "you" statements.
▪ Be nonjudgmental.	▪ Judge the child.
▪ Set clearly defined limits and reinforce them.	▪ Set no known limits or boundaries.
▪ Share quality time together.	▪ Give time grudgingly.
▪ Be honest.	▪ Be dishonest.
▪ Describe behaviors observed when praising and disciplining.	▪ Use coercion and power as discipline.
▪ Compliment the child.	▪ Belittle, blame, or shame the child.
▪ Smile.	▪ Use sarcastic, caustic, or cruel "humor."
▪ Touch and hug the child.	▪ Avoid coming near child even when the child is open to touching, holding, or hugging. Touch and hold only when performing a task.
▪ Rock the child.	▪ Avoid comforting through rocking.

From James SR, Ashwill JW: *Nursing care of children,* Philadelphia, 2007, Saunders.

    4. Various needs to develop and preserve self-esteem
      a. To feel worthwhile
      b. Recognition for achievements
      c. Approval of parents and peers
      d. Stress inappropiate behavior as unacceptable
      e. Constructive communication
         (1) Use of "I" messages
         (2) Conveys feelings and needs
         (3) Does not destroy child's self-esteem
    5. Positive experiences during developmental phases
      a. Child successful in early motor/verbal experiences
      b. Develops positive self-concept and high self-esteem
      c. Receives encouragement and positive recognition form others
      d. Exposed to appropriate role models
      e. Permitted to experience fear, disappointment, and frustration
      f. Encouraged to finish tasks and reach goals
      g. Results in an individual with sturdy identity and high level of self-actualizing behavior
    6. Negative experiences during developmental phases
      a. Leads to negative self-concept and low self-esteem
      b. Receives insufficient or negative recognition from others.
      c. Expose to inappropriate role models
      d. Prevent from finishing tasks and reaching goals
      e. Results in an individual with frail identity and self-destructive behavior

BIBLIOGRAPHY

1. Bantz DL, Siktberg L: Teaching families to evaluate age-appropriate toys. *J Pediatr Health Care* 7(3):111–114, 1993.
2. Burden N, DeFazio Quinn DM, O'Brien D, et al: *Ambulatory surgical nursing*, ed 2, Philadelphia, 2000, Saunders.
3. Carter AS, Briggs-Gowan MJ, Davis NO: Assessment of young children's social-emotional development and psychopathology: Recent advances and recommendations for practice. *J Child Psychol Psychiatry* 45(1):109–134, 2004.
4. Chez Z, Siegler RS: Across the great divide: Bridging the gap between understanding of toddlers' and older children's thinking. *Monogr Soc Res Child Dev* 65(2):i-vii, 1–96, 2000.
5. Chouinard MM: Children's questions: A mechanism for cognitive development. *Monogr Soc Res Child Dev* 72(1):vii–ix, 1–112; discussion 113–126, 2007.
6. Hockenberry MJ: *Wong's essentials of pediatric nursing*, ed 6, St Louis, 2005, Mosby.
7. James SR, Ashwill JW: *Nursing care of children principles and practice*, ed 3, Philadelphia, 2007, Saunders.
8. Johanson LS: Teaching using G.R.O.W.T.H. *Nurse Educ* 25(1):7, 2000.
9. Kliegman RM, Behrman RE, Jenson HB, et al: *Nelson textbook of pediatrics*, ed 18, Philadelphia, 2007, Saunders.
10. McDowell BM: Using toy critiques to teach growth and development. *Nurse Educ* 27(5):199–200, 2002.
11. Morrongiello BA, Corbett M, Bellissimo A: "Do as I say, not as I do": family influences on children's safety and risk behaviors. *Health Psychol* 27(4):498–503, 2008.
12. Overbay JD: Comics and childhood development. *Nurse Educ* 26(6):262–263, 2001.
13. Phippen ML, Wells MP: *Patient care during operative and invasive procedures*, Philadelphia, 2000, Saunders.
14. Savedra MC, Tesler MD, Holzemer WL, et al: *Adolescent pediatric pain tool (APPT): Preliminary user's manual*, San Francisco, 1989, University of California.
15. Sieving R, Zirbel-Donish S: Development and enhancement of self-esteem in children. *J Pediatr Health Care* 4(6):290–296, 1990.
16. Vandell DL, Pierce KM, Dadisman K: Out-of-school settings as a developmental context for children and youth. *Adv Child Dev Behav* 33:43–77, 2005.

11 The Pediatric Patient

MAUREEN SCHNUR
KERRIE TALBOT

OBJECTIVES

At the conclusion of this chapter, the reader will be able to:

1. Identify six anatomic and physiologic differences to consider when caring for infants and children.

2. Identify four precautionary measures for prevention and treatment of hypothermia in the pediatric patient.

3. Identify two pain assessment scales used for pediatric patients.

4. Identify two reasons for under treatment of pain in infants and children.

5. Identify three stressors associated with hospitalization in the infant, toddler, preschooler, and school-age child.

6. Identify three nursing interventions to lessen the stress associated with separation and hospitalization.

7. State two elements of family centered care.

I. CLASSIFICATION BY AGE
    A. Newborn: less than 72 hours old
    B. Neonate: first 28 days of life
    C. Infant: neonatal period through 12 months
    D. Toddler: 1 to 3 years
    E. Preschooler: 3 to 6 years
    F. School-age child: 6 to 12 years
    G. Adolescent: 12 years and older
II. ANATOMY AND PHYSIOLOGY CONSIDERATIONS
    A. Respiratory system
        1. Infants
            a. Head is larger in proportion to body.
            b. Larynx is high and funnel shaped.
            c. Trachea is located downward and posterior with small diameter.
            d. Epiglottis is short, stiff, U-shaped.
                (1) Difficult intubation
                (2) Swelling narrows opening, leading to potential for airway obstruction
            e. Obligatory nose breather
            f. Cartilage of larynx easily compressed, causing narrowing of airway
                (1) Occurs when neck is flexed or extended
            g. More susceptible to spasm
                (1) Active laryngeal reflexes
            h. Diaphragmatic breathing in neonates
                (1) Predisposed to hypoventilation due to
                    (a) gastric distention
                    (b) bowel obstruction
                    (c) improper positioning
                (2) Accessory and intercostal musculature poorly developed

2. Infants and children
   a. Large tongue, narrow nares, smaller airway opening, shorter neck
   b. Potential for compromised or obstructed airway and difficult intubation
   c. Narrowing of trachea at cricoid cartilage ring
   d. Edema due to infection or irritation may lead to significant narrowing of the airway.
      (1) Reduction in airway radius causes potential increase in airflow resistance.
      (2) Small amount of mucus, edema, or foreign body may cause airway obstruction and compromise gas exchange.
      (3) Limits size of endotracheal tube (ETT) used
      (4) Uncuffed ETT allowing slight leak used for children until age 8 to 10 years
   e. Tonsillar tissue normally enlarged until early school age
   f. Abdominal muscles used to inhale
   g. Intercostal musculature poorly developed
   h. Accessory muscles do not contribute to inspiration.
   i. Child more dependent on effective movement of diaphragm for ventilation
   j. Respiratory rate decreases with increasing age.
B. Cardiovascular system
   1. Blood volume
      a. Neonate: 85 to 90 milliliters/kilogram (mL/kg)
      b. Infant: 75 to 80 mL/kg
      c. Child: 70 to 75 mL/kg
   2. Infants
      a. Myocardium of neonate less compliant
      b. Minimal cardiac reserve
      c. Cardiac output of infant 30% to 50% greater than that of adults
      d. Heart rate major determining factor of cardiac function
      e. High vagal tone predisposes to bradycardia.
      f. Hypotension not apparent until 50% of circulating volume lost
         (1) Due to myocardial depression, most often from inhalation anesthesia
         (2) Poorly equipped to compensate for conditions such as hypoxemia, acidosis, myocardial depression
   3. Infants and children
      a. Chest wall thin in infants and young children
      b. Less subcutaneous fat and muscle tissue than older child
      c. Heart rate decreases with increasing age.
      d. Blood pressure (BP) levels increase with age.
      e. Adult levels reached in adolescence (Table 11-1 for normal vital signs by age)
C. Renal system
   1. Infants
      a. Newborns prone to dehydration and fluid overload
      b. Limited but increasing ability to conserve sodium
      c. Low glomerular filtration rate and limited tubular function
      d. By age 20 weeks, maturation nearly complete
      e. Higher percentage of extracellular fluid
      f. Decreased excretion of drugs eliminated by renal clearance
   2. Infants and children
      a. Water distribution impacts volume of drug distribution.
      b. Complete maturation of renal function at 2 to 3 years of age
D. Thermoregulation
   1. Infants
      a. Large head, large body surface area, less subcutaneous fat, decreased ability to produce heat
      b. Lose up to 75% of body heat through exposure of head to room air

  c. At risk for hypothermia (core temperature <36° C [96.8° F])
     (1) At less than 3 months of age, there is no shiver response.
     (2) Neonate response is nonshivering thermogenesis mediated by brown fat.
     (3) When hypothermic, anesthetic agents are metabolized more slowly.
         (a) Prone to respiratory depression
         (b) Slow emergence
III. DEVELOPMENTAL CONSIDERATIONS
   A. More than 5 million children in the United States undergo surgery annually.
      1. Preoperatively, 50% to 75% experience significant fear and anxiety.
      2. Higher levels of anxiety and fear occur with:
         a. Venipuncture
            (1) The major fear of children related to hospitalization is pain from needles and injections.
         b. Long wait time between admission and induction of anesthesia
         c. Separation from parents at time of transport to the OR
            (1) Infant or child may display behaviors associated with separation (e.g., protest, despair, detachment) (Box 11-1).
                (a) Educate parents that reactions are normal responses to separation.

■ TABLE 11-1
■ ■ **Normal Vital Signs by Age**

Age	Temperature*		Pulse Rate (beats/ min)	Respiratory Rate (breaths/ min)	Blood Pressure (mm Hg)
	Degrees Fahrenheit	Degrees Celsius			
Newborn	96.8-99 (axillary)	36-37.2 (axillary)	120-160	30-60	Systolic: 46-92 Diastolic: 38-71
3 yr	97.5-98.6 (axillary)	36.4-37 (axillary)	80-125	20-30	Systolic: 72-110 Diastolic: 40-73
10 yr	97.5-98.6 (oral)	36.4-37 (oral)	70-110[†]	16-22	Systolic: 83-121 Diastolic: 45-79
16 yr	97.5-98.6 (oral)	36.4-37 (oral)	55-90	15-20	Systolic: 93-131[‡] Diastolic: 49-85

*The normal range of the child's temperature will depend on the method used. Temperatures exhibit circadian rhythms at all ages.
[†]After age 12 years, a boy's pulse rate is 5 beats/min slower than a girl's.
[‡]After age 14 years, blood pressure in boys is higher than in girls.
From James SR, Ashwill JW, Droske SC: *Nursing care of children*, ed 2, Philadelphia, 2002, WB Saunders.

■ BOX 11-1
■ **STAGES OF SEPARATION**

Protest: Child is agitated, resists caregivers, cries, and is inconsolable.
Despair: Child experiences hopelessness and becomes quiet, withdrawn, and apathetic.
Detachment: Child becomes interested in the environment, plays, and seems to form relationships with caregivers and other children. If parents reappear, the child may ignore them.

From James SR, Ashwill JW, Droske SC: *Nursing care of children*, ed 2, Philadelphia, 2002, WB Saunders.

   (b) Minimizing separation may enhance resilience of child.
   (c) Older toddlers generally protest most vigorously.
   (d) Detachment stage is more common in long-term separation.
  d. Anesthesia induction
 B. Preparation of child
  1. Essential that child is prepared
  2. Deceiving information or lack of explanation regarding surgery may lead to:
   a. Feelings of betrayal towards those that protect them
   b. Feelings of terror towards health care team and in daily life
   c. Altered emotional state to one of being fearful and timid
  3. Lessens with time and most often disappears within 2 weeks
 C. Infant response to surgery/hospitalization
  1. Stressors
   a. Separation
   b. Pain
   c. Fear
  2. Reactions
   a. Protest (crying)
   b. Despair
   c. Detachment
  3. Interventions
   a. Meet needs promptly
   b. Liberal visiting for parents
   c. Comfort measures (e.g., pacifier, special toy or blanket, swaddling, holding)
 D. Toddler response to surgery/hospitalization
  1. Stressors
   a. Separation
   b. Loss of control
   c. Physical restrictions, change in routine, dependency on others
   d. Bodily injury and pain
  2. Reactions
   a. Intensity of response affected by:
    (1) Memory
    (2) Physical restraint
    (3) Emotional reactions of others
    (4) Lack of preparation
    (5) Separation from loved ones
   b. Protest, despair
    (1) Resistance, verbal uncooperativeness
    (2) Regression
    (3) Negativism, physical aggression, temper tantrums
    (4) Intrusive experiences may be as anxiety provoking as painful ones (e.g., taking temperature).
   c. Detachment
  3. Interventions
   a. Provide safe limits for allowing expression of negative feelings.
   b. Expect and accept regressive behavior.
    (1) Reassure parent(s) that behavior is normal.
   c. Incorporate aspects of home routine, as possible.
   d. Comfort objects (special toy or blanket)
   e. Optimize parental visiting and involvement.
   f. Comfort measures (held by parent)
   g. Consider Parent-Present Induction (PPI)
 E. Preschooler response to surgery/hospitalization
  1. Stressors
   a. Separation
   b. Loss of control

        c. Bodily injury and pain

        d. Intrusive procedures threatening

        e. Fear of bleeding and punctures, insides will "leak out"

    2. Reactions

        a. Specific and goal-directed physical and verbal aggression

        b. Avoidance

        c. Regression

        d. Despair

        e. Detachment

    3. Interventions

        a. Acknowledge and accept fears and anxieties.

        b. Encourage hands-on practice with equipment.

        c. Encourage verbalization.

        d. Simple explanations minimize misinterpretation. Examples:

           (1) "We will give you medicine to drink that will help you relax."

           (2) "We will be able to help you fall asleep by asking you to breathe in special smells from a soft mask, like this one. You can pick the special smell that you like best."

           (3) "You will have three stickers on your chest with wires that will help us see the beats of your heart on a computer screen."

        e. Use distraction (e.g., singing a favorite song, reading a book).

        f. Consider PPI.

        g. Optimize parental visiting.

  F. School-age child response to surgery/hospitalization

    1. Stressors

        a. Separation

        b. Loss of control

        c. Bodily injury and pain

        d. Death, disfigurement, mutilation, procedures involving genitals

    2. Reactions

        a. Disinterest, isolation, withdrawal

        b. Inquisitiveness

        c. Active interest in health or illness

        d. Frustration

        e. Try to act brave

        f. Able to express concerns about pain

    3. Interventions

        a. Respond honestly to requests for factual information.

        b. Want to know what a procedure is for, if it will hurt, how it will make them well, and what injury or harm could result

        c. Attentively listen, perceive lies or half truths.

        d. Encourage verbalization and questions.

        e. Acknowledge fears.

        f. Encourage presence of comfort objects (stuffed animal, toy, music).

        g. Offer choices to provide measure of control (flavors of anesthetic gas, which book to read while waiting, wearing a cap into the operating room).

        h. Encourage hands-on practice with equipment.

        i. Respect increasing need for privacy.

        j. Consider PPI.

        k. Optimize parental visiting.

IV. FAMILY-CENTERED CARE

  A. Philosophy of care adopted by pediatric nursing

    1. Families are partners in care.

  B. Core concepts

    1. Dignity and respect

    2. Sharing of information

    3. Involvement of patient and family in care and decision-making

    4. Collaboration between health care team, patient, and family

C. Elements
   1. Family is at the center as the constant in child's life.
   2. Illness or injury affects all members of the family system.
   3. Crucial to assess family and establish therapeutic relationship with family to ensure support, compliance, and therapeutic change
   4. Parents encouraged to participate in child's care as much as possible
   5. Care practiced with respect for wide range of families with varied values and beliefs
      a. Families vary (e.g., may be single parent, blended, three generational).
      b. May be traditional or nontraditional primary caregiver and decision-maker (e.g., biological parent(s), adoptive or foster parent(s), grandparents, other family members, or other involved individuals)
D. Parents feel secure when they:
   1. Have established trust with the professional(s) caring for their child
   2. Have some control over what is happening to their child
   3. Are respected as knowing their child best and are influential in care
   4. Are allowed to stay for procedures
      a. Both children and parents tend to benefit.
E. Siblings
   1. When sibling becomes ill or injured
      a. Fear of uncertainty for sibling and parents
      b. Fear of acquiring the illness or having same injury
      c. Fear or guilt that they are responsible
      d. Jealousy
      e. Increased sibling rivalry
      f. Interventions
         (1) Provide information consistent with developmental level.
         (2) Encourage questions, provide honest answers.
F. Perioperative considerations for care of family
   1. Manifestations of the stress of procedure/surgery are multifactorial and unique to the individual family member regardless of complexity of surgery (e.g., parent of patient having myringotomy may demonstrate and/or experience more anxiety than a parent of a baby having cardiac surgery).
   2. Daily family routine is interrupted.
      a. Arrangements for care of siblings and pets, rides have often been made.
         (1) For day of procedure/surgery, making arrangements for other siblings enables parent(s) to focus on the child having surgery as well as their own needs.
            (a) Parents are encouraged to eat since they may opt not to eat while their child is not able to eat or drink.
            (b) They may have gotten up early in the morning or not slept because of anticipatory stress and may appreciate having a quiet place to lie down while their child is undergoing the procedure/surgery.
            (c) Parent with multiple children and limited support network may find no alternative but to bring siblings of the patient on the day of surgery.
      b. Delays in surgery/recovery may add additional stress related to outside concerns and the need to make additional arrangements.
V. PHASES OF PERIOPERATIVE CARE FOR PEDIATRIC PATIENT
   A. Preoperative physiologic and psychological preparation of child and family
   B. Safe and efficient management of child's procedure or surgery and anesthesia
   C. Provision of optimal postoperative care minimizing complications
VI. PREOPERATIVE TEACHING
   A. Providing information to patient and family about inpatient process
      1. Child admitted for surgery from:
         a. Home on the morning of surgery
         b. An inpatient unit

        c. Emergency department

        d. Other facilities

   2. Undergoes procedure

   3. Recovers from procedure

   4. Transferred to nursing unit or returns to original facility for continued recovery

B. Outpatient process at hospital or freestanding facility

   1. Child admitted to facility on morning of procedure

   2. Undergoes procedure

   3. Recovers from procedure

   4. Discharged home same day

   5. May need transport to hospital from freestanding facility for further care if necessary

C. Methods

   1. Preoperative on-site tours

        a. Waiting area, operating room area, postanesthesia care unit (PACU), discharge area

        b. Play therapy with Child Life Specialist (CLS)

        c. Provide coloring books about surgery.

        d. Encourage role play using surgical masks, stethoscopes, hats, booties.

   2. Preoperative web-based tours

   3. Preoperative phone interview

        a. Encourage questions.

   4. Preoperative assessment and teaching

D. Developmental considerations

   1. Preparation for procedures/surgery for child varies (Box 11-2).

        a. Age

           (1) Timing of preparation

              (a) For children 6 years or older, best to provide preparation 5 to 7 days before surgery

                  (i) Least beneficial is 1 day before surgery

           (2) Children 1 to 5 years of age at higher risk for significant preoperative anxiety

        b. Temperament

           (1) Those with tendency towards being anxious or shy or use passive coping methods are at higher risk for preoperative anxiety.

        c. Past exposure to hospital

           (1) Conditioned by previous positive or negative health care provider encounters

               (a) Positive experiences lessen subsequent anxiety.

               (b) Negative experiences may result in high levels of preoperative anxiety.

        d. Growth and development

        e. Cognitive development

        f. Parental anxiety influences anxiety level of child.

E. Family considerations

   1. Coping abilities

   2. Sociocultural environment

   3. Support systems

   4. Prior experience with hospitalization

   5. Additional stresses on family

   6. Religious beliefs

   7. Family communication patterns

F. Educational strategies

   1. Parental presence

   2. Limit teaching to 5 to 10 minutes.

   3. Provide clear explanations of which body part(s) will be affected.

■ BOX 11-2
■ **PREPARATION OF CHILDREN FOR PROCEDURES AND SURGERY***

Infants
Major fears: Separation and strangers

Preparation

- Minimize separation from parents.
- Provide consistent caretakers.
- Decrease parents' anxiety.

Toddlers
Major fears: Separation and loss of control

Characteristics of Toddlers' Thinking

- Egocentric, primitive, magical, little concept of body integrity

Preparation

- Prepare child hours or even minutes before procedures, because preparation too far in advance produces even more intense anxiety.
- Keep explanations very simple and choose wording carefully, avoiding words with multiple meanings.
- Let the toddler play with equipment, e.g., put mask on teddy bear.
- Minimize separation from parents; keep security objects at hand.
- Recognize that any intrusive procedure is likely to provoke an intense reaction.
- Use restraints judiciously.

Preschoolers
Major fears: Bodily injury and mutilation, loss of control, the unknown, the dark, and being left alone.

Characteristics of Preschoolers' Thinking

- Preoperational: egocentric, magical, animistic, transductive
- Highly literal interpretation of words, inability to abstract
- Primitive ideas about their bodies
- Difficulty in differentiating a "good" hurt (beneficial treatment) from a "bad" hurt (illness or injury)

Preparation

- Prepare the preschooler days in advance for major events (hours for minor ones). Tie explanations to known events (e.g., lunchtime).
- Keep explanations simple and concrete, and choose wording carefully.
- Emphasize that the child will wake up after surgery, because anesthesia described as "being put to sleep" may be frightening.
- Use pictures, models, actual equipment, or hospital play and behavioral rehearsal. Describe what child will feel, hear, and taste. Assess comprehension.
- Repeat many times that the child has not done anything wrong and is not being punished.
- Repeat explanations every time something is done; do not assume the child remembers. Anxiety may interfere with memory.
- Do not tell the children they will feel better after surgery, because they will undoubtedly feel worse in the immediate postoperative period.
- Give the child choices whenever possible.
- Do not tie evaluations of the child to behavior during procedures (e.g., he is not "a good boy" for holding still, but rather, "That was helpful to hold still!").
- Teach the child some simple coping skills such as distraction techniques in advance of the procedure, and then guide the child in use during the procedures.
- After the procedure, play sessions are important to help the child understand and integrate experience.

School-Age Children
Major fears: Loss of control, bodily injury and mutilation, failure to live up to expectations of important others, and death

*It is important to remember that the child's psychosocial developmental stage may not always match his or her chronologic age. Development may be delayed, particularly in chronically ill children. For example, an adolescent who is delayed in development may need to be approached more like a school-age child.

■ BOX 11-2
■ **PREPARATION OF CHILDREN FOR PROCEDURES AND SURGERY—cont'd**

Characteristics of Thinking of School-Age Children

- Concrete operational period
- Beginning of logical thought but continuing tendency to be literal
- Vague, false, or nonexistent ideas about illness and body construction and function
- Ability to listen attentively to all that is said without always comprehending
- Reluctance to ask questions or admit not knowing something they think they are expected to know
- Better ability to understand relationship between illness and treatment
- Increased awareness of the significance of various illnesses, potential hazards of treatments, lifelong consequence of injury, and the meaning of death

Preparation

- Prepare days to weeks in advance for major events because it is extremely important to the child's ability to cope effectively, to cooperate, and to comply with treatment; in addition, preparation gives the child a greater sense of control.
- Ask children to explain what they understand.
- Use body diagrams, pictures, and models; this age group of children enjoys learning scientific terminology and handling actual equipment because their thinking is concrete (although some older school-age children object to being seen looking at a doll).
- Stress that peer group contact can be maintained.
- Emphasize the "normal" things the child will be able to do after hospitalization.
- Give as many choices as possible to increase the child's sense of control.
- Reassure the child that he or she has done nothing wrong and that necessary procedures and surgery are not punishments.
- Standardized multimedia education may be helpful.
- Anticipate and answer questions regarding the long-term consequences (e.g., what the scar will look like, how long activities may be curtailed).
- Sessions conducted after the procedure are important to help the child "work through" and master the experience.

From Hazinski MF: *Manual of pediatric critical care,* St Louis, 1999, Mosby.

    a. Use play as a method of expression.
      (1) Describe equipment and allow hands-on demonstration.
      (2) Use visual aids, books, models, dolls to explain procedures.
      (3) When available, collaborate with a certified CLS.
      (4) Use behavioral distraction techniques.
      (5) If the child cries, tell him or her it is okay to cry
G. Communication
   1. Introduce yourself, including role.
   2. Ask the name of each family member present.
   3. Address adults by appropriate titles such as "Mr." and "Mrs." unless otherwise indicated.
   4. Use an interpreter employed by the facility if indicated and available.
   5. Use a developmental approach in communicating with the child (Table 11-2).
H. Optimizing privacy
   1. Verbal communication
     a. Use consult room when possible for discussion, information gathering.
     b. Maintain low speaking voice in crowded areas.
   2. Personal information
     a. Protect medical and sensitive information including electronic and/or hard copies.

■ TABLE 11-2
■ **Developmental Milestones and Their Relationship to Communication Approaches**

Development	Language Development	Emotional Development	Cognitive Development	Suggested Communication Approach
INFANTS (0-12 MO) Infants experience the world through the sense of hearing, seeing, smelling, tasting and touching.	Crying, babbling, cooing, single word production, able to name some objects	Dependent on others; high need for cuddling and security Responsive to environment (e.g., sounds, visual stimuli). Distinguish between happy and angry voices as well as between familiar and strange voices. Beginning to experience separation anxiety	Interactions largely reflexive Beginning to see repetition of activities and movements. Beginning to initiate interactions intentionally Short attention span (1-2 minutes)	Use calm, soft soothing voice. Be responsive to cries. Engage in taking turns vocalizing (adult imitates baby sounds). Talk and read regularly to infants. Prepare infants as you are about to perform care. Talk to infant about what you are about to do. Use a slow approach and allow child time to get to know you.
TODDLERS (1-3 YR) Toddlers experience the world through the senses of hearing, seeing, smelling, tasting, and touching.	Two-word combinations emerge. Participate in taking turns in communication (speaker/listener). "No" becomes a favorite word. Able to use gestures and verbalize simple wants and needs	Strong need for security objects Separation/stranger anxiety heightened Participate in parallel play Thrive on routines Beginning development of independence: "Want to do by self." Still very dependent on significant adults	Experiment with objects Participate in active exploration. Begin to experiment with variations on activities Begin to identify cause-and-effect relationships. Short attention span (3-5 minutes)	Learn the toddler's words for common items, and use them in conversations. Describe activities and procedures as they are about to be done. Use picture books. Use play for demonstrations. Be responsive to child's receptivity toward you, and approach cautiously. Preparation should occur immediately before the event.

PRESCHOOL CHILDREN (3-6 YR)

Preschool children use words they do not fully understand, nor do they accurately understand many words used by others. Further development and expansion of word combination (able to speak in full sentences) Growth in correct grammatical usage. Use pronouns Clearer articulation of sounds Vocabulary rapidly expanding; may know words without understanding meaning.	Like to imitate activities and make choices. Strive for independence but need adult support and encouragement Demonstrate purposeful attention-seeking behaviors Learn cooperation and taking turns in game playing Need clearly set limits and boundaries	Begin developing concepts of time, space, and quantity. Magical thinking prominent World seen only from child's perspective. Short attention span (5-10 minutes)	Seek opportunities to offer choices. Use play to explain procedures and activities. Speak in simple sentences, and explore using relative concepts. Use picture and story books, puppets. Describe activities and procedures as they are about to be done. Be concise: limit length of explanations (<5 minutes). Engage in preparatory activities 1 to 3 hours before the event.

SCHOOL-AGE CHILDREN (6-12 YR)

School-age children communicate thoughts and appreciate viewpoints of others. Words with multiple meanings and words describing things they have not experienced are not thoroughly understood. Expanding vocabulary enables child to describe concepts, thoughts, and feelings. Development of conversational skills	Interact well with others Understand rules to games Very interested in learning Build close friendships Beginning to accept responsibility for own actions Competition emerges. Still dependent on adults to meet needs	Able to grasp concepts of classification, conversation Concrete thinking emerges. Become very oriented to "rules" Able to process information in serial format Lengthened attention span (10-30 minutes)	Use photographs, books, diagrams, charts, videos to explain. Make explanations sequential. Engage in conversations that encourage critical thinking. Establish limits and set consequences. Use medical play techniques. Introduce preparatory materials 1 to 5 days in advance of the event.

From James SR, Ashwill JW, Droske SC: *Nursing care of children*, ed 2, Philadelphia, 2002, WB Saunders.

VII. PREOPERATIVE PHASE
    A. Goals of preoperative assessment
        1. Identify potential risks for and plans to prevent complications.
            a. Primary care provider performs/provides complete history and physical.
            b. Anesthesiologist is responsible for clearing patient for anesthesia.
        2. Educate and prepare patient and family.
        3. Reduce anxiety level for child and caregivers.
        4. Establish trusting relationship with child and family.
    B. Methods for preoperative assessment
        1. Multiple ways to gather information depending on patient status and facility protocol/policy
            a. Medical record review
            b. Phone assessment
                (1) Healthy patients having minor to moderately complex procedures
                (2) Patients with stable medical conditions having low-risk procedures
                (3) Assessment criteria necessitating presence of patient deferred until day of surgery
            c. Preanesthetic consult before day of surgery
                (1) Complex patients
                (2) Moderately complex to complex procedures in healthy patients or patients with stable medical conditions
                (3) Goals
                    (a) Minimize cost and optimize outcomes.
                    (b) Ensure optimal condition of patient for surgery.
                    (c) Review and address all medical conditions, including newly discovered or chronic issues.
            d. Day of surgery assessment and validation of information gathered
    C. Preadmission assessment
        1. Medical record review
            a. Pediatric comorbidities (Table 11-3)

■ TABLE 11-3
■ ■ **Specific Pediatric Diseases and Their Anesthetic Implications**

Disease	Implications
RESPIRATORY SYSTEM	
Asthma	Intraoperative bronchospasm that may be severe Pneumothorax Optimal preoperative medical management essential; may require preoperative steroids
Difficult airway	May require special equipment and personnel Should be anticipated in children with dysmorphic features or acute airway obstruction as in epiglottitis or laryngotracheobronchitis or with airway foreign body Patients with Down syndrome may require evaluation of atlanto-occipital joint. Patients with storage diseases may be at high risk.
Bronchopulmonary dysplasia	Barotrauma with positive pressure ventilation Oxygen toxicity, pneumothorax a risk
Cystic fibrosis	Airway reactivity, bronchorrhea Risk of pneumothorax, pulmonary hemorrhage Atelectasis Assess for cor pulmonale.
Sleep apnea	Must rule out pulmonary hypertension and cor pulmonale Requires careful postoperative observation for obstruction
Cardiac	Need for antibiotic prophylaxis for subacute bacterial endocarditis Use of air filters; careful purging of air from intravenous equipment Need to understand effects of various anesthetics on the hemodynamics of specific lesions

Disease	Implications
	Preload optimization and avoidance of hyperviscous states in cyanotic patients
	Possible need for preoperative evaluation of myocardial function and pulmonary vascular resistance
	Provide information about pacemaker function and ventricular device function.
HEMATOLOGIC	
Sickle cell	Possible need for simple or exchange transfusion based on preoperative Hgb and percent Hgb S
Oncology	Pulmonary evaluation of patients who have received bleomycin, bis-chloroethyl-nitrosourea, chloroethyl-cyclohexyl-itrosourea, methotrexate, or radiation to the chest
Rheumatologic	Limited mobility of temporomandibular joint, cervical spine, arytenoids cartilages
	Requires careful preoperative evaluation
	May be difficult airway
GASTROINTESTINAL	
Esophageal, gastric	Potential for reflux and aspiration
Liver	High overall morbidity and mortality in patients with hepatic dysfunction
	Altered metabolism of some drugs
	Potential for coagulopathy
Renal	Altered electrolyte and acid-base status
	Altered clearance of some drugs
	Need for preoperative dialysis with selected cases
	Succinylcholine to be used with extreme caution and only when serum potassium level is recently shown to be normal
NEUROLOGIC	
Seizure disorder	Avoid anesthetics that may lower threshold.
	Ensure optimal control preoperatively.
	Preoperative anticonvulsant levels
Increased intracranial pressure	Avoid agents that increase cerebral blood flow.
	Avoid hypercarbia.
Neuromuscular disease	Avoid depolarizing relaxants; at risk for hyperkalemia
	May be at risk for malignant hyperthermia
Development delay	May be uncooperative at induction
Psychiatric	Monoamine oxidase inhibitor (or cocaine) may interact with meperidine, resulting in hyperthermia and seizures.
	Selective serotonin reuptake inhibitors may induce or inhibit various hepatic enzymes that may alter anesthetic drug clearance.
	Illicit drugs may have adverse effects on cardiorespiratory homeostasis and may potentiate the action of anesthetics.
ENDOCRINE	
Diabetes	Greatest risk is unrecognized intraoperative hypoglycemia; if insulin is administered, monitor blood glucose level intraoperatively; must provide glucose and insulin with adjustment for fasting condition and surgical stress
SKIN	
Burn	Difficult airway
	Risk of rhabdomyolysis and hyperkalemia from succinylcholine
	Fluid shifts
	Bleeding coagulopathy
Immunologic	Retroviral drugs may inhibit benzodiazepine clearance.
	Immunodeficiency requires careful infection control practices.
	May require cytomegalovirus-negative blood products, irradiation, or leukofiltration
Metabolic	Careful assessment of glucose homeostasis in infants

Hgb, hemoglobin.

From Behrman RE, Kliegman RM, Jenson HB: *Nelson textbook of pediatrics,* ed 17, Philadelphia, 2004, WB Saunders.

      b. Current state of health (e.g., rhinitis, cough, fever, rash, gastritis)

      c. Allergies and sensitivities (e.g., medications, latex, environmental, foods)

      d. Medications

      e. Assess need for preoperative consults (e.g., endocrine, cardiac, pulmonary).

          (1) Follow-up with anesthesiologist regarding need for consult(s).

      f. Determine need for laboratory, x-ray, or other requirements from physician.

          (1) Routine laboratory or diagnostic testing not necessary for preanesthetic evaluation

          (2) Vary per hospital or facility policy/practice, physician preference and/or procedure

      g. Review prior surgeries and hospitalizations.

          (1) Assess risk for malignant hyperthermia.

             (a) Personal and family history

             (b) Previous administration of anesthesia

                (i) Related complications

             (c) Partial list of conditions placing pediatric patient at higher risk

                (i) King Denborough syndrome

                (ii) Evans myopathy, muscular dystrophies

                (iii) Central core disease, multicore disease

                (iv) Kyphoscoliosis

                (v) Osteogenesis imperfecta

                (vi) Myotonia congenita

      h. Arrange for interpreter for phone call if need known.

  2. Phone assessment

      a. Medications including dose, route, and frequency

          (1) Follow facility policy/protocol or confer with anesthesiologist regarding how best to advise parent about holding medications before surgery.

          (2) May be helpful for family to bring medications on day of procedure/surgery to clarify dosages and determine last dose given

      b. Elicit information about any special needs of the child or family that may necessitate additional planning.

          (1) Language barrier

             (a) May need to plan for interpreter as indicated if previously not known

          (2) Developmental

             (a) Parents may choose to bring comfort objects such as special toy, blanket, doll, sippy cup, or favorite book

          (3) Behavioral

             (a) May benefit from admission to quieter area

          (4) Social

          (5) Safe transportation

             (a) Ensure transportation plan is established.

             (b) Recommend additional caregiver to be with child while going home.

      c. Assist family to understand process, preoperative routines, and expected time frames

          (1) Preoperative, intraoperative, and postoperative phases

             (a) Combination of written information from physician offices and verbal information provided during preoperative assessment phone call may optimize understanding of perioperative process.

          (2) Nothing by mouth (NPO) and feeding guidelines per facility policy/protocol

             (a) Minimum fasting periods recommended by the American Society of Anesthesiologists (ASA) are:

                (i) 2 hours for clear liquids

                (ii) 4 hours for breast milk

                (iii) 6 hours for infant formula

                (iv) 6 hours for nonhuman milk

                (v) 6 hours for light meal

        (3) Check-in time and location

    d. Verify guardianship and ensure guardian will be available for consent(s).

        (1) Consult with legal resources to clarify guardianship as needed.

    e. Report concerns to anesthesiologist.

    f. Document and communicate pertinent information per facility policy/protocol.

D. Additional criteria for preanesthesia consult with patient present

  1. Assessment

    a. Vital signs including oxygen saturation

    b. Physical assessment including height and weight per facility policy/protocol

    c. Safety needs as indicated by facility policy/protocol:

        (1) Medication reconciliation

        (2) Fall risk

        (3) Patient identification

        (4) Site verification

        (5) Others as indicated by facility policy/protocol

    d. Pain assessment:

        (1) Obtain history from family and child.

        (2) Determine current pain location, severity, and duration if applicable.

        (3) Identify child's normal words to communicate pain.

        (4) Identify child's normal response to pain.

        (5) Identify age and cognitively appropriate pain scale.

E. Day of surgery

  1. Admission to preoperative area

    a. Validate previously reviewed information.

    b. Identify patient per facility policy/protocol.

    c. Verify procedure and site with patient/family.

    d. Identify/verify allergies including potential for latex sensitivity if indicated as per facility policy/protocol.

        (1) Children with chronic illnesses and hospitalizations at higher risk for latex sensitivity

    e. Obtain accurate weight and height per facility policy/protocol (recommend on admission).

    f. Obtain vital signs including temperature and oxygen saturation.

    g. Obtain urine sample if indicated.

        (1) Human chorionic gonadotropin per facility policy/protocol, if indicated

    h. Establish and document NPO time.

        (1) Enables accurate calculation of fluid requirements

        (2) Verify with family that child has been NPO as required.

           (a) Stomach should be free of solids before anesthesia.

           (b) Clear liquids up to 2 to 4 hours preoperatively per facility policy/protocol

    i. Review, validate, and/or complete preadmission assessment as appropriate.

    j. Review and verify current medications, including dose, frequency, and last dose administered.

    k. Review feeding history, special needs (e.g., cleft palate feeder, sippy cup or straw, breast-fed, gastrostomy tube).

    l. Establish baseline pain assessment.

        (1) Consider child's previous pain experiences.

           (a) Determine appropriate pain scale for postoperative use and provide teaching.

    m. Verify safe transport home.

    n. Notify anesthesia provider of concerns (e.g., anxiety, symptoms of cold, wheezing, fever, rash).

    o. Document and communicate per facility policy/protocol.

  2. Preanesthesia evaluation (Box 11-3)

■ BOX 11-3
■ **THE PREANESTHETIC HISTORY**

Child's Previous Anesthetic and Surgical Procedures
Review anesthetic record for information about mask and endotracheal tube size, type and size of laryngoscope used, difficulties with mask ventilation or intubation, history of hyperthermia or acidosis.

Perinatal Problems (Especially for Infants)
Need for prolonged hospitalization
Need for supplemental oxygen or intubation
History of apnea and bradycardia

Other Major Illnesses and Hospitalizations
Family History of Anesthetic Complications, Malignant Hyperthermia, or Pseudocholinesterase Deficiency
Respiratory Problems
Chronic exposure to environmental tobacco smoke
Obstructive apnea, breathing irregularities, or cyanosis (especially in infants younger than 6 months)
History of snoring or obstructive breathing pattern
Recent upper respiratory tract infection
Recurrent respiratory infections
Previous laryngotraches bronchitis (croup)
Asthma or wheezing during respiratory infections

Cardiac Problems
Murmurs
Dysrhythmia
Exercise intolerance
Syncope
Cyanosis

Gastrointestinal Problems
Reflux and vomiting
Feeding difficulties
Failure to thrive
Liver disease

Exposure to Exanthems or Potentially Infectious Pathogens
Neurologic Problems
Seizures
Developmental delay
Neuromuscular diseases
Increased intracranial pressure

Hematologic Problems
Anemia
Bleeding diathesis
Tumor
Immunocompromise
Prior blood transfusions and reactions

Renal Problems
Renal insufficiency, oliguria, anuria
Fluid and electrolyte abnormalities

Psychosocial Considerations
Posttraumatic stress
Drug abuse, use of cigarettes or alcohol

■ BOX 11-3
■ **THE PREANESTHETIC HISTORY—cont'd**

Physical or sexual abuse
Family dysfunction
Previous traumatic medical and surgical experiences
Psychosis, anxiety, depression

Gynecologic Considerations
Sexual history (sexually transmitted diseases)
Possibility of pregnancy

Current Medications
Prior administration of corticosteroids

Allergies
Drugs
Iodine
Latex products
Surgical tapes
Food allergies (especially soy and egg albumin)

Dental Condition (Loose or Cracked Teeth)
When and What the Child Last Ate (Especially in Emergency Procedures)

From Behrman RE, Kliegman RM, Jenson HB: *Nelson textbook of pediatrics,* ed 17, Philadelphia, 2004, WB Saunders.

a. Performed by anesthesia provider
b. Precedes delivery of anesthesia
c. Clinical assessment includes:
  (1) Review of previous medical records
  (2) Interview with parents and the patient
  (3) General observations of patient
  (4) Physical examination
    (a) Review of systems
      (i) Special attention to heart, lungs, upper airways
        [a] Airway assessed for potential difficulty with mask induction or intubation
        [b] Note and document loose teeth.
        [c] Note birthmarks, bruises, rashes, skin discolorations.
      (ii) Identify new symptoms.
      (iii) Evaluate for recent exposure to communicable and infectious diseases (e.g., chickenpox, human immunodeficiency virus, hepatitis).
      (iv) Evaluate for preexisting conditions with implications for anesthesia (e.g., gastroesophageal reflux, sleep apnea, asthma).
  (5) Verify ASA physical status classification.
  (6) Determine additional medical tests, lab work, consults needed.
  (7) Assess need for premedication.
  (8) Assess ability to perform venous access after induction.
  (9) Consider PPI.
  (10) Develop plan for perianesthesia care, including postoperative pain management.
  (11) Counsel patient and parents regarding anesthesia and surgery.
  (12) Perform painful procedures last.

3. Premedication

    a. Provides sedation

    b. Decreases fear, anxiety, emotional trauma

    c. Allows easier transition of child from parents to anesthesia provider

    d. Techniques to assist in preparation of the child preoperatively (based on child's cognitive development)

        (1) Explain purpose of procedure.

        (2) Use pictures, diagrams, dolls, video.

        (3) Use words child can understand.

        (4) Describe sequence of events.

        (5) Describe potential discomfort.

        (6) Allow time for ample questions and discussion.

    e. Premedication is not a substitute for preoperative visit and discussion with patient and family.

    f. Since child's major fear related to hospitalization is pain from needles, intramuscular (IM) route is least preferred.

    g. Options for premedication

        (1) Midazolam

            (a) Most common pediatric premedication in the United States

            (b) Dosing guideline

                (i)   0.25 to 1 mg/kg by mouth (PO) up to maximum of 20 mg (onset 20–30 minutes)

                (ii)   0.025 to 0.1 mg/kg intravenous (IV)

                    [a] Dosing recommendations for infants younger than 6 months not clear

                (iii) 0.1 to 0.15 mg/kg IM

                    [a] May give up to 0.5 mg/kg for very anxious patients

                    [b] Maximum IM dose: 10 mg

            (c) Nursing considerations

                (i)   May cause respiratory depression

                (ii)   May cause paradoxical excitement

        (2) Ketamine

            (a) Indications

                (i)   Reserved for sedation of children with behavioral disorders or who are highly distressed and/or uncooperative

            (b) Dosing guideline

                (i)   3 to 5 mg/kg IM

                (ii)   5 to 10 mg/kg PO

                (iii) 1 mg/kg IV

                (iv) 5 to 10 mg/kg per rectum (PR)

            (c) Adverse reactions

                (i)   Hypersalivation

                    [a] Accumulation of pharyngeal secretions may cause laryngospasm.

                (ii)   Dysphoria

                (iii) Hallucinations

                (iv) Postoperative nausea and vomiting (PONV)

                (v)   Increases heart rate and blood pressure (BP)

            (d) Contraindicated in patients with increased intracranial pressure

            (e) When used alone, associated with dysphoria and hallucinations

                (i)   May be combined with midazolam

                    [a] Prevents or reduces preoperative and separation anxiety

                (ii)   May be administered with glycopyrrolate or atropine

                    [a] Inhibits salivation and secretions

            (f) Formulate plan with anesthesia team before medicating.

                (i)   Ensure appropriate staff to safely manage patient for IM injection.

        (3) Methohexital

            (a) Dosing guideline

(i)   20 to 35 mg/kg/dose PR

(ii) Maximum dose: 500 mg/dose as 10% aqueous solution

  (b) Safety and efficacy not established in infants younger than 1 month

 (4) Nursing interventions for premedication

  (a) Monitor patient per facility policy/protocol.

(i)   Oxygen saturation

(ii) Respiratory rate

(iii) Heart rate

(iv) Level of consciousness

  (b) Ensure resuscitation equipment immediately available

  (c) Nursing staff skilled in airway management

  (d) Provide safety measures:

(i)   Side rails up

(ii) Family at bedside

(iii) Personal items within reach

F. Intraoperative anesthetic considerations

 1. Placement of IV catheter (Figure 11-1)

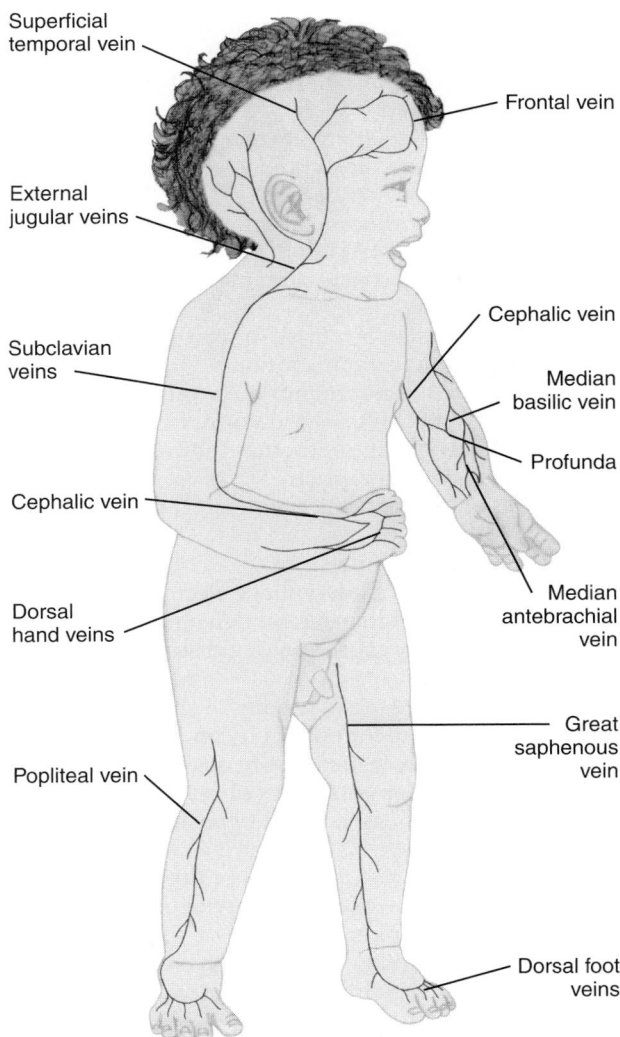

FIGURE 11-1 ■ Venous access sites in children. (From James SR, Ashwill JW, Droske SC: *Nursing care of children*, ed 2, Philadelphia, 2002, WB Saunders.)

    a. Avoid use of dominant hand or arm.

      (1) Consider thumb or finger sucking in infant.

    b. Usually inserted in the OR after mask induction on younger or fearful child

      (1) Children exhibit significant fear and distress associated with procedures involving needles, and phobia may last a lifetime.

      (2) Repeated experience of pain with procedure may result in anticipatory anxiety and increased perception of pain.

    c. May be inserted before induction with older or cooperative child

      (1) Ensure that child is comfortable with being awake for IV insertion.

        (a) Determine comfort level of accompanying adult(s) to stay for procedure and encourage them to sit down while providing support for patient.

      (2) May use behavioral distraction techniques, guided imagery

      (3) Topical methods are available to reduce discomfort such as:

        (a) Eutectic mixture of lidocaine and tetracaine (Synera, S-Caine Patch)

          (i) Controlled heating system quickens delivery and analgesic effect of local anesthetic.

            [a] Vasodilatory effect may enhance IV insertion.

          (ii) Application time of 20 minutes adequate to achieve analgesia

        (b) 4% lidocaine cream (L.M.X.4)

          (i) Average application time of 30 minutes necessary to achieve analgesia

        (c) 4% tetracaine gel (Amethocaine)

          (i) Average application time of 45 minutes necessary to achieve analgesia

        (d) 5% lidocaine-prilocaine cream (Eutectic Mixture of Local Anesthetics [EMLA])

          (i) Initial vasoconstriction may result in more difficulty obtaining vascular access.

          (ii) Infants may be at risk for methemoglobinemia due to prilocaine administration.

            [a] Not recommended for infants younger than 1 month or those younger than 12 months receiving methemoglobin-inducing agents such as acetaminophen

          (iii) Average application time of 60 minutes necessary to achieve analgesia

        (e) Lidocaine iontophoresis

          (i) Noninvasive low-voltage electrical current applied to skin, enhancing transdermal delivery of medication

          (ii) May rarely cause stinging discomfort and skin burns due to electrodes

            [a] Distressing especially to children

            [b] Prepare for possibility and be ready to stop treatment as soon as patient expresses difficulty with tolerating it.

    d. Ensure IV site is secure per facility policy/protocol.

      (1) Padded armboard may be used to position extremity and protect IV from movement.

        (a) Ensure neutral position of extremity.

        (b) Minimize tape to skin contact where possible to minimize discomfort upon removal.

          (i) One method is "backing" tape with shorter and/or narrower piece of tape to hold extremity in place while minimizing area that sticks to skin.

2. Anesthesia induction
   a. Technique dependent on:
      (1) Specific patient risks
      (2) Disease status
      (3) Preoperative medical condition
      (4) Presence or absence of IV line
      (5) Outcome of preoperative discussion with parents and child regarding options
   b. Options
      (1) IV induction
         (a) Medically indicated if child coming in for emergency surgery
            (i) Child at increased risk for aspiration of gastric contents
      (2) Rapid sequence induction
         (a) Patient inhales 100% oxygen before induction.
            (i) Prolongs the time to arterial desaturation with apnea
         (b) Anesthesia induced with rapid-acting hypnotic and a muscle relaxant
         (c) Cricoid pressure applied to occlude the esophagus
            (i) Prevents reflux of gastric contents into the pharynx
         (d) Risks associated with rapid sequence induction
            (i) Unknown whether muscle paralysis will cause inability to intubate the trachea or ability to ventilate by mask
            (ii) The fixed dose of hypnotic may cause hypertension or hypotension.
            (iii) The younger the infant, the shorter the time before child becomes hypoxic after preoxygenation induction.
            (iv) Cricoid pressure does not protect against aspiration.
      (3) Inhalation induction technique
         (a) Medically indicated in situations where spontaneous breathing needs to be preserved
            (i) Foreign body in the airway
         (b) Most widely accepted technique of induction in the United States
         (c) Technique
            (i) Proceed in quiet surroundings.
            (ii) Avoid delays once in operating room.
            (iii) Use flavored aromas on mask (e.g., cherry, orange, bubble gum).
            (iv) Administer nitrous oxide (odorless) in conjunction with oxygen first.
            (v) Introduce more aromatic vapor anesthetics.
3. Anesthetic agents (see Chapter 22)
4. Emotional responses to anesthetic induction (Table 11-4)
   a. Identified as most stressful point throughout the surgical experience
   b. Developmental considerations
   c. New onset negative postoperative responses to anxiety at 2-week period after elective surgery may occur in up to 55% of children, may persist in 19% and 6% of children up to 6 months and 1 year postoperatively, respectively
      (1) Nightmares
      (2) Separation anxiety
      (3) Eating disturbances
      (4) Enuresis
      (5) Increased fear of doctors
      (6) Long-lasting psychological effects may occur.
   d. Positive correlation between preoperative anxiety and postoperative pain and analgesia requirements.
   e. Goal is to minimize distress.

■ TABLE 11-4
■ ■ **Emotional Responses to Anesthetic Induction**

Age	Typical Responses and Implications
0-8 mo	Fewer anticipatory responses Generally calm with strangers Mask induction well tolerated
8 mo-2 yr	Separation anxiety is high. Most difficult for mask induction Premedication, preinduction useful
3-7 yr	Separation anxiety still present Mask induction aided by parental presence
7-11 yr	Generally calm with mask induction Fear of needles Fear of loss of control
12-18 yr	Generally prefers intravenous to mask induction

From Behrman RE, Kliegman RM, Jenson HB: *Nelson textbook of pediatrics,* ed 16, Philadelphia, 2000, WB Saunders.

      (1) Environmental considerations
         (a) Control acoustic and visual disturbances as much as possible.
            (i) Keep potentially frightening objects out of view (e.g., syringes, medications).
            (ii) Optimize calm environment.
      (2) Allow children to practice beforehand with selected equipment (inhalation mask) to familiarize them with equipment.
      (3) Consider PPI.
         (a) Hospital or facility policies/protocols vary.
         (b) Practice strongly supported by many clinicians
         (c) Remains controversial
         (d) Potential advantages
            (i) Decrease fear and anxiety for child and parent(s)
            (ii) Reduce need for premedication
            (iii) Improve compliance of child
         (e) Potential disadvantages
            (i) Parental anxiety may negatively affect child's level of anxiety.
            (ii) Parent may be upset by the events of induction (e.g., child may be upset, may go limp when anesthesia administered).
         (f) Education is vital for positive experience.
            (i) Know what to expect and how to behave during induction.
            (ii) Enhance ability to help child.
            (iii) May be emotional experience
            (iv) Communicate as an option, rather than recommendation or expectation (Box 11-4).
      (4) Alternative methods to lessen anxiety
         (a) Music, singing a favorite song, reading
         (b) Dimmed lights
         (c) Limit numbers of staff interacting with child.
   G. Perianesthesia considerations
     1. Metabolism
       a. Infants have greater nutritional requirements to minimize loss of body protein.
         (1) Develop disturbances more rapidly than adults
         (2) Complications increase proportionately with increase in time of fluid restriction.

■ BOX 11-4
■ **EDUCATION WORKSHEET FOR PARENT/CAREGIVER/LEGAL GUARDIAN ACCOMPANYING THEIR CHILD FOR ANESTHESIA INDUCTION**

The goal of this program is to provide emotional security to children and to prevent psychological trauma during stressful times by allowing a parent to be present for emotional support during the administration of anesthesia.

- Think about what helps your child to relax or cope in stressful situations and how you can help. Quiet talking, singing, counting, holding hands, or lightly touching the child's face is helpful for some children. Some children may cry to relieve tension. This is all right and can be a natural response for some children.
- One parent may be allowed to accompany their child into the operating room/treatment room/radiology room/Pediatric Outpatient Treatment Center anesthesia room/MRI suite, etc.
- Your child may receive medication to help him or her relax before going back to the operating room.
- If you are accompanying your child into the operating room for induction, you will be required to wear scrubs, shoe covers, and a hat and mask because the room is germ free. Everyone walking into the operating room is required to wear this clothing.
- Your child may either walk, be carried by you, ride in a pediatric car or on a hospital bed with wheels to the operating room.
- There will be a bed in the operating room. You may help your child get comfortable. The nurses and anesthesiologists will apply several monitors before your child falls asleep.
- During this time, the parent will have the opportunity to be right next to his or her child, comforting and talking until he or she falls asleep.
- Anesthesia medicine is given either through a mask or into a vein. This will be decided by the anesthesiologist when you meet him or her before the surgery or procedure.
- Falling asleep happens very quickly. Common reactions include the following: Stage I (excitability): arms and legs may move around, eyes may become unfocused and roll around, rapid breathing may occur; Stage 2: child's body appears limp looking. This is a normal and expected part of anesthesia induction.
- The anesthesiologist will let us know when the patient has fallen asleep, and the parent will be accompanied out of the operating room/procedural room and back to the preop/waiting room.

Safety Precautions:
- Touching or handling medical equipment and supplies is strictly prohibited.
- Picking up your child or moving your child during the induction of anesthesia is also strictly prohibited.

From Eaton S, Everson C, Jirava J, et al. Parents influence and advance pediatric policy. *Nurs Adm Q* 30(2):156, 2006.

    b. Infants and small children should have priority on surgery schedule in order to limit food and fluid deprivation to as short a time as possible.
    c. NPO requirements
        (1) May vary according to facility policy/protocol
    d. Thermoregulation (see Chapter 24)
        (1) Heat loss occurs by:
            (a) Evaporation: skin becomes wet; evaporative heat loss can occur.
            (b) Radiation: heat transfers from body surface to surfaces in room not in direct contact with body.
            (c) Conduction: air currents pass over skin.
                (i) May be accentuated by cold diapers and blankets
            (d) Convection: heat loss at a surface caused by fluid flowing across at a lower temperature
        (2) Most common methods for measurement of temperature in infants and children are peripheral and noninvasive.
            (a) Axillary

            (i) Infants and children younger than 4 to 6 years

            (ii) Uncooperative, immunosuppressed, neurologically impaired

            (iii) Patient who has undergone oral surgery

            (iv) Reading is approximately 1 degree lower than the body's core temperature.

      (b) Tympanic

            (i) Infrared radiation emission detector measures thermal radiation emitted from the tympanic membrane and the walls of the auditory external canal.

            (ii) Frequently used for pediatric patients

               [a] Consider alternative method if patient has had ear surgery or ear drops were administered in the OR.

            (iii) Provides quick measurement

            (iv) Preferred route of temperature measurement preoperatively and postoperatively based on survey results

               [a] Proper technique essential to obtain accurate readings

               [b] Pull pinna down and back for younger child and up and back for older child to expose tympanic membrane and ensure that probe is placed fully into auditory canal for most accurate reading.

      (c) Temporal artery

            (i) Infrared sensor probe captures heat from temporal artery blood flow along with ambient temperature and synthesis of the two readings.

            (ii) Well tolerated

            (iii) Provides quick measurement

            (iv) Limited studies providing evidence for its use in pediatric perianesthesia population to date

            (v) Gaining popularity in perianesthesia care based on ease of use, patient tolerance, and anecdotal observations

      (d) Oral

            (i) Children older than 6 years

            (ii) Avoid liquids 30 minutes before oral temperature assessment.

            (iii) Taken in sublingual pocket provides most reliable measure

               [a] May be inaccurate in children who are mouth breathing

      (e) Rectal

            (i) Avoid in patients who are neutropenic, have had rectal surgery or have compromised immune systems.

            (ii) Taken only when no other route is feasible

      (f) Digital

            (i) May be used for oral, axillary, or rectal readings

            (ii) Disposable covers over probe prevent cross-contamination.

    (3) Documentation

      (a) Document method used to obtain reading.

      (b) Provides health care professional with consistent measurement when evaluating fluctuations in temperature

H. Postoperative assessment (see Chapter 50)

  1. Before arrival: pediatric considerations

    a. Oxygen source and suction available with appropriate size self-inflating Ambu bag, masks, suction catheters (Table 11-5)

    b. Prepare bed space with appropriate equipment based on age/size/special needs.

      (1) Age- and size-specific BP cuff(s)

        (a) Based on midpoint limb circumference

        (b) Inappropriate size will cause BP to be artificially elevated or decreased.

TABLE 11-5

Selection of Proper Pediatric Resuscitation Equipment

Color on Brosolow Pediatric Resus Tape	Infant (3-7 kg) Red	Small Child (8-11 kg) Purple	Child (12-14 kg) Yellow	Child (14-17 kg) White	Child (18-22 kg) Blue	Young Adult (24-30 kg) Orange	Young Adult (32-34 kg) Green
Bag valve device	Infant	Child	Child	Child	Child	Child/adult	Adult
O$_2$ mask	Newborn	Pediatric	Pediatric	Pediatric	Pediatric	Adult	Adult
Oral airway	Infant/small child	Small child	Child	Child	Child/small adult	Child/small adult	Medium adult
Laryngoscope blade	0 to 1 straight	1 straight	2 straight or curved	2 straight or curved	2 straight or curved	2 to 3 straight or curved	3 straight or curved
ET tubes	Premie: 2.5-mm uncuffed Term: 3.0-mm uncuffed Infant: 3.5-mm uncuffed	4.0-mm uncuffed	4.5-mm uncuffed	5.0-mm uncuffed	5.5-mm uncuffed	6.0-mm cuffed	6.5-mm cuffed
Suction	8 Fr	8 Fr	8-10 Fr	10 Fr	10 Fr	10 Fr	12 Fr
BP cuff	Newborn to infant	Infant to child	Child	Child	Child	Child to adult	Adult
IV catheter	22-24 G	20-24 G	18-22 G	18-22 G	18-20 G	18-20 G	16-20 G
Nasogastric tube	5-8 Fr	8-10 Fr	10 Fr	10-12 Fr	12-14 Fr	14-18 Fr	18 Fr
Urinary catheter	5-8 Fr	8-10 Fr	10 Fr	10-12 Fr	10-12 Fr	12 Fr	12 Fr

ET, endotracheal; Fr, French; BP, blood pressure; IV, intravenous; G, gauge.
Adapted from Hazinski MF: *Manual of pediatric critical care*, St Louis, 1999, Mosby.

             (2) Cold, wet facecloths, emesis basin, iced saline

             (3) Pillows, padding for siderails, need for quieter or more private area

             (4) Rocking chair at bedside for parents of infants and young children

                 (a) Providing a foot stool and pillow will make holding infant or child more comfortable for parent.

     c. Pre-arrival review of patient chart if possible

             (1) Overview of patient

             (2) Review of physician orders

2. Patient arrival to PACU

     a. Rapid initial assessment with focus on airway, breathing, circulation, and placement on appropriate monitors

     b. Full admission report from anesthesia provider

     c. Admission procedure per facility policy/protocol

             (1) Based on stability of patient

             (2) Developmental needs considered if stable and safe

                 (a) For example, parent visit may be expedited if patient's condition is stable and patient is calling for "Mommy."

     d. Patient-specific additions for anesthesia report

             (1) Birth history, if applicable (e.g., born prematurely, congenital conditions)

             (2) Preoperative behavior

                 (a) Calm and cooperative, anxious, combative

             (3) Developmental considerations

                 (a) Ensure that personal comfort items are securely transferred and available for infant or child upon waking up (e.g., stuffed animal, blanket, religious items).

             (4) Special needs (e.g., hearing aid, glasses, needle phobia)

             (5) Any loose teeth removed may be saved for "tooth fairy."

3. Comprehensive and ongoing assessment

     a. Monitor respiratory rate, heart rate, BP, and oxygen saturation, and document at least every 15 minutes during initial postoperative period.

             (1) Apical pulse rate recommended for infants and children younger than 2 years

             (2) Radial pulse may be used for children older than 2 years.

             (3) Potential to auscultate innocent murmurs

             (4) Compare vital signs with preoperative and intraoperative measurements.

     b. Initial monitoring

             (1) Respiratory rate

             (2) BP

             (3) Pulse oximetry

                 (a) Avoid extremity with BP cuff, IV line, arterial catheter, congenital defect, or operative site.

                 (b) Finger, toe, ear lobe placement most common

                 (c) May be placed on hand or foot in infants

                     (i) Ensure that sensor is placed in an area where the pulse may be tracked reliably (e.g., over site of radial or ulnar arterial distribution in the hand, or of the dorsalis pedis in foot).

             (4) Electrocardiogram

                 (a) Lead placement

                     (i) May place on extremities to decrease artifact from breathing

                     (ii) Do not place leads on bony prominences.

                     (iii) To decrease potential of trauma on fragile ribs, snap leads to electrodes before placing on child.

                     (iv) When leads no longer necessary, prepare child and remove leads gently.

(b) Waveforms
  (i) T waves in infants much larger because electrodes are situated much closer to the heart
  (ii) May be same size as QRS complex
  (iii) Accurate assessment to avoid erroneous or double counting
  (iv) Monitor in lead II for best P-wave configuration.
(5) Temperature control
  (a) Assess temperature.
    (i) Avoid/minimize invasive techniques.
(6) Pain assessment
  (a) Fifth vital sign
  (b) Age-appropriate pain scale
  (c) Special postoperative considerations
    (i) If a patient is unable to use the planned self-report scale during initial postoperative period, document observations rather than pain score (e.g., patient sleeping, restless, grimacing) until the patient is able to self-report.
    (ii) Sleep does not indicate a pain score of "0"; document that child is sleeping, not a zero for pain.
(7) Level of consciousness
  (a) Alert, responsive, cooperative, asleep, unresponsive, agitated
(8) Fluid balance
  (a) Determined based on NPO status, crystalloid and colloid fluids received in the OR, blood loss, weight-based maintenance fluid requirements
  (b) Fluid replacement per anesthesia provider or facility policy/protocol
    (i) Consider underlying conditions (e.g., renal, neurologic, cardiac).
    (ii) Consider procedure/surgery (e.g., tonsillectomy patient may have sore throat).
    (iii) Consider wakefulness, likelihood of drinking, and presence of IV.
  (c) Monitor urine output.
(9) IV fluids
  (a) Infuse IV fluids via an infusion pump.
    (i) Preset volume
    (ii) Hourly rate based on maintenance requirements
    (iii) May be used in conjunction with volume control sets and tubing
      [a] Usually 100- to 150-mL capacity
  (b) Assess IV site per facility policy/protocol.
    (i) Observe and gently palpate in area of IVs to identify signs of phlebitis, infiltration, extravasation, infection early.
      [a] Skin soft or taut, scalp site boggy
      [b] Edema, erythema, pain, blanching, coolness, streaking of skin above vein, leaking
    (ii) If resistance met when flushing:
      [a] Assess patency of catheter.
      [b] Do not forcibly flush.
    (iii) Assess stability of IV site and secure as needed to prevent removal by infant, toddler, or small child.
      [a] Maintain extremity in neutral position.
      [b] Consider protection for site in infants and children who may attempt to remove the IV.
      [c] Secure in manner following facility policy/protocol that preserves circulation and allows easy visibility of site (clear IV dressing, soft armboard, gauze wrap, plastic IV site protectors).

      (10) Patient safety needs
         (a) Infant or child in stretcher, crib, or bed with protection/design that prevent falls
           (i) Ideal for distance between vertical siderails or slats to be narrow enough to prevent patient from slipping through
           (ii) Siderail pads may be used to establish additional protection.
           (iii) Ensure that mattresses are secured to stretchers.
         (b) Assess level of consciousness and protect from injury.
           (i) Responsive, unresponsive, restless, alert, combative
           (ii) Pad siderails if indicated (e.g., history of seizures, combative).
           (iii) Restrain only if necessary per facility policy/protocol.
      (11) Surgical site assessment
         (a) Check dressing if present.
           (i) Note and record quantity and quality of drainage if present.
           (ii) Reinforce if necessary.
           (iii) Inspect areas underneath bed linens to identify potential bleeding sites.
         (b) Assess for bleeding in areas without dressing.
           (i) Throat after tonsillectomy, oral, dental procedures
           (ii) Genitourinary area
      (12) Skin assessment
         (a) Observe for any abnormalities that may not have been present preoperatively (e.g., scratches, bruises, pressure areas).
         (b) Wash antiseptic from skin if present (e.g., Betadine).
      (13) Developmental considerations
         (a) Talk softly to and reassure the disoriented child.
         (b) Communicate in an age-appropriate way to the awake child to prepare the child for interventions before touching him or her.
           (i) For BP: "You'll feel a firm hug on your arm, then it will go away."
         (c) Bundle hands on care to minimize disturbances to patient while completing necessary assessments.
      (14) Accommodate and include family member(s) at bedside as soon as safely manageable per patient needs and facility policy/protocol.
  4. Complications (see Chapter 28)
  5. Airway/respiratory
    a. Airway problems are most common upon emergence and in immediate postoperative period.
    b. Risk factors for adverse outcomes (e.g., breath holding and major desaturation, in children with active or recent upper respiratory infections) include:
      (1) Tracheal intubation for children younger than 5 years
      (2) History of prematurity
      (3) Reactive airway disease
      (4) Parents that smoke
      (5) Airway surgery
      (6) Nasal congestion and copious secretions
    c. Observe for signs of respiratory distress (Box 11-5).
      (1) Increased respiratory rate
         (a) Response to respiratory distress is an increase in respiratory rate.
         (b) Tachypnea is often the first sign of respiratory distress in infant.
      (2) Oxygen desaturation
      (3) Increased heart rate one of first signs
      (4) Nasal flaring
         (a) Significant finding in infant
      (5) Retractions, use of accessory muscles, increased work of breathing, cyanosis

■ BOX 11-5
■ SIGNS OF RESPIRATORY DISTRESS AND POTENTIAL RESPIRATORY FAILURE

Tachypnea, tachycardia
Retractions
Nasal flaring
Grunting
Stridor or wheezing
Mottled color
Change in responsiveness
Hypoxemia, hypercarbia, decreased Hemoglobin saturations
Late: Poor air entry, weak cry
   Apnea or gasping
   Deterioration in systemic perfusion
   Bradycardia

From Hazinski MF: *Manual of pediatric critical care,* St Louis, 1999, Mosby.

       (6) Apnea
         (a) Lack of respirations for more than 15 to 20 seconds or associated with bradycardia, cyanosis, or pallor
         (b) More common in infants with a history of apnea
         (c) Infrequent after 44 weeks postconceptual age
           (i) Recommend to admit and monitor former premature infants of less than 44 to 46 weeks postconceptual age overnight after general anesthesia.
             [a] Based on evaluation by surgeon and anesthesiologist and facility policy/protocol on case by case basis
       (7) Head bobbing in an infant
       (8) Grunting
         (a) May also be sign of pain in older children
       (9) Shallow, slow, ineffective respirations
      (10) Wheezing
      (11) Stridor
   d. Respiratory dysfunction
      (1) Causes
         (a) Excess fluid volume
         (b) Pain
         (c) Hypothermia or hyperthermia
         (d) Residual effects of anesthetic agents
         (e) Narcotic, barbiturate, sedative administration
         (f) Preexisting pulmonary disease
      (2) Nursing interventions
         (a) Stimulate patient.
         (b) Encourage coughing and deep breathing.
         (c) Crying in infants and younger children fosters airway clearance.
         (d) Reposition airway (e.g., neck roll, chin lift, or jaw thrust)
         (e) Administer oxygen.
           (i) Blow-by tolerated best when responsive
             [a] End of oxygen hose may be wrapped in a towel to provide mist near patient's nose and mouth.
         (f) Notify anesthesiologist.
         (g) Insertion of oral or nasal airway may be considered if unresponsive.
           (i) Follow facility policy/protocol (e.g., oral or nasal surgery patients).

(h) Suction if needed
(i) Be prepared for endotracheal intubation.
(j) Airway obstruction
  (i) Causes
    [a] Tongue
    [b] Soft tissue edema
    [c] Retained packs, sponges
    [d] Secretions
  (ii) Signs and symptoms
    [a] Snoring
    [b] Use of accessory muscles
    [c] Nasal flaring
    [d] Abdominal, diaphragmatic contractions
    [e] Decrease in inhaled air
    [f] Gurgling indicates secretions.
  (iii) Nursing interventions:
    [a] Reposition airway (e.g., chin lift or jaw thrust maneuver, position on side, place in "sniffing" position).
    [b] Administer oxygen.
    [c] Suction
    [d] Notify anesthesiologist.
    [e] Be prepared to insert oral or nasal airway.

e. Stridor
  (1) Definition: a high-pitched sound produced by turbulent airflow through a narrowed segment of the upper airway
  (2) Causes
    (a) Tracheal irritation and edema
  (3) Signs and symptoms
    (a) Crowing respirations
    (b) Shrill, harsh sound
    (c) Heard during inspiration, expiration, or both
      (i) Inspiratory indicates tracheal, laryngeal, or pharyngeal obstruction
      (ii) Expiratory indicates tracheal or bronchial obstruction
      (iii) Biphasic suggests glottic or subglottic obstruction
  (4) Nursing interventions
    (a) Provide calm reassurance.
    (b) Administer cool humidified mist/oxygen.
    (c) Elevate head of bed.
    (d) Notify anesthesiologist, surgeon if indicated.
    (e) Physician may order racemic epinephrine nebulizer treatment.
      (i) Associated with rebound effect
        [a] Within 2 hours edema may resume and worsen.
        [b] Observe patient for up to 4 hours per facility policy/protocol.
      (ii) Dosing guideline
        [a] Younger than 2 years: 0.25 mL of a 2.25% solution in 2.5 mL of normal saline
        [b] Older than 2 years: 0.5 mL of a 2.25% solution in 2.5 mL of normal saline
      (iii) Follow facility policy/protocol for further monitoring.
      (iv) Consider admission if indicated.
    (f) Physician may order corticosteroids (e.g., dexamethasone 0.5 to 1 mg/kg IV, maximum 16-20 mg).
      (i) To lessen laryngeal inflammation
      (ii) Use remains controversial

    f. Croup
      (1) Definition: a group of conditions involving inflammation of the upper airway
        (a) Postintubation croup common in children
          (i) More common in presence of upper respiratory infection
          (ii) Usually occurs within 1 hour after extubation
          (iii) May intensify within 4 hours
          (iv) Completely resolved in 24 hours
          (v) Increased incidence in children from 1 to 4 years old
            [a] Small laryngeal lumen
      (2) Causes
        (a) Traumatic, prolonged, or repeated intubations
          (i) Tight-fitting ETT
          (ii) Subglottic injury and edema
        (b) Coughing with ETT in place
        (c) Change of patient position while intubated
        (d) Surgical procedure greater than 1 hour in duration
        (e) Surgical trauma
      (3) Signs and symptoms
        (a) Barklike cough
          (i) May or may not be accompanied by stridor
        (b) Hoarseness
        (c) Varying degrees of respiratory distress
      (4) Nursing interventions
        (a) Similar to treatment for bronchospasm
    g. Laryngospasm
      (1) Definition: involuntary muscle contraction of the laryngeal muscles causes the vocal cords to close.
      (2) Causes
        (a) Preexisting irritable airway
        (b) Inadequate depth of anesthesia with sensory stimulation
        (c) Secretions or blood on vocal cords
        (d) Manipulation of the airway
        (e) Irritation from the ETT or oral airway
        (f) Surgical stimulation
        (g) Excessive or aggressive suctioning
        (h) Irritant trigger (e.g., anesthetic gases)
      (3) Signs and symptoms
        (a) Dyspnea
        (b) Crowing sound on inspiration
        (c) Rocking motion of chest indicating use of accessory muscles
        (d) Aphonia (no sound)
      (4) Nursing interventions
        (a) Administer humidified 100% oxygen.
        (b) Continuous positive pressure by mask maintaining end-expiratory pressure to open vocal cords
        (c) Oropharyngeal suctioning if secretions present
        (d) Notify anesthesiologist.
          (i) Airway and ventilatory support
          (ii) Be prepared for intubation.
        (e) May administer muscle relaxants (e.g., succinylcholine)
    h. Bronchospasm
      (1) Definition: sudden constriction of the muscles in the walls of the bronchioles
      (2) Causes
        (a) Preexisting airway disease (asthma)
        (b) Allergy, anaphylaxis
        (c) Histamine release

     (d) Aspiration

     (e) Mucous plug

     (f) Foreign body

     (g) Pulmonary edema

    (3) Signs and symptoms

     (a) High-pitched wheezing, inspiratory and expiratory

     (b) Coarse rales

     (c) Increased respiratory rate

     (d) May have mild, moderate, or severe dyspnea

     (e) Intercostal retractions

    (4) Nursing interventions

     (a) Administer oxygen.

     (b) Suction secretions.

     (c) Notify anesthesiologist.

     (d) Administer bronchodilators as ordered.

      (i) Albuterol 0.15 mg/kg in 2 mL normal saline solution nebulized

     (e) Support ventilation; reintubation as indicated.

     (f) Consider overnight admission or longer stay to observe after treatment.

  i. Aspiration

   (1) Definition: inhalation of gastric or oropharyngeal contents that may cause irritation to trachea or bronchi

   (2) Causes

    (a) Residual gastric volume

    (b) Inability to protect airway

    (c) Inhalation of foreign body (e.g., loose tooth)

   (3) Signs and symptoms

    (a) Tachypnea

    (b) Dyspnea

    (c) Bronchospasm

    (d) Cyanosis

    (e) Shock

    (f) Pulmonary edema

   (4) Interventions

    (a) Position with head down and turned to side to promote drainage.

    (b) Administer humidified oxygen via face mask.

    (c) Suction as needed (prn).

    (d) Notify anesthesiologist.

    (e) Chest x-ray to document

    (f) Be prepared to reintubate if necessary.

 6. Circulation (Box 11-6)

  a. Bradycardia

■ BOX 11-6
■ **SIGNS OF POOR SYSTEMIC PERFUSION**

Tachycardia
Mottled color, pallor
Cool skin, prolonged capillary refill
Oliguria (urine volume <1-2 mL/kg/h)
Diminished intensity of peripheral pulses
Metabolic acidosis
Change in responsiveness
Late: Hypotension, bradycardia

From Hazinski MF: *Manual of pediatric critical care,* St Louis, 1999, Mosby.

      (1) Sign of decompensation in infants and younger children
      (2) Causes
         (a) Respiratory distress (late sign)
         (b) Hypoxia
         (c) Vagal response
         (d) Increased intracranial pressure
         (e) Administration of morphine, neostigmine
  b. Tachycardia
      (1) Causes
         (a) Elevated temperature
         (b) Pain
         (c) Hypovolemia
         (d) Early respiratory distress
         (e) Medications (e.g., atropine, glycopyrrolate, epinephrine, ketamine)
         (f) Decreased perfusion caused by impending shock
      (2) Normal method of increasing cardiac output
  c. Hypertension
      (1) Causes
         (a) Excess intravascular fluid
         (b) Carbon dioxide retention
         (c) Pain
         (d) Increased intracranial pressure
         (e) Medications (e.g., ketamine, epinephrine)
  d. Hypotension
      (1) Causes
         (a) Anesthetic agents
         (b) Opioids (e.g., morphine)
         (c) Sedatives
         (d) Hypovolemia
         (e) Late sign of shock
7. Fluid and electrolyte balance
  a. Infants and young children more vulnerable to changes (Box 11-7)
      (1) Hypovolemia (fluid volume deficit)
         (a) Due to decrease in fluid intake, fluid loss, blood loss
         (b) Results in electrolyte imbalance
         (c) Causes cellular dysfunction
         (d) May result in hypovolemic shock and death
         (e) Signs and symptoms
            (i) Negative fluid balance
               [a] May be misleading in instances of sequestration of interstitial fluid
            (ii) Concentrated, amber urine
            (iii) Flushed dry skin, dry furrowed tongue, cool extremities, thirst
            (iv) Vital signs
                [a] Tachycardia
                [b] Decreased BP
                [c] Narrow pulse pressure
                [d] Sluggish capillary refill
                [e] Peripheral vasoconstriction
                [f] May be irritable, lethargic, confused; infant cry may be high pitched and weak
         (f) Interventions
            (i) Assess fluid balance.
            (ii) Correct imbalance.
            (iii) Treat underlying cause.
            (iv) Treatment is based on maintenance fluid requirements (Box 11-8).

■ BOX 11-7
■ **PEDIATRIC DIFFERENCES RELATED TO FLUID AND ELECTROLYTE BALANCE**

Infants
- Because of the higher percentage of water in the extracellular fluid (ECF), infants can lose fluids equal to their ECF within 2 to 3 days.
- Infants are less able to concentrate urine because of immature renal function.
- Infants have a higher rate of peristalsis than older children.
- Infants have an immature lower esophageal sphincter, making them more prone to gastroesophageal reflux, which can lead to dehydration and electrolyte disturbances.
- Infants have a harder time compensating for acidosis because of their decreased ability to acidify urine.

Infants and Young Children
- Infants and young children have a higher metabolic turnover of water relative to adults because of a higher metabolic rate. (If losses are not replaced rapidly, imbalance occurs.)
- Infants and young children are unable to verbalize or communicate thirst.

Infants and Children
- In comparison with adults, infants and children have a proportionately greater body surface area in relation to body mass, resulting in a greater potential for fluid loss via the skin and gastrointestinal tract.
- Infants and children have a higher proportionate water content (premature infants have 90%, full-term infants 75% to 80%, preschool children 60% to 65%, and adolescents and adults approximately 55% to 60%), with a larger proportion of fluid in the extracellular space.
- The immune system of infants and children is not as robust as an adult's immune system, rendering young children more susceptible to infectious diseases, fever, gastroenteritis, and respiratory infections, all of which can result in fluid and electrolyte disturbances and fluid-volume deficit.
- Infants and children are at higher risk because of increased exposure to infections in a day care or nursery setting.

From James SR, Ashwill JW, Droske SC: *Nursing care of children*, ed 2, Philadelphia, 2002, WB Saunders.

■ BOX 11-8
■ **MAINTENANCE FLUID REQUIREMENTS AND MINIMUM URINE OUTPUT**

Daily Fluid Requirements by Body Weight
- ≤10 kg: 100 mL/kg
- 10-20 kg: 1000 mL ± 50 mL/kg for each additional kilogram between 10 and 20 kg
- 20 kg: 1500 mL ± 20 mL/kg for each additional kilogram over 20 kg

Minimum Urine Output by Age/Group
- Infants and toddlers: >2-3 mL/kg/h
- Preschoolers and young school-age children: >1-2 mL/kg/h
- School-age children and adolescents: 0.5-1 mL/kg/h

From James SR, Ashwill JW, Droske SC: *Nursing care of children,* ed 2, Philadelphia, 2002, WB Saunders.

(2) Hypervolemia (fluid volume excess)
    (a) Infants and toddlers at increased risk
    (b) Excessive IV fluid administration
    (c) Increase in antidiuretic hormone and aldosterone being produced in response to stress of surgery
    (d) Signs and symptoms
        (i)   Headache
        (ii) Behavior changes such as restlessness, agitation
        (iii) Tachycardia, hypertension

(iv) Tachypnea, dyspnea
  [a] Grunting respirations
  [b] Adventitious lung sounds
(v) Periorbital edema
  [a] May be more prominent on dependent side (side child is lying on)
(e) Interventions
  (i) Notify physician and adjust IV fluids as ordered.
  (ii) Monitor intake and output.
  (iii) Note periorbital edema and report to physician.
(3) Disturbances in acid-base balance (see Chapter 21)
8. Hypothermia (see Chapter 24)
  a. Occurs rapidly in child because of:
    (1) High ratio of body surface area to weight
      (a) Greatest loss occurs from exposed head.
    (2) Decreased mass
    (3) Lack of insulating subcutaneous fat
    (4) Immature temperature-regulating mechanism in infants
      (a) May exhibit mottling
  b. Potential causes of hypothermia
    (1) Vasodilating anesthetic agents (e.g., halothane, isoflurane, enflurane)
    (2) Muscle relaxants
    (3) Environmental causes (e.g., cool environment of OR, transport to PACU)
    (4) Administration of cool IV fluids
  c. Danger to small child
    (1) Increased oxygen consumption
    (2) Increased vasoconstriction
      (a) Results in hypoxemia, hypoglycemia, and metabolic acidosis
      (b) Depletes metabolic energy stores
      (c) Causes fluid and electrolyte imbalance
  d. Assessment
    (1) Core temperature less than 36° C (96.8° F)
    (2) May observe shivering, peripheral vasoconstriction, and piloerection
      (a) Neonatal shivering not determined to correlate with thermoregulation
    (3) Monitor temperature every half hour until normothermic (36° C to 38° C [96.8° F to 100.4° F]).
  e. Interventions
    (1) Maintain warm room temperature.
    (2) Apply warmed blankets.
      (a) Consider wrapping head in warm blanket.
    (3) Apply slipper socks.
    (4) Use forced air warming devices as indicated.
    (5) Use radiant heat lamps as indicated.
    (6) Special considerations for infants
      (a) Cover head with cap and apply booties to feet.
      (b) Swaddle in warm blankets, maintaining optimal accessibility to IV site(s) and dressing(s).
      (c) Hold close to body for benefit of body heat.
      (d) If severe hypothermia, consider infant incubator or warmer.
9. Hyperthermia (a core temperature >38° C [100.4° F])
  a. Causes
    (1) Fever
    (2) Dehydration
    (3) Infection
    (4) Environmental causes (e.g., warm operating room)
    (5) Overwarming in operating room, excessive drapes

        (6) Medications that disturb temperature regulation such as general anesthetics (e.g., malignant hyperthermia)
- **b.** Assessment
  - (1) Warm, flushed skin
  - (2) Tachycardia
  - (3) Increased respiratory rate
  - (4) Diaphoresis
- **c.** Interventions
  - (1) Notify physician.
  - (2) Administer antipyretic as directed.
  - (3) Expose skin to air.
  - (4) Reduce room temperature.
  - (5) Apply cool, wet compresses.
  - (6) If severe, apply ice packs to groin and axillary area.
- **10.** Nonrespiratory complications (see Chapter 28)
  - **a.** PONV
    - (1) Risk factors in children
      - (a) Surgery length greater than 30 minutes
      - (b) Otorhinolaryngologic, ophthalmologic, testicular, dental surgery
      - (c) Age 3 years or older
      - (d) May be associated with motion sickness
      - (e) History of PONV in mother, father, or siblings
    - (2) Positive correlation between number of risk factors and incidence of PONV
      - (a) With all above risk factors, incidence as high as 70%
  - **b.** Postoperative agitation
    - (1) Agitated behavior in the postoperative patient may indicate:
      - (a) Pain
        - (i) Incidence similar for painful and nonpainful procedures
      - (b) Emergence delirium
        - (i) Characterized by state of excitement upon emergence from general anesthesia
        - (ii) Highest incidence within first 10 minutes of PACU arrival
        - (iii) Incidence as high as up to 13% upon PACU admission
        - (iv) Dissociative state, child amnesic
        - (v) May last less than 10 minutes up to 45 minutes
        - (vi) Increased risk in otorhinolaryngologic and ophthalmologic populations
        - (vii) Associated with certain anesthetic agents such as sevoflurane, desflurane, isoflurane, or halothane
      - (c) Physiologic causes (e.g., hypoxemia, hypercarbia, hypovolemia)
        - (i) Must be considered although may be rare and difficult to differentiate
      - (d) Anxiety
    - (2) Assessment
      - (a) Consider physiologic causes.
      - (b) Evaluate the expected painfulness of a condition/procedure/ surgery.
        - (i) Pain can be ruled out as cause if patient is emerging from anesthesia after a non-painful procedure.
        - (ii) Most reliable way to differentiate emergence delirium from pain-related agitation after non-painful procedure
      - (c) Expression of distress symptoms is similar whether due to pain or emergence delirium.
      - (d) Challenge in identifying cause may interfere with provision of timely and optimal treatment.

(3) Signs and symptoms
  (a) Severe restlessness
  (b) Combativeness
  (c) Crying, screaming, moaning
  (d) Kicking, flailing, non-purposeful movements
  (e) Disorientation, incoherence, unresponsiveness
(4) Adverse effects
  (a) Increased bleeding
  (b) Accidental removal of tubes and IV lines
  (c) Injury to care providers (e.g., nurses, unlicensed assistive personnel)
(5) Interventions via simultaneous, multifaceted and collaborative team approach
  (a) Protect from injury.
    (i) If small child, may hold
    (ii) Surround with pillows, pad siderails.
    (iii) Gently prevent extremities from flailing to avoid patient or caregiver injury.
  (b) Initiate appropriate treatment for physiologic causes.
  (c) Reunite with parent(s) as soon as possible.
    (i) May correlate with shorter period of agitation
    (ii) Provide information about emergence delirium and how the child will appear and behave.
    (iii) Provide support to parent(s).
      [a] Provide reassurance that postoperative agitation is not uncommon.
      [b] Provide information about expected outcome that patient will fall asleep and wake up calmly with no memory of episode.
  (d) Assess need for medication for pain or anxiety.
    (i) Children will fall asleep on own or with medication and upon waking will be calm and not recall incident.
  (e) Provide comfort measures.
  (f) Postanesthesia agitation algorithm may support decision-making (Figure 11-2).
c. Malignant hyperthermia
  (1) Rare, genetic, autosomal dominant, life threatening
  (2) Predisposing conditions
    (a) Young athletic males most at risk
    (b) Occurs more often in children
    (c) Individuals with myopathies and musculoskeletal disorders
  (3) Incidence in children is 1 in 15,000.
  (4) Mean age of occurrence is 15 years.
    (a) Cases have occurred in infant population.
  (5) Most cases occur during onset or within 1 hour of general anesthesia.
    (a) Delayed onset has been reported.
  (6) Signs and symptoms
    (a) Unexplained and progressive tachycardia
      (i) Consistent and early indicator
    (b) Increased end-tidal carbon dioxide
    (c) Tachypnea in spontaneously breathing patient
    (d) Masseter muscle rigidity
      (i) Affects 1% of pediatric surgical patients after induction with halothane and succinylcholine
        [a] Routine use of succinylcholine in children is contraindicated.
      (ii) Be alert to report of masseter muscle spasm or limited jaw opening upon intubation.

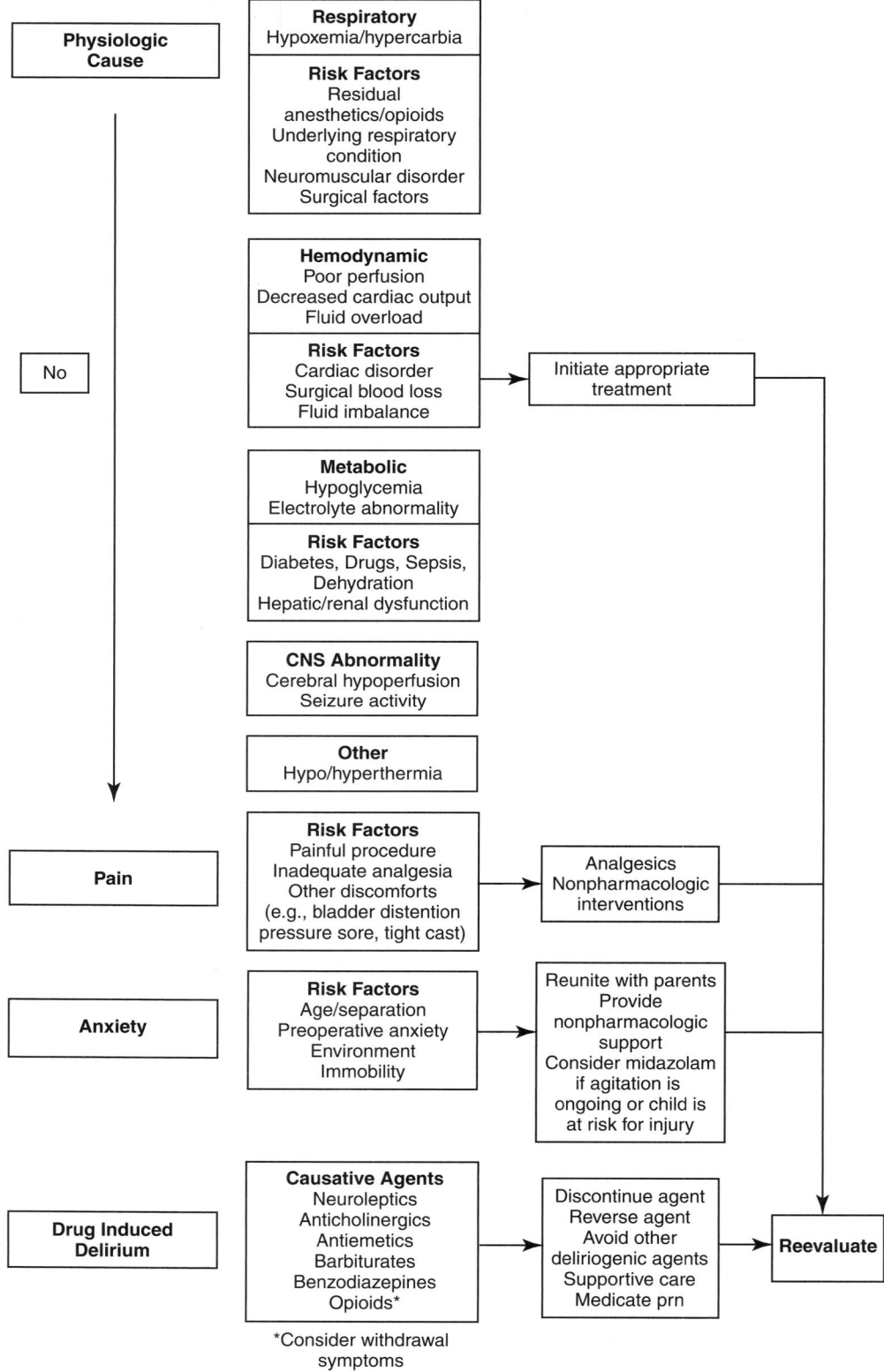

FIGURE 11-2 ■ Postoperative agitation algorithm. (Modified from Voepel-Lewis T, Burke C, Hadden SM, et al: Nurses' diagnoses and treatment decisions regarding care of the agitated child. *J Perianesth Nurs* 20(4):245, 2005.)

(e) Evidence of temperature increase may or may not occur.
  (i) Maximum temperature reached correlates with mortality rate due to damage to internal organs.
(7) Interventions
  (a) Most successful when treated promptly by quickly assembled team
    (i) Immediate administration of dantrolene sodium
      [a] Initial bolus is 2 to 3 mg/kg (suggested dose).
      [b] Repeat every 5 to 10 minutes until symptoms under control.
      [c] Total dose may reach 10 mg/kg or more.
    (ii) Administer 100% oxygen.
    (iii) Aggressive cooling measures (e.g., cooling blankets, ice packs)
    (iv) Obtain bloodwork as ordered, and treat underlying electrolyte or acid-base imbalances.
  (b) Provide education to family regarding patient's condition.
    (i) At appropriate time, family will need to be educated regarding the importance of testing for family members.
(8) Diagnosis
  (a) Caffeine halothane contracture test
    (i) Children must weigh greater than 20 kg.
11. Pain assessment (see Chapter 26)
  a. McCaffery defines pain as: "whatever the experiencing person says it is, existing whenever he says it does."
  b. Pain in children has historically been undertreated.
    (1) Children who are younger, nonverbal, combative, or agitated are more at risk.
  c. If unrelieved, can worsen respiratory complications
  d. Common causes of unrelieved pain and unnecessary suffering
    (1) Failure to ask patient about their pain
    (2) Failure to accept and act on reports of pain
    (3) Fear of opioid-induced respiratory depression in pediatric patients
  e. Misconceptions (Box 11-9)
12. Assessment of pain
  a. Assess according to developmental level (Box 11-10).
  b. Age-appropriate assessment tools provide means for:
    (1) Child to communicate about pain
    (2) Health care provider to communicate about pain to advocate for child and to determine effectiveness of interventions
  c. Take into account pain at rest (static pain) and pain on activity (dynamic pain).
  d. Use the following hierarchy to assess pain in children:
    (1) Patient's self-report
      (a) Self-report of pain is the gold standard for pain assessment, when possible.
        (i) Single most reliable indicator of pain
        (ii) Children as young as 3 years are able to rate pain intensity with an appropriate pain scale.
    (2) Knowledge of presence of pathology or condition associated with pain
    (3) Behavioral indicators of pain
    (4) Parent proxy rating
      (a) Consider with caution.
        (i) May be fearful of safety of narcotics
        (ii) Unfamiliar with postanesthesia emergence
        (iii) May underestimate or overestimate pain on day of surgery
    (5) Physiologic indicators of pain
      (a) Elevated vital signs are least sensitive and specific indicators of pain.
        (i) May be associated with hypovolemia, anxiety, oxygen desaturation
      (b) Absence of increased heart rate or BP should not be considered to indicate absence of pain.

■ BOX 11-9
■ **MISCONCEPTIONS ABOUT PAIN IN INFANTS AND CHILDREN**

Fallacy	Fact
Neonates and infants are incapable of feeling pain.	All infants, including neonates and preterm infants, have the ability to feel pain.
Infants are not as sensitive to pain.	Anything that causes pain in adults also causes pain in infants. Some things that do not cause pain in adults may cause pain in infants.
Neonates and infants cannot express pain.	Infants respond to pain with a variety of physiological and behavioral indicators. Lack of response does not mean lack of pain.
Assessment of pain is inaccurate and unreliable with neonates and infants and is questionable in the nonverbal toddler.	Pain must be assessed with the use of multiple indicators, with special attention when indicators change. Ongoing open communication must take place between staff and parents about infant's pain so that accurate assessments and insights will occur.
Neonates and infants are incapable of remembering pain.	Neonates and infants experiencing long-term pain, repeated pain, and/or the stress of traumatic repeated procedures show an increase in depression, insomnia, change in feeding patterns, and impaired coping responses.
Opioid analgesics and anesthetics cannot be safely given to neonates and infants because of their immature capacity to metabolize and eliminate drugs and their sensitivity to opioid-induced respiratory depression.	The appropriate opioid dose is the amount of opioid that controls pain with the fewest adverse effects. By 3 to 6 months of age, healthy infants can metabolize opioids similarly to other children.
Fear of addiction.	Narcotics are no more dangerous for children than they are for adults. Addiction to opioids used to treat pain is extremely rare in children.

From Ireland D: Overview for pediatric pain management. In Krenzischek DA, Wilson L, eds: *ASPAN pain and comfort resource manual*, Cherry Hill, NJ, 2004, ASPAN.

13. Developmental considerations
    a. Infant
        (1) Stores memories of acute pain, resulting in greater behavioral responses to subsequent episodes of pain
        (2) Older infants may react intensely with physical resistance.
            (a) Refuse to lie still
            (b) Attempt to push health care provider away
            (c) Try to escape
        (3) Distraction is of little benefit.
        (4) Physiologic indicators of pain
            (a) Increased heart rate, respiratory rate, and BP
            (b) Palmar sweating
            (c) Autonomic changes
                (i) Skin color
                (ii) Nausea/vomiting
                (iii) Gagging
                (iv) Hiccupping
                (v) Diaphoresis
                (vi) Dilated pupils

■ BOX 11-10
■ **PAIN ASSESSMENT ACCORDING TO DEVELOPMENTAL LEVEL**

Neonate and Infant
- Changes in facial expression, including frowns, grimaces, wrinkled brow, expression of surprise, and facial flinching
- Increases in blood pressure and heart rate and decrease in arterial saturation
- High-pitched, tense, harsh crying
- Generalized or total body response in neonate and young infant that becomes more purposeful as the infant matures
- May thrash extremities; may exhibit tremors
- Older infants: rub painful area, pull away, or guard the involved part

Toddler
- Loud crying
- Verbalizes words that indicate discomfort ("ouch," "hurt," "boo boo")
- Attempts to delay procedures perceived as painful
- Generalized restlessness
- Guards the site
- Touches painful areas
- May run from the nurse

Preschooler
- May think the pain is punishment for some deed or thought
- Crying, kicking
- Describe the location and intensity of pain (e.g., "ear hurts bad")
- Regression to earlier behaviors (e.g., loss of bladder and bowel control)
- Withdrawal
- Denies pain to avoid a possible injection
- May have been told to "be brave" and deny pain even though it is present

School-age Child
- Able to describe pain and quantify pain intensity
- Fears bodily harm
- Has an awareness of death
- Stiff body posture
- Withdrawal
- Procrastinates or bargains to delay procedure

Adolescent
- Perceives pain at a physical, emotional, and mental level
- Understands cause and effect
- Describes pain and quantifies pain intensity
- Increased muscle tension
- Withdrawal and decreased motor activity
- Uses words such as "sore," "ache," or "pounding" to describe pain

From James SR, Ashwill JW, Droske SC: *Nursing care of children*, ed 2, Philadelphia, 2002, WB Saunders.

(d) Responses due to activation of the sympathetic nervous system
  (i) Not sustainable over time
(e) Must be assessed in combination with other contextual and behavioral indicators
(5) Behavioral indicators
  (a) Facial expression
    (i) Most consistent indicator of pain in an infant
    (ii) Typical expression

                    [a] Bulging brow and forehead

                    [b] Eyes squeezed tightly shut

                    [c] Cheeks raised to form a nasolabial furrow

                    [d] Mouth opened and stretched both vertically and horizontally

        (b) Cry

             (i) Typical pain cry is high pitched, tense, harsh, short, sharp, and loud.

             (ii) Absence of cry cannot be interpreted as absence of pain.

                  [a] Silent cry in intubated infant

                  [b] Premature infant may be conserving energy.

        (c) Gross motor movement

        (d) Flexor reflex threshold

        (e) Changes in behavioral state and functions

             (i) Eating patterns

             (ii) Sleeping patterns

  b. Toddler

    (1) Reacts intensely to actual or perceived painful experiences

    (2) Behavioral indicators of pain

        (a) Grimacing

        (b) Clenching teeth or lips

        (c) Opening eyes wide

        (d) Rocking, rubbing

        (e) Aggressiveness

        (f) Running away

        (g) Overactive and restless

  c. Preschooler

    (1) May be able to verbalize pain

    (2) May be able to use pain assessment tools

    (3) Will relate a negative experience with one caregiver to similar caregivers

    (4) Behavioral indicators of pain

        (a) Crying

        (b) Restlessness

        (c) Whimpering

        (d) Active resistance

        (e) Screaming

  d. School-age child

    (1) Able to communicate about pain and its location, intensity, and description

    (2) Less active resistance to pain

    (3) Crying or pulling away may be embarrassing.

    (4) Behavioral indicators of pain

        (a) Surface composure may mask pain.

        (b) Hold rigidly still, clench teeth or fists

        (c) Try to act brave

        (d) Nonverbal cues

             (i) Serious facial expression

             (ii) Silence

             (iii) Lack of activity

14. Examples of pain assessment methods

  a. Behavioral pain assessment tool

    (1) FLACC Behavioral Pain Scale (Table 11-6)

        (a) Acronym stands for face, legs, activity, cry, consolability.

        (b) Child rated from 0 to 2 in each of the above five categories

        (c) Score ranges from 0 to 10.

        (d) Useful for measuring pain/distress in infants and children up to 7 years

■ TABLE 11-6
■ ■ **FLACC Pain Assessment Tool**

	0	1	2
Face	No particular expression or smile	Occasional grimace or frown, withdrawn, disinterested	Frequent to constant frown, clenched jaw, quivering chin
Legs	Normal position or relaxed	Uneasy, restless, tense	Kicking or legs drawn up
Activity	Lying quietly, normal position, moves easily	Squirming, shifting back and forth, tense	Arched, rigid or jerking
Cry	No cry (awake or asleep)	Moans or whimpers, occasional complaint	Crying steadily, screams or sobs, frequent complaints
Consolability	Content, relaxed	Reassured by touching, hugging, talking	Difficult to console or comfort

Each of the five categories (F) Face; (L) Legs; (A) Activity; (C) Cry; (C) Consolability is scored from 0-2, which results in a total score between zero and ten.
From *Pediatr Nurs* 23(3):294, 1997. With permission of Jannetti Publications, Inc.
Merkel S, Voepel-Lewis T, Shayevitz J, et al: The FLACC: a behavioral scale for scoring postoperative pain in young children. *Ped Nurs 23* (3):294, 1997.

    b. Self-report
        (1) FACES Pain Rating Scale (Figure 11-3)
            (a) For children as young as 3 years
            (b) Consists of drawings or pictures of faces ranging from smiling to crying
        (2) Ask child to answer yes or no or to squeeze eyes shut to questions about pain.
            (a) For children unable to use a scale, or who can't move or speak
        (3) Numerical Pain Intensity Scale (Figure 11-4)
            (a) For 0 to 10 scale, patient indicates pain score along a line with numbers 0 to 10, with 0 meaning no pain and 10 meaning the worst possible pain.
            (b) Patient may be asked to provide 0 to 10 pain score verbally.
    c. Tools for cognitively impaired children
        (1) Non-communicating Children's Pain Checklist—Postoperative Version (Figure 11-5)

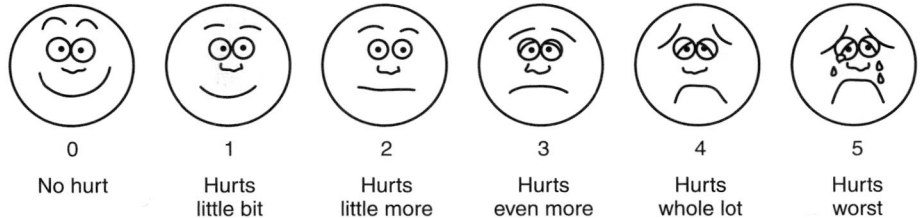

0	1	2	3	4	5
No hurt	Hurts little bit	Hurts little more	Hurts even more	Hurts whole lot	Hurts worst

FIGURE 11-3 ■ FACES Pain Rating Scale. (From Hockenberry MJ, Wilson D, Winkelstein ML: *Wong's essentials of pediatric nursing*, ed 8, St Louis, 2009, Mosby. Used with permission.)

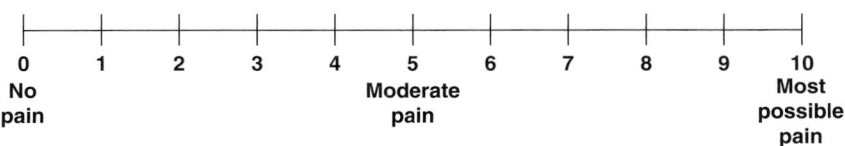

FIGURE 11-4 ■ 0 to 10 Numerical Pain Intensity Scale. (Agency for Healthcare Research and Quality.)

Non-Communicating Children's Pain Checklist—Postoperative Version (NCCPC-PV)

Name: _____ Unit/file #: _____ Date: _____ (dd/mm/yy)

Observer: _____ Start time: _____ AM/PM Stop time: _____ AM/PM

How often has this child shown these behaviors in the last 10 minutes? Please circle a number for each behavior. If an item does not apply to this child (for example, this child cannot reach with his/her hands), then indicate "not applicable" for that item.

I. Vocal

1. Moaning, whining, whimpering (fairly soft)	0	1	2	3 NA
2. Crying (moderately loud)	0	1	2	3 NA
3. Screaming/yelling (very loud)	0	1	2	3 NA
4. A specific sound or word for pain (e.g., a word, cry, or type of laugh)	0	1	2	3 NA

II. Social

5. Not cooperating, cranky, irritable, unhappy	0	1	2	3 NA
6. Less interaction with others, withdrawn	0	1	2	3 NA
7. Seeking comfort or physical closeness	0	1	2	3 NA
8. Being difficult to distract, not able to satisfy or pacify	0	1	2	3 NA

III. Facial

9. A furrowed brow	0	1	2	3 NA
10. A change in eyes, including: squinching of eyes, eyes opened wide, eyes frowning	0	1	2	3 NA
11. Turning down of mouth, not smiling	0	1	2	3 NA
12. Lips puckering up, tight, pouting, or quivering	0	1	2	3 NA
13. Clenching or grinding teeth, chewing, or thrusting tongue out	0	1	2	3 NA

IV. Activity

14. Not moving, less active, quiet	0	1	2	3 NA
15. Jumping around, agitated, fidgety	0	1	2	3 NA

V. Body and Limbs

16. Floppy	0	1	2	3 NA
17. Stiff, spastic, tense, rigid	0	1	2	3 NA
18. Gesturing to or touching part of the body that hurts	0	1	2	3 NA
19. Protecting, favoring or guarding part of the body that hurts	0	1	2	3 NA
20. Flinching or moving the body part away, being sensitive to touch	0	1	2	3 NA
21. Moving the body in a specific way to show pain (e.g., head back, arms down, curls up, etc.)	0	1	2	3 NA

VI. Physiological

22. Shivering	0	1	2	3 NA
23. Change in color, pallor	0	1	2	3 NA
24. Sweating, perspiring	0	1	2	3 NA
25. Tears	0	1	2	3 NA
26. Sharp intake of breath, gasping	0	1	2	3 NA
27. Breath holding	0	1	2	3 NA

SCORE SUMMARY

Score							

FIGURE 11-5 ■ Non-communicating Children's Pain Checklist—Postoperative Version (NCCPC-PV). (From Hockenberry MJ, Wilson D, eds: *Wong's nursing care of infants and children*, ed 8, St Louis, 2007, Mosby.)

USING THE NCCPC-PV

The NCCPC-PV was designed to be used for children, aged 3 to 18 years, who are unable to speak because of cognitive (mental/intellectual) impairments or disabilities. It can be used whether or not a child has physical impairments or disabilities. Descriptions of the types of children used to validate the NCCPC-PV can be found in: Breau, L.M., Finley, G.A., McGrath, P.J. & Camfield, C.S. (2002). Validation of the Non-Communicating Children's Pain Checklist—Postoperative Version. Anesthesiology, 96 (3), 528-535. The NCCPC-PV was designed to be used without training by parents and caregivers (carers), or by other adults who are not familiar with a specific child (do not know them well).

The NCCPC-PV may be freely copied for clinical use or use in research funded by not-for-profit agencies. For-profit agencies should contact Lynn Breau: Pediatric Pain Research, IWK Health Centre, 5850 University Avenue, Halifax, Nova Scotia, Canada, B3J 3G9 (lbreau@ns.sympatico.ca).

The NCCPC-PV was intended for use for pain after surgery or due to other procedures conducted in hospital. If short- or long-term pain is suspected for a child at home or in a long-term residential setting, the **Non-Communicating Children's Pain Checklist—Revised** may be used. It can be obtained by contacting Lynn Breau. Information regarding the NCCPC-R can be found in: Breau, L.M., McGrath, P.J., Camfield, C.S. & Finley, G.A. (2002). Psychometric Properties of the Non-Communicating Children's Pain Checklist—Revised. *Pain, 99,* 349-357.

ADMINISTRATION

To complete the NCCPC-R, base your observations on the child's behavior over ***10 minutes***. **It is not necessary to watch the child continuously for this period.** However, it is recommended that the observer be in the child's presence for the majority of this time (e.g., be in the same room with the child). Although shorter observation periods may be used, the cut-off scores described below may not apply.

At the end of the observation time, indicate how frequently (how often) each item was seen or heard. This should not be based on the child's typical behavior or in relation to what he or she usually does. A guide for deciding the frequency of items is below:

> 0=Not present at all during the observation period. (Note: If the item is not present
>   because the child is not capable of performing that act, it should be scored as "NA").
> 1=Seen or heard rarely (hardly at all). but is present.
> 2=Seen or heard a number of times, but not continuous (not all the time).
> 3=Seen or heard often, almost continuous (almost all the time); any one would easily
>   notice this if they saw the child for a few moments during the observation time.
> NA=Not applicable. This child is not capable of performing this action.

SCORING

1. Add up the scores for each subscale and enter below that subscale number in the Score Summary at the bottom of the sheet. Items marked "NA" are scored as "0" (zero).
2. Add up all subscale scores for Total Score.
3. Check whether the child's score is greater than the cut-off score.

CUT-OFF SCORE

Based on the scores of 24 children aged 3 to 18 (Breau, Finley, McGrath, & Camfield, 2002), a Total **Score of 11 or more** indicates a child has **moderate to severe pain**. Based on unpublished data from this same sample, a **Total Score of 6-10** indicates a child has **mild pain**. When parents and caregivers completed the NCCPC-PV in hospital for the study group, this was accurate 88% of the time. When other observers completed the NCCPC-PV, this was accurate 75% of the time. A Total Score of 10 or less indicates less than moderate/severe pain. This was correct in the study group for parents and caregivers 81% of the time, and for other observers 63% of the time.

USE OF CUT-OFF SCORES

As with all observational tools, caution should be taken in using cut-off scores, because they may not be 100% accurate. They should not be used as the only basis for deciding whether a child should be treated for pain. In some cased children may have lower scores when pain is present. For more detailed instructions for use of the NCCPC-PV in such situations, please refer to the full manual, available from Lynn Breau: Pediatric Pain Research, IWK Health Centre, 5850 University Avenue, Halifax, Nova Scotia, Canada, B3J 3G9 (lbreau@ns.sympatico.ca).

FIGURE 11-5—cont'd.

The following scale will help us assess and manage your child's pain.

Directions:
1. Think about your child's past painful events. How does your child act when in mild pain, moderate pain, or severe pain?

2. In the diagram below, write in your child's typical pain behaviors on the line that corresponds to its pain intensity where 0 = no pain and 10 = worst possible pain.

3. When describing your child's pain, think about changes in:
   1. Facial expression
         Squinting eyes, frowning, distorted face, grinds teeth, thrusts tongue
   2. Leg or general body movements
         Tense, gestures (more or less) or touches part of body that hurts
   3. Activity, or social interaction
         Not cooperative, cranky, irritable, unhappy; Not moving, less active, quiet or more active, fidgety
   4. Cry or vocalization
         Moaning, whimpering, crying, yelling
   5. Consolability
         Less interaction, seeks comfort or physical closeness, difficult to distract/satisfy
   6. Other changes: Tears, sweating, holds breath, gasping

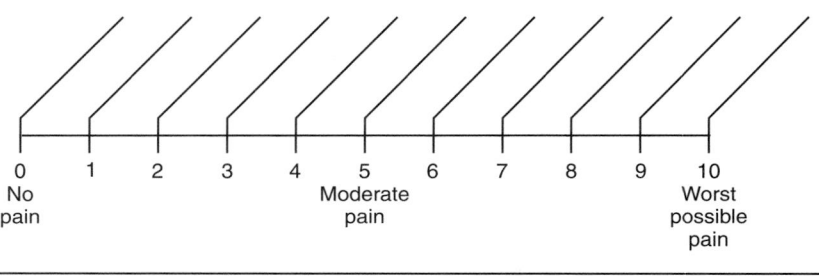

| 0 | 1 | 2 | 3 | 4 | 5 | 6 | 7 | 8 | 9 | 10 |
| No pain | | | | | Moderate pain | | | | | Worst possible pain |

FIGURE 11-6 ■ Individualized Numeric Rating Scale (INRS). (From Solodiuk J, Curley MAQ: Pain assessment in nonverbal children with severe cognitive impairments: The Individualized Numeric Rating Scale [INRS]. *J Pediatr Nurs* 18(4):297, 2003.)

        (a) Twenty-seven items, each scored from 0 to 3, total possible score 81
    (2) Revised—Face, Legs, Activity, Cry, Consolability (r-FLACC)
        (a) 10-point scale based on the FLACC scale
        (b) Includes space to record specific behaviors unique to the child for each of the five areas of the FLACC scale
    (3) Individualized Numeric Rating Scale (INRS)
        (a) 10-point scale adapted from the numeric rating scale
        (b) Provides parent/caregiver a place to document typical behaviors that correspond to levels of pain for the child
           (i) FLACC acronym may be used by nurses to guide parents in identifying past pain behaviors (Figure 11-6).
  I. Pain management
    1. Treatment plan begins preoperatively.
      a. Age-appropriate education before procedure
      b. Discussion of proposed plan
        (1) Selection of appropriate pain tool
      c. Hands-on play with medical equipment
    2. Multimodal approach unless contraindicated
      a. Analgesic therapy (Table 11-7)
        (1) Consider age, weight, comorbidities.
        (2) Dosages are based on weight and not a standard dose.
           (a) Calculated based on milligrams per kilogram

■ TABLE 11-7
■ ■ **Commonly Used Medications in the Pediatric PACU Setting**

Medications	General Dosing Guideline
ANALGESIA	
Acetaminophen	10 to 15 mg/kg every 4 hours Maximum: 3 g/24 hours or 60 to 80 mg/kg/24 hours, 4 to 6 doses
Ibuprofen	10 mg/kg every 6 to 8 hours Maximum: 40 mg/kg/day
Keterolac	0.5 mg/kg every 6 hours, PO or IV Maximum: 40 mg/kg/day PO, 120 mg/day IV
Codeine	0.5 to 1 mg/kg PO every 3 to 4 hours
Fentanyl	1 to 5 micrograms/kg IV May cause chest muscle rigidity related to high dose and rapid administration
Hydromorphone	0.03 to 0.08 mg/kg/dose every 4 to 6 hours PO Maximum: 5 mg 0.015 mg/kg/dose every 4 to 6 hours IV
Meperidine	0.05 to 1.5 mg/kg IV every 2 to 4 hours Maximum: 100 mg Normeperidine, an active metabolite, can accumulate after repeated doses, resulting in central nervous system symptoms (e.g., seizures).
Methadone	0.1 to 0.2 mg/kg IV THEN 0.05 to 0.1 mg/kg 0.2 mg/kg every 6 to 24 hours PO Maximum: 10 mg
Morphine	0.05 to 0.1 mg/kg IV every 1 to 2 hours
OPIOID ANTAGONIST	
Naloxone	Full narcotic reversal <20 kg: 0.1 mg/kg IV push >20 kg: 2 mg IV push Partial narcotic reversal 0.005 to 0.01 mg IV
BENZODIAZEPINES	
Diazepam	0.04 to 0.3 mg/kg IV every 2 to 4 hours 0.2 to 0.3 mg/kg PO or PR Maximum: 0.6 mg/kg over 8 hours DO NOT ADMINISTER IM
Lorazepam	0.025 to 0.05 mg/kg IV or PO Maximum: 4 mg/dose MAY BE ADMINISTERED IM if IV route not available
Midazolam	0.05 to 0.2 mg/kg IV 0.03 to 0.75 mg/kg for PO, PR, and intranasal use
BENZODIAZEPINE ANTAGONIST	
Flumazenil	0.01 to 0.015 mg/kg IV Maximum: 2 mg

Adapted from Hazinski MF: *Manual of pediatric critical care*, St Louis, 1999, Mosby.

VIII. INTRAOPERATIVE TREATMENT
   A. Opioid analgesics
   B. Nonopioid analgesics including nonsteroidal anti-inflammatory drugs
   C. Regional blocks
   D. Local infiltration
   E. Continuous infusion of local anesthetics
       1. Wound catheters
           a. Catheter placed into wound to infuse local anesthetic for up to several days

    2. Peripheral nerve blocks
       a. Local anesthetics injected near peripheral nerves (e.g., brachial plexus, femoral)
       b. Anesthetic effect occurs distally to injection site.
       c. May be administered in preoperative area
         (1) Use personal protective equipment because of potential for needle to dislodge from skin and cause risk to health care providers for mucous membrane exposure.
       d. Signs of toxicity
         (1) Metallic taste, tinnitus, blurred vision
         (2) Dysrhythmias, cardiac arrest
         (3) Confusion, seizures
         (4) Nausea, vomiting, diarrhea
         (5) Neurologic injury
       e. Safety considerations:
         (1) Prevent injury to affected area.
           (a) Maintain neutral positioning.
           (b) Protect and monitor pressure points.
           (c) Avoid use of cold or heat to affected area.
           (d) Check return of sensation to area.
       f. Anticipate, evaluate and plan for need to administer systemic analgesia as block wears off to prevent escalation of pain.
   F. Spinal anesthesia
     1. Epidurals
       a. Single or intermittent bolus
       b. Continuous infusion
       c. Patient-controlled epidural analgesia
     2. Caudal
       a. Single dose at either the beginning or the end of surgery
   G. Muscle relaxants
IX. PACU
   A. Obtain adequate pain control as quickly as possible to decrease postoperative anxiety.
     1. Current literature indicates relationship between inadequately treated acute pain and long-term detrimental effects.
     2. Assess for surgical pain and other causes of distress (e.g., tight casts or bandages, distended bladder, Foley catheter).
   B. Immediate postoperative pain management
     1. For perioperative therapeutic plan for pain control, around-the-clock regimen preferred over prn.
     2. Guidelines may not accurately determine dose requirements for all pediatric patients.
     3. Opioid doses should be titrated to pain relief/prevention.
       a. Morphine IV
         (1) Gold standard for opioids
         (2) Infants younger than 3 months clear morphine three to five times slower than adults.
         (3) More prone to respiratory depression
         (4) Infants older than 3 months metabolize morphine similarly to adults.
         (5) Infants younger than 6 months receiving opioid analgesia must be closely monitored, including use of pulse oximetry.
         (6) Suggested dosing guideline
           (a) 0.025 to 0.05 mg/kg IV in incremental doses to achieve analgesia during initial postoperative period as needed as intermittent doses
           (b) 0.05 to 1 mg/kg every 3 to 4 hours as needed as intermittent doses
           (c) 10 to 30 micrograms/kg/h for continuous infusion
           (d) For young opioid-naive infants, using doses one fourth to one half of suggested doses recommended

      b. Patient-controlled analgesia (PCA)

         (1) In children as young as 5 years based on manual dexterity and ability to understand the concept

         (2) Nurse-assisted PCA for younger children

    4. Nonsteroidal anti-inflammatory agent

      a. Keterolac

         (1) Dosing guideline

            (a) 0.25 to 0.5 mg/kg IV every 6 hours

C. Oral medications

    1. Opioid analgesics

      a. Codeine

         (1) Dosing guideline

            (a) 1 mg/kg/dose every 3 to 4 hours as needed

         (2) Often in combination with acetaminophen

         (3) Side effect profile (nausea, vomiting, constipation) has led to increase in use of hydrocodone and oxycodone for first-line opioid analgesia.

      b. Hydrocodone and acetaminophen

         (1) Dosing guideline

            (a) 2 to 13 years old or less than 50 kg: Hydrocodone 0.135 mg/kg/dose every 4 to 6 hours not to exceed 6 doses per day or maximum dose of acetaminophen

      c. Oxycodone

         (1) Dosing guideline

            (a) 6 to 12 years: 1.25 mg PO every 6 hours as needed

            (b) Older than 12 years: 2.5 mg PO every 6 hours as needed

    2. Nonopioid analgesics

      a. Acetaminophen 10 to 15 mg/kg PO

    3. Nonsteroidal anti-inflammatory medications

      a. Ibuprofen

         (1) 10 to 15 mg/kg/dose every 6 hours as needed (suggested dose)

D. Nursing considerations

    1. Assure "seven rights" with each medication administration.

      a. Right client with two identifiers

      b. Right drug

      c. Right dose

      d. Right time

      e. Right route

      f. Right reason

      g. Right documentation

    2. Double-check calculations of narcotics, including those obtained from pharmacy, with another nurse as specified by facility policy/protocol.

    3. Whenever possible, administer medications through a noninvasive route.

      a. Existing IV line

      b. Orally in cooperative child

         (1) Infants

            (a) May be administered through a nipple or a small syringe into the side of the mouth

         (2) Unpleasant tasting medicines

            (a) Incorporate developmental approach.

            (b) Be honest and patient with child, expressing support for the child to get ready for a difficult task he or she needs to do or something unpleasant.

            (c) "It's important that you take this medicine because it will help you, but it tastes yucky. Some kids do best taking little sips, others like to take it all at once. What do you think will work best for you?"

      c. Fear of injections makes IM and invasive routes aversive.

      (1) If there is no alternative, it is imperative that child is prepared truthfully and patiently, and that methods to decrease discomfort such as topical anesthetics or behavioral distraction techniques are optimized.

4. Plan pain management strategy using anticipatory approach and based on procedure and medications given.
5. Assess pain as fifth vital sign using pain scale.
    a. Upon admission
    b. Before and after interventions
    c. At time of discharge
6. Administer analgesics as prescribed, to maintain optimal analgesia.
7. Reassess pain score before and after interventions.
    a. Goal is for child to evidence reduced pain score.
       (1) Calm, relaxed facial expression
       (2) Relaxed posture
       (3) Decreased crying, fussiness, restlessness, stiffness
       (4) Interaction with others
8. Medicate before performing nursing activities that could be painful (e.g., dressing change, deep breathing, ambulation).
    a. If something will hurt, let them know to ensure that trust is maintained. For example:
       (1) "I will wipe your arm with a small, cold wet cloth and then there will be a pinch."
       (2) "We will need to remove this tape. It will be like taking off a Band-Aid, but I will be as gentle as I can be; it might help if I wet it. Should we try that?"
       (3) "It helps some kids to count to 10. Maybe you could look at Mom and she could count with you."
9. Anticipate, monitor for, prevent, and treat side effects associated with narcotics.
    a. Respiratory depression and somnolence
       (1) Naloxone 0.01 mg/kg every 2 to 3 minutes prn (suggested dose)
       (2) Duration 20 to 60 minutes
          (a) Be prepared to administer additional dose(s) if patient has had longer-acting narcotics in the event that initial symptoms reappear.
          (b) Anticipate potential need to judiciously medicate for pain as narcotic is reversed.
    b. Nausea and vomiting
       (1) Ondansetron 0.15 mg/kg/dose every 6 hours as needed to maximum dose of 4 mg/dose (suggested dose)
    c. Constipation
    d. Pruritus
       (1) Diphenhydramine 0.5 mg/kg/dose (suggested dose)
    e. Urinary retention
       (1) Consider indwelling urinary catheter.
10. Involve parents in care.
11. Use nonpharmacologic interventions for pain management (Box 11-11).
    a. Provide distraction.
       (1) Playing, singing, taking a deep breath, blowing bubbles, watching television, reading
    b. Provide relaxation opportunities.
       (1) Hold baby in comfortable position, rock, assist child to get into a comfortable position, ask child to take a deep breath and hold it, then to go "limp as a rag doll" while exhaling slowly.
    c. Use guided imagery.
       (1) Child imagines and describes the details of a pleasurable experience, enabling the child to concentrate on pleasurable experience during painful procedures.

■ BOX 11-11
■ **NONPHARMACOLOGIC STRATEGIES FOR PAIN MANAGEMENT**

General Strategies
- Use nonpharmacologic interventions to supplement, not replace, pharmacologic interventions, and use for mild pain and pain that is reasonably well controlled with analgesics.
- Form a trusting relationship with child and family. Express concern regarding their reports of pain and intervene appropriately. Take an active role in seeking effective pain management strategies.
- Use general guidelines to prepare child for procedure.
- Prepare child before potentially painful procedures but avoid "planting" the idea of pain.

  For example, instead of saying, "This is going to (or may) hurt," say, "Sometimes this feels like pushing, sticking, or pinching, and sometimes it doesn't bother people. Tell me what it feels like to you."

  Use "non-pain" descriptors when possible (e.g., "It feels like heat" rather than "It's a burning pain"). This allows for variation in sensory perception, avoids suggesting pain, and gives the child control in describing reactions.

  Avoid evaluative statements or descriptions (e.g., "This is a terrible procedure" or "It really will hurt a lot").
- Stay with the child during a painful procedure.

  Allow parents to stay with child if child and parent desire; encourage parent to talk softly to child and to remain near child's head.

  Involve parents in learning specific nonpharmacologic strategies and in assisting child with their use.
- Educate child about the pain, especially when explanation may lessen anxiety (e.g., that pain may occur after surgery and does not indicate something is wrong); reassure children that they are not responsible for the pain.
- For long-term pain control, give child a doll, which represents "the patient," and allow child to do everything to the doll that is done to the child; pain control can be emphasized through the doll by stating, "Dolly feels better after the medicine."
- Teach procedures to child and family for later use.

Specific Strategies
Distraction
- Involve parent and child in identifying strong distracters.
- Involve child in play; use radio, tape recorder, CD player, or computer game; have child sing or use rhythmic breathing.
- Have child take a deep breath and blow it out until told to stop.
- Have child blow bubbles to "blow the hurt away."
- Have the child concentrate on yelling or saying "ouch," with instructions to "yell as loud or soft as you feel it hurt; that way I know what's happening."
- Have child look through kaleidoscope (type with glitter suspended in fluid-filled tube) and encourage the child to concentrate by asking, "Do you see the different designs?"
- Use humor, such as watching cartoons, telling jokes or funny stories, or acting silly with child.
- Have child read, play games, or visit with friends.

Relaxation
- With an infant or young child:

  Hold in a comfortable, well-supported position, such as vertically against the chest and shoulder.

  Rock in a wide, rhythmic arc in a rocking chair or sway back and forth, rather than bouncing child.

  Repeat one or two words softly, such as "Mommy's here."
- With slightly older child:

  Ask child to take a deep breath and "go limp as a rag doll" while exhaling slowly; then ask child to yawn (demonstrate if needed).

  Help child assume a comfortable position (e.g., pillow under neck and knees).

  Begin progressive relaxation: starting with the toes, systematically instruct child to let each body part "go limp" or "feel heavy"; if child has difficulty relaxing, instruct child to tense or tighten each body part and then relax it.

Continued

■ BOX 11-11

■ **NONPHARMACOLOGIC STRATEGIES FOR PAIN MANAGEMENT—cont'd**

Allow child to keep eyes open, since children may respond better if eyes are open rather than closed during relaxation.

Guided Imagery

- Have child identify some highly pleasurable real or imaginary experience.
- Have child describe details of the event, including as many senses as possible (e.g., "feel the cool breezes," "see the beautiful colors," "hear the pleasant music").
- Have child write down or tape record script.
- Encourage child to concentrate only on the pleasurable event during the painful time; enhance the image by recalling specific details through reading the script or playing the tape.
- Combine with relaxation and rhythmic breathing.

Positive Self-Talk

- Teach child positive statements to say when in pain (e.g., "I will be feeling better soon," When I go home, I will feel better, and we will eat ice cream").

Thought Stopping

- Identify positive facts about the painful event (e.g., "It does not last long").
- Identify reassuring information (e.g., "If I think about something else, it does not hurt as much").
- Condense positive and reassuring facts into a set of brief statements and have child memorize them (e.g., "Short procedure, good veins, little hurt, nice nurse, go home").
- Have child repeat the memorized statements whenever thinking about or experiencing the painful event.

Behavioral Contracting

- Informal—May be used with children as young as 4 or 5 years of age:
  Use stars, tokens, or cartoon character stickers as rewards.
  Give a child who is uncooperative or procrastinating during a procedure a limited time (measured by a visible timer) to complete the procedure.
  Proceed as needed if child is unable to comply.
  Reinforce cooperation with a reward if the procedure is accomplished within specified time.
- Formal—Use written contract, which includes:
  Realistic (seems possible) goal or desired behavior
  Measurable behavior (e.g., agrees not to hit anyone during procedures)
  Contract written, dated, and signed by all persons involved in any of the agreements
  Identified rewards or consequences that are reinforcing
  Goals that can be evaluated
  Commitment and compromise requirements for both parties (e.g., while timer is used, nurse will not nag or prod child to complete procedure)

From Hockenberry MJ, Wilson D, eds: *Wong's nursing care of infants and children,* ed 8, St Louis, 2007, Mosby.

      d. Comfort measures
         (1) Warm blankets, pillows
         (2) Security objects from home
         (3) Fluids or food when appropriate
X. DISCHARGE (Box 11-12)
   A. Planning process usually begins before admission.
     1. Encourage parental participation in child's care.
     2. Encourage child to participate in own care based on physical and developmental abilities.
       a. Involvement helps maintain and improve coordination, muscle tone, and circulation.
       b. Fosters positive self-esteem and self-control
       c. Assists child to view hospitalization in a more positive manner
     3. Seek child's input when developing plan of care.

■ BOX 11-12
■ **INFORMATION FOR DISCHARGE**

After assessing the family's knowledge, provide the information families need to know to help the child's transition from hospital to home:

- Information about the procedure, surgery, illness and/or trauma and expected outcomes. Tell the parents when they should consult the primary care physician or nurse.
- Medications or treatments to be given at home and information about times, route, side effects, and any special care to be taken when giving the medication. Providing written information is valuable.
- Information about any special nutritional needs
- Specific activities the child may, may not, and sometimes should participate in
- The date when the child may return to school
- The date to bring the child back to the hospital, clinic, or office for follow-up care
- Information about any referral agency needed for the child or family
- The unit phone number and primary nurse's name

  Explain, demonstrate, and request a return demonstration of any treatments or procedures that will be done at home. This teaching should be an ongoing process and not left until the time of discharge, because learning takes place at different rates.

From James SR, Ashwill JW, Droske SC: *Nursing care of children*, ed 2, Philadelphia, 2002, WB Saunders.

    B. Criteria
        1. Ensure postanesthesia score or discharge criteria are met as determined by facility specific policy/protocol.
            a. Airway patent, vital signs and respiratory function stable
            b. Pain and nausea adequately controlled
            c. Adequately hydrated
            d. Awake and appropriate
        2. Provide instructions.
            a. Procedure specific
            b. Anesthesia specific
            c. Provide written instruction with appropriate contacts should questions arise regarding anesthesia-related concerns or potential surgical complications.
        3. Safe transport
            a. Optimal for two adults to accompany child on discharge, one to drive and one to attend to needs of the child
            b. Child safely secured in restraint device or seat of car as appropriate for age
   C. Nurse's role
        1. Assess parental capability to meet child's needs.
        2. Reinforce physician's instructions.
        3. Plan time for questions and answers.
        4. Clarify misconceptions for both parent and child.
        5. Include child in discussion as able and as tolerated by child.
        6. Review necessary information, including but not limited to:
            a. Necessary physical care
            b. Instructions on activities of daily living (e.g., play activities, sports, return to school or day care)
            c. Diet
            d. Medication administration
                (1) Encourage to be honest with child about medications with unpleasant taste and make suggestive plans with child (e.g., take it all at once or small sips at a time and follow the gulp or each sip with a drink or soft snack of his or her choice).

        (2) Provide tips to make administration of ear drops less distressing (e.g., warm ear drops in pan of warm water, instill ear drops in more comfortable ear first, time administration for one-half hour after oral analgesia to minimize discomfort).

        (3) Consider procedure and determine whether it may be beneficial to wake child once during the night to maintain optimal analgesia (e.g., tonsillectomy patients, patients undergoing orthopedic procedures).

    e. Necessary equipment and/or supplies needed to care for child (e.g., crutches, dressings)

    f. Potential complications

        (1) Expected

        (2) Unexpected

    g. Emergency contact information

    h. Follow-up appointment with physician(s)

    i. Necessary home health agency referrals

  7. Return demonstration assists in verifying child and/or parental understanding.

D. Postoperative telephone evaluation

  1. Usually performed the day after surgery

  2. Assess patient's progress.

  3. Reinforce discharge instructions.

  4. Answer questions or concerns.

  5. Identify postoperative complications.

  6. Evaluate need for referral to physician.

BIBLIOGRAPHY

1. American Society of Anesthesiologists Task Force on Preoperative Fasting: Practice guidelines for preoperative fasting and use of pharmacologic agents to reduce the risk of pulmonary aspiration: Application to healthy patients undergoing elective procedures. *Anesthesiology* 90(3):896-905, 1999.

2. American Society of Anesthesiologists Task Force on Acute Pain Management: Practice guidelines for acute pain management in the perioperative setting. *Anesthesiology* 100(6):1573-1581, 2004.

3. American Society of PeriAnesthesia Nurses: *Standards of perianesthesia nursing practice 2008-2010*, Cherry Hill, NJ, 2009, American Society of PeriAnesthesia Nurses.

4. Eaton S, Everson C, Jirava J, et al: Parents influence and advance pediatric policy. *Nurs Adm Q* 30(2):147-152, 2006.

5. Finley A, McGrath PJ, Chamber CT, eds: *Bringing pain relief to children: Treatment approaches*, Totowa, NJ, 2006, Humana Press.

6. Hazinski MF: *Manual of pediatric critical care*, St Louis, 1999, Mosby.

7. Hicks R, Wenzer LJ, Reilly CA, et al. *Drug information handbook for perioperative nursing*, Hudson, OH, 2006, LexiComp.

8. Hockenberry MJ, Wilson D, editors: *Wong's nursing care of infants and children*, ed 8, St Louis, 2007, Mosby.

9. Hommertzheim R, Steinke EE: Malignant hyperthermia—The perioperative nurse's role. *AORN J* 83(1):151-164;quiz 167-170, 2006.

10. Ireland D: Pediatric pain management competencies. In Krenzischek DA, Wilson L, eds: *ASPAN pain and comfort resource manual*, Cherry Hill, NJ, 2004, American Society of PeriAnesthesia Nurses.

11. Ireland D: Unique concerns of the pediatric surgical patient: Pre-, intra, and postoperatively. *Nurs Clin North Am* 41:265-298, 2006.

12. James SR, Ashwill JW, Droske SC: *Nursing care of children: Principles and practice*, ed 2, Philadelphia, 2002, WB Saunders.

13. Johnson DL: Care of the pediatric patient. In Drain CB: *Perianesthesia nursing: a critical care approach*, ed 4, St Louis, 2003, Saunders.

14. Kain ZN, Caldwell-Andrews AA: Preoperative psychological preparation of the child for surgery: an update. *Anesthesiol Clin N Am* 23:597-614, 2005.

15. Kain ZN, Mayes LC, Caldwell AA, et al: Preoperative anxiety, postoperative pain, and behavioral recovery in young children undergoing surgery. *Pediatrics* 118(2):651-658, 2006.

16. Kamerling SN, Cunningham Lawler L, Lynch M, et al: Family-centered care in the pediatric post anesthesia care unit: Changing practice to promote parental visitation. *J Perianesth Nurs* 23(1):5-16, 2008.

17. Krenzischek DA, Dunwoody CJ, Polomano RC, et al: Pharmacotherapy for acute pain: Implications for practice. *Pain Manag Nurs* 9(suppl 1):S22-S32, 2008.

18. Lewandowski LA, Tesler MD, eds: *Family-centered care: Putting it into action: The SPN/ANA guide to family-centered care*, Washington, DC, 2003, American Nurses Association.

19. Manworren RC, Paulos CL, Pop R: Treating children for acute agitation in the PACU: Differentiating pain and emergence delirium. *J Perianesth Nurs* 19(3):183-193, 2004.

20. McCaffery M, Pasero C: *Pain: Clinical manual*, ed 2, St Louis, 1999, Mosby.

21. McCarthy EJ: Malignant hyperthermia: Pathophysiology, clinical presentation, and treatment. *AACN Clin Issues* 15(2):231-237, 2004.

22. Muscari ME: *Pediatric nursing*, ed 4, Philadelphia, 2005, Lippincott Williams & Wilkins.

23. Pasero C: Lidocaine iontophoresis for dermal procedure analgesia. *J Perianesth Nurs* 21(1):48-52, 2006.

24. Romino SL, Keatley VM, Secrest J, et al: Parental presence during anesthesia induc-tion in children. *AORN J* 81(4):780-792, 2005.

25. Sethna NF, Verghese ST, Hannallah RS, et al: A randomized controlled trial to evaluate S-Caine Patch for reducing pain associated with vascular access in children. *Anesthesiology* 102(2):403-408, 2005.

26. Solodiuk J, Curley MAQ: Pain assessment in nonverbal children with severe cognitive impairments: The Individualized Numeric Rating Scale (INRS). *J Pediatr Nurs* 18(4): 295-299, 2003.

27. Stanhope N: Temperature measurement in the phase I PACU. *J Perianesth Nurs* 21(1): 27-33, quiz 34-36, 2006.

28. Taketomo CK, Hodding JH, Kraus D: *Pediatric dosage handbook*, ed 13, Hudson, OH, 2006, Lexi-Comp.

29. Voepel-Lewis T, Burke C, Hadden S, et al: Nurses' diagnoses and treatment decisions regarding care of the agitated child. *J Perianesth Nurs* 20(4):239-248, 2005.

30. Voepel-Lewis T, Malviya S, Tait AR, et al: A comparison of the clinical utility of pain assessment tools for children with cognitive impairment. *Pediatr Anesthesiol* 106(1):72-78, 2008.

The Adolescent Patient

MAUREEN SCHNUR
KERRIE TALBOT

OBJECTIVES

At the conclusion of this chapter, the reader will be able to:

1. Identify the stages of adolescence and three developmental considerations for each one.

2. Identify two legal issues related to the adolescent patient.

3. List two common responses of the adolescent to surgery/hospitalization and effective communication techniques to use in caring for them.

4. Name two interventions that may enhance care of the adolescent patient with sensory challenges.

5. Identify two suggested approaches to performing a physical examination in an adolescent.

6. Identify two potential risks related to the perianesthesia care of adolescents with body piercing(s).

7. Identify an optimal postoperative position for the obese patient.

8. Identify two safety concerns to discuss with the adolescent upon discharge.

I. CLASSIFICATION BY AGE
   A. Eleven through 21 years of age
   B. Transition from childhood to adulthood
      1. Biologic changes
      2. Psychosocial changes
   C. Three stages
      1. Early adolescence
      2. Middle adolescence
      3. Late adolescence
II. GROWTH AND DEVELOPMENTAL CONSIDERATIONS (Table 12-1)
   A. Early adolescence
      1. Eleven to 14 years of age
      2. Period of growth acceleration
         a. Increase in appetite in response to rapid growth
      3. Biologic development
         a. Girls
            (1) Development of breast tissue
            (2) Begin to put on fat
            (3) Slightly taller and heavier than boys
            (4) Beginning of hair growth
               (a) Pubic
               (b) Axillary
            (5) Menarche
         b. Boys
            (1) Enlargement of testes
            (2) Transient gynecomastia
            (3) Spermatogenesis

■ TABLE 12-1
■ ■ **Growth and Development during Adolescence**

	Early Adolescence (11-14 yr)	Middle Adolescence (15-17 yr)	Late Adolescence (18-20 yr)
Growth	▪ Rapidly accelerating growth ▪ Reaches peak velocity ▪ Secondary sexual characteristics appear	▪ Growth decelerating in girls ▪ Stature reaches 95% of adult height ▪ Secondary sexual characteristics well advanced	▪ Physically mature ▪ Structure and reproductive growth almost complete
Cognition	▪ Explores newfound ability for limited abstract thought ▪ Clumsy groping for new values and energies ▪ Comparison of "normality" with peers of same sex	▪ Developing capacity for abstract thinking ▪ Enjoys intellectual powers, often in idealistic terms ▪ Concern with philosophic, political, and social problems	▪ Established abstract thought ▪ Can perceive and act on long-range options ▪ Able to view problems comprehensively ▪ Intellectual and functional identity established
Identity	▪ Preoccupied with rapid body changes ▪ Trying out of various roles ▪ Measurement of attractiveness by acceptance or rejection by peers ▪ Conformity to group norms	▪ Modifies body image ▪ Very self-centered, increased narcissism ▪ Tendency toward inner experience and self-discovery ▪ Has rich fantasy life ▪ Idealistic ▪ Able to perceive future ▪ implications of current behavior and decisions; variable application	▪ Body image and gender role definition nearly secured ▪ Mature sexual identity ▪ Phase of consolidation of identity ▪ Stability of self-esteem ▪ Comfortable with physical growth ▪ Social roles defined and articulated
Relationships with parents	▪ Defining independence and dependence boundaries ▪ Strong desire to remain dependent on parents while trying to detach ▪ No major conflicts over parental control	▪ Major conflicts over independence and control ▪ Low point in parent and child relationship ▪ Greatest push for emancipation; disengagement ▪ Final and irreversible emotional detachment from parents; mourning	▪ Emotional and physical separation from parents completed ▪ Independence from family with less conflict ▪ Emancipation nearly secured
Relationships with peers	▪ Seeks peer affiliations to counter instability generated by rapid change ▪ Upsurge of close, idealized friendships with members of same sex ▪ Struggle with mastery within peer group	▪ Strong need for identity to affirm self-image ▪ Behavioral standards set by peer group ▪ Acceptance by peers extremely important—fear of rejection ▪ Exploration of ability to attract opposite sex	▪ Peer group recedes in importance in favor of individual friendship ▪ Testing of romantic relationships against possibility of permanent alliance ▪ Relationships characterized by giving and sharing
Sexuality	▪ Self-exploration and evaluation ▪ Limited dating, usually group ▪ Limited intimacy	▪ Multiple plural relationships ▪ Internal identification of heterosexual, homosexual, or bisexual attractions ▪ Exploration of "self-appeal" ▪ Feeling of "being in love" ▪ Tentative establishment of relationships	▪ Forms stable relationships and attachment to another ▪ Growing capacity for mutuality and reciprocity ▪ Dating as a romantic pair ▪ May publicly identify as gay, lesbian, or bisexual ▪ Intimacy involves commitment rather than exploration and romanticism

Continued

■ TABLE 12-1
■ ■ **Growth and Development during Adolescence—cont'd**

	Early Adolescence (11-14 yr)	Middle Adolescence (15-17 yr)	Late Adolescence (18-20 yr)
Psychological health	• Wide mood swings • Intense daydreaming • Anger outwardly expressed with moodiness, temper outbursts, verbal insults and name calling	• Tendency toward inner experiences, more introspective • Tendency to withdraw when upset or feelings are hurt • Vacillation of emotions in time and range • Feelings of inadequacy common, difficulty asking for help	• More constancy of emotion • Anger more likely to be concealed

From Hockenberry MJ, Wilson D, eds: *Wong's nursing care of infants and children*, ed 8, St Louis, 2007, Mosby.

4. Motor development
   a. Increase in gross muscle mass
   b. Increase in fine motor coordination
   c. Prone to ligament tears
   d. Awkward, gangly period
5. Psychosocial development
   a. Erikson theory
      (1) Stage of identity versus role confusion (12-18 years of age)
         (a) Corresponds to Freud's genital stage
         (b) Characterized by rapid physical changes
         (c) Adolescents become preoccupied with appearance (how they look to others).
   b. Freud theory
      (1) Genital stage (age 12 and older)
         (a) Begins with puberty
         (b) Reproductive system and sex hormones mature.
         (c) Genital organs become major source of sexual tensions and pleasures.
         (d) Period of forming relationships and preparing for marriage
   c. Other characteristics
      (1) Shy, awkward
      (2) Adjusting to middle school
      (3) Move from operational thinking to formal, logical operations and increasingly able to:
         (a) Manipulate abstractions
         (b) Reason from principles
         (c) Weigh multiple points of view according to varying criteria
      (4) More at ease with same sex
         (a) Increased activity with peers
            (i) Conformity and cliques
         (b) Less activity with family
      (5) Increase in self-consciousness
         (a) Adolescents meticulous about their appearance
         (b) Think everyone is looking at them
      (6) Low self-esteem
      (7) Increase in rebellious behavior
      (8) Increase in independence
      (9) Increase in sexual interest
         (a) Interest is greater than sexual activity
         (b) Often have questions about sexual changes they are experiencing

B. Middle adolescence
   1. Fifteen to 17 years of age
   2. Biologic development
      a. Girls
         (1) Height increases.
         (2) Breast size increases.
         (3) Growth of pubic hair increases.
         (4) Sexual maturation occurs.
         (5) Shoulder-to-hip proportions are becoming those of an adult woman.
         (6) Growth acceleration declines.
         (7) Appetite decreases.
      b. Boys
         (1) Voice changes.
         (2) Larynx enlarges.
         (3) Muscle mass enlarges.
         (4) Strength increases.
         (5) Shoulders widen.
         (6) Facial hair growth begins.
         (7) Height increases rapidly.
         (8) Appetite increases.
         (9) Size of genitalia increases.
         (10) Transient gynecomastia decreases.
      c. Both sexes
         (1) Acne may develop and be a problem.
         (2) Body odor increases as sweat glands further develop.
         (3) Dentition is completed.
         (4) Sensory and language development are complete.
         (5) Capacity of cardiovascular pump increases.
            (a) Heart size doubles.
            (b) Blood pressure, blood volume, and hematocrit increase.
         (6) Lung capacity doubles.
         (7) Physiologic need for sleep increases.
   3. Motor development
      a. Physical endurance increases.
      b. Skill in sports increases.
      c. Fine and gross muscle coordination increases.
   4. Psychosocial development
      a. Increased conflicts with parents
      b. Mood swings
         (1) Impulsive
         (2) Impatient
         (3) Narcissistic
         (4) Moody
      c. Test established limits
      d. Privacy very important
      e. Peer group very important
      f. Abstract thoughts increase.
         (1) Tend to question and analyze everything
         (2) Become more self-centered
   5. Sexual development
      a. Sexual experimentation begins.
      b. Degree of sexual activity varies.
      c. Begin to sort out sexual identity
         (1) Form beliefs regarding love, honesty, and propriety
      d. May choose monogamous or polygamous experimentation, or celibacy
      e. Knowledgeable regarding risk of pregnancy, acquired immunodeficiency syndrome, and other sexually transmitted diseases
         (1) Knowledge does not necessarily influence behavior.

6. Development of self-concept
    a. Period of experimentation
        (1) Peers less important
        (2) Change style of dress
        (3) May change group of friends
    b. Deal with inner turmoil
7. Development of relationships
    a. Parental relationship strained
        (1) May become distant
        (2) Dating may become source of conflict.
    b. Physical attractiveness remains important.
    c. Acceptance by a peer group promotes positive peer relationships and self-esteem.
    d. Begin to identify career path
        (1) Life skills
        (2) Opportunities
    e. Positive role models crucial at this stage of development
C. Late adolescence
    1. Eighteen to 20 years of age or beyond
    2. Biologic development
        a. Growth slows
        b. No neurological developmental changes apparent
        c. Cardiopulmonary capacity relatively mature
    3. Psychosocial development
        a. Aware of own strengths and limitations
        b. Establish own value system
        c. Cognition tends to be less self-centered.
            (1) Able to express thoughts and feelings about various aspects of life (e.g., justice, patriotism, history)
            (2) Idealistic about love, social issues, ethics and lifestyles
        d. Social relationships more mature
        e. Conformity less important
        f. Turbulence with parents decreases.
        g. Prepare to leave home
    4. Sexual development
        a. More commitment to intimate relationships
        b. More realistic concept of a partner's role
    5. Self-concept
        a. Self-esteem increases.
            (1) More stable body image
        b. Social roles defined and articulated
            (1) Career decisions become important.
            (2) Self-concept increasingly tied to role in society (e.g., student, worker, parent)
    6. Relationships
        a. Separation from parents
            (1) Emotional and physical
        b. Gain independence from family
III. ADOLESCENT RESPONSE TO SURGERY/HOSPITALIZATION
    A. Loss of control
        1. A planned procedure (scheduled surgery) allows a greater sense of control than an unplanned (emergency) procedure.
        2. Want to be in control
        3. May resist dependence
        4. May react to loss of control with anger, withdrawal, uncooperativeness, or refusal to follow rules
        5. Often feel isolated and unable to obtain adequate support

B. Fear
   1. Fear bodily injury, pain and how illness is viewed by peers
      a. Activity limitations
      b. Appearance
   2. May refuse to cooperate if treatment does not fit into lifestyle
   3. May project image of "calm and cool" even though they are anxious and/or scared
   4. May question everything or appear confident
   5. Able to describe degree of pain
C. Separation anxiety
   1. May or may not want parents involved
   2. May become more dependent on parents
   3. Separation from friends increases anxiety.
D. Emotional and behavioral considerations
   1. Adolescents use a range of modalities from sophisticated verbal or written expression to motor activity.
   2. May regress in behavior
   3. Thoughts, feelings, and fears may be shared with friends, especially peers.
   4. Major fears and worries
      a. Uncertainty about self as a person
      b. Concerned about whether or not body, thoughts, and feelings are normal
IV. FAMILY-CENTERED CARE (see Chapter 11)
   A. Support system
      1. Recognize the increasing maturity and independence of the adolescent, respecting his or her wishes for involvement of family/accompanying significant others as appropriate.
      2. Determine the responsible adult accompanying the adolescent.
      3. Provide education that it is not unusual for the adolescent to regress, withdraw, or act out.
   B. Emergency situations
      1. Parents experience stress.
         a. Fear and anxiety most common emotions
         b. Parent fears that adolescent may:
            (1) Experience pain
            (2) Suffer permanent changes
            (3) Be diagnosed with chronic or terminal illness, or even die
      2. Cause of stress is unique to circumstances.
      3. Parents may experience guilt.
         a. Feel responsible
         b. May be submitting adolescent to a painful experience
      4. Include family members/support system in adolescent's care to reduce feelings of helplessness.
         a. May choose to access community support (e.g., religious leader, primary physician)
   C. Legal issues (see Chapter 5)
      1. Bill of Rights (Box 12-1)
         a. Facilities may develop and post "bill of rights" for patients and their families.
      2. Verify guardianship.
      3. Consent of minors (Box 12-2)
         a. Governed by state laws
         b. Exemptions to parental consent for medical treatment
            (1) Emancipated minors
               (a) Have a child of their own
               (b) Married
               (c) Live away from home
               (d) No longer subject to parental control

■ BOX 12-1
■ **BILL OF RIGHTS FOR CHILDREN AND TEENS**

In this hospital, you and your family have the right to:
- Respect and personal dignity
- Care that supports you and your family
- Information you can understand
- Quality health care
- Emotional support
- Care that respects your need to grow, play, and learn
- Make choices and decisions

Adapted from Association for the Care of Children's Health: *A pediatric bill of rights.* Mt Royal, NJ, 1998, Association for the Care of Children's Health.

■ BOX 12-2
■ **LEGAL AND ETHICAL CONSIDERATIONS**

The nurse or physician must obtain informed consent before any procedure or treatment that is potentially harmful to the child. These include immunizations and participation in research. A parent, an adolescent older than 18 years, or an emancipated minor (a minor child who is no longer dependent upon parents for either emotional or financial support) may give consent. Children able to understand the procedure and its implications should be included in the decision making. In certain cultures, the primary caregiver is not the child's legal guardian and cannot give consent. To give culturally sensitive care, include all the child's significant caregivers in the decision-making process.

From Luckmann J: *Saunders manual of nursing care,* Philadelphia, 1997, WB Saunders.

         (e) Economically self-supporting
         (f) Member of military service
      (2) Emergencies
         (a) May be treated without parental consent during medical emergency
            (i) Physician judgment
            (ii) Delay would jeopardize health or life of minor
      (3) Mature minor rule
         (a) Emerging trend in law
         (b) Recognizes minor is mature enough to understand nature of illness and risks and benefits of therapy
         (c) Should receive treatment at their own request
   4. Child abuse and neglect reporting
     a. Governed by each state
     b. Nurses are mandated reporters in every state.
   5. Reproductive health rights
     a. Governed by state laws
       (1) Disclosure of reproductive health information to parent(s) may or may not be legal (e.g., pregnancy, sexually transmitted diseases).
V. PHASES OF PERIOPERATIVE/PROCEDURAL CARE FOR THE ADOLESCENT PATIENT
  A. Preadmission/preprocedural assessment (Box 12-3) (see Chapter 15)
    1. Medical record review
    2. Phone assessment
      a. Patients younger than 18 years
        (1) Parent/guardian interview
      b. Patients 18 years or older
        (1) Interview with adolescent
        (2) Parent interview with knowledge/agreement of adolescent

■ BOX 12-3
■ PREPARATION OF ADOLESCENTS FOR PROCEDURES AND SURGERY

Major Fears
- Loss of control
- Altered body image
- Separation from peer group

Characteristics of Adolescents' Thinking
- Beginning of formal operational thought and ability to think abstractly
- Existence of some magic thinking (e.g., feeling guilty for illness) and egocentrism
- Tendency toward hyperresponsiveness to pain
- Little understanding of the structure and workings of the body

Preparation
- Prepare them in advance, preferably weeks before major events. Advance preparation is vital to adolescents' ability to cope, cooperate, and comply.
- Provide tours and equipment and models to examine. Audiovisual and multimedia computer-based programs may be helpful.
- Allow adolescents to be an integral part of decision making about their care, because they can project the future and see long-term consequences and thus are able to understand much more.
- Give information sensitively, because adolescents react not only to *what* they are told but to the *manner* in which they are told. Explore tactfully what adolescents know and what they do not know.
- Stress how much adolescents can do for themselves and how important their compliance and cooperation are to their treatment and recovery; be honest about the consequences.
- Allow the adolescent as many choices and as much control as possible. Respect adolescents' need to exert independence from parents, and remember that they may alternate between dependence and a wish to be independent.
- Assure ability to maintain contact with peer group if adolescent desires.
- Teach adolescent coping techniques such as relaxation, deep breathing, self-comforting talk and/or the use of imagery.

It is important to remember that the child's psychosocial developmental stage may not always match his or her chronologic age. Development may be delayed, particularly in chronically ill children. For example, an adolescent who is delayed in development may need to be approached more like a school-age child.
Adapted from Hazinski MF: *Manual of pediatric critical care*, St Louis, 1999, Mosby.

      (a) Optimizes obtaining more complete history
  c. Assess communication barriers (e.g., language, hearing impaired).
    (1) Develop plan for resources needed.
  d. Determine, plan, and communicate with the health care team for special needs such as:
    (1) Disorders with sensory challenges (e.g., autism, attention-deficit/hyperactivity disorder, pervasive developmental delay)
      (a) Plan to minimize stimulation.
        (i) Admit to quiet area or room.
        (ii) Minimize number of interactions/interventions with patient by organizing care.
          [a] Develop plan with accompanying caregiver(s).
      (b) Provide option to family to bring favorite familiar comfort objects and/or activities that will help patient cope while waiting for surgery (e.g., music, books, games).
        (i) Educate patient/family about potential for risks of damage/loss of personal items, and communicate strategies to minimize possibility.
      (c) Determine need for premedication to optimize ability to cope with change in routine.

(2) Obesity
    (a) Large wheelchair, appropriate size bed, trapeze on bed, lifting devices, larger-size hospital attire
    (b) Plan for need for teaching regarding coughing, deep breathing, and use of incentive spirometry to optimize postoperative respiratory status.

B. Day of surgery
  1. Admission to preoperative/preprocedural area
    a. Role of family/accompanying adult(s)
      (1) Ascertain and be sensitive to degree to which adolescent wants parent(s)/accompanying adult present.
      (2) Be aware that questions may not be answered truthfully in presence of parent(s)/accompanying adult.
        (a) Choose time to ask adolescent about sensitive questions that will optimize telling the truth (e.g., when providing adolescent private space to change into hospital attire, this may be an optimal time to ask about use of drugs, alcohol, and smoking).
      (3) Encourage parent(s)/responsible adult to accompany adolescent to holding area if requested.
      (4) Inform parent(s)/responsible adult of necessity to remain at facility.
    b. Developmental considerations (Box 12-4)
      (1) Interviewing adolescents (Box 12-5)

■ BOX 12-4
■ **DEVELOPMENTAL MILESTONES AND THEIR RELATIONSHIP TO COMMUNICATION APPROACHES (12 YEARS AND OLDER)**

Development	Language Development	Emotional Development	Cognitive Development	Suggested Communication Approach
■ Adolescents are able to create theories and generate many explanations for situations. ■ They are beginning to communicate like adults.	■ Able to verbalize and understand most adult concepts	■ Beginning to accept responsibility for own actions ■ Perception of "imaginary audiences" ■ Need independence ■ Competitive drive ■ Strong need for group identification ■ Frequently have small group of very close friends ■ Question authority ■ Strong need for privacy	■ Able to think logically and abstractly ■ Attention span up to 60 minutes	■ Engage in conversations about adolescent's interests. ■ Use photographs, books, diagrams, charts, and videos to explain. ■ Use collaborative approach and foster and support independence. ■ Introduce preparatory materials up to 1 week in advance of the event. ■ Respect privacy needs.

Adapted from James SR, Ashwill JW, Droske SC: *Nursing care of children*, ed 2, Philadelphia, 2002, WB Saunders.

(a) Communication approaches
  (i) Optimize privacy for interactions.
  (ii) Communicate in open and respectful manner.
  (iii) Involve in decision-making.
  (iv) Provide information sensitively.
  (v) Encourage questions regarding fears, options, and alternatives.
  (vi) Answer all questions truthfully and honestly.
(2) Privacy considerations
  (a) Inform adolescent that certain procedures will be conducted only after induction of anesthesia (e.g., hair removal, skin preparation, insertion of urinary catheters).
  (b) If appropriate for procedure, allow adolescent to leave undergarments on.
(3) Emotional considerations
  (a) May show false bravery to nurse
  (b) May be very anxious but not able to verbalize concerns
c. Nursing interventions to minimize stress
  (1) Give information about proposed procedure to reduce psychological stress and elicit cooperation.
    (a) May be concerned regarding cause of illness/need for surgery
  (2) Provide information about:
    (a) Reasons for tests and procedures
    (b) What to expect (e.g., what the adolescent will be asked to do, how long it will take, if discomfort is or isn't involved)
    (c) How the adolescent will feel during and after tests/procedures
    (d) When results of tests will be known
  (3) Discuss approximate length of time in each phase of hospitalization (e.g., preadmission, OR, Post Anesthesia Care Unit [PACU]).
  (4) Inform about when the adolescent/accompanying adult will speak with the surgeon, anesthesia care provider and/or other physician(s).
d. Patient education (see Chapter 3)
  (1) Comfort
    (a) Teach concepts of interventions they may experience/participate in postprocedure to enhance comfort such as:
      (i) Distraction
      (ii) Imagery
      (iii) Breathing techniques
      (iv) Positive self-talk

■ BOX 12-5
■ **INTERVIEWING ADOLESCENTS**

- Ensure confidentiality and privacy; interview adolescent without parents.
- Show concern for the adolescent's perspective; "First, I'd like to talk about your main concerns" and "I'd like to know what you think is happening."
- Offer a nonthreatening explanation for the questions you ask: "I'm going to ask a number of questions to help me better understand your health."
- Maintain objectivity; avoid assumptions, judgments, and lectures.
- Ask open-ended questions when possible; move to more directive questions if necessary.
- Begin with less sensitive issues and proceed to more sensitive ones.
- Use language that both the adolescent and you understand.
- Restate: reflect back to the adolescent what he or she has said, along with feelings that may be associated with the descriptions.

From Hockenberry MJ, Wilson D, eds: *Wong's nursing care of infants and children*, ed 8, St Louis, 2007, Mosby.

      (v)   Moving as one unit (e.g., log rolling after spinal fusion surgery)

      (vi) Pillows placed for comfort (e.g., under knees after abdominal surgery to reduce tension on abdomen, to support extremities, for positioning, for splinting abdomen, for coughing exercises)

      (vii) Techniques for getting out of bed and turning to reduce pressure on incisions

(2) Allow choices when possible.

  (a) Induction of anesthesia

  (b) Intravenous insertion

     (i)   In OR

     (ii) In preprocedural area

        [a] Interventions to minimize discomfort and anxiety include:

            [1] Topical anesthetic agents

            [2] Alternative methods (e.g., guided imagery, music, reiki)

  (c) Parental/responsible adult presence

     (i)   Adolescent's anxiety may be decreased by presence of trusted adult(s) who provide comfort, protection, and encouragement.

(3) Provide information and teaching about intraoperative experience.

  (a) Monitoring devices that will be applied (e.g., electrocardiogram, pulse oximeter, blood pressure cuff)

  (b) Invasive lines, tubes, or drains that may be inserted as part of the procedure; safety strap that may be secured for transport to PACU

     (i)   May wake up with these in place

  (c) Sensations from anesthetics administered

  (d) Endotracheal intubation after "asleep" or loss of consciousness obtained

     (i)   Inform patients they may experience "sore throat" postoperatively.

  (e) Only surgical area exposed for staff to view

     (i)   Sterile drapes applied around site

  (f) Will remain unconscious throughout procedure

     (i)   Provide reassurance to the adolescent that they do not need to worry about talking or doing anything embarrassing while under anesthesia.

2. Admission assessment (see Chapter 15)

  a. Anticipate postoperative complications.

    (1) Review and assess body systems.

    (2) Note recent or current cold, asthma exacerbation, rash, fever, vomiting, or diarrhea.

    (3) Observe verbal and nonverbal behavior before surgery.

    (4) Assess for child abuse and neglect.

      (a) Follow state law regarding reporting.

      (b) Follow facility protocol/policy.

    (5) Check vital signs, including heart rate, respirations, blood pressure, oxygen saturation, and temperature.

    (6) Obtain weight and height.

      (a) Optimize privacy.

        (i)   May be focused on being overweight or underweight

    (7) Document allergies and sensitivities (e.g., food, drugs, latex).

    (8) Determine use of alcohol, tobacco, recreational drugs, or other substances per facility policy/protocol.

      (a) Maintain privacy when obtaining history of smoking, drug use, body art, last menstrual period, and other potentially sensitive information.

    (9) Ask adolescent about contact lenses, oral appliances, and other cosmetic or medical devices.

   (10) Ask adolescent about jewelry, including body piercings, and assess need to insulate or remove.

    (a) To insulate:

     (i) Tape down with surgical tape.

      [a] May apply soft dressing over piercing and tape

    (b) Remove if indicated due to potential risks.

     (i) Infection

     (ii) Obstruction

      [a] May be dislodged (e.g., tongue stud)

      [b] With tongue studs, may be best to remove in holding area and reinsert as soon as possible in the PACU to avoid interfering with patency

     (iii) Increased magnetic pull

      [a] Magnetic resonance imaging procedures

     (iv) Serve as metal conductor

      [a] Risk for burns

     (v) May catch on items

      [a] Electrocardiogram leads, drapes, accidental tearing of pierced site

     (vi) Interference with routine procedures if undisclosed (e.g., unknown genital piercing may interfere with intraoperative insertion of urinary catheter)

     (vii) Risk of loss (e.g., navel stud)

   (11) Secure personal belongings.

    (a) Follow facility policy on safe keeping of personal belongings.

    (b) Family/responsible adult may hold items for patient while in tests/procedure/surgery.

 C. Physical assessment (see Chapter 15)

  1. Approach

   a. Use straightforward approach.

   b. Involve adolescent in decision of who should be present for exam.

  2. Technique

   a. Move from head to toe.

   b. Perform genital exam in the middle of exam.

    (1) Allow ample time for questions and answers.

   c. Assure adolescent regarding normal growth and development.

   d. Answer questions or concerns regarding what is happening to their bodies.

   e. Drape appropriately to preserve dignity.

  3. Nursing considerations

   a. Admission to hospital or facility may be viewed as a threat to adolescent's independence, resulting in sense of loss of control.

    (1) May react by not cooperating or withdrawing

   b. May resent dependency on others and have difficulty accepting restrictions (e.g., dietary)

    (1) Explain consequences of not telling the truth regarding eating and/or drinking before procedure.

   c. Involve in decision-making and planning.

   d. Accept childish methods of coping.

   e. Provide support and reassurance as necessary.

   f. Provide explanations and consequences of decisions.

  4. Conduct sexual assessment.

   a. Determine possible pregnancy.

    (1) Document last menstrual period.

    (2) Conduct pregnancy testing if indicated per facility protocol/policy.

    (3) Refer to individual state laws regarding disclosure of reproductive health information.

D. Preoperative teaching (see Chapter 15)
  1. Provide information about what will happen.
    a. Estimated time frames
      (1) Preempt anxiety related to expectations about estimated time frames by educating patient/family about the often dynamic nature of the perioperative environment.
    b. Postoperative routine in PACU
      (1) Oxygen
      (2) Position
      (3) Monitoring
      (4) Dressing checks
      (5) Tubes
        (a) Intravenous and/or arterial line(s)
        (b) Drainage collection devices
        (c) Urinary catheter
        (d) Chest tube(s)
      (6) Respiratory interventions
        (a) Deep breathing
        (b) Coughing
        (c) Incentive spirometry
          (i) May be helpful to practice in patient populations more at risk (e.g., patients having abdominal surgery, obese patients, smokers)
      (7) Pain assessment and treatment
        (a) Review pain scales.
        (b) Identify goal for pain relief.
        (c) Coach to help develop coping strategies.
          (i) Deep breathing
          (ii) Guided imagery
          (iii) Positive self-talk statements (e.g., "I can make it through this.")
      (8) Visitation
        (a) Provide information on visiting guidelines per facility policy/protocol.
        (b) Encourage patient/family to use caution keeping small items on bed during provision of care to patient (e.g., electronic devices may fall to floor while turning patient and be damaged).
      (9) Resumption of oral intake
  2. Teaching strategies
    a. Determine most effective way to communicate necessary information to both adolescent and responsible adult caregiver.
      (1) Assess whether it is best to teach adolescent and the adult who will be responsible for care together or separately.
      (2) Determine preferred method(s) of learning of adolescent and responsible adult caregiver.
      (3) Promote collaborative decision-making.
    b. Clearly explain how the body is affected by surgery or procedure.
      (1) Provide information openly and honestly.
      (2) Use scientific names with explanations.
      (3) Use diagrams and printed materials.
    c. Provide opportunities for adolescent to express anxieties.
      (1) Consider that some adolescents may be embarrassed about peers finding out about certain procedures and may benefit from planning a communication strategy (e.g., patients undergoing circumcision may be more comfortable indicating to peers that they had a similar procedure such as a hernia repair).
E. Intraoperative considerations
  1. Provide reassurance before induction.
    a. Hold hand.
    b. Offer verbal support.

      c. Assure preservation of privacy and dignity.

      d. Provide for patient safety.

F. Postoperative assessment (see Chapter 50)

  1. Respiratory assessment

      a. Position airway for optimal ventilation.

        (1) Semirecumbent position suggested for obese patients to decrease abdominal pressure on diaphragm

      b. Monitor rate and depth of ventilation.

      c. Monitor oxygen saturation.

      d. Observe for tongue obstruction.

      e. Observe for respiratory depression from narcotics and muscle relaxants.

  2. Cardiovascular assessment

      a. Assess vital signs and perfusion.

      b. Heart rate

        (1) Awake: 60 to 90 beats per minute

        (2) Sleeping: 50 to 90 beats per minute

        (3) May be lower if adolescent is athletic

      c. Blood pressure (BP)

        (1) Systolic: 112 to 128 mm Hg

        (2) Diastolic: 66 to 80 mm Hg

  3. Thermoregulation (see Chapter 24)

      a. Responds to cold environment by increasing metabolism

        (1) Increase in oxygen consumption

        (2) Shivering

      b. Hypothermia

        (1) Monitor:

          (a) Vital signs including core temperature, pulse rate, respiratory rate

          (b) Degree of emergence from anesthesia

          (c) Continuous electrocardiogram

            (i) Dysrhythmias and cardiovascular depression associated with hypothermia

      c. Hyperthermia

        (1) Overheating

        (2) Infection

          (a) Preexisting fever versus new onset

        (3) Malignant hyperthermia (see Chapters 11, 24, and 28)

      d. Emergence delirium (see Chapter 11)

  4. Pain assessment (see Chapter 26)

      a. Perceive pain on three levels

        (1) Physical

        (2) Emotional

        (3) Mental

      b. Able to understand cause and effect of pain

      c. Able to describe pain

        (1) Verbalize with words such as "ache," "sore," "pounding."

        (2) Describe pain intensity and quality.

          (a) Express feelings regarding pain.

          (b) Identify strategies that have helped with past experiences of pain.

      d. Not unusual for adolescents to deal with pain through regressive behavior

        (1) Increased dependence on parent

        (2) Expect the nurse to know they are in pain.

        (3) Believe they should not have to ask for pain medication

      e. Concerned with maintaining composure and are embarrassed and ashamed if lose control

      f. Observed symptoms of pain include:

        (1) Increased muscle tension

          (a) Facial grimacing

          (b) Muscle rigidity

      (2) Withdrawal
         (a) Decreased interest in environment and usual activities
      (3) Physical response
         (a) Decreased motor activity
            (i) Reluctant to move
         (b) Physical resistance and aggression—unusual unless the adolescent is totally unprepared for the procedure
      (4) Vocalization
         (a) May grunt, groan, sigh, or use inappropriate language
         (b) Rarely cry or scream
g. Pain assessment scales (see Chapters 11 and 26)
      (1) Self-report
         (a) Visual analog scale
            (i) Mark on a line (no pain to worst pain) a point that corresponds to the adolescent's pain level.
         (b) Verbal numerical score
            (i) Choose a number from 0 to 10 that corresponds to their pain level (0, no pain; 10, worst pain imaginable).
         (c) Adolescent and Pediatric Pain Tool (Figure 12-1)
            (i) Patient draws on front and back of body outlines to locate pain.
            (ii) Indicates pain intensity on a Word Graphic Rating Scale
            (iii) Circles words that describe the quality of pain
h. Pharmacologic interventions: Analgesics (see Table 11-6)
      (1) Opioids
         (a) For moderate to severe pain
         (b) Routes
            (i) Intravenous
               [a] Preferred route after major surgery and/or if intravenous line in place
               [b] May be administered continuously and/or intermittently
               [c] Used for patient-controlled analgesia
                  [1] Provides steady level of analgesia
                  [2] Increased risk for respiratory depression
                  [3] Risk for dependence or addiction very low in patients without a history of prior substance abuse
                  [4] Not routinely used in outpatient setting
            (ii) Epidural, intrathecal
               [a] Provides effective analgesia
               [b] Increased risk of respiratory depression
               [c] May have delayed onset
               [d] Requires careful monitoring
               [e] Not routinely used in outpatient setting
            (iii) Oral
               [a] Route of choice for mild to moderate pain when tolerating oral intake
               [b] May be as effective as parenteral in appropriate doses
               [c] Assess ability to swallow or chew pills and/or swallow liquids.
            (iv) Intramuscular or subcutaneous injections
               [a] Painful and emotionally upsetting
               [b] Absorption unreliable
               [c] Avoid injections if possible.
      (2) Nonsteroidal anti-inflammatory drugs (NSAIDs)
         (a) Contraindicated in patients with renal disease and those with, or at risk for, actual coagulopathy
         (b) May mask fever

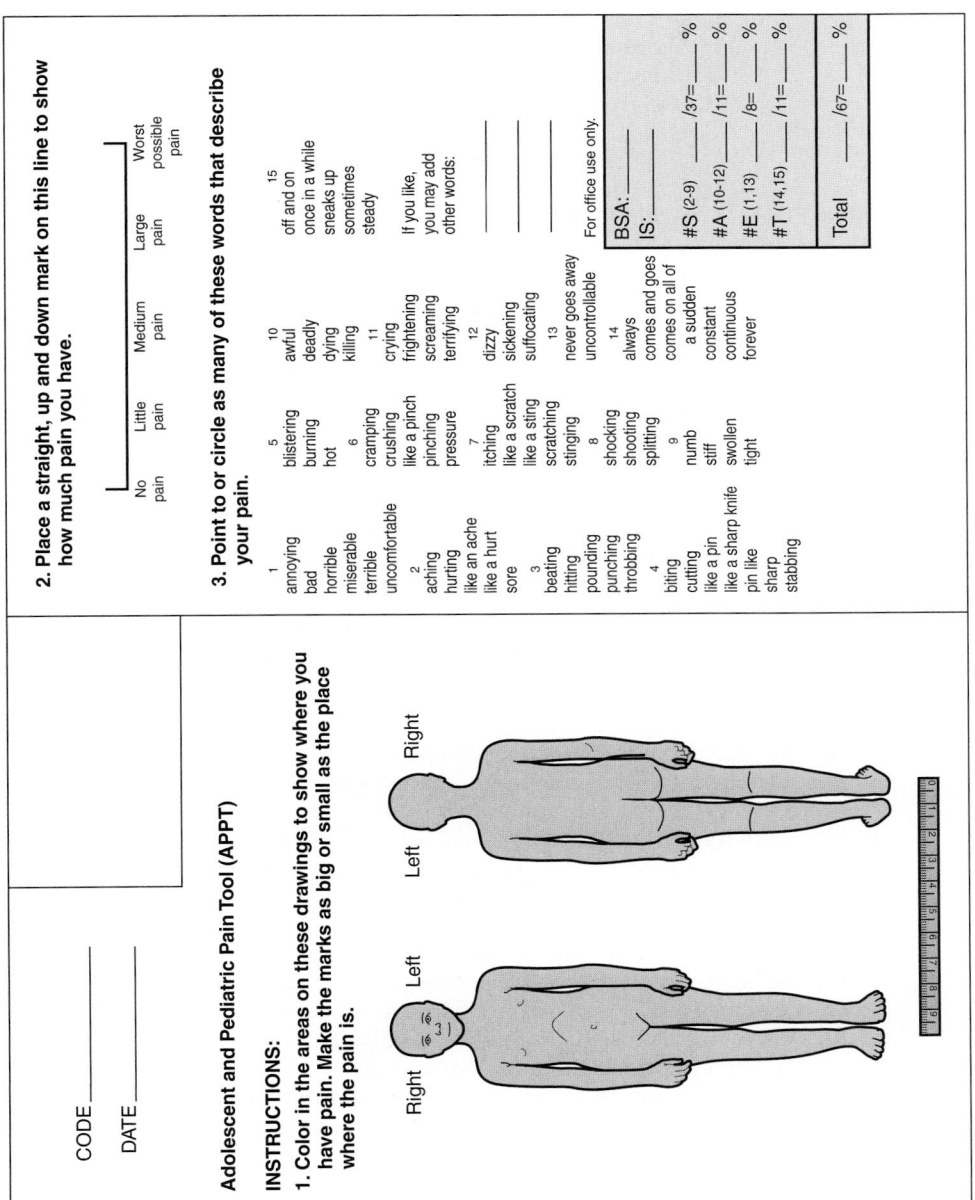

FIGURE 12-1 ■ Adolescent and Pediatric Pain Tool. (From James SR, Ashwill JW, Droske SC: *Nursing care of children*, ed 2, Philadelphia, 2002, WB Saunders.)

(c) May be given in conjunction with opioid(s)

(d) Parenteral

    (i) Ketorolac

        [a] For moderate to severe pain

        [b] May be useful when opioids contraindicated

        [c] Only NSAID approved for parenteral analgesia

        [d] Limit use to 48 to 72 hours.

(e) Oral

    (i) For mild to moderate pain

    (ii) May be administered preoperatively

    (iii) Naproxen

        [a] Longer half-life than other NSAIDs

        [b] Suggested dosage: 5 mg/kg orally, every 12 hours as necessary

VI. POSTPROCEDURAL CONSIDERATIONS FOR ADOLESCENTS (see Chapters 11 and 50)

A. Nursing interventions

  1. PACU phase I

    a. Use safety measures.

      (1) Side rails up

      (2) When adolescent is emerging from anesthesia:

        (a) Provide reassurance.

        (b) Speak in strong voice.

        (c) Orient to place.

        (d) Set limits on unacceptable behavior (e.g., inappropriate language).

    b. Equipment

      (1) Generally same as adult

  2. PACU phase II

    a. Anxiety of patient and family/responsible adult

      (1) Maintain calm, reassuring manner.

      (2) Provide privacy.

      (3) Encourage expression of feelings.

      (4) Give encouragement and positive feedback.

      (5) Encourage parental/responsible adult presence if agreed by patient.

    b. Assess patient for readiness for discharge to home, extended observation, or to extended care environment per facility policy/protocol.

    c. Use discharge criteria as established by facility policy/protocol.

      (1) Comply with standards set by American Society of PeriAnesthesia Nurses, state, and regulatory agencies.

  3. Extended observation

    a. Optimize privacy and comfort for extended stay.

      (1) Assess environment for quieter, less busy area.

      (2) Offer oral intake per ordered diet when appropriate.

      (3) Assess need to use bathroom frequently.

        (a) Offer assistance to bathroom as needed.

    b. Provide options for interested adolescents for entertainment per availability (e.g., movies, hand-held electronic games, books or magazines, card games, music).

B. Postprocedural patient education

  1. Extended observation/intervention

    a. Include adolescent and accompanying adult(s) in patient education and discharge instructions as appropriate.

  2. Ambulatory

    a. Postprocedural instructions

      (1) Provide written instructions to home care provider.

      (2) Younger than 18 years

        (a) Review instructions with the accompanying responsible adult(s), including the adolescent as much as possible in teaching.

(3) Eighteen years and older or emancipated/mature minors
  (a) Review discharge instructions with the adolescent and assess understanding.
  (b) Review instructions with the accompanying adult(s) to optimize postoperative care.
  b. Follow-up visits as indicated (e.g., surgeon, physical therapy, postoperative teaching for equipment)
  c. Provide information regarding procedure findings.
  d. Provide instructions regarding home care.
  (1) Activity
    (a) Discuss impact of tests/procedures/surgery on daily living (e.g., expected return to work or school, driving, sports).
  (2) Diet
  (3) Medications
    (a) Drug and food interactions
  (4) Procedure-specific instructions
  e. Enforce importance of compliance with postoperative instructions.
  f. Confirm safe transport from facility with responsible adult.
  g. Confirm that responsible adult will stay with patient upon return home.

BIBLIOGRAPHY

1. American Society of PeriAnesthesia Nurses: *2008-2010 Standards of perianesthesia nursing practice*, Cherry Hill, NJ, 2009, American Society of PeriAnesthesia Nurses.
2. Chelley JE, ed: *Peripheral nerve blocks*, ed 2: Philadelphia, 2004, Lippincott Williams & Wilkins.
3. DeFazio Quinn DM, Schick L, eds: *Perianesthesia nursing core curriculum: Preoperative, phase I and phase II PACU nursing*, St Louis, 2004, Saunders.
4. Dreger VA, Tremback TF: Management of preoperative anxiety in children. *AORN J* 84(5):778-790; quiz 805-808, 2006.
5. Hazinski MF: *Manual of pediatric critical care*, St Louis, 1999, Mosby.
6. Hicks R, Wenzer LJ, Reilly CA, et al: *Drug information handbook for perioperative nursing*, Hudson, OH, 2006, LexiComp.
7. Hockenberry MJ, Wilson D, eds: *Wong's nursing care of infants and children*, ed 8, St Louis, Mosby, 2007.
8. Ireland D: Unique concerns of the pediatric surgical patient: Pre-, intra-, and postoperatively. *Nurs Clin North Am* 41:265-298, 2006.
9. James SR, Ashwill JW, Droske SC: *Nursing care of children: Principles and practice*, ed 2, Philadelphia, 2002, Saunders.
10. Justus R, Wyles D, Wilson J, et al: Preparing children and families for surgery: Mount Sinai's multidisciplinary perspective. *Pediatr Nurs* 32(1):35-43, 2006.
11. LaMontagne L, Hepworth JT, Salisbury MH, et al: Effects of coping instruction in reducing young adolescents' pain after major spinal surgery. *Orthop Nurs* 22(6):398-403, 2003.
12. Lewandowski LA, Tesler MD, eds: *Family-centered care: Putting it into action: The SPN/ANA guide to family-centered care*, Washington, DC, 2003, American Nurses Association.
13. Marenzi B: Body piercing: a patient safety issue. *J Perianesth Nurs* 19(1):4-10, 2004.
14. Neacsu A: Malignant hyperthermia. *Nurs Stand* 20(28):51-57, 2006.
15. Romino SL, Keatley VM, Secrest J, et al: Parental presence during anesthesia induction in children. *AORN J* 81(4):780-792; quiz 793-796, 2005.
16. Smith JL, Meldrum DJ, Brennan LJ: Childhood obesity: a challenge for the anaesthetist? *Paediatr Anaesth* 12(9):750-761, 2002.
17. Tutag Lehr V, BeVier P: Patient-controlled analgesia for the pediatric patient. *Orthop Nurs* 22(4):298-304; quiz 305-306, 2003.

The Adult Patient

VALLIRE D. HOOPER
JACQUELINE M. ROSS

OBJECTIVES
At the conclusion of this chapter, the reader will be able to:

1. Identify developmental issues associated with each stage of adulthood.
2. Define health, wellness, and illness.
3. List three types of health and illness behaviors.
4. Identify the effects of the stress response on the body's adaptation to surgery.
5. List three characteristics unique to the adult learner.

I. DEFINITIONS
  A. Growth
    1. Increase in body size
    2. Change in structure, function, or complexity of body cell content and metabolic and biochemical processes
    3. Occurs up to some point of optimum maturity
  B. Development
    1. Growth responsibility arising at a certain time in the course of development
      a. Successful achievement
        (1) Satisfaction
        (2) Continued success in future tasks
      b. Failure
        (1) Unhappiness
        (2) Disapproval by society
        (3) Difficulty with later developmental tasks and functions
  C. Maturation and learning
    1. Maturation: emergence of genetic potential for changes in
      a. Form
      b. Structure
      c. Complexity
      d. Integration
      e. Organization
      f. Function
    2. Learning
      a. The process of gaining specific knowledge or skill
      b. Acquiring habits and attitude
      c. Results from experience, training, and behavioral changes
    3. Adequate maturation must be present for learning to occur.
  D. Young adulthood
    1. Age
      a. Young-young adult: 25 to 30 years of age
      b. Old-young adult: 31 to 45 years of age
    2. Birth date and generation
      a. Nexters/Generation Y: born between 1980 and 2000, although dates of generational cohort differ among authors

        (1) Racially and ethnically diverse and tolerant
        (2) Indulged as children; parents spent more time with children
        (3) Blunt with opinions and expressions
        (4) Sense of entitlement
        (5) Techno-savvy; multitasking
        (6) Adaptable to situations and change
        (7) College education expected
        (8) Defining moments
            (a) Oklahoma City bombing—April 19, 1995
            (b) Columbine High School shooting—April 20, 1999
            (c) World Trade Center (9/11)—September 11, 2001
    b. Generation X: born between 1964 and 1979, although dates of generational cohort differ among authors
        (1) A very educated group of individuals in the United States
        (2) Come from families with the highest divorce rate in the country; drastic increase in single-parent homes
        (3) The largest group of latchkey children ever known
            (a) Adept at self-management because of lack of attention in childhood
            (b) Adept at managing their environments
            (c) Comfortable with independent decision-making
        (4) Less optimistic about the future; pragmatic
        (5) Never feel financially secure
        (6) View authority as on same level as self
        (7) Value work-life balance
        (8) Communicate directly, sometimes almost abruptly
        (9) Defining moments
            (a) Challenger explosion—January 28, 1986
            (b) End of Cold War—1985-1991
            (c) Economic turmoil; downsizing and layoffs
            (d) Acquired immunodeficiency syndrome (AIDS)—1981
E. Middle age
  1. Covers ages 45 to 65
    a. Consider the physiologic age and condition of the body
    b. Consider psychological age: how old the person acts and feels
  2. Age divisions
    a. Early middle age: 40 to 55
    b. Late middle age: 56 to 64
  3. Social class will affect age assignment.
    a. Poorer person will perceive prime or midpoint as occurring at an earlier age.
  4. Birth date and generation
    a. Baby Boomers: born between 1946 and 1964, although definition of years vary among authors
        (1) Most were raised in a two-parent home.
            (a) Mother's responsibilities were caring for the children and the home.
            (b) Father was the breadwinner, authority figure, and rarely questioned.
            (c) Most doted on generation by parents; seek personal gratification; considered the "me" generation
        (2) Experienced many social reforms
            (a) Civil rights movement
            (b) Antiwar protests
        (3) Experienced a lot of gains from a thriving economy
        (4) Embrace the attitude of "only the best for me"
        (5) Classified as workaholics
            (a) Take great interest in material rewards
            (b) Value promotion and recognition
        (6) Committed to making the world a better place; fight for causes

    F. Health
       1. Defined by the World Health Organization, 1947, as a state of complete physical, social, and mental well-being; not merely the absence of disease
       2. Often described on a continuum of wellness and illness
    G. Wellness
       1. The ability to adapt, relate effectively, and to function at near maximum capacity
       2. Need to examine functioning in four areas
         a. Physiologic factors: structures and functions of the body
         b. Psychological factors: self-concept as affected by various demographic variables
           (1) Age
           (2) Sex
           (3) Race
           (4) Education
           (5) Economic status
           (6) Other
         c. Sociocultural factors
           (1) Interrelationships with others
           (2) Environmental factors
           (3) Lifestyle
         d. Developmental factors: related to completion of developmental tasks
    H. Disease
       1. A state of non-health
       2. Biological dysfunction present
       3. Major focus of the medical model
       4. Can be legitimized by the health care provider
    I. Illness
       1. The patient's personal perspective of the disease state
       2. Related to the psychosocial impact of the disease on the individual
       3. Individual influences on perception of illness severity
         a. Personality
         b. Demographic characteristics
         c. Presence of support systems
    J. Learning
       1. Process of acquiring wisdom, knowledge, or skill
       2. Overt changes in behavior may be observed.
    K. Teaching
       1. Process of sharing knowledge and insight
       2. Facilitating another to learn knowledge, insight, and skills
    L. Health education
       1. Transmits information, motivates, and helps people adopt and maintain healthful practices and lifestyles
       2. Is concerned with the environment, professional training, and research to maintain and evaluate the process
       3. Traditionally focuses on what the professional thinks is good or needed by the patient
       4. Positive approaches generally more effective than fear
II. STAGES OF ADULTHOOD
    A. Young adulthood
       1. Developmental issues
         a. Settling down
         b. Must enter and successfully manage multiple new roles simultaneously
           (1) Work
           (2) School
           (3) Marriage
           (4) Home
           (5) Child rearing

       c. Primary tasks
         (1) Finding an occupation
         (2) Establishing a new family
           (a) Often done without extended family in area
           (b) Will change jobs and locations more frequently than previous generations
    2. Sociocultural issues
       a. Consistent positive influences
         (1) Abundance of material goods and technology
         (2) Rapid social changes
         (3) Sophisticated medical care
         (4) Accepting of diversity
       b. Constant threats
         (1) Terrorist attacks
         (2) Pollution
         (3) Overpopulation
         (4) Loss of natural resources
       c. Instant media coverage and internet access make the world small and outer space a not-so-distant place.
         (1) All information is easily accessible and readily available.
         (2) Instant, up close, and continuous coverage of traumatic events may cause psychological stress.
           (a) Depression
           (b) Panic and anxiety disorders
           (c) Posttraumatic stress disorder
           (d) Information overload
       d. Other influences
         (1) Changes in women's roles
         (2) Decreasing birth rates
         (3) Increasing longevity
         (4) Cultural and ethnic diversity
    3. Issues affecting response to ambulatory surgery (Box 13-1)
  B. Middle age
    1. Developmental and sociocultural issues
       a. Becoming one of the largest segments of the population
         (1) Earn the most money
         (2) Pay a major portion of the bills and taxes
       b. Yield much power in
         (1) Government
         (2) Politics
         (3) Education
         (4) Religion
         (5) Science
         (6) Business
         (7) Communication

■ BOX 13-1
■ **DEVELOPMENTAL ISSUES AS RELATED TO AMBULATORY SURGERY**

Young Adulthood	Middle Age
▪ Little or no insurance coverage	▪ Physical condition often better indicator of surgical/anesthesia response than chronological age
▪ Needs to return to work or school as soon as possible	▪ More financially stable
▪ May need help with care of home, children, or parents	▪ Better insurance coverage
▪ May expect sophisticated medical technology to be able to fix anything with very little "down" time	▪ May be balancing many professional, civic, and family responsibilities

        c. Common experiences
           (1) Good physical and mental health
           (2) Personal freedom
           (3) Good command of self and the environment
     2. Issues affecting response to ambulatory surgery (Box 13-1)

III. HEALTH, WELLNESS, AND ILLNESS

    A. Health care and prevention

      1. Levels of health care

        a. Health promotion: activities to improve or maintain optimum health

        b. Disease prevention: actions to prevent disease or disability

        c. Diagnosis and treatment: emphasizes early recognition and treatment of health problems

        d. Rehabilitation: designed to limit incapacity caused by health problems as well as to prevent recurrences

      2. Levels of prevention

        a. Primary prevention: ways to prevent illness

        b. Secondary prevention: early identification and treatment of health problems

        c. Tertiary prevention: activities designed to return the physically or emotionally compromised person to the highest possible level of health

      3. Ambulatory arena now involved in all levels of health care and prevention

IV. HEALTH AND ILLNESS BEHAVIOR

    A. Health behavior

      1. Activities undertaken by those believing themselves to be healthy

      2. Purpose: to prevent disease or detect it in an asymptomatic stage

      3. Examples

        a. Breast self-exam

        b. Regular exercise

        c. Prudent heart living

        d. Routine checkups

        e. Ambulatory procedures

           (1) Routine screening colonoscopy

           (2) Follow-up cardiac catheterization in nonsymptomatic patient

    B. Illness behavior

      1. Activities carried out in response to a set of symptoms by those who feel ill

      2. Allow individuals to determine their state of health and need for treatment

      3. Limited to health-seeking behavior to identify and/or assess the changes occurring or to search for a solution

      4. Influences affecting illness behavior

        a. Recurrence of symptoms

           (1) The more frequent or severe the symptoms, the more likely that outside help will be sought.

        b. Visibility and consequences

           (1) The more apparent the symptoms, the more illness behavior exhibited

           (2) If the disorder is attached to stigma, the individual will be less likely to seek help.

           (3) Help will usually be sought for life-threatening symptoms.

        c. Perceived seriousness or severity

           (1) Disorders perceived as serious lead to earlier illness behavior.

           (2) Influences on perception of symptom severity

              (a) Social class

              (b) Health belief system

              (c) Hierarchy of other needs and desires

d. Availability of treatment and the medical care system
  (1) Distance, costs, convenience, time, effort, and fear of outcome affect willingness to seek help.
  (2) Individual subordination by the health care system also affects willingness to seek treatment.
e. Knowledge and significance of symptoms
  (1) Lack of knowledge of symptom significance often influences the individual to seek help.
f. Cultural and social expectations
  (1) Cultural and ethnic backgrounds affect symptom interpretation and notion of when it is acceptable to seek health care.
  (2) Lower classes are more influenced by symptoms interfering with important roles.
  (3) The elderly use more health care services.
  (4) Women seek medical attention more frequently than men.
  (5) Those with a lack of access to care encounter issues with prevention and detection.

C. Sick role behavior
  1. Activities undertaken by individuals who consider themselves ill for the purpose of getting well
  2. Learned and influenced by evaluation and legitimization from others
  3. Assumed when one accepts being ill, initiates some form of action, and demonstrates a desire to be well again
  4. Major role components divided into rights and obligations
    a. Rights
      (1) Exemption from normal responsibilities
        (a) Dependent on the nature and severity of the illness
        (b) Requires validation or legitimization by others and the physician
        (c) Once legitimized, person obligated to avoid responsibilities
      (2) Right to be cared for
        (a) Person not expected to recover by an act of will or decision
        (b) Is not responsible for becoming sick and therefore has a right to be cared for
        (c) Physical dependency and the need for emotional support are acceptable.
    b. Obligations
      (1) Obligation to want to become well
        (a) Being ill is seen as undesirable.
        (b) The sick role can result in secondary gains.
        (c) Motivation to recover is of primary importance.
      (2) Obligation to seek and cooperate with technically competent help
        (a) The individual needs the technical expertise that health care professionals can provide.
        (b) Cooperation with these professionals for the goal of getting well is mandatory.
  5. Ambulatory implications
    a. Patient may need to be educated that sick role behavior is acceptable and often expected after ambulatory procedures.
    b. Ambulatory procedures often reduce the amount of time spent in the sick role.

V. STRESS RESPONSE SYNDROME
  A. Definitions
    1. Stress
      a. A socio-psychophysiologic phenomenon
      b. A composite of intellectual, behavioral, metabolic, and other physiologic responses to a stressor or stressors of internal or external origin
      c. Influenced by environmental, psychological, and social factors
      d. Uniquely perceived by the individual

    2. Stressors (stress agents)

      a. May be internal or external

      b. Examples

        (1) Cold

        (2) Heat

        (3) Infectious organisms

        (4) Disease processes

        (5) Fever

        (6) Pain

        (7) Imagined events

        (8) Intense emotional involvement

    3. Stress response

      a. Initiated in response to a stressor

      b. Is protective and adaptive by nature

      c. Regulated by the nervous and endocrine systems

        (1) Sympathetic nervous system (SNS)

        (2) Pituitary gland

        (3) Adrenal gland

      d. The magnitude of the response depends on the perceived severity of the threat.

    4. Survival depends on one's ability to balance between stressors and adaptive capacities.

B. General adaptation syndrome

    1. Developed by Hans Selye

    2. Most widely accepted and frequently used physiologic theory of stress and adaptation

    3. Three stages

      a. Alarm stage

        (1) Begins with the first exposure to the stressor

        (2) Fight or flight mechanism activated

          (a) Heart rate increases.

          (b) Cardiac output increases.

          (c) Stroke volume increases.

          (d) Peripheral vasoconstriction

          (e) Increased perspiration

          (f) Gastrointestinal upset

        (3) In most situations, the body's defensive forces are mobilized to deal with the stressor.

        (4) Death can occur if the stressor is strong enough to result in exhaustion of the body's adaptive mechanisms and energy supply.

      b. Stage of resistance or adaptation

        (1) Reflects "adaptation" as the body fights back

        (2) Psychological mobilization occurs.

        (3) Influences on ability to adapt

          (a) Physical functioning

          (b) Coping skills

          (c) Total number of stressors experienced

      c. Stage of exhaustion

        (1) A progressive breakdown of compensatory mechanisms and homeostasis

        (2) Occurs only if the stress becomes overwhelming, is not removed, or if the individual is ineffective in coping with it

        (3) All energy for adaptation exhausted

        (4) Physiologic and psychological collapse will ensue.

C. Physiologic responses to stress

    1. The initial response is stimulated by the central nervous system.

    2. Information is then forwarded to the hypothalamus, which integrates and coordinates the homeostatic adjustments.

     3. Hypothalamus stimulates the autonomic nervous system and the anterior and posterior pituitary.

     4. The physiologic responses to hypothalamic stimulation and their effects on the surgical patient are listed in Table 13-1.

D. Psychosocial responses to stress

     1. Primary theory is the stress-appraised event theory by Lazarus.

       a. Looks at stress and adaptation from the viewpoint of cognition, perception, and transaction

         (1) The way the individual interprets the situation will determine whether he or she perceives it as stressful.

       b. Positive and negative events can result in stress.

       c. Emphasis is on the process or dynamics of what is happening.

     2. Cognitive appraisal

       a. The mental process used by the person to assess an event in relation to his or her well-being and available coping resources and options

       b. Evaluative forms

         (1) Irrelevant appraisal

           (a) Occurs if the event is considered to be of no concern or impact on the current level of well-being

         (2) Benign-positive appraisal

           (a) Occurs if the event is considered as indicative of a positive state of affairs

           (b) The event shows that all is well.

         (3) Stressful appraisal

           (a) Occurs with a negative evaluation of the present or future state of well-being

           (b) Occurs in three forms

             (i) Harm–loss: damage or injury has already taken place.

             (ii) Threat: harm or loss has not yet occurred but is expected.

             (iii) Challenge

               [a] The possibility for growth or mastery is perceived.

               [b] The opportunity for gain outweighs the possible risk of harm.

     3. Coping modes

       a. Defined as those efforts used to manage the environmental and internal demands exceeding personal resources; mobilized in response to an event perceived as stressful

       b. Accomplished by eight coping modes

         (1) Escape–avoidance

           (a) Wishful thinking and other behavioral efforts to escape or avoid the problem

         (2) Confrontive

           (a) Aggressive efforts to alter the situation

           (b) Involves some degree of hostility and risk taking

         (3) Distancing

           (a) Attempt to detach from the situation and thus minimize the significance

         (4) Self-control

           (a) Strive to regulate one's feelings and actions

         (5) Seeking social support

           (a) Seek information, tangible and emotional support

         (6) Accepting responsibility

           (a) Acknowledge one's own role in the problem

           (b) Attempt to rectify the situation

         (7) Planful problem solving

           (a) Deliberate and analytical approach to altering the situation

         (8) Positive reappraisal

           (a) An effort to focus on the positive side or opportunity for personal growth

■ TABLE 13-1
■ ■ **Physiologic Responses to Hypothalamic Stimulation**

Responding Organ/ System	Organ/ System Action	Physiologic Response	Surgical Adaptation	Surgical Maladaptation
Autonomic nervous system	Triggers the SNS to stimulate exocrine glands	Sweating	No impact	No impact
	Triggers the SNS to stimulate epinephrine and norepinephrine release	Decreases insulin and increases glucagon release	Increased amino acids for wound healing; increased wound healing	Negative nitrogen balance that may negatively impact tissue repair unless reversed Development of excessive scar tissue and adhesions Increased blood sugar is detrimental to diabetics. Increased heat loss may result in hypothermia, shivering, and increased oxygen demand.
		Constriction of vascular smooth muscle Increase in BP	Shifts blood away from periphery to the vital organs Decreases blood loss by increasing clotting	May decrease renal perfusion Increased thrombus formation
		Increased heart rate and contractility Bronchodilation	Increased myocardial perfusion Increased oxygen and perfusion to vital organs Increased oxygen exchange Improved ventilation	Increased workload for heart; may lead to heart failure Hypertension No maladaptation as a result of bronchodilatation

	Kidneys are stimulated to release renin Converted to aldosterone by angiotensin II. Aldosterone results in sodium and water retention at the renal tubules, resulting in increased blood volume.	Increased blood volume helps to reduce hypovolemia Maintenance of BP and cardiac output	Hypervolemia Hypertension Circulatory overload Heart failure Prolonged anti-inflammatory response may lead to infection. See above for other maladaptive responses.
Anterior pituitary	Releases ACTH Stimulates the adrenal cortex to release aldosterone and cortisol	Aldosterone results in increased blood volume. Cortisol results in increase in blood glucose and protein and fat catabolism.	Increased blood sugar Increased wound healing Increased energy Increased anti-inflammatory responses
Posterior pituitary	Stimulates the release of vasopressin/ADH	Causes sodium and water retention at the renal tubules: Results in increased blood volume	See above

SNS, sympathetic nervous system; BP, blood pressure; ACTH, adrenocorticotropin hormone; ADH, antidiuretic hormone.

    E. Behavioral responses to stress
        1. Anger, hostility, antagonism, noncompliance
        2. Depression, apathy, crying, inability to concentrate
        3. Grief, shock, denial, withdrawal
        4. Acceptance, information seeking, planning, decision-making
    F. Factors affecting response to stressors
        1. Nature of specific stressors encountered
        2. What the stressors mean to the patient
            a. May differ based on past experience and development
            b. Ill patients may become less mature, less discriminating, and less reality oriented.
        3. Patient's characteristic mode of coping with stress
            a. Depends on personality
            b. Threat of hospitalization or surgery may be responded to by:
                (1) An aggressive manner
                (2) Resignation
                (3) Seeking constant information
        4. Patient's current psychological resources
            a. Determines the person's resiliency and ability to endure the stress without decompensation
            b. Affected by:
                (1) Level of self-esteem and social support
                (2) Presence or absence of any underlying depression or chronic anxiety
        5. Hardiness factor
            a. A personality characteristic
                (1) A sense of control over one's life
                (2) Involvement and commitment to productive activities
                (3) Anticipation of change as an exciting positive challenge
            b. Acts as a buffer between stress and illness
VI. STRESS MANAGEMENT
    A. Assessment of current level of stress
    B. Intervention
        1. Physical relaxation and stress management
            a. Progressive relaxation
            b. Acupuncture and acupressure
            c. Biofeedback
            d. Massage
            e. Therapeutic touch
        2. Cognitive methods of relaxation and stress management
            a. Thought stopping
            b. Positive self-talk
            c. Assertive communication training
            d. Laughter, humor, play, tears
            e. Guided imagery
        3. Time and resource management
        4. Other nursing interventions
            a. Acknowledge individual feelings and behaviors.
            b. Develop trusting relationship.
            c. Involve family and significant others.
VII. HEALTH PROMOTION AND PREVENTION
    A. Activities designed to improve or maintain optimum health
    B. Likelihood to participate in such behaviors influenced by internal and external cues
        1. Internal cues include bodily states such as feeling good or energetic.
        2. External cues
            a. Interactions with significant others
            b. Impact of media communication

       c. Visual stimuli from the environment
  C. Strategies include:
    1. Physical, physiologic
      a. Proper nutrition
      b. Balance of exercise and rest
      c. Cessation of destructive health habits (smoking, alcohol, or drug abuse)
      d. Health screening
    2. Emotional
      a. Effective communication
      b. Promotion of self-esteem, self-confidence, security
      c. Anxiety reduction measures
      d. Crisis resolution
    3. Cognitive
      a. Coping methods
      b. Visualization and imagery
      c. Health education
    4. Social
      a. Family, friend, peer relations
      b. Group associations and processes
      c. Maintenance of cultural ties
    5. Spiritual and moral
      a. Values clarification
      b. Acknowledgment of meaning and purpose of life
      c. Establishment of belief system
      d. Establishment of moral and ethical behaviors
VIII. PREOPERATIVE HEALTH HISTORY INTERVIEW (see Chapter 15)
  A. Should focus on age-specific issues in addition to general preoperative assessment and preparation
  B. Young adulthood
    1. Generally a healthy population
    2. Pertinent health problems include:
      a. Upper respiratory infection
      b. Influenza
      c. Essential hypertension
      d. Mitral valve prolapse
      e. Iron deficiency anemia
      f. Simple diarrhea
      g. Cystitis
      h. Acute pyelonephritis
      i. Chronic fatigue syndrome
      j. AIDS
      k. Hepatitis B
      l. Cervical, breast, and testicular cancer
  C. Middle age
    1. Variety of health problems may begin to develop.
    2. Pertinent health problems include:
      a. Sinusitis
      b. Hiatal hernia
      c. Duodenal peptic ulcer disease
      d. Angina pectoris
      e. Secondary hypertension
      f. Hyperthyroidism
      g. Hyperuricemia or gout
      h. Diabetes mellitus type II
      i. Acute and chronic prostatitis
      j. Lumbosacral strain

IX. HEALTH TEACHING–LEARNING (see Chapter 3)
   A. Teaching is a critical nursing intervention that is crucial to successful outcomes in the ambulatory setting.
      1. Teaching and learning processes are related.
      2. Teaching–learning process is easily integrated into the nursing process.
   B. Phases of the teaching–learning process
      1. Assessment
         a. Begins with an assessment of the nurse's teaching abilities
         b. Gather information about the patient, his or her learning needs, and his or her readiness to learn.
            (1) Patient's level of understanding, ability to comprehend, and any obstacles to learning (sensory losses, language barriers) should be identified during the general psychosocial assessment.
            (2) Assessment should also include patient's interest level, attentiveness, and current understanding about upcoming procedure.
         c. A realistic teaching plan should be established based on:
            (1) Patient's current level of knowledge
            (2) Nurse's ability to provide the new information needed by the patient
         d. A plan to identify and dispel patient misconceptions should also be included
      2. Diagnosis
         a. Diagnose the patient's learning needs.
         b. Set teaching priorities.
      3. Planning
         a. Set goals with the patient.
         b. Determine behavioral objectives.
         c. Select teaching and evaluation methods.
            (1) Content and type of information
            (2) Type of media used
            (3) Who will be involved?
            (4) The environment and time frame in which it will be provided
      4. Intervention
         a. Use appropriate strategies for instruction.
      5. Evaluation
         a. Evaluate patient outcomes.
         b. Revise and reevaluate as needed.
   C. Characteristics of the adult learner
      1. Readiness to learn is determined by life tasks, roles, and immediate problems.
      2. Application of learning is related to the relevancy of the problems.
      3. Orientation to learning is independent and self-directed.
      4. Value of experiences
         a. Experiences are internalized.
         b. Experiences provide a foundation for further learning.
         c. May contribute to resistance to change
      5. Rate of learning
         a. Resistant to learning nonrelevant material
         b. Aging process increases time needed to complete some learning tasks.
      6. Barriers to learning
         a. Family, work, or community responsibilities may compete with learning time and energy.
         b. Anxieties about self-image may also threaten ability to learn.
      7. Cultural differences
         a. Unique beliefs should be respected.
         b. Use interpreters and/or audiovisual aids for persons who do not speak English.

c. Be knowledgeable of cultures, ethnic groups, and religions commonly encountered in your environment.
8. Educational background
    a. Identify level of formal education attained by the patient.
    b. Remember that level of formal education does not equate with one's ability to learn.
    c. Determine patient's reading level.
    d. Determine patient's health knowledge.
    e. Determine patient's feelings about education and learning.
    f. Use pictures for patients with low literacy skills.
D. Domains of learning
    1. Cognitive: concerns the learner's knowledge and understanding
    2. Affective: concerned with the learner's attitudes, emotions, and ways of adjusting to an illness
    3. Psychomotor: concerned with motor skills
E. Goals of teaching
    1. To forewarn or provide information
    2. To teach skills (Foley catheter care, dressing changes, etc.)
    3. Assist in decision-making and planning.
    4. Family involvement in patient care
    5. Reinforcement of existing knowledge
    6. Explain procedures, follow-up, and medications.
    7. Discuss future events, expectations.
    8. Advice about home health follow-up, home management
    9. Encourage change, provide alternative behaviors or thoughts.
F. Maximizing teaching–learning effectiveness
    1. Allow sufficient time.
    2. Choose appropriate time and environment.
    3. Confirm patient readiness.
        a. Preoperative: admission details taken care of
        b. Postoperative: pain controlled, stable, awake, family present
    4. Actively involve the learner.
    5. Use creativity in approaches.
    6. Encourage learner to contribute to ideas.
    7. Use humor or novelty to help learner relax and retain the content.
    8. Organize material logically and present it in manageable amounts.
    9. Highlight or point out important information.
    10. Differentiate between similar concepts and contrasting information.
    11. Allow practice as much as possible, giving constructive feedback.
G. Common barriers to effective teaching–learning
    1. Providing false reassurance
    2. Invading privacy
    3. Minimizing or ignoring feelings
    4. Not listening
    5. Giving wrong information
    6. Violating trust relationship
    7. Noisy environment
    8. Lack of privacy
    9. Physiologic distraction (pain, nausea, vomiting, etc.)
    10. Health literacy issues
        a. Refers to individuals' ability to understand their health care issues and effectively care for themselves within the health care system
        b. Encompasses the skills that patients require to improve their health and navigate within the health care environment
        c. Assume that literacy level 3 to 4 years below last completed year of education.
        d. Lower income and blue-collar workers tend to have lower health literacy.
        e. Essential in promotion of self-care

BIBLIOGRAPHY

1. Berman A, Snyder SJ, Kozier B, et al: *Kozier & Erb's fundamentals of nursing: Concepts, process, and practice*, ed 8, 2008, Pearson Education.
2. Burmeister WL: *Hiring/developing future leaders*. Presented at Southern Company training session, Birmingham, AL, 2000.
3. Cutilli CC: Health literacy in geriatric patients: An integrative review of the literature. *Orthop Nurs* 26(1):43-48, 2007.
4. Hooper VD: The next generation. *J Perianesth Nurs* 17(3):219-221, 2002.
5. Kupperschmidt BR: Understanding generation X employees. *J Nurs Adm* 28(12):36-43, 1998.
6. Lancaster L, Stillman D: *When generations collide: Who they are. Why they clash. How to solve the generational puzzle at work*, New York, 2003, Harper Business.
7. Lubkin IM, Larson PD, eds: *Chronic illness: Impact and interventions*, ed 5, Boston, 2002, Jones & Bartlett.
8. McCance KL, Huether SE: *Pathophysiology: The biologic basis for disease in adults and children*, ed 5, St Louis, 2006, Mosby.
9. Meisenhelder JB: Anniversary responses to terrorism. *Am J Nurs* 102(9):24AA-24EE, 2002.
10. Mitchell S: *American generations: Who they are, how they live, what they think*, ed 3, Ithaca, NY, 2000, New Strategist Publications.
11. Nielsen-Bohlman L, Panzer AM, Kindig DA, the Committee on Health Literacy: *Health literacy: A prescription to end confusion*, Washington, DC, 2004, National Academies Press.
12. Strauss W, Howe N: *Generations*, New York, 1990, William Morrow & Company.
13. Taylor CR, Lillis C, LeMone P, et al: *Fundamentals of nursing: The art & science of nursing care*, ed 6, Philadelphia, 2008, Lippincott Williams & Wilkins.
14. Taylor RB, David AK, Johnson TA, et al: *Family medicine: Principles & practice*, ed 6, New York, 2003, Springer-Verlag.
15. Tulgan B: *Managing generation X: How to bring out the best in young talent*, New York, 2000, W.W. Norton & Company.
16. Watson DS: Wanted: a few good nurses. *AORN J* 76(1):8-11, 2002.
17. White L: *Foundations of nursing*, ed 2, 2005, Thomson Delmar.
18. Zemke R, Raines C, Filipczak B: *Generations at work*, New York, 2000, Amacon.
19. Zimmerman PG: Generation X staff. *J Emerg Nurs* 26:492–495, 2000.

14 The Geriatric Patient

JENNIFER ALLEN*

OBJECTIVES
At the conclusion of this chapter, the reader will be able to:

1. Identify changes that occur with aging using a systems approach.
2. Describe the demographics of the geriatric patient.
3. Identify potential problems that may occur after a surgical procedure.
4. Discuss the purpose of a preoperative assessment.
5. Identify postoperative priorities in consideration of the physiologic changes that occur with aging.

I. OVERVIEW
    A. Geriatric patients present a unique challenge.
    B. Physiological changes and pathological conditions mandate utilization of the nursing process.
II. DEFINITION OF GERIATRIC OR OLDER ADULT
    A. Age 65 years or older and when one qualifies for retirement income
        1. 65 to 74 years: "young-old"
        2. 75 to 84 years: "old"
        3. ≥85 years: "old-old"
    B. Life expectancy
        1. Men: 81 years
        2. Women: 84 years
    C. Number of older adults in United States is increasing.
        1. By 2030, the older population will double to about 72 million people.
            a. One in five will be 65 or older.
            b. The age group 85 years and older is the fastest growing cohort of the United States population.
            c. The 85 and older population is projected to increase from 4.7 million in 2003 to 9.6 million in 2030.
        2. Members of minority groups are projected to represent 26.4% of the older population in 2030.
        3. More than 2 million Americans celebrated their sixty-fifth birthday in 2003 (5574 per day).
        4. Older adults account for one third of all health care costs.
            a. Focus is shifting to health promotion and health maintenance.
            b. Nurses need to be aware of what health promotion and maintenance practices will benefit the older adult.
            c. Recommended health practices

---

* The views expressed in this chapter are those of the author and do not necessarily reflect the official policy or position of the Department of the Navy, Department of Defense, nor the United States Government.

(1) Diet
(2) Exercise
(3) Tobacco cessatation and alcohol reduction
(4) Physical examinations and preventive care
(5) Dental examinations and preventive care

5. There were 50,639 persons aged 100 or more in 2003 (0.17% of total population).
6. Number of centenarians is expected to grow quickly, with estimates of 381,000 by 2030.

D. The Silent Generation, also known as the Veteran Generation (people born before 1946)
   1. Comprise 10% of today's work force
   2. Rely on tried and true ways of doing things
   3. Core values include:
      a. Dedication and sacrifice
      b. Hard work
      c. Conformity
      d. Law and order
      e. Respect for authority
      f. Patience
      g. Duty before reward
      h. Adherence to rules
         (1) Honor
            (a) A keen sense of ethical conduct
            (b) One's word given as a guarantee of performance
   4. Veteran generational personality
      a. Likes consistency and uniformity
      b. Likes things on a grand scale
      c. Are conformers
      d. Believe in "logic" not "magic"
      e. Are disciplined
      f. Are past oriented and history absorbers
      g. Believe in law and order

E. The Baby Boomers (people born from 1946 though 1964)
   1. Comprise approximately 45% of today's work force and one third of all Americans in 2007
   2. Due to size, this group has had and will continue to have a great influence in all areas of society.
   3. By 2030, all the baby boomers will be 65 years or older.
   4. Unprecedented implications for all areas of society, especially health care
   5. There is no typical baby boomer; they are extremely diverse and differ by:
      a. As much as 19 birth years
      b. Race
      c. Culture
      d. Socioeconomic status
   6. Baby boomers paid their dues and climbed the ladder under the old rules.
   7. Core values include:
      a. Optimism
      b. Team orientation
      c. Personal gratification
      d. Health and wellness
      e. Youth
      f. Personal growth
      g. Involvement
      h. Work

8. Baby Boomer generational personality
   a. Dedicated and driven
   b. Equate work with self-worth
   c. Define themselves through their jobs, achieve identity by work performed
   d. Arrive early and leave late
   e. Chose profession with intent to make the world a better place
   f. Believe you must pay your dues
   g. Believe they do not have to grow old and be sedentary
   h. Also called the Sandwich Generation, responsible for aging parents while still caring for teenage and college-age children

III. THEORIES OF AGING
   A. Biological theories
      1. Cellular functioning
      2. Stochastic (error) theories
         a. Wear and tear theory
         b. Cross-linkage theory
         c. Free radical theory
            (1) Free radical and antioxidants
      3. Nonstochastic theories
         a. Programed aging theory
         b. Gene theory
         c. Immunity theory
      4. Emerging biological theories
         a. Neuroendocrine control or pacemaker theory
         b. Caloric restriction (metabolic) theory
   B. Sociological theories
      1. Role theory
      2. Activity theory
      3. Disengagement theory
      4. Continuity theory
      5. Age stratification theory
      6. Social exchange theory
      7. Modernization theory
   C. Psychological theories
      1. Jung's theories of personality
      2. Developmental theories of Erikson and Peck
         a. Theory of psychosocial development most widely used
         b. Emphasis on healthy personality rather than pathologic approach
            (1) Stresses rational and adaptive natures of individual
            (2) Explains child's behaviors in mastering developmental tasks
         c. Stages of development
            (1) Each stage has two components—favorable and unfavorable aspect of conflict.
            (2) Progression to next stage depends on resolution of conflict.
            (3) Conflict never mastered completely—remains a recurrent problem throughout life.
         d. Stage VIII relates to the older adult.
            (1) Ego integrity versus despair stage (stage VIII)
               (a) Old age
               (b) Results from satisfaction with life and acceptance of what has been
               (c) Despair is a result of remorse for what might have been.
               (d) Ego integrity results in renunciation and wisdom and concern with life in the face of death.
               (e) Process achieved through introspection
         e. Peck expanded on the original work of Erikson.
            (1) Identification of discrete tasks of late life
            (2) Achievement of tasks will result in ego integrity.
            (3) Tasks represent a movement toward Erikson's final stage.

3. Maslow's Hierarchy of Human Needs

    a. Focuses on attributes or characteristics that contribute to healthy personality development

    b. Concerned with uniqueness and potential of individuals

        (1) Humans motivated by two need systems

            (a) Basic

                (i) Food, water, and shelter

            (b) Growth needs—internally motivated and reinforced

                (i) Beauty

                (ii) Self-fulfillment

        (2) Needs arranged in a hierarchy

            (a) Lower-level needs assume dominance.

            (b) When one level need is satisfied, the next becomes predominant.

            (c) Theory does not address developmental stages or shaping of human behaviors.

IV. PHYSIOLOGIC CHANGES OF AGING: CHANGES IN BOTH STRUCTURE AND FUNCTION

    A. Changes that occur with aging are not incidental, they are expected.

        1. Changes begin the moment life begins.

        2. Changes become more apparent in the fifth or sixth decade.

        3. In seventh and eighth decades, physiologic changes are significant and no longer deniable.

        4. Changes in aging are predictable, but not the exact time they occur.

        5. The timing and degree of aging is affected by heredity, environment, and health maintenance.

    B. Functional age is impacted by:

        1. Chronic disease processes

        2. Personal attitudes and outlook

        3. Family and friends network

    C. Nervous system

        1. Divided in two systems

            a. Central nervous system (CNS)

                (1) Consists of brain and spinal cord

            b. Peripheral nervous system

                (1) Consists of cranial nerves and spinal nerves

                (2) Includes the somatic nervous system and the autonomic nervous system

            c. Many functions occur at an unconscious level.

            d. Other activities are done at a conscious level.

        2. Neurogenic atrophy and reduction of peripheral nerve fibers

            a. Decreased blood flow and CNS activity

                (1) Causing slower reaction times

                (2) Reduced ability to cope with body stressors

                (3) Diminished ability to respond to demands on cardiovascular systems

                (4) Prolonged emergence from pharmacologic interventions (e.g., benzodiazepines) and decreased pain perception

            b. Decreased cognitive function

                (1) Loss of memory and decreased understanding

                (2) Lengthening of learning speed

                (3) Higher risk of confusion

                (4) Short attention span

                (5) Decreased sensory abilities

                    (a) Impaired hearing acuity

                        (i) Men especially lose high-frequency sounds.

                        (ii) Deafness

                        (iii) Decrease in acoustic acuity

                    (b) Vestibular changes may also alter balance and/or cause vertigo.

                    (c) Visual precision is reduced.

(i) Lenses fail (as in cataracts).
(ii) Glaucoma
(d) Decreased tactile perception
(e) Acuity of smell diminished
(i) May impair hygiene
(6) Postoperative cognitive dysfunction in the elderly may persist at least 3 months after otherwise uncomplicated surgery.

c. Homeostatic mechanism slows, altering sympathetic and parasympathetic responsiveness.
(1) Decreased sensitivity to baroreceptors
(2) Change in thermoregulation
(a) Affected by autonomic impairment
(b) Changes to skin and blood vessels
(c) Impaired by many chronic medications
(d) Elderly vulnerable to heat stroke and hypothermia

d. Compromised perfusion caused by arteriosclerotic changes
(1) Increased incidence of organic brain syndrome
(2) Increased incidence of cerebrovascular accidents (strokes)
(3) Increased incidence of microemboli
(4) Decreased cerebral blood flow
(5) Decreased cerebral metabolic oxygen consumption
(6) Decreased CNS activity

3. Common disorders
a. Cerebral arteriosclerosis
b. Cerebral vascular accident
c. Parkinson's disease
d. Dementia
e. Alzheimer's disease

4. Nursing implications
a. Allow additional time to assimilate information and give responses.
b. Prepare for possible increased length of stay in ambulatory surgery.
c. Encourage use of sensory aids.
(1) Hearing aids
(2) Visual aids
(a) Glasses
(b) Contacts
(c) Magnifying glass
d. Include family member or responsible adult in instructions.
e. Verbal communication
(1) Face patient when speaking.
(2) Raise speaking volume, not pitch.
(3) Speak slowly and clearly.
f. Observe for prolonged or toxic effects of drugs.
(1) Encourage lower doses.
g. Safety measures
(1) Handrails
(2) Other assistive devices
(a) Canes, walkers, nonslip shower chairs
(3) Nonskid footwear
(4) Physical support by caretaker
(5) Observation

D. Respiratory system
1. Includes the nose, pharynx, larynx, trachea, bronchi, bronchioles, alveolar ducts, and alveoli
a. Provides for ventilation and gas exchange
b. Facilitates transfer of oxygen into and removal of carbon dioxide from the blood
c. Depends on the musculoskeletal system and CNS to function

2. Airway
   a. Edentia
      (1) Impacts patency of airway
      (2) Creates difficulty in intubation
   b. Decreased bone mass of jaw
3. Anatomic changes
   a. Increased anteroposterior diameter
   b. Progressive flattening and decreased muscle strength of diaphragm
   c. Increased chest wall rigidity
      (1) Arthritic changes in rib cage
   d. Reduction in alveolar surface
   e. Narrowing of intervertebral disks
      (1) Reduces total lung capacity by 10%
   f. Loss of skeletal muscle mass, leading to wasting of diaphragm and skeletal muscles
   g. Loss of teeth changes jaw structure, leading to difficult airway maintenance.
4. Physiologic changes
   a. Reduction in pulmonary elasticity
   b. Decreased chest wall mobility
   c. Loss of alveolar septa, leading to air trapping
   d. Decreased pulmonary compliance
   e. Increased airway resistance
   f. Decreased cough and gag reflex, leading to risk of aspiration
   g. Ventilation and perfusion alterations develop.
      (1) Decreased tidal volume
      (2) Decreased vital capacity
      (3) Decreased inspiratory reserve
      (4) Decreased cardiac output
      (5) Decreased aerobic capacity
      (6) Increased dead space
      (7) Decreased oxygen and carbon dioxide exchange
      (8) Decreased oxygen content of blood
         (a) $Pao_2 = 100 - (0.4 \times \text{Age in years}) = \text{mm Hg}$
         (b) For example, in an 80 year old: $Pao_2 = 100 - (0.4 \times 80) = 68 \text{ mm Hg}$ (vs normal Pao_2 of 100 mm Hg)
   h. Environmental changes impact the respiratory system.
      (1) Smoke
      (2) Dust
         (a) Air pollution
5. Common disorders
   a. Chronic obstructive pulmonary disease (COPD)
   b. Influenza
   c. Pneumonia
   d. Tuberculosis
   e. Lung cancer
6. Nursing considerations
   a. Airway
      (1) Assess airway constantly.
      (2) Protect unconscious airway.
         (a) Suction oropharynx as needed.
         (b) Support and position.
      (3) Provide appropriate airways and oxygen delivery supplies.
      (4) Inserting dentures can help support the airway.
   b. Secretions and effective cough
      (1) Position
         (a) With head elevated when possible
         (b) To maximize chest expansion

  (2) Encourage coughing and deep breathing.

  (3) Ensure reflexes have returned before administering oral fluids.

 c. Oxygenation

  (1) Monitor oxygen saturation (e.g., pulse oximeter).

  (2) Support with oxygen as necessary.

 d. Pain

  (1) Alleviate pain.

  (2) Use anxiety- and stress-reduction tactics.

E. Cardiovascular system

 1. Comprises the heart, blood, blood vessels, and the lymphatics

  a. Transports oxygen- and nutrient-enriched blood to the organs

  b. Transports waste products to the excretory organs

 2. Cardiovascular disease is the leading cause of death of older adults in the United States.

 3. Most changes are caused by arteriosclerotic changes.

  a. Loss of large artery elasticity

   (1) Coronary

   (2) Aorta

   (3) Carotid

   (4) Iliac

   (5) Femoral

   (6) Popliteal

   (7) Renal

  b. Decreased organ perfusion and decreased compensatory regulation from loss of elasticity

  c. Vessel fragility

  d. Increase in systolic blood pressure

 4. Loss of tissue elasticity

  a. Organ perfusion decreases

   (1) Myocardium

   (2) Decreases optimal regulation of all body systems

  b. Peripheral circulation impaired

   (1) Lowers tolerances to stress response (heart workload increases)

   (2) Along with decreased collagen, increases difficulty of venipuncture

    (a) Aging collagen makes tough "rolling" veins.

    (b) Loss of elasticity is likely to cause bleeding around site during and after venipuncture.

   (3) Higher risk for bruising

   (4) Increases peripheral vascular resistance

    (a) Restricts left ventricular ejection

    (b) Promotes cardiac hypertrophy

   (5) Potential for orthostatic hypotension

  c. Increased susceptibility to clotting disorders

   (1) Stroke

   (2) Thrombosis

   (3) Embolism

 5. Cardiac conduction system

  a. Decreased heart rate

   (1) Resulting from increased parasympathetic activity

   (2) Resulting from degenerative changes in conduction system

  b. Dysrhythmias and blocks occur more frequently.

  c. Can lead to CNS changes

  d. Myocardial changes

   (1) Left ventricular hypertrophy

   (2) Increased myocardial irritability, leading to dysrhythmias

   (3) Fibrosis of endocardial lining, leading to endocardial thickening and rigidity, decreased contractility

   (4) Calcification of valves, leading to valve incompetence

6. Altered hemodynamics
   a. Pump effectiveness diminishes because of atrophy of myocardial fibers.
   b. Decrease in cardiac output (1% per year after 30 years of age)
   c. Slower circulation time
   d. Prolonged onset of action and clearing times for drugs
   e. Increased blood pressure
   f. Systolic blood pressure increases with aging, reflecting development of poorly compliant arterial walls.
   g. Heart rate decreases, suggesting increase in activity of parasympathetic nervous system.
   h. Slowed circulation time, leading to slower onset of drug effects
   i. Decreased cardiac reserve; stressors
      (1) Fever
      (2) Tachycardia
      (3) Exertion
      (4) Anxiety
      (5) Hypoxemia
      (6) Pain
7. Orthostatic hypotension
   a. Decreased blood vessel tone, leading to peripheral pooling of blood, increased risk for deep vein thrombosis
   b. Baroreceptor failure
   c. Medications (most common cause)
      (1) Antihypertensives
      (2) Diuretics
      (3) Tricyclic antidepressants
      (4) Phenothiazines
      (5) Alcohol
   d. Decreased tolerance to volume changes
8. Common disorders
   a. Coronary artery disease
   b. Coronary valve disease
   c. Congestive heart failure
   d. Peripheral vascular disease
9. Nursing considerations
   a. Observe responses to medications.
      (1) Allow adequate time for response before repeating.
      (2) Use lower range of medication dosage and encourage team to use lower dosages.
   b. Monitor for cardiac inadequacy.
      (1) Lungs
         (a) Provide adequate oxygenation.
            (i) Encourage deep breathing.
            (ii) Watch for fluid overload while ensuring adequate hydration.
      (2) Heart
         (a) Assess heart sounds.
         (b) Cardiac monitoring for arrhythmias
         (c) Assess lung sounds.
         (d) Avoid extremes of blood pressure.
            (i) Watch for orthostatic changes.
         (e) Encourage slow position changes.
         (f) Vascular considerations
            (i) Gentle venipunctures
         (g) Avoid tourniquets where possible.
            (i) Minimize use of automatic blood pressure devices.
            (ii) Adequate pressure on sites after venipuncture or catheter removal
         (h) Encourage early ambulation.

F. Integumentary system
1. The largest organ of the body, includes the skin, hair, and nails
2. Loss of subcutaneous fat
   a. Compromises thermoregulation
   b. Increased risk of hypothermia
   c. Loss of padding for bony prominences
3. Increase in overall body fat (especially women)
   a. Increased availability of lipid storage sites
      (1) Reservoir for lipid-soluble (fat-soluble) drugs: diazepam, midazolam, enflurane
      (2) Prolongs drug action
4. Loss of sweat glands
5. Decreased skin pigmentation caused by decreased production of melanocytes; pallor does not equal anemia
6. Epidural atrophy and loss of collagen
   a. Increases risk of skin breakdown and injury
   b. Decreases skin elasticity and turgor
7. Common disorders
   a. Basal cell carcinoma
   b. Pressure ulcers
   c. Inflammation and infection
   d. Hypothermia
8. Nursing considerations
   a. Provide warmed blankets and warm environment during and after operative event.
   b. Protect skin with:
      (1) Proper positioning
      (2) Padding on bony prominences
      (3) Use paper or other nontearing skin tape.
   c. Remember, loss of pigmentation mimics pallor.
      (1) Do not rely on skin color to assess for anemia or cardiac distress.
   d. Provide careful positioning and safety instructions.
G. Musculoskeletal system
1. Multifunctional and complex system made up of bones, joints, tendons, ligaments, and muscles
   a. Age-related changes are not life-threatening, but may affect the ability to function and ultimately the quality of life.
2. Osteoporosis: inappropriately low bone mass for age, gender, and race
   a. Leads to decline in bone matrix
   b. Peak bone mass around 30 to 40 years of age
   c. Mineral content of bone (bone density) decreases.
      (1) After 40 years of age
      (2) For men, 0.5% per year
      (3) About 1.0% per year for women
   d. Skeletal support compromised
   e. Bone reabsorption exceeds bone formation.
   f. Increased risk of fractures, pain, skeletal deformities
      (1) Repair of hip fractures is one of top five surgeries done in elderly patients.
   g. Decrease in flexibility
   h. Risk factors
      (1) Age
      (2) Female
      (3) Low body weight
      (4) White race
      (5) Cigarette smokers

3. Degenerative changes in vertebrae increase difficulty of spinal anesthesia and intubation.
   a. Degeneration of bone causes
      (1) Pathologic changes
         (a) Vertebral degeneration
4. Kyphoscoliosis
   a. Limits chest expansion and capacity
   b. Limits success in establishing spinal or epidural injection
   c. Compression fractures
   d. Increased potential for pathologic fracture
   e. Higher incidence of traumatic fractures (falls especially)
5. Osteoarthritis
   a. Specific cause unknown, but there is demonstrated relationship with:
      (1) Advancing age
      (2) Wear and tear of joints throughout life span
   b. Structural changes in the joint
      (1) Probably starts in cartilage
      (2) Leads to:
         (a) Reduced mobility of joint
         (b) Difficult ambulation
         (c) Potential for falls
         (d) Pain
         (e) Less flexibility
   c. May compromise intraoperative positioning
6. Common disorders
   a. Osteoporosis
   b. Degenerative joint disease
   c. Fractures
7. Nursing considerations
   a. Careful positioning throughout perioperative experience
      (1) Support for back
      (2) Alignment
      (3) Protection of bony processes
   b. Observe for prolonged or toxic effects of regional agents.
   c. Provide for pain relief.
   d. Assist patient with physical tasks related to strength.
      (1) Moving
      (2) Ambulation
      (3) Exercise
         (a) Gentle movement
         (b) Encourage frequent activity.
   e. Safety concerns
      (1) Concerted fall prevention program
         (a) Fall risk assessment with individualized plan
         (b) Environmental assessment
            (i) Floor surfaces may be slippery, wet, or uneven.
            (ii) Poor lighting or blinding light
            (iii) Bathrooms not fall proof
            (iv) Cluttered hallways and patient rooms
         (c) Support when walking: cane, walker, rails
         (d) Treaded (skid-resistant) footwear
         (e) Education for patient and caretakers
            (i) Potential for accidental falls: use skid-resistant slippers, handrails
            (ii) Other safety measures: side rails, bed alarms
H. Digestive system
   1. Includes the GI tract and accessory organs that assist in the digestive process

    a. Begin to identify age-related changes in the fifth decade

    b. GI tract includes the mouth, pharynx, esophagus, stomach, small and large intestine.

    c. Accessory organs include the liver, gall bladder, and exocrine pancreas.

2. Decreased salivation

3. Decreased peristalsis

    a. Gastric emptying delayed

    b. Increased risk of aspiration

    c. Increased problem of constipation

4. Decreased hepatic blood flow resulting from arteriosclerotic changes

5. Decreased microsomal enzyme activity

    a. Delayed drug metabolism (e.g., fentanyl, vecuronium)

6. Decreased absorption of orally administered drugs and nutrients (e.g., ferrous sulfate iron and calcium)

7. Malnutrition possible

    a. Can increase perioperative morbidity

    b. Can compromise postoperative recovery and wound healing

    c. Most reliable indicator of malnutrition is hypoalbuminemia.

8. Common disorders

    a. Hiatal hernia

    b. Gastroesophageal reflux disease

    c. Diverticulitis

    d. Hemorrhoids

    e. Colon cancer

9. Nursing considerations

    a. Careful administration of oral fluids and food

        (1) Start with small amounts.

        (2) Begin when sitting up if possible.

    b. Elevate head of bed for most effective gastric emptying.

    c. Consider ulcers with complaint of chest pain.

        (1) Observe for prolonged or toxic drug effects.

I. Renal and genitourinary systems

    1. Includes two kidneys, two ureters, bladder, and urethra

        a. The urinary system is responsible for the removal of waste and excess fluid from the body.

        b. The kidneys are highly vascular.

            (1) Produce the hormone erythropoietin, which stimulates red blood cell production.

            (2) Produce the enzyme renin, which helps regulate blood pressure.

            (3) Continuously filter blood and regulate water, salts, and maintain acid-base balance.

    2. Decreased bladder capacity (200 mL)

    3. Decreased muscle tone and weakened sphincters

        a. Especially in women after multiple obstetric deliveries

        b. May result in incontinence

        c. Increased residual urine

    4. Enlarged prostate (men) may result in urinary incontinence and retention.

    5. Atrophic changes of vagina and urethral mucosa in women

    6. Decreased renal plasma flow

    7. Decreased glomerular filtration rate

        a. Resulting from decreased blood flow

        b. Decreases 1% to 1.5% per year after 30 years of age

        c. Results in decreased renal metabolism

            (1) Decreased clearance of medications and metabolites

            (2) Examples: fentanyl, vecuronium, midazolam

    8. Response time to correct fluid and electrolyte balance increased

        a. May increase risk of fluid overload

        b. Decreased ability to concentrate urine

c. Inability to conserve sodium, leading to hyponatremia

d. Decreased activity of renin or aldosterone, leading to hyperkalemia

9. Common disorders

a. Urinary incontinence

b. Urinary tract infection

c. Chronic renal failure

10. Nursing implications

a. Observe for fluid imbalance.

(1) Monitor intake and output.

(2) Encourage oral fluids postoperatively.

b. Observe for effects of electrolyte imbalance.

(1) Monitor and/or observe for cardiac dysrhythmias, electrocardiogram (ECG) changes.

(2) Consider that hyponatremia may be a cause of confusion.

c. Observe for prolonged medication effect.

(1) Use lower dosage range of medications, and encourage smaller medication dosage by team.

(2) Provide support for toileting needs.

(a) Toilet frequently (offer urinal or bedpan).

(b) Assist to bathroom.

(c) Facilitate genitourinary hygiene.

(d) Provide protection for bedding and clothing.

(e) Reassure and support emotionally.

(f) Regard privacy to diminish embarrassment.

J. Endocrine system

1. The endocrine system works in conjunction with the neurological system to regulate and integrate body activities.

2. Includes the pituitary gland, thyroid gland, parathyroid gland, adrenal glands, and endocrine pancreas

3. Decreased ability to metabolize glucose

a. Results in glucose intolerance

b. Pancreatic function declines.

(1) Increased incidence of adult-onset diabetes mellitus

(2) Greatest between 60 and 70 years of age

c. Plasma renin concentrating ability decreases 30% to 50%.

4. Decreased production of renin, aldosterone, and testosterone

5. Decreased vitamin D absorption

6. Increased activation and increased plasma concentration of antidiuretic hormone

7. Common disorders

a. Diabetes mellitus

b. Hypoglycemia

c. Hypothyroidism

10. Nursing implications

a. Monitor laboratory values.

b. Educate the patient.

(1) Dietary requirements

(2) Blood glucose self-testing

K. Hematologic and immune system

1. Decreased bone marrow production

2. Decreased T-cell function

3. Increased autoantibodies

4. May see anemia and autoimmune diseases (see Chapter 29)

L. Sensory changes

1. Visual changes

a. Decreased visual acuity

b. Decreased peripheral vision

c. Decreased accommodation (presbyopia)

      d. Retinal vascular changes

      e. Cataract formation

      f. Increased incidence of glaucoma

    2. Auditory changes

      a. Decreased sensitivity to sound (presbycusis)

      b. Loss of high-pitched sound perception

      c. Impairment of sound localization

    3. Tactile changes

      a. Decreased sensation

      b. Decreased response to pain

    4. Taste and smell acuity decreases.

M. Laboratory changes

    1. Decreased potassium

      a. Medications, diuretics

      b. Diet deficient in potassium

    2. Decreased sodium

      a. Dilutional

      b. True decrease

      c. Renal failure

    3. Decreased hemoglobin

      a. Blood loss (GI and postmenstrual uterine bleeding)

      b. Malabsorption of iron

      c. Malnutrition

N. Neuropsychiatric changes

    1. Acute brain syndrome

      a. Physiologic

      b. Rapid onset

      c. Reversible

      d. Possible causes—always rule out hypoxemia first!

        (1) Medication intolerance

        (2) Metabolic disturbance

        (3) Electrolyte imbalance

          (a) Hypernatremia and hyponatremia

        (4) Nutritional deficit

        (5) Depression

        (6) Stress, fear, anxiety

    2. Chronic brain syndrome

      a. Associated with arteriosclerosis

      b. Degenerative changes

        (1) Alzheimer's disease

        (2) Cerebrovascular accident (stroke)

        (3) Dementia

    3. Depression

      a. Causes: isolation, illness, loss, biochemical changes

      b. Symptoms: fatigue, insomnia, anorexia, somatic changes

O. Pathophysiologic conditions in elderly

    1. Of people 75 years of age, 86% have one or more of the following chronic conditions

      a. Cardiovascular: hypertension, atherosclerosis, dysrhythmias, valve disease

      b. Cerebral: cerebrovascular accident, cognitive degeneration

      c. Pulmonary: COPD, asthma

      d. Endocrine: diabetes mellitus, hypothyroidism

      e. Neurologic: Parkinson's disease

      f. Musculoskeletal: arthritis

      g. Sensory: visual and hearing loss

      h. Hepatic: cirrhosis

    2. Physical status changes increase anesthetic and surgical risk.

   V. PSYCHOSOCIAL CONSIDERATION FOR THE ELDERLY
- **A.** Maintain and promote autonomy.
  - **1.** Independence
    - **a.** Encourage performance of self-care.
    - **b.** Address issues of concern.
      - (1) Advance directives
      - (2) Quality-of-life issues
    - **c.** Talk with, not "around," the patient.
    - **d.** Inquire about preferences.
      - (1) Name use (e.g., "What do you prefer that I call you?")
      - (2) Time schedules (eating, sleeping, etc.)
  - **2.** Competence
    - **a.** Reduced ability to provide self-care leads to depression and reduced self-worth
    - **b.** Abilities to perform may alter with time of day, health status, and life events
    - **c.** Elders require more practice with new skills.
    - **d.** Repetition and clarification enhance learning
- **B.** Encourage self-acceptance.
  - **1.** Maintain patient dignity.
  - **2.** Invite expression of fears.
    - **a.** Death and dying
    - **b.** Change in body image and function
  - **3.** Review coping mechanisms.
  - **4.** Present patient with decision alternatives when possible.
- **C.** Time concept is altered.
  - **1.** Employ tactics for time orientation.
    - **a.** Time perception of elapsed time
    - **b.** Past, present, and future
- **D.** Social awareness
  - **1.** Older adults are experiencing life role changes.
    - **a.** May outlive friends and family (especially old-old)
    - **b.** Caregivers become the patients (drastic role change when other party is already ill and debilitated).
  - **2.** Encourage participation of significant others.

  VI. ELDER ABUSE (USUALLY RELATED TO FAMILY OR OTHER CAREGIVER)
- **A.** Types
  - **1.** Material and financial
  - **2.** Physical
    - **a.** Sexual
    - **b.** Beating, slapping, kicking
    - **c.** Neglect
      - (1) Passive
      - (2) Active (especially old-old)
      - (3) Self
    - **d.** Emotional
    - **e.** Verbal
      - (1) Threatening physical abuse or isolation
      - (2) Humiliation
      - (3) Intimidation
    - **f.** Withholding (e.g., care, food, company)
    - **g.** Abandonment
- **B.** Detection
  - **1.** Physical assessment and evidence of bodily harm
    - **a.** Bruises
    - **b.** Skin tears
    - **c.** Burns
    - **d.** Evidence of restraint

      2. Emotional abuse (difficult to assess)
         a. Fear of violence
         b. Social isolation
   C. Mandatory reporting
      1. Different laws in each state
   D. Resources
      1. Adult protection programs
      2. Domestic violence programs
      3. Services
         a. Financial advocacy
         b. Social advocacy
         c. Religious groups
VII. PHARMACOLOGIC ALTERATIONS IN AGING
   A. Pharmacokinetics
      1. Study of drug actions; includes absorption, distribution, metabolism, and excretion
      2. Determines the concentration of drugs in the body
   B. Pharmacodynamics
      1. Describes the interaction of chemicals in medications being consumed and the receptors in the body
         a. Responses to medications are less predictable in the older adult.
         b. Pathologic changes may affect the response to medications.
         c. Receptors may respond normally to some medications and not to others.
         d. Receptors may be more sensitive and lead to an increased risk for toxicity.
   C. The Beers criteria are guidelines for nurses to use to increase awareness of potentially inappropriate medications and possible adverse drug reactions in geriatric patients.
   D. Alterations in organs responsible for drug metabolism and clearance
      1. Lungs
      2. Kidneys
      3. Liver
   E. Protein binding of medications impaired
      1. Increases amount of available (free, unbound) drug
         a. Free drug is active drug, increasing drug effects.
   F. Storage of lipid-soluble medications increased
      1. Unpredictable clearance and elimination
   G. Prolonged action and elimination of medications
      1. Require decreased doses of medications
      2. Increased risk of cumulative drug effects
      3. Increased risk of adverse drug reactions
   H. Issues and trends in medication usage
      1. Polypharmacy is a situation when multiple medications are taken at the same time.
         a. May be multiple medications of the same class for chronic illness
         b. May be related to multiple chronic illnesses
         c. May be due to the addition of over-the-counter medications and supplements added to the prescribed medications
      2. Financing medication use
      3. Self-prescribing
      4. Drug-herbal interactions
      5. Drug-food interactions
      6. Drug-drug interactions
      7. Adverse drug reactions
VIII. CONSIDERATIONS BEFORE SURGERY (Box 14-1)
   A. Advantages of ambulatory surgery for the elderly
      1. Decreased risk of nosocomial infections
         a. Wound infections
         b. Respiratory infections

■ BOX 14-1
■ **COMMON SURGICAL PROCEDURES PERFORMED ON THE GERIATRIC PATIENT**

- Ophthalmic: cataract, vitrectomy
- Genitourinary: cystoscopy, transurethral resection of the prostate
- Orthopedic: open reduction and internal fixation—hip, joint replacement
- Cardiovascular: pacemaker, carotid endarterectomy
- General: herniorrhaphy

    2. Decreased incidence of mental confusion
      a. Environment less disruptive
      b. Decreased disruption in personal routine
    3. Minimized length of stay away from home environment
    4. Cost-effectiveness
  B. Disadvantages of ambulatory surgery for the elderly
    1. Compliance to the plan of care
      a. Diminishing abilities
        (1) Cognitive (e.g., forgetfulness)
          (a) Unable to complete care regimen
          (b) Unable to cope with changes in routine
            (i) New medication protocols
            (ii) Care related to procedure
        (2) Physical
          (a) Diminished stamina and strength for self-care
          (b) Increased potential for falls
          (c) Unaware of wound contamination
      b. Lack of support system at home
        (1) Transportation issues and other logistic issues
        (2) Financial concerns (unable to obtain medications, supplies)
        (3) Lack of caregiver or significant other
        (4) Reduced or nonexistent circle of friends (especially in the old-old)
  C. Preoperative assessment (see Chapter 15)
    1. To obtain precise baseline
      a. Consider physiologic not chronologic age.
      b. Age alone does not determine risk.
    2. To obtain information about preexisting disease
      a. Especially with ambulatory patients
      b. Includes medications used and appropriateness of use
      c. Acute versus chronic conditions
      d. Skin and pressure ulcer risk assessment
      e. Previous surgical history
        (1) Allow patient enough time to discuss history.
        (2) Past tolerance to surgical procedures
        (3) History of nausea and vomiting
        (4) History of malignant hyperthermia
        (5) Include accompanying adult in discussion as appropriate.
      f. Risk assessment
        (1) Coexisting diseases increase with age.
        (2) General health status
          (a) American Society of Anesthesiologists Status Classification
        (3) Functional health status
          (a) Complications more common in inactive patients
        (4) Nutritional status
          (a) Healing is delayed if undernourished.
          (b) Decreased albumin level is a risk for increased complications and mortality.
          (c) Serum albumin is warranted if poor nutrition is suspected.

(5) Psychological status
   (a) Social support systems
   (b) Will to live
   (c) Dementia
(6) Heart disease
   (a) Cardiac complications such as myocardial infarction and heart failure increase risk of complications and possible deaths.
   (b) Any rhythm other than sinus rhythm
   (c) Risk increased if premature atrial contractions are present
   (d) Symptoms of heart failure (e.g., jugular vein distention, a third heart sound)
   (e) Hypertensive and cardiac medications should not be withdrawn before surgery.
(7) Carotid artery disease
(8) Pulmonary disease
   (a) Increases the risk of perioperative complications
   (b) Smoking history
   (c) Severe COPD increases risk of surgery.
       (i) Ineffective cough
       (ii) Inability to clear secretions
   (d) Emphysema
(9) Liver disease
   (a) Poor surgical outcome likely
   (b) Coagulopathies
(10) Renal disease
   (a) Assess by measuring blood urea nitrogen and serum creatinine.
   (b) Dehydration should be corrected preoperatively.
(11) Sleep disorders
   (a) Obstructive sleep apnea
       (i) Characterized by repetitive cessation of respiration (>10 seconds) during sleep
       (ii) May experience hypopnea
       (iii) Excessive daytime sleepiness
       (iv) Assessment should include information from sleeping partner.
       (v) Therapy is dependent on the severity of sleep apnea.
   (b) Insomnia
3. To review or obtain laboratory information
   a. Anemia common
   b. Electrolyte imbalance
      (1) Hypokalemia resulting from diuretics
      (2) Hyponatremia resulting from inability to conserve sodium
      (3) Glucose levels in diabetic patients
4. To identify special needs
   a. Prostheses
   b. Language and communication barriers
   c. Mobility aids
   d. Barriers to ambulatory patient returning home
      (1) Transportation
      (2) Caregiver availability, ability to care for self
      (3) Access to follow-up care
5. To anticipate postoperative sequelae and to reduce risk factors
6. To begin patient teaching
7. To maximize preoperative physical status
   a. Pulmonary function
   b. Nutritional status, including hydration
   c. Medication protocol

8. Perioperative beta-blockade management
   a. Beta-blocker use is appropriate when:
      (1) Prescribed preoperatively, continue beta-blockers perioperatively
      (2) High or intermediate risk of cardiac complications undergoing emergent, vascular, or other major surgery
      (3) Consider beta-blockade for older adults at low risk of cardiac complications undergoing vascular surgery.
      (4) Begin beta-blockade several days to 1 week before surgery to achieve heart rate less than 70 beats per minute.
      (5) Continue after surgery with a goal of less than 80 beats per minute in the postoperative period.
      (6) Withhold if:
         (a) Heart rate less than 55 beats per minute or systolic blood pressure less than 100 mm Hg
         (b) Patient has asthma, decompensated heart failure, or third-degree heart block.
   D. Multidisciplinary assessment
      1. PACU nurse
      2. Anesthesiologist
      3. Surgeon
      4. Medical consultation as needed
IX. INTRAOPERATIVE CONSIDERATIONS FOR THE OLDER ADULT
   A. Sensory
      1. Avoid loud noises.
         a. Music
         b. Conversation not including the patient
      2. Allow patient to keep sensory aids if possible.
      3. Maintain voice, tactile, or visual contact with awake patient.
   B. Environment
      1. Remember thermostatic needs.
         a. Increased risk when core body temperature falls below 96.8° F (36° C)
      2. Protective measures
         a. Raise room temperature.
         b. Use warming blankets or devices.
         c. Warm anesthetic gases, solutions, IV fluids.
         d. Cover patient's head.
   C. Positioning
      1. Change slowly and gently; avoid extremes.
      2. Lift patient! Do not pull!
      3. Support back of neck (e.g., prevent discomfort from kyphosis or arthritis).
      4. Pad and support to protect pressure points.
   D. Circulation: remember that hypotension and slowed circulation predispose patient to thrombus formation and emboli.
      1. Use antiembolitic stockings or sequential compression devices.
         a. Especially high-risk patient
         b. Prolonged (greater than 2 hours) procedures
      2. Observe for points of pressure that might inhibit blood flow to extremities.
   E. Nurse-monitored local anesthesia; monitoring notes
      1. Older adults do not tolerate fluid or blood loss well.
         a. When patient approaches hypovolemia, small changes can have large impact.
         b. Monitor fluid loss and output carefully.
      2. Impending crisis may be indicated by fluctuations in cardiac rate and rhythm.
X. ANESTHETIC OPTIONS FOR OLDER ADULT PATIENT (see Chapter 22)
   A. General anesthesia
      1. Smooth induction and rapid recovery
      2. Inhalation requirements less
         a. Minimum alveolar concentration decreases by 4% per year after 40 years of age.

      3. Delayed clearance or metabolism of IV anesthetic agents
        a. Decrease dose of barbiturates, benzodiazepines, opioids.
      4. Increased risk of hypothermia
      5. If edentulous, may be difficult to ventilate by mask
      6. Arthritis may limit cervicospinal mobility for intubation.
   B. Regional anesthesia
      1. Minimal physiologic alterations
      2. Decreased cardiopulmonary complications
      3. Less postoperative confusion
      4. Provides postoperative analgesia
      5. Spinal anesthesia
        a. Lower abdomen and lower extremity surgery
        b. Duration prolonged in older adult
        c. Hypotension may be pronounced.
        d. May be complicated by musculoskeletal changes
        e. Low incidence of spinal headaches
      6. Epidural anesthesia
        a. Less hypotension
        b. Greater cardiovascular stability
        c. Reduced anesthetic dose requirements
   C. Intravenous sedation and analgesia
      1. Increased sedating effects of benzodiazepines
      2. Increased respiratory depressant effects of narcotics
      3. Because of coexisting diseases, may not be appropriate for RN to administer intravenous moderate sedation
   D. Ambulatory surgery
      1. Minimizes separation from family and environment
      2. May be appropriate depending on type of surgery
        a. Must consider risks of anesthetic, surgery, home care
XI. POSTANESTHESIA PRIORITIES FOR THE OLDER ADULT PATIENT IN PHASE I (Box 14-2)
   A. Reduction of morbidity and mortality
   B. Ventilation
      1. Promote optimal gas exchange.
        a. Provide high-humidity oxygen.
        b. Promote deep breathing and coughing.
        c. Prevent atelectasis.
        d. Elevate head of bed to facilitate lung expansion.

■ BOX 14-2
■ **EXAMPLES OF RELATED NURSING DIAGNOSIS CATEGORIES**

- Impaired gas exchange
- Potential for infection
- Ineffective breathing pattern
- Alteration in fluid volume (excess or deficiency)
- Ineffective thermoregulation: hypothermia
- Knowledge deficit: preoperative/postoperative information
- Alteration in comfort: pain; nausea/vomiting
- Sensory-perceptual alteration
- Ineffective airway clearance
- Impaired physical mobility
- Self-care deficit
- Impaired communication: hearing loss/verbal/foreign language barrier

2. Prevent respiratory infections.
  a. Sterile suctioning of endotracheal tube
  b. Protect patient from aspiration.
  c. Promote deep breathing (prevent pneumonia).
3. Monitor for compromised function.
  a. Observe for residual drug effects.
  b. Maintain artificial airways.
  c. Use pulse oximetry monitoring.
  d. Consider preexisting disease.
C. Fluid balance (see Chapter 21)
  1. Correct preoperative dehydration.
    a. Nothing by mouth status
    b. Diuretic therapy
    c. Poor nutritional status
    d. Presence of nausea and vomiting
  2. Prevent fluid overload.
    a. Assess preexisting cardiopulmonary disease.
    b. Monitor intake and output.
    c. Assess breath sounds.
  3. Monitor urine output.
    a. Decreased bladder capacity
    b. Urinary retention (men), incontinence (women)
    c. Perioperative diuretics
    d. Perioperative fluid intake
    e. Decreased awareness of distension
D. Activity—"stir-up" routine
  1. Promotes circulation and ventilation
  2. Permits assessment of neurologic status
    a. Deviations from preoperative status
  3. Monitor for orthostatic hypotension when mobilizing outpatients.
    a. Mobilize more slowly than younger adults.
E. Thermoregulation (see Chapter 24)
  1. Rewarm patient.
  2. Document temperature.
  3. Normothermia promotes cardiovascular stability.
F. Comfort (see Chapter 26)
  1. Positioning
    a. Care in turning; turn frequently
    b. Anatomic and surgical alignment
    c. Pad bony prominences
  2. Skin care
    a. Avoid excessive tape application.
    b. Remove tape and ECG leads carefully.
    c. Dry wet skin promptly.
    d. Hold venipuncture sites after removal of needle.
    e. Remove skin preparation solutions to decrease irritation.
  3. Pain management
    a. Titrate narcotics
    b. Pain increases myocardial oxygen demand.
    c. Consider decreased sensory response to pain.
    d. Evaluate presence of residual preoperative or anesthetic drugs.
  4. Psychological support
    a. Reorientation
    b. Avoid sensory deprivation and overload.
    c. Avoid use of restraints.

      d. Continue verbal and tactile communication.

      e. Provide hearing aids, glasses, and dentures.

      f. Provide simple, clear instructions—ascertain patient's level of understanding.

      g. Rule out hypoxemia as cause of postoperative agitation.

      h. Maintain dignity and respect.

    5. Social support

      a. Family visitation in PACU phase I

XII. POSTANESTHESIA PHASE II AND EXTENDED OBSERVATION PHASE (see Chapter 52)

  A. Physical status

    1. Ensure safety.

      a. Orient/reorientation

      b. Ambulate carefully.

        (1) Sit on edge of stretcher to gain balance.

        (2) Provide physical support for walking.

          (a) Use orthopedic and prosthetic devices as necessary.

          (b) Lower stretcher

          (c) Step stool with caution (they tip!)

        (3) Encourage, while allowing patient to find own pace of movement.

      c. Return all sensory aids before ambulation.

      d. Monitor neuromuscular status.

    2. Psychological interventions

      a. Promote wellness concept.

        (1) Return clothes and belongings promptly.

        (2) Reunite with family members, responsible adult, significant others.

      b. Communicate with patient expecting:

        (1) Slower thought processes, movements, and responses

        (2) Old does not mean stupid!

    3. Home preparation

      a. Include support persons when reviewing home instructions.

      b. Verify plans for home support.

        (1) Ascertain patient, family, or responsible adult's understanding of and ability to comply with discharge instructions.

        (2) Older adult caring for older adult may not be adequate or responsible.

        (3) Arrange time and place for postoperative contact.

          (a) Recovery issues evaluation

            (i) Consider tool easily understood by patient.

            (ii) Introducing a Likert-type scale to patient before surgery would be beneficial.

            (iii) Discuss possible topics of postoperative telephone contact.

      c. Instruct on return to normal preoperative medication regimen.

      d. Instructions

        (1) Avoid sedating medications.

        (2) Provide clear verbal instructions.

        (3) Provide large-print written instructions.

          (a) Large, simple diagrams or pictures

        (4) Ascertain understanding (patient and other care providers as necessary).

          (a) By demonstration

          (b) Return demonstration

        (5) Repeat instructions.

BIBLIOGRAPHY

1. American Society of Anesthesiologists: *Syllabus on geriatric anesthesiology*. Available at: www.asahq.org/clinical/geriatrics/syllabus.htm. Accessed January 6, 2008.

2. Ang P, Knight H, Matadial C, et al: Managing acute postoperative pain: Is 3 hours too long? *J Perianesth Nurs* 19(5):312-330; quiz 331-333, 2004.

3. Beers MH, Berkow R: *The Merck manual of geriatrics*, Whitehouse Station, NJ, 2000, Merck Research Laboratories.

4. Capezuti E, Zwicker D, Mezey M, et al: *Evidence-based geriatric nursing protocols for best practice*, ed 3, New York, 2008, Springer Publishing.

5. Centers for Disease Control and Prevention–National Center for Health Statistics: *Health, United States, 2006: Special excerpt: Trend tables on 65 and older population*. Available at: www.cdc.gov/nchs/data/hus/hus06_SpecialExcerpt.pdf. Accessed January 27, 2008.

6. Drain C, Odom-Forren J: *PeriAnesthesia nursing: A critical care approach*, Philadelphia, 2008, WB Saunders.

7. Ebersole P, Hess P, Touhy TA, et al: *Toward healthy aging*, ed 7, St Louis, 2008, Mosby.

8. Gould E: Tips for effective communication with older adults. *Breathline* 25(2):15, 2005.

9. Hart SM: Generational diversity impact on recruitment and retention of registered nurses. *J Nurs Adm* 36(1):10-12, 2006.

10. Hartford Institute for Geriatric Nursing, New York University College of Nursing: *ConsultGeriRn*. Available at: www.consultgerirn.org. Accessed January 27, 2008.

11. Iacono M: Osteoporosis: A national public health priority. *J Perianesth Nurs* 22(3):175-180; quiz 181-182, 2007.

12. Laney M, Bayley E: Incidence of adult immunization for influenza and pneumonia in a preadmission testing unit. *J Perianesth Nurs* 17(5):325-336, 2002.

13. Mamaril M: The epidemiology of our aging population. *Breathline* 23(4):2, 2003.

14. Mamaril M: Assessing neurological changes in the aging patient. *Breathline* 24(2):7, 2004.

15. Mamaril M: Cardiac changes in the aging patient. *Breathline* 24(2):7, 2004.

16. Mamaril M: Polypharmacy in the geriatric population. *Breathline* 24(6):5, 2004.

17. Mamaril M: Advocating cultural sensitivity in older adults. *Breathline* 25(5):3, 2005.

18. Mamaril M: Nursing considerations in the geriatric surgical patient: the perioperative continuum of care. *Nurs Clin North Am* 41(2):313-328, 2006.

19. Mamaril M, Saufl N, editors: Focus Issue: Geriatric Care. *J Perianesth Nurs* 19(6):371-443, 2004.

20. Martin C: Bridging the generation gap. *Nursing* 34(12):62-63, 2004.

21. McKenney K: Anesthesia considerations in older adults. *Breathline* 24(5):7, 2004.

22. Mezey MD, Berkman BJ, Callahan CM, et al: *The encyclopedia of elder care*, Amherst, NY, 2004, Prometheus Books.

23. Molony SL: *Beers' criteria for potentially inappropriate medication use in the elderly*. Try This Series Issue 16, 1999. Available at: www.hartfordign.org/publications/trythis/issue16.pdf. Accessed January 21, 2008.

24. Rakel B, Herr K: Assessment and treatment of postoperative pain in older adults. *J Perianesth Nurs* 19(3):194-208, 2004.

25. Reuben DB, Herr KA, Pacala JT, et al: *Geriatrics at your fingertips 2007-2008*, ed 9, New York, 2007, American Geriatrics Society.

26. Swearingen S, Liberman A: Nursing generations expanded look at the emergence of conflict and its resolution. *Health Care Manag (Frederick)* 23(1):54-64, 2004.

27. US Census Bureau: *65+ in the United States: 2005: Current population reports*. Available at: www.census.gov/prod/2006pubs/p23-209.pdf. Accessed January 6, 2008.

28. US Department Health and Human Services: *A profile of older Americans: 2004*. Available at: www.aoa.gov/prof/Statistics/profile/2004/2004profile.pdf. Accessed January 4, 2008.

28. US Department of Health and Human Services, US Census Bureau: *Population (2000)*. Available at: www.aoa.dhhs.gov/agingstatsdotnet/Main_Site/Data/2000_Documents/Population.pdf. Accessed December 30, 2007.

29. Wold GH: *Basic geriatric nursing*, St Louis, 2008, Mosby.

COMPETENCY OF PREOPERATIVE ASSESSMENT

15 Preoperative Assessment

KATHLEEN P. DONOHUE
SUSAN M. ANDREWS

OBJECTIVES

At the conclusion of this chapter, the reader will be able to:

1. List three options available for conducting preoperative assessments and interviews.
2. Identify essential components of preadmission assessment.
3. Explain how the psychological and emotional assessment of a patient will help reduce anxiety on day of surgery.
4. Analyze the learning needs of ambulatory surgery patients.

I. TIMING OF PREOPERATIVE ASSESSMENT
   A. Far enough in advance to ensure time for an appropriate evaluation
      1. Obtain diagnostic testing and consultative services if needed.
      2. Alter current medical regimen if necessary (e.g., anticoagulant therapy, glycemic control, hypertension).
      3. Obtain equipment, supplies, and other items necessary for postoperative care.
      4. Make arrangements in family schedule (home care, day care, transportation, etc.).
      5. Prepare patient physically and emotionally for surgery.
   B. Not too far in advance
      1. Patient forgets preoperative instructions.
      2. Diagnostic test results are outdated.
II. PURPOSE OF PREOPERATIVE ASSESSMENT AND PROGRAMS
   A. Decrease potential delays and cancellations on day of surgery.
      1. Provide for comprehensive assessments (nursing and anesthesia).
         a. Potential problems identified and addressed before surgery
         b. Nursing discharge plan
         c. Complete systems review
         d. Prior surgery, medical, and anesthesia history
         e. American Society of Anesthesiologists (ASA) physical status identified
            (1) ASA 1 or (P1): healthy patient
            (2) ASA 2 or (P2): healthy patient with mild systemic disease
               (a) Well-controlled chronic bronchitis
               (b) Moderate obesity
               (c) Diet-controlled diabetes mellitus
               (d) Mild hypertension
               (e) Old myocardial infarction (MI)
            (3) ASA 3 or (P3): patients with severe systemic disease that limits activity but is not incapacitating
               (a) Coronary artery disease with angina
               (b) Type I diabetes mellitus
               (c) Morbid obesity

(d) Moderate to severe pulmonary insufficiency
(4) ASA 4 or (P4): patients with severe systemic disease that is a constant threat to life
    (a) Organic heart disease with marked cardiac insufficiency
    (b) Persisting angina
    (c) Intractable dysrhythmia
    (d) Advanced pulmonary, renal, hepatic, or endocrine insufficiency
(5) ASA 5 or (P5): moribund patients who are not expected to survive without surgery
    (a) Ruptured abdominal aortic aneurysm
    (b) Major multi-system or cerebral trauma
(6) ASA 6 or (P6): patients declared brain dead whose organs are being harvested
(7) E: the E suffix denotes an emergency surgical procedure.
(8) Ambulatory surgery patients usually fall into the first three categories.

2. Provide for perioperative and perianesthesia teachings.
  a. Physician and anesthesia providers are the chief source of information.
  b. Preoperative nurse is the primary educator and teacher of the provided information.
  c. Encourage patient and family to openly and honestly communicate their:
    (1) Needs
    (2) Emotions
    (3) Concerns
  d. Promote patient safety.
    (1) Clear understanding of preoperative instructions

3. Provide patient and family opportunity for questions.
  a. Clarify patient's understanding of:
    (1) Procedure
    (2) Informed consent
    (3) Anesthetic approach
    (4) Goals/expected outcomes
    (5) Personal responsibilities
    (6) Comprehensive instructions
      (a) Assist with understanding and compliance.
      (b) Allow for preparation for transport and postoperative home needs.
        (i) Caregiver
        (ii) Practice techniques (e.g., emptying drains, dressing changes, crutch walking, injections, etc.)
      (c) Physician follow-up care

4. Reduce patient anxiety.
  a. Provide clear and concise explanations.
  b. Inaccuracies or misinformation may cause fear.
    (1) Induction of anesthesia smoother in calm persons
    (2) Recovery enhanced when patient less stressed
  c. Promote the wellness concept.

III. BENEFITS OF A PREOPERATIVE ASSESSMENT PROGRAM
  A. Identify issues needing further work-up before admission to avoid costly delays and cancellations.
  1. History and physical
    a. Performed within 30 days of the scheduled surgery
    b. Completed
    c. Updated within 24 hours of surgery
  2. Advance directive
    a. Need to bring a copy on the day of surgery
    b. Opportunity to convey patient's decision about end of life care, if so desires
  3. Identify needed laboratory, diagnostic testing, and/or additional work-ups.

4. Identify any postoperative care needs.
  a. Supplies, prescriptions, medication teaching and demonstration (e.g., enoxaparin sodium [Lovenox])
  b. Equipment for home use (crutches, walker, continuous passive motion, continuous positive airway pressure, etc.)
  c. Arrange for home care services (visiting nurse, home care aide, etc.).
  d. Transportation home if outpatient surgery
    (1) Avoid unnecessary postoperative stays.
    (2) Potential unsafe transportation plans
  e. Responsible adult (18 years or older), especially for first 24 hours
B. Allows for preoperative diagnostic screening
  1. Based on specific individualized clinical indicators or risk factors (Figure 15-1)
    a. Age
    b. Preexisting disease or illness
    c. Surgical procedure being performed
C. Allows for identification of potential safety issues
  1. Patient and family history
    a. Malignant hyperthermia
    b. Pseudocholinesterase deficiency
    c. Allergies including latex allergy/sensitivity
      (1) Notify operating room (OR) before of day of surgery.
    d. Use of narcotics for chronic pain
    e. Use of street drugs/herbals
    f. History of postoperative/postdischarge nausea and vomiting (PONV/PDNV)
  2. Mobility issues
  3. Ability to care for self if lives alone
  4. Quality and amount of caregiver assistance
  5. Ability and willingness to comply with preoperative instructions
    a. Fasting and nothing by mouth (NPO) requirements
    b. Smoking cessation
    c. Necessary preoperative preparations

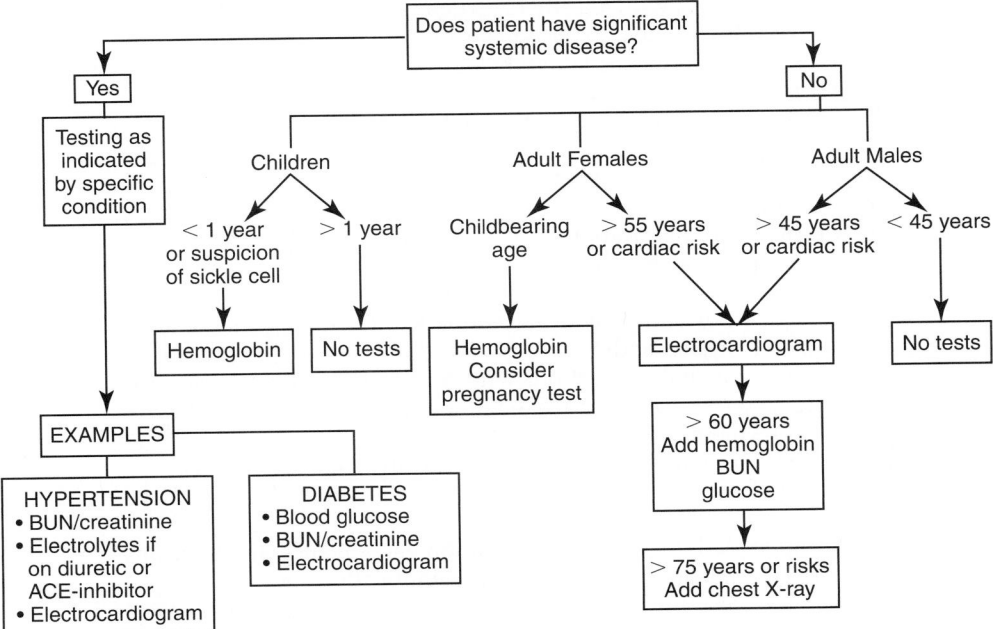

FIGURE 15-1 ■ Preadmission testing algorithm.

    D. Allows for medication review and education

        1. Current medications reviewed

            a. Medication reconciliation starts preoperatively.

            b. Name, dose, frequency

            c. Herbals, supplements and over-the-counter medications

                (1) Ask about specific supplements used. Patients often do not consider these "medications."

        2. Preoperative medication instructions

            a. Some medications may be stopped before surgery as determined by surgeon and/or anesthesia provider.

                (1) Anticoagulant therapy and nonsteroidal anti-inflammatory drugs, aspirin

                    (a) How handled may be procedure or physician specific

                (2) Aspirin can affect platelet adhesiveness for up to 7 days.

                (3) Coumadin often discontinued 48 hours before surgery.

                    (a) Clotting studies done immediately before surgery

                    (b) Closely monitor patients receiving long-term therapy for signs of bleeding.

                (4) Dipyridamole (Persantine) usually stopped 2 days before surgery

                (5) Indomethacin, tricyclic antidepressants, phenothiazines, furosemide, and steroids can interfere with platelet function.

                (6) Herbals and supplements

                    (a) Feverfew, garlic, ginger, ginkgo, ginseng, and vitamin E may increase bleeding, particularly in patients already taking anticoagulants.

                    (b) Ginseng may cause an increase in heart rate and blood pressure.

                    (c) Licorice, some mixture types may increase blood pressure.

                    (d) Goldenseal and vitamin E may exacerbate high blood pressure in people who already have hypertension.

        3. Some medications may be held the day of surgery as determined by surgeon and/or anesthesia provider.

            a. Diuretics, insulin, oral hypoglycemic medications, etc.

            b. Monoamine oxidase inhibitor (MAOI) antidepressants

                (1) Usually discontinued before anesthesia

                (2) Interaction with anesthetic drugs can result in a release of epinephrine and dopamine.

        4. Medications that may be taken the day of surgery as determined by surgeon and/or anesthesia provider

            a. Cardiac, antihypertensive (may be held if contain diuretics)

            b. Beta-blockers

            c. Calcium channel blockers

            d. Anticonvulsants

            e. Chronic pain medications

    E. Provide preoperative teaching.

        1. Procedure-specific instructions in nonmedical jargon

            a. Provide information in easy-to-understand language at the level of the patient's understanding.

            b. Reinforce verbal instructions with written handouts whenever possible.

            c. Video aids for patients to take home are an excellent teaching reinforcement tool.

        2. Need for compliance with preoperative instructions

            a. Arrival time

            b. Leave valuables at home.

            c. Bring needed documents (medication list, advance directive, any paperwork from surgeon, picture identification, etc.).

            d. Need for responsible adult, at least first 24 hours postoperative

            e. Transportation

            f. Diet, NPO, and smoking restrictions

(1) No gum or hard candy
    (a) Increases stomach acid secretions
(2) Small amounts of clear liquids morning of surgery can reduce stomach acid secretions.
(3) Refrain from smoking for at least 8 hours or per facility policy.
    (a) Reduces amount of carbon monoxide in blood
    (b) Promotes better oxygenation during anesthesia
    (c) Reduces upper airway irritation
    (d) Reduces bronchospastic tendency
    (e) Reduces gastric volumes
  3. What type of clothing to wear
    a. Front button-down shirt for eye cases, skirt or loose fitting pants for leg surgery, etc.
    b. Refrain from wearing makeup, nail polish.
  4. Need for surgical preoperative preparations (e.g., bowel prep, antiseptic shower, no shaving of operative site, etc.)
  5. Review of preoperative and postoperative expectations
  6. Importance of caregiver support
  7. Postoperative pain management
F. Patient/family satisfaction
  1. Convenient for patient
  2. Informative
  3. Allows patient and family to ask questions and express concerns

IV. TYPES OF PREOPERATIVE ASSESSMENTS AND PROGRAMS
  A. Hospital or freestanding ambulatory surgery center in-person interview
    1. Advantages
      a. Formal program
      b. May have nursing, anesthesia, other health care team and diagnostic testing at same time and place
      c. Decreases delays and cancellations day of surgery
        (1) Able to take corrective actions on recognized complications or problems
      d. Allows patient and families the opportunity to see facility, meet staff, ask questions
      e. Allows interviewer to assess patient's level of understanding, apprehension, etc.
      f. Able to identify potential issues (e.g., language, other communication barriers, physical disabilities that may affect preparation time day of surgery)
    2. Disadvantages
      a. Some patients precluded
        (1) Time constraints
        (2) Transportation issues
        (3) Travel distance
        (4) Physical limitations
        (5) Emergent or add-on cases
      b. Cost
        (1) Staff
        (2) Physical space
  B. Surgeon or primary care provider (PCP) office in-person interview
    1. Advantages
      a. Saves patient's time
      b. Decreases need to repeat information
        (1) Preoperative interview done at time of history and physical, consent.
      c. Allows patient to ask surgeon questions directly at time of preoperative work-up
      d. PCP may perform clearance for comorbidities at the same time as preoperative work-up.

        e. Diagnostic testing may be completed during visit.

        f. Consultations performed, if needed

    2. Disadvantages

        a. No opportunity for patient and family to visit surgical facility

        b. Preoperative staff does not meet patient before the day of surgery.

C. Phone interview

    1. Advantages

        a. May be screening tool to identify high-risk patients

        b. Potential to be done at patient's convenience

        c. Saves any patient inconvenience of an in-person visit

        d. Patient able to ask questions

    2. Disadvantages

        a. Potential of required testing not being completed

        b. May have difficulty in contacting patients at a convenient time and location where they can speak freely

        c. May be difficult to assess patient's level of understanding

        d. Unable to perform a physical assessment

        e. Anesthesia interview may not be performed until immediately before surgery.

        f. Patient may not be a proper candidate for a phone interview.

D. Web-based assessment and teaching programs

    1. Facility based

        a. Specifically designed by facility

            (1) Forms and format

        b. May include virtual preoperative tour

    2. Independent web based

        a. Purchased service

    3. Process

        a. Patient accesses a designated secure website to complete a medical history.

        b. RN reviews questionnaire for completeness and need to follow-up with patient.

        c. Program may offer preoperative teaching module.

    4. Advantage (Box 15-1)

        a. Patient convenience

            (1) Completes information at own time and pace

            (2) No travel or lost work time

    5. Disadvantages

        a. Decreased opportunity to build rapport with patient

            (1) No one available to answer questions or provide explanations

        b. Possible lack of Internet access

        c. Potential anxiety over privacy issues

■ BOX 15-1

■ **ADVANTAGES OF COMPUTER-BASED PREOPERATIVE EDUCATION**

- Consistency: Quality and content is standardized.
- Individualized instruction: Patients proceed at their own paces and can repeat and review information.
- Privacy: Only the patients see incorrect answers, avoiding embarrassment over incorrect or personal answers.
- Time efficiency: It reduces professional time spent presenting information common to most patients.
- Accessibility: It can be used at any time, for inpatients as well as outpatients.

From Burden N, Quinn DMD, O'Brien D, et al: *Ambulatory surgical nursing,* Philadelphia, 2000, WB Saunders, p. 349.

        d. Potential for actual breech of privacy

        e. Web instructions unfriendly to user

E. Questionnaires

    1. Advantages

        a. Patient completes an abbreviated history.

            (1) RN reviews to determine whether an in-person interview and/or diagnostic testing is warranted.

            (2) Healthy patients are contacted by phone to review preoperative instructions.

    2. Disadvantages

        a. Same disadvantages as with phone interview

F. Preoperative group sessions

    1. Advantages

        a. May be general or pertinent to specific patient populations

        b. May include various team departments

            (1) Admissions

            (2) OR

            (3) Perianesthesia care units

            (4) Anesthesia

            (5) Social services

            (6) Case manager

            (7) Financial counselor

            (8) Rehabilitation

            (9) Visiting nurse services

        c. Patients may benefit from talking with patients who are having same procedure and/or who have undergone same procedure (major surgeries).

        d. Allows nurse to instruct multiple patients at one time

        e. Use of return demonstration of any postoperative equipments (e.g., pain management pumps)

        f. Helpful to review clinical pathway and expectations for the specific surgical procedure

        g. Patient and family have opportunity to ask questions and express concerns.

    2. Disadvantages

        a. Patient may be unable to attend.

        b. Length of time for group session

        c. Patient may feel uncomfortable asking questions in group setting.

        d. Attention to and time spent with individual patients may be limited.

G. Preoperative tours for pediatric population

    1. Benefits of program

        a. Provides information to patient and family

        b. Allows for education to be personalized as needed

        c. Decreases anxiety by reviewing perioperative process and answering questions

        d. Allows child to see and become familiar with the area before the day of surgery

        e. Opportunity for child to practice "leaving parents" to go into procedure room and then reunite

            (1) Builds trust

            (2) Many children's hospitals allow parents to accompany child in the OR until after induction is completed.

    2. Types of programs

        a. May be group or individual

        b. Tour includes hands-on familiarization with common equipment.

            (1) Blood pressure cuff

            (2) Thermometer

            (3) Face mask (able to select "flavor" of mask)

            (4) Casting materials, slings, crutches, etc.

      c. Theme tours through perioperative areas (safari, circus, etc.)
      d. "Dress-up" programs
      e. Role playing
      f. Procedure specific (e.g., cardiac, urological, orthopedic, etc.)
  H. Preoperative tours for adult population
    1. Benefits of program
      a. Useful for patients undergoing major surgery
      b. May be individual or as a group
      c. Review of preoperative and postoperative expectations
      d. Allows for patient and family to ask questions
      e. Allows patient and family to see where family will wait
  I. Additional alternatives
    1. Preoperative videos
      a. Can be generalized or surgery specific
      b. Can focus on specific population (pediatric or adult)
      c. Allows viewing at own home in familiar surroundings
      d. Can be reviewed numerous times until patient is comfortable with content
    2. Educational pamphlets and brochures
      a. Distribute to patient at time of preoperative assessment.
      b. Can be brief or detailed
      c. Provide pictures for ease of understanding.

V. IMPORTANCE OF PREOPERATIVE ASSESSMENT
  A. Goals
    1. Provide patient and family with necessary information for a positive surgical experience; may be verbal and/or written.
    2. Assess patient's understanding of and potential compliance with instructions.
    3. Obtain vital information to avoid delays or cancellations on day of surgery.
    4. Provide for a smoother, more efficient patient flow on day of surgery.
  B. Does not matter which method is used as long as end result of a patient ready for surgery is achieved
    1. Different approaches may meet varied patient and family needs.

VI. SCHEDULING SURGERY
  A. Based on:
    1. Surgeon's availability
    2. Slots available in OR schedule
    3. Patient's needs
      a. Emotional and physical
        (1) May not want a prolonged delay for someone extremely anxious
        (2) Children and diabetic patients need to maintain nutrition and medication schedules.
        (3) Procedures requiring prolonged postoperative observation should be done early in the day.
      b. Urgency of surgical procedure
      c. Third-party reimbursement
      d. Patient's and family's schedule
      e. Completeness of the preoperative process before the day of surgery
        (1) If incomplete should not be scheduled as a first case
          (a) Need for completion of work-up day of surgery may delay OR start time.

VII. PATIENT TYPES
  A. Morning (AM) admissions, outpatient observation patients (short stays: 23:59) extended recovery, and day surgery patients
    1. Cost savings for institution
    2. Diagnostic testing and preoperative assessment done as outpatient
    3. AM admissions and outpatient observation patients
      a. Admitted to hospital either before or after surgery

      b. Transferred from PACU to an inpatient, extended recovery, or observation room
    4. Day surgery patients
      a. Discharged day of surgery

VIII. DAY OF SURGERY GENERAL PREPARATION

  A. Expedite processes to avoid OR delays or cancellations.

  B. Nursing process
    1. Follow regulatory guidelines (see Chapter 7).
    2. Complete patient's assessment, obtain actual height and weight.
    3. Assess patient for changes since preoperative evaluation interview.
      a. Some changes may result in case being cancelled.
        (1) Abnormal vital signs including pulse oximetry
        (2) Upper respiratory infections (cough, congestion, fever)
        (3) Skin disruptions, bruises
          (a) Especially on or near surgical site
      b. Assess for risk of PONV/PDNV.
    4. Emotional support
      a. Atmosphere
        (1) Ensure privacy.
        (2) Calm and unhurried demeanor
        (3) Soft music
        (4) Subdued lighting, warm colors, painting on the walls
      b. Familiarize patient and family with area.
        (1) Patient's room
        (2) Waiting area
        (3) Where family can go for food and drinks
        (4) Approximate length of procedure
        (5) How often and how family will be updated on patient's status
        (6) Liaison person/nurse, if available
        (7) PACU visitation policy
    5. Assess patient for compliance with preoperative instructions.
      a. Notify surgeon and/or anesthesia care provider of any noncompliance issues.
        (1) NPO status
        (2) Smoking status
        (3) Current patient's medical condition (e.g., fever)
        (4) Medications taken and/or held
        (5) Availability of home caregiver
        (6) Transportation if outpatient
    6. Nursing has role of primary educator.
      a. Clarify patient's understanding of:
        (1) Procedure
        (2) Anesthetic approach
        (3) Goals/expected outcomes
        (4) Personal responsibilities
    7. Preparation for the OR
      a. Hospital gowns required for most procedures
        (1) Some institutions make exceptions for minor surgery (e.g., eye, breast biopsies, hand surgery can keep on undergarments or pants).
        (2) Some allow patients to wear undergarments.
          (a) No nylon due to static electricity
      b. Dentures, partials, eyeglasses, hearing aides
        (1) Some institutions allow these items to go with patient to OR holding area.
      c. Jewelry
        (1) Instruct to remove all jewelry.
          (a) Be aware body piercings can be on any body part.
            (i) May cause arcing—electrosurgical burns

d. Securing of clothes and personal items
   (1) Give any valuables to family to keep.
   (2) Some institutions have lockers for clothing.
   (3) Others give to family or stay on the patient's bed.
e. Surgical Care Improvement Project (SCIP) recommend whenever possible hair should be left at the surgical site.
   (1) There is a relationship between shaving and increased wound infections.
   (2) If hair removal is necessary, remove with clippers or depilatories.
      (a) Electrical or battery powered
      (b) Disposable or disinfect between patients
      (c) Perform outside the OR (e.g., preoperative area).
f. IV access
   (1) Policies vary from facility to facility.
   (2) May be responsibility of preoperative admitting nurse, anesthesia provider, intravenous team, etc.
   (3) Needle gauge dependent on patient need
      (a) Outpatients usually 20 gauge
      (b) Patients with small, fragile veins may require a smaller gauge.
      (c) AM admit patients who may require blood transfusion, an 18 gauge may be recommended.
g. Preoperative medications
   (1) May be used to reduce anxiety
   (2) May be used to reduce risk for nausea, vomiting, and gastric acidity
   (3) Standards for antibiotic prophylaxis
      (a) SCIP recommendations
         (i) Within 60 minutes of incision
         (ii) Selection according to surgical procedure
         (iii) Time challenge due to changes in surgery schedule
         (iv) Some must be given over 1 to 2 hours.
         (v) Discontinuation within 24 hours
         (vi) Collaborative effort between nursing and anesthesia
   (4) Prophylaxis for preventing subacute bacterial endocarditis
      (a) Generally give before dental, gastrointestinal, genitourinary, oral, and respiratory procedures.
   (5) SCIP recommendations for beta-blockers
   (6) SCIP recommendations for glucose control
C. Documentation
   1. Essential that initial assessment be complete and accurate
      a. Some ambulatory surgery centers use abbreviated assessments (focused assessments).
   2. Update information with specific day-of-surgery assessment.
      a. Specific and unusual findings, actions taken, disposition of patient's belongings, family contact information, IV information including missed attempts, vital signs including pulse oximetry, height, weight, etc.
   3. Essential that history and physical be complete and updated within 24 hours of surgical procedure
   4. Essential that surgery consent be complete, accurate, dated, and signed by all individuals
      a. Legal responsibility of surgeon and anesthesia providers (if separate anesthesia consent)
         (1) Accurately identifies procedure being performed
         (2) Include explanation of procedure, risks, benefits, outcomes, potential complications, and options to proposed surgery/anesthesia.
         (3) Words and names should be spelled correctly.
         (4) Avoid abbreviations.
         (5) No blank areas

                (6) No erasures, white outs, or obliterations
                (7) Language that patient understands
                (8) Changes or additions should be written clearly.
                (9) Person making change should initial and date changed area(s).
                (10) Patient should also initial and date changed area(s).
                    (a) Significant changes are best done with new consent form.
        b. Role of the nurse in obtaining consents
            (1) Actual consent for surgery occurs when the surgeon and patient agree to proceed.
            (2) Explanation of the procedure, including risks, benefits, outcomes, and potential complications, is the surgeon's responsibility.
            (3) Some institutions require that the nurse facilitates the process of obtaining the patient's consent on the form as well as witnessing the patient's signature.
            (4) According to the American Nurses Association, the nurse has a moral and ethical obligation to ensure that:
                (a) Patients do not feel pressured or forced into treatment.
                (b) Patients receive accurate information that is understood by them.
                (c) Patients understand that the consent can be withdrawn at any time.
                (d) Patients understand what is being done.
                    (i) If patient understands, the nurse may obtain signature on consent form and witness that signature.
                    (ii) If patient does not indicate understanding or is unsure about other aspects of surgery or anesthesia, notify the surgeon or anesthesia provider before obtaining signature.
                    (iii) Document incident and subsequent conversation in patient's record.
        c. Special consents
            (1) Anesthesia consents should be obtained by the anesthesia provider.
            (2) Additional consents may be required for:
                (a) Sterilization procedures
                (b) Termination of pregnancy
                (c) Implantation of investigational devices
                (d) Photographing procedure
                (e) Laparoscopic procedures
                (f) Release of information to another physician and/or facility
                (g) Study patients
        d. More institutions using computerized charting
            (1) Provides for more continuity
            (2) Information easier to share between providers
D. Handoff to anesthesia, holding or operating room
    1. The Joint Commission (TJC) National Patient Safety Goals (NPSG)
        a. Communication between caregivers
        b. Method determined by facility
            (1) Face to face
            (2) Phone
            (3) Written report
            (4) Combination of above
        c. Process includes opportunity to ask questions.
    2. Seen by anesthesia provider before surgery
        a. May be done in preoperative department or preoperative holding
            (1) Regional anesthesia (nurse's role)
                (a) Provide emotional support.
                (b) Position so patient can see nurse.
                (c) Maintain eye contact.
                (d) Hold hand for physical contact or support as needed.
                (e) Supportive conversation

(2) Monitored anesthesia care
(3) Local anesthesia
(4) General anesthesia
3. Prevention of hypothermia
a. SCIP recommendations
b. Starts in preoperative area
c. Start with normothermia.
d. Use warming techniques.
(1) Warmed blankets
(2) Warmed IV fluids
(3) Increased ambient room temperature
(4) Socks, head coverings
(5) Limited skin exposure
IX. REGULATORY
A. The Joint Commission
1. NPSGs
a. Change yearly
(1) Goals that directly impact preoperative phase
(a) Patient identification
(b) Correct site surgery
(c) Medication reconciliation
(d) Communications, handoffs
(e) Infections
(f) Surgical fires
(g) Medication safety
(h) Patient involvement in their care
(i) Falls
(2) Some goals dropped off the list and others added each year
2. Core measures
a. SCIP
(1) Antibiotic timing
(a) Within 1 hour of surgical incision
(b) Discontinue within 24 hours after surgery end time; 48 hours for cardiac procedures.
(2) Cardiac patients with controlled 6 AM postoperative serum glucose
(3) Appropriate hair removal
(a) Clipping or depilatory
(b) No shaving
(4) Normothermia for immediate postoperative colorectal patients
(5) Beta-blocker therapy
(6) Venous thromboembolism
B. Patient Self-Determination Act
1. An amendment to the Omnibus Budget Reconciliation Act of 1990
a. Medicare and Medicaid providers such as hospitals must provide adult patients written information about their rights under state law.
(1) To participate in and direct their health care choices
(2) To agree to or refuse medical or surgical treatment
(3) To prepare an advance directive
(a) Living will
(b) Durable power of attorney
(c) Right to direct end-of-life decisions
b. Providers must supply information on their policies that govern the utilization of these rights.
c. Currently freestanding surgical centers are not required to participate.
(1) Some are supplying this information.
C. Health Insurance Portability and Accountability Act
1. Took effect April 2003

      2. Involves three separate sets of rules to protect patients' health information

         a. Transactions

         b. Security

         c. Privacy

   D. National Standards on Culturally and Linguistically Appropriate Services

      1. Culturally competent

      2. Access services

         a. Currently mandated federal requirements for all recipients of federal funds

            (1) Standard 4: health care organizations must offer and provide language assistance services, including bilingual staff and interpreter services, at no cost to each patient/consumer with limited English proficiency at all points of contact, in a timely manner during all hours of operation.

            (2) Standard 5: health care organizations must provide to patients/consumers in their preferred language both verbal offers and written notices informing them of their right to receive language assistance services.

            (3) Standard 6: health care organizations must assure the competence of language assistance provided to limited English-proficient patients/consumers by interpreters and bilingual staff.

            (4) Standard 7: health care organizations must make available easily understood patient-related materials and post signage in the languages of the commonly encountered groups and/or groups represented in the service area.

      3. Organizational supports for cultural competence

BIBLIOGRAPHY

1. American Society of Anesthesiologists: *ASA physical status classification system.* Available at: www.asahq.org/clinical/physicalstatus.htm. Accessed February 11, 2008.

2. American Society of Anesthesiologists: *What you should know about your patients' use of herbal medicine and other dietary supplements.* Available at: www.asahq.org/patientEducation/herbPhysician.pdf. Accessed February 11, 2008.

3. American Society of PeriAnesthesia Nurses: *Standards of perianesthesia nursing practice 2008-2010,* Cherry Hill, NJ, 2009, American Society of PeriAnesthesia Nurses.

4. Ascension Health: *Patient self-determination act (PSDA).* Available at: www.Ascensionhealth.org/ethics/public/issues/patient_self. Accessed February 17, 2008.

5. Association of Operating Room Nurses: *AORN standards: Recommended practice and guidelines,* Denver, CO, 2007, Association of Operating Room Nurses.

6. Burden N, Quinn DMD, O'Brien D, et al: *Ambulatory surgical nursing,* ed 2, Philadelphia, 2000, WB Saunders.

7. Michigan Health and Hospital Association Service Corporation Core Options: *The Joint Commission/core measures.* Available at: www.coreoptions.com/new_site/jcahocore.html. Accessed February 17, 2008.

8. Ireland D: *Redi-Ref 2004 ambulatory/PACU/pediatrics,* Cherry Hill, NJ, 2004, American Society of PeriAnesthesia Nurses.

9. Oshodi T: Clinical skills: an evidence based approach to preoperative fasting. *Br J Nurs* 13:958-962, 2004.

10. Spaulding NJ: Reducing anxiety by preoperative education: make the future familiar. *Occup Ther Int* 10(4):278-293, 2003.

11. The Joint Commission: *National patient safety goals.* Available at: www.jointcommission.Org/PatientSafety/NationalPatientSafetyGoals/08. Accessed February 6, 2008.

12. U.S. Department of Health and Human Services, OPHS Office of Minority Health: *National standards for culturally and linguistically appropriate services in health care.* Available at: www.Omhrc.gov/assets/pdf/checked/Executive.pdf. Accessed February 11, 2008.

History and Physical Examinations

ROSE FERRARA-LOVE

OBJECTIVES

At the conclusion of this chapter, the reader will be able to:

1. State goals of preoperative history and physical exams.

2. Plan a subjective and objective patient exam.

3. Discuss the importance of completing a system review.

I. THE NURSING HISTORY AND PHYSICAL EXAMINATION
   A. General health
      1. Questions and observations regarding overall health include:
         a. General appearance
         b. Height
         c. Weight
            (1) Often converted to kilograms to facilitate rapid calculation of medication doses in milligram per kilogram (mg/kg) format
                (a) Weight in pounds (divided by 2.2 equals weight in kilograms)
                (b) Weight in kilograms (multiplied by 2.2 equals weight in pounds)
            (2) Obesity
                (a) Many freestanding surgical centers enforce weight restrictions because of increased risk of anesthesia complications.
                    (i) Usually 300 lb (136.4 kg)
            (3) Recent unplanned weight loss
         d. Recent or current infection
            (1) Upper respiratory infections
            (2) Lower respiratory infections
         e. Allergies
            (1) Food
            (2) Drugs
            (3) Environment
         f. Nutritional habits
         g. Physical handicaps
            (1) Use of adjuncts for walking
      2. Family history
         a. Problems with anesthesia
            (1) Malignant hyperthermia (MH)
                (a) Anesthetic-related deaths
                (b) MH testing
                    (i) Caffeine-halothane contracture test
      3. Physical examination includes observation.
         a. Skin
            (1) Color
            (2) Turgor
            (3) Elasticity

        (4) Presence of bruises
           (a) May necessitate report to authorities if abuse is suspected
        (5) Other injuries
        (6) Dryness
        (7) Lesions
           (a) Mucous membrane
        (8) Cleanliness
        (9) Dental hygiene
  b. Abnormalities
        (1) Posture
        (2) Gait
        (3) Mobility
           (a) Use of wheelchair, walker, or cane should be noted.
        (4) Pain at rest
  c. Physical characteristics
        (1) Potential complications for intubation
           (a) Short, stocky neck
           (b) Cervical fusion or arthritis
           (c) Thick tongue
           (d) Temporal mandibular joint disease
           (e) Dental or orthopedic abnormalities
  d. Vital signs should be obtained to identify aberrancies and for baseline measurements.
        (1) Blood pressure
           (a) Dynamic measurements that change minute to minute
               (i) Response to:
                  [a] Environment
                  [b] Physiologic demands
           (b) Average ranges
               (i) 100 to 135 mm Hg systolic
               (ii) 60 to 80 mm Hg diastolic
           (c) Orthostatic measurements with underlying cardiac or hypertensive history
        (2) Pulse rate
           (a) Average range 60 to 100 beats per minute
        (3) Respirations
           (a) Average rate
               (i) 12 to 20 breaths per minute
               (ii) 16 to 25 breaths per minute in elderly
           (b) Use of accessory muscles of respiration
           (c) Shape and symmetry
           (d) Sternal abnormalities
               (i) Pectus carinatum
                  [a] Chicken breast or pigeon breast
               (ii) Pectus excavatum
                  [a] Breastbone caves in resulting in sunken chest appearance
               (iii) Anterior-posterior diameter increased
                  [a] May be normal with:
                    [1] Age
                    [2] Hyperinflation
           (e) Abnormal breathing patterns
               (i) Küssmaul
               (ii) Cheyne-Stokes
               (iii) Biot's
        (4) Temperature (see Chapter 24)
           (a) Oral temperatures are considered normal at 96.4° F (35° C).
           (b) Rectal temperatures average slightly less than 1° F higher.
           (c) Axillary temperatures are approximately 0.5° F to 1° F lower.

      (d) Tympanic thermometer readings are approximately 0.5° F to 1° F higher than oral readings.

      (e) Temporal thermometer readings are more accurate than tympanic thermometer readings.

      (f) Variances in normal ranges

        (i) Normal physiologic status

      (g) Extrinsic forces

        (i) Medication

        (ii) Recent exercise

        (iii) Effort

        (iv) Anxiety

        (v) Fear

B. Medication history

  1. Medication protocol affects types of medications and anesthetic agents used.

    a. Helps avoid untoward drug interactions or withdrawal episodes

  2. Include in history form

    a. Names

    b. Dosages

    c. Frequency

      (1) Date and time of last dose

        (a) Medication reconciliation upon admission and before discharge

    d. Length of time prescribed

    e. Effects

    f. Nonprescription drugs

      (1) Aspirin

        (a) Prolongs bleeding time

    g. Herbal preparations

    h. Habit-forming drugs used

      (1) Tobacco

        (a) Number of pack years

          (i) Number of packs per day × number of years

          (ii) Attempts to stop

        (b) Smokeless tobacco

          (i) Amount per day

      (2) Alcohol

        (a) Type

        (b) Amount

        (c) Frequency

        (d) Changes in reaction to alcohol intake

      (3) Recreational

      (4) Prescription

    i. Side effects

    j. Allergic reactions

      (1) Specific drug

        (a) May know only category of drug (i.e., antibiotic)

        (b) Identify if related categories will be used in the ambulatory surgery center (ASC).

      (2) Specific reaction

        (a) True allergy or expected side effect

      (3) Usually documented in red

        (a) Highly visible

          (i) On medical record

        (b) On patient identification band

      (4) Environmental and food allergies

        (a) Allergy to eggs may have possible cross-sensitivity with propofol.

        (b) Allergy to bananas, kiwis, peaches, water chestnuts may have link with latex allergies.

(i) Cutaneous exposure (i.e., latex)
[a] Anesthesia masks, head straps, rebreathing masks, tourniquets, ECG patches, adhesive tape, surgical gloves
[b] Other sources: elastic bandages, rubber positioning rings, rubber shoes, elastic clothing, balloons, Koosh balls, sporting equipment
(ii) Mucous membrane
[a] Nasogastric tubes, balloons, nipples, pacifiers, products used in dentistry, urinary catheters, glove contact with vaginal mucosa, enema kits, rectal pressure catheters (especially in patients with spina bifida and impaired bowel control)
[b] Other sources: condoms
(iii) Inhalation
[a] Often associated with glove powder
(iv) Internal tissue
[a] Intraoperative resulting from surgical gloves contacting the peritoneum or internal organs
(v) Intravascular
[a] Disposable syringes, medication aspirated from vials with latex stoppers, injection of medication via ports of intravenous tubing (latex can leech into solutions injected)

C. Nutrition status
  1. Weight history
    a. Typical day's diet
      (1) Salt
      (2) Saturated fats
      (3) Food habits
        (a) Ethnicity
      (4) Dentition
  2. Physiologic processes dependent upon proper nutrition
    a. Wound healing
    b. Oxygen transport
    c. Enzyme synthesis
    d. Clotting factors
    e. Resistance to infection
  3. Diseases associated with poor nutrition
    a. Crohn's disease
    b. Malignancies
    c. Chronic obstructive pulmonary disease
    d. Ulcerative colitis
  4. Indications of malnutrition
    a. Anorexia
    b. Recent weight loss
    c. Dull hair
    d. Brittle nails
    e. Diagnostic tests
      (1) Decreased lymphocytes
      (2) Decreased serum albumin and transferrin levels
  5. Obesity complicates:
    a. Administration of anesthesia
      (1) Requires higher-than-normal levels of anesthetic agents
        (a) Fat-soluble agents tend to prolong effects.
      (2) Increased stress on cardiovascular system
        (a) Increased oxygen needs
        (b) Increased carbon dioxide production
          (i) Associated with increased body mass

    b. Technical aspects of performing procedure
      (1) Often difficult to intubate
        (a) Difficult to maintain airway
          (i) Increased risk of aspiration
          (ii) Increased intra-abdominal pressures
        (b) Gastric contents higher in volume and more acidic
      (2) Problems with positioning
        (a) Weight of abdominal and chest contents can cause respiratory embarrassment when in Trendelenburg position.
      (3) Difficult to perform venipuncture
    c. Patient's recovery
      (1) Electrolyte and fluid balance essential for homeostasis (see Table 16-1)
        (a) Regulates cardiac rhythm
        (b) Muscle strength
        (c) Distribution and metabolism of drugs
          (i) Mental alertness

■ TABLE 16-1
■ ■ **Signs and Symptoms of Electrolyte Imbalance**

Electrolyte Normal Value	Physiologic Functions	Excess	Deficiency
Potassium (K) 3.5-5.5 mEq/L	—Nerve conduction —Muscle contraction —Enzyme action for cellular energy production —Regulates intercellular osmolality	—Generalized muscle weakness, flaccidity; can affect respiratory muscles, paresthesia —Cardiac: bradycardia, ventricular ectopy and fibrillation, third degree heart block, asystole (>7.0 mEq/L) —ECG changes: flat or absent P wave, wide ORS, peaked T wave, prolonged PR interval	—Muscle weakness, flaccidity, fatigue, leg cramps, ↓ deep tendon reflexes, shallow respirations, weak, thready pulse, hypotension —Cardiac: atrial dysrhythmias, premature ventricular contractions (PVCs), atrioventricular (AV) blocks, cardiac arrest (<2.5 mEq/L) —ECG changes: flat or inverted T wave, depressed ST segment, U wave present, potentiates digitals toxicity, premature atrial contractions (PACs) or PVCs —Abdominal cramping, anorexia, malaise, nausea and vomiting, muscle weakness, headache, confusion, lethargy, convulsions, coma
Sodium (Na) 135-145 mEq/L	—Transmission and conduction of nerve impulses —Regulates vascular osmolality —Regulates neuromuscular activity via sodium pump	—Excitement; thirst; dry, sticky tongue and mucous membranes; oliguria; flushed skin; confusion; lethargy; coma; convulsions; hypo- or hypertension; elevated temperature	—Abdominal cramping, anorexia, malaise, nausea and vomiting, muscle weakness, headache, confusion, lethergy, convulsions, coma

■ TABLE 16-1
■ ■ **Signs and Symptoms of Electrolyte Imbalance—cont'd**

Electrolyte Normal Value	Physiologic Functions	Excess	Deficiency
Calcium (Ca) 8.5-10.5 mg/dl	—Nerve and muscle activity —Myocardial contractility —Maintains cell permeability —Converts prothrombin to thrombin —Formation of teeth and bones	—Lethargy, depression, apathy, anorexia, nausea and vomiting, muscle weakness, headache, confusion, decreased attention span, slurred speech, hypertension —Cardiac: heart block, PVCs, idioventricular rhythms, cardiac arrest —ECG changes: shortened QT interval	—Anxiety, excitement, hyperreflexia, grimacing, numbness and tingling of lips or fingers, muscle cramps and spasms, laryngospasm, convulsions, tetany, dysrhythmias including ventricular tachycardia (VT) —Positive Trousseau's sign: carpal spasm after inflation of blood pressure cuff on upper arm to 20 mm Hg over systolic for 3 minutes, shows tetany —Positive Chvostek's sign: abnormal facial spasm when facial nerve is tapped at the angle of the jaw —ECG changes: prolonged QT interval

From Quinn DMD: *Ambulatory surgical nursing core curriculum*, Philadelphia, 1999, WB Saunders.

(2) Signs of dehydration
    (a) Loss of skin turgor
    (b) Listlessness
    (c) Orthostatic hypotension
    (d) Rapid and thready pulse
    (e) Dryness of mucous membranes
    (f) Thirst
(3) Cardiovascular
    (a) Symptoms of cardiac disease
        (i) Chest pain or tightness
    (b) Palpitations
    (c) Chronic fatigue
    (d) Loss of appetite
    (e) Angina
    (f) Swelling of the ankles
    (g) Paroxysmal nocturnal dyspnea
    (h) Exhaustion
(4) Particular importance
    (a) Recent cardiac surgery
    (b) Myocardial infarction (MI)
        (i) Considered most important indicator of anesthesia morbidity
    (c) Generally elective, non-urgent surgery postponed for at least 6 months after an MI
    (d) Angina
    (e) Aortic stenosis

           (f) Poorly controlled dysrhythmias

           (g) Congestive heart failure (CHF)

           (h) Extremes in blood pressure (high or low)

               (i) Presence of pacemaker

        (5) Physical examination parameters

           (a) Apical pulse

               (i) Rate

           (b) Rhythm

           (c) Quality

           (d) At least one blood pressure reading

           (e) Palpation of peripheral pulses

           (f) Observation for edema

           (g) Clubbing of fingers

           (h) Cyanosis

           (i) Distention of neck veins

           (j) General energy level

           (k) Respiratory ease

           (l) Auscultation of heart for murmurs

               (i) Systolic murmur over right sternal border, second intercostal space may indicate presence of aortic stenosis.

               (ii) Associated with unexpected dysrhythmias

           (m) Diminished stroke volume

    6. Cardiac drugs

      a. Maintain normal routine preoperatively.

        (1) Do not skip doses.

           (a) Beta-blockers

           (b) Calcium channel blockers

           (c) Antihypertensives

D. Peripheral vascular disease

    1. Inspection

      a. Skin color

      b. Hair distribution

      c. Edema

      d. Varicosities

        (1) Stasis ulcers

        (2) Capillary refill time

    2. Palpation

      a. Peripheral pulses

        (1) Characteristics

           (a) Absent = 0

           (b) Weak, thready = 1+

           (c) Normal = 2+

           (d) Full, bounding = 3+

      b. Rigidity of vessels

        (1) Palpable vibration (thrill)

    3. Auscultation

      a. Bruit

        (1) Humming sound from narrow or bulging artery

    4. Symptoms

      a. Peripheral cyanosis

      b. Pain

      c. Cold

      d. Intermittent claudication

      e. Central vessel involvement

        (1) Confusion

        (2) Transient blindness

        (3) Hemiparesis

5. Nursing interventions
   a. Intraoperative passive range of motion
   b. Use of padding of bony prominences intraoperatively
      (1) Heels
      (2) Elbows
      (3) Shoulders
      (4) Hips
      (5) Coccyx
   c. Encouragement of active exercises before and after surgery
   d. Use of antiembolism stockings
   e. Explanation of symptoms of thrombophlebitis
   f. Encouragement of adequate fluid intake
   g. Have patient immediately report any of the following symptoms postoperatively:
      (1) Pain in the leg, especially increased calf pain when foot is dorsiflexed (positive Homans' sign)
      (2) Fever
      (3) Chills
      (4) Swelling
      (5) Redness
      (6) Heat
      (7) Tenderness in leg
E. Respiratory (see Chapter 31)
   1. History
      a. Infectious or chemical influences
      b. Smoking habits
      c. Chronic cough
      d. Previous lung surgery
      e. Emphysema
         (1) Patients may not admit to emphysema as a disease.
         (2) Look for symptomatology.
            (a) Dyspnea
               (i) Minimal exertion
            (b) Rest
            (c) Chronic cough
            (d) Barrel chest
            (e) Elevation of shoulders
            (f) Pursed lip breathing
            (g) Cyanosis
            (h) Clubbing of fingers
            (i) Tachypnea
            (j) Predisposition to respiratory infections
         (3) Shortness of breath
         (4) Current or past episodes of:
            (a) Pneumonia
            (b) Tuberculosis
            (c) Bronchitis
            (d) Asthma
   2. Physical examination
      a. Auscultation of the chest
         (1) Crackles
            (a) Typically short, explosive, discontinuous sounds
            (b) May be heard in patients with:
               (i) Pulmonary emphysema
            (c) Bronchiti
            (d) Asthma
            (e) Pulmonary congestion
               (i) Caused by CHF

(2) Rhonchi
   (a) Coarser, rattling sounds with lower pitch
      (i) Generally heard over large airways
(3) Wheezes
   (a) Continuous, musical sound
      (i) Asthma or emphysema
   (b) Particularly expiration
   b. Baseline breath sounds
      (1) Comparison for postanesthetic findings
         (a) Aspiration
         (b) Fluid overload
         (c) Bronchospasm
   c. Baseline oximetry readings
      (1) Observation of:
         (a) Rate
         (b) Depth
         (c) Ease of breathing
   d. Cyanosis
   e. Symmetry of chest movements
   f. Use of accessory muscles
   g. Production of sputum
   h. Upper airway including anatomic structures
      (1) Short, stocky neck
      (2) Excessive skin or fat on back of neck
      (3) Thick tongue
      (4) Previous cervical fusion
      (5) Temporal mandibular joint disease
      (6) Down syndrome
         (a) Thick, protruding tongue
         (b) Skin folds on posterior neck
         (c) Instability of atlantalaxial joint in cervical spine
            (i) Found in approximately 10% to 20% of persons with Down syndrome
            (ii) Dislocation or subluxation of this joint can occur with hyperextension of neck.
         (d) Cervical cord compression with nerve damage and possible death in 5% to 10% of those predisposed
F. Neurologic (see Chapter 33)
   1. Assessment
      a. General affect
         (1) Behavior
         (2) Speech patterns
         (3) Orientation
         (4) Gait
      b. Fine motor movements
         (1) Writing
         (2) Cough
         (3) Blink
         (4) Swallow
         (5) Pupil reflexes
      c. Motor abilities
         (1) Muscle strength
         (2) Vision
         (3) Hearing
      d. Presence of:
         (1) Headache
         (2) Dizziness
         (3) Paralysis

(4) Seizures

(5) Loss of motor control

    e. Preexisting neurologic deficit

        (1) More complete examination

            (a) Cerebral

            (b) Motor

            (c) Cranial nerves (see Chapter 33)

                (i) Table 16-2 describes abnormalities in function of the cranial nerves.

            (d) Reflex functions

G. Sensory and prosthetic

    1. Patients may not provide accurate information about sensory deficits.

        a. Embarrassment

        b. Vanity

        c. Assessment skills

            (1) Hearing loss

                (a) Patient may lean or turn toward conversation.

                (b) Answer questions inappropriately or not at all

---

■ **TABLE 16-2**

■ ■ **Abnormalities in Cranial Nerve Function**

	Name	Type*	Function	Test Abnormality
I	Olfactory	S	Smell	Coffee, tobacco
II	Optic	S	Vision	Visual acuity, pupillary reaction, visual fields
III	Oculomotor	M	Eye movement	Ptosis; lateral and downward deviation of eye
IV	Trochlear	M	Eye movement	Medial and upper deviation of eye
V	Trigeminal (3 branches—	S	From skin of face and cornea	Loss of sensation on one side of face
	opthalmic, maxillary, mandibular)	M	Muscle movement	Temporal and masseter muscles movement loss
VI	Abducens	M	Eye movement	Medial deviation of eyeball
VII	Facial	S	Tastes—anterior tongue	Inability to grimace on one side of face
		M	Muscles of facial expression	
VIII	Acoustic auditory	S	Hearing	Watch ticking; whispered voice
	vestibulocochlear	S	Equilibrium	Vertigo; nystagmus
IX	Glossopharyngeal	S	Taste of posterior portion of tongue	Loss of gag reflex; deviation of uvula toward the unaffected side
		M	Pharyngeal muscles	
X	Vagus	S	From thoracic and abdominal organs	As with IX plus hoarseness
		M	Pharyngeal and laryngeal muscles plus thoracic and abdominal organs	
XI	Spinal accessory	M	Sternocleidomastoid and trapezius muscles	Inability to shrug one shoulder or to move chin to one side against pressure of examiner's hand
XII	Hypoglossal	M	Tongue movement	Deviation of tongue to affected side

*S, sensory; M, motor.

From Quinn DMD: *Ambulatory surgical nursing core curriculum*, Philadelphia, 1999, WB Saunders.

(c) Watch interviewer's lips
(d) Provide interpreter in American Sign Language if patient is knowledgeable in use.
    (i) Provide information and answers to questions that patient can understand.
  (2) Visual impairment
    (a) Difficulty seeing documents
    (b) Should have instructions, consents, and other forms read to them before having them signed

2. Note that this occurred on patient record.
  a. Emphasis is to ensure effective communication and understanding between patient and staff throughout surgical experience.
  b. Patient must be able to understand instructions and explanations.
    (1) May need sensory aids such as:
      (a) Hearing aids
      (b) Glasses or contact lenses
      (c) Electronic voice stimulator
      (d) Historically banned from operating room
        (i) Current wellness-centered care approach brings more liberal policy.
        (ii) As long as there is no threat to patient safety, potential for loss or harm to device, these devices are often allowed to remain with the patient.
        (iii) Decision usually made by anesthesiologist
      (e) Reassures patients that they may retain these devices and promotes psychological health
      (f) May retain dentures, wigs, prosthetic limbs, and bras
        (i) Essential for self-image and security
        (ii) If they must be moved, reassure patients that they will be returned as soon as possible.
        (iii) Personal privacy and dignity will be maintained.
        (iv) Some ASCs are reevaluating the policy of removing dentures from all patients.
          [a] Unless having general anesthesia, usually not necessary
  c. Documentation of presence of:
    (1) Loose or chipped teeth
    (2) Permanent bridgework
      (a) Avoid accidental injury during airway or tube insertion.
      (b) Identify potential complications of airway management.
      (c) Establish preexisting problems for legal reasons.

H. Musculoskeletal (see Chapter 42)
  1. History
    a. Arthritis
    b. Scoliosis
    c. Osteoporosis
    d. Sciatica
    e. Vertebral disc problems
    f. Amputations
    g. Prior fractures
    h. Frequent falls
  2. Physical assessment
    a. Muscle strength
    b. Gait
    c. Mobility
    d. Range of motion
    e. Use of orthopedic appliances or prostheses
    f. Need for assistive devices

        (1) Walker
        (2) Cane
        (3) Wheelchair

I. Integumentary
  1. Assessment
    a. Observation
      (1) Color
      (2) Temperature
      (3) Texture
      (4) Dryness
      (5) Turgor
      (6) Loss of elasticity
        (a) Normal change in aging
        (b) Can also indicate dehydration
      (7) Integrity
        (a) Easy bruising or petechiae
          (i) Could indicate hematologic problems
      (8) Jaundice
        (a) Could indicate history of hepatitis
      (9) Cyanosis or mottling
        (a) May indicate serious vascular or cardiac disease

J. Communicable diseases
  1. Scabies
  2. Pediculosis (lice)
  3. Impetigo
    a. Presence of rash, especially in children
  4. Tuberculosis
    a. Making a comeback with advent of human immunodeficiency virus
    b. Newer strains often drug resistant
  5. History of:
    a. Recent fever
    b. Upper respiratory symptoms
    c. Measles (rubeola)
    d. German measles (rubella)
    e. Chickenpox (varicella)
      (1) Treatment before admission to ASC
      (2) Isolation
      (3) Other people, including patients in contact, could contract disease or infestation.
      (4) Wound infection potential as result of self-contamination

K. Gastrointestinal (see Chapter 35)
  1. History
    a. Previous surgery
      (1) Diversional surgery
      (2) Colostomy
    b. Gastrointestinal bleed
    c. Cancer
    d. Hiatal hernia
    e. Chronic diarrhea or constipation
    f. Presence of postoperative nausea and vomiting (PONV)
      (1) If predisposition known, psychological and pharmacological interventions can be initiated to prevent occurrence.
      (2) PONV unpleasant but potential for aspiration strong
    g. Aspiration risk
    h. Pyloric obstruction
    i. Intestinal obstruction
    j. Esophageal diverticula
    k. Diminished pharyngeal reflexes

      l. Obesity

      m. Advanced pregnancy

      n. Unknown compliance with nothing by mouth (NPO) requirements

  2. Assessment

      a. Mouth

      b. Pharynx

      c. Esophagus

      d. Stomach

      e. Large intestine

      f. Small intestine

      g. Pancreas

      h. Liver

      i. Gallbladder

L. Renal and hepatic (see Chapter 37)

  1. Many anesthetic drugs are metabolized in the kidneys and liver.

  2. History or presence of renal or hepatic disease is of great concern.

      a. Pseudocholinesterase

        (1) Enzyme necessary for metabolism of succinylcholine and ester-type local anesthetics

  3. Kidney function

      a. Excretion of urine

      b. Influences fluid and electrolyte and acid–base balance

      c. Nitrogenous wastes from protein metabolism are excreted.

      d. Electrolytes are maintained.

        (1) Sodium, potassium, chloride

        (2) Excretion of some drugs also dependent on kidney function

  4. Liver function

      a. Metabolism of bilirubin

      b. By-products of red blood cell breakdown

      c. Protein synthesis

        (1) Particularly albumin

        (2) Patients with chronic liver disease have decreased serum protein levels.

      d. Drug biotransformation

        (1) Protein-bound drugs (thiopental and bupivacaine) have fewer sites to bind.

        (2) Unbound portions remain active in bloodstream, creating prolonged or enhanced effects.

  5. Physical assessment

      a. Renal disease

        (1) May not be evident until 50% or more function is lost

      b. Liver disease

        (1) Jaundice

        (2) Spider angiomata

        (3) Ecchymosis

        (4) Ascites

        (5) Pedal edema

        (6) Scleral icterus

  6. History

      a. Cirrhosis

        (1) Chronic alcohol or drug abuse

        (2) Idiopathic

      b. Hepatitis

      c. Immune disorders

      d. Extreme forms of dieting

      e. Liver or kidney insufficiency or failure

      f. Extremes in blood pressure

      g. Anemia

      h. Electrolyte imbalance

      i. Depression

   M. Endocrine (see Chapter 34)
   1. Diverse diseases; can affect many processes necessary for tolerance of anesthesia and surgery
   2. Hormones regulate:
      a. Response to stress
      b. Rate of metabolism
      c. Blood pressure
      d. Pulse rates
      e. Blood glucose levels
      f. Urine production
      g. Electrolyte balance
      h. Table 16-3 lists principal hormones and symptoms from imbalances.
   3. Diabetes
      a. Complications secondary to diabetic condition
        (1) Delayed wound healing
        (2) Retinopathy
        (3) Kidney failure
        (4) Peripheral artery disease
        (5) Potential for:
          (a) Ketoacidosis
          (b) MI
          (c) Severe hypoglycemia
      b. Requires special instructions especially with regard to insulin and diet on day of surgery
        (1) Often asked to bring own insulin to ASC
        (2) May be asked to bring own food if ASC does not serve food or serves only donuts or sweet rolls for postoperative nourishment
   N. Hematologic (see Chapter 29)
   1. Disorders of the blood may involve:
      a. Red blood cells
        (1) Anemia
        (2) Sickle cell anemia
        (3) Thalassemia
        (4) Polycythemia
      b. Lymphocytes and plasma cells
        (1) Agranulocytosis
        (2) Leukemia
        (3) Multiple myeloma

■ **TABLE 16-3**
■ ■ **Endocrine Imbalances**

Hormone	Hyposecretion	Hypersecretion
Thyroid hormone	Children—cretinism Adults—myxedema, ↓ BMR, tiredness, mentally slow, bradycardia	Hyperthyroidism, ↑ BMR, always hungry, irritable, tachycardia, weight loss
Parathyroid hormone	Spontaneous discharge of nerves, spasms, tetany, death	Weak, brittle bones; kidney stones
Insulin	Diabetes mellitus	Hypoglycemia
Adrenocortical hormones	Addison's disease (body does not synthesize enough glucose, unable to deal with stress, sodium loss in urine may lead to shock)	Cushing's disease (edema gives full moon face, fat around trunk, ↑ blood glucose levels, depressed immune response)

BMR, basal metabolic rate.
From Quinn DMD: *Ambulatory surgical nursing core curriculum*, Philadelphia, 1999, WB Saunders.

      c. Lymph nodes and spleen
        (1) Lymphoma
        (2) Infectious mononucleosis
      d. Platelets and clotting factors
        (1) Hemorrhagic disorders
        (2) Purpura
        (3) Coagulation disorders
          (a) Hemophilia
          (b) Hypoprothrombinemia
  2. Physical examination
    a. Observation
      (1) Petechiae and bruising
      (2) Pallor and cyanosis
        (a) Skin and mucous membranes
      (3) Hepatomegaly
      (4) Splenomegaly
  3. History of:
    a. Fatigue
    b. Lassitude
    c. Easy bruising
    d. Frequent nosebleeds
    e. Hematuria
    f. Blood in stools
    g. Excessive bleeding after minor injuries or dental extractions
  4. Leukemia and acquired immunodeficiency syndrome
    a. May be scheduled in ASC to avoid hospitalization and subsequent nosocomial infections

II. PSYCHOSOCIAL ASSESSMENT
  A. Evaluation of emotional, cognitive, social, and cultural assessments occurs during physical assessment.
  B. Emotional assessment
    1. Most patients express a moderate to high degree of anxiety and fear facing surgery.
      a. Patients have a right to feel anxiety.
        (1) Placating or belittling the situation seen as demeaning to the patient
        (2) Credibility of staff undermined by this approach
    2. Anxiety and fear are similar but different.
      a. Anxiety is described as a vague, unknown, or unidentified source evoked by a threat to one's existence or personality.
      b. Fear is related to a more specific person or occurrence.
        (1) Some common fears related to surgery are:
          (a) Possibility of not waking up after anesthesia
          (b) Having a mask placed on the face
          (c) Regaining consciousness during the surgery
          (d) Making a fool of oneself
          (e) Feeling the operation
          (f) Anticipated postoperative pain
          (g) Outcome of surgery
      c. Ambulatory surgery would seem to provoke less fear and anxiety, but this is not the case.
        (1) Home recuperation can add additional pressure.
          (a) Fear of facing emergencies at home without medical attention
          (b) Concern about family members who would have to care for them
          (c) Inadequate pain medication
          (d) Need to have another adult for transportation and home support
            (i)   Threat to independence
          (e) Embarrassment at having to ask for help

(f) Problems of obtaining other person to provide support
(g) Pressure of arriving on time
    (i) Many people do not sleep the night before for fear of not waking in time.
(h) May be primary caregiver for spouse
    (i) Concern over their care while in surgery and during recuperation period

3. Preoperative interview important
  a. Assess emotional state.
    (1) Objective observations
      (a) General appearance
      (b) Nervousness
      (c) Decreased attention span
      (d) Lack of eye contact
      (e) Increase heart rate
      (f) Lack of self-confidence
      (g) Decreased concentration
      (h) Rapid speech patterns
      (i) Diaphoresis
      (j) Dry mouth
      (k) Clammy skin
      (l) Pressure of arriving on time
      (m) Nausea
      (n) Urinary frequency
      (o) Hyperventilation
      (p) Precordial chest pain
    (2) Subjective information
      (a) Patient
      (b) Family
    (3) Provide answers to questions.
      (a) Information and support allow patient to gain understanding of upcoming surgery.
      (b) Trust develops with surgical staff.
      (c) By allowing patient to express feelings, staff can help patients to identify coping mechanisms to deal with rational and irrational fears.
      (d) Anxiety can influence amount of teaching patients understand.
        (i) Mildly anxious patients receive the most complete instructions.
        (ii) Moderately anxious patients receive less information.
        (iii) Give more attention to their specific areas of concern.
        (iv) Severely anxious patients should receive only basic information.
        (v) Need encouragement to verbalize fears
      (e) Patients in state of panic are unable to learn.
      (f) No instructions should be given.
      (g) Physician should be notified of patient's status.
    (4) Cognitive assessment
      (a) Evaluate patient's understanding of procedure.
      (b) Ask open-ended questions to elicit and encourage patient's response in own words.
      (c) Avoid yes and no answers.
      (d) Evaluate before having patient sign consent.
      (e) Patient and/or family must be sufficiently intelligent and responsible to provide care.
      (f) Understand and comply with preoperative and postoperative instructions.
      (g) Knowledge of hygiene

(h) Nutrition requirements
(i) Complying with NPO status
C. Illiteracy
1. Written instructions of no use to person who cannot read or understand what is read
2. Estimated more than 23 million Americans are illiterate
a. Cannot read at the level most health care information is written (fifth-grade level)
(1) Many may be able to sign name without reading form.
(a) Clear verbal instructions particularly important
b. Language barrier
(1) English as a second language
(a) Need for interpreter to provide information
(i) Preferably not a family member
(ii) May be protecting patient by withholding information they feel patient should not know
D. Social assessment
1. Concept of ambulatory surgery is family based and home based.
a. Patients need strong support system.
b. Equally important are those persons responsible for aftercare.
2. Evaluation of home situation important during preoperative planning process
a. Elderly patients
(1) Surgical patient may be healthier of couple (spouse/companion).
(a) Often require outside help
(i) Neighbors
(b) Other family members
(c) Home health provider
(d) Physical environment of home
(i) Number of stairs
(e) Bathroom location
(f) May need to use social services to provide discharge planning
(g) Proximity of home to surgical center
E. Cultural assessment
1. Cultural and ethnic beliefs play role in patient's attitudes about health care.
a. Difficult to separate beliefs from modern health care
b. May be considered superstitions by health care workers
(1) Spiritual control over body
(2) Faith healing
(3) Being one with the environment
c. Health care workers must respect patient's cultural beliefs.
III. DIAGNOSTIC ASSESSMENT
A. 1970s and 1980s
1. Many ASCs cared for essentially healthy individuals.
a. Diagnostic practices were limited to few tests.
(1) Fingerstick hemoglobin and hematocrit screen
(2) Dipstick urinalysis
(a) Provided sufficient data to safely administer anesthesia
B. Today—sicker patients having surgery on an outpatient basis
1. Diagnostic requirements now include a variety of basic and complex testing.
a. Often same requirements as hospitalized counterparts
2. Preoperative testing is done to reduce risks associated with anesthesia and surgery.
a. Provides information about whether the patient can tolerate surgical procedures
C. Debate over amount and type of preoperative testing
1. Cost-effectiveness
a. Current trend toward ordering only those tests specifically indicated by abnormal clinical symptoms or history

2. Clinical thoroughness
   a. Diagnostic testing is expensive.
      (1) Benefit thought to outweigh expense
         (a) Offers early detection of previously undiagnosed diseases
         (b) Provides information regarding patient's general health and ability to tolerate surgery

BIBLIOGRAPHY

1. Allen GC, for the North American Malignant Hyperthermia Registry of MHAUS: The sensitivity and specificity of the caffeine-halothane contracture test: a report from the North American Malignant Hyperthermia Registry. *Anesthesiology* 88(3):579-588, 1998.
2. Burden N, Quinn DMD, O'Brien D, et al: *Ambulatory surgical nursing*, Philadelphia, 2000, WB Saunders.
3. Delgan JH, Vallerand AH: *Davis's drug guide for nurses*, ed 20, Philadelphia, 2009, Davis.
4. Dennison, RD: *Pass CCRN*, ed 3, St Louis, 2007, Mosby.
5. Drain C, Odom-Forren J: *Perianesthesia nursing: A critical care approach*, ed 5, Philadelphia, 2009, WB Saunders.
6. Fagerlund K, Salwyc E, Temple M: A national survey of certified registered nurse anesthetists knowledge, beliefs, and assessment of herbal supplements in the anesthesia setting. *AANA J* 73(5):368-377, 2005.
7. Fischback F: *Manual of laboratory and diagnostic tests*, ed 8, Philadelphia, 2008, Lippincott.
8. Flanagan K: Preoperative assessment: safety considerations for patients taking herbal products. *J Perianesth Nurs* 16(1):19-26, 2001.
9. Hooper T: *Mosby's pharmacy technician: Principles and practice*, ed 2, Philadelphia, 2007, Saunders.
10. Lewis SM, Heitkemper MM, Dirksen SR: *Medical-surgical nursing: Assessment and management of clinical problems*, ed 7, St Louis, 2008, Mosby.

Preexisting Medical Conditions

LOIS SCHICK

OBJECTIVES

At the conclusion of this chapter, the reader will be able to:

1. Identify patients with an increased perioperative risk.
2. State the specific perioperative nursing care priorities for the high-risk patient.
3. Describe techniques to reduce perioperative morbidity and mortality.

I. PREEXISTING MEDICAL CONDITIONS
  A. Increases American Society of Anesthesiologists classification
  B. Increases perioperative risk, morbidity, and mortality
  C. May require multiple medications
    1. Increased potential for drug interactions
    2. Increased potential for laboratory test alterations
    3. Increased potential for noncompliance
  D. May jeopardize ambulatory status
II. CARDIOVASCULAR DISEASES (see Chapter 32)
  A. Hypertension
    1. Definition: systolic blood pressure (BP) >140 mm Hg and/or diastolic BP >90 mm Hg on three separate readings
      a. Ideal BP of 120/80 mm Hg or less
      b. Hypertensive crisis: BP >180/110 mm Hg or mean arterial pressure >150 mm Hg
    2. Incidence: 24% of U.S. population; greater in males than females
    3. Significance
      a. Risk factor for coronary artery disease, cerebrovascular accidents, congestive heart failure, arterial aneurysm, and end-stage renal failure
      b. Common in diabetics associated with diabetic neuropathy
    4. Etiology and findings
      a. Severe hypertension (diastolic BP >110 mm Hg): immediate evaluation with surgery cancelled because of increased cardiac morbidity
      b. Primary (essential hypertension): untreated or inadequate treatment
        (1) Accounts for >95% of patients
        (2) Risk factors (Box 17-1)
        (3) Poor compliance
          (a) Lack of symptoms (silent myocardial infarction [MI])
          (b) Side effects of pharmacological agents
          (c) Cost of pharmacological agents
        (4) Mechanisms
          (a) Hyperactivity of sympathetic nervous system: epinephrine and norepinephrine increase cardiac contractility and vasoconstriction.
          (b) Hyperactivity of renin-angiotensin-aldosterone system
          (c) Endothelial dysfunction: vasoconstriction leads to hypertrophy of vascular smooth muscles.
      c. Secondary (Box 17-2)
        (1) Accounts for <5% causes

■ BOX 17-1
■ **PRIMARY RISK FACTORS FOR HYPERTENSION**

Family history
Black race
Obesity
Hyperlipidemia
Diabetes
Tobacco use
Excessive alcohol use
Stress
Sedentary lifestyle
Aging
Oral contraceptives
High-fat diet, high-sodium diet, or both

■ BOX 17-2
■ **SECONDARY RISK FACTORS FOR HYPERTENSION**

Increased renin-angiotensin levels
Acute and chronic glomerulonephritis
Eclampsia or preeclampsia of pregnancy
Central nervous system injuries (head, spinal cord)
Burns
Drug side effects: oral contraceptives, steroids, cocaine, amphetamines, methamphetamine, decongestants
Drug interactions: monoamine oxidase inhibitors, ethyl alcohol
Drug withdrawal: clonidine, beta-blockers, alcohol
Pheochromocytoma
Polycythemia
Coarctation of the aorta
Pituitary or adrenocortical hyperfunction: Cushing's syndrome and primary hyperaldosteronism
Vasculitis
Scleroderma

    5. Perianesthesia considerations
      a. Advise patient to take routine prescription antihypertensive medication on day of surgery with sip of water.
      b. Ask about presence of heart disease during preoperative interview.
      c. Postoperative systemic hypertension warrants prompt assessment and treatment to minimize risks of myocardial ischemia, heart failure, stroke, and bleeding.
        (1) Assess for pain.
        (2) Assess for fluid overload.
  B. Coronary artery disease (CAD)
    1. Definition: accumulation of plaque within coronary arteries resulting in narrowing or obstruction
    2. Incidence: common in men; predominantly younger than 55 years; equal in men and women older than 55
    3. Significance: increased risk for MI, diabetes, hypertension, renal disease, dysrhythmias, high cholesterol, hyperlipidemia, congestive heart failure (CHF), familial incidence, and sudden death
    4. Etiology
      a. Atherosclerosis with obstructive deposits in coronary arteries

      b. Common factors:
- (1) Genetics
- (2) Diet
- (3) Environment
- (4) Hypertension
- (5) Diabetes

      c. Myocardial ischemia may occur when there is an increase in oxygen demand in the following conditions:
- (1) Increased sympathetic activity
- (2) Surgical stress and pain
- (3) Interruption of beta-blocker medications
- (4) Use of sympathomimetic drugs

      d. MI may occur because of reduced oxygen supply in the following conditions:
- (1) Hypotension
- (2) Vasospasm
- (3) Anemia
- (4) Hypoxia

5. Perianesthesia considerations

      a. Requires evaluation and clearance from a cardiologist

      b. May increase intraoperative monitoring requirements

      c. Assess for any of following signs of CHF and if present, surgery may be cancelled.
- (1) Shortness of breath
- (2) Dyspnea on exertion or nocturnal
- (3) Jugular venous distention
- (4) Crackles
- (5) Edema

      d. Assess incidence and triggers of chest pain.
- (1) If new onset (<2 months) or unstable, postpone surgery pending cardiologist evaluation.
- (2) All prescription medications to be taken on morning of surgery with sip of water

      e. Treatment:
- (1) Coronary vasodilators (nitrates)
- (2) Exercise
- (3) Diet
- (4) Weight loss
- (5) Antihyperlipidemia drugs
- (6) Aspirin
- (7) Patient education

      f. Second and third postoperative days are most common time for MI in noncardiac surgical patients.

      g. Intraoperative ischemia designates patient as "high risk" in postoperative period.

C. Heart failure

  1. Definition

      a. Heart cannot pump enough blood to meet the body's metabolic needs.

      b. CHF is an interruption in circulation.
- (1) Failure of heart to function normally
- (2) Impairment of heart to fill or empty the left ventricle
- (3) Congestion in lung and peripheral beds
  - (a) Respiratory symptoms
  - (b) Peripheral edema

  2. Incidence

      a. Most common inpatient diagnosis for patients older than 65 years

      b. Complication of most cardiac disease: 4 to 5 million cases in United States

      c. Primary diagnosis for 1 million hospitalizations

        d. Medium survival after onset for men is 1.7 years and 3.2 years for women.
    3. Significance: increased risk for pulmonary edema, dyspnea, peripheral edema
    4. Etiology: CAD, myocardial infarction, rheumatic heart disease, volume overload, congenital heart disease, noncompliance with medications
        a. Acquired acute or chronic cardiac disease
        b. Congenital heart disease
        c. Multiple precipitating causes
            (1) Noncompliance with medications
            (2) Excessive sodium
            (3) Excessive intravenous (IV) fluids
            (4) Drugs
                (a) Beta-blockers
                (b) Corticosteroids
                (c) Nortriptyline
                (d) Disopyramide
                (e) Nonsteroidal anti-inflammatory drugs (NSAIDs)
                (f) Androgens
                (g) Estrogens
                (h) Doxorubicin
            (5) High-output states
                (a) Pregnancy
                (b) Fever
                (c) Hyperthyroid
                (d) Sepsis
                (e) Arteriovenous fistula
                (f) Anemia
    5. Perianesthesia considerations
        a. If symptomatic (see section II.B), surgery cancelled
        b. Auscultate breath sounds on arrival, on admission to post anesthesia care unit phase I, and before discharge.
        c. Obtain chest x-ray.
        d. Obtain cardiologist clearance before surgery.
        e. Increased mortality rate by 40% during first 4 years after diagnosis
        f. Strict intake and output records
        g. Aggressive pain management to avoid sympathetic activation of pulmonary edema intraoperatively and postoperatively
        h. Regional anesthesia acceptable for peripheral operations
        i. May need postoperative mechanical ventilatory support
        j. Treatment:
            (1) Diuretics
            (2) Inotropic therapy
            (3) Oxygen
            (4) Low-sodium diet
            (5) Ventricular assist devices
D. Mitral valve disease
    1. Definition: prolapse or stenosis of mitral heart valve that results in resistance to left ventricular emptying (increased afterload)
        a. Prolapse: billowing of posterior mitral leaf into the left atrium during systole
        b. Regurgitation: the mitral valve does not close tightly which allows the blood to flow backward to the heart.
        c. Stenosis: mechanical obstruction to left ventricular filling secondary to progressive decreases in the mitral valve orifice
    2. Incidence: age <30 congenital; age >70 degenerative
    3. Significance:
        a. Increased risk of angina
        b. Syncope
        c. Fatigue

    d. Dyspnea

    e. Heart murmur on auscultation

    f. Pulmonary embolism

    g. Dysrhythmias

4. Etiology:

    a. Congenital

    b. Rheumatic heart disease

    c. Aging

5. Perianesthesia considerations

    a. It is suggested patients at greatest risk for a bad outcome from infective endocarditis take short-term preventive antibiotics before dental work.

    b. Patients at greatest risk for bad outcomes include

      (1) Artificial heart valves

      (2) History of previous infective endocarditis

      (3) Certain specific, serious congenital heart conditions

      (4) Cardiac transplant that develops a problem in a heart valve

    c. May be anticoagulated on warfarin; check prothrombin time/international normalized ratio (PT/INR)

      (1) Patient may be asked to stop warfarin 3 days before surgery.

    d. Risk of pulmonary edema

    e. Avoid hypertension and acute increases in sympathetic tone.

    f. Treatment

      (1) Prolapse often requires no treatment.

      (2) Regurgitation often requires valve replacement if ejection fraction <0.6.

      (3) When symptoms increase or pulmonary hypertension develops, stenosis requires:

        (a) Valve reconstruction

        (b) Commissurotomy

        (c) Valve replacement

        (d) Prophylaxis against endocarditis

        (e) Diuretics

        (f) Anticoagulant therapy

        (g) Low-sodium diet

        (h) Controlling heart rate, because tachycardia impairs left ventricular filling and increases left atrial pressure

          (i) Digoxin

          (ii) Beta-blockers

          (iii) Calcium channel blockers

E. Aortic valve disease (Table 17-1)

    1. Insufficiency: also described as aortic regurgitation, aortic incompetence

    2. Aortic stenosis

F. Dysrhythmias

    1. Definition: alteration in conduction system requiring pharmacological or surgical (automatic implantable cardiac defibrillator [AICD], pacemaker) intervention

    2. Incidence: very common (dysrhythmias)

      a. Use of pacemakers and AICDs increases with age.

      b. Common outcome of coronary artery disease

    3. Significance: increased risk of MI and progression to lethal dysrhythmias

    4. Etiology:

      a. CAD

      b. CHF

      c. Valve disease

      d. Myocardial infarction

      e. Hypoxia

      f. Hypercarbia

      g. Electrolyte imbalance

■ TABLE 17-1
■ ■ **Aortic Valve Disease**

	Insufficiency	**Stenosis**
Definitions	Aortic valve leaflets do not close properly Blood flows back into left ventricle during systole	Stiff and fibrotic valve Narrowing of aortic valve
Incidence	Manifests in third to sixth decade	Manifests in third to sixth decade
Significance	Dyspnea Syncope Congestive heart failure ECG changes Pulmonary edema Exercise intolerance	Dyspnea on exertion Chest pain (angina) Syncope Congestive heart failure Exercise intolerance Risk for bacterial endocarditis
Etiology	Rheumatic heart disease Congenital Marfan syndrome Acquired disease (syphilis, aortic dissection) Infection (endocarditis) Trauma	Congenital defect Rheumatic heart disease Calcification
Perianesthesia considerations	**PREPROCEDURE** Continue preoperative medications Monitor atrial fibrillation Check INR Antibiotic therapy **POST PROCEDURE** Suppress catecholamines on emergence May have delayed emergence Monitor cardiac output Treat atrial dysrhythmias Restart preoperative medications (digoxin, diuretics) Maintain or increase contractility (use dopamine) Decrease afterload (nicardipine, nitroprusside) Anticoagulate	**PREPROCEDURE** Continue preoperative medications (anticoagulant therapy) Suppress catecholamines (control pain) **POST PROCEDURE** Avoid tachycardia Avoid histamine and catecholamine release Consider dexmedetomidine infusion (provides analgesia without respiratory depression; can delay awakening; can potentiate beta-blockers) Restart preoperative medications (Digoxin, diuretics, anticoagulants if chronic atrial fibrillation)

ECG, Electrocardiogram; *INR*, international normalized ratio.

  h. Acid-base alterations
  i. Altered activity of the autonomic nervous system
  j. Drugs (i.e., volatile anesthetics, catecholamines)
5. Perianesthesia considerations
  a. Treatment: pharmacological, patient education, pacemaker (heart block, asystole), cardioversion, AICD (ventricular fibrillation)
  b. Perioperative significance
    (1) Patient to take anti-dysrhythmic medications on day of surgery
    (2) Inquire about type of pacemaker and setting (patient may have pacer identification card); document in chart (may need to call cardiologist).
    (3) Have external pacemaker readily available.
    (4) Have cardiologist available, although not necessarily in the operating room (OR).
    (5) If patient has AICD, bovie or cautery should not be used during surgery.
      (a) If bovie or cautery must be used, AICD is turned off.
      (b) External defibrillator must be available in OR suite for immediate use if needed.

III. PULMONARY DISEASES (see Chapter 31)
    A. Chronic obstructive pulmonary disease (COPD)
        1. Definition: term includes chronic bronchitis and emphysema.
            a. Bronchitis
                (1) Chronic productive cough caused by excess bronchial mucus secretions
                (2) Reduction in expiratory flow rate
                (3) Signs include cough, increased sputum production, dyspnea, wheezing.
            b. Emphysema
                (1) Characterized by abnormal permanent enlargement air spaces distal to terminal bronchioles
                (2) Destruction of parenchyma
                (3) Increased minute ventilation to compensate for hypercapnia
                (4) Signs include barrel chest, pursed lip breathing, decreased breath sounds, dyspnea.
        2. Incidence: 20% to 30% of adults younger than 40 years; greater in males than in females
        3. Significance: hypoxia, hypercapnia, pneumonia, respiratory failure, bronchospasm, atelectasis
        4. Etiology: cigarette smoking, air pollution, occupational exposure to smoke
        5. Perianesthesia considerations
            a. Treatment: bronchodilators, possibly anticholinergics and corticosteroids, patient education to stop smoking at least 8 to 10 weeks before surgery
            b. General anesthesia may exacerbate symptoms and disease; regional anesthesia avoids intubation and use of controlled ventilation.
            c. Patient's respirations controlled by hypoxic drive.
                (1) High flow, high concentration of oxygen may produce apnea.
                (2) Nasal cannula <3 L oxygen preferred delivery system unless unable to maintain saturation
            d. Encourage deep breathing and coughing after general anesthesia; postoperative pulmonary infections common
            e. Ask patient to bring inhalers used to the facility on day of surgery.
            f. Pulmonary function tests may be ordered preoperatively.
            g. Consider impact of neuraxial blockade and/or sedation if COPD.
                (1) COPD patients rely on intercostals and abdominal muscles.
                    (a) Clearing of secretions affected
                    (b) Coughing ability impacted
                    (c) Avoid techniques that provide sensory anesthesia above T6.
    B. Asthma
        1. Definition: tracheobronchial disorder characterized by obstruction to airflow secondary to narrowing of airways, edema, and inflammation
        2. Incidence: 22 million cases in United States; affects 6 million children
        3. Significance: increased risk of laryngospasm and bronchospasm on induction, hypoxemia, decreased peak flow rates
        4. Etiology: allergic factors, genetic predisposition, smoke, infection, cold air, exercise, and occupational exposures such as grain dust, plastics, and fumes
        5. Perianesthesia considerations
            a. Treatment: oxygen, bronchodilators (beta-2 agonists), corticosteroids (acute asthma), mast cell stabilizers, education, mechanical ventilation
            b. Encourage patient to avoid known irritants to minimize wheezing.
            c. Question patient on the frequency, severity, and management of attacks.
            d. Auscultate breath sounds preoperatively and postoperatively.
            e. Increased risk of bronchospasm on intubation and emergence
            f. Halothane, sevoflurane, and ketamine may be used because they cause bronchodilation during administration.
            g. Ask patient to use and to bring any inhalers used to the facility on day of surgery.
            h. If receiving steroids, determine last use and dose; may need steroid preoperatively.

(1) Steroids by inhalation diminish systemic affects.

(2) If steroid-resistant asthma, IV immunoglobin may be administered.

(3) If patient with severe asthma receiving long-term oral corticosteroid therapy, a burst of corticosteroids may need to be administered to prevent adrenal insufficiency.

    i. Cancel surgery if patient has an upper respiratory infection.

C. Smoking

    1. Definition: use of inhaled tobacco

    2. Incidence: extremely common; teenagers, adults, and elderly. Young females fastest growing group

    3. Significance: increased risk of COPD, heart disease, hypertension, peripheral vascular disease, hypoxia, poor tissue healing, postoperative pulmonary complications six times greater than that of nonsmoker, hyper-reactive airway, higher rate of prolonged mechanical ventilation

    4. Etiology: access to and use of product, habituation

    5. Perianesthesia considerations

        a. Treatment: cessation, nicotine patch, Smokers Anonymous, self-withdrawal

        b. Patient has elevated carboxyhemoglobin levels.

        c. Carbon monoxide has greater affinity for hemoglobin than does oxygen.

        d. Increased risk of bronchospasm and laryngospasm on induction, intubation, emergence

        e. Encourage patient to stop smoking 8 weeks before surgery; be aware that most will not comply. No smoking on day of surgery.

        f. If chronic productive cough, preoperative antibiotics may be used.

        g. Consider deep extubation if severe reactive airway disease.

        h. Epidural analgesia may be beneficial

            (1) To decrease hypercoagulability

            (2) In patients with CAD

            (3) In patients with COPD

        i. Risks associated with cigarette smoking (Table 17-2)

D. Obstructive sleep apnea

    1. Definition: repetitive episodes of upper airway occlusion during sleep often with oxygen desaturation; apnea defined as cessation of airflow at mouth for >10 seconds

    2. Incidence

        a. Middle-aged women, 2%; middle-aged men, 4%

        b. Suspected that 80% of cases undiagnosed

    3. Significance:

        a. Obesity with body mass index >30 and large neck circumference

        b. High risk of postoperative complications when undergoing general anesthesia

        c. Systemic and pulmonary hypertension

    4. Etiology: chronic decrease in partial pressure of oxygen in arterial blood (Pao_2) during apneic episodes, pharyngeal fat deposits, obesity exacerbate upper airway obstruction

    5. Perianesthesia considerations

        a. Preoxygenation because of reduced functional residual capacity

        b. Extubation when breathing spontaneously

        c. Repetitive apnea can occur with opioid and benzodiazepine administration.

        d. Bring in continuous positive airway pressure for postoperative usage.

        e. Assess cardiovascular status.

        f. Preoperative histamine (H_2) blockers and antacids for morbidly obese

        g. Potential for airway obstruction at induction and on extubation

        h. Aspiration risk

        i. Postoperative thromboembolism

        j. Worsening pulmonary hypertension and right-sided heart failure

        k. Consider candidate for apnea even several hours postoperatively, especially after epidural anesthesia.

■ TABLE 17-2
■ ■ **Risks Associated with Cigarette Smoking**

Cardiovascular	Coronary artery disease
	Peripheral vascular occlusive disease
	Cerebrovascular disease
	Stroke
Respiratory	Chronic obstructive pulmonary disease
	Reduced lung function
Gastrointestinal	Peptic ulcer disease
	Esophageal reflux
	Gum disease
	Tooth loss
Cancer	Lung
	Oral cavity
	Larynx
	Esophagus
	Stomach
	Pancreas
	Kidney
	Urinary bladder
	Colon
Gestational	**PERINATAL**
	Increases in miscarriage; stillbirth; low birth weight
	Sudden infant death syndrome
	Impaired intellectual development
	MATERNAL
	Increases in abruptio placenta and placenta previa
Ophthalmic	Macular degeneration
	Cataracts
Musculoskeletal	Osteoporosis
	Spinal disc disease
Reproductive	Infertility
Immune	Inhibited immune function
Dermatologic	Premature facial wrinkling

From Nagelhout J, Zaglaniczny KL: *Nurse anesthesia*, ed 3, Philadelphia, 2005, Saunders.

IV. RENAL DISEASES (see Chapter 37)
   A. Acute renal failure (ARF)
      1. Definition: impairment or cessation of kidney function characterized by accumulation of nitrogenous waste and fluid and electrolyte imbalance
      2. Significance: patient will experience derangement in fluid-electrolyte balance, acid-base homeostasis, calcium/phosphate metabolism, BP regulation, and erythropoiesis.
      3. Incidence: 5% of hospitalized patients have coexisting renal disease that could contribute to perioperative morbidity.
      4. Etiology
         a. Prenal: decreased renal blood flow leads to hypoperfusion.
            (1) Hypovolemia
            (2) Hypotension
            (3) Vasoconstriction
            (4) Inadequate cardiac output
         b. Renal (intrinsic): damage to filtering structure of kidneys
            (1) Ischemia

           (2) Nephrotoxins

           (3) Inflammation

     c. Postrenal: urinary tract obstruction

        (1) Prostatic hypertrophy

        (2) Cancer of prostate or cervix

        (3) Congenital anomalies

     d. ARF pass through three distinct phases.

        (1) Oliguric phase

           (a) Necrosis of tubules

           (b) Retrograde increase in pressure

           (c) Decrease in glomerular filtration rate (GFR)

           (d) Inability to conserve sodium

           (e) Fluid volume excess

           (f) Azotemia

           (g) Electrolyte imbalance

           (h) Renal failure can occur within 24 hours

        (2) Diuretic phase

           (a) Increased urine secretion of >400 mL/24 hours

           (b) GFR increased or normal

           (c) Increased blood urea nitrogen (BUN) produces osmotic diuresis, deficits of sodium and potassium.

           (d) May last days or weeks

        (3) Recovery phase

           (a) Gradual return to normal or near normal

           (b) Occurs in 3 to 12 months

  5. Perianesthesia considerations

     a. Patient inappropriate for ambulatory surgery

     b. Assess hemoglobin and hematocrit levels.

     c. Measure intake and output accurately.

     d. Maintain proper electrolyte balance.

     e. Use sterile technique because highly susceptible to infections.

B. Chronic renal failure (CRF)

  1. Definition: progressive, irreversible disruption of the excretory and regulatory function of the nephron; inability to eliminate waste products and maintain fluid and electrolyte balance. When renal replacement therapy is required, the patient has end-stage renal disease (ESRD).

  2. Incidence: 500,000 patients affected by ESRD in United States; 1.4 times higher for males than females, and 4 times higher for African Americans. CRF will develop in 25% to 30% of patients with ARF.

  3. Significance: patients commonly diabetic with multiple laboratory alterations, hypertension and anemia

  4. Etiology: pyelonephritis, polycystic kidneys, autoimmune, diabetes mellitus, drug-induced nephropathy (antibiotics, NSAIDs), hypertension, congenital

  5. Perianesthesia considerations

     a. All anesthetic techniques have potential to reduce renal perfusion.

     b. Obtain preoperative weight.

     c. Obtain preoperative glucose level in diabetic patients.

     d. Determine date of last dialysis; if off schedule, anticipate fluid and electrolyte imbalance.

     e. Instruct patient to take antihypertensive medications on day of surgery.

     f. Anemia may compromise oxygenation, especially with hematocrit <18%.

     g. Monitor electrolytes (potassium, BUN, serum creatinine) and renal function (urinalysis) preoperatively, as well as complete blood count and bleeding time.

     h. Careful intake and output; may be on fluid restriction

     i. Use of lactated Ringer's or dextrose in lactated Ringer's may lead to acidosis; use 0.9% normal saline or 5% dextrose in one-half normal saline.

     j. Avoid same-arm venipunctures and BPs if patient has arteriovenous fistula for hemodialysis.

     k. Avoid nephrotoxic drugs.

     l. Consider decreased doses of medications eliminated through kidneys; avoid meperidine and potassium-containing solutions.

     m. Increased risk for infection

     n. Poor tolerance for physiological stress

     o. Treatment: renal replacement therapy, hemodialysis, peritoneal dialysis, ultrafiltration, renal transplantation, diet, patient education

V. LIVER DISEASES

  A. Key functions of liver

    1. Detoxifies chemicals

    2. Makes bile

    3. Stores energy

    4. Manufactures new proteins

    5. Produces plasma

  B. Hepatitis

    1. Definition

     a. Diffuse inflammation of liver

     b. Infectious or noninfectious

     c. Acute hepatitis is an inflammatory disease of hepatocytes.

      (1) Most often caused by a virus

      (2) May be from drugs and toxins

      (3) Lasts less than 6 months

     d. Chronic hepatitis (active): widespread destruction of hepatocytes causing cirrhosis and hepatic failure

      (1) Nonprogressive inflammatory disease confined to portal areas

      (2) Lasts more than 6 months

    2. Incidence (varies with cause)

     a. Hepatitis A: 25% of cases

      (1) Active viral hepatitis associated with high morbidity and mortality

      (2) Elective surgery should not be performed on patients until 4 weeks after blood tests normalized.

     b. Hepatitis B: 3% to 5% of population has disease, whereas 0.3% to 1% are carriers.

     c. Hepatitis C: most common cause of acute viral hepatitis; greater in males than in females

    3. Significance: hepatitis in presence of alcoholism increases risk of cirrhosis and depending on extent of disease, may have alterations in:

     a. Coagulation

     b. Fluid and electrolytes

     c. Wound healing

    4. Etiology: viral

     a. Hepatitis A: transmitted enterically (fecal-oral route)

      (1) Contaminated water

      (2) Raw or partially cooked shellfish

      (3) Infectious

       (a) Two weeks before jaundice

       (b) One week after jaundice

     b. Hepatitis B: carried in and spread by blood and body fluid including sexual contacts

     c. Hepatitis C: transmitted via blood transfusions and body fluids, although in 50% of cases route of transmission unknown

      (1) Fifty percent of infected cases become chronic.

      (2) No immunity is developed.

      (3) Leading cause of liver transplantation in United States

     d. Chronic infection from hepatitis leads to cirrhosis and liver cancer.

5. Perianesthesia considerations
   a. Treatment: supportive because disease is viral
      (1) Hepatitis A: immune globulin, hepatitis A vaccine, treat at home unless dehydrated
      (2) Hepatitis B: hepatitis B vaccine for prevention, hepatitis B immune globulin for passive immunization, bed rest, and orthotopic liver transplantation for liver failure
      (3) Hepatitis C: type 1 interferon with or without ribavirin; orthotopic liver transplantation for liver failure
   b. Patients with acute hepatitis are inappropriate for ambulatory surgery.
   c. Patients with chronic persistent hepatitis should be evaluated by a gastroenterologist before surgery.
   d. Consider obtaining preoperative liver enzymes to compare with previous levels.
      (1) Increases reflect worsening of disease.
      (2) Requires medical evaluation before surgery
   e. Anticipate hypoglycemia and potential fluid overload postoperatively.
   f. Be cognizant of potential for delayed awakening from prolonged drug metabolism or encephalopathy.
   g. Vigilance to universal precautions

C. Cirrhosis—liver failure
   1. Definition: hepatic fibrosis producing portal hypertension including ascites, variceal bleeding, hepatic encephalopathy
   2. Incidence: 30,000 deaths per year; greater in males than in females
   3. Significance: inappropriate for ambulatory surgery
   4. Etiology: excessive alcohol ingestion, chronic viral hepatitis
   5. Perianesthesia considerations
      a. Volatile anesthetics decrease hepatic blood flow.
      b. At risk for aspiration
      c. Treatment
         (1) Parenteral vitamin K if PTs prolonged
         (2) Monitor arterial blood gases, pH.
         (3) Monitor intake and urine output.
         (4) Monitor for hypoglycemia.
      d. Ensure adequate hydration.

D. Alcohol abuse (Table 17-3)
   1. Definition: illness characterized by significant impairment associated with persistent and excessive use of alcohol
      a. Physiological impairment
      b. Psychological impairment
      c. Social impairment
   2. Incidence: 10% of men; 3.5% of women; 11% to 15% of all adults; highest incidence between 18 and 39 years of age
   3. Significance: associated with malnutrition, poor compliance, hypertension, pulmonary disease with concomitant cigarette use, stroke, diabetes, gastrointestinal (GI) disease
   4. Etiology: biological, psychological, and sociocultural factors
   5. Perianesthesia considerations
      a. Compliance with preoperative and postoperative instructions may be poor.
      b. Determine usual consumption, time, and amount of last drink.
      c. Patients arriving intoxicated for ambulatory procedures should have surgery cancelled.
      d. Malnutrition may compromise wound healing.
      e. Correct hyponatremia and hypokalemia slowly (over 24-48 hours).
      f. Aberrant responses to narcotics and benzodiazepines
      g. At risk for cirrhosis, alterations in coagulation, and bleeding
      h. Delirium tremens may require heavy sedation or restraints to prevent patient self-injury.

■ TABLE 17-3
■ ■ **Alcohol Withdrawal Syndrome**

Early manifestations	Generalized tremor
	Autonomic nervous system hyperactivity
	Insomnia
	Agitation
Delirium tremens (2-4 days after cessation of alcohol ingestion)	Hallucinations
	Combativeness
	Hyperthermia
	Tachycardia
	Hypotension/hypertension
	Seizures
Treatment	Diazepam (5-10 mg IV every 5 minutes until patient becomes calm)
	Esmolol until heart rate <100 beats/min
	Correction of electrolyte (magnesium) and metabolic (thiamine) derangements
	Lidocaine
	Physical restraining

Stoelting R, Dierdorf S: *Handbook for anesthesia and co-existing disease*, ed 2, New York, 2002, Churchill Livingstone.

(1) First sign of delirium tremens in patient still sedated after general anesthesia may be tachycardia.
(2) Occurrence of delirium tremens in perioperative period associated with high incidence of morbidity and mortality
  i. Increased incidence of aspiration pneumonitis
    (1) Concomitant pulmonary disease will require aggressive postoperative pulmonary hygiene.
  j. Long-term consumption impairs hepatic metabolism; short-term consumption inhibits drug metabolism.
  k. Polyneuropathy is a relative contraindication to regional anesthesia.
VI. NEUROMUSCULAR, SKELETAL, CONNECTIVE TISSUE DISEASES
  (see Chapters 33 and 42)
  A. Spine Curvature
    1. Definition: C-shaped or S-shaped lateral curvature of vertebral spine
      a. Kyphosis: anterior flexion of vertebral column
      b. Scoliosis: lateral curvature of vertebral column
    2. Incidence: greater in women than in men (80% women)
    3. Significance: most commonly diagnosed and treated in childhood during maximal growth period
    4. Etiology: idiopathic, congenital, neuropathic, myopathic, or traumatic
    5. Perianesthesia considerations
      a. Severe deviations (>50°) can compromise cardiopulmonary function.
      b. Any significant curvature involving the thoracic spine may alter lung function: obtain preoperative pulmonary function tests and institute aggressive pulmonary care postoperatively.
      c. Curvature can cause lower back pain.
      d. Deformity may compromise intraoperative positioning.
      e. Patients with concomitant myopathies likely to require postoperative ventilation; inappropriate as outpatients
      f. In childhood and adolescence: exercises, weight reduction, bracing, casting, surgery (spinal fusion with rod placement)
      g. In adults: spinal fusion
      h. Avoid depressant drugs.

B. Arthritis: rheumatoid and osteoarthritis
   1. Definitions
      a. Rheumatoid: chronic inflammatory disease of multiple joints producing disability and disfigurement
      b. Osteoarthritis: degenerative disease of articular cartilage with minimal inflammation
   2. Incidence
      a. Rheumatoid: 1 in 1000 children; greater in females than in males; most common between ages of 30 and 50 years
      b. Osteoarthritis: 63% to 85% of Americans older than 65 years; 20 million patients
   3. Significance
      a. Rheumatoid: increased incidence of cardiopulmonary involvement
      b. Osteoarthritis: most common form of joint disease with stiffness, discomfort, pain
   4. Etiology
      a. Rheumatoid: unknown, includes genetics, altered immune response, trauma
      b. Osteoarthritis: aging, genetics
   5. Perianesthesia considerations
      a. Rheumatoid arthritis
         (1) Joint stiffness worse in morning; consider afternoon scheduling.
         (2) Pericardial effusion, thickening present in one third of adults
         (3) Pleural effusion is the most common pulmonary alteration.
      b. Osteoarthritis
         (1) Corticosteroids not recommended; increased risk of degenerative joint changes
      c. Arthritis (both types)
         (1) Cervical spine and temporomandibular joint involvement may restrict neck mobility for intubation; may require use of fiberoptic bronchoscopy.
         (2) Limited joint mobility may compromise intraoperative positioning.
         (3) NSAIDs can alter platelet function and coagulation and cause mild anemia.
         (4) Obtain preoperative coagulation studies, hemoglobin, and hematocrit.
         (5) Treatment: goal is to maintain joint function and to minimize disability.
            (a) Rheumatoid: symptomatic, NSAIDs, gold, methotrexate, corticosteroids, and newer treatment with combination of tumor necrosis factor (TNF) blocking drugs with methotrexate for patients who failed traditional disease modifying anti-rheumatic drugs
            (b) Osteoarthritis: NSAIDs and heat
C. Muscular dystrophy (MD)
   1. Definition
      a. Progressive disease of muscle resulting in painless degeneration and atrophy of skeletal muscles
         (1) Caused by increased permeability of skeletal muscle membranes and presents with decreased cardiopulmonary reserve
         (2) Ten different varieties, with Duchenne's MD most common and severe
         (3) Inappropriate for ambulatory surgery because of late respiratory depression
      b. Incidence: 1:544,000 in United States, which is 500 newborn boys per year; Duchenne's most prevalent in children, whereas myotonic MD more common in adults. Becker's MD is a milder form of Duchenne's MD.

      c. Significance: gait problems, waddling gait, falls, difficulty standing up, difficulty climbing stairs, difficulty descending stairs, lordosis, firm-looking muscles, enlarged muscles, enlarged calf muscles

      d. Etiology: various genetic mechanisms involving enzymatic or metabolic defect, X- linked recessive disorders

      e. Perianesthesia considerations

        (1) Provide limited sedation.

        (2) Succinylcholine is contraindicated because of hyperkalemia.

        (3) Encourage coughing, deep breathing exercises including diaphragmatic breathing.

D. Myasthenia gravis (see Chapter 19)

    1. Definition: chronic autoimmune disease of neuromuscular junction

      a. Causes disturbance in transmission of impulses between motor neurons and innervated muscle cells

      b. Results in fatigue and diminished muscle strength

    2. Incidence: 5-14 people per 100,000 with incidence of women aged 20 to 30 years, older than 60 years

    3. Significance: disease classified as type I to IV based on skeletal muscle involvement and severity of symptoms

      a. Type I: involvement of only extraocular eye muscles

      b. Type IIA: slow, progressive mild skeletal muscle weakness without respiratory muscle involvement

      c. Type IIB: severe, rapidly progressive form of skeletal muscle weakness with respiratory muscle weakness

      d. Type III: acute onset, rapid deterioration of skeletal muscle strength with high mortality

      e. Type IV: severe skeletal muscle weakness that results from progression of type I or type II

    4. Etiology: unknown; thymus gland abnormality; autoimmune disease of neuromuscular junction mediated by reduction in number of acetylcholine receptors at neuromuscular junction

    5. Perianesthesia considerations

      a. Not appropriate for ambulatory surgery if type IIB, III, or IV

      b. Will likely require prolonged postoperative ventilatory support

      c. Anticholinesterase drugs alter effects of nondepolarizing muscle relaxants with variable responses.

      d. Susceptible to respiratory depression

      e. Consider epidural analgesics.

      f. Treatment: anticholinesterase drugs pyridostigmine (Mestinon), corticosteroids, immunosuppressants, plasmapheresis, thymectomy

E. Parkinson's disease (paralysis agitans) (see Chapter 19)

    1. Definition: slow adult-onset, progressive disease of central nervous system (CNS) degeneration characterized by classic triad of resting tremor, muscle rigidity, and bradykinesia (slow movement)

    2. Incidence: 50,000 new cases per year; greater in men than in women; onset >40 years of age

    3. Significance: do not assume presence of mental status changes.

    4. Etiology: possible genetic predisposition

    5. Perianesthesia considerations

      a. Physical limitations may increase need for assistive devices.

      b. Continue levodopa on day of surgery—interruption of drug for 6 to 12 hours can result in loss of drug's therapeutic effect, including difficulty in maintaining ventilation.

      c. Levodopa may produce orthostatic hypotension, dysrhythmias, hypertension.

      d. Use of phenothiazines (Compazine) and butyrophenones (Droperidol) contraindicated—may produce extrapyramidal effects

      e. Depression common in advanced stages of disease (if monoamine oxidase [MAO] inhibitors being used, notify anesthesiologist)

    f. Intravascular volume depletion and inadequate response to hypotension make BP and heart rate fluctuate.

    g. Ketamine may cause exaggerated sympathetic response.

    h. Potential hyperkalemic response to succinylcholine

    i. Postoperative period

        (1) Close attention to respiratory status

        (2) Close attention to CNS state

        (3) Begin anti-Parkinson's therapy immediately after surgery.

    j. Treatment: no cure

        (1) Goal is to control symptoms and to slow disease course.

        (2) Dopaminergics

            (a) Levodopa

            (b) Levodopa in combination with Carbidopa (Sinemet, Parcopa)

            (c) Bromocriptine mesylate (Parlodel)

            (d) Pramipexole (Mirapex)

            (e) Amantadine hydrochloride (Symmetrel)

            (f) Ropinirole (Requip)

            (g) Dopaminergics are contraindicated with:

                (i) Glaucoma

                (ii) Within 2 weeks of administration of MAO inhibitors

        (3) Stereotaxic surgery

        (4) Experimental treatment with fetal adrenal implantation

F. Multiple sclerosis (MS) (see Chapter 19)

    1. Definition: autoimmune demyelinating disease that affects both the spinal cord and brain

    2. Incidence: MS usually begins between ages of 20 and 40 years; 8:1 women to men; occurs in temperate climates.

    3. Significance: injuries from falls, urinary tract infection, joint contractures, pressure ulcers

    4. Etiology: unknown

    a. Slow-acting or latent viral infection, an autoimmune response, environmental and genetic factors

    b. Emotional stress, overwork, fatigue, pregnancy, and acute respiratory tract infections exacerbate or precede onset

    5. Perianesthesia considerations

    a. Document preoperative neurologic status.

    b. May need premedication with benzodiazepines

    c. Provide adequate volume status.

    d. Consider steroid supplementation.

    e. Exacerbation of MS with hyperthermia

    f. Hyperkalemia with succinylcholine

G. Lupus erythematosus

    1. Definition

    a. Chronic inflammatory disorder of connective tissues

        (1) Discoid lupus erythematosus (skin)

        (2) Systemic lupus erythematosus

    b. Characterized by recurring remissions and exacerbations

    2. Incidence 1:1000; females greater than males; majority of patients aged 30 to 40 years at time of diagnosis

    3. Significance: respiratory obstruction, systemic vascular collapse

    4. Etiology: unknown; autoimmune process possibly after trauma to mast cells

    5. Perianesthesia considerations:

    a. Steroid dose if receiving long-term steroid therapy

    b. Careful titration of fluid; accurate intake and output

    c. Assess respiratory, renal, cardiovascular status before extubation.

    d. Treat with rest, steroids, salicylates.

    H. Systemic sclerosis
        1. Definition
            a. Disease state causing changes in connective tissue that affect synovium, skin, blood vessels, and internal organs
            b. Scleroderma: disorder affects only skin
            c. Rare chronic autoimmune condition
        2. Incidence
            a. Women greater than men: 3:1 to 7:1
            b. More prevalent in women between ages of 35 and 54 years
            c. More prevalent in Native Americans and African Americans
        3. Significance
            a. Painless edema in hands and fingers
            b. Taut and shiny skin that lacks elasticity
            c. Loss of range of motion in joints, leading to contractures
            d. As sclerosis progresses, process of hardening and fibrosis adversely affects internal organs and structures, including heart and lungs.
        4. Etiology: autoimmune, hormones, and environment play a role.
        5. Perianesthesia considerations:
            a. Proton pump inhibitors to reduce gastric acid preoperatively
            b. Skin temperature may be 1.5° C lower than core temperature.
            c. Maintain fluid and electrolyte balance; may be hypovolemic due to vasoconstriction.
            d. May initially see hypertension followed by vasodilatation and hypotension
            e. Anticipate potential for difficult airway, hypoxemia, and hypotension.
            f. Treatment includes antifibrinolytic agents, anti-inflammatory drugs, immunosuppressive therapy, and vascular drugs.
VII. ENDOCRINE DISEASES (see Chapter 34)
    A. Characterized by an overproduction or underproduction of single or multiple hormones
    B. Diabetes mellitus (DM)
        1. Definition: metabolic dysregulation of glucose metabolism related to insulin deficiency, resistance, and/or abnormal gluconeogenesis
            a. Chronic, systemic disease producing altered glucose metabolism and hyperglycemia
            b. Insulin-dependent DM (IDDM, type I, ketosis prone) commonly develops in childhood and adolescents.
                (1) Patient produces no insulin.
                (2) Requires insulin to sustain life
            c. Non–insulin-dependent DM (NIDDM, type II nonketosis prone)
                (1) Commonly managed with diet and oral hypoglycemic agents
                (2) May require insulin
                (3) Federal health statistics revealed in 2005
                    (a) 57 million Americans have prediabetes.
                    (b) About 2 million U.S. adolescents have prediabetes.
        2. Incidence: 23.6 million people in the USA (7.8% of population) have diabetes.
        3. Significance: increased risk of macroangiopathy (CAD, cerebrovascular disease, peripheral vascular disease), microangiopathy (retinopathy, nephropathy), and CNS disorder (autonomic nervous system neuropathy, peripheral neuropathy)
        4. Etiology
            a. IDDM: autoimmune, viral, genetic, environmental
            b. NIDDM: genetic, obesity
        5. Perianesthesia considerations
            a. Treatment: diet, oral hypoglycemic agents (not with IDDM), insulin, exercise, BP control; pancreatic transplant optional if renal disease is end stage in IDDM cases.
            b. Ultimate goal: to mimic normal metabolism, avoid hypoglycemia, excessive hyperglycemia, ketoacidosis, and electrolyte disturbances

     c. Patients will require glucose-containing IV solutions to prevent hypoglycemia and insulin to prevent ketosis and hyperglycemia.
      (1) Goal: blood glucose level of 80 to 110 mg/dL
     d. Diabetic patients ideally scheduled early in day to avoid prolonged fasting.
     e. Continue insulin on day of surgery (some physicians request half-normal dose—check facility policy); alternative is to hold insulin on day of surgery and to monitor blood glucose levels during surgery.
     f. Oral hypoglycemic agents commonly held because hypoglycemia common without caloric intake
     g. Obtain preoperative electrocardiogram, electrolytes, glucose (may vary with facility policy).
      (1) Most common cause of perioperative morbidity in diabetic patients is ischemic heart disease.
     h. Presence of autonomic nervous system dysfunction may increase risk of aspiration and cardiovascular instability.
     i. Peripheral neuropathy may influence selection of regional anesthesia.
     j. Regional: diabetic nerves may be more prone to edema and ischemia, especially if the vasoconstrictor epinephrine is used. There is decreased perfusion of an already compromised nerve.
     k. IV solutions commonly contain potassium.
     l. All supplemental insulin to be given IV to prevent unpredictable subcutaneous absorption
     m. Limited joint mobility and obesity may make intubation difficult.
     n. Infections and end-organ risk substantially increased with blood sugar >250 mg/dL.
  C. Adrenocortical insufficiency (Addison's disease)
    1. Definition: absence of cortisol and aldosterone owing to destruction of adrenal cortex
    2. Incidence: 1 in 100,000 in United States; affects all ages; no race or gender predominance
    3. Significance: endocrine or hormonal disorder and metabolic alterations
    4. Etiology: autoimmune, tuberculosis (TB), acquired immunodeficiency syndrome (AIDS), adrenal hemorrhage in anticoagulated patient
    5. Perianesthesia considerations
     a. Steroid dose may be increased for patients undergoing surgical procedure because patients are unable to increase release of endogenous cortisol to meet physiologic stress; can lead to cardiovascular collapse.
     b. Most minor ambulatory procedures require no change of steroid dose.
     c. Instruct patient to take steroid medication on morning of surgery.
     d. Correct hypovolemia, hyperkalemia, hyponatremia, hypoglycemia.
     e. May administer benzodiazepine before surgery
     f. Chest x-ray for pneumothorax if adrenalectomy
     g. Increased pancreatitis seen with left adrenalectomy
     h. Cardiac dysrhythmias with hyperkalemia
     i. Perioperative steroids may:
      (1) Decrease wound healing
      (2) Increase infections
      (3) Increase stress ulcers
      (4) Increase glucose intolerance
      (5) Increase BP
     j. Treatment: corticosteroid replacement
VIII. HEMATOLOGIC DISEASES (see Chapter 29)
  A. Anemia
    1. Definition: deficiency of erythrocytes (red blood cells)
     a. Females: hemoglobin <11.5 g/dL (hematocrit 36%)
     b. Males: hemoglobin <12.5 g/dL (hematocrit 40%)

    2. Incidence: common

    3. Significance: will compromise oxygen delivery to cells

    4. Etiology

       a. Iron deficiency anemia: due to inadequate intake of iron rich foods or absorption deficiency; seen most commonly in premenopausal women, infants, children, and adolescents

       b. Pernicious anemia: caused by a deficiency of intrinsic factor, which is necessary for absorption of vitamin B_{12}

       c. Folic acid deficiency anemia

       d. Acute blood loss anemia: seen with gastrointestinal or genitourinary trauma and coagulopathies

       e. Chronic disease in adults (renal failure and cancer)

       f. Aplastic anemia: bone marrow fails to produce blood cells.

       g. Sickle cell anemia: hereditary; affects primarily persons of African, Hispanic, Mediterranean, or Middle East descent

    5. Perianesthesia considerations

       a. No minimally accepted standard of hemoglobin concentration required for surgery

       b. Low hemoglobin level does not require transfusion.

       c. Low hemoglobin level does not compromise wound healing.

       d. Low hemoglobin level does not increase risk of infection.

       e. Decision to transfuse intended only to increase oxygen-carrying capacity

       f. Patients with compromised oxygenation not candidates for ambulatory surgery

       g. Keep patient warm postoperatively, prevent shivering.

       h. Maintain high PaO_2.

       i. Avoid hyperventilation or acute alkalosis.

B. Sickle cell anemia

    1. Definition: chronic hemoglobinopathy with varying quantities of hemoglobin S (normal is hemoglobin A), resulting in vascular occlusion and compromised tissue oxygenation

    2. Incidence:

       a. 8% to 10% of all African Americans with sickle cell trait (defined as hemoglobin S concentration <50%)

       b. 0.2% of all African Americans with sickle cell disease (hemoglobin S 70%-98%)

       c. 1 in 500 African Americans

       d. Also present in persons from India and Saudi Arabia

    3. Significance: characterized by chronic hemolysis (anemia) and acute vasoocclusive crisis that causes organ failure and can be life threatening

    4. Etiology: inherited, autosomal recessive

    5. Perianesthesia considerations

       a. Patients in sickle cell crisis inappropriate for ambulatory surgery

       b. Patients with sickle cell trait not at increased risk during perioperative period

       c. Patient with sickle cell disease must be free of infection, hydrated, and hemodynamically stable preoperatively.

       d. Obtain sickle cell lab test in all African Americans younger than 15 years.

          (1) If by age 15, patient has never been tested nor had sickle cell disease diagnosed, can omit lab test.

          (2) Most commonly diagnosed in childhood

       e. Anesthetic goal: avoid acidosis secondary to hypoventilation, maintain oxygenation, prevent circulatory stasis, maintain body temperature.

       f. Treatment: minimize factors that cause sickling, including hypoxia, acidosis, hypothermia, hemoglobin concentration <8.5 g/dL, dehydration, pain, and infection.

  g. Postoperative goal: maintain oxygenation, maintain intravascular fluid volume, maintain body temperature, use analgesics.
(1) Palliative care for painful crisis
(2) Simple and exchange transfusions
(3) Hydroxyurea to increase fetal hemoglobin
C. The anticoagulated patient
  1. Definition: administration of oral anticoagulant to induce alterations in coagulation to prevent thrombus formation
  2. Incidence: 600,000 cases of pulmonary embolism, with 10% resulting in death
  3. Significance: used in patients with thromboembolism, hypercoagulable states, cancer, mechanical heart valves, and atrial fibrillation
  4. Etiology: balance between risk of bleeding and thromboembolism, with risk increasing in major and emergency surgeries
  5. Perianesthesia considerations
    a. Increased risk of surgical bleeding
    b. Heparin or low-molecular-weight heparins (LMWHs) used acutely for short-term action
      (1) LMWHs have the same effect on factor X as heparin but less effect on thrombin.
      (2) LMWHs are given subcutaneously or IV, and onset of action is rapid. Patients can administer LMWHs to themselves.
    c. Oral anticoagulants ideally stopped 4 to 5 days before elective procedure
      (1) May not be possible for patients with prosthetic valves
      (2) INR should be 1.5 or less.
      (3) Used for long-term therapy
    d. Obtain PT day of surgery.
    e. Consider bleeding time and platelet count.
    f. Inquire about use of aspirin and NSAIDs in addition to Coumadin use.
    g. Increased risk of cerebrovascular accident in patients with atrial fibrillation off Coumadin
IX. INFECTIOUS DISEASES
  A. Human immunodeficiency virus (HIV) infection, AIDS
    1. Definition: destruction of lymphocytes with decline in immune function
    2. Incidence: 2006 Statistics show per 100,000 population; black male, ages 30-39 with highest incidence
    3. Significance: increased risk of opportunistic infections in CNS, GI tract, lungs
    4. Etiology: HIV spread via sexual activity, blood transfusions, IV drug use, fetal transmission, needlestick
    5. Perianesthesia considerations
      a. Meticulous attention to universal precautions
      b. Chest x-ray to rule out interstitial pneumonitis
      c. Must consider extent of organ system involvement when approving ambulatory status (pneumonia, dementia, cardiomyopathy, renal dysfunction)
      d. Treatment: supportive, antiretroviral drugs either alone or in combination with other antiretrovirals, prophylaxis against opportunistic infections by administering pneumococcal vaccine, hepatitis B vaccine, influenza vaccine, isoniazid, trimethoprim-sulfamethoxazole
      e. Asymptomatic patient who is HIV positive will respond in normal manner to anesthetic agents.
  B. TB
    1. Definition: bacterial pulmonary infection characterized by asymptomatic conversion of a TB skin test or presence of fever and nonproductive cough in an "at-risk" patient

2. Incidence: 100 in 100,000 population; greater in males than in females; increased risk with elderly in nursing homes, HIV-positive patients, homeless, prisoners, Asian and Latin American immigrants
3. Significance: can affect bones, joints, meninges, kidney, and skin
4. Etiology: *Mycobacterium tuberculosis* via droplet aerosol transmission (coughing and sneezing)
5. Perianesthesia considerations
    a. Highest risk of disease within 8 to 12 weeks of exposure
    b. Treatment: isoniazid, rifampin, and ethambutol in combination, varying with severity of disease
    c. Rifampin colors urine, tears, and secretions orange.
    d. Isoniazid can cause peripheral neuritis and hypersensitivity—can prevent with pyridoxine.
    e. Compliance issues predominate with number of drugs and length of treatment.
    f. Not infectious after 2 weeks of therapy and negative acid-fast bacilli culture
    g. Chest x-ray will show infiltrate with or without effusion.
    h. Homeless patients will have significant discharge limitations.
    i. Patients with active TB require respiratory isolation.
    j. Limit traffic, use disposable equipment, wear protective clothing, and remove nonessential equipment in surgical suite when patients done.

X. SUBSTANCE ABUSE
  A. Illicit drug use
    1. Definition: self-administration of drug(s) that deviate(s) from accepted medical or social use, which, if sustained, can lead to physical and psychological dependence
    2. Incidence: varies with drug; includes alcohol, cocaine, opioids, barbiturates, benzodiazepines, amphetamines, marijuana, hallucinogens
    3. Significance: physical withdrawal requires inpatient hospitalization—should not be attempted in perioperative period.
    4. Etiology: biological, social, environmental, psychological factors
    5. Perianesthesia considerations
        a. Can manifest cross-tolerance to drugs, making it difficult to predict anesthetic and/or analgesic requirements; usually increased
        b. May have concomitant problems of HIV, hepatitis, TB, malnutrition
        c. Frequently has associated personality disorders
        d. Patients acutely affected by substances not candidates for ambulatory surgery
        e. Treatment: medical management of withdrawal, behavioral, and supportive counseling

XI. OBESITY (see Chapter 48)
  A. Definition: weight >20% above ideal body weight
    1. Morbidly obese: double normal body weight
  B. Incidence: 20% to 30% of adult men, 30% to 40% of adult women; greater in females than in males; all ages
  C. Significance: may have concomitant heart disease, diabetes, pulmonary insufficiency
  D. Etiology: food intake greater than energy expenditure; genetic, endocrine, acquired disease
  E. Perianesthesia considerations
    1. Increased risk of aspiration; administer metoclopramide, H_2 antagonist.
    2. Decreased use of positive pressure ventilation to preoxygenate to prevent distention and vomiting
    3. Increased difficulty in intubation
    4. May be chronically hypoxemic and hypercarbic; sleep apnea common
    5. Increased duration of action of lipid-soluble drugs

6. Increased morbidity from cardiovascular disease
7. Increased risk of deep venous thrombosis—consider antiembolism precautions.
8. Increased risk of wound infection
9. Respiratory insufficiency, pneumonia, and thromboembolic phenomena avoided postoperatively by:
   a. Minimal sedation
   b. Appropriate pain control
   c. Early ambulation
10. Treatment: medically supervised weight loss with nutritional counseling, increase exercise and activity; surgical: gastric stapling or bypass or intestinal bypass

BIBLIOGRAPHY

1. Atlee J: *Complications in anesthesia*, ed 2, Philadelphia, 2007, Saunders.
2. Burden N, Quinn D, O'Brien D, et al: *Ambulatory surgical nursing*, Philadelphia, 2000, Saunders.
3. Cole D, Schlunt M: *Adult perioperative anesthesia: The requisites in anesthesiology*, Philadelphia, 2004, Mosby.
4. Dennison R: *Pass CCRN*, ed 3, St Louis, 2007, Mosby.
5. Drain C, Odom-Forren J: *Perianesthesia nursing: A critical care approach*, Philadelphia, 2009, Saunders.
6. Faust R: *Anesthesiology review*, ed 3, New York, 2002, Churchill Livingstone.
7. Fleisher L: *Evidence-based practice of anesthesiology*, Philadelphia, 2004, Saunders.
8. Gutierrez K, Peterson P: *Saunders nursing survival guide: Pathophysiology*, ed 2, St Louis, 2007, Saunders.
9. Moore K, Dalley A: *Clinically oriented anatomy*, ed 5, Philadelphia, 2006, Lippincott Williams & Wilkins.
10. Morton P, Fontaine D, Hudak C, Gallo B: *Critical care nursing: A holistic approach*, ed 8, Philadelphia, 2005, Lippincott Williams & Wilkins.
11. Nagelhout J, Zaglaniczny KL: *Nurse anesthesia*, ed 3, Philadelphia, 2005, Saunders.
12. Rathmell J, Neal J, Viscomi C: *Regional anesthesia: The requisites in anesthesiology*, Philadelphia, 2004, Saunders.
13. Roisen M, Fleischer L: *Essence of anesthesia practice*, ed 2, Philadelphia, 2002, Saunders.
14. Sladen R, Coursin D, Ketzler J, Playford H: *Anesthesia and co-existing disease*, Cambridge, N.Y., 2007, Cambridge University Press.
15. Springhouse: *Critical care nursing made incredibly easy*, Philadelphia, 2004, Lippincott Williams & Wilkins.
16. Springhouse: *Pathophysiology: A 2-in-1 reference for nurses*, Philadelphia, 2005, Lippincott Williams & Wilkins.
17. Stoelting R, Dierdorf S: *Handbook for anesthesia and co-existing disease*, ed 2, New York, 2002, Churchill Livingstone.
18. Stoelting R, Miller R: *Basics of anesthesia*, ed 5, Philadelphia, 2007, Churchill Livingstone.

18 Complementary Therapies

SUSAN A. GOODWIN
JANE C. DIERENFIELD

OBJECTIVES

At the conclusion of this chapter, the reader will be able to:

1. Define the terms complementary therapies (CTs) and integrative medicine.
2. Discuss the influence of Eastern medicine, including Traditional Chinese Medicine and East Indian contributions.
3. Compare and contrast 27 commonly used herbs, vitamins, and dietary supplements.
4. Summarize six CTs that could be used in the perianesthetic period.
5. Briefly define additional CTs.

I. OVERVIEW OF COMPLEMENTARY THERAPIES (CTs)
   A. Definitions
      1. Conventional medicine—practiced by medical doctors or doctors of osteopathy, and other allied health professionals (e.g., registered nurses, psychologists, or physical therapists)
         a. Taught at United States (U.S.) medical schools, and generally provided at U.S. hospitals
         b. Commonly known as Western medicine and is based on biology and pathology
      2. CTs: group of diverse medical and health care systems, practices, and products that are not presently considered to be a part of conventional medicine
         a. Used in conjunction with conventional medicine, or used by themselves without conventional medicine
         b. Based on Eastern philosophy, which is based on balance and harmony
         c. Oriental medicine began approximately 5000 years ago. The *Yellow Emperor's Classic of Internal Medicine* was written 2000 years ago.
      3. Integrative medicine—the eventual combination of CT and medicine
      4. Reliable evidence of complementary medicine efficacy is needed before its integration into clinical practice.
   B. Clinical trial articles of complementary medicine increased from 1987 through the present.
II. CURRENT UTILIZATION OF CTS
   A. Terms
      1. "Complementary and alternative medicines" (CAMs) commonly used.
         a. In the medical literature
         b. By the National Center for Complementary and Alternative Medicine (NCCAM)
      2. The term CAMs will be used when referring to medical practice.
      3. In this chapter, CTs will be used to describe these interventions, as this term more appropriately describes nursing practice.

B. Current use
  1. Searches conducted in 2008 on Ovid, Cumulative Index to Nursing and Allied Health Literature (CINAHL), PubMed, and Google Scholar revealed a plethora of articles on CAM. Diverse patient and ethnic populations represented, and treatment of a variety of diseases and conditions was detailed.
  2. When health insurance plans offered CT coverage, it varied by state and was often limited. Most CTs were paid out-of-pocket.
  3. Health insurance covers the following:
      a. Chiropractic
      b. Acupuncture
      c. Massage
      d. Biofeedback
      e. Naturopathy
C. NCCAM
  1. In 1992, the National Institutes of Health established the Office of Alternative Medicine (OAM).
      a. Mission: to provide the Americans with reliable information about the CAM safety and effectiveness
      b. Budget for 1992 was $2 million.
  2. Congress expanded the OAM into the NCCAM in 1998.
  3. The annual budget was increased to $121.6 million in 2008.
  4. CAM is defined by the NCCAM as a group of diverse medical and health care systems, practices, and products that are not presently considered to be part of conventional medicine.
  5. A review of clinical trials listed on the NCCAM website lists 235 completed clinical trials, (90 that are beginning the recruiting process, and over 100 that are in progress as of March 2009).
D. Partial listing of CTs
  1. Acupuncture/acupressure
  2. Aromatherapy
  3. Ayurveda
  4. Chiropractic
  5. Dietary supplements
  6. Energy healing
  7. Guided imagery
  8. Herbal therapies
  9. High-dose vitamin or megavitamin therapies
  10. Homeopathy
  11. Magnetic therapy
  12. Massage
  13. Meditation
  14. Music
  15. Naturopathy
  16. Osteopathic
  17. Prayer
  18. Qigong
  19. Reiki
  20. Relaxation techniques
  21. Therapeutic touch
  22. Yoga
E. Recent trends in CTs in the U.S.
  1. National surveys indicate that CTs are widely used and increasing in popularity.
  2. Use of CTs tends to be higher among patients who are:
      a. Female
      b. Middle aged or younger, 35 to 49 years of age
      c. White

      d. Married

      e. Employed

      f. More affluent

      g. Better educated, with some college education

      h. Have more insurance

      i. Live in the western part of the U.S.

   3. People who use CTs also use medical doctors.

      a. The more visits made to a medical doctor, the more likely he or she was to use CAM.

   4. CTs are used less frequently by:

      a. African Americans

      b. Persons 65 years or older

   5. CTs are used most frequently for:

      a. Chronic pain

      b. Anxiety and/or depression

      c. Urinary tract problems

      d. Back problems

      e. Headaches

      f. Allergies

      g. Arthritis

      h. Digestive problems

      i. Cancer

      j. Diabetes

      k. Acquired immunodeficiency syndrome

      l. Preventing future illness from occurring

      m. Maintaining health and vitality

   6. Unsupervised use, which is a form of expanded self-care, is the usual method of use for most CTs. There is usually no involvement of either a medical doctor or a complementary medicine practitioner.

   7. The increasing use of CTs has occurred despite the fact that the majority of costs have been paid out-of-pocket.

F. Use of CTs throughout the world

   1. In Denmark in 1987, 10% of the population used CTs.

   2. In Australia in 1993, 49% of the population used CTs.

   3. The United Kingdom spent $94 million on herbal remedies and $30 million on homeopathic remedies.

   4. Germany spent $541 million on herbal remedies and $528 million on homeopathic remedies.

   5. In Germany, herbal medicine is well integrated into the medical culture.

      a. Tens of millions of prescriptions written by physicians for herbal medicines each year

G. Reasons for use of CTs

   1. Dissatisfaction with conventional treatment

   2. Desire to try all options, especially among cancer patients

   3. Anecdotal information from friends or acquaintances

   4. Belief that CTs are less harmful than conventional therapies

   5. Many CTs are holistic and encompass a spiritual component, which is lacking in conventional medicine.

H. Implications for further study

   1. The use of traditional randomized, double-blind, placebo-controlled clinical trials with CTs presents certain challenges.

   2. It would be extremely difficult to design and implement randomized, double-blind, placebo-controlled clinical trials of all the CTs that are in use today.

   3. Many of the CTs have been in use for thousands of years, with vast anecdotal success.

   4. Treatment plans with CTs are often individualized and are thus hard to replicate.

5. CTs are increasingly being integrated with conventional medicine, rather than being used alone or in the place of conventional medicine.
6. Pharmaceutical companies invest between $350 and $500 million in a 10-year period to bring a new drug to market; when the drug is marketed, the money is recouped.
7. Obtaining financial support for research on herbs is difficult because there is no financial incentive for investment by pharmaceutical companies.
   a. The herb is readily available, cannot be patented, and is thus not financially lucrative.

III. PREOPERATIVE ASSESSMENT OF PERIANESTHETIC PATIENTS
   A. Lack of report of CTs
      1. A study of older adults residing in Minnesota revealed that 62.9% used CAMs, while only 53% disclosed their CAM use to their primary care providers.
      2. The flourishing use of herbal preparations increases the need to question preoperative patients about their use of herbals.
      3. Many people do not view herbals as "medicine" or may be reluctant to disclose their uses of CT to conventional practitioners, such as nurses or doctors.
      4. The preoperative nurse must make specific and repeated inquires to the patient about the potential use of herbals.
   B. Herbals
      1. Are plant-derived products used for medicinal and health purposes (Table 18-1).
      2. Thirty percent of all modern drugs derived from plants
      3. The use of herbals has increased significantly in the past 10 years.
      4. Herbals may have many allergic reactions as well as interactions with prescription drugs.
      5. Perioperative patients are exposed to a great number of pharmacological agents during their surgical experience.
         a. Potential for adverse drug interactions is much higher than during their everyday life.
         b. Potential interactions with anesthetic drugs
            (1) Coagulation disturbances
            (2) Prolongation of anesthetic sedation
            (3) Adverse cardiovascular effects
            (4) The American Society of Anesthesiologists recommends that patients discontinue herbal medicines at least 2 weeks before surgery.
   C. Regulation of herbals in the U.S.
      1. In 1994, herbal medications were classified as dietary supplements in the Dietary Supplement Health and Education Act.
      2. This law exempts herbals from the safety and efficacy requirements that must be met by prescription and over-the-counter drugs. It requires:
         a. No proof of efficacy
         b. No proof of safety
         c. Sets no standards for quality control
         d. That supplements not promise a specific cure on the label
      3. There is no guarantee that the herb(s) listed on the packaging are actually present, that the ingredient is bioavailable, the dosing is appropriate, or whether the next bottle will have the same composition.
         a. The same herb marketed by different manufacturers can vary greatly.
         b. Herbs manufactured from outside the U.S. may contain heavy metals, pesticides, and even pharmaceuticals.
      4. The Food and Drug Administration must show that an herbal product is unsafe before it can be removed from the market.
      5. There is no mechanism for reporting of herbal adverse effects, or herbal and drug interactions; thus, they are grossly underreported.

◼ TABLE 18-1
◼ **Herbs**

Herb	Actions	Uses	Side Effects	Perianesthetic Implications	Preoperative Precautions
Aloe vera	Anti-inflammatory. Relieves pain, decreases inflammation and swelling, and may encourage wound contraction. May increase blood flow. Useful for first- and second-degree burns. May be useful in the treatment of psoriasis.	*Topical:* Emollient. Encourages healing of a wound, burn, hemorrhoids, insect bites, poison ivy or oak, rashes, sunburn, and yeast infections. *Oral:* Treats or prevents constipation.	Rare topical allergic reactions. Oral gel can reduce absorption of many drugs.	Oral use may cause hypokalemia due to cathartic effects.	Not necessary
Arnica	An immunostimulant. May increase macrophage activity and blood circulation to injured area. Has anti-inflammatory and mild analgesia properties. Is frequently combined with goldenseal.	*Topical and Oral:* Relieves muscle, joint, and cartilage pain from bruises, contusions, hyperextensions, bursitis, and arthritis.	Long-term topical use can lead to toxic skin reactions. Internal use has a very narrow dosing range. The FDA classifies arnica as unsafe for internal use. The German Commission E does not recommend internal use because of potentially toxic effects.	May be the source of preoperative skin irritations. May have minimal anticoagulant effects.	2 weeks
Black cohosh	Estrogenic activity. Causes hypotensive effects via decreased vascular spasm. Has sedative, anti-inflammatory, and antispasmodic effects.	Approved by the German Commission E for the treatment of PMS, dysmenorrhea, and menopausal symptoms, including mood changes.	GI discomfort, frontal headache, nausea, heaviness in the legs,	May cause hypotension and bradycardia. May potentiate antihypertensive medications.	2 weeks

	May inhibit bone loss caused by menopause. Appears to increase the normal growth of vaginal cells, thereby reducing vaginal dryness and dyspareunia. Alleviates insomnia. Used as an anti-inflammatory for arthritis. (Remifemin, a European form of black cohosh, is available in the United States.)	weight problems, dilated pupils, and flushed face. Avoid use during pregnancy or lactation.		
Chamomile	Mild sedative. Has antispasmodic, antibacterial, antipyretic, and anti-inflammatory activity.	Used as an antiemetic, for indigestion, to decrease cramping secondary to diarrhea, and as an aid for sleep. Used for dysmenorrhea and to treat arthritis.	Allergic reactions are common, especially in patients who are allergic to ragweed, and include contact dermatitis and pharyngeal edema.	May potentiate sedation. Anticoagulant effects due to platelet inhibition.	2 weeks
Cranberry	Prevents *Escherichia coli* from adhering to bladder wall and the urinary tract. Acidifies the urine.	To acidify the urine and treat urinary tract infections. Decreases the incidence of urinary stones.	None with normal doses. Very large doses may result in diarrhea.	None known	Not necessary

Continued

■ TABLE 18-1
■ Herbs—cont'd

Herb	Actions	Uses	Side Effects	Perianesthetic Implications	Preoperative Precautions
Echinacea	Anti-inflammatory, immunostimulating, bacteriostatic, bactericidal, and free-radical scavenging effects. Causes activation of cell-mediated immunity. Enhances phagocytosis. Decreases the activity of viruses.	Used for the prophylaxis and treatment of bacterial and fungal infections. Begin use at the first sign of a cold to decrease cold symptoms and duration. If used for longer than 8 weeks, the effectiveness declines. Also used to treat chronic wounds, ulcers, and arthritis. Used in Germany along with chemotherapy to treat cancer.	Use longer than 8 weeks could cause immunosuppression and hepatotoxicity (some controversy exists about this). Should not be used with other hepatotoxic drugs, such as anabolic steroids, amiodarone, methotrexate, or ketoconazole. Do not give concomitantly with immunosuppressants. Can cause transplant rejection. Use with caution in patients with asthma or allergic rhinitis. May cause allergic responses in individuals allergic to ragweed.	Causes inhibition of hepatic enzymes. May affect many anesthetic agents.	2 weeks
Evening primrose oil	Chemical constituents are prostaglandin precursors, which have anti-inflammatory properties.	Used for PMS symptom relief, diabetic neuropathy, numerous skin conditions, and chronic autoimmune diseases such as rheumatoid arthritis, Raynaud's syndrome, and multiple sclerosis.	Lowers seizure threshold and increases anticonvulsant requirements. Nausea, softening of stools, and headache.	May interact with drugs that are anticonvulsants. Inhibits platelet aggregation.	2 weeks

Feverfew	A prostaglandin inhibitor. Has been shown to suppress 86%-88% of prostaglandin production.	Used to treat migraines, other types of headaches. Can reduce the number as well as severity of migraines. Also used to treat fever, dizziness, stomachache, and rheumatoid arthritis.	NSAIDs may negate the effects of feverfew in the treatment of migraines. May cause mouth ulcers.	Anticoagulant effects due to platelet inhibition.	2 weeks. Discontinuation after prolonged use can cause a rebound effect, resulting in symptoms of migraine, insomnia, and anxiety. A slow withdrawal may reduce these effects.
Garlic	Can lower the risk of developing atherosclerosis through its antihypertensive and anticholesterolemic effects, as well as platelet inhibition. Has antibacterial and antiviral properties. Appears to prevent some cancers.	Used to treat hypertension, hypercholesterolemia, atherosclerosis, and infection.	Inhibits platelet function and fibrinogen. Concomitant use with aspirin, NSAIDs, or anticoagulants is not recommended. May cause nausea, hypotension, and allergy. Bad breath is a common side effect.	Anticoagulant effects due to platelet inhibition. Can cause hypotension.	2 weeks
Ginger	Has antiemetic, antispasmodic, and anti-inflammatory properties. A potent inhibitor of thromboxane synthetase.	Used to treat PONV, motion sickness, hyperemesis gravidarum, intestinal gas, indigestion, and arthralgias.	Inhibits platelet function. May cause GI upset when taken on an empty stomach.	Anticoagulant effects due to platelet inhibition. May cause hypotension or bradycardia.	2 weeks. However, there have been studies in which ginger was given just before surgery to reduce PONV, and no increased bleeding was seen.
Ginkgo biloba (also sold under Bai Guo Ye, Baiguo, & Fossil Tree)	Its components act as antioxidants, alter vasoregulation, alter neurotransmitter and receptor activity, and inhibit platelet-activating factor.	Stabilizes and perhaps improves cognitive function in patients with dementia. Used for peripheral vascular disease, vertigo, tinnitus, and erectile dysfunction. Promotes vasodilation, improves mental function and sexual functioning. Slows macular degeneration and protects the retina, especially in diabetic retinopathy.	Mild GI upset and headache. Inhibits platelet function and fibrinogen. Concomitant use with aspirin, NSAIDs, or anticoagulants is not recommended. May diminish effectiveness of anticonvulsants.	Anticoagulant effects due to platelet inhibition.	2 weeks

Continued

■ TABLE 18-1
■ ■ Herbs—cont'd

Herb	Actions	Uses	Side Effects	Perianesthetic Implications	Preoperative Precautions
Ginseng	A number of ginseng products exist, whose effects vary widely. It is important to be familiar with which ginseng is used. In general, acts as an adaptogen, protecting the body against stress and restoring homeostasis. The underlying mechanism appears to be similar to steroids. Acts as an immunostimulant. Has a hypoglycemic effect.	Used to reduce stress and improve vitality. Can also be used for mild depression, chronic fatigue syndrome, fibromyalgia, and stress-induced asthma. Improves cognitive function, attention span, psychomotor performance, and concentration.	May cause headache, tremulousness, and insomnia. Avoid in patients with bipolar syndrome and psychosis. Avoid concurrent use with estrogens and corticosteroids due to additive effects. May lower blood glucose levels; should not be used in patients with diabetes. Concomitant use with aspirin, NSAIDs, or anticoagulants is not recommended due to inhibition of platelet function.	Anticoagulant effects due to platelet inhibition. Can cause hypertension or tachycardia. May potentiate sedation and hypoglycemia.	2 weeks
Goldenseal	Has antibacterial properties. May reduce gastric inflammation. Frequently combined with arnica.	Used for its antibacterial and antifungal properties to treat conjunctivitis, gastric and duodenal ulcers, thrush, and strep throat.	Excessive doses can cause jaundice and elevated liver enzymes. Contraindicated with diarrhea, GI cramping, and nausea and vomiting.	Use cautiously with heparin. May augment or diminish effects of antihypertensives.	2 weeks

Continued

Kava-kava	Acts as a sedative-hypnotic possibly by potentiating GABA inhibitory neurotransmission. Has mild analgesic and muscle-relaxing effects. Has abuse potential.	Alleviates stress, anxiety, tension, and nervousness. Used as an anxiolytic and sedative. Relieves tension headaches and muscle spasms (restless leg syndrome, TMJ pain).	Avoid concomitant use with barbiturates, alcohol, and benzodiazepines as excessive sedation can occur. Do not use with antiparkinsonian drugs. Decreases platelet function. Heavy use produces kava dermopathy, characterized by reversible, scaly, cutaneous eruptions accompanied by jaundice. The sale of kava has recently been banned in Canada and the United Kingdom because of reported liver damage.	Excessive sedation can occur with anesthetic drugs. Anticoagulant effects due to platelet inhibition.
				24 hours
Ma huang (ephedra)	Known as ephedra. Ephedrine, a sympathomimetic amine, is the predominant active compound. It increases heart rate and blood pressure, bronchodilates, has anti-inflammatory properties, and inhibits prostaglandins.	Commonly used as a decongestant for allergies and hay fever. Used to promote weight loss, increase energy, and treat bronchospastic disorders such as asthma or bronchitis. Also used as an aphrodisiac.	Cause dose-dependent increases in blood pressure and heart rate. Can cause palpitations, coronary spasm, MI, and stroke. Concomitant use of ephedra and MAOIs can result in hyperpyrexia and hypertension. The American Medical Association has called for a ban of ephedra in supplements.	May cause hypertension or arrhythmias. When given halothane, may cause ventricular dysrhythmias.
				7 days
Peppermint	Relaxes the lower esophageal sphincter. Antispasmodic, smooth muscle relaxant.	Used for nausea, rhinitis, heartburn, and flatulence.	Avoid in patients with hiatal hernia and GERD, as the relaxation of the lower esophageal sphincter may worsen symptoms.	None known
				Not necessary

■ TABLE 18-1
■ ■ Herbs—cont'd

Herb	Actions	Uses	Side Effects	Perianesthetic Implications	Preoperative Precautions
Saw palmetto (also called American dwarf palm tree, cabbage palm or ju-zhong)	Increases urinary flow, decreases nocturia, and decreases postvoid residual volumes. Acts as a urinary antiseptic.	Relief of BPH symptoms, such as frequent urination, difficulty in initiating urination, and high residual volume. Useful in chronic pelvic pain, bladder disorders, decreased sex drive, hair loss, and hormone imbalance.	Side effects uncommon, but may include mild GI distress, bleeding, and headache. Because of its antiplatelet effect, the use of aspirin on NSAIDs may increase bleeding risk.	May increase INR in patients receiving warfarin.	2 weeks
St. John's Wort	Acts similarly to MAOIs or SSRIs by inhibiting serotonin, norepinephrine, and dopamine reuptake by neurons.	Licensed in Germany for the treatment of anxiety, depression, nerve pain, and sleep disorders. Use for moderate depression may be more effective than a placebo. A 2005 study found that St. John's Wort was more effective than fluoxetine (Prozac).	Avoid concomitant use with MAOIs and SSRIs, which could result in a serotonin syndrome. May inhibit the absorption of iron. Causes photosensitivity. Through enzyme induction, increases the metabolism of many drugs, including cyclosporine, alfentanil, midazolam, lidocaine, calcium channel blockers, warfarin, and SSRIs. Avoid in pregnancy.	May potentiate anesthetic effects. May affect blood pressure.	7 days. Discontinuation is especially important in patients awaiting organ transplantation or who may require anticoagulation therapy postoperatively.

| Valerian | Causes a significant decrease in sleep latency. Causes dose-dependent sedation and hypnosis. | Used for insomnia, anxiety, headache, irregular heartbeat, depression, or trembling. | Avoid concomitant use with barbiturates, alcohol, and benzodiazepines as excessive sedation can occur. Can cause "morning hangovers." May cause paradoxical stimulation, GI upset, nervousness, disturbed sleep, and rare liver toxicity. | May potentiate sedation caused by anesthesia. | 7 days. Abrupt discontinuation in patients who are physically dependent may cause benzodiazepine-like withdrawal. Taper over several weeks. |

BPH, Benign prostatic hypertrophy; *FDA*, Food and Drug Administration; *GABA*, gamma-aminobutyric acid; *GERD*, gastroesophageal reflux disease; *GI*, gastrointestinal; *INR*, international normalized ratio; *MAOIs*, monoamine oxidase inhibitors; *MI*, myocardial infarction; *NSAIDs*, nonsteroidal anti-inflammatory drugs; *PMS*, premenstrual syndrome; *PONV*, postoperative nausea and vomiting; *SSRIs*, selective serotonin reuptake inhibitors (such as nefazodone, sertraline, or paroxetine); *TMJ*, temporomandibular joint.

   D. Regulation of herbals in Europe
      1. In Germany, France, the United Kingdom, and Canada, regulating agencies enforce standards of herb quality and safety assessment of manufacturers.
      2. The *German Commission E Monographs* are a comprehensive study of herbals.
      3. Significant numbers of studies are being conducted in Germany, France, Japan, China, and India.
   E. Vitamins and dietary supplements
      1. Vitamins are complex organic substances found in most foods that are essential for the normal function of the body.
      2. Dietary supplements correct a dietary deficiency.
      3. A number of commonly used vitamins and dietary supplements interact with perianesthetic drugs in similar ways to herbals (Table 18-2).
IV. CTs USEFUL IN PERIANESTHESIA
   A. Nursing and CT
      1. Nurses are in a unique position to combine conventional Western medicine and CTs.
      2. Integrative and holistic nature of nursing lends to the esoteric nature of many complementary interventions.
      3. Forty-seven percent of state boards of nursing permit the practice of some CAMs (Arizona, Arkansas, California, Connecticut, Illinois, Iowa, Kansas, Louisiana, Maine, Maryland, Massachusetts, Mississippi, Missouri, New Hampshire, New York, Nevada, North Carolina, North Dakota, Ohio, Oregon, Pennsylvania, Texas, Vermont, and West Virginia).
      4. The practice of CAMs is under discussion in seven states: Delaware, District of Columbia, Georgia, Minnesota, New Jersey, New Mexico, and Washington.
      5. The remaining 40% of states have no formal position on CAMs (Alabama, Alaska, Colorado, Florida, Georgia, Hawaii, Idaho, Indiana, Kentucky, Michigan, Montana, Oklahoma, Puerto Rico, Rhode Island, South Carolina, Tennessee, Utah, Virgin Islands, Virginia, Wisconsin, and Wyoming).
   B. Six CTs practiced by nurses in the perianesthetic setting
      1. Aromatherapy
        a. Use of essential oils (EOs) for therapeutic or medical purposes
        b. Used throughout history in many cultures, including ancient Egypt in 3000 B.C.
        c. EOs are steam distillates from aromatic plants and can be used with massage, friction, inhalation, compresses, and baths.
        d. EOs can have sedative, stimulatory, analgesic, antispasmodic, and antibacterial properties.
        e. The effects of the EO depend on the therapeutic actions of the oil as well as the learned smell memory of the patient.
        f. Inhaled peppermint and ginger can be used to treat postoperative nausea and vomiting.
        g. Inhaled lavender, Roman chamomile, lemongrass, and rose can be used to treat pain.
        h. Topical lemon, clove, cinnamon bark, eucalyptus, rosemary, and melaleuca (also known as tea tree oil) have antiviral, antiseptic, antibacterial, and anti-infectious properties.
      2. Massage
        a. An ancient technique; a Chinese medical work written in 2760 B.C. contains descriptions of massage techniques.
        b. Modern massage developed by Henrik Ling from Sweden (1776-1839)
        c. A series of soothing and energizing stroking techniques that stimulate the muscles, increasing their ability to absorb nutrients and eliminate waste products
        d. Nonpharmacological and holistic intervention

■ TABLE 18-2
■ Dietary Supplements

Dietary Supplements	Actions	Uses	Side Effects	Perianesthetic Implications	Preoperative Discontinuation
Chondroitin	Usually given in conjunction with glucosamine. Contains glycosaminoglycans, which increase proteoglycan concentration, a substance that forms cartilage in joints. Reduces collagen breakdown. Has anti-inflammatory effects.	May improve joint pain and function in osteoarthritis.	Mild GI symptoms. Concomitant use with warfarin should be avoided.	None	Not necessary
Coenzyme Q$_{10}$	A fat-soluble chemical present in all tissue used to make ADP. Acts as an antioxidant, removing free radicals. Improves immune function.	Used to treat cancer, heart failure, cardiomyopathy, hypertension, angina, and dysrhythmias.	Mild GI distress. Works synergistically with antihypertensives. Concomitant use with warfarin should be avoided. May diminish the effects of aspirin, NSAIDs, and other anticoagulants.	May augment hypotensive effects of anesthesia. May have anticoagulant effects.	2 weeks
Fish oil	Has anti-inflammatory and antiembolus effects. Promotes vasodilation. Reduces cholesterol production.	Used to treat coronary artery disease, hyperlipidemia, hypertension, and diabetes.	Belching, bad breath, heartburn, and nosebleeds. May increase bleeding time. Works synergistically with antihypertensives.	Anticoagulant effects due to inhibition of platelet aggregation. May augment the hypotensive effects of anesthesia.	2 weeks
Glucosamine	Usually given with chondroitin. An aminomonosaccharide, which stimulates the production of glycosaminoglycans, a component of cartilage. Has anti-inflammatory effects.	May improve joint pain and function in osteoarthritis. Slow acting; may have to take it for up to 2 months before benefits are seen.	Mild GI distress. Avoid if allergic to shellfish or iodine. May raise blood sugar levels.	None	Not necessary

Continued

■ TABLE 18-2
■ **Dietary Supplements—cont'd**

Dietary Supplements	Actions	Uses	Side Effects	Perianesthetic Implications	Preoperative Discontinuation
Melatonin	A hormone produced by the pineal gland during sleep. Produced from tryptophan.	Used to treat insomnia and sleeplessness caused by jet lag or working the night shift.	Headaches, vivid dreams or nightmares, and morning hangovers. Contraindicated in severe mental illness or autoimmune disease.	May potentiate sedation.	24 hours
Vitamin C	An essential nutrient needed for collagen and tissue formation, hormone production, carbohydrate metabolism, and immune system function.	A wide variety of uses, including treatment and prophylaxis of colds, fractures, immune system stimulation, wound healing, and periodontal disease.	Rare side effects. May cause GI distress.	May decrease the effects of heparin or warfarin.	Not necessary
Vitamin E	An essential fat-soluble vitamin. Acts as an antioxidant, binding to free radicals. A component of the immune system, maintains healthy eyes and skin, and promotes normal clotting.	A wide variety of uses, including diabetes, Alzheimer's disease, fibrocystic breast disease, immune system integrity, skin disorders, and menopause.	Rare side effects. As a fat-soluble vitamin, is stored in the liver.	Anticoagulant effects due to inhibition of platelet aggregation. May augment the hypotensive effects of anesthesia.	2 weeks
Zinc	Acts as an immunostimulant.	Used to decrease the symptoms and longevity of the common cold.	Do not give with immuosuppressants. May cause nausea and a bad taste.	None known	Not necessary

ADP, Adenosine diphosphate; *GI,* gastrointestinal; *NSAIDs,* nonsteroidal anti-inflammatory drugs.

        e. Relieves muscle tension, stimulates the nervous system, enhances skin condition, improves circulation, aids digestion and intestinal function, increases mobility in joints, relieves chronic pain and especially low back pain, and reduces swelling and inflammation

        f. Used to ease childbirth; with asthmatic children to improve breathing; with terminally ill, homebound, and nursing home residents; and with preoperative and postoperative patients

        g. Do not use massage with fever, infections, open wounds, contagious skin conditions or diseases, phlebitis, or acute strains or sprains; wait 48 hours after a strain or sprain to massage.

    3. Music

        a. Uses melody to effect changes in behavior, emotions, and physiology

        b. Lowers anxiety, provides distraction, promotes relaxation, and increases pain tolerance; helps the body release energy used for healing

        c. Used in the perioperative period, and many patients feel less anxious when listening to music before and after surgery.

        d. A trained sound therapist uses a wide range of tools (i.e., musical instruments, tapes, tuning forks, and machines that release sound waves at specific frequencies to help heal the body).

    4. Relaxation therapy

        a. Encompasses a variety of stress-reduction techniques

        b. Can be done with yoga, meditation, guided imagery, hypnosis, positive suggestions, and breathing techniques

        c. Elicits a relaxation response, which results in reduced muscle tension, decreased blood pressure, heart rate, and respiration, and reduced oxygen consumption

        d. Surgical patients who use relaxation exercises recover more quickly, use less pain medication, have lower blood pressure, and have fewer postoperative complications than those who do not use them.

    5. Therapeutic touch

        a. First developed in the early 1970s by Dolores Kreiger, PhD, RN, and psychic Dona Kunz

        b. Similar to qigong

        c. Based on an ancient technique called laying-on of hands

        d. The healing force of the therapist positively affects the patient's recovery.

        e. Practitioner scans the patient's energy field by moving his or her hands in a sweeping motion above the body, clears the energy field to blockages of energy, and facilitates the flow of energy from his or her hands to the patient's energy field.

        f. Used to promote relaxation and reduce stress, pain, anxiety, and restlessness—can also promote a sense of well-being

        g. Used in acute situations to treat sprains or muscle spasms, to sooth and relax, and to decrease heart rate and blood pressure

        h. Enhances the onset of pain medications as well as the effectiveness

    6. Guided imagery

        a. A form of self-hypnosis that uses directed thoughts and suggestions; based on the concept that your body and mind are connected

        b. Used to relieve physical, mental, and emotional stress, as well as many of the medical conditions associated with stress

        c. Used to stimulate the immune system and promote healing

V. BRIEF DEFINITIONS OF SELECTED CTS

  A. Acupuncture/acupressure

    1. Based on traditional Chinese medical theory, and has been in existence for at least 2500 years

    2. Involves inserting thin-gauged needles into specific anatomical points in the body for therapeutic purposes

    3. Disrupted patterns of energy flow (qi) that travel in meridians are rebalanced by acupuncture

4. Insertion points tend to correspond to areas where connective tissue is the thickest.
5. Acupressure uses the fingers, hands, elbows, or other devices to press on the surface of the skin on the same anatomical points used in acupuncture; no needles are involved.
6. Acupressure and acustimulation devices may be used to treat postoperative nausea and vomiting.

B. Ayurvedic
   1. Ayurvedic medicine is traditional Hindu medicine, and was developed more than 5000 years ago.
   2. Ayurveda means the "science of life."
   3. The physician prevents or treats diseases by restoring the balance of body, mind, and spirit with diet, exercise, meditation, herbs, massage, and controlled breathing.

C. Balneotherapy involves the use of baths in the treatment of health conditions.

D. Chiropractic
   1. Focuses on the relationship between bodily structure and function
   2. Focuses on how that relationship affects the preservation and restoration of health
   3. Uses spinal manipulation and adjustments to bring about healing

E. Homeopathy
   1. A Western system of care based on the belief that very dilute substances are able to stimulate a healing response in the body
   2. Developed by Samuel Hahnemann, a German physician who practiced medicine in the late 1700s
   3. Stimulates the body's defense mechanisms to cure symptoms by administering minute doses of medicinal substances; these same substances at higher doses would actually cause symptoms or disease.

F. Magnetic therapy
   1. Electromagnetic fields are invisible lines of force that are present in the earth and are believed to be produced by electric currents flowing at the earth's core.
   2. Often used to relieve pain

G. Meditation
   1. A cultivation of the mind through quieting, and observing one's inner state
   2. Learning to slow down and examine passing sensations in minute detail
   3. The practitioner allows pain, emotions, and bodily sensations to be experienced as a natural progression of life.
   4. Results in:
      a. Reduction of stress activity
      b. Lowers heart rate
      c. Lowers blood pressure
      d. Lowers respirations
      e. Evokes the "relaxation response"

H. Naturopathy
   1. Arose in the late nineteenth century in America
   2. Works with natural healing forces within the body to restore health through nutrition, exercise, homeopathy, acupuncture, herbal medicine, hydrotherapy, massage, counseling, and/or pharmacology

I. Osteopathic medicine
   1. A form of conventional medicine that emphasizes that diseases arise in the musculoskeletal system
   2. Its paradigm is that all the body's systems work together, and a disturbance in one system may affect functioning in other body systems.

J. Prayer
   1. Addresses a "Supreme Being" or a "Higher Power" and implies a relationship between the individual and the "Higher Power"
   2. Control of healing is given to a higher being.
   3. Resembles meditation, bringing similar benefits such as lowered blood pressure and a strengthened immune system

K. Qigong—"Qi"
    1. Pronounced "chee kung"
    2. An ancient term denoting the vital energy of the body, and gong is the skill to work with qi
    3. Part of traditional Chinese medicine
    4. Combines movement, meditation, and regulation of breathing to remove blockages that stop or slow the flow of qi and to ensure an equal balance of qi within the body
    5. Qigong masters can treat organ systems or body areas with or without physical contact.
    6. Used to enhance the immune system, treat heart disease, stroke, hypertension, osteoporosis, cancer, and senility

L. Reflexology
    1. Practiced by Egyptians as early as 2330 B.C.
    2. A touch modality based on the principle that reflexes exist on each foot and hand that correspond to the glands, organs, and parts of the body.
    3. Three different methods exist.
        a. Foot—the most commonly practiced
        b. Hand
        c. Zone therapy
    4. Used to reduce anxiety, stress and tension, and facilitate sleep

M. Reiki
    1. A Japanese word denoting "Universal Life Energy"
    2. Based on a belief that when spiritual energy is channeled through a Reiki practitioner, the patient's spirit is healed, which heals the body

N. Yoga
    1. An East Indian practice that has existed for 5000 years
    2. The word yoga comes from the Sanskrit word yui, which means to unite.
    3. A central belief of yoga is that a healthy body, mind, and spirit are needed for a healthy person.
    4. Involves stretching exercises, breathing control, and meditation
    5. Yoga training results in decreased sympathetic tone, decreased peripheral vascular resistance, improved cardiac output, and lowered blood pressure and heart rate.
        a. Can help many conditions, including diabetes, epilepsy, obesity, asthma, depression, osteoarthritis, and cardiovascular disease

BIBLIOGRAPHY

1. American Massage Therapy Association: *ASPAN's evidenced-based clinical practice guideline for the prevention and/or management of PONV/PDNV.* Available at: www.amtamassage.org. Accessed November 25, 2008.
2. American Society of PeriAnesthesia Nurses PONV/PDNV Strategic Work Team: ASPAN's evidence-based clinical practice guideline for the prevention and/or management of PONV/PDNV. *J Perianesth Nurs* 21(4):230–250, 2006.
3. Barnes J, Abbot NC, Harkness EF, et al: Articles on complementary medicine in the mainstream medical literature: An investigation of MEDLINE, 1966 through 1996. *Arch Intern Med* 159(15):1721–1725, 1999.
4. Buckle J: *Clinical aromatherapy in nursing,* London, 1997, Arnold.
5. Cheung CK, Wyman JF, Halcon LL: Use of complementary and alternative therapies in community-dwelling older adults. *J Altern Complement Med* 13(9):997–1006, 2007.
6. Cumulative index for nursing and allied health literature (CINAHL). Available at: www.cinahl.com. Accessed November 25, 2008.
7. Gach MR: *Acupressure.* Available at: www.acupressure.com. Accessed January 13, 2008.
8. *HerbMed.* Available at: www.herbmed.org. Accessed November 25, 2008.
9. Hulisz DT, Wiebe C, Hart CA: *Top herbal products: Efficacy and safety concerns.* Available at: www.medscape.com/viewprogram/8494_pnt. Accessed January 1, 2008.
10. Kuhn MA, Winston D: *Herbal therapy and supplements,* Philadelphia, 2000, Lippincott.
11. National Center for Complementary and Alternative Medicine. Available at: http://nccam.nih.gov. Accessed August 7, 2008.

12. National Center for Complementary and Alternative Medicine: *Paying for CAM treatment*. Available at: http://nccam.nih.gov/health/financial/. Accessed August 11, 2008.

13. National Center for Complementary and Alternative Medicine. Available at: http://nccam.nih.gov. Accessed November 25, 2008.

14. Ness J, Cirillo DJ, Weir DR, Nisly NL, Wallace RB: Use of complementary medicine in older Americans: Results from the health and retirement study. *Gerontologist* 45(4):516–524, 2005.

15. Office of Dietary Supplements, National Institutes of Health: *Black cohosh*. Available at: http://ods.od.nih.gov/factsheets/black-cohosh.html. Accessed October 3, 2008.

16. *PDR for essential oils*, USA, 1999, Essential Science Publishing.

17. Prioreschi P: Alternative medicine in ancient and medieval history. *Med Hypotheses* 55(4):319–325, 2000.

18. PubMed. Available at: www.ncbi.nlm.nih.gov/pubmed. Accessed November 25, 2008.

19. RJ Buckle Associates. Available at: www.rjbuckle.com. Accessed November 25, 2008.

20. The Nurse Healers–Professional Associates International and Therapeutic Touch. Available at: www.therapeutic-touch.org. Accessed November 25, 2008.

21. Weil A: *Guided imagery therapy*, 2008, Weil Lifestyle, LLC. Available at: www.drweil.com/drw/u/id/ART00468. Accessed January 13, 2008.

22. Working to get ephedra banned. *Consum Rep* 68(2):6, 2003.

23. Wren KR, Kimball S, Norred CL: Use of complementary and alternative medications by surgical patients. *J Perianesth Nurs* 17(3):170–177, 2002.

24. Wren KR, Norred CL: *Complementary and alternative therapies*, Philadelphia, 2003, WB Saunders.

19 The Mentally and Physically Challenged Patient

THERESA CLIFFORD

OBJECTIVES

At the conclusion of this chapter, the reader will be able to:

1. List special considerations in interviewing the mentally challenged patient.
2. List different stages of Alzheimer's disease and manifestation of limitations in each stage.
3. State effective communication techniques to use with the hearing impaired.
4. Identify techniques to facilitate learning and reduce apprehension for visually impaired patients.
5. Identify manifestations of select physical disabilities and incorporate management of these symptoms and risks in the nursing plan of care.
6. Identify effective techniques related to caring for the pediatric patient with intellectual and/or physical challenges.

I. OVERVIEW
  A. According to the Americans with Disabilities Act (ADA) of 1990, a person is considered to have a "disability" if that individual has:
    1. A physical and/or mental impairment that substantially limits one or more major life activities
    2. A recorded history of such impairments
    3. Perceived by others as having such impairments
  B. Health care providers and institutions are required to offer the disabled patient full and equal access to the facility's:
    1. Goods
    2. Services
    3. Programs
    4. Activities
  C. Patients with disabilities present significant challenges in providing quality nursing care.
  D. Perianesthesia standards for ethical practice require that quality care be given to all patients regardless of their disabilities.
II. THE MENTALLY CHALLENGED PATIENT
  A. Communication considerations
    1. Communication: an act by means of which one person conveys to another his or her ideas, thoughts, needs, or feelings
    2. A person must have some communication channel open to convey information to those around him or her.
    3. Communication involves:
      a. Getting information to the brain
      b. Processing the information
      c. Transmitting the brain's response
    4. Normal channels of communication may not be available.

5. Mental ability may be impaired from birth or acquired as a result of disease or injury.
   a. Congenital defect
   b. Infectious process
   c. Trauma
   d. Manifestation of a medical problem
   e. Psychiatric disorder
6. Level of impairment of developmentally disabled
   a. Mild—85%
      (1) Slow learner
      (2) Rarely asks questions
      (3) Answers questions with a minimum of words
      (4) Usually functions at a 10-year-old level
      (5) Minimal impairment in sensorimotor areas
      (6) Usually achieves academic skills necessary for minimum self-support
   b. Moderate—10%
      (1) Has little or no speech
      (2) Understands and can follow simple commands
      (3) Can learn simple tasks; may need supervision to perform
      (4) May be able to function at a 2- to 6-year-old level
      (5) May perform unskilled or semiskilled work under supervision
   c. Severe and profound—5%
      (1) May learn to perform simple self-care tasks with supervision
      (2) Shows basic emotional response
      (3) May cause self harm
      (4) May function at a 2-year-old level or less
7. Cognitive considerations of the mentally challenged patient
   a. Degree of impairment will determine method of instruction.
   b. Simple words and phrases are more likely to be understood than complex words and ideas.
   c. Common traits
      (1) Short attention span
      (2) Decreased retention capability
      (3) Decreased sensory capability
   d. Instructions may be taken very literally.
      (1) May need to have basic concepts deconstructed to the essence
      (2) Instructions should build on this basic essence.
   e. Becomes confused and distracted easily
   f. Fearful of changes in environment, loss of familiar routine
   g. May have a history of previous bad experiences with health care
8. Mental status—patient may:
   a. Be agitated
   b. Show aggression
   c. Not exhibit any response
   d. Have delusions, hallucinations, and/or paranoia
9. Sensory function—patient may have:
   a. Visual deficits
   b. Auditory deficits
   c. Asthenia
10. Communication problems
    a. Poor articulation, especially consonants
    b. More inarticulate when upset, frustrated, or discussing emotionally charged information
    c. Use words that he or she does not really understand.
    d. Be eager to please and say what thinks interviewer wants to hear.
    e. Need extra time to formulate answers
    f. Use sign language, read lips.
    g. Use nonverbal forms of communication.

B. Improving communication successes
  1. Determine the patient's strengths and weaknesses.
  2. Show respect to the patient.
    a. Do not talk down to the patient.
    b. Determine the "age appropriateness" of words, remembering not only the "calendar age" of a person but the "mental age" as well.
    c. Maintain good eye contact.
  3. Be sensitive to nonverbal communication.
    a. Do not cover or hide your mouth.
    b. Do not mimic how the patient pronounces words.
  4. Allow adequate time.
    a. Remain calm, relaxed, and unhurried.
    b. Maintain a low volume.
    c. May need to repeat information
    d. May need to reformulate the question
  5. Use the name to which the patient is accustomed.
  6. Be aware that some patients may have delusions, hallucinations, and/or paranoia.
    a. Approach in a calm, nonthreatening, reassuring manner.
    b. Avoid activities that may feed into abnormal thinking.
      (1) No sudden movement
      (2) Avoid standing too close.
      (3) Do not whisper or joke in patient's presence.
      (4) Do not show signs of impatience.
      (5) Do not touch the patient.
      (6) Challenge or agree with patient's delusions, hallucinations, or paranoia.
  7. Communicate slowly and clearly.
    a. Use open-ended questions.
    b. Be prepared to reword questions if the patient does not grasp the meaning of what is being asked.
    c. Avoid running words together.
    d. Provide a small pause between words if the patient seems to be struggling.
    e. Opt for simple words instead of ones that are complex. The more basic a word is, the better the chance is that it will be understood.
    f. Maintain eye contact when possible.
  8. Encourage and allow patient independence according to abilities.
  9. Include family and caregiver in planning care and instructions as appropriate.
  10. Demonstration may be more effective than verbal explanations.
  11. Provide frequent reinforcement.
C. Preadmission, preoperative interview and management
  1. An in-person interview is preferable to a telephone interview.
    a. Nonverbal communication may be as important as verbal communication.
    b. Face to face may be a good way to communicate with the person.
    c. Allow adequate time for the interview and assessment.
      (1) Engage patient to increase desensitization to setting.
  2. Determine the patient's functional ability and needs.
    a. Conduct developmental assessment if appropriate.
    b. Include the family's and caregiver's perceptions about the patient's abilities.
    c. Assess family's and caregiver's successful management techniques.
    d. Assess use of assistive devices (i.e., glasses, braces, hearing aid).
    e. Identify most effective means of communication for the patient.
    f. Determine willingness and capability of family and caregiver to participate in preoperative preparation and postoperative care.

3. Determine the patient's, the family's, and the caregiver's knowledge and expectations of the proposed procedure.
4. Complete health history per protocol.
   a. Cause of disability
      (1) At birth or acquired
      (2) Degree of disability
         (a) Retains self-determination capabilities
         (b) Caregiver shares decision-making.
         (c) Durable power of attorney for health care
         (d) Appointed legal guardian
   b. Consider common health conditions associated with multiple disabilities.
      (1) Alimentary—dental caries, high arched palate, gum disease, facial asymmetry, mandible subluxation, jaw and tongue asymmetry, oral sensitivity, inadequate nutrition
      (2) Sensory—limited communication abilities, visual and hearing impairment
      (3) Cardiovascular—reduced cardiac and lung functions linked to spinal curvature, conduction defects, cardiac anomalies
      (4) Respiratory—possible history of aspiration, chronic pneumonitis, and chronic respiratory infections
      (5) Musculoskeletal—spinal curvatures such as scoliosis; hyperlordosis; hyperkyphosis; deformities of shoulders, elbows, wrists and hands, knees and feet; hypertonia; hypotonia; fluctuating muscular tone; athetosis
      (6) Skin—damage to skin integrity from pressure and incontinence
      (7) Elimination—urinary and fecal incontinence, urinary tract infection (UTI), constipation, urinary retention, bowel impaction
      (8) Central nervous system—epilepsy, seizures
   c. Past illnesses—especially those for which the patient was hospitalized
      (1) Coping mechanisms to handle illness-related stress
      (2) Length of recuperative period
      (3) Frequency of respiratory infections
      (4) Normal response to pain
      (5) Bladder function difficulties
      (6) Bowel function difficulties
   d. Other health problems
      (1) Congenital heart defect and other cardiovascular disorders
      (2) Diabetes—mellitus, insipidus
      (3) Seizures
         (a) Time of last seizure
         (b) Frequency of seizures
         (c) Description of seizures
      (4) Elicit if any other problems.
   e. Medications
      (1) Current medication use
         (a) Prescription
         (b) Over-the-counter
         (c) Herbal preparations
         (d) Dietary supplements
      (2) Behavior changes caused by medications
      (3) Previous response to medications
   f. Allergies
      (1) Medications
      (2) Environmental
      (3) Food
      (4) Latex
      (5) Tape
      (6) Type of reactions to allergies

    g. Nutritional requirements and modifications
        (1) Special dietary restrictions
        (2) Food consistency
        (3) Preferences
        (4) Ability to swallow
        (5) Ability to eat independently or amount of assistance needed
    h. Usual behavior
        (1) Patient's interaction with people and environment
        (2) Orientation to time and place
        (3) Emotional stability
            (a) Mood swings
            (b) Potential for violence
            (c) Panic attacks
            (d) Hallucinations, delusions, paranoia
        (4) State of consciousness
        (5) Language ability
5. Physical assessment per protocol
    a. Vital signs and oxygen saturation (vital signs usually within expected range for size and age)
        (1) Past tendency for pronounced temperature deviations
    b. Body size
        (1) Obese
        (2) Emaciated
    c. Skin color and blemishes may provide clues to other illnesses.
        (1) Pallor may indicate anemia.
        (2) Uneven coloring and/or mottling may indicate poor neural functioning of the autonomic system.
        (3) Excessive pigmentation (freckles) could indicate pathology.
        (4) Multiple café au lait spots indicate neurofibromatosis (von Recklinghausen's disease).
        (5) Port wine stain on the face along the trigeminal nerve may indicate Sturge-Weber syndrome.
    d. Differences in skin temperature, skin turgor
    e. Defects of the craniofacial area
        (1) Anatomical deformities that interfere with intubation
        (2) Weakness of pharyngeal muscles
        (3) Large tongue
    f. Joint deformities
        (1) Pain on movement
        (2) Muscle strength
        (3) Involuntary movements or spasms
        (4) Altered stance, gait, or posture
        (5) Contractures
    g. Deficits in hearing or vision
6. Psychosocial assessment per protocol
    a. Anxiety
        (1) Fear of strange environment
        (2) Loss of independence
        (3) Change in daily routine
    b. Support system
        (1) Ensure competent and willing adult to assist with preoperative care and after discharge.
        (2) May need early social service referral for discharge care
7. Develop a plan of care based on the assessment of the patient's and caregiver's knowledge and needs.
8. Preoperative teaching per protocol and using techniques listed in prior sections
    a. Explain what will happen in simple terms.
    b. Explain what to expect preoperatively and immediate postoperatively.

    c. Determine the patient's regular schedule and incorporate that schedule into the hospital routine whenever possible.

    d. Include family and caregiver in the preoperative and postoperative preparations.

    e. Encourage the patient to bring some familiar comfort item from home.

    f. Demonstrate preoperative preparation or postoperative exercises and/or treatments and have the patient or caregiver do a return demonstration.

    g. Nothing by mouth (NPO) requirements—consider harm of extensive NPO time element to patient's emotional well-being.

    h. Medications to take or hold
        (1) Maintain regular dose schedule as much as possible.
        (2) Keep in mind the interactions with anesthesia of tricyclic antidepressants and monoamine oxidase inhibitors when giving instructions—seek clarification from the anesthesia provider if necessary.

    i. Pain scale (modify to suit patient's learning ability)
        (1) Demonstrate use of pain scale to patient.
        (2) Have patient return demonstration.

    j. Ensure that appropriate person will be available to sign necessary consents.

    k. Ensure arrangements for safe transport to and from the hospital.

    l. Ensure that there will be a responsible adult to assist with care after discharge.

  9. Complete preparation for admission per protocol.
    a. Make referrals as necessary.
    b. Preoperative testing as ordered
    c. Document and communicate special needs to the perianesthesia staff.

D. Day of admission (Box 19-1)

E. Preoperative holding and intraoperative (Box 19-2)

F. Phase I (Box 19-3)

G. Phase II (Box 19-4)

H. Postdischarge (Box 19-5)

■ BOX 19-1
■ **ADMISSION PROCEDURE**

- Review data collected during preadmission interview.
- Verify compliance to preoperative instructions with patient, family, and caregiver.
- Verify safe transportation home and competent adult help at home.
- Verify consents are appropriately signed.
- Perform physical assessment (history and physical per policy).
- Provide emotional support to patient and family and caregiver.
- Institute appropriate nursing measures to decrease anxiety.
- Decrease stimulation in the waiting area.
- Limit number of personnel who interact with the patient while providing continuity.
- Allow family and caregiver to remain with the patient as long as possible.
- Allow patient to use assistive devices as long as possible.
- Consider preoperative medications to decrease anxiety.
- Consider applying topical anesthetics at least 1 hour before IV insertion.
- Maintain a calm, unhurried, and accepting attitude.
- Call patient by name he or she is most familiar with.
- Allow patient to take comfort item to surgery if permissible.
- Prepare patient for procedure per protocol.
- Communicate patient's special needs to all members of the health care team (surgical, anesthesia, and perianesthesia team members).

IV, Intravenous line.

■ BOX 19-2
■ **PREOPERATIVE HOLDING AND INTRAOPERATIVE**

- Whenever possible, have the PACU nurse meet the patient beforehand so that the patient will recognize and be comforted by a familiar face in an unfamiliar and frightening environment.
- Review collected data.
- Provide routine care per protocol.
- Provide emotional support.
- Use the name with which the patient is familiar.
- Reassure the patient you are with him or her; touch patient if it will provide comfort.
- Allow patient to keep comfort item.
- Whenever possible, allow patient to keep hearing aid, glasses, etc.
- Maintain normothermia, taking care not to overheat.
- When moving patient, lift rather than pull, especially if joint deformities are present.
- Communicate the patient's special needs to the PACU staff.

PACU, Post anesthesia care unit.

■ BOX 19-3
■ **PHASE I**

- Review collected data.
- Provide routine care per PACU protocol and ASPAN Standards.
- Be alert for agitation, disorientation, or combative behavior.
- Minimize risk of aspiration.
- Observe for return of gag and swallowing reflexes.
- Elevate head of bed if not contraindicated.
- Suction as necessary.
- Position on side if not contraindicated.
- Provide for safety—use restraints for protection only as a last resort to prevent injury (refer to facility policy on restraint use).
- Assess frequently for pain, administer medication, and monitor response as indicated.
- Recognize patient may not be able to tell you pain is present.
- Be attuned to nonverbal communication.
- Provide emotional support.
- Use the name with which the patient is familiar.
- Provide reassurance to the patient that you are present.
- Allow use of comfort item if sent with a patient.
- Reorient patient to surroundings.
- Allow use of assistive devices as soon as possible.
- Have a family member and caregiver with the patient if possible.
- Communicate patient's special needs to phase II team.

ASPAN, American Society of PeriAnesthesia Nurses; *PACU,* post anesthesia care unit.

III. ALZHEIMER'S DISEASE
  A. Background information
    1. Alzheimer's disease (AD): a complex progressive, ultimately fatal, neurodegenerative disorder.
      a. Certain types of nerve cells in particular areas of the brain degenerate and die.
      b. Affected cells include cortical pathways involved in:
        (1) Catecholaminergic
        (2) Serotonergic
        (3) Cholinergic transmission

■ BOX 19-4
■ **PHASE II**

- The patient may return to phase II directly from the operating room (fast-tracking).
- Patient may be disoriented, combative, or agitated.
- Review collected data.
- Provide routine care per protocol and ASPAN *Standards*.
- Minimize risk of aspiration.
- Observe for return of gag and swallowing reflexes.
- Elevate the head of bed if not contraindicated.
- Suction as necessary.
- Position on side if not contraindicated.
- Use caution when giving liquids or solids.
- Assess for pain level per protocol.
- Use a pain scale that is appropriate for the patient.
- Medicate as needed and observe for response.
- Use relaxation methods as appropriate.
- Document reactions to interventions.
- Provide emotional support.
- Allow family and caregiver to be with patient as soon as possible.
- Allow use of assistive devices as soon as possible.
- Reorient to surroundings.
- Prepare for discharge.
- Verify safe transportation home and competent adult to care for patient at home.
- Include family and caregiver when reviewing instructions; if a procedure is to be done at home, have patient or caregiver perform a return demonstration.
- Recognize the possible need to give instructions to protect operative site based on patient's psychological needs.
- Provide written as well as verbal home care instructions.
- Use large type if necessary for written instructions.
- It may be necessary to use a tape recorder if reading skills are inadequate.
- Obtain a phone number to reach the patient and caregiver for postoperative follow-up phone call.
- Give appropriate phone numbers so the patient and caregiver can obtain assistance if questions or problems arise at home.

ASPAN, American Society of PeriAnesthesia Nurses.

■ BOX 19-5
■ **POSTDISCHARGE**

- Contact patient and caregiver within 24 hours of discharge.
- Identify yourself and state purpose of the call.
- Identify compliance with postoperative instructions.
- Identify potential complications:
  - Unrelieved pain and nausea
  - Unexpected or excessive bleeding or swelling
  - Elevated temperature
  - Redness or drainage from operative site
  - Other adverse occurrences
- Refer to appropriate physician or agency as necessary.
- Complete postdischarge assessment per facility protocol.

    c. Advancing pathology leads to the classic clinical symptoms.

      (1) Memory loss

      (2) Changes in personality

      (3) Noticeable decline in cognitive abilities (including speech and understanding)

      (4) Loss of executive function (decision-making)

      (5) Losses impairing activities of daily living (ADLs; dressing, eating, toileting, etc.)

    d. Most common cause of dementia in people 65 years or older

2. Stages of progression

    a. Forgetful stage—changes in:

      (1) Short-term memory

      (2) Depression

      (3) Conflict with others

      (4) Expressive aphasia

      (5) Frustration

    b. Confused stage:

      (1) Agnosia (inability to recognize common objects)

      (2) Decreased time sense

      (3) Withdrawn

      (4) Impaired reading abilities

      (5) Difficulty managing daily activities (money, driving, cooking, cleaning)

      (6) Wandering, night walking, walking without lifting feet

      (7) Belligerence

      (8) Confusion

      (9) Paranoia

      (10) Agitation

      (11) Delusions

      (12) Aggression

    c. Demented stage:

      (1) Loss of ability to perform ADLs

      (2) Decreased awareness

      (3) Repetitive behaviors

      (4) Decline in language ability

    d. End-stage dementia—loss of purposeful mobility, loss of communication, dependence in ADLs. Patient is at risk for:

      (1) Contractures

      (2) Weight loss

      (3) Skin breakdown

      (4) Repeated infections

      (5) Aspiration

3. Treatment—stabilize symptoms and minimize or prevent behavioral problems.

    a. Acetylcholinesterase inhibitor drugs temporarily delay worsening cognitive symptoms.

      (1) Donepezil hydrochloride (Aricept)

      (2) Rivastigmine (Exelon)

      (3) Galantamine (Reminyl)

    b. Vitamin E—may delay the progression from one stage to the next

      (1) Antioxidant properties

      (2) Doses prescribed range from 400 to 1200 IU twice per day.

    c. Behavioral modification for agitation

4. Symptoms are exacerbated by:

    a. Illness, disease

    b. Increased temperature

    c. Dehydration

    d. Medications, including anesthesia

    e. Tests, treatments

      f. Changes in routine

      g. Unfamiliar people, sights, sounds, smells

B. Preadmission and preoperative interview and management

  1. Patient may not be able to provide information.

  2. Determine the patient's level of ability with input from family and caregiver.

  3. Determine the patient's and family's understanding of AD.

  4. Determine the family's willingness and ability to participate in preoperative preparation and postoperative care.

  5. Provide a safe, comfortable environment without distraction and allow enough time for interview and assessment.

    a. Include family and caregiver to decrease anxiety and agitation and increase compliance.

    b. Include the patient in discussions about his or her procedure.

      (1) Establish eye contact, talk in a low-pitched, reassuring tone using patient's name.

      (2) Speak slowly and clearly using short, simple sentences with familiar words.

      (3) Ask one question at a time.

      (4) Ask yes or no questions.

      (5) Allow 20 to 30 seconds for patient to answer question.

      (6) Give simple directions, one step at a time.

      (7) Because of patient's short-term memory loss, be prepared to repeat information frequently.

      (8) Patient may respond to mood of situation more than words spoken.

      (9) Overstimulation of environment or pressure to answer questions may make patient more confused, agitated, aggressive.

      (10) Be alert to patient's nonverbal communication.

      (11) Do not leave patient alone because he or she may wander away.

  6. Assessment per protocol

    a. Abilities and needs of the patient

      (1) Caregiver's and family's successful management techniques

      (2) Use of assistive devices

      (3) Effective method of communication

      (4) Normal daily routine for patient

    b. Degree of disability

      (1) Retains self-determination capabilities

      (2) Family shares decision-making.

      (3) Has durable power of attorney for health care

      (4) Legal guardian appointed

  7. Complete health history per protocol

    a. Swallowing problems

    b. History of aspiration

    c. Triggers for agitation

  8. Physical assessment per protocol

    a. At risk for aspiration caused by:

      (1) Decreased level of consciousness

      (2) Decreased cough and gag reflexes

      (3) Impaired swallowing mechanism

    b. Patients treated with *Ginkgo biloba* or vitamin E may be at increased risk of bleeding.

      (1) Observe for bruising.

      (2) Consult with primary care physician about stopping or adjusting dosage before surgery.

  9. Psychosocial assessment per protocol

    a. Support system

      (1) Possible lack of support system related to:

        (a) Personality changes

        (b) Altered behavior patterns

(c) Depression
(d) Inability to interact in an adult manner
(e) Delusions
(f) Socially unacceptable behavior
(2) Consider early referral to social services for discharge planning.
(3) Arrangements for safe transportation to and from the hospital
(4) Arrangements for willing, competent adult in home for postdischarge care
   b. Anxiety—symptom for all stages of AD
    (1) One nurse as much as possible for continuity of care and familiarity
    (2) State name and purpose of encounter every time.
    (3) Orient patient frequently.
 10. Develop a plan of care based on patient's and family's and caregiver's knowledge and needs.
 11. Preoperative teaching per protocol
   a. Include family and caregiver—patient is likely to forget instructions.
   b. Present small amount of information at one time.
   c. Give written as well as verbal instructions.
 12. Complete preparation for admission per protocol.
   a. Referrals as necessary
   b. Preoperative tests as ordered
C. Admission for procedure (see Box 19-1)
  1. Provide safe, calm, unhurried environment.
   a. Use one nurse for care and approach as outlined in previous section.
    (1) State name and what is happening every time.
    (2) Orient patient to surroundings frequently.
    (3) Explain actions before proceeding.
    (4) If becomes agitated, pat or hold hand gently—avoid physical contact that could seem restraining.
   b. Keep bed low, side rails up, family and caregiver at bedside.
  2. Cognitive assessment
   a. Memory loss
   b. Confusion and disorientation
   c. Agitation
D. Preoperative holding and intraoperative (see Box 19-2)
  1. Use care when moving the patient.
   a. Lift rather than pull to protect skin.
   b. Protect bony prominences by positioning and use of padding.
  2. Restraints are likely to cause agitation.
   a. May need sedation before applying restraints necessary for procedure
   b. Will need distraction from restraints if awake
  3. Patient may be at risk for aspiration—more common in the later stages of AD.
   a. Elevate the head of the bed if possible.
   b. Suction as needed.
   c. Position on side if possible.
  4. May have an impaired cholinergic system. Avoid anticholinergic medicines such as atropine and scopolamine that may result in untoward behavioral activity.
E. Phase I (see Box 19-3)
  1. Pain frequently undertreated because of cognitive disability
   a. Pay attention to nonverbal clues.
   b. Observe carefully for response to pain medication.
  2. Increased risk of bleeding if has been taking *Ginkgo biloba* or vitamin E supplements
  3. May be agitated, combative, confused
   a. Repeated orientation to surroundings
   b. Use one nurse for care.
   c. Use nasal cannulas rather than mask.

  d. Turn down sound from bedside monitors.
  e. May need to wrap intravenous line in gauze or put on stockinette sleeve
  f. If nasogastric tube in place, tape behind ear and fasten to gown's shoulder.
  g. Consider dehydration as contributing cause.
  h. Observe for bladder distention.
  i. Allow use of assistive devices as soon as possible.
  j. Return to area with family and caretaker as soon as possible.
  k. Avoid restraints if at all possible.
 F. Phase II (see Box 19-4)
  1. May be at risk for aspiration
   a. May need to remind the patient to swallow
   b. Elevate the head of the bed if possible.
   c. Suction as needed.
   d. Position on side if not contraindicated.
   e. Use caution when giving liquids and solids.
  2. Patient may be confused and/or combative.
   a. Frequently orient patient to surroundings.
   b. Allow family and caregiver to be with patient.
   c. Allow use of assistive devices as soon as possible.
   d. Provide safe environment, nursing interventions as listed in prior sections.
  3. Pain is frequently undertreated because of cognitive disability.
   a. Pay attention to nonverbal clues.
   b. Observe carefully for response to pain medication.
  4. Discharge
   a. Patient will benefit from returning to familiar environment as soon as possible.
   b. Verify safe transportation home.
 G. Postdischarge (see Box 19-5)
IV. HEARING IMPAIRMENT
 A. Background information
  1. Estimated 28 million U.S. citizens have hearing impairments.
   a. Leading disability in America
   b. Affects 30% of patients 65 years and older
   c. Affects more than 50% of those older than 75
  2. Definitions
   a. Deaf: unable to hear or understand oral communications with or without the aid of amplification devices
   b. Hard of hearing: a hearing loss severe enough to necessitate use of amplification devices to hear oral communication
  3. Types of hearing impairment
   a. Conductive hearing loss—reduced ability of sound to be transmitted to middle ear
   b. Sensorineural—reduced hearing resulting from damage to inner ear or neural brain pathways
   c. Mixed—combination of conductive and sensorineural impairments
   d. Central—auditory compromise at the level of the brain
  4. Hearing deficit is not reflective of low intelligence.
  5. Not all hearing impaired people can read lips or use sign language.
  6. Only about 20% to 30% of words are readable on the lips.
 B. Techniques for effective communication with the hearing impaired in any setting
  1. Provide an environment for effective communication.
   a. Provide a quiet, distraction-free area.
   b. Provide adequate lighting.
   c. Provide interpreter if necessary.
   d. Supply a battery-powered microphone with earpiece if applicable.
   e. Allow patient to choose appropriate seating arrangement.

   2. Get patient's attention before speaking.
      a. Approach within the patient's line of vision; face patient directly.
      b. Wave hand.
      c. Touch gently as to avoid startling the patient.
   3. Determine the patient's preferred method of communication.
      a. Hearing aid
      b. Lip reading
      c. Sign language
      d. Written messages
      e. Alphabet, picture, word or phrase board
      f. Combination of methods
   4. For lip reading and/or hearing augmented by hearing aids
      a. Sit or stand directly in front of the patient.
      b. Keep mouth visible when speaking.
      c. Do not chew gum or food.
      d. Maintain comfortable voice volume.
      e. Speak slowly and distinctly; do not exaggerate your pronunciation.
      f. Use smallest number of words to convey the message.
      g. Maintain eye contact.
   5. Working with an interpreter
      a. The interpreter is used to transmit information, not to explain information or give opinions.
      b. Stand or sit across from the patient with the interpreter beside you.
      c. Speak at a normal tone and face the patient directly.
      d. Ask the patient, not the interpreter, to clarify information if not understood.
C. Preadmission and preoperative interview and management
   1. An in-person interview facilitates the patient's participation, especially if he or she relies on lip reading or gestures.
      a. Determine whether an interpreter for sign language will be needed to communicate with the patient.
      b. Determine whether the patient has access to a telecommunications relay service for phone messages.
   2. Incorporate communication techniques for hearing impairment.
   3. Include family member in preoperative visit if possible.
   4. Identify level and duration of disability.
      a. Totally deaf
      b. Able to hear with hearing aids in place
      c. Severe decrease in hearing
        (1) Is one ear better than the other?
        (2) Is hearing improved by using a supplemental microphone with earpiece?
   5. Provide adequate time for interview and assessment.
   6. Use patient's method of communication; provide an interpreter if necessary.
   7. Determine the patient's and family's knowledge and expectations of the proposed procedure.
   8. Assessment per protocol
      a. Abilities and special needs
      b. Willingness of family to participate in preparation for procedure and postoperative care
      c. Use of hearing aid or other assistive devices
      d. Be alert to nonverbal communication.
   9. Complete health history per protocol
   10. Physical assessment per protocol
   11. Psychosocial assessment per protocol
      a. Anxiety
        (1) Feeling of isolation because of disability
        (2) Fear of not understanding what is happening in a strange environment
        (3) History of bad experiences in health care settings

        b. Support system
- (1) Arrangements made for safe transportation to and from hospital
- (2) Arrangements made for competent adult help after discharge
- (3) Arrangements to communicate messages to the patient
  - (a) Before the procedure—time changes if necessary
  - (b) Interpreter on hand day of surgery if needed
  - (c) Follow-up postoperatively
- (4) If patient is primary caregiver of another person, have arrangements for help been made while patient recovers?

    12. Develop a teaching plan based on patient's and family's knowledge and needs.

    13. Preoperative teaching per protocol
- **a.** Verify that the patient understands instructions.
  - (1) Ask the patient directly.
  - (2) Repeat or reinforce information as necessary.
  - (3) Provide written information to take home.
- **b.** Explain that family can be with patient as long as possible before surgery and as soon as possible after surgery.
- **c.** Hearing aid and/or assistive devices will be used as long as safely possible before surgery and returned as soon as possible after surgery.
- **d.** If patient wears a hearing aid, instruct to check hearing aid battery and that aid is clear of earwax before admission.

    14. Complete preparation for admission.
- **a.** Referrals made as necessary
- **b.** Preoperative tests as ordered
- **c.** Arrange for interpreter day of procedure if necessary.

    15. Document and communicate special needs to other members of perioperative team.

  D. Admission for procedure (see Box 19-1)
- **1.** Use communication techniques for hearing impairment.
  - **a.** Know patient's method of communication.
  - **b.** Provide interpreter if necessary.
  - **c.** Inform patient that hearing aid or communication device will be returned as soon as possible after surgery.

  E. Preoperative holding and intraoperative (see Box 19-2)
- **1.** Use communication techniques for hearing impairment.
- **2.** If possible, avoid covering face with mask when speaking to patient.
- **3.** Allow use of hearing aid, communication, or other assistive devices if possible.
- **4.** Use gestures or written messages if necessary.

  F. Phase I (see Box 19-3)
- **1.** Approach patient in his or her line of sight.
- **2.** Gently touch patient to get his or her attention.
- **3.** If protective lubricant used, clear from patient's eyes.
- **4.** Return hearing aid or other assistive devices as soon as possible.
- **5.** Speak slowly and distinctly.
  - **a.** Remain in patient's line of vision when speaking.
  - **b.** Keep your mouth visible when speaking.
  - **c.** Recognize that the patient will hear and understand less when tired and/or ill.

  G. Phase II (see Box 19-4)
- **1.** Return hearing aid and assistive devices as soon as possible.
- **2.** Use communication techniques for hearing impairment.
- **3.** Recognize that the patient will hear and understand less when tired and/or ill.

  H. Postdischarge (see Box 19-5)

V. VISION IMPAIRMENT
  A. Background information
- **1.** Estimated 10 million people affected in United States
  - **a.** Seventy percent of the estimate are 65 years or older.
  - **b.** Complete blindness—no vision
  - **c.** Legal blindness—unable to see at 20 feet what normal vision can see at 200 feet

        d. Partially sighted—need adaptive methods to read and write

        e. Hemiplegics—may have loss of half of visual field in each eye

        f. Macular degeneration—loss of sight in the center vision field, accounts for 54% of all blindness

   2. May or may not have other disabilities

B. Preadmission and preoperative interview and management

   1. Identify yourself and state purpose of visit.

        a. Use a normal tone of voice.

           (1) Sense of hearing in a blind patient is often very acute.

           (2) Ask the patient if he or she can hear you before speaking louder.

        b. Provide a safe environment.

           (1) If moving to another area, offer arm to patient.

               (a) Patient takes arm from behind, just above the elbow.

               (b) Expect the patient to keep a half step behind you so he or she can anticipate if a step is coming.

           (2) Orient to environment.

               (a) Give specific directions such as "straight in front of you" and "directly to your left."

               (b) Introduce everyone in the room.

               (c) Let the patient know what you are doing if there is silence in the room for awhile: "I need to write this down now."

        c. Assure patient his or her needs will be communicated to perianesthesia team members.

   2. Identify level and duration of disability.

        a. Totally blind

        b. Partial vision

        c. Light perceptive

        d. Patient's management skills

   3. Ask the patient how much assistance he or she needs and wants in performing ADLs.

   4. Determine patient's and family's knowledge of proposed procedure.

   5. Assessment per protocol

        a. Abilities, special needs

        b. Desired method of communication

           (1) Braille

           (2) Special glasses or contacts

           (3) Large print

           (4) Audiotape

           (5) Computer disk

        c. For other disabilities

   6. Complete health history per protocol

   7. Physical assessment per protocol

   8. Psychosocial assessment per protocol

        a. Support system

           (1) A competent adult who can assist at home after discharge

           (2) If the patient and/or caregiver is a primary caregiver for another person, arrangements made for someone else to provide care for that person.

           (3) Safe transportation to and from the hospital

        b. Anxiety

           (1) Isolation because of disability

           (2) Fear of being left alone

   9. Develop plan of care based on patient's needs and knowledge.

C. Preoperative teaching and preparation per protocol

   1. Provide instructions.

        a. Verbal

        b. Written—use large bold letters with black felt tip markers on white paper.

        c. Audiotape—preferred method to take home

  d. Need for a safe environment at the facility
   (1) Side rails for safety; keep bed low.
   (2) Call light will be within reach.
   (3) Encourage support person to be available to stay with patient the day of surgery.
  e. Assure patient of emotional support.
   (1) Explain what will happen preoperatively and in the immediate postoperative period.
    (a) Describe what surroundings will sound and feel like: "group room with curtain dividers," "cold," and so forth.
    (b) Explain who will be present in the different stages of care.
   (2) Availability of preoperative medications for relaxation
   (3) Assure patient that staff will be within calling distance.
 2. Prepare for procedure per protocol.
  a. Referrals as necessary
  b. Preoperative testing as ordered
 3. Document and communicate patient's special needs to perioperative team members.
D. Admission for the procedure (see Box 19-1)
 1. Use communication technique in which patient is comfortable.
  a. Verbal only, Braille, combination of methods
  b. Get patient's attention before speaking.
   (1) Speak in normal tone of voice.
   (2) Provide a quiet area to prevent distraction.
 2. Promote independence based on patient history.
 3. Provide description of new surroundings.
  a. Identify those present.
  b. Allow time and opportunity for patient to explore new environment.
 4. Include patient in discussions about his or her procedure.
 5. Inform patient that communication device will be returned as soon as possible after the procedure.
E. Preoperative holding and intraoperative (see Box 19-2)
 1. Avoid confusion and too many people speaking at once.
 2. Let the patient know who is in the room.
 3. Let the patient know what is being done before touching him or her.
 4. Keep the environment safe.
  a. Use safety devices such as side rails and straps for stretchers.
   (1) Explain to patient where the devices are located.
   (2) Explain the purpose of and how the straps feel before applying.
  b. Have a means for the patient to call for assistance.
  c. Assure patient he or she will not be left alone.
F. Phase I (see Box 19-3)
 1. Speak in a normal tone of voice.
 2. Touch patient gently to get his or her attention.
 3. Resume use of assistive devices if possible.
 4. Maintain calm, quiet environment to decrease confusion.
G. Phase II (see Box 19-4)
 1. Speak softly and gently touch patient to get his or her attention.
 2. Use safety devices such as side rails.
  a. Keep call light within reach at all times.
  b. Allow family or caregiver in as soon as possible.
 3. Discharge (see Box 19-5)
  a. Provide clear discharge instructions.
   (1) Provide written copy of instructions for caregiver.
   (2) May need to provide audiotape of instructions
  b. Instruct caregiver on visual assessment of the operative site.

VI. SPEECH IMPAIRMENT
  A. Background information
    1. Aphasia: language disorder that impairs the expression and understanding of language as well as reading and writing
      a. Receptive: an inability to understand the spoken word due to damage of Wernicke's area; can speak but the words do not make sense
      b. Expressive: an inability to speak or write due to damage of Broca's area; can understand what is being said
      c. Usually occurs suddenly—stroke or brain injury
      d. May also develop slowly—brain tumor
      e. Patient may also suffer from:
        (1) Dysarthria: difficult, poorly articulated speech caused by paralysis of the muscles that control speech
        (2) Apraxia: inability to correctly position and sequence speech muscles to produce understandable speech
        (3) Aphonia: loss of ability to produce normal speech sounds from vocal cords
    2. Mutism: inability to speak caused by a physical defect or emotional problem
    3. Neurological diseases can cause speech disorders.
      a. Parkinson's disease
      b. AD
      c. Stroke
      d. Brain tumors
    4. Malignant conditions may require the removal of speech apparatus.
      a. May use a voice synthesizer
      b. Laryngectomy patient may use controlled breathing or belching to speak.
  B. Techniques for effective communication with the speech impaired
    1. Keep distractions to a minimum (turn off radio, television).
    2. Maintain a natural conversational manner appropriate for an adult.
    3. Include the speech-impaired person in conversations.
    4. Simplify language using short and simple sentences.
    5. Maintain a normal voice volume.
    6. Allow enough time for a response.
      a. Avoid correcting the person's speech.
      b. Encourage any type of communication.
        (1) Speech
        (2) Gestures
        (3) Pointing
        (4) Drawing
  C. Preadmission and preoperative interview and management
    1. An in-person interview is more effective than a telephone interview and allows the patient a greater opportunity to participate.
    2. Use techniques for effective communication with the speech impaired.
    3. Determine the patient's effective means of communication.
      a. Use of assistive devices (i.e., glasses, hearing aid)
      b. Story board, writing tablet, or slate
    4. Encourage but do not pressure the patient to respond in whatever way he or she can.
      a. Encourage patient to write responses, if he or she can write and spell.
      b. Encourage the use of gestures if that is most effective means to communicate.
    5. Allow adequate time for the interview and assessment.
      a. Allow for differences in accuracy and articulation when soliciting patient's response.
      b. Present a relaxed attitude by mannerisms, patience, and acceptance.
      c. One person speaking at a time helps to decrease confusion.
      d. Ask direct questions requiring one-word answers.

6. Encourage family and caregiver to be present.
   a. May better understand patient's gestures and speech patterns
   b. Continue to include patient in discussions.
7. Complete health history per protocol
   a. Cause and duration of disability
   b. Concurrent diseases that contribute to speech impairment
8. Physical assessment per protocol
9. Psychosocial assessment per protocol
   a. Anxiety level—concern over ability to communicate with staff
   b. Support system
      (1) Willingness of family and caregiver to be present the day of surgery to assist with communication
      (2) Arrangements made for patient to communicate with hospital staff from home concerning questions or changes
         (a) Contact person via phone
         (b) Internet and e-mail access
10. Determine the patient's and family's knowledge of the proposed procedure.
11. Develop a teaching plan based on the patient's and family's knowledge and needs.
12. Preoperative teaching per protocol
    a. Use techniques for effective communication with the speech impaired.
    b. Give written instructions to review at home.
13. Complete preparation for admission.
    a. Preoperative tests as ordered
    b. Referrals as necessary
    c. Document and communicate patient's special needs to perioperative team members.
D. Day of procedure admission (see Box 19-1)
   1. Use techniques for effective communication with the speech impaired.
   2. Provide enough time for the patient to communicate concerns.
E. Preoperative holding and intraoperative (see Box 19-2)
   1. Allow the patient to continue to use assistive devices as long as possible.
   2. Discuss with patient how he or she can make needs known or answer questions if he or she is without his or her normal communication tools.
      a. Squeeze hand—once for yes, twice for no.
      b. Raise hand if appropriate.
      c. Give patient a bell to ring.
      d. Provide writing board.
   3. Reassure the patient that you are with him or her.
F. Phase I (see Box 19-3)
   1. May be at higher risk for aspiration
      a. Observe for return of swallowing and gag reflexes.
      b. Position on side, if allowed, until return of gag and swallowing reflexes.
      c. Elevate head of bed after return of reflexes if not contraindicated.
      d. Suction as needed.
   2. Reduce apprehension.
      a. Reorient to surroundings.
      b. Provide means of communicating.
      c. Reunite patient and family as soon as possible.
G. Phase II (see Box 19-4)
   1. Use techniques for effective communication with the speech impaired.
   2. Return assistive devices as soon as possible.
   3. Arrange for a contact person to phone or how to communicate with patient at home for postoperative follow-up.
H. Postdischarge (see Box 19-5)

VII. SPINAL CORD INJURY (see Chapter 33)
 A. Background information
  1. Classification
   a. Complete—total paralysis and loss of sensation below the zone of injury, resulting in quadriplegia or paraplegia
    (1) Paraplegia: the result of injury to the thoracolumbar region (T2 to L1), causing loss of motor and sensory function of the lower extremities while upper extremity function remains intact
    (2) Quadriplegia: the result of injury to cervical or thoracic regions (C1 to T1), with impaired function of the arms, trunk, legs, and pelvic organs occurring
   b. Incomplete—with partial preservation of function below the zone of injury
   c. Measurement of functional ability: Functional Independence Measurement
    (1) Seven-point scale measures 18 items in six categories:
     (a) Self-care
     (b) Continence of bowel and bladder
     (c) Mobility
     (d) Locomotion
     (e) Communication
     (f) Social cognition
    (2) Scale of 1 equals total dependence on caregiver.
    (3) Scale of 7 indicates independence.
  2. Consequences of level of injury
   a. C1 to C4—results in quadriplegia with complete loss of motor and sensory function from the neck down and loss of respiratory function
   b. C5—results in quadriplegia and loss of all functions below the upper shoulder level; the phrenic nerve is intact but not the intercostal muscles.
   c. C6—results in quadriplegia and loss of all functions below the shoulders and upper arms; no use of intercostal muscles
   d. C7—results in incomplete quadriplegia with loss of motor control to parts of the arm and hand, and loss of sensation below the clavicle and parts of the arms and hands; no use of intercostal muscles
   e. C8—results in incomplete quadriplegia with loss of motor control to parts of the arms and hands and loss of sensation below the chest and part of the hands; no use of intercostal muscles
   f. T1 to T6—results in paraplegia with loss of motor function below the midchest, including the trunk muscles, and loss of sensation from the midchest downward, including the lower limbs; the phrenic nerve functions independently; there is some impairment of the intercostal muscles.
   g. T6 to T12—results in paraplegia with loss of motor control and sensation below the waist; there is no interference with respiratory function.
   h. L1 to L3—results in paraplegia with loss of most of the control of the legs and pelvic area, and loss of sensation to the lower abdomen and legs
   i. L3 to L4—results in incomplete paraplegia with loss of control and function of part of the lower legs, ankles, and feet
   j. L4 to S2—results in incomplete paraplegia with varying degrees of motor and sensory loss; can walk with braces or may use a wheelchair, and can be relatively independent
  3. May be at a higher risk for mobility, perfusion, and reflex activity complications
   a. Cardiac arrhythmias and cardiac arrest
   b. Deep vein thrombosis from peripheral vasodilation related to decreased muscle function
   c. Orthostatic hypotension (especially above level of T7)
   d. Autonomic hyperreflexia (possible only at or above the level of T6)

    e. Sleep apnea
    f. UTI and bladder dysfunction
    g. Skin breakdown
    h. Spasticity, contractures, and deformity
    i. Difficult pain management related to dysesthetic or phantom pain
    j. Depression, social isolation

B. Preadmission/preoperative interview and management
  1. Provide a comfortable space for the interview.
  2. Recognize that a physical disability alone does not affect intelligence.
    a. Refer to the patient as a person with a disability not as a disabled person.
    b. Speak directly to the patient.
    c. Ask the patient the type of physical assistance he or she prefers.
  3. Identify the level and duration of the disability.
  4. Determine patient's and family's management and coping strategies.
  5. Conduct interview and assessment per protocol.
    a. Physical abilities, special needs
    b. Use of assistive devices—braces, splints, ADL modifications
    c. Willingness and ability of family to participate in preoperative preparation and postoperative care
  6. Complete health history per protocol
    a. Cardiac arrhythmias and cardiac arrest
      (1) Electrolyte imbalance
      (2) Response to vagal stimulation
    b. Orthostatic hypotension—history of hypotension when the head of the bed is raised or when the patient is gotten out of bed
    c. Autonomic hyperreflexia—previous response to noxious stimulation of the sensory receptors
      (1) Urinary calculi, severe bladder infections, urinary retention or bladder distention/spasms
      (2) Bowel impaction and stimulation of anal reflex
      (3) Temperature changes
      (4) Tight, irritating clothes
      (5) Decubiti
      (6) Pain and operative incisions
    d. Pain
      (1) Spinal cord injury pain most common type of pain in this population
        (a) Mild, tingling to severe, intractable
        (b) Usually unresponsive to standard pain treatments
      (2) Transitional zone pain
        (a) Felt at the level of injury
        (b) Bandlike pattern over the trunk or upper arms
      (3) Pain can be felt above or below the level of injury.
      (4) Pain management techniques patient has found most helpful
    e. Spasticity
      (1) A state of increased tonus in a weak muscle
      (2) Usually peaks 1.5 to 2 years after the injury
      (3) Gradual regression
    f. Pressure sores
      (1) Usual skin care routine
      (2) Positioning routine
    g. Bladder and bowel management—recognize increased risk for latex sensitivity if indwelling catheter present.
    h. Nutrition
      (1) Type of diet
      (2) Amount of assistance needed to eat
      (3) Mechanical consistency of foods
      (4) Methods used to prevent aspiration
  7. Physical assessment per protocol

8. Psychosocial assessment per protocol
   a. Anxiety
      (1) Losing independence
      (2) Suffering greater disability caused by complications from procedure
      (3) Inadequate pain relief postoperatively
   b. Support system
      (1) Availability and willingness of responsible adult to provide care at home
      (2) Arrangements for safe transport to and from the facility
      (3) Referrals to social services if needed
         (a) Make arrangements for additional equipment in the home.
         (b) May need home health care for postoperative discharge care
9. Develop a plan of care based on the knowledge and needs of the patient and family.
10. Preoperative instructions per protocol—include family and caregiver if possible.
11. Complete preparation for admission.
    a. Preoperative tests as ordered
    b. Referrals as necessary
    c. Document and communicate the patient's special needs to the perioperative team members.

C. Admission (see Box 19-1)
   1. Use latex precautions if the patient is on a bladder program or has indwelling catheter.
   2. Laboratory values within acceptable range
      a. Electrolytes, especially potassium
      b. Blood coagulation studies
      c. Urinalysis—evaluate for evidence of UTI

D. Preoperative holding and intraoperative (see Box 19-2)
   1. Use latex precautions if necessary.
   2. Maintain normothermia.
   3. Be aware of potential for:
      a. Cardiac arrhythmias
         (1) Electrolytes, especially potassium within normal range
         (2) Avoid excessive vagal stimulation.
      b. Autonomic hyperreflexia symptoms
         (1) Hypertension
         (2) Superficial vasodilatation
         (3) Flushing
         (4) Profuse sweating
         (5) Piloerection (gooseflesh) occurring above the level of injury, often seen in patients with upper thoracic and cervical injuries
      c. Pain, paresthesia, and hyperesthesia
      d. Spasticity
         (1) May result from a slight touch on the skin
         (2) Aggravated by cold or staying in one position for a prolonged period
   4. Move patient with care, lifting rather than pulling.
   5. Avoid pressure on bony prominences by positioning or use of padding.

E. Phase I (see Box 19-3)
   1. Continue use of latex precautions if necessary.
   2. Keep patient warm.
   3. Be aware that even slight touch could trigger spasticity.
   4. Monitor for signs of bladder distention.
   5. Monitor for signs of autonomic hyperreflexia.
      a. Paroxysmal hypertension
      b. Pounding headache
      c. Vasodilatation

        d. Flushing

        e. Profuse sweating

        f. Piloerection

    6. Increased potential for orthostatic hypotension exists.

        a. Be cautious when elevating the head of the bed if caring for a patient with quadriplegia.

    7. Be aggressive with pain management.

  F. Phase II (see Box 19-4)

    1. Keep patient warm without overheating.

    2. Be aware that light touch on the skin may trigger spasticity.

    3. Monitor for bladder distention.

    4. Monitor for autonomic hyperreflexia.

    5. Monitor for orthostatic hypotension.

        a. Be cautious when elevating the head of the bed of the patient.

        b. Provide assistance when increasing activity.

    6. Be aggressive with pain management.

    7. Return assistive devices as soon as possible.

  G. Discharge (see Box 19-5)

VIII. TRAUMATIC BRAIN INJURY

  A. Background information

    1. Approximately 600,000 new traumatic brain injuries (TBIs) occur in the United States each year.

        a. Nearly 100% of persons with severe head injury and two thirds of those with mild injury will be permanently disabled.

        b. Greatest cause of TBI is motor vehicle accidents.

        c. Most severe head injuries occur in adolescents and young adults.

    2. May have motor impairment

        a. Spasticity, tremors, ataxia

        b. Weakness

        c. Apraxia: the inability to perform a skilled motor act in the absence of paralysis

        d. Paralysis

        e. Poor breathing patterns

    3. May have sensory impairment of:

        a. Sense of position

        b. Spatial judgment

        c. Vision, hearing, touch, smell, and taste

        d. Increased or decreased pain sensitivity

    4. May have communication impairment

        a. Aphasia: inability to communicate

        b. Dysarthria: defective articulation caused by motor deficits of the tongue or muscles used for speech

    5. May have cognitive impairment

        a. Abstract thinking

        b. Judgment

        c. Generalization and planning abilities

        d. Memory

        e. Decreased concentration ability

        f. Reduced tolerance for stress, irritability, impatience—labile emotions

  B. Preadmission and preoperative interview and management

    1. An in-person interview may be more beneficial than a telephone interview; the patient may use nonverbal forms of communication.

    2. Provide a calm, quiet environment; limit stimulation factors.

    3. Include family and caregiver whenever possible.

    4. Allow adequate times for interview and assessment; recognize that the patient's attention span may be limited.

    5. Remember to include patient in the conversation.

    6. Complete health history per protocol

    a. Cause and duration of disability

    b. Type of limitations caused by disability

    c. Seizure activity, if appropriate

        (1) Manifestation of seizure

        (2) Frequency

        (3) Aura, triggers

        (4) Effective treatment

  7. Assessment per protocol

    a. Abilities, special needs

        (1) Level reached on a rehabilitation scale

            (a) Rancho Los Amigos, a cognitive functioning scale; Level I—no response, total assistance, to Level X—modified independent

            (b) Disability Rating Scale—point system to estimate general level of disability from none to extreme vegetative state

        (2) Patient's and family's or caregiver's successful management techniques

    b. Use of assistive devices

  8. Physical assessment per protocol

    a. Swallowing difficulty because of poor muscle control

    b. Positioning problems caused by paralysis, contractures, spasticity

  9. Psychosocial assessment

    a. Anxiety

        (1) Be alert to nonverbal communication.

        (2) Level of ability to cope with hospital environment

    b. Emotional lability

    c. Support system

        (1) Arrangements for safe transport to and from the facility

        (2) Willingness and ability of family to participate in preoperative preparation and postoperative care

    d. Make referrals as necessary.

  10. Develop a plan of care based on the knowledge and needs of the patient and family.

  11. Preoperative teaching per protocol

    a. Provide verbal and written preoperative instructions.

    b. Include family and caregiver in instructions if at all possible.

    c. Adjust teaching to patient's level of disability.

        (1) Recognize patient may have short attention span.

        (2) Patient may have short-term memory problems.

        (3) Use short, clear instructions; do not use abstract ideas.

    d. Emphasize pain management.

        (1) Determine which pain scale is most appropriate for the patient.

        (2) After instruction, have patient demonstrate the use of the pain scale.

  12. Complete preparation for admission.

    a. Preoperative tests as ordered

    b. Referrals as needed

    c. Document and communicate special needs to the perioperative team members.

C. Admission (see Box 19-1)

  1. Limit stimulation in room.

D. Preoperative holding and intraoperative (see Box 19-2)

  1. Recognize that the patient may be emotionally labile.

  2. Provide a calm, quiet environment.

E. Phase I (see Box 19-3)

  1. If swallowing difficulty exists, minimize risk for aspiration.

    a. Observe for return of swallowing and gag reflexes.

    b. Suction as needed.

    c. Elevate the head of the bed if allowed.

    d. Position on side if not contraindicated.

      2. Allow use of assistive devices as soon as possible.

   F. Phase II (see Box 19-4)

      1. Verify competent adult help at home after discharge.

   G. Postdischarge (see Box 19-5)

IX. PARKINSON'S DISEASE (see Chapter 17)

   A. Background information

      1. Parkinson's disease (PD) is a common, slowly progressive neurological disease.

         a. Peak onset at age 55 to 60

         b. Affects men more than women: 55 men to 45 women

         c. Affects Hispanics/Latinos and Non-Hispanic Whites more than African Americans

         d. Progresses from diagnosis to major disability over 10 to 20 years

      2. Symptoms result primarily from loss of dopamine in the brain.

      3. Primary clinical symptoms

         a. Rigidity of the limbs—appreciated as stiffness of the joints simulating arthritis

         b. Tremor of the limbs—more prominent in the hands and is asymmetrical, often occurring while at rest

         c. Bradykinesia of the limbs and body—most prominent and disabling symptom of PD

            (1) Difficulty initiating movement

            (2) Slowness in movement

            (3) Paucity or incompleteness of movement

         d. Postural instability—results from impairment of postural reflexes

            (1) Patient perceives as unsteadiness or lack of balance.

            (2) When patients trip, they are unable to stop falling or ease their fall.

      4. Secondary symptoms

         a. Difficulty walking resulting from a combination of bradykinesia and postural instability

            (1) Short steps and shuffling gait

            (2) Festinating gait—a manner of walking in which speed increases to catch up with a displaced center of gravity

            (3) Anteropulsion—be propelled forward, or backward (retropulsion)

            (4) Freeze—a difficulty turning, and a tendency to stop abruptly and inexplicably

            (5) Stooped posture

         b. Masklike features

            (1) Diminished facial expression

            (2) Stares straight ahead

            (3) Has decreased blinking of eyes

         c. Speech changes

            (1) Difficulty initiating speech

            (2) Difficulty coordinating expiration and articulation

         d. Autonomic symptoms

            (1) Drooling

            (2) Excessive perspiration

            (3) Constipation

            (4) Orthostatic hypotension

            (5) Dysphasia

         e. Changes in behavior and mental ability

            (1) Depression

            (2) Slowness of information processing

            (3) Social withdrawal

            (4) Generalized apathy and loss of appetite

            (5) Dementia—occurs in 15% of patients with PD as they age

         f. General weakness and muscle fatigue

        (1) Complications can include injuries from falls, skin breakdown, UTIs, aspiration pneumonia.

    g. Hypersensitivity to heat

        (1) Treatment

    h. Antiparkinson drugs to restore dopamine or mimic dopamine's actions; partial list

        (1) Antiparkinson: levodopa (Larodopa), carbidopa-levodopa (Sinement)

        (2) Dopamine agonists: pergolide (Permax), pramipexole (Mirapex), ropinirole (Requip)

        (3) Antivirals: amantadine

        (4) Anticholinergics: benztropine mesylate (Cogentin) and trihexyphenidyl (Artane)

    i. Surgical treatment

        (1) Thalamotomy, pallidotomy

        (2) Deep brain stimulation

B. Preadmission and preoperative interview and management

  1. An in-person interview affords the opportunity to observe the patient's abilities and interaction with family members.

  2. Maintain a calm, unhurried, accepting attitude in a safe, comfortable environment.

    a. Provide assistance with ambulation.

    b. Recognize that information processing may be slowed.

  3. Speak to the patient and encourage to respond in whatever manner he or she can.

    a. PD does not affect patient's intelligence.

    b. Respect patient's level of independence.

  4. Include the family and caregiver in preoperative preparation when possible.

  5. Assessment per protocol

    a. Abilities and special needs of the patient

        (1) Determine the patient's and/or family's understanding of PD.

        (2) Length of time disease has been present

        (3) Manifestations of PD

        (4) Effects of PD on patient

           (a) Patient's usual routine to cope with limitations

           (b) Consider using ADL scoring system for PD.

           (c) Patient's and family's successful management techniques

        (5) Use of assistive devices

        (6) Sleep disturbances

    b. Willingness and ability of family and caregiver to participate in preoperative preparation and postoperative care

  6. Complete health history per protocol

  7. Physical assessment per protocol

    a. Vital signs and oxygen saturation

    b. Muscle strength

    c. Location of tremors

    d. History of dysphagia

  8. Cognitive assessment

    a. Memory loss

    b. Depression

    c. Information processing speed may be slowed down.

  9. Psychosocial assessment per protocol

    a. Anxiety

        (1) Prominent feature in 40% of PD patients

        (2) Many PD patients have panic attacks.

        (3) Determine patient's coping mechanisms.

    b. Support system

      (1) Competent adult help at home after discharge

      (2) Arrangements made for safe transportation to and from the hospital

  10. Develop plan of care based on the patient's and family's knowledge and needs.

  11. Preoperative teaching per protocol

    a. Provide verbal and written preoperative instructions.

    b. Patients should be instructed to take normal PD medications the day of surgery.

      (1) Prevent muscle weakness and tremors that make self-care difficult.

      (2) Rigidity may contribute to a difficult intubation.

      (3) Rigidity predisposes to venous thrombosis.

  12. Complete preparation for admission per protocol.

    a. Referrals as necessary

      (1) May require physical therapy and occupational therapy to maintain function postoperatively

    b. Preoperative testing as ordered

    c. Document and communicate patient's special needs to the perianesthesia team.

C. Admission (see Box 19-1)

  1. Verify competent adult help at home after discharge.

  2. Physical assessment per protocol

    a. Muscle strength

    b. Tremors, rigidity

    c. Swallowing problems

  3. Prepare patient per protocol.

    a. Verify PD drugs have been taken as instructed.

    b. Drugs that exacerbate extrapyramidal symptoms should be avoided.

      (1) Metoclopramide

      (2) Droperidol

      (3) Phenothiazines

      (4) Alcohol

  4. Provide emotional support for family and patient.

    a. Use measures to decrease anxiety.

    b. Provide safe environment.

      (1) Assist patient in getting out of bed.

      (2) Keep side rails up and bed position low.

      (3) Do not leave patient unattended.

    c. Maintain comfortable temperature.

D. Preoperative holding and intraoperative (see Box 19-2)

  1. Recognize potential for aspiration.

  2. Avoid overheating.

  3. Recognize patient is at greater risk for hypotension and cardiac arrhythmias.

E. Phase I (see Box 19-3)

  1. Increased risk for aspiration because of difficult or ineffective swallowing

    a. Elevate head of the bed if allowed.

    b. Suction as necessary.

    c. Observe for return of gag and swallowing reflexes.

    d. Position on side if not contraindicated.

  2. Prevent overheating.

F. Phase II (see Box 19-4)

  1. Increased risk for aspiration because of difficult or ineffective swallowing

    a. Elevate head of the bed if allowed.

    b. Suction as necessary.

    c. Observe for return of gag and swallowing reflexes.

    d. Position on side if not contraindicated.

  2. Prevent overheating.

3. Increased risk of orthostatic hypotension
   a. Ambulate gradually and with assistance.
   b. Evaluate vital signs after activity progression.
G. Postdischarge (see Box 19-5)

X. MULTIPLE SCLEROSIS (see Chapter 17)
A. Background information
   1. Multiple sclerosis (MS): a chronic, unpredictable neurological disease that affects the white matter of the brain and the spinal cord.
   2. Myelin is lost in multiple areas, leaving scar tissue—sclerosis.
      a. Damaged areas—plaques or lesions
      b. Disrupts ability of the nerves to conduct electrical impulses to and from the brain
   3. Usually diagnosed between the ages of 20 and 50
   4. Each year, 25,000 new cases diagnosed
   5. Two to three times as many women as men have MS.
   6. Clinical courses—each may be mild, moderate, or severe.
      a. Benign MS—affects 20% of patients; causes mild disability with infrequent, mild, and early attacks followed by near-complete recovery
      b. Exacerbating-remitting MS—affects 25% of patients with frequent attacks that start early in the course of the illness, followed by less-than-complete clearing of signs and symptoms than in benign MS
      c. Chronic relapsing MS—affects approximately 40% of patients; has fewer, less-complete remissions after an exacerbation than has exacerbating-remitting MS. Chronic relapsing MS has a cumulative progression, with more symptoms occurring during each new attack.
      d. Chronic progressive MS—affects approximately 15% of patients and is similar to chronic relapsing MS except that the onset is more subtle and the disease progresses slowly without remission
   7. Symptoms are unpredictable; vary from person to person and from time to time in the same person.
      a. Sensory—numbness, paresthesia, pain, dysesthesia, trigeminal neuralgia, Lhermitte's sign, chronic pain from other symptoms, decreased proprioception and sense of temperature, depth, and vibration
      b. Motor—paresis, paralysis, dragging of foot, dysphagia, spasticity, diplopia, bowel and bladder dysfunction (incontinence or retention)
      c. Cerebellar—ataxia, staggering, loss of balance and coordination, nystagmus, speech disturbances, tremors, vertigo
      d. Other symptoms—optic neuritis, impotence or decreased genital sensation, depression or euphoria, fatigue or decreased energy level
   8. Factors that may cause a relapse
      a. Infections
      b. Trauma—accidental or planned (i.e., surgery)
      c. Pregnancy
      d. Undue fatigue or excessive exertion
      e. Overheating or excessive chilling or cold
      f. Emotional stress
   9. Treatment
      a. Immunomodulators—beta-interferon (Avonex) and glatiramer (Copaxone)
      b. Monoclonal antibodies—natalizumab (Antegren)
      c. Steroids given to decrease inflammation and increase periods of remission
      d. Antispasmodics—baclofen (Lioresal) and dantrolene (Dantrium)
      e. Fatigue controlled with amantadine (Symmetrel)
B. Preadmission and preoperative interview and management
   1. Provide a comfortable, safe environment.
      a. Allow adequate time—patient fatigue may be a factor.
      b. May need extra time to formulate questions and responses
   2. Assessment per protocol

  a. Abilities, special needs
   (1) Determine level and duration of disease.
   (2) Determine patient's and family's understanding of MS.
   (3) Determine patient's and family's routine to minimize symptoms.
  b. Use of assistive devices
  c. Willingness and capability of family to participate in preoperative preparations and postoperative care
 3. Complete health history per protocol
  a. Identify previous events triggering relapses.
  b. Determine patient's response to physical and psychological stresses.
 4. Physical assessment per protocol
  a. Evaluate ability to swallow.
  b. Evidence of infectious process present
 5. Psychosocial assessment per protocol
  a. Anxiety
   (1) Surgery may cause relapse.
   (2) Loss of independence
  b. Support system
   (1) Competent adult help at home on discharge
   (2) Arrangements made for safe transport to and from the hospital
 6. Develop plan of care based on patient's and family's knowledge and needs.
 7. Preoperative teaching per protocol
  a. Provide verbal and written instructions.
  b. Include family in instructions if at all possible.
 8. Complete preparation for admission per protocol.
  a. Make referrals as necessary.
  b. Preoperative tests as ordered
  c. Document and communicate special needs to the perianesthesia team.
C. Admission (see Box 19-1)
 1. Provide comfortable, safe environment.
  a. Assist patient in getting out of bed if needed.
  b. Keep side rails up and bed in low position.
 2. Use measures to reduce stress.
  a. Explain what will be happening.
  b. Allow patient to verbalize concerns.
  c. Allow family to be with patient as long as possible.
  d. Allow use of assistive devices as long as possible.
  e. Allow extra time for patient to answer or formulate questions.
 3. Avoid undue fatigue; provide periods of rest.
 4. Physical assessment per routine protocol
  a. Sensory deficit
  b. Motor deficit
  c. Cerebellar disturbances
D. Preoperative holding and intraoperative (see Box 19-2)
 1. Maintain normothermia.
 2. If swallowing deficits, may be at increased risk for aspiration
  a. Elevate head of bed if possible.
  b. Suction as needed.
  c. When possible, position on side.
E. Phase I (see Box 19-3)
 1. Provide specialized care based on patient's symptoms.
 2. May be at higher risk for aspiration
  a. Elevate head of bed if not contraindicated.
  b. Suction as needed.
  c. Observe for return of swallowing and gag reflexes.
  d. Position on side if not contraindicated.
 3. Maintain normothermia.
 4. Reduce stress.

      a. Reorient patient to surroundings.

      b. Medicate for pain or anxiety as necessary.

F. Phase II (see Box 19-4)

  1. May be at increased risk for aspiration

    a. Elevate head of bed if not contraindicated.

    b. Suction as needed.

    c. Observe for return of swallowing and gag reflexes.

    d. Position on side if not contraindicated.

  2. Provide comfortable, safe environment.

    a. Reorient patient to surroundings.

    b. Allow use of assistive devices as soon as possible.

    c. Assist patient with ambulation.

  3. Reduce stress.

    a. Reunite patient and family as soon as possible.

    b. Avoid fatigue; provide periods of rest.

G. Postdischarge (see Box 19-5)

XI. MYASTHENIA GRAVIS (see Chapter 17)

A. Background information

  1. Myasthenia gravis (MG): a chronic, progressive autoimmune disease causing voluntary muscle weakness.

  2. Two thirds of patients first present with oculomotor disturbances, ptosis, or diplopia.

  3. Most other patients first have oropharyngeal muscle weakness, difficulty chewing, swallowing, or talking.

  4. Severity of weakness fluctuates, being the most severe after prolonged use of affected muscles.

  5. As progression occurs, the patient may exhibit:

    a. Increased weakness of certain voluntary muscles

    b. Improvement of muscle strength with rest

    c. Dramatic improvement in muscle strength with use of anticholinesterase drugs

    d. Difficulty with speech

    e. Difficulty swallowing

    f. Respiratory insufficiency

    g. Drooping head

    h. Fatigue

    i. Bowel and bladder dysfunction

    j. Depression

    k. May develop myasthenia crisis (weakness from MG exacerbation) or a cholinergic crisis (weakness from too much anticholinesterase medication)

      (1) Acute respiratory difficulty

      (2) Acute motor weakness of voluntary muscles, including those for swallowing, speaking, and moving parts of the body

      (3) Treatment for either crisis is respiratory assistance.

  6. Symptoms worsen with:

    a. Emotional upset

    b. Systemic illness

    c. Viral respiratory infections

    d. Hypothyroidism and hyperthyroidism

    e. Pregnancy, menstrual cycle

    f. Drugs affecting neuromuscular transmission

    g. Increased body temperature

B. Preadmission and preoperative interview and management

  1. Provide a calm environment.

  2. Allow for periods of rest if necessary.

  3. Include family in preoperative preparations whenever possible.

  4. If patient has difficulty talking, provide with alternative communication tools.

     5. Assessment per protocol
       a. Patient's abilities and special needs
         (1) Determine patient's and family's understanding of MG.
         (2) Patient's successful management techniques
         (3) Use of assistive devices
         (4) If patient has had any myasthenia crisis episodes—treatment needed.
       b. Willingness and capability of family to participate in preoperative preparation and postoperative care
     6. Complete health history per protocol
       a. Progression of disease
       b. Normal routine to avoid exacerbating factors
       c. Particularly note anticholinesterase medications patient is taking for MG.
         (1) Pyridostigmine (Mestinon)
         (2) Neostigmine (Prostigmin)
         (3) Cholinergic effects can be reversed by common perioperative medications such as mycin-type antibiotics, aminoglycosides, nondepolarizing muscle relaxants, morphine, procainamide.
     7. Physical assessment per protocol
       a. Respiratory assessment—ease of breathing, depth of respirations, auscultation
       b. Muscle strength—identify which muscles are involved with the disease.
     8. Psychosocial assessment per protocol
       a. Anxiety
         (1) Determine patient's coping mechanisms.
         (2) Fear of respiratory difficulties during surgery and recovery
       b. Support system
     9. Develop a plan of care based on patient's and family's knowledge and needs.
    10. Preoperative teaching per protocol
    11. Complete preparation for admission per protocol.
       a. Referrals as necessary
       b. Preoperative tests as ordered
       c. Document and communicate patient's special needs to the perianesthesia team.
  C. Admission (see Box 19-1)
     1. Physical assessment per protocol
       a. Respiratory function assessment
         (1) Auscultation
         (2) Observation
       b. Muscle strength—note which muscles are affected by the disease at this time.
     2. Monitor patient closely after any medication for signs of interaction with routine MS medications.
       a. Increased muscle weakness
       b. Decreased respirations
       c. Agitation
  D. Preoperative holding and intraoperative (see Box 19-2)
     1. Observe for myasthenia crisis, manifested with:
       a. Increased muscle weakness
       b. Respiratory distress
       c. Difficulty talking or swallowing
     2. Potential for aspiration
       a. Elevate head of bed if possible.
       b. Suction as necessary.
       c. Monitor for swallowing difficulty.
     3. At increased risk for infection
       a. Maintain aseptic technique.
       b. Use care to avoid skin tears.

        (1) Protect bony prominences by positioning and padding.

        (2) Use care when removing adhesive pads.

        (3) Lift rather than pull when moving patient.

  4. Maintain normothermia.

  5. Use measures to reduce stress.

  6. Monitor closely after any medication for signs of interaction with routine MG medications.

    a. Increased muscle weakness

    b. Respiratory difficulty

    c. Agitation

  7. Protect eyes from injury.

    a. Lubricant

    b. Tape eyelids closed.

E. Phase I (see Box 19-3)

  1. Greater risk for aspiration

    a. Observe for return of gag and swallowing reflexes.

    b. Elevate head of bed if allowed.

    c. Suction as necessary.

    d. Watch for weakness in throat.

      (1) Difficulty speaking

      (2) Difficulty swallowing

    e. Position on side if not contraindicated.

  2. Greater risk for respiratory distress

    a. Auscultation of lungs

    b. Observe respiratory pattern and effort.

    c. Monitor oxygen saturation.

  3. Risk for myasthenia crisis

    a. Maintain normothermia.

    b. Monitor patient closely after any medication for signs of interaction with routine MG medications.

      (1) Increased muscle weakness

      (2) Respiratory difficulty

      (3) Agitation

    c. Observe for symptoms that may indicate crisis.

      (1) Acute respiratory distress

      (2) Acute motor weakness of voluntary muscles, including those for swallowing, speaking, and moving parts of the body

    d. Assess muscle strength frequently.

  4. Monitor vital signs and temperature frequently.

F. Phase II (see Box 19-4)

  1. Risk for respiratory distress

    a. Auscultate lungs.

    b. Observe respiratory pattern and effort.

    c. Monitor oxygen saturation.

    d. Avoid fatigue.

  2. Higher risk for aspiration

    a. Elevate head of bed.

    b. Suction as necessary.

    c. Assess for weakness of throat muscles.

    d. Position on side if not contraindicated.

    e. Exercise caution when giving fluids or solids.

  3. Risk for myasthenia crisis—observe for symptoms that may indicate an impending myasthenia crisis.

    a. Acute respiratory distress

    b. Acute motor weakness of voluntary muscles, including those used for swallowing, speaking, and moving parts of the body

  4. Monitor patient closely after any medication for signs of interaction with routine MG medications.

        a. Increased muscle weakness

        b. Respiratory difficulty

        c. Agitation

    5. Assess muscle strength frequently.

    6. Reduce psychological stress.

        a. Reorient patient to surroundings.

        b. Allow use of assistive devices as soon as possible.

        c. Allow family to be with patient as soon as possible.

    7. Keep patient comfortable.

        a. Have room at comfortable temperature—prevent overheating the patient.

        b. Medicate for pain or nausea and observe for desired or adverse medication reactions.

        c. Provide nourishment with care.

        d. Check for bladder distention.

  G. Postdischarge (see Box 19-5)

XII. AUTISM SPECTRUM AND INTELLECTUAL DISORDERS IN THE PEDIATRIC PATIENT (see Chapter 11)

  A. Autism spectrum disorders

    1. Cause: unknown but thought to be a result of an interaction between genes and the environment

    2. Incidence: mean prevalence is 6.6 per 1000 children.

    3. Symptoms: involve three types of behaviors

        a. Impaired speech

        b. Problems interacting socially

        c. Tendency towards repetitive behavior and interests

    4. Disorders include:

        a. Autism

          (1) Symptoms include:

            (a) Persistence of unusual reflexes

            (b) High rates of seizure disorders (25% in most cases)

            (c) Marked problems in social interaction

            (d) Delayed and deviant communication development

            (e) Other behaviors:

              (i) Stereotyped motor behaviors (hand flapping, body rocking)

              (ii) Insistence on sameness

              (iii) Resistance to change

        b. Asperger's syndrome

          (1) Symptoms include:

            (a) Deficits in social interaction and unusual responses to the environment

            (b) Cognitive and communicative development within the normal or near-normal range in the first years of life

            (c) Fewer deficits noted in terms of verbal skills compared to other autism spectrum disorders

        c. Childhood disintegrative disorder

          (1) Symptoms resemble autism but only after a relatively prolonged period (usually 2-4 years) of clearly normal development; differs from autism in the pattern of onset, course, and outcome.

          (2) May mimic childhood schizophrenia

        d. Rett's disorder

          (1) Affects girls almost exclusively

          (2) Symptoms follow normal early development:

            (a) The first few months of life: head growth begins to decelerate with a loss of purposeful hand movements and striking motor involvement.

            (b) Profound mental retardation is typical.

        e. Pervasive developmental disorder

(1) Also referred to as "atypical personality development" or "atypical autism"

(2) Encompasses cases where there is marked impairment of social interaction, communication, and/or stereotyped behavior patterns or interest

(3) Full features of autism are not met.

f. Intellectual disability

(1) Symptoms include significantly subaverage general intellectual functioning manifested before 18 years of age.

(2) Limited adaptive skills in at least two or more areas of functioning:

(a) Communication

(b) Self-care, home living

(c) Use of community resources

(d) Social/interpersonal skills

(e) Self-direction

(f) Functional academic skills

(g) Health and safety

(h) Work

(i) Leisure

(3) Degrees of severity

(a) Mild mental retardation (most common)

(i) Often not noticed by observers

(ii) May note developmental delays (achievement of developmental milestones later than expected) in language acquisition, social development, and motor skills

(iii) Can acquire these skills to the third- to sixth-grade level, and can be guided toward social appropriateness

(b) Moderate mental retardation

(i) Obvious delays in motor development and speech

(ii) Can learn basic self-help activities

(iii) Seldom progress academically beyond the second-grade level

(c) Severe mental retardation

(i) Typically acquire little if any communicative speech during preschool years

(ii) Education focuses on the basics of independent living skills, such as toileting, bathing, simple communication, self-feeding, and rules of behavior.

B. Perianesthesia considerations

1. When speaking to the child: speak clearly, simply, and slowly.

a. Allow ample time for the child to process information.

b. Do not insist on eye contact—some children with autistic tendencies find eye contact distressing.

c. Provide for language tools as required by the child including communication boards and sign language.

2. Obtain information from the caregivers about the child's routines, likes, dislikes, rituals, skills and abilities regarding self-care, such as feeding, dressing, bathing, and toileting.

3. Assessment should also include the child's communication skills, interactive patterns, and response to others.

4. Assess the method the caregivers use to give the child medications.

5. Assess family's support system.

6. Determine utilization of nontraditional alternative treatments, which may or may not impact care.

a. Several nutritional supplements have been used such as high-dose pyridoxine (vitamin B_6), magnesium, and ascorbic acid (vitamin C).

b. Dietary requirements including certain foods that have been eliminated from the diet such as gluten (e.g., wheat and barley) and casein (found in milk) products

7. Arrange for continuity of care settings and care providers whenever possible.

XIII. PEDIATRIC MOTOR/NEUROLOGICAL DISABILITIES (see Chapter 11)

A. Cerebral palsy

1. Chronic motor dysfunction caused by damage to the motor areas of the brain before, during, or after birth
   a. Alterations in muscle tone such as abnormal posturing and movements
   b. Delay in gross motor skills (i.e., sitting, crawling, cruising, or walking)
   c. Fine motor coordination may be affected, hampering the ability to perform ADLs including self-feeding and dressing.
   d. Many infants and children have other deficits (i.e., poor vision, strabismus or nystagmus, hearing loss, cognitive impairments, speech or language delays, seizures, and growth problems).
2. Incidence is estimated to be 7 per 1000 live births per year.
3. Many have additional cognitive and language delays ranging from mild to severe.

B. Down syndrome

1. Congenital chromosomal disorder characterized by varied degrees of mental retardation and a characteristic appearance
   a. Common features of Down syndrome include:
      (1) Muscle weakness and hypotonia
      (2) Oblique palpebral fissures and an upward slant to the eyes
      (3) A small nose and a depressed nasal bridge
      (4) A large tongue in a small mouth
      (5) A high-arched palate
      (6) Square hands with short fifth finger, and a simian (single transverse) crease across the palm of the hand
      (7) A wide space between the great and second toe
      (8) Epicanthic folds (small skin folds at the inner corners of the eyes)
2. Incidence for women older than 30 years is 1 in 1500; in women older than 40 it increases to 1 in 100 live births.
3. Associated conditions include congenital heart defects (especially septal defects), respiratory tract infections and chronic otitis media, altered immune system, gastrointestinal conditions (Hirschsprung's megacolon, tracheoesophageal fistula), hypothyroidism, ocular cataract, leukemia.

C. Spina bifida (SB)

1. Neural tube defect where there is an incomplete closure of the vertebrae and neural tube
   a. Saclike protrusion on the neonate's back noted at birth
   b. Clinical manifestations depend on the location of the lesion—the higher the deformity, the more neurological deficits will be present.
      (1) Lower extremities may be partially or completely paralyzed.
      (2) Bowel and bladder may or may not be affected.
      (3) Renal impairment may occur secondary to faulty kidney innervation.
      (4) Orthopedic complications such as flexion or extension contractures, talipes valgus, or varus contractures may also be present at birth.
      (5) Approximately 90% of infants with the most severe form of SB also develop hydrocephalus.
2. Incidence is approximately 1 in every 2000 births in the United States each year; higher in families with Hispanic or white European ancestries.
3. Complications associated with the defect include:
   a. UTIs
   b. Orthopedic problems such as kyphosis, scoliosis, tethering of the spinal cord
   c. Back pain
   d. Spasticity
   e. Skin breakdown.
   f. Loss of sensation secondary to interrupted nerve pathways

 D. Perianesthesia considerations

 1. Obtain information from the caregivers about the child's routines, likes, dislikes, rituals, skills and abilities regarding self-care, such as feeding, dressing, bathing, and toileting.
 2. Assessment should also include the child's communication skills, interactive patterns, and response to others.
 3. Assess the method the caregivers use to give the child medications.
 4. Assess family's support system.
 5. Determine utilization of nontraditional alternative treatments, which may or may not impact care.
 6. Ensure the infant's or child's body is in the best possible alignment, using pillows and bolsters as supports.
 7. Special care should be taken to protect bony prominences because they are prone to breakdown.
 8. Postoperatively, monitor carefully for aspiration, cardiac abnormalities, and respiratory complications due to congenital anomalies associated with physical disabilities.
 9. If the infant or child is hospitalized, the at-home regime should be followed as much as possible, and physical, occupational, and speech therapy department referrals should be made so that therapy sessions can be initiated.
 10. Infants, children, and adolescents with SB are 41% more likely to have latex allergy than the general public.
    a. Signs and symptoms
       (1) Urticaria
       (2) Wheezing
       (3) Watery eyes
       (4) Rash
       (5) Anaphylaxis, in extreme cases
    b. Ensure equipment such as tourniquets, intravenous tubing, urinary and intravenous catheters, and tapes are latex free.

BIBLIOGRAPHY

1. Bay E, McLean SA: Mild traumatic brain injury: An update for advanced practice nurses. *J Neurosci Nurs* 39(1):43-51, 2007.
2. Blackwell J, Niederhauser C: Diagnose and manage autistic children. *Nurse Pract* 28(6):36-43; quiz 44-45, 2003.
3. Blann LE: Early intervention for children and families with special needs. *MCN Am J Matern Child Nurs* 30(4):263-267; quiz 268-269, 2005.
4. Browne MF: Communicating with the child who has autistic spectrum disorder: A practical introduction. *Paediatr Nurs* 18(1):14-17, 2006.
5. Buchman AS, Boyle PA, Wilson RS, et al: Frailty is associated with incident Alzheimer's disease and cognitive decline in the elderly. *Psychosom Med* 69(5):483-489, 2007.
6. Burke KM, LeMone P, Mohn-Brown EL, et al: *Medical-surgical nursing care*, ed 2, Upper Saddle River, NJ, 2007, Pearson Education.
7. Desai AK, Grossberg GT: Diagnosis and treatment of Alzheimer's disease. *Przegl Lek* 55(12):676-682, 1998.
8. Guzofski S, Peralta R: Mental retardation. In Domino FJ, ed: *5-Minute clinical consult*, Philadelphia, 2008, Lippincott Williams & Wilkins.
9. Hayes C: Down syndrome: Caring holistically in primary health care. *Br J Community Nurs* 12(9):404-410, 2007.
10. McGuinness TM, Hardeman SM: Update on autistic spectrum disorders. *J Psychosoc Nurs Ment Health Serv* 45(4):27-31, 2007.
11. Meitzner MC, Skurnowicz JA: Anesthetic considerations for patients with Down syndrome. *AANA J* 73(2):103-107, 2005.
12. National Institute on Aging: *Alzheimer's disease fact sheet*. Available at: www.nia.nih.gov/Alzheimers/Publications/adfact.htm. Accessed February 18, 2008.
13. Palmieri RL: Is it myasthenia gravis or Guillain-Barre syndrome? *Nursing* 35(12):32hn1-32hn4, 2005.
14. Potts NL, Mandleco BL: *Pediatric nursing: Caring for children and their families*, Clifton Park, NY, 2007, Thomson Learning.
15. Rice C: Prevalence of autism spectrum disorders—Autism and Developmental Disabilities

Monitoring Network, 14 sites, United States, 2002. *MMWR* 56(SS01):12-28, 2007.

16. Seow D, Gauthier S: Pharmacotherapy of Alzheimer disease. *Can J Psychiatry* 52(10): 620-629, 2007.

17. Snoweling MJ, Hayiou-Thomas ME: The dyslexia spectrum: Continuities between reading, speech, and language impairments. *Top Lang Disord* 26(2):110-126, 2006.

18. Sommers MS: *Diseases and disorders: A nursing therapeutics manual*, ed 3, Philadelphia, 2007, F.A. Davis.

19. Sorrell JM: Listening in thin places. Ethics in the care of persons with Alzheimer's disease. *ANS Adv Nurs Sci* 29(2):152-160, 2006.

20. Thurgate C: Living with disability: Part 3. Communication and care. *Paediatr Nurs* 18(5):40-44, 2006.

21. U.S. Department of Justice: *Americans with Disabilities: Americans with Disabilities Act of 1990*. Available at: www.usdoj.gov/crt/ada/pubs/ada.htm. Accessed February 18, 2008.

22. Van Cleve S, Cohen W: Part I: Clinical practice guidelines for children with Down syndrome from birth to 12 years. *J Pediatr Health Care* 20(1):47-54, 2006.

23. Wagner KD, Johnson KL, Kidd PS: *High acuity nursing*, ed 4, Upper Saddle River, NJ, 2006, Pearson Education.

24. Wallhagen MI, Pettingil E, Whiteside M: Sensory impairment in older adults: Part 1: Hearing loss. *Am J Nurs* 106(10):40-48; quiz 48–49, 2006.

25. Watkinson S: Visual impairment in older people: The nurse's role. *Nurs Stand* 19(17):45-52; quiz 54–55, 2005.

26. Whiteside MM, Wallhagen MI, Pettengill E: Sensory impairment in older adults: Part 2: Vision loss. *Am J Nurs* 106(11):52-61; quiz 61-62, 2006.

20 Transcultural Nursing: Care of Culturally Diverse Patients

MEG BETURNE
MYRNA MAMARIL

OBJECTIVES
At the conclusion of this chapter, the reader will be able to:

1. Identify key perianesthesia transcultural concepts of cultural competence.
2. Define transcultural nursing.
3. Describe seven major components of a perianesthesia cultural assessment.
4. Discuss the importance of communication as it relates to assessment of culturally diverse patients.
5. Discuss the significance of verbal and nonverbal communication in dealing with culturally diverse patients.
6. Summarize important life events that concern culturally diverse patients in their perianesthesia hospitalizations.

I. DEFINITIONS
  A. Culture
    1. Integrated system that is shaped by learned values, beliefs, norms, and practices
    2. Characteristic of a society
    3. Guides individual behavior
      a. Thoughts
      b. Feelings
      c. Actions/patterns of expressions
      d. Decision-making that facilitates self-worth and self-esteem
    4. Passed down from one generation to the next generation
  B. Transcultural nursing
    1. Used interchangeably with cross-cultural, intercultural, or multicultural nursing
      a. "Trans" means across, "inter" means between, and "multi" means many.
      b. Goes across cultural boundaries in search for scientific theory of nursing
    2. Integrates the concept of culture into all aspects of nursing
    3. A humanistic and scientific area of formal study and practice
      a. Focuses on differences and similarities among cultures with respect to:
        (1) Human care
        (2) Health (or well-being)
        (3) Illness
      b. Based on individual's:
        (1) Cultural values
        (2) Beliefs
        (3) Practices

    C. Cultural competence

        1. Definition

            a. Dynamic, continuous process

            b. Individual and/or organizational process that continually finds meaningful and useful care delivery strategies based on:

                (1) Knowledge of the cultural heritage

                (2) Beliefs

                (3) Attitudes

                (4) Skills

                (5) Encounters

                (6) Behaviors of those to whom care is rendered

        2. Health care professionals need to use knowledge gained from conceptual and theoretical models of culturally appropriate care.

        3. Cultural competence assists the nurse to devise meaningful interventions to promote optimal health among individuals regardless of race, ethnicity, gender identity, sexual identity, or cultural heritage.

II. CULTURE

    A. Values, norms, beliefs, and practices of a society

    B. Develops over time

    C. Learned responses, actions, words, and thoughts

    D. Passed down through the generations

    E. Not genetic in nature

    F. Guides behavior

    G. Affects health care practices

III. THE TRANSCULTURAL NURSING SOCIETY

    A. Founded in 1974: Madeline Leininger, founder

    B. Publications on transcultural nursing

    C. Annual transcultural nursing conferences

    D. Certification available

IV. MAJOR WORLD VIEWS OF HEALTH AND ILLNESS

    A. Biomedical (scientific)

        1. Life is regulated by biomedical and physical processes.

        2. Health is absence of disease.

        3. Illness is alteration in structure and function of body.

        4. Treatment focuses on physical and chemical interventions.

    B. Magicoreligious (supernatural)

        1. All that exists is dependent on supernatural forces.

            a. Includes good and evil

        2. Health means person is blessed or favored by the supernatural.

        3. The cause of disease is mystical.

            a. Not based on scientific fact

            b. Foreign object or spirit enters the body.

            c. Sign of punishment or possession by the supernatural

        4. Treatment aimed at removing foreign object or spirit

    C. Holistic

        1. Everything governed by laws of nature

        2. Health achieved by adapting to constantly changing environment

        3. Illness is imbalance or lack of harmony between forces.

        4. Treatment aimed at restoring harmony or balance

V. MAJOR SECTORS OF HEALTH CARE

    A. Types

        1. Popular

            a. Lay; nonprofessional, non–folk healer

                (1) Define and treat illness.

            b. Determine whether additional care is needed (folk or professional).

            c. Activities

                (1) Self-care is administered using home remedies.

                (2) Consult with family, friends, clergy, neighbors, others who have had same condition.

      (3) Remedies include over-the-counter medications.

      (4) Care provided by self, family, and/or friends

  2. Folk

    a. May be consulted when home remedies and self-care methods fail

    b. Ethnomedical and traditional

    c. Ethnomedical

      (1) The study of non-Western, traditional, or folk medicine

      (2) Encompasses cultural traditions, beliefs, and practices related to health and illness

      (3) Not related to biomedical theory

    d. Characteristics

      (1) Defines and removes supernatural causes

      (2) Works to restore balance

      (3) Strives to restore health and prevent illness

    e. Activities

      (1) Holistic approach

      (2) Treatment of illnesses caused by:

        (a) Imbalances in individual, physical, social, and metaphysical environments

        (b) Supernatural forces

      (3) Treatment of:

        (a) Culture-specific illnesses

        (b) Illnesses not controlled by home remedies or professional medicine

      (4) Rituals

        (a) Incorporated to prevent illness, misfortune, and to enhance effects of biomedicine

    f. Acts as intermediary between popular and professional sectors

    g. May be the only sector consulted, depending on cause, signs, and symptoms

    h. Care provided by:

      (1) Folk healers

        (a) Secular

        (b) Sacred

        (c) Combination of both

  3. Professional

    a. Types

      (1) Biomedicine—United States

      (2) Traditional Chinese medicine—China

      (3) Ayurvedic medicine—India

    b. Goal: to define, treat, and prevent disease and illness

    c. May be consulted when home remedies or folk sector treatments are ineffective

    d. Initially consulted if acute trauma, surgery, or restoration of body part necessary

B. Characteristics

  1. Each explains and treats illness differently.

  2. Each defines who should be the health care provider.

  3. Each defines how the provider and patient should interact.

  4. Sectors are used individually, in combination, or simultaneously.

C. Use of different sectors

  1. Folk sector

    a. New immigrants and refugees use as primary source.

    b. Used by individuals from all socioeconomic groups

    c. Use dependent on cause of illness and availability of healers in other sectors

D. Nurse's role

  1. Understand why different sectors are used

    a. Enables nurse to better explain goals of nursing intervention and treatments

    b. Ensures patient understands advantages and disadvantages and potential incompatibilities of treatments from multiple sectors

VI. TRADITIONAL HEALERS
 A. Description
  1. Not part of popular or professional health sector
  2. Specialize in forms of healing characteristic of ethnomedicine
  3. Deal with secular, sacred, or both
  4. Combine methods from both sacred and secular
 B. Secular
  1. Use organic and technical means to treat conditions resulting from natural causes
  2. Types of healers
   a. Herbalist
   b. Bone setters
   c. Granny midwives
   d. Tooth extractors
   e. Injectionists
 C. Sacred
  1. Use nonorganic methods to treat supernatural and natural causes.
  2. Nonorganic
   a. Semimystical and religious practices
   b. Influence mind and faith of individual
   c. Examples
    (1) Chants
    (2) Prayers
    (3) Rituals
    (4) Amulets—object worn or cherished to ward off evil or attract good fortune
   d. Types of healers
    (1) Sorcerers
    (2) Shamans
    (3) Spiritualists
    (4) Voodoo priests, priestesses
    (5) Diviners
 D. Nurse's role
  1. Determine whether patient receiving treatment from traditional healer.
  2. Inform patient if traditional treatments and biomedical treatments are incompatible (Table 20-1).
  3. Consult with traditional healer, if necessary, to ensure all have understanding of same goal: assisting the patient to recovery.
  4. Modify plan of care if no compromise is reached.
VII. PREOPERATIVE INTERVIEW AND NURSING ASSESSMENT (see Chapter 15)
 A. Develop culture sensitivity.
  1. Clarify own culture and value systems.
   a. Reflect on actions, thoughts, communications, and beliefs of own culture.
  2. Examine personal negative opinions of different cultures.
  3. Increase awareness of other cultures through churches and schools.
 B. Do not project own views on patients through verbal and nonverbal communication cues (Box 20-1).
  1. Verbal communication
   a. Voice quality
   b. Intonation
   c. Rhythm
   d. Speed
   e. Pronunciation used
  2. Nonverbal communications
   a. Facial expressions
   b. Gestures
   c. Posture
 C. Observe client's family and support system.

■ TABLE 20-1
■ ■ **Traditional Healers, Preparation, and Area of Practice**

	Healer	Preparation	Practice
African American (southern urban)	Family members, especially grandmother	Word of mouth Practical experience	Secular: Common, everyday self-limiting illness that respond to home remedies Illness prevention
	Wise woman ("old day")	Practical experience of caring for and raising own children, grandchildren, and other kin Develops reputation among family, friends, and neighbors of being knowledgeable about home remedies for common illnesses	Secular: Treatment and prevention of common, everyday illnesses Advice about child care and child rearing
	Herbalist	No formal training	Secular: Diagnose a variety of natural illnesses Dispense herbs to neutralize or eliminate harmful substances that impair the power of body to heal or protect itself
	Spiritualist	No formal training Power may be present at birth (twins) or given by God later in life Usually associated with fundamentalist Christian religion (Holy Ghost, Pentecostal)	Sacred: Cure illnesses sent by God as punishment Cure ailments beyond the power of biomedical practitioners (e.g., arthritis, hypertension, diabetes mellitus) Power of God is present in the body of the spiritualist and transferred to the ill person through laying on of the hands Draws on the faith of the individual Sacred or secular: May combine laying on of the hands with herbal therapy, massage, and life counseling
	Root doctor (root worker, conjure man or woman, voodoo priest or priestess)	Apprenticeship May be born with magical powers	Sacred or secular: Serves as intermediary between supernatural and natural worlds Enact or remove spells Counteract or protect against witchcraft or sorcery Combine magical powers with use of herbs Read omens and signs and prescribe therapy or preventive measures Counseling and magical powers with use of herbs

Continued

■ TABLE 20-1
■ ■ **Traditional Healers, Preparation, and Area of Practice—cont'd**

	Healer	Preparation	Practice
African Caribbean (Haitian)	Family members, primarily female	Word of mouth generation to generation Practical experience	Secular: Prevention and treatment of common, everyday illnesses
	Doctor feuilles, bocars, dokte feuilles (leaf doctors, herbalists)	Apprenticeship training Hands-on experience Learn "formulas" for healing	Secular: Treats patients with herbs, roots, medical plants, and rituals Bone setting, burn treatments, and massage
	Droquistes	Apprenticeship	Secular: Make and sell potions to prevent or treat illnesses of natural causation
	Houngan (voodoo priest) Mambo (voodoo priestess)	Apprenticeship training in rituals Knowledge of prayers and herbal remedies from elders Long training in and study of mythology of spirits	Sacred or secular: Treatment of illnesses due to supernatural causation (angry voodoo spirits; dead ancestors; or magic, witchcraft, or sorcery) Treatment of illnesses that are long lasting or fail to respond to biomedicine
	Sages-femme, fam saj, matrone (lay midwife, wise woman)	Apprenticeship	Secular: Performs deliveries, prepartum and postpartum care, treats other "female" conditions related to reproduction Uses herbs, massage, rituals, baths, and diet
	Piqurestes (injections)	Training in missions and other medical facilities	Secular: Give injections, change dressings
Hispanic (Puerto Rican)	Family member, especially oldest female	Word of mouth Practical experience	Secular: Common, everyday illnesses that respond to home remedies
	Curandero or curandera	Apprenticeship Gift from God	Sacred or secular: Knowledge of herbs, diet, massage, and ritual Commune with supernatural Conduct religious curing ceremonies
	Partera (lay midwife)	Apprenticeship training from older female relatives	Secular: Prepartum and postnatal care, herbal remedies, massage, treatment of natural illness affecting women
	Yerbero (herbalist)	No formal training	Secular: Preventive and curative care Treats both ethnomedical and biomedical illnesses

■ TABLE 20-1
■ ■ **Traditional Healers, Preparation, and Area of Practice—cont'd**

	Healer	Preparation	Practice
	Santiguadore (sabador)	Apprenticeship	Secular: Massage and manipulation of body for illness affecting the musculoskeletal and gastrointestinal systems Treats both ethnomedical and biomedical illnesses
	Spiritualist (espiritualista, brujera, santero)	May be born with gift to fortell future Perfect skills through apprenticeship	Sacred: Prevention and diagnosis of witchcraft, or sorcery; uses amulets, prayers, and other artifacts Some limited curative functions
Moslem (Iranian)	Family members, especially older women	Knowledge handed down generation to generation	Secular: Self-care measures such as bed rest, diet, herbs, home remedies, and childbirth assistance
	Dais (traditional midwife)	Apprenticeship Older women who have raised their own families	Secular: Prepartum and postpartum care Childbirth Newborn care Herbal therapies Massage
	Mullah (religious healer)	Religious training	Sacred: Prevention of illness via preparation of tawiz (amulet with verses from the Koran) Treat illness due to evil spirits Treat emotional problems, nervousness, excessive anxiety, and mental illness
	Injectionists	Self-taught	Secular: Administer medications prescribed by physicians Purchase and prescribe injectable medications on their own
	Hakimji (traditional healer)	Apprenticeship	Sacred or secular: Combine procedures and medicines from Urani and Greco-Arabic medical traditions
	Bonesetters	Apprenticeships	Secular: Sets broken bones Treats sprains, strains, dislocations, and generalized body pains

Continued

■ TABLE 20-1
■ ■ **Traditional Healers, Preparation, and Area of Practice—cont'd**

	Healer	Preparation	Practice
Native American (Navajo Indian)	Family members	Knowledge handed down from generation to generation	Secular: Common, everyday illnesses of natural origin Prevention of illnesses Herbal remedies
	Medicine man	Born with power to heal Acquire power to heal via vision or quest Apprenticeship with medicine man once power to heal is known	Sacred or secular: Diagnosis and treatment of supernatural or natural illness (meditation, trance state, divination, or star gazing) Use combination of herbs and curing ceremonies
	Diagnostician	As per medicine man	Sacred: Diagnose underlying cause of illness via divination
	Herbalists	Knowledge passed down generation to generation Apprenticeship	Secular: Diagnose and treat common illnesses of natural causation

From Luckman J, ed: *Saunders manual of nursing care*, Philadelphia, 1997, WB Saunders.

■ BOX 20-1
■ **VERBAL AND NONVERBAL COMMUNICATION**

Language or Verbal Communication
- Vocabulary
- Grammatical structure
- Voice qualities
- Intonation
- Rhythm
- Speed
- Pronunciation
- Silence

Nonverbal Communication
- Touch
- Facial expression
- Eye movement
- Body posture

Communications That Combine Verbal and Nonverbal Elements
- Warmth
- Humor

From Giger JN, Davidhizar RE: *Transcultural nursing: Assessment and intervention,* ed 4, St Louis, 2004, Mosby.

    D. Respect the patient.
        1. All cultures are unique.
        2. All individuals are unique.
    E. Tips for effective communication
        1. Introduce yourself.
            a. Exhibit confidence; avoid arrogance.
            b. Shake hands if appropriate.
            c. Explain reason for your presence.
            d. Explain upcoming sequence of events (admission assessment, preoperative holding, intraoperative, postoperative).
        2. Avoid assuming where the patient comes from; the patient will tell you if he or she wants you to know.
        3. Show respect, especially to males.
            a. Males are often the decision-makers.
            b. If patient is child or woman, male may be the one making decisions regarding care and follow-up.
        4. In some cultures, it is customary for children to go everywhere with parents.
            a. Poorer families may not have childcare options available to them.
            b. Include children in perioperative experience.
        5. Understand traditional health-related practices.
            a. Do not show disapproval of them.
            b. If practice is potentially harmful, inform patient.
        6. Be cognizant of folk illnesses and remedies for the cultural population in your service area.
        7. When possible, involve leaders of local groups.
            a. Leader may have understanding of problem.
            b. May be able to assist in offering acceptable interventions
            c. Ensure confidentiality is maintained.
        8. Accept diversity as an asset, not a liability.
            a. Listening and verbal interactions need to be made with an appreciation of cultural differences (Box 20-2).
        9. Culturally sensitive interactions
VIII. HEALTH HABITS
    A. Western
        1. Care providers
            a. Physician is most common care provider.
            b. Physician assistants
            c. Nurse practitioners
            d. Chiropractors
            e. Doctors of osteopathy
            f. Doctors of podiatry
        2. Causes for illness
            a. Genetic
        3. Toxins
            a. Cigarettes
            b. Asbestos
            c. Environmental
        4. Dietary
            a. Inappropriate diet
            b. Excessive fat intake
            c. Excessive alcohol intake
        5. Illness is treatable or curable.
        6. Focus on prevention of illness
    B. Non-Western (folk medicine)
        1. Care providers
            a. Indigenous healers
                (1) Surgeons
                (2) Spiritualists
                (3) Herbalists

■ BOX 20-2
■ **GUIDELINES FOR CULTURALLY SENSITIVE INTERACTIONS**

Nonverbal Strategies
- Invite family members to choose where they would like to sit or stand, allowing them to select a comfortable distance.
- Observe interactions with others to determine which body gestures (e.g., shaking hands) are acceptable and appropriate. Ask when in doubt.
- Avoid appearing rushed.
- Be an active listener.
- Observe for cues regarding appropriate eye contact.
- Learn appropriate use of pauses or interruptions for different cultures.
- Ask for clarification if nonverbal meaning is unclear.

Verbal Strategies
- Learn proper terms of address.
- Use a positive tone of voice to convey interest.
- Speak slowly and carefully, not loudly, when families have poor language comprehension.
- Encourage questions.
- Learn basic words and sentences of family's language, if possible.
- Avoid professional terms.
- When asking questions, tell families why the questions are being asked, the way in which the information they provide will be used, and how it might benefit their child.
- Repeat important information more than once.
- Always give the reason or purpose for a treatment or prescription.
- Use information written in family's language.
- Offer the services of an interpreter when necessary.
- Learn from families and representatives of their culture methods of communicating information without creating discomfort.
- Address intergenerational needs (e.g., family's need to consult with others).
- Be sincere, open, and honest and, when appropriate, share personal experiences, beliefs, and practices to establish rapport and trust.

From Wong DL: *Wong's essentials of pediatric nursing*, ed 8, St Louis, 2009, Mosby.

        2. Causes for illness

           a. Evil spirits

           b. Witches

           c. Dysfunction within the harmony of the body

IX. CULTURAL BELIEFS OF ASIANS (CHINESE AMERICANS)

    A. Basis for health culture beliefs and practices is holistic.

        1. Oneness of all things with nature, the universe, and the divine

    B. Health

        1. Results when body works in rhythmic and finely balanced manner

        2. Body adjusts to external environment.

        3. Functions and emotions are in harmony.

    C. Traditional Chinese medicine (TCM)

        1. System of preventive medicine

        2. Components

           a. Tao

               (1) Way of life, virtue, heaven, and death

               (2) Individuals should:

                   (a) Flow with nature.

                   (b) Avoid excesses and extremes.

                   (c) Maintain a middle position.

                   (d) Practice moderation.

           b. Ch'i (vitality)

(1) "Universal energy"
(2) Fundamental concept of entire system of TCM
(3) Origin of all disease
(4) Health is balance of harmony in the flow of ch'i; illness results from imbalance.

  c. Yin and yang

    (1) Represents duality and unity of universe and Tao
    (2) Balance of yin and yang
      (a) The negative and positive energy forces
      (b) Gift from prior generations
      (c) Harmony and balance of physical and spiritual with nature

  d. Law of five elements

    (1) Association between external physical worlds and internal milieu of body
    (2) Includes fire, earth, metal, water, and wood

  e. Meridians and pulses

    (1) Invisible systems or pathways that carry ch'i through the body
    (2) Regulate organs, blood flow, and connect internal and external organs
    (3) Pulses
      (a) Present in each organ
      (b) Pulse indicates status of organ.
        (i) Balance
        (ii) Imbalance
      (c) No difference among pulses indicates perfect balance.

  f. Causative factors of disease

    (1) Internal
      (a) Excess or lack of emotion
      (b) Constitution
      (c) Anxiety
      (d) Irregularity of food and drink
    (2) External
      (a) Cold, heat, humidity, fire, dryness, dampness, and wind
    (3) Illness results from:
      (a) Excess or deficiency of internal or external causative factors
      (b) Interruption in flow of ch'i
      (c) Loss of ch'i
      (d) Imbalance of yin and yang

D. Illness

  1. Prevented by:
    a. Conforming with nature
    b. Wearing of jade charms to prevent harm
  2. Disruption of yin and yang energy forces caused by:
    a. Overexertion
    b. Lying or sitting for prolonged periods
  3. Treatment
    a. Herbs such as ginseng
    b. Acupuncture
    c. Curing methods
      (1) Cold treatments
      (2) Hot treatments (moxibustion—application of heat to skin)

E. Grief handled stoically and internalized

F. Family

  1. Is valued
  2. Act as caregivers
  3. Respect and value elders

G. Language and communication

  1. Official language: Mandarin
  2. Many dialects; not all are understood by other groups

  3. Silence is valued.
  4. Do not verbalize disagreements.
  5. Unacceptable to display affection to opposite sex in public
  6. Excessive eye contact may be interpreted as rude.
 H. Death: viewed as religious experience
 I. Medical conditions linked to Asians
  1. Thalassemia
  2. Lactose intolerance
 J. Medical care provided by healers
 K. Nursing implications
  1. Expect use of multiple sectors; attempt to accommodate alternative therapies.
  2. Patient will use self-care measures; support and encourage patient.
  3. Incorporate family in planning care.
  4. Patient tends to be submissive, quiet, and agreeable.
   a. Ability to maintain harmonious relationship supersedes disagreement.
   b. Impolite to disagree with authority figures
   c. Will say "yes" even when patient does not fully understand to prevent disruption in harmony
   d. Will not openly express pain
   e. Will not ask for assistance
  5. Do not draw large amounts of blood from patient.
   a. Blood contains ch'i.
   b. Vital energy for TCM
  6. Avoid lengthy conversations and questioning of patient.
   a. May confuse patient or convey incompetence
   b. Combine health teaching with interactive techniques and demonstration.
X. CULTURAL BELIEFS OF HISPANICS (PUERTO RICAN AMERICANS)
 A. Basis for health culture beliefs and practices is holistic.
 B. Health
  1. Luck or gift from God
  2. Balance and harmony among mind, body, spirit, and nature
   a. Forces of "hot" and "cold," "wet" and "dry"
  3. Maintain equilibrium through:
   a. Proper balanced diet
   b. Avoiding conflict
   c. Moderate lifestyle
   d. Sharing resources with others
   e. Honoring God
  4. Maintain health by:
   a. Praying to God
   b. Consumption of herbs and spices
   c. Wearing amulets
   d. Keeping religious materials in home
   e. Proper conduct
   f. Proper nutrition
 C. Illness
  1. Caused by God as punishment for misconduct
  2. Cause may be natural or supernatural
  3. Cause determined by:
   a. Previous social behavior
   b. Religious behavior
  4. Spiritism
   a. Supernatural illness
   b. Cause is external force.
   c. Individual is "passive" instrument in treatment.
   d. Failure of patient to respond to biomedical treatment may confirm presence of supernatural cause.

   D. Family
       1. Respect for one another is important.
       2. Plays key role in health care
       3. Strong sense of family, both nuclear and extended
          a. Needs of family supersede needs of individual.
          b. Men are dominant providers; women are homemakers.
          c. Female health consultant is oldest female in family.
   E. Treatment
       1. Medical care provided by healers
       2. Healer (curandero)
          a. Cures hot illness with cold medicine and vice versa
          b. Uses massage and cleanings
          c. May use herbs and spices for prevention and healing
       3. Brujo: uses witchcraft for healing illnesses related to jealousy and envy
   F. Medical conditions linked to Hispanics
       1. Diabetes mellitus
       2. Tuberculosis
   G. Language and communication
       1. Primary language: Spanish
       2. Direct confrontation considered rude and disrespectful
   H. Death
       1. Predominantly Catholic
       2. Believe in heaven and hell
       3. Administration of sacraments of the sick is important.
   I. Nursing implications
       1. Key cultural concepts
          a. Respect
             (1) Treat others and expect to be treated with dignity and respect.
                (a) Professional attire
                (b) Correct tone of voice
                (c) Professional image
                (d) Providing proper explanations for treatments
                (e) Answering all questions completely
                (f) Allowing patient opportunity to express his or her feelings
             (2) Personalismo: treating each patient as an individual
                (a) Establish rapport with patient initially.
                (b) Touch arm, shoulder, or back during interactions.
                (c) Allow patient opportunity to express concerns.
                (d) Take initiative to learn a few words in Spanish.
       2. Expect full physical for any complaint or problem.
       3. Very expressive, dramatic
          a. Cultural norm
       4. Difficult to express degree or location of pain
       5. Prefer Hispanic health care professional
          a. Understand and respect traditional health care beliefs.
XI. CULTURAL BELIEFS OF NATIVE AMERICANS (NAVAJO INDIANS)
   A. Basis of traditional Navajo health culture beliefs and practices is holistic.
       1. Health achieved by living in harmony with universe
       2. Individuals have spiritual and physical dimensions.
       3. Physical dimension
          a. Individuals treat bodies and nature with respect.
       4. Spiritual dimension
          a. Individuals participate in development of own potential through will or volition.
       5. World governed by supernatural powers and holy people
          a. Failure to honor supernatural results in lack of harmony.
          b. Harmony essential for good health

B. Cultural traditions
  1. Emphasize cooperation rather than competitiveness.
  2. Share and give to others.
  3. Continue to develop self throughout lifetime.
  4. Believe nature is more powerful than humans.
  5. Respect elders.
  6. Welfare and security of family more important than individual success
  7. Strive to live in balance with nature.
C. Health
  1. Harmony within self and environment
  2. Ability to survive under difficult circumstances
D. Illness
  1. Caused by disharmony within self and environment
    a. Action of witches
    b. Disturbing physical world
    c. Angering the spirit world
    d. Failure to follow established rituals
    e. Not taking care of self
    f. Failure to observe moderation and balance in all things
    g. Being disrespectful
  2. Do not believe in infection, communicable agents, or physiological processes.
  3. Do not believe in germ theory.
  4. Prevention by rituals
E. Healing
  1. Occurs when ill person becomes one with holy people
  2. Establishes harmony with universe
F. Treatment
  1. Biomedical and ethnomedical systems sought for treatment
  2. Medical care provided by Medicine Man
    a. Healing achieved only through ethnomedicine
    b. Healing cannot be separated from religion and individual spirituality.
    c. Chanting used at traditional healing ceremonies
      (1) Used to diagnose and restore balance
  3. Nature is powerful force.
  4. Medicine, rest, diet, isolation, and sweat baths
  5. Medications made of herbs and plants
  6. For medication to be effective, it must be administered according to proper ceremony.
G. Family
  1. Should be included for nursing care
  2. Strong sense of community and extended family
H. Prevention of illness
  1. Wearing of amulets to ward off illness or witchcraft
  2. Amulets can be bags of herbs, fetishes, or other symbolic objects that are believed to have curative or protective powers.
  3. Blessing occurs at important events.
    a. Enhance good fortune, happiness, and health
I. Medical conditions associated with Native Americans
  1. Lactose intolerance
  2. Tuberculosis
J. Language and communication
  1. Navajo or English
  2. Silence shows respect.
  3. Eye contact avoided

XII. CULTURAL BELIEFS OF AFRICAN AMERICANS
  A. Basis of health culture beliefs and practices is magicoreligious and holistic.
    1. Perceptions about health and illness come from popular, ethnomedical, and biomedical health culture.
    2. Little distinction between science and religion, or body and mind
    3. Good health equates to good fortune.
    4. Illness viewed as misfortune
  B. Health is:
    1. Synonymous with good luck
    2. Harmony with nature
  C. Illness
    1. Causes
      a. Disharmony with nature
      b. Demons
      c. Personal tragedy
    2. Classified as natural and unnatural
    3. Natural illness caused by failure to follow three laws of nature (God's law)
      a. Humans are bound by same laws of nature.
      b. Humans are to know, love, and serve God.
      c. Humans are to love each other.
    4. Unnatural illness caused by God withdrawing divine protection
      a. Makes person vulnerable to evil influences
      b. Devil is in control.
      c. Evil influences not responsive to treatment
    5. Individuals vulnerable to illness
      a. Elderly
      b. Young
      c. Women
      d. Unborn fetus
  D. Treatment
    1. Medical care by healers
    2. Cannot be separated from religious beliefs and practices
    3. Occurs around practice of religious ceremonies
    4. Prevention by:
      a. Proper nutrition
      b. Adequate rest
      c. Taking care of relationship with God, nature, and others
  E. Family
    1. Strong family ties
    2. Extended family assists with health care
  F. Medical conditions linked to African Americans
    1. Sickle cell anemia
    2. Hypertension
XIII. CULTURAL BELIEFS OF HAITIAN AMERICANS (CARIBBEAN)
  A. Basis of health culture beliefs is magicoreligious and holistic.
    1. Believe in healing power of Christian God
    2. Believe in traditional folk religion such as voodoo
      a. Maintaining health and recovery from illness depends on faith.
      b. Power of supernatural works in conjunction with traditional healers and biomedical health care providers.
      c. Usually seek biomedical care after appropriate rituals performed
  B. Health
    1. Ability to carry out activities of daily living
      a. Looks well
      b. Good appetite
      c. Shiny skin

      d. Bright eyes

      e. Good color

      f. Able to move about without pain

  C. Illness

    1. Natural

      a. Dominant illnesses

    2. Supernatural

      a. Rare

      b. Suspected when:

        (1) Child becomes ill or dies.

        (2) Home remedies, biomedicine, or treatments from secular healers do not work.

        (3) Social conflict occurs before symptoms.

        (4) Sudden onset

        (5) Illness becomes life-threatening.

        (6) Other misfortunes occur at same time.

        (7) Occurs after one has good fortune; caused by envy and anger of others

  D. Family

    1. Rely on family, kin, and friends.

    2. Usually use extended family

    3. Health care is home managed by grandmother, mother, or maternal aunt.

    4. Older siblings care for younger siblings.

  E. Nursing implications

    1. Patient may regard questions with suspicion.

      a. Keep questions to a minimum.

      b. Explain reason for questions.

      c. If health care practitioner asks too many questions, may be viewed as lacking competence

    2. Oral medications not so effective as parenteral

    3. View vitamin injections as important for maintaining blood.

    4. Explain reason for all blood tests; very concerned about status of their blood.

    5. Commonly use purgatives with castor oil.

      a. Assess for signs and symptoms of dehydration, especially in children.

    6. Have difficulty expressing location of pain.

      a. Have patient point to area.

      b. Give opportunity for patient to describe pain.

      c. Not accustomed to using pain rating scales to describe intensity.

XIV. CULTURAL BELIEFS OF WHITE AMERICANS OR ANGLO-AMERICANS

  A. Basis of health culture beliefs and practices is scientific.

    1. Incorporate variety of self-care measures and home remedies.

    2. Number of illness episodes brought to health care practitioner is limited.

    3. Faith in God

      a. Assists in protecting from illness

      b. Aids in recovery

      c. Assists in coping with illness

      d. May consider illness as punishment from God

    4. Supernatural causes

      a. Evil eye and curses

  B. Health

    1. Absence of illness

    2. Ability to function in acceptable manner

  C. Illness

    1. Interferes with ability to function in acceptable manner

    2. Experienced when:

      a. Pain occurs.

      b. Changes in bodily feelings or functions occur.

    3. Most illnesses result from natural causes.

    4. Dominant theory is germ theory.

    D. Prevention
        1. Diet and nutrition
        2. Taking vitamins, minerals, and tonics
        3. Exercising
        4. Maintaining normal bowel function
        5. Moderate lifestyle
        6. Adequate sleep and rest
    E. Family
        1. Structure usually nuclear family only
        2. Spouse generally main health consultant
        3. Mother or wife as primary caregiver
            a. Diagnoses of illness when it occurs
    F. Nursing implications
        1. Wide variation among groups
        2. Some groups have difficulty expressing signs and symptoms.
        3. May not openly express pain
XV. ASPECTS OF COMMUNICATION
    A. Factors that can have an effect on communication (Box 20-3)
        1. Although communication is universal, styles and types of feedback may be unique to certain cultural groups.
    B. Communication techniques
        1. Use open-ended questions.
        2. Approach in nonthreatening manner.
        3. Allow time for patient's responses.
        4. Do not hurry through interview.
        5. Use professional interpreters whenever possible; patient may be more willing to give important health history information through stranger than family member (especially information regarding sexual matters).
        6. Avoid use of medical terms.
        7. Use language appropriate to patient's level of understanding.
        8. Use language dictionary appropriate to culture.
        9. Use pictures and gestures.
      10. Speak slowly.
    C. Culture specific—verbal
        1. Chinese Americans
            a. Soft tone
            b. Slow speech with silence at times
            c. Silence valued

■ BOX 20-3
■ **FACTORS INFLUENCING COMMUNICATION**

- Physical health and emotional well-being
- The situation being discussed and its meaning
- Distractions to the communication process
- Knowledge of the matter being discussed
- Skill at communicating
- Attitudes toward the other person and toward the subject being discussed
- Personal needs and interests
- Background, including cultural, social, and philosophical values
- The senses involved and their functional ability
- Personal tendency to make judgments and be judgmental of others
- The environment in which the communication occurs
- Past experiences that relate to the current situation

From Giger JN, Davidhizar RE: *Transcultural nursing: Assessment and intervention*, ed 5, St Louis, 2008, Mosby.

     2. Hispanics
       a. Loud tone
       b. Rapid speech
     3. Native Americans
       a. Soft tone
       b. Slow speech with silence at times
     4. African Americans
       a. Loud tone
       b. Rapid speech
  D. Culture specific—nonverbal
     1. Chinese Americans
       a. Avoid eye contact.
       b. Discomfort expressed privately
       c. Avoid excessive touch.
     2. Hispanics
       a. Maintain eye contact.
       b. Discomfort expressed openly
       c. Tactile culture
     3. Native Americans
       a. Respect indicated by avoiding eye contact
       b. Respect indicated by periods of silence
       c. Discomfort expressed privately
       d. Light touch or hand passing
     4. Orthodox Jews
       a. Eye contact may have sexual connotation.
       b. Older male to female other than wife
       c. Tactile culture
     5. African Americans
       a. Maintain eye contact (avoid prolonged eye contact).
       b. Open display of discomfort

XVI. NUTRITIONAL CONCERNS
  A. Ethnic and religious food preferences
     1. Chinese Americans
       a. Prefer rice with all meals
     2. Native Americans
       a. Usually consists of corn, beans, and squash
     3. African Americans
       a. Prefer salted and spiced foods
       b. High intake of yellow and dark green leafy vegetables
     4. Hispanics
       a. Foods and illness have varying degrees of "hot" and "cold" (not related to temperature of food).
       b. Easier to digest hot foods—chili peppers, onions, garlic
       c. Cold foods include fresh vegetables, corn, beans, squash, tropical fruits.
     5. Jehovah's Witnesses
       a. No food that contains blood as an additive, such as lunch meats
     6. Seventh-Day Adventists
       a. Avoid meat or foods with shells.
       b. Avoid caffeine.
       c. Vegetarian diet encouraged
       d. Protein deficiency may need to be considered.
     7. Jews
       a. Consider pigs unholy or unclean
       b. Pork products not allowed
       c. Cannot mix meat with milk
       d. Kosher products

        8. Muslim
          a. No pork or food products made with pork
          b. No animal fat shortening
  B. Manner of preparation
      1. Identify any cultural preconditions.
  C. Frequency
      1. Identify any cultural requisites.
  D. Nursing implications
      1. Incorporate normal diet into postoperative plan of care.
      2. Consult with nutritionist if areas of concern are identified.

XVII. SPIRITUAL AND RELIGIOUS NEEDS
  A. Practices pertaining to health care
      1. Availability of spiritual resources
      2. Pray before meals
      3. Religious articles made available
  B. Chinese
      1. Taoism
      2. Buddhism
      3. Islam
      4. Christianity
  C. Hispanics
      1. Catholicism
  D. Christian Science
      1. Prayer heals the body.
      2. Children treated by Christian Science practitioners only
  E. Jehovah's Witnesses
      1. Opposed to homologous blood transfusions
      2. May submit to autologous blood transfusions
      3. May refuse surgery if blood transfusion is required
      4. Do not partake in national holidays including Christmas
  F. Seventh-Day Adventists
      1. Belief that their bodies are temples of God
      2. Avoidance of meat, caffeine, drugs, tobacco, and alcohol
      3. May refuse foods with shells (lobster, crab)
  G. Nursing implications
      1. Be cognizant of patient's religious needs.
      2. Patient may request private time before procedure (preoperative holding).

XVIII. PERIOPERATIVE NURSING CONSIDERATIONS
  A. Preoperative teaching
      1. Be alert and sensitive to cultural differences (Box 20-4).
      2. Differences may:
        a. Dictate type of teaching method based on patient's learning style
        b. Show variation in patient's educational needs
        c. Cause variation in patient's response to teaching
        d. Cause variations in patient's discharge plan
  B. Consent
      1. Decision for surgery may be made by head of family or group of elders in a religious community.
      2. Decision-maker and patient must understand importance of surgery.
      3. Ensure consent forms signed appropriately, according to facility policy.
  C. Body hair
      1. Shaving may violate some cultural beliefs and practices.
        a. Sikh religion (East India): forbids shaving of hair
        b. Greece: manhood is linked to body hair.
        c. Native Americans: body hair sign of health and strength

■ BOX 20-4
■ **GUIDELINES FOR RELATING TO PATIENTS FROM DIFFERENT CULTURES**

1. Assess your personal beliefs surrounding persons from different culture.
   a. Review your personal beliefs and past experiences.
   b. Set aside any values, biases, ideas, and attitudes that are judgmental and may negatively affect care.
2. Assess communication variables from a cultural perspective.
   a. Determine the ethnic identity of the patient, including generation in America.
   b. Use the patient as a source of information when possible.
   c. Assess cultural factors that may affect your relationship with the patient and respond appropriately.
3. Plan care based on the communicated needs and cultural background.
   a. Learn as much as possible about the patient's cultural customs and beliefs.
   b. Encourage the patient to reveal cultural interpretation of health, illness, and health care.
   c. Be sensitive to the uniqueness of the patient.
   d. Identify sources of discrepancy between the patient's and your own concepts of health and illness.
   e. Communicate at the patient's personal level of functioning.
   f. Evaluate effectiveness of nursing actions and modify nursing care plan when necessary.
4. Modify communication approaches to meet cultural needs.
   a. Be attentive to signs of fear, anxiety, and confusion in patients.
   b. Respond in a reassuring manner in keeping with the patient's cultural orientation.
   c. Be aware that, in some cultural groups, discussion concerning the patient with others may be offensive and may impede the nursing process.
5. Understand that respect for the patient and communicated needs is central to the therapeutic relationship.
   a. Communicate respect by using a kind and attentive approach.
   b. Learn how listening is communicated in the patient's culture.
   c. Use appropriate active listening techniques.
   d. Adopt an attitude of flexibility, respect, and interest to help bridge barriers imposed by culture.
6. Communicate in a nonthreatening manner.
   a. Conduct the interview in an unhurried manner.
   b. Follow acceptable social and cultural amenities.
   c. Ask general questions during the information-gathering stage.
   d. Be patient with a respondent who gives information that may seem unrelated to the patient's health problem.
   e. Develop a trusting relationship by listening carefully, allowing time, and giving the patient your full attention.
7. Use validating techniques in communication.
   a. Be alert for feedback that the patient is not understanding.
   b. Do not assume meaning is interpreted without distortion.
8. Be considerate of reluctance to talk when the subject involves sexual matters.
   a. Be aware that in some cultures, sexual matters are not discussed freely with members of the opposite sex.
9. Adopt special approaches when the patient speaks a different language.
   a. Use a caring tone of voice and facial expression to help alleviate the patient's fears.
   b. Speak slowly and distinctly, but not loudly.
   c. Use gestures, pictures, and play-acting to help the patient understand.
   d. Repeat the message in different ways if necessary.
   e. Be alert to words the patient seems to understand and use them frequently.
   f. Keep messages simple and repeat them frequently.
   g. Avoid using medical terms and abbreviations that the patient may not understand.
10. Use interpreters to improve communication.
    a. Ask the interpreter to translate the message, not just the individual words.
    b. Obtain feedback to confirm understanding.
    c. Use an interpreter who is culturally sensitive.

From Giger JN, Davidhizar RE: *Transcultural nursing: Assessment and intervention*, ed 4, St Louis, 2004, Mosby.

   D. Removal of jewelry
      1. Some cultures view as religious articles.
      2. Not permitted to be removed from body
         a. If site interferes with surgery, may consent to placement of article on another part of body
         b. May need to be secured (taped) on person before procedure
         c. Document presence of article in nursing record.
   E. Pain
      1. Emphasize that it is acceptable to express pain.
         a. Patient may not verbalize or may continue to deny pain.
         b. Incorporate nonverbal patient reactions into nursing assessment of pain.
         c. Medicate as necessary.
      2. Cultural belief to express stoic attitude toward pain
         a. Patient may refuse pain medication.
      3. Meditation
         a. Used by Eastern religions
         b. Relaxation techniques may be helpful in minimizing postoperative pain.
   F. Postoperative dietary needs
      1. Incorporate cultural food practices into dietary teaching for the postoperative patient.
   G. Geriatric considerations
      1. Nursing approach
         a. Elderly person is unique individual.
         b. Avoid imposing own attitude and belief toward aging on the patient.
XIX. LOSS OF PRIVACY THROUGHOUT PERIOPERATIVE EXPERIENCE
   A. History and physical (Table 20-2)

■ TABLE 20-2
■ ■ **Culturally Sensitive Interview**

Traditional Western Health Care History Model	Interview Example: Blending Explanatory Model and Traditional Model	Culture-Sensitive Listening: Listening for Illness (Cultural Perception) and Disease (Biomedical Perception)
Introduction	Mr. Smith? Hi, I'm J. P., a primary care clinician. I will be working with you today. How would you like to be addressed? or What name would you like me to use?	In every culture, your name has special significance, and the way you are addressed may have great meaning. Never assume that it is acceptable to use the person's first name, or for them to use yours. Age, gender, and cultural norms all play a role in how individuals wish to be addressed.
Chief complaint	What brought you in today? (Ascertain what symptom is of concern.) What is the name of your problem?	Asking a patient to name the problem will give you clues to the patient's beliefs about the origin of the illness.
SYMPTOM ANALYSIS Onset/duration	When did it start? Can you think of anything that brought this on? What do you think caused your problem? Why do you think it started then? How long do you think it will last?	This will provide information about the patient's insight into the problem and may reveal underlying beliefs.
Location	What parts of your body are affected? How does it work in your body?	Actively listen to understand the patient's perception of the condition.

Continued

■ TABLE 20-2
■ ■ **Culturally Sensitive Interview—cont'd**

Traditional Western Health Care History Model	Interview Example: Blending Explanatory Model and Traditional Model	Culture-Sensitive Listening: Listening for Illness (Cultural Perception) and Disease (Biomedical Perception)
Frequency/chronology	How often do you notice it in your body? Have you noticed it before? Are you generally getting better? Worse? About the same? What is it like?	This may add information regarding previous episodes and treatment modalities as well as patient expectations for treatment.
Quality	Is it dangerous?	Show empathy, interest, and respect for the patient's concerns.
Quantity	Will this last a long time? How much of a problem is it?	Encourage the patient to explain.
Aggravating or alleviating factors	Is there anything that makes it better? Makes it worse? (Ask about various common cultural practices.)	This shows interest and gives the patient permission to talk about the illness and his or her conceptualization of the condition.
Associated symptoms	Do you have any other symptoms with this? Is this causing any other problems in your body?	Again, this gives insight into the patient's perceptions.
Treatments tried	Have you talked with anyone else about this? Did they make any suggestions? Have you tried any other medicines or home remedies? Did these help? Are there any special remedies that you have been advised to try or that are recommended by your healers? Who recommended the remedies you have tried?	Knowing, understanding, and accepting culturally determined treatments and respecting those who utilize them often enables you to develop treatment plans that blend traditional healing measures with allopathic health care practices.
Effects on ADLs	What bothers you most about this illness? How has it affected your daily life?	Provides insight into the patient's illness and allows interpretation of the disease effects.
Patient perceptions	What do you think is going on? Is there anything you fear about your illness? What would you like me to do today?	Positions the clinician to better provide a culturally appropriate plan of care.
Conclusion	Is there anything else I should know or that you would like to tell me? What would you like me to do today?	Patients may or may not be able to tell you what they would like you to do. In some cultures, it may be presumptuous to tell a provider what to do or to express an opinion.

ADLs, Activities of daily living.
From Meredith PV, Horan NM: *Adult primary care*, Philadelphia, 2000, WB Saunders.

      1. Use of touch during assessment: respect individual's cultural practice.

      2. Need to remove clothing: respect individual's cultural practice; accommodate patient's requests.

      3. Communication with physician regarding "taboo" topics

        a. Incorporate cultural practices into plan of care if appropriate.

    B. Exposure during perioperative experience

      1. Reinforce confidentiality; respect cultural practices; accommodate patient requests.

      2. Keep personnel to a safe minimum.

      3. Avoid overexposure.

XX. PERSONAL SPACE

    A. Determined by individual cultures

      1. Close personal space

        a. Chinese Americans

        b. Hispanics

        c. Native Americans

        d. African Americans

      2. Distant personal space

        a. Whites

BIBLIOGRAPHY

1. Andrews MM, Boyle JS: *Transcultural concepts in nursing,* ed 5, Baltimore, MD, 2008, Kluwer Lippincott Williams & Wilkins.
2. Campesino M: Commentary: Problematic issues in cultural comparisons. *J Prof Nurs* 18(6):343-345, 2002.
3. Campinha-Bacote J: The process of cultural competence in the delivery of healthcare services: A model of care. *J Transcult Nurs* 13(3):181-184; discussion 200-201, 2002.
4. Chang MK, Harden JT: Meeting the challenge of the new millennium: Caring for culturally diverse patients. *Urol Nurs* 22(6):372-376, 390; quiz 377, 2002.
5. Cioffi RN: Communicating with culturally and linguistically diverse patients in an acute care setting. *Int J Nurs Stud* 40(3):299-306, 2003.
6. Dawood M, James J: Cross-cultural care: What are you afraid of? *Nurs Times* 97(40):24-25, 2001.
7. Geissler EM: *Cultural assessment,* ed 2, St Louis, 1998, Mosby.
8. Giger J, Davidhizar RE: *Transcultural nursing: Assessment and intervention,* ed 5, St Louis, 2008, Mosby.
9. Kearns CJ, Meehan NK, Carr RL, et al: Using cross-cultural definitions of health care. *Nurse Pract* 28(1):61-62, 2003.
10. Krau SD: Working toward cultural competence in the workplace. *SCI Nurs* 19(4):193-194, 2002.
11. Leininger M: Transcultural nursing: The study and practice field. *Imprint* 38(2):55-59, 1991.
12. Leininger M: Founder's focus: Transcultural nursing care makes a big outcome difference. *J Transcult Nurs* 14(2):157, 2003.
13. Luckman J, editor: *Saunders manual of nursing care,* Philadelphia, 1997, WB Saunders.
14. Martsolf DS: Cultural aspects of orthopaedic nursing. *Orthop Nurs* 18(2):65-71, 1999.
15. McEvoy M: Culture and spirituality as an integrated concept in pediatric care. *MCN Am J Matern Child Nurs* 28(1):39-43; quiz 44, 2003.
16. Narayanasamy A: Transcultural nursing: How do nurses respond to cultural needs? *Br J Nurs* 12(3):185-194, 2003.
17. Sharma SB, Smith MK: The importance of cultural assessment. *SCI Nurs* 19(4):177-180, 2002.
18. Stacciarini JM: Experiencing cultural differences: Reflections on cultural diversity. *J Prof Nurs* 18(6):346-349, 2002.
19. Wong DL, Hockenberry-Eaton M, Wilson D, et al: *Wong's essentials of pediatric nursing,* ed 6, St Louis, 2001, Mosby.

CORE COMPETENCIES OF PACU NURSING

21 Fluid, Electrolyte, and Acid-Base Balance

KIM A. NOBLE

OBJECTIVES
At the conclusion of this chapter, the learner will be able to:

1. Identify the three primary fluid compartments of the body and the volume and distribution of fluid in each.

2. Differentiate between the individual forms of crystalloid and colloid solutions and their indications for use.

3. Identify fluid and electrolyte imbalances and the nursing assessment and management for each.

4. Describe the primary mechanisms responsible for the regulation of fluid and electrolyte balance.

5. Identify the physiological origination of acid-base balance in the body and the potential implications of abnormalities in the perianesthetic patient.

6. Describe the components of arterial blood gas (ABG) results specific to acid-base interpretation and their physiological rationale for analysis.

7. Identify common abnormalities in acid-base balance and their application to the perianesthetic population.

I. FLUID AND ELECTROLYTE BALANCE OVERVIEW
  A. Body cells function in a tightly regulated fluid- and electrolyte-filled environment.
    1. Fluid and electrolyte homeostasis
      a. Maintained via hormonal mechanisms
      b. Maintained via neural mechanisms
    2. Alterations in fluid and electrolyte homeostasis impact cellular function.
      a. Change the electrical potential of excitable cells
      b. Lead to intracompartmental fluid shifts
      c. Directly impact organ system function
    3. There is a constant flux or movement of water and solutes between the three primary body fluid compartments.
      a. Extracellular fluid compartment
        (1) Intravascular fluid
        (2) Interstitial fluid
      b. Intracellular compartment
      c. Transcellular compartment
    4. Fluid flux is constrained by:
      a. Compartmental membranes
      b. Solute and plasma protein concentrations
    5. Sodium/potassium (Na^+/K^+) adenosine triphosphatase (ATPase) pump
      a. Active (energy dependent) pump on cell membranes
      b. Functions in the maintenance of solute concentration gradients across the cell membranes
  B. Fluid balance requires both:
    1. Normal volume of water
    2. Normal concentrations of particles in solution (Table 21-1)

■ TABLE 21-1

Primary Electrolytes of the ECF and ICF*

ECF Ion	Normal Serum Value	Indicators	
		Deficit (Hypo-)	Excess (Hyper-)
Sodium (Na⁺) Regulates ECF osmolality and vascular fluid volume ↓ICF content; ↑ECF content maintained by Na⁺/K⁺ ATPase pump	135-145 mEq/L	***Hyponatremia*** <130 mEq/L, ↓serum osmolality Salt diluted by excess retained water Bladder irrigations, electrolyte-free IV infusions, ADH oversecretion (SIADH) ***Outcomes:*** Weak muscles Confusion Nausea/vomiting Hypotension Seizure Coma if <115 mEq/L	***Hypernatremia*** >145 mEq/L, ↑serum osmolality Excess salt from water losses Inadequate osmotic diuresis; poor fluid intake; lack of ADH (DI) ***Outcomes:*** Thirst Flushed skin Hypotension Oliguria Seizures, coma if extreme
Chloride (Cl⁻) Preserve acid-base balance Reciprocal: if Cl⁻ depleted, HCO₃⁻ rises Combines with Na⁺ to maintain osmolality	96-106 mEq/L	***Hypochloremia*** ~<98 mEq/L Prolonged Cl⁻ loss: gastric suction, diuresis ***Metabolic Alkalosis*** Patient hypoventilates	***Hyperchloremia*** ~>108 mEq/L Cl⁻ gain; NSS resuscitation ***Metabolic Acidosis*** Patient hyperventilates
Bicarbonate (HCO₃⁻)	22-28 mEq/L	***Metabolic Alkalosis*** pH >7.45 Acid loss/HCO₃⁻ gain: N/V; ↑GI suction Patient hypoventilates; compensatory ↓K⁺	***Metabolic Acidosis*** pH <7.35 Acid gain/HCO₃⁻ loss: renal failure; DKA Patient hyperventilates; compensatory ↑K⁺

Osmolality (mOsm)	**Dehydration**	**Overhydration**
280-300 Osm/kg	ECF concentrated (DI) ↑ Risk of thrombosis	ECF dilute (SIADH)

Potassium (K+)	*Hypokalemia*	*Hyperkalemia*
3.5-5.0 mEq/L ↓ECF content; ↑ICF content maintained by Na+/K+ ATPase pump Potent effect on cell and neuromuscular irritability Acidosis, catabolism: move K+ to serum Insulin, glucose shift K+ back to cell ↑ Concentration in ECF maintained by Na+/K+ ATPase pump	~ <3.5 mEq/L Reflects ECF loss: diuretics, diarrhea, N/V, digitalis, bowel preps ↓ECF K+ → ↓ICF K+ Muscle weakness Hypoventilation Flaccid paralysis Cardiac arrhythmias: more PVCs, U wave classic, conduction blocks *Slow KCl doses: 10 mEq/h peripheral; 20 mEq/h central line*	~ >5.0 mEq/L ↑ Serum K+: tissue lysis, acidosis (renal or DKA) Malignant hyperthermia: LETHAL Muscle weakness Hypoventilation Paralysis Cardiac arrhythmias: peaked T waves; wide QRS; asystole Stat insulin (glucose), bicarbonate and Ca+ drives K+ back into ICF Dialyze renal patients Stop any K+ intake

Magnesium (Mg+)	*Hypomagnesemia*	*Hypermagnesemia*
1.5-2.5 mEq/L Promotes acetylcholine release at neuromuscular junction Regulates K+ Opposes Ca++	<1.5 mEq/L *Causes:* Diarrhea Mal-absorption Long-term N/V ↑ Aldosterone *Signs:* Neuromuscular irritability, seizures Cardiac: long PR, wide QRS, flat T, torsades risk Affects serum K+, Ca++, and PO_4^-	>2.5 mEq/L *Causes:* $MgSO_4$ infusion (eclampsia) Ketoacidosis Chronic renal failure *Signs:* CNS depression, sedation, muscle weakness, ↓ reflexes ↓BP, ↓heart rate If Mg+ >12 → ↓RR

*Electrolytes found in high concentration in ECF are in low concentration in ICF; similarly, the primary electrolytes of the ICF are present, but in low concentrations, in the ECF. *ADH*, Antidiuretic hormone; *ATPase*, adenosine triphosphatase; *BP*, blood pressure; *CNS*, central nervous system; *DI*, diabetes insipidus; *DKA*, diabetic ketoacidosis; *ECF*, extracellular fluid; *ECG*, electrocardiogram; *GI*, gastrointestinal; *ICF*, intracellular fluid; *NSS*, normal saline solution; *N/V*, nausea/vomiting; *PTH*, parathyroid hormone; *PVCs*, premature ventricular contractions; *RR*, respiratory rate; *SIADH*, syndrome of inappropriate secretion of ADH.

Continued

■ TABLE 21-1
■ Primary Electrolytes of the ECF and ICF*—cont'd

ECF Ion	Normal Serum Value	Indicators	
		Deficit (Hypo-)	Excess (Hyper-)
Phosphate (PO_4^-) Most stored in bone Essential for energy and acid-base balance Inverse relationship with calcium: if PO_4^-↑, Ca^{++}↓ Need parathyroid hormone (PTH) to excrete	1-2 mEq/L (3-4.5 mg/dL)	*Hypophosphatemia* <1.5 mg/dL *Causes:* Aspirin overdose Ketoacidosis Steroids Malabsorption *Outcome:* ↑Ca^{++} Energy depletion: weak muscle, seizures, cardio-respiratory failure	*Hyperphosphatemia* >4.5 mg/dL *Causes:* Laxative excess Supplement in diet Trauma *Outcome:* Cell death, renal failure, PTH decreases
Calcium (Ca^{++}) Critical for impulse conduction, contraction, and coagulation Is stored in bone Present in blood (ECF): ionized (50%), protein bound Inverse relationship with PO_4^-: when Ca^{++}↑, PO_4^-↓	4.5-5.3 mEq/L (8.5-10.5 mg/dL)	*Hypocalcemia* <4.5-5.3 mEq/L *Causes:* Low albumin Renal failure (chronic) Hypoparathyroidism **Signs and symptoms:** Tingling/weakness Twitching/tetany Low BP ECG change Postoperative laryngospasm	*Hypercalcemia* >4.5 mEq/L *Causes:* Immobility Malignancy Low PO_4^- Hyperparathyroidism *Signs and symptoms:* Lethargy Short QT

II. BODY FLUID DISTRIBUTION
- **A.** Body water accounts for:
    - **1.** Approximately 60% of adult total body weight
    - **2.** As much as 75% to 77% of infant total body weight
    - **3.** Average male (154 lb or 70 kg) has 42 L of total body water.
        - **a.** Extracellular fluid (ECF) accounts for approximately 14 L of fluid.
            - (1) Intravascular fluid: accounts for approximately one third of total ECF
            - (2) Interstitial fluid: accounts for approximately two thirds of total ECF
        - **b.** Intracellular fluid (ICF) accounts for approximately 28 L of fluid.
    - **4.** Percentage of water varies with percentage of body fat.
        - **a.** Muscle: high water content
        - **b.** Fat: low water content
        - **c.** Female body contains a higher proportion of fat than male.
- **B.** Body fluid compartments
    - **1.** ECF compartment: accounts for one third of total body water.
        - **a.** Fluid circulating outside of cells
        - **b.** Volume: 33% to 40% of adult's total body weight, nearly 75% of a young child's body weight
        - **c.** Three subcomponents of ECF
            - (1) Intravascular fluid: fluid within the vascular system
                - (a) Crucial for cardiovascular function
                - (b) Accounts for one third of ECF volume or 8% of total body water
            - (2) Interstitial fluid: fluid between the cells
                - (a) Returns to circulation via lymphatics
                - (b) Controlled by capillary cell wall integrity, oncotic and hydrostatic pressures
                - (c) About two thirds of ECF volume (20% of adult total body water
            - (3) Transcellular fluid
                - (a) Includes:
                    - (i) Synovial
                    - (ii) Cerebrospinal
                    - (iii) Intestinal, hepatic
                    - (iv) Biliary
                    - (v) Pancreatic
                    - (vi) Sweat
                    - (vii) Pleural
                    - (viii) Pericardial
                    - (ix) Peritoneal
                    - (x) Intraocular fluids
                - (b) Accounts for about 1% of adult total body weight
        - **d.** Anesthetic medications dilate vasculature and expand ECF capacity.
            - (1) Ease fluid overload and improve diastolic filling in the heart.
            - (2) If ECF volume insufficient, significant hypotension results.
    - **2.** ICF compartment: accounts for two thirds of total body water
        - **a.** Volume accounts for 66% to 75% of total body water.
        - **b.** Fluid found within cells
- **C.** Three processes that govern water movement
    - **1.** Osmosis
        - **a.** The movement of water from a dilute space with few particles across a semipermeable membrane to a more densely concentrated space; "salt sucks"
        - **b.** Osmosis seeks to establish equilibrium between ECF and ICF.
        - **c.** The unequal numbers and size of particles controls fluid movement between ECF and ICF.

(1) Glucose, urea, and protein are large molecules that normally cannot pass from blood (ECF) through selectively permeable cell walls.

(2) Because of large particles in the blood, ECF contains more particles, and is therefore more concentrated, than in cells (ICF).

(3) Water shift is constant.

    (a) Net movement of water is towards the ECF.

    (b) Prevents cells from becoming:

        (i)   Waterlogged

        (ii) Edematous

        (iii) Bursting

  d. Factors influencing osmosis or the movement of water

    (1) Cell wall permeability (integrity)

    (2) Serum sodium levels

    (3) Na^+/K^+ ATPase pump

        (a) Active pump found on cell membranes

        (b) Functions in the maintenance of intracellular to extracellular ion concentration gradients

2. Oncotic pressure

  a. Also called colloid osmotic pressure

  b. Colloids are large particles, such as protein, that normally cannot cross cell membrane.

  c. Plasma colloid osmotic pressure: primarily contained in serum and pulls fluid from interstitial space into capillaries across a pressure gradient

3. Hydrostatic pressure

  a. Pump pressure exerted by blood against blood vessel (capillary) walls

    (1) Elevated capillary hydrostatic pressure with rise in arterial pressure or vessel resistance

    (2) Low capillary resistance or low arterial pressure reduces capillary hydrostatic pressure.

  b. Principal force causing capillary filtration, or the movement of fluid out of the capillary into the interstitial space

  c. Greater at arterial end of the capillary (32 mm Hg) than venous (15 mm Hg)

  d. Opposes oncotic or osmotic pressure

III. PHYSIOLOGICAL PARTICLE (SOLUTE) DISTRIBUTION

  A. Components (solute) distributed within body water

    1. Electrolytes: electrically active ions with either a positive or negative charge when dissolved in solution (Box 21-1). NOTE: A measure of the serum (ECF) concentration of an electrolyte does not necessarily reflect the electrolyte content of intracellular electrolytes (ICF).

      a. Primary extracellular (ECF) electrolytes

        (1) Cation: positively charged ion

          (a) Sodium (Na^+)

            (i)   Reflects serum osmolality

            (ii) Regulates fluid balance

            (iii) The cation in highest concentration in the ECF

          (b) Expect fluid imbalance if serum sodium increased or decreased.

          (c) Inverse relationship with serum potassium

            (i)   If Na^+ rises, expect low K^+.

          (d) Na^+ concentration gradient (ICF: ECF) maintained by the activity of the Na^+/K^+ ATPase pump

        (2) Anion: negatively charged ion

          (a) Chloride (Cl^-) competes with bicarbonate (HCO_3^-) to combine with sodium.

          (b) Bicarbonate: immediately available acid-base buffer

      b. Primary ICF electrolytes: cannot directly measure; reflected by ECF values. NOTE: Status of ICF electrolytes is not necessarily reflected by a laboratory measure of an electrolyte in the serum (ECF).

■ BOX 21-1
■ **TONICITY OF REPLACEMENT IV SOLUTIONS**

Normal Serum Osmolarity: 290 mOsm/L
Tonicity
Hypotonic: Osmolality <240 mOsm/L
ECF concentration < ICF
Causes water to move from serum into cells
Isotonic: Osmolality 240-340 mOsm/L
Concentration of dissolved particles in ECF = ICF
Hypertonic: Osmolality >340 mOsm/L
ECF concentration > ICF
Causes water to move from cell to serum

IV Solution Tonicity
Half normal saline (0.45 NS): 154 mOsm/L
5% dextrose in water (D_5W): 252 mOsm/L
2.5% dextrose in one-half NS ($D_{2.5}$ 0.45NS): 265 mOsm/L
Lactated Ringer's (LR): 5% dextrose in one-half normal saline: 310 mOsm/L
0.9 normal saline (NS): 308 mOsm/L
5% dextrose in one-fourth NS (D_5 0.225 NS): 326 mOsm/L
5% dextrose in one-half NS (D_5 0.45 NS): 406 mOsm/L
10% dextrose in water ($D_{10}W$): 505 mOsm
5% dextrose in LR (D_5LR): 524 mOsm/L
5% dextrose in NS (D_5 0.9 NS): 560 mOsm/L

ECF, Extracellular fluid; *ICF,* intracellular fluid.

    (1) Cations: positively charged ions, critical for cardiac function
       (a) Potassium (K^+): poorly stored, deficits occur quickly with loss or reduced intake; cation in highest concentration in ICF
       (b) Magnesium (Mg^+)
       (c) Calcium (Ca^{++}); stored in ICF; released for cellular activity
       (d) Replace all cations slowly.
          (i)   Always in diluted solution
          (ii) Never intravenous (IV) push
    (2) Anions: negatively charged ions
       (a) Phosphorus (P), present in body fluid as phosphate (PO_4)
  2. Nonelectrolyte particles, undissolved
    a. Large, osmotically active molecules
    b. Influence movement of water across permeable cell membranes
    c. Examples
       (1) Sugar
       (2) Urea
       (3) Protein
  3. Buffers: physiological controls to regulate acids and bases
    a. Bicarbonate: immediate chemical buffer
       (1) Present in ECF
       (2) Regulate (buffer) pH by accepting or releasing acidic hydrogen ions (H^+).
       (3) Maintain serum's chemical neutrality, specifically pH - 7.4: a mathematic representation of hydrogen ion in ECF.
       (4) Maintain bicarbonate-to–carbonic acid ratio of 20:1.
    b. Phosphate, hemoglobin, and protein: chemical buffers
       (1) Present in all body fluids to help maintain acid-base balance and coagulation
       (2) Proteins create colloid osmotic pressure to regulate fluid distribution.

      (a) Low-protein conditions include:
         (i)   Hemorrhage (red blood cell loss)
         (ii)   Malnutrition
         (iii) Severe infections
         (iv) Fistulas
         (v) Fluid imbalances
      (b) Low-protein conditions allow fluid to leak from vascular space (ECF) to ICF because of loss of oncotic pressure.
      (c) Need serum albumin level greater than 4 g/dL for adequate protein level
   4. Salts: potassium chloride (KCl) is one example.
B. Osmolality is a measure of the amount of solute per volume of solution.
   1. An index of the body's hydration status
   2. Normal value: 280 to 294 milliosmoles (mOsm)/kg
   3. Total number of "osmotically active" particles in solution
      a. Determined by total of electrolyte and nonelectrolyte particles
      b. Creates osmotic pressure per liter of solution to maintain water in appropriate compartment
      c. Serum sodium is the most important determinant.
         (1) Water follows sodium to equalize concentration and establish equilibrium; "salt sucks."
         (2) When serum sodium elevated, water shifts into serum (ECF) by osmosis, diluting sodium and normalizing osmolality.
         (3) When serum sodium low, water shifts from serum by osmosis to concentrate sodium and normalize osmolality.
   4. Serum osmolality monitored by the hypothalamus
      a. Increased osmolarity (increased Na^+; decreased water) causes thirst and the negative feedback release of antidiuretic hormone (ADH).
         (1) ADH causes the kidney to:
            (a) Reabsorb water from the distal tubule
            (b) Expand the water in the ECF
            (c) Normalize the osmolarity
         (2) The normal osmolarity leads to the negative feedback (decreased) release of ADH.
      b. Decreased osmolarity (decreased Na^+; increased water) decreases the release of ADH.
         (1) As ADH secretion decreases:
            (a) The water reabsorbed from the distal tubule decreases, causing an increased urinary output.
            (b) This leads to decreased water in the ECF and normalizes the osmolarity.
   5. Osmolality, in the form of volume or pressure, is also sensed by baroreceptors in the right atrium, leading to the release of atrial natriuretic peptide (ANP).
      a. Osmolality high
         (1) Low volume and pressure
         (2) ECF-concentrated (hypertonic) patient is dehydrated.
      b. Osmolality low
         (1) High volume and pressure
         (2) ECF-dilute (hypotonic) patient is overhydrated.
      c. Primarily adjusted by titrating the release of ADH
C. Mechanisms of solute transport
   1. Passive or non–energy-expending transport
      a. Diffusion: results in the movement of particles in solution across a selectively permeable cell membrane "down" the concentration gradient, or from an area of high solute concentration to an area of lower solute concentration

(1) Purpose: try to equalize concentration of particles between compartments
(2) Electrolytes are small; pass easily across cell walls
(3) Larger particles inhibited from crossing selectively permeable membrane
(4) Although individual ions move constantly, passively, and randomly between ECF and ICF mostly towards the dilute solution
(5) Particle concentration dissolved in ECF or ICF determines water movement (osmosis) and fluid balance.
(6) Solute concentration difference between areas is a concentration gradient.
  b. Facilitated diffusion: a substance (for example, insulin) facilitates the diffusion of particles (e.g., glucose) across the semipermeable membrane.
  c. Filtration: transfer of water and dissolved substances through the semipermeable gradient via a pressure gradient from higher to lower pressure (hydrostatic pressure).
(1) Pressure created by the weight of the solute-laden solution
(2) Glomerular filtration in kidney's nephron is an example
    (a) Arterial blood pressure is greater than intrarenal pressure.
    (b) This pressure gradient forces blood into the glomerulus for filtration.
(3) A force opposing oncotic pressure
  d. Osmotic pressure: pressure exerted within a compartment by osmotically active particles in solution
(1) Differences in particle concentration between two compartments create a concentration gradient.
(2) Pressure across this gradient moves (redirects) water across the gradient to equalize water between cells or fluid compartments.
(3) After water equilibrates:
    (a) Concentrations of particles in solution equalize.
    (b) Volume of water in the compartments may not be equal.
(4) Opposes interstitial fluid pressure
2. Active or energy-dependent solute transportation; primarily through the action of the Na^+/K^+ ATPase pump
  a. Metabolic energy in the form of adenosine triphosphate (ATP) is consumed to move substances against their concentration gradient(s) through semipermeable cell membranes.
  b. Oxygen also required
(1) During cellular processes, Na^+ diffuses down concentration gradient, through cell wall and into ICF; K^+ moves passively in opposite fashion out of the cell.
(2) Na^+/K^+ ATPase (active, energy-dependent pump) returns Na^+ (against concentration gradient; uphill) to ECF and K^+ (uphill) to ICF.

IV. HORMONAL REGULATORS OF BLOOD VOLUME
  A. ADH: adjusts serum osmolality, concentrates electrolytes
    1. Regulates reabsorption or elimination of water, but not Na^+, in the distal renal tubules, thereby concentrating or diluting Na^+
    2. Released by the pituitary's posterior (hypophysis) in response to a 1% to 2% increase or decrease in serum osmolality, as sensed by osmoreceptors in hypothalamus
    3. Increased ADH secretion: response to increased serum osmolality
      a. Prompts water reabsorption at kidney's collecting ducts: urine concentrates and output decreases.
(1) Normal urine specific gravity: 1.010-1.025
(2) Specific gravity increases: more concentrated with dissolved solutes

      b. Secretion stimulated by stress such as:
- (1) Pain
- (2) Trauma
- (3) Surgery
- (4) Hypovolemia
- (5) Opioids
- (6) Hypoxia
- (7) Hypercapnia

  4. Decreased ADH secretion: response to decreased serum osmolality
      a. Promotes water elimination through collecting ducts
- (1) Urine dilutes.
- (2) Output increases.

      b. Secretion halted by:
- (1) Mechanical ventilation
- (2) Pulmonary disease, such as pneumonia
- (3) Central nervous system pathology, such as:
  - (a) Cranial trauma
  - (b) Tumors
  - (c) Surgery
  - (d) Infection

      c. Diabetes insipidus may follow pituitary hypophysectomy
- (1) Observe for dilute, unconcentrated urine (may be up to 1000 mL/h).
- (2) Thirst
- (3) Dehydration

      d. Urine specific gravity decreases: fewer solutes dissolved in urine

B. Renin-angiotensin-aldosterone: regulates circulating blood volume and peripheral vascular resistance to sustain blood pressure (Figure 21-1)

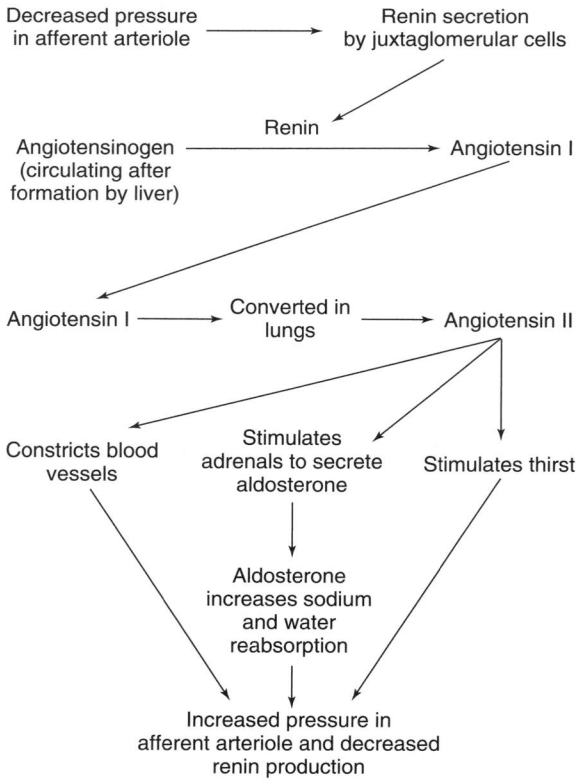

FIGURE 21-1 ■ The renin-angiotensin-aldosterone system. (From Dennison RD: *Pass CCRN!* ed 3, St Louis, 2007, Mosby.)

1. Secretion via feedback mechanism to the renal nephron's distal tubule; senses blood flow changes (pressure or flow) at the glomerulus impacting glomerular filtration rate (GFR).
2. Renin, an enzyme, is released by the juxtaglomerular apparatus in the distal tubule of the nephron to raise blood pressure and GFR. Renin converts the plasma protein angiotensinogen to angiotensin I, an inactive substance.
3. Angiotensin I circulates in the plasma and is converted to angiotensin II primarily in the lung by angiotensin-converting enzyme.
4. Angiotensin II has two effects:
    a. Vasoconstriction from contraction of arterial vascular smooth muscle
    b. Release of aldosterone from the adrenal cortex, leading to increased Na^+ reabsorption by the distal tubule
    c. Renin release increases pressure in the glomerulus by increasing peripheral vascular resistance, and increases volume through the action of aldosterone. This increased pressure and flow then decrease the release of renin (negative feedback).
C. Aldosterone
    1. Primary mineralocorticoid hormone of adrenal cortex
    2. Acts at the kidney's distal renal tubule
    3. Actively increases total body water by:
        a. Regulating sodium reabsorption in response to:
            (1) Serum osmolality
            (2) Serum K^+
            (3) Renin secretion
    4. Renal tubule excretes K^+ or H^+ into the urine in exchange for Na^+.
    5. Water migrates with Na^+.
        a. Water is retained.
        b. Vascular volume increases.
    6. Aldosterone regulation does not alter ECF sodium concentration.
        a. Regulates only about 2% of total body sodium
        b. Sufficiently prevents hypovolemia and hypotension
    7. Decrease in aldosterone secretion leads to:
        a. Excretion of Na^+ and water
        b. Retention of K^+
D. Atrial natriuretic peptide
    1. Secreted by cardiac atrium when stretched by increased venous return (preload)
    2. Leads to the excretion of Na^+, followed by water excretion
V. FLUID AND ELECTROLYTE-RELATED PERIANESTHESIA ISSUES
A. Clinical status alters fluid status.
    1. Cell function requires an exquisite yet dynamic fluid and solute balance.
    2. Normal required daily fluid intake is approximately 2 L.
        a. Altered normal fluid requirements by:
            (1) Stress
            (2) Food and fluid restrictions
            (3) Preexisting chronic conditions
            (4) Acute illness
            (5) Trauma
            (6) Surgically induced losses
            (7) Medications
        b. Extent of preoperative dehydration undervalued for patients with limited fluid reserves.
            (1) Healthy ambulatory surgery patient is mildly dehydrated (by 5%), because of nothing by mouth (NPO) restrictions.
            (2) Children can become significantly:
                (a) Dehydrated
                (b) Hypoglycemic

        (3) Percentage of body water decreases with age
           (a) Muscle decreases
           (b) Fat increases
           (c) Kidneys less able to conserve fluid (concentrate) and regulate Na^+
        (4) Percentage of body water less in obese patients: fat contains little water.
        (5) Malnutrition alters protein intake and use, altering oncotic pressure and water balance.
        (6) Preanesthesia NPO rules relaxed: clear liquids permitted 2 to 4 hours preprocedure
    3. Preoperative deficit, surgical blood loss replaced with an isotonic crystalloid solution
      a. Consider fluid spacing when managing fluid infusions.
        (1) First spacing: normal distribution of body fluids (⅓ ECF; ⅔ ICF).
        (2) Second spacing: excess accumulation of interstitial fluid with edema, with puffy:
           (a) Eyelids
           (b) Fingers
           (c) Ankles
        (3) Third spacing: fluid migration from vascular space (ECF) to areas normally with minimal or no fluid; also known as the transcellular spaces
           (a) Examples: ascites, or bowel after peritonitis, injury, or surgery
           (b) Depletes vascular circulation: hypovolemia, ongoing hypotension
B. Before day of surgery, determine stable biochemical status, organ function.
    1. Clinically relevant laboratory tests are within normal limits.
      a. Selectively assess preoperative laboratory values only when warranted by a patient's:
        (1) Health needs
        (2) Medications
        (3) Coexisting disease
        (4) Medical history
        (5) Age
        (6) Physical examination (Table 21-2)
        (7) If no new clinical events:
           (a) Lab results acceptable for 3 to 6 weeks; or as per institution policy
        (8) Preoperative renal assessment with blood urea nitrogen and creatinine:
           (a) Indicated if elderly
           (b) Systemic disease
           (c) Uses nephrotoxic medications as per policy
        (9) Verify stable fluid status, update specific tests (K^+, glucose) on the day of surgery if indicated.
      b. For ambulatory surgery, no extensive physiological fluid or electrolyte shifts
        (1) No increased risk of perianesthetic crisis is foreseen.
        (2) Aged, American Society of Anesthesiologists classification III and IV patients increasingly accepted or as per policy or physician order
        (3) Anticipated need for blood transfusion is a debatable issue.
           (a) Some surgeons transfuse autologous blood after liposuction.
           (b) Large blood loss often results in unplanned hospital admission.
        (4) For preterm infants younger than 60 weeks, hematocrit less than 30% increases risk of apnea.
      c. "Routine" laboratory tests: need versus cost in ambulatory surgery

■ TABLE 21-2
■ ■ **Clinical Indicators for Preanesthetic Laboratory Assessment**

Obtain Preoperative Test	To Assess
POTASSIUM* IF	
Potassium-depleting diuretics; digoxin, especially with toxicity; corticosteroids; preoperative colon preparation, or laxative; acid-base disorders: alkalosis	*Hypokalemia:* lethal cardiac tachydysrhythmia
Chronic renal failure; acid-base disorders: acidosis; MVA or crushing injuries; acute tubular necrosis	*Hyperkalemia:* lethal cardiac bradydysrhythmia; muscle weakness, including respiratory; metabolic dysfunction
ELECTROLYTE PANEL AND CHEMISTRIES IF	
Renal failure or renal insufficiency; diabetes; cardiopulmonary disease; chemotherapy	*Hyperkalemia:* acidosis; BUN and creatinine increases; dilutional hyponatremia
GLUCOSE* IF	
Metabolic syndrome, insulin resistance; diabetes mellitus (type 1 or type 2)	Baseline preoperative blood sugar; day of admission preoperative blood sugar (type 1) or elevation; monitor intraoperatively (type 1); postoperative blood sugar
Chronic corticosteroid use	Possible hyperglycemia, need for insulin; baseline preoperative blood sugar as indicated
HEMOGLOBIN, HEMATOCRIT	
Infants younger than 1 year	Normal physiological anemia
Anticoagulants	Unrecognized bleeding potential and determine baseline status
Malignancy, radiation/chemotherapy, use of nonsteroidal anti-inflammatories	Suppressed bone marrow function; potential for decreased red blood cell count, white blood cell count, and platelets, mild anemia
COAGULATION: PT/PTT/INR/PLATELETS	
Chronic anticoagulation	Great risk of excessive or prolonged bleeding
Warfarin stopped at least 3-7 days preoperatively	Increased bleeding risk for spinal/epidural anesthetic; risk of operative bleeding and puncture sites. Verify return to normal with PT/INR parameters.
Chronic aspirin	Altered platelet function for the life of the platelet
Anti-inflammatory drugs (NSAIDs)	Potential for prolonged postsurgical bleeding

*Some recommend potassium and glucose values be updated on day of surgery.
BUN, Blood urea nitrogen; *INR,* international normalized ratio; *MVA,* motor vehicle accident; *NSAIDs,* nonsteroidal anti-inflammatory drugs; *PT,* prothrombin time; *PTT,* partial thromboplastin time.

> (1) A controversial, well-scrutinized issue
> (2) No lab measures truly required for healthy, asymptomatic patients for either ambulatory or inpatient surgery
> (3) A battery of "routine" laboratory tests costly, frequently medically unnecessary
> (4) Studies demonstrate even new abnormal lab findings in asymptomatic patients rarely cause surgery to be canceled.
> (5) False-positive abnormal results in healthy, asymptomatic patients create undue concern, increase costs, and/or cause surgical delays.
> C. Postanesthetic hydration and chemical concerns
> > 1. Postoperative nausea and vomiting (PONV). (See Chapter 25 for ASPAN's PONV/PDNV guideline for patient risk stratification and treatment recommendations.)
> > > a. Increases potential for hypovolemia
> > > b. Significantly delays discharge to home and increases cost of care

     c. Infants, children, and elderly patients dehydrate easily.

     d. Unrelenting, protracted vomiting can result in clinically significant chemical imbalances and hospital readmission.

     e. Highly associated with laparoscopy, strabismus correction, and ear surgery

  2. Replace preoperative deficit and surgical blood loss with an isotonic crystalloid solution and colloids as required.

  3. In perianesthesia care unit (PACU), measure and replace postoperative electrolytes, magnesium, calcium, particularly when intraoperative blood loss is high, fluid and colloid replacement is large (see Box 21-1).

VI. FLUID IMBALANCES (Box 21-2)

  A. Fluid spacing may be:

    1. Localized: migration to single area or organ, as with a sprained ankle or blister

    2. Multisystem: postoperative migration to abdominal spaces after organ removal, repair of obstructions, or fluid leakage from sites of severe burns: third spacing

    3. Caused by:

     a. Decreased plasma proteins: insufficient to maintain oncotic osmotic pressures and ECF fluid volumes—renal protein losses

     b. Increased capillary permeability: alteration from sepsis, allergic reaction, radiation, and trauma allows fluid leakage.

     c. Lymphatic blockage: lymph system is an accessory route to return excess interstitial fluid and leaked proteins into vascular space.

    4. Related to anesthetic issues

     a. Anesthetic depth and medications, sepsis, or fever can mask fluid volume excess or deficit until the postoperative period.

     b. Rewarming after intraoperative hypothermia may cause peripheral vasodilation, thereby expanding the vascular compartment (ECF); transient but significant hypotension results, requiring fluid volume expansion.

     c. Spinal and epidural anesthetic techniques expand the ECF by blocking sympathetic tone and dilating peripheral vasculature.

      (1) Vasopressors and fluid volume expansion are needed until anesthetic effects have resolved and normal vessel tone has returned, often in phase I PACU.

      (2) Excess interstitial fluid and leaked proteins can flow back into vascular space.

    5. Surgical shifts: third-space fluid loss

     a. Shifts begin immediately after massive trauma or surgery.

      (1) Capillary permeability increases.

       (a) Protein leaks from cell into inflamed or traumatized areas.

       (b) Fluid shifts through leaky cell walls from vascular to interstitial space.

      (2) Ongoing hypotension common

■ BOX 21-2
■ **REGULATORS OF FLUID AND ELECTROLYTE EQUILIBRIUM**

Diffusion: Movement of particles such as potassium or calcium through a cell's permeable wall from an area of high concentration to a lower concentration.

Osmosis: Movement of water from a dilute solution toward a more concentrated fluid.

Concentration gradient: Difference in concentration (osmolality) between two solutions that causes fluid or electrolyte movement.

Osmotic pressure: A physical force, determined by the number (or concentration) of particles in a solution, causing the movement of fluid (osmosis) toward the concentrated solution.

Oncotic pressure: Osmotic force produced in vascular spaces by molecules such as plasma proteins.

Antidiuretic hormone (ADH): Hypothalamic hormone released by the posterior pituitary gland in response to increased serum osmolality; ADH regulates sodium concentration and thereby the passive movement of water with sodium.

      b. Reabsorption phase: within 72 hours after injury or trauma
         (1) Injured tissues heal.
            (a) Capillaries repair; normal permeability restored
            (b) Lymph blockage clears.
            (c) Plasma proteins return to normal.
            (d) Capillary pressures, filtration, reabsorption restored
         (2) Fluid volume returns (shifts) to vascular compartment.
            (a) Urine volume increases as excess fluid excreted
            (b) Low urine specific gravity
            (c) Fluid output exceeds intake.
            (d) Water weight loss
         (3) Monitor electrolyte homeostasis (see Box 21-1).
  B. ECF volume deficit (hypovolemia): ECF shift to ICF, or total loss from body
    1. Caused by:
      a. Abrupt decrease in fluid intake such as NPO status
      b. Acute loss: blood loss (hemorrhage), fluid shifts caused by altered capillary membrane permeability, diuretics, excess fistula drainage, burns, vomiting, diarrhea
      c. Bowel preparation with large fluid losses through the gastrointestinal (GI) tract
      d. Third spacing
    2. Assess and monitor:
      a. Dehydration and hemoconcentration
         (1) Increased serum osmolality and sodium: thirst
         (2) Impaired renal perfusion: oliguria (<15 mL/h)
            (a) Low-volume concentrated urine, high specific gravity
            (b) Acute tubular necrosis and renal failure if protracted
         (3) Poor skin turgor: dry skin and mucous membranes
         (4) Decreased cardiac output
            (a) Hypotension and tachycardia
            (b) Decreased central venous pressure (CVP), pulmonary artery pressure
         (5) Clear lung fields
         (6) Inadequate cerebral perfusion: confusion, lethargy
    3. Intervene and evaluate (Tables 21-3 and 21-4)
      a. Generous fluid replacement with isotonic solutions and/or colloid
      b. Treat underlying cause
         (1) Blood losses: return to operating room to reexplore, cauterize bleeding vessels, or repair anastomoses.
         (2) Replace large urine losses hourly, caused by diabetes insipidus, for example, and monitor electrolytes.
         (3) Replace large fluid and electrolyte losses via surgical wound drains, nasogastric tube, vomiting, and diarrhea hourly.
  C. ECF volume excess (hypervolemia): shift from ICF to ECF (serum) or second spacing
    1. Caused by:
      a. Fluid intake, either oral or parenteral, beyond physiological tolerance
         (1) Renal failure: inability to excrete fluid
         (2) Congestive heart failure: circulatory overload
         (3) Remobilization of third-space fluid 48 to 72 hours postoperatively
      b. Excess Na^+ intake
         (1) Intravenous Na^+
         (2) Hyperaldosteronism: Na^+ retention
         (3) Seawater ingestion
      c. Sodium hemodilution: relative fluid excess
         (1) Intraoperative absorption of fluid through vascular "beds" during transurethral resection of prostate (TURP):

■ TABLE 21-3
■ ■ **Symptoms Associated with Chemical and Fluid Imbalances**

Symptom	Possible Clinical Significance
CARDIOVASCULAR	
Bounding pulse, neck vein distention	Fluid overload, increased ECF
Weak or thready pulse	Dehydration, decreased ECF volume
Increased heart rate	May reflect fever, acidosis, or ECF volume deficit
Irregular pulse	Cardiac dysrhythmia—may signal K^+ abnormality
Hypotension, orthostatic	ECF volume deficit
RESPIRATORY	
Increased rate and depth	Anxiety with hyperventilation→respiratory alkalosis
	Perhaps compensation for acidosis or $\uparrow CO_2$
Decreased rate and depth	Perhaps compensation for alkalosis and $\downarrow CO_2$
	With somnolence, may signal oversedation
"Crackles" and rales at lung bases	Overhydration, cardiac congestion or failure; atelectasis
NEUROLOGICAL	
Altered level of consciousness	Abnormal Na^+, dehydration, acid-base imbalance; $\downarrow$BS
Vertigo	ECF volume deficit
Muscle weakness	Severely elevated or low potassium, hypercalcemia, hypermagnesemia
	May reflect volume losses
Altered reflexes	Magnesium or calcium imbalance
Tingling	Hyperventilation with respiratory alkalosis
	Suspect calcium elevation
Excitability	Decreased calcium or magnesium
SKIN	
Turgor at sternum	Dehydration if remains "tented" when pinched
	Not reflective of fluid status in elderly patients
Mucous membranes	Dryness may indicate ECF deficit

BS, Blood sugar; *CO₂,* carbon dioxide; *ECF,* extracellular fluid.

      (a) Confusion
      (b) Hyponatremia
      (c) Possibly seizures
  2. Assess and monitor: overhydration, hemodilution, low osmolality
    a. Circulatory overload: observe
      (1) Increased CVP, pulmonary artery pressures
      (2) Congestive heart failure
        (a) Pulmonary congestion
        (b) Respiratory compromise
          (i) Rales
          (ii) Dyspnea
          (iii) S3 heart sound
      (3) Peripheral edema—pitting edema at:
        (a) Ankles
        (b) Fingers
        (c) Eyelids
      (4) Jugular vein distention
      (5) Pleural effusion
      (6) Hypertension or hypotension, perhaps tachycardia
      (7) Renal perfusion and urinary output

■ TABLE 21-4
■ ■ **ECF Volume Expanders**

Solution	Considerations
COLLOID	Raise oncotic pressure in ECF
Synthetic protein replacement fluids	Blood products refused, contraindicated
Hydroxyethyl starch (Hetastarch)	Most Jehovah Witness beliefs allow use
	Variety of suspensions available (70/.05 to 450/0.7)
	Effect on vascular volume medium to long depending on suspension
Dextran (40 or 60)	High antibody titers: cannot cross-match
	Less expensive than blood products
	Caution: Can interfere with clotting
	Effect on VASCULAR volume medium too long depending on suspension
Gelatins	Inexpensive; similar effectiveness to hetastarch
Albumin: 5%, 25%	Expensive; short effect on vascular volume
	Limited availability, replaces low albumin
Blood products	Exposure to blood-transmitted diseases
	Need indicated by laboratory measures
	Anemia: Hemoglobin, hematocrit decrease
	Coagulopathy: Elevated INR, PTT
CRYSTALLOID	
Hypertonic electrolyte solutions	Rarely used; acute treatment for ↑ICP by reducing cerebral edema
	Administration of concentrated Na^+/Cl^-
Isotonic fluids	Restore circulating fluid volume, electrolytes
	Maintenance fluid: 100-200 mL/h
	Operative: 1-2 L to replace NPO and replace surgical, insensible losses
	Critical hypovolemia, massive burns: replace up to 8-10 L
Hypotonic fluids	Rehydrate cells
	Hyperosmolar diabetes

ECF, Extracellular fluid; *ICP,* intracranial pressure; *INR,* international normalized ratio; *NPO,* nothing by mouth; *PTT,* partial thromboplastin time.

      (8) Skin: plump, moist, and perhaps weeping through pores
      (9) X-ray evidence of pulmonary congestion, enlarged cardiac silhouette
     (10) Hypoxia, hypercapnia per ABGs, electrolyte measures
     (11) Mental status
  3. Intervene and evaluate: remove excess fluid, maintain electrolyte balance.
    a. Treat underlying cause.
    b. Diuretics
    c. Fluid restriction
D. Volume replacement
  1. Crystalloids: electrolytes in dextrose- or water-based solutions (see Box 21-1)
    a. Advantages of crystalloids:
      (1) Inexpensive
      (2) Promote urinary output and restore third-space losses
      (3) Good for maintenance IV fluid administration, to replace insensible fluid losses and for replacement of fluid and electrolyte losses
    b. Disadvantages of crystalloids: can dilute plasma proteins and decrease oncotic pressure, leading to a net outward filtration of fluid from vascular space to interstitial space

    2. Colloids: solutions containing natural or synthetic protein impermeable to the vascular membrane (see Table 21-4)

      a. Advantages: restore vascular colloid pressure and ECF fluid balance between interstitial and intravascular spaces, and smaller amounts required for fluid replacement.

      b. Disadvantages: expensive, protein basis may trigger coagulation abnormalities and anaphylaxis, and protein movement into interstitial space and increased edema.

    3. Fluid replacement calculation: Adults

      a. Replacement of NPO status: replace

      b. Fluid maintenance dependent on the surgery type

    4. Fluid replacement calculation: Pediatrics (Box 21-3)

      a. Fluid maintenance is weight dependent.

  E. Blood loss replacement

    1. Healthy patients

      a. Blood loss replaced 3 mL crystalloid for each 1 mL blood loss

      b. Blood loss replaced 1 mL colloid or blood solution for each 1 mL blood loss

VII. ACID-BASE CONCEPTS: PHYSIOLOGY OF CHEMICAL BALANCE

  A. Body cells: extremely sensitive to the chemical environment

    1. Cell wall protects environment to maintain life-sustaining intracellular functions.

    2. Minor changes in acidity or alkalinity alter cellular function, cause cell death.

    3. Chemical imbalance affects:

      a. Electrolyte charge

      b. Changes ion concentrations in solution

    4. Carbonic acid (H_2CO_3), the body's dynamic chemical buffer system, compensates for moment-to-moment acid-base shifts to maintain acid-base "harmony" in a normal ratio of 20 base to 1 acid (Table 21-5).

■ BOX 21-3
■ **FLUID REPLACEMENT FOR PEDIATRIC PATIENT**

0-10 kilogram (kg): 4 mL/kg/hr for each kg body weight
10-20 kg: 40 mL bolus + 2 mL/kg/hr for each kg >10 kg
>20 kg: 60 mL bolus + 1 mL/kg/hr for each kg >20 kg

■ TABLE 21-5
■ ■ **Carbonic Acid Regulation of Acid-Base Balance**

Immediate response as directed by Henderson-Hasselbach equation*:
Hydrogen + Bicarbonate → Carbonic Acid → Water + Carbon Dioxide

$$H^+ \quad \rightarrow \quad HCO_3^- \quad \rightarrow \quad H_2CO_3 \quad \rightarrow H_2O + \quad CO_2$$

ACIDIC CONDITIONS (PH <7.35):	ALKALOTIC CONDITIONS (PH >7.45):
Bicarbonate ion reabsorbed	Bicarbonate ion excreted
Recombines with hydrogen ion	Relative excess of hydrogen ion
Forms more carbonic acid	Less carbonic acid formed
H_2CO_3 dissociates to water and CO_2.	
Respiratory rate and depth increase (↑)	Respiratory rate and depth decrease (↓)
CO_2 is exhaled (↓ Pco_2).	CO_2 accumulates (↑ Pco_2).
pH restored toward 7.4 (↑)	pH restored toward 7.4 (↓)

*Henderson-Hasselbach equation: describes a dynamic buffer of body fluids. Hydrogen ion is regulated by combining with or dissociating from bicarbonate.

5. Oxygen
   a. Critical component of acid-base balance
   b. Metabolism occurs even during oxygen lack—termed anaerobic metabolism.
   c. Anaerobic metabolism leads to an acidic environment.
6. Adequate hemoglobin is necessary for effective oxygen transport to cells.
7. ECF
   a. Accessible for measurement by serum analysis
   b. Means for treatment for acid-base disharmony
   c. Semipermeable cell walls allow some equilibration of ions—ICF affected.
8. Carbon dioxide (CO_2) more soluble in cool temperature
   a. Hypothermia
   b. $\uparrow CO_2$
   c. Acidity increases
B. Perianesthesia concerns
   1. Acid-base disruption relatively common among preoperative and postoperative perianesthesia patients due to:
      a. Ability to sustain acid-base balance is disturbed
         (1) Trauma
         (2) Acute or chronic illness
         (3) Surgical fluid shifts
         (4) Anesthetic effects
      b. The body of a healthy patient "automatically" compensates to sustain normal acid-base parameters.
      c. The perianesthesia nurse must:
         (1) Anticipate conditions that disrupt a patient's acid-base balance
         (2) Analyze ABG results
         (3) Quickly initiate nursing and medical treatment
      d. Acidosis is likely:
         (1) With hypothermia
         (2) With hypoxia
         (3) Corrected by active rewarming techniques
         (4) Corrected with delivery of supplemental oxygenation
      e. Anesthetic agents can cause myocardial depression $\rightarrow \downarrow$ tissue perfusion
         (1) $\downarrow$ Oxygen (O_2) supply $\rightarrow$ anaerobic metabolism $\rightarrow$ lactic acidosis
         (2) $\uparrow CO_2$ levels $\rightarrow$ respiratory acidosis
C. Definitions
   1. Acid: a hydrogen ion (H^+) donates a hydrogen ion when in solution.
      a. Binds with a base to form an inert compound
      b. The body's primary acid is hydrogen ion (H^+).
   2. Base: a hydrogen ion (H^+) acceptor when a compound is in solution
      a. Synonymous with the term alkali
      b. The body's primary base is bicarbonate (HCO_3^-).
   3. Acidosis: abnormal increase of acid content within body fluids from:
      a. Accumulation of acid (H^+)
      b. Loss of base (HCO_3^-)
      c. May arise from respiratory or metabolic causes
      d. Acidemia refers to an acid condition in the blood.
   4. Alkalosis: abnormal decrease in acid content within body fluids from:
      a. Loss of acid (H^+)
      b. Accumulation of base (HCO_3^-)
      c. Alkalemia refers to an alkaline status of blood.
D. Determinants of acid-base homeostasis
   1. pH: a mathematical calculation reflecting the concentration of H^+ in solution
      a. An abbreviation for "potential hydrogen"
      b. Negative algorithm of the amount of H^+ in a solution
      c. Describes the relative balance between acids and bases in solution

      d. pH of a neutral, neither acid nor alkaline, solution is 7.0.

         (1) Increasing a solution's acidity (adding acid [H^+] or decreasing the base [HCO_3]) decreases pH to <7.0.

         (2) Decreasing a solution's acidity (adding base [HCO_3^-] or losing acid [H^+]) increases pH to >7.0.

      e. Body's buffer systems normally maintain the pH of blood in a range of 7.35 to 7.45.

      f. Initiate treatment pH

         (1) Decreased (7.30-7.35)

         (2) Increased (7.45-7.50)

      g. Definitive therapy indicated when pH <7.15 or >7.60

      h. Death is imminent if no intervention

         (1) pH <6.90

         (2) pH >7.90

  2. Partial pressure of carbon dioxide in arterial blood (Pco_2): respiratory component

      a. Represents the amount of CO_2 dissolved in arterial blood

      b. CO_2 dissolves in plasma and reversible

         (1) Binds with water (H_2O) to create carbonic acid (H_2CO_3)

         (2) Considered a nonfixed or volatile acid

      c. Carbonic acid forms in tissue capillaries to transport CO_2 to the lungs for excretion.

      d. Regulated by breathing to exhale CO_2 (acid) from body

         (1) Encourage a groggy perianesthesia patient with a purely respiratory acidosis (elevated $Paco_2$) to deep breathe.

         (2) Correct this acid-base disturbance by exhaling excess CO_2.

         (3) Add supplemental oxygen.

      e. Unresponsiveness may render the patient unable to follow the request to deep breathe due to:

         (1) Residual muscle relaxant

         (2) Sedation

      f. To excrete CO_2 it may be necessary for:

         (1) Reintubation

         (2) Positive pressure ventilation

         (3) Manually/mechanical ventilator

      g. A patient with severe metabolic acidosis will "automatically" compensate by:

         (1) Increasing respirations to exhale excess acid in the form of CO_2

         (2) An example is Kussmaul respiration, the deep, blowing respiratory compensation seen in diabetic ketoacidosis.

  3. Bicarbonate (HCO_3^-): metabolic component

      a. Represents amount of HCO_3^- available to buffer acids

      b. Regulated at kidney: excreted or reabsorbed at the collecting tubule

      c. Influenced by amount of fixed or nonvolatile acid

         (1) Infuse sodium bicarbonate to increase HCO_3^- levels and buffering capacity.

         (2) Correct other electrolyte disturbances.

  4. Anion gap: expressed as base excess

      a. Calculated difference between serum cations and anions

$$\text{Anion Gap} = (Na^+ + K^+) - (HCO_3^- + Cl^-)$$

      b. Used to determine the potential cause of metabolic acidosis

      c. Formula: Serum sodium value minus sum of bicarbonate and chloride

      d. Normal anion gap = 10 to 12 mOsm/L

      e. Increased anion gap: associated with metabolic acidosis with H^+ gain

         (1) Ketoacidosis: diabetic, alcoholic, starvation

         (2) Lactic acidosis: hypoxia (anaerobic metabolism), shock, sepsis

         (3) Rhabdomyolysis: acute, massive tissue destruction

(4) Acute renal failure: acute tubular necrosis, shock

f. Normal anion gap: associated with metabolic acidosis due to HCO_3^- losses with retention of Cl^- to maintain ionic balance

(1) Diarrhea, intestinal or biliary fistulas

(2) Excessive sodium chloride (NaCl) intake

5. Temperature: pH decreases (produces acidosis) as temperature decreases.

a. Pco_2 decreases by 4.5% per degree Celsius.

b. Hemoglobin, one of the body's acid-base buffers, accepts more H^+ in cool temperatures, so pH increases.

6. Oxygenation: Po_2, percent saturation, and hemoglobin

a. Pao_2: measure of partial pressure of dissolved oxygen in arterial blood

b. Oxygen loosely bound to hemoglobin (saturation) or dissolved in blood (Pao_2)

c. Oxyhemoglobin dissociation: relationship between Po_2 and saturation

(1) Po_2 >70 mm Hg is the critical point: at >70 mm Hg, hemoglobin saturation is nearly 100%.

(2) As Po_2 dips <70 mm Hg, small decrease in Pao_2 correlates with large decrease in oxygen saturation as hemoglobin quickly releases oxygen tissues.

(a) When Po_2 ≥40 mm Hg, hemoglobin approximately 70% saturated

(b) Temperature, pH, and Pco_2 are indicators of metabolism and affect oxygen binding to hemoglobin and the release of oxygen from hemoglobin.

(i) ↑ Temperature; ↓ pH; ↑ Pco_2 indicate ↑ metabolism and ↓ affinity or strength of oxyhemoglobin bond and ↑ release of O_2 from hemoglobin to tissues (e.g., fever with hypermetabolism).

(ii) ↓ Temperature; ↑ pH; ↓ Pco_2 indicate ↓ metabolism and ↑ affinity or strength of bond and ↓ release of O_2 from hemoglobin to tissues (e.g., hypothermia with hypometabolism).

VIII. PRIMARY ACID-BASE IMBALANCE

A. Acidosis

1. Respiratory: $Paco_2$ >45 mm Hg and pH <7.35

a. Results from alveolar hypoventilation: failure to excrete carbonic acid (CO_2)

b. Metabolic state normal

c. Clinical causes

(1) Depression of central respiratory centers

(a) Effects of residual anesthetic agents, such as muscle relaxants that render the patient unable to breathe effectively

(b) Consider pseudocholinesterase deficiency if respiratory effort ineffective after succinylcholine.

(c) Sedation from narcotics or hypnotic (intentional or as part of conscious sedation) or caused by overmedication

(d) Compression of medullary centers from increases in intracranial pressure

(i) Edema from surgical intervention or trauma

(ii) Intracranial masses caused by lesions

(iii) Increased Pco_2, a potent intracerebral vasodilator

(e) Hypothermia: slows metabolism of depressant medications

(f) Exhaustion from ineffective respiratory effort

(2) Interference with muscles of respiration

(a) Residual effects of neuromuscular blocking agents

(b) Pain causes splinting and limited chest expansion; more pronounced after thoracic and abdominal surgery

(c) Physical limitation of chest expansion from:
  (i) Tight chest binders
  (ii) Chest tubes
  (iii) Dressings
  (iv) From burn eschar
  (v) Kyphosis
(d) Obesity: lung expansion especially hampered in supine position
(e) Neuromuscular diseases: myasthenia gravis, poliomyelitis
(f) Inadequate mechanical ventilation: rate or tidal volume too low to exhale CO_2

(3) Airway obstruction
  (a) Oropharynx
    (i) Secretions
    (ii) Relaxed tongue
    (iii) Pharyngeal edema, tracheal or subglottic stenosis
  (b) Laryngospasm or bronchospasm
  (c) Pulmonary aspiration
  (d) Endotracheal tube (ETT)
    (i) Malpositioned resulting in single-lung ventilation
    (ii) Blocked ETT by secretions or kinks

(4) Pulmonary disease
  (a) Chronic obstructive pulmonary disease
  (b) Pulmonary fibrosis
  (c) Atelectasis and pneumonia
  (d) Bronchospasm or asthma

d. Therapeutic interventions to correct alveolar hypoventilation
  (1) Stimulate! Stir up! Remind patient to breathe.
  (2) Ensure airway patency.
    (a) Jaw lift
    (b) Head reposition
    (c) Suction
    (d) Insert oral or nasal airway.
    (e) Intubation if stimulation ineffective
    (f) Mechanical ventilation as needed
  (3) Provide oxygen.
  (4) Reverse muscle relaxants and/or sedatives or narcotics as appropriate.
  (5) Rewarming measures if patient is hypothermic

2. Metabolic: HCO_3^- <22 mEq/L and pH <7.35
  a. Results from accumulated ionized acid (H^+) or depletion of base
  b. Respiratory status normal, except as in compensation
  c. Clinical causes
    (1) Acid overproduction: promotes K^+ release from cells
      (a) Ketoacidosis: type 1 diabetes or starvation with protein catabolism
      (b) Anaerobic metabolism: lactate production (acidosis)
      (c) Renal failure, acute and chronic
      (d) Muscle destruction: rhabdomyolysis
      (e) Overdose: salicylic acid (aspirin) or ferrous sulfate (iron)
        (i) Salicylate metabolites increase fixed acids.
        (ii) Directly stimulates respiratory chemoreceptors to cause hyperventilation
        (iii) Respiratory alkalosis predominates in adults.
        (iv) Metabolic acidosis predominates in infants, young children.
      (f) Fevers caused by infection
    (2) Severe bicarbonate loss
      (a) GI: diarrhea, small bowel or pancreatic fistulas

(b) Excessive doses: acetazolamide (Diamox) or ammonium chloride
   d. Therapeutic interventions to correct
     (1) Encourage deep breathing ($\uparrow$ respiratory rate and depth) so CO_2 is exhaled.
     (2) Administer sodium bicarbonate, usually 1 mEq/kg.
     (3) Remonitor ABGs, K^+ retreat as needed: aim for slow resolution.
     (4) Give insulin (+ dextrose) to return potassium to cells as acidosis resolves.
     (5) Monitor cardiac rhythm (electrocardiogram) for dysrhythmia, peaked T waves.
     (6) Frequently monitor vital signs, neurologic and respiratory status.
  B. Alkalosis
    1. Respiratory: Pco_2 <35 mm Hg and pH >7.45
      a. Results from alveolar hyperventilation: $\uparrow$ excretion of CO_2
      b. Respirations increased, metabolic status normal
      c. Clinical causes
        (1) Psychogenic causes: pain, anxiety, and panic
        (2) Respiratory center overstimulation: tumors at level of medulla or pons; surgical manipulation of brainstem
        (3) Overzealous mechanical ventilation: rate, tidal volume too high.
        (4) Normal finding in pregnancy
      d. Patient reports headache, dizziness, tingling, paresthesias.
      e. Therapeutic interventions to correct
        (1) Sedate or provide analgesia.
        (2) Coach breathing: slow, regular, moderate depth.
        (3) Emotional support and calming reassurance
        (4) Adjust mechanical ventilator settings to reduce rate, tidal volume.
        (5) Monitor ABGs, labs, clinical status.
    2. Metabolic: HCO_3^- >26 mEq/L and pH >7.45
      a. Results from excessive loss of acid (H^+) or accumulation of bases
      b. Respirations normal, though may be shallow as compensatory means
      c. Clinical causes
        (1) Excessive loss of gastric acid from upper GI tract, or insufficient replacement
          (a) Protracted vomiting
          (b) Gastric suction
          (c) Gastric lavage
        (2) Excessive circulating HCO_3^-
          (a) Chemical response relative to chloride loss
          (b) Overcorrection of acidosis with bicarbonate
          (c) Overingestion of antacid or baking soda
          (d) Overinfusion of lactated solution
        (3) Overretention of base ions
          (a) Diuretics
            (i)   Furosemide (Lasix)
            (ii) Thiazides
          (b) Excessive administration of corticosteroids
        (4) Systemic diseases: Cushing's syndrome, aldosteronism
      d. Therapeutic interventions to correct
        (1) Treat or eliminate cause.
        (2) Monitor lab values, particularly hypokalemia as K^+ moves to cell.
        (3) Observe clinical status, reporting confusion, muscle cramps, twitching, tingling.
IX. MIXED ACID-BASE IMBALANCES
  A. Inadequate compensation: several concurrent acid-base disorders
    1. For example, if pH <7.35 (acidosis), $Paco_2$ – 55 mm Hg (respiratory acidosis), and HCO_3^- = 14 mEq/L (metabolic acidosis), then have a mixed acidosis

a. Could occur in patient with chronic lung disease (chronic respiratory acidosis, usually compensated) who develops diarrhea with large HCO_3^- losses

B. pH change is dramatic with mixed acidosis or mixed alkalosis disorders.

C. pH change less severe if mixed acidosis-alkalosis: opposing disorders balance.

X. PHYSIOLOGICAL COMPENSATION OF ACID-BASE IMBALANCES

A. The body's natural effort to restore acid-to-base ratio toward 1:20 and pH toward 7.40

1. Compensation occurs when pH is within normal range.

2. Partial compensation results when $Paco_2$ or HCO_3^- changes but pH changes minimally.

3. Rarely overcompensates

B. Compensation via three mechanisms

1. Cellular acid-base compensation

a. Compensation begins immediately with the accumulation of acid (H^+).

(1) H^+ moves into the cell and intracellular K^+ moves out of cell; any acidotic state will be accompanied by hyperkalemia.

(2) H^+ is buffered by intercellular protein.

b. Effective but limited compensation

2. Pulmonary acid-base compensation

a. Compensation begins within minutes with the accumulation of acid (H^+).

(1) ↓ pH is monitored by respiratory center in the medulla.

(2) Causes an ↑ in the rate and ↑ depth of ventilation; ↓ CO_2 → normalizing pH

b. Effective but limited compensation

3. Renal acid-base compensation

a. Compensation begins within days with the accumulation of acid (H^+).

b. Single mechanism has two effects.

(1) H^+ excreted into the urine

(2) In the same mechanism causes reabsorption of HCO_3^-

c. Effective long-term compensation

C. Compensation for common acid-base derangements

1. Respiratory acidosis

a. [Acute] Immediate rise in serum K^+ (K^+/H^+ exchange)

b. [Chronic] Occurs slowly in kidneys over days

(1) Excretion of H^+: acidic urine results

(2) Reabsorption of HCO_3^-

2. Respiratory alkalosis

a. Immediate decline in serum K^+ as K^+ enters cell in exchange for H^+ (K^+/H^+ exchange)

b. [Chronic; as seen in pregnancy] Occurs slowly in kidneys over days

(1) ↓ in renal excretion of H^+: ↓ acidity of urine

(2) ↓ in the reabsorption of HCO_3^-

3. Metabolic acidosis

a. Immediate rise in serum K^+ (K^+/H^+ exchange)

b. Within minutes, ↑ rate and ↑ depth of breathing (hyperventilation) to eliminate CO_2

c. Occurs slowly in kidneys over days

(1) Excretion of H^+: acidic urine results

(2) Reabsorption of HCO_3^-

4. Metabolic alkalosis

a. Immediate decline in serum K^+ as K^+ enters cell in exchange for H^+ (K^+/H^+ exchange)

b. Within minutes, ↓ rate and ↓ depth of breathing (hypoventilation) to retain CO_2

c. Occurs slowly in kidneys over days

(1) ↓ excretion of H^+: alkalotic urine results

(2) ↓ reabsorption of HCO_3^-

XI. INTERPRETING ABGs
  A. Purpose for measuring ABGs
    1. Determine status of alveolar ventilation and arterial oxygenation.
      a. Determine acid-base status of patient.
      b. Guide respiratory and metabolic interventions.
      c. Must interpret in the context of the patient's clinical status.
  B. Systematic ABG analysis: name the disorder.
    1. Consider pH, the acidosis/alkalosis component—normal: 7.35 to 7.45.
      a. If <7.35 (low), condition is acidosis.
      b. If >7.45 (high), condition is alkalosis.
      c. If in normal range, condition is "normal pH," and patient either has normal acid-base balance or acidosis or alkalosis is compensated.
    2. Next, consider Pco_2, the respiratory component—normal: 35 to 45 mm Hg.
      a. If <35 mm Hg ($\downarrow$) and pH $\uparrow$, condition is respiratory alkalosis.
      b. If >45 mm Hg ($\uparrow$) and pH $\downarrow$, condition is respiratory acidosis.
      c. If normal, move on to consider HCO_3^- as cause of high or low pH.
    3. Then, consider HCO_3^-, the metabolic component—normal: 22 to 26 mEq/L.
      a. If <22 mEq/L ($\downarrow$) and pH $\downarrow$, condition is metabolic acidosis.
      b. If >26 mEq/L ($\uparrow$) and pH $\uparrow$, condition is metabolic alkalosis.
    4. Consider Po_2: Is patient hypoxic? Normal: 80 to 100 mm Hg
      a. If <80 mm Hg: Stimulate patient to increase respiratory effort, treat airway obstructon, pulmonary congestion, obstruction or bronchospasm, or measure hemoglobin level.
      b. If >100 mm Hg: Monitor status.
      c. If >150 mm Hg: Adjust oxygen delivery.
      d. Is percent saturation >95%? Verify respiratory quality and adequacy of circulating hemoglobin to transport oxygen.
      e. Remember that hypoxemia contributes to acidosis.
    5. Determine abnormality and determine whether acute (primary abnormality) or compensated.
      a. Assess pH to identify the trend.
      b. If pH within normal range but not exactly 7.40
        (1) If pH is 7.35 to 7.39, leans toward acidosis
        (2) If pH is 7.41 to 7.45, leans toward alkalosis
      c. Determine processes Pco_2 and HCO_3^- as in steps 2 and 3 above.
        (1) Primary process: signified by component that supports leaning tendency of pH
        (2) Compensation: signified by component that supports opposite tendency before treatment is initiated
      d. Now state your decision based on the ABG facts.
        (1) Does decision mesh with the patient's history or clinical status?
          (a) Respiratory acidosis or metabolic acidosis?
          (b) Respiratory alkalosis or metabolic alkalosis?
        (2) Report ABG results to physician; plan interventions.

BIBLIOGRAPHY

1. Agodoa L: Acute renal failure in the PACU. *J Perianesth Nurs* 17:377-383, 2002.
2. Ard JL, Prough DS: Perioperative electrolyte and acid-base abnormalities. In Benumof JL, Saidman LG, eds: *Anesthesia and perioperative complications*, ed 2, St Louis, 1999, Mosby, pp 503-535.
3. Berry BE, Pinard AE: Assessing tissue oxygenation. *Crit Care Nurse* 22:22-40, 2002.
4. Boldt J, Priebe HJ: Intravascular volume replacement therapy with synthetic colloids: Is there an influence on renal function? *Anesth Analg* 96:376-382, 2003.
5. Chernecky C, Butler SW, Graham P, et al: *Real-world nursing survival guide: Fluids and electrolytes*, Philadelphia, 2002, WB Saunders.
6. Chernecky C, Macklin D, Murphy-Ende K: *Saunders nursing survival guide: Fluids and electrolytes*, St. Louis, 2006, Saunders.
7. Cowling GE, Haas RE: Hypotension in the PACU: An algorithmic approach. *J Perianesth Nurs* 17:159-163, 2002.

8. Czekaj LA: Promoting acid-base balance. In Kinney MR, Brooks-Brunn JA, Molter N, et al, eds: *AACN clinical reference for critical care nursing*, ed 4, St Louis, 1998, Mosby, pp 135-145.

9. Drain CB, Odom-Forren J: *Perianesthesia nursing: A critical care approach*, ed 5, St Louis, 2009, Saunders.

10. Ferrara-Love R: Immediate postanesthesia care. In Burden N, DeFazio Quinn DM, O'Brien D, eds: *Ambulatory surgical nursing*, ed 2, Philadelphia, 2000, WB Saunders, pp 442-448.

11. Golembiewski JA, O'Brien D: A systematic approach to the management of postoperative nausea and vomiting. *J Perianesth Nurs* 17:364-376, 2002.

12. Goskowicz R: Complications of blood transfusions. In Benumof JL, Saidman LG, eds: *Anesthesia and perioperative complications*, ed 2, St Louis, 1999, Mosby, pp 536-574.

13. Grocott MP, Mythen MG, Gan TJ: Perioperative fluid management and clinical outcomes in adults. *Anesth Analg* 100:1093-1106, 2005.

14. Heitz UE, Horne MM, Webber KS, et al: *Guide to fluid, electrolyte and acid-base balance*, St Louis, 2001, Mosby.

15. Josephson D: *Intravenous infusion therapy for nurses: Principles & practice*, ed 2, Clifton Park, NY, 2003, Thomson Delmar Learning.

16. Matthias J, Chappel D, Rehm M: Clinical update: Perioperative fluid management, *Lancet* 369:1984-1986, 2007.

17. Nisanevich V, Felsenstein I, Almogy G, et al: Effect of intraoperative fluid management on outcome after intraabdominal surgery. *Anesthesiology* 103:25-32, 2005.

18. O'Brien D: Acute postoperative delirium: Definitions, incidence, recognition, and interventions. *J Perianesth Nurs* 17:384-392, 2002.

19. O'Flaherty JE, Berry FA: Anesthesia complications occurring primarily in the very young. In Benumof JL, Saidman LG, eds: *Anesthesia and perioperative complications*, ed 2, St Louis, 1999, Mosby, pp 606-625.

20. Roth S, Gillesberg I: Injury to the visual system and other sensory organs. In Benumof JL, Saidman LG, eds: *Anesthesia and perioperative complications*, ed 2, St Louis, 1999, Mosby, pp 377-408.

21. Simpson PJ, Popat M: *Understanding anaesthesia*, ed 4, Boston, 2002, Butterworth/Heinemann.

22 Anesthetic Agents and Adjuncts

COURTNEY BROWN

Note: Dosage guidelines presented in this chapter are for healthy adults unless otherwise stated.

OBJECTIVES

At the conclusion of this chapter, the reader will be able to:

1. Describe anesthetic options used.
2. Recognize the local anesthetics used for regional anesthesia.
3. Review the perianesthesia nursing care implications for patients who have received epidural and spinal anesthetics.
4. Differentiate between thiopental, methohexital, etomidate, ketamine, and propofol as intravenous (IV) anesthetics.
5. Identify perianesthesia nursing care implications for patients who have received benzodiazepines.
6. Identify common pharmacologic properties of opioids.
7. Describe the physiological and pharmacological differences between depolarizing and nondepolarizing muscle relaxants.
8. Define the mechanism of action of anticholinesterase reversal agents.
9. Describe the use of anticholinergic agents in anesthesia.
10. Identify properties specific to each inhalation anesthetics.
11. Describe implications for the perianesthesia nurse in caring for patients who have received inhalation agents.

I. ANESTHESIA AS A CONTINUUM (Box 22-1)
   A. Awake
   B. Minimal sedation (anxiolysis)
      1. Patient remains conscious.
      2. Responds normally to verbal commands
      3. Ventilatory and cardiovascular functions unaffected
   C. Moderate sedation and analgesia or monitored anesthesia care (MAC)
      1. Drug-induced minimally depressed level of consciousness
      2. Patient maintains patent airway independently and continuously.
      3. Patient responds to verbal commands.
      4. Cardiovascular function usually maintained
      5. Patient does not lose consciousness.
      6. When provided by anesthesiologist or nurse anesthetist, known as MAC
   D. Deep sedation and analgesia
      1. Patient may sleep and may be aroused.
      2. Respond purposefully after repeated or painful stimulation
         a. Reflex withdrawal not considered a purposeful response
      3. May require assistance in maintaining a patent airway
      4. Ability to independently maintain ventilatory function may be impaired.
      5. Cardiovascular function usually maintained

■ BOX 22-1
■ **CONTINUUM OF ANESTHETIC OPTIONS**

Awake-Conscious	Awake/Moderate Sedation	Moderate Sedation/Deep Sedation	Deep Sedation	General Anesthesia
None	**Local anesthesia**	**Intravenous**	**Gaseous inhalation anesthetic**	**Sedatives/Hypnotics**
▪ Oxygen	▪ Topical	▪ Droperidol	▪ Nitrous oxide	▪ Etomidate (Amidate)
	▪ EMLA	**Anticholinergics**		▪ Propofol (Diprivan)
	Regional anesthesia	▪ Atropine	**Dissociative**	**IV barbiturates**
	▪ IV regional blocks	▪ Scopolamine	▪ Ketamine (Ketalar)	▪ Thiopental
	▪ Bier	▪ Glycopyrrolate (Robinul)		▪ Methohexital
	▪ Peripheral nerve block	**Benzodiazepines**		**Inhalation**
	▪ Cervical plexus	▪ Diazepam (Valium)		▪ Halothane
	▪ Brachial plexus	▪ Midazolam (Versed)		▪ Enflurane (Ethrane)
	▪ Digital	▪ Lorazepam (Ativan)		▪ Isoflurane (Forane)
	▪ Intercostal	**Benzodiazepine antagonist**		▪ Desflurane (Suprane)
	▪ Lower extremity	▪ Flumazenil		▪ Sevoflurane (Ultane)
	▪ Sympathetic block	**IV opioids**		**Depolarizing muscle relaxants**
	▪ Stellate ganglion	▪ Morphine		▪ Succinylcholine
	▪ Celiac plexus	▪ Meperidine		**Nondepolarizing muscle relaxants**
	▪ Lumbar	▪ Dilaudid		▪ Atracurium (Tracrium)
	▪ Regional blocks	▪ Alfentanil		▪ Cisatracurium (Nimbex)
	▪ Caudal	▪ Fentanyl		▪ Curare (d-tubocurarine)
	▪ Epidural	▪ Remifentanil		▪ Doxacurium (Nuromax)
	▪ Spinal	▪ Sufentanil		▪ Gallamine
		Opioid Antagonist		▪ Metocurine
		▪ Naloxone (Narcan)		▪ Pancuronium (Pavulon)
		Alpha₂-Agonists		▪ Pipecuronium (Arduan)
		▪ Dexmeditomidine (Precedex)		▪ Rocuronium (Zemuron)
		▪ Clonidine		▪ Vecuronium (Norcuron)
				▪ Nondepolarizing muscle relaxant reversals
				▪ Anticholinesterases
				▪ Neostigmine
				▪ Edrophonium (Enlon)
				▪ Pyridostigmine
				▪ Anticholinergics
				▪ Atropine
				▪ Scopolamine
				▪ Glycopyrrolate (Robinul)

EMLA, Eutectic Mixture of Local Anesthetics.

E. General anesthesia
   1. Patient not arousable
   2. Ability to independently maintain ventilatory function often impaired
   3. Assistance to maintain a patent airway often required
   4. Positive pressure ventilation may be required because of depressed spontaneous ventilation or drug-induced depression of neuromuscular function.

       5. Cardiovascular function may be impaired.

       6. Reversible state providing:

         a. Analgesia

         b. Sedation

         c. Appropriate muscle relaxation

         d. Appropriate control of autonomic nervous system

         e. Partial or complete loss of protective reflexes

II. PHARMACOKINETICS AND PHARMACODYNAMICS

  A. Pharmacokinetics

    1. Relationship between:

      a. Dose of drug administration

      b. Concentration of drug delivered to site of action

    2. What the body does to the drugs (i.e., drug uptake, distribution, biotransformation, excretion of drugs)

      a. How the body:

        (1) Absorbs

        (2) Distributes

        (3) Metabolizes

        (4) Excretes

  B. Pharmacodynamics (i.e., additive, synergistic, antagonistic effect)

    1. Relationship between:

      a. Concentration of drugs at site of action

      b. Intensity of effect produced

    2. What the drugs do to the body

      a. Examples

        (1) Central nervous system (CNS) depression

        (2) Respiratory depression

        (3) Cardiovascular changes

III. STAGES OF ANESTHESIA

  A. Stage I: stage of anesthesia and amnesia

    1. Begins with initiation of anesthesia and ends with loss of consciousness

      a. Patient can follow simple commands.

      b. Protective reflexes remain intact.

  B. Stage II: stage of delirium

    1. Starts with loss of consciousness and ends with disappearance of lid reflex

      a. Respirations irregular

      b. May be passed through quickly with newer anesthetic agents

      c. High risk for aspiration, laryngospasm, and bronchospasm

  C. Stage III: stage of surgical anesthesia

    1. Cessation of spontaneous respirations

      a. Absence of:

        (1) Eyelash response

        (2) Blink

        (3) Swallowing reflexes

    2. Airway management essential

  D. Stage IV: cessation of respiration to circulatory collapse

    1. Considered overdose of anesthetic

IV. LOCAL ANESTHESIA OPTIONS

  A. Common property general facts

    1. Agents that impair conduction of neurally mediated impulses

    2. Two chemical groups

      a. Esters: cocaine, procaine, chloroprocaine, tetracaine

      b. Amides: prilocaine, lidocaine, mepivacaine, bupivacaine, etidocaine, ropivacaine, levobupivacaine

  B. Physiology

    1. Three major classes of nerves (Table 22-1)

      a. A fibers: myelinated somatic nerves

      b. B fibers: myelinated preganglionic autonomic nerves

      c. C fibers: unmyelinated postganglionic autonomic nerves

■ TABLE 22-1
■ ■ **Classification of Nerve Fibers**

Fiber Type	Myelin	Diameter (μm)	Function
Aα	+++	10-20	Motor neurons (efferent: to skeletal muscle)
Aβ	++	5-10	Touch, pressure, and proprioception neurons (afferent: from skin)
Aγ	++	5-10	Motor neurons (efferent: to muscle spindles)
Aδ	++	1-5	Pain (sharp/fast) and temperature neurons (efferent: from skin)
B	+	1-2.5	Preganglionic sympathetic neurons (efferent: to vascular smooth muscle)
C	0	0.5-1	Pain (dull/slow) and temperature neurons (afferent from skin) Postganglionic sympathetic neurons (efferent: to vascular smooth muscle)

2. Pharmacodynamics
   a. Impair conduction of impulses along axons
      (1) Effect mediated by blocking sodium channels
      (2) Communication between CNS and peripheral nervous system impaired
      (3) Block is reversible and dose dependent.
   b. Rank order of nerve fiber sensitivity to local anesthetic blockade
      (1) B > C and Aδ > Aγ > Aß > Aα
   c. Rank order of nerve fiber diameters
      (1) C < B < Aδ < Aß and Aγ < Aα (thinnest/least myelinated nerves blocked first)
   d. Two separate pain-conducting pathways (both blocked by same tissue concentration of agent)
      (1) C fibers (slow pain)
      (2) Aδ fibers (fast pain)
3. Pharmacokinetics (Table 22-2)
   a. Esters: hydrolyzed by plasma cholinesterase
   b. Amides: metabolized in liver
   c. Onset related to:
      (1) Amides have a faster onset.
      (2) Lipid solubility (directly proportional)
      (3) Infection or acidosis at site slows onset (increased toxicity with hypoxia and acidosis)
      (4) Adding bicarbonate speeds onset.
   d. Absorption related to:
      (1) Dosage
      (2) Vasoconstrictor additives (slows absorption)
      (3) Protein binding: helps local stay at injection site
      (4) Blood flow: highly vascular sites have faster systemic absorption.
      (5) Physiologic
         (a) Age
         (b) Cardiovascular function: decreased cardiac output means slower washout
         (c) Hepatic function: liver metabolizes amides, decrease administered dose by one-half
   e. Site of injection related to toxicity in order of most common
      (1) Intercostal (most common)
      (2) Caudal

■ TABLE 22-2

Local Anesthetics Used for Regional Techniques

Drug	Onset	Duration (min)	Local	Topical	IV Block	Peripheral	Epidural	Spinal	Maximum Dose/Extra Information
ESTERS									
Cocaine	Rapid	10-55	No	Yes	No	No	No	No	150 mg or 3 mg/kg Only local that constricts
Procaine (Novocain)	Slow	15-30	Yes	No	No	Yes	No	Yes	1000 mg Increased incidence allergic reactions
Chloroprocaine (Nesacaine)	Rapid	15-30	Yes	No	No	Yes	Yes	No	600-800 mg Permanent neural damage with EDTA additive (SAB)
Tetracaine (Pontocaine)	Slow	120-240	No	Yes	No	No	No	Yes	100 mg 20 mg max in SAB Most potent local
AMIDES									
Prilocaine (Citanest)	Slow	60-120	Yes	No	Yes	Yes	Yes	No	>600 mg leads to methemoglobinemia High lung uptake
Lidocaine	Rapid	60-120	Yes	Yes	Yes	Yes	Yes	Yes	300 mg or 5 mg/kg (7 mg/kg with epinephrine); CNS toxic; CES
Mepivacaine (Carbocaine)	Slow	45-90	Yes	No	No	Yes	Yes	No	300 mg Great for peripheral nerve blocks

Continued

■ TABLE 22-2

Local Anesthetics Used for Regional Techniques—cont'd

Drug	Onset	Duration (min)	Local	Topical	IV Block	Peripheral	Epidural	Spinal	Maximum Dose/Extra Information
Bupivacaine (Marcaine, Sensorcaine)	Slow	120-240	Yes	No	No	Yes	Yes	Yes	175 mg or 3 mg/kg 20 mg max SAB CV toxic
Etidocaine (Duranest)	Slow	240-480	Yes	No	No	Yes	Yes	No	300 mg Profound motor (not for OB) Surgical usage only
Ropivacaine (Naropin)	Rapid	240-360	Yes	No	Yes	Yes	Yes	Yes	200 mg Less motor block than bupivacaine; less CV toxic as well
Levobupivacaine (Chirocaine)	Slow	240-480	Yes	No	No	Yes	Yes	Yes	Structurally related to bupivicaine

CES, Cauda equina syndrome; *CNS*, central nervous system; *CV*, cardiovascular; *EDTA*, ethylenediaminetetracetic acid; *max*, maximum; *OB*, obstetrics; *SAB*, subarachnoid block.

(3) Para-cervical
(4) Epidural
(5) Brachial plexus
(6) Spinal
(7) Femoral/sciatic
(8) Tracheal—equates to IV injection of lidocaine in 10 to 15 minutes
  f. Tissue distribution related to:
    (1) Lungs: prilocaine/bupivacaine have increased pulmonary uptake.
    (2) Lipid solubility into fatty tissues
    (3) Placenta: local anesthetics diffuse through placenta, become more ionized in fetus' higher acidic environment; once ionized, cannot easily pass back through placenta (phenomenon called *ion trapping* and leads to local anesthetic build-up in fetus)
  g. Clearance
    (1) Esters
      (a) Metabolized by pseudocholinesterase in the blood
      (b) This releases para-aminobenzoic acid (PABA), an active antigen responsible for allergic reactions to esters.
    (2) Amides
      (a) Metabolized by liver
      (b) Allergy to amides rare
  h. Duration directly proportional to lipid solubility + protein binding
  i. Additives
    (1) Vasoconstrictors (epinephrine): increase duration and enhance block
    (2) Carbonation: increases onset inside cell
    (3) Bicarbonate: speeds onset outside cell, increases duration
    (4) Local + local = additive effects
    (5) Opioids: increase intensity and duration of block (synergistic)
    (6) Alpha$_2$-agonist (clonidine): central and peripheral effects
    (7) Neostigmine
    (8) Ephedrine
4. Local anesthetic toxicity (hypercarbia/hypoxia potentiate toxic effects of all local anesthetics)
  a. CNS toxicity
    (1) Apply oxygen (O_2) to help prevent seizure activity.
    (2) Symptoms in order of appearance
      (a) Circumoral numbness
      (b) Lightheadedness
      (c) Tinnitus
      (d) Visual disturbance
      (e) Slurred speech
      (f) Muscle twitch
      (g) Irrational conversation
      (h) Grand mal
      (i) Coma
      (j) Apnea then cardiovascular depression
      (k) Grand mal: treat with Versed, Valium, thiopental
      (l) Coma
  b. Cardiovascular toxicity
    (1) More resistant to treat than CNS toxicity; sodium (Na^+) channels of heart blocked
    (2) Signs and symptoms: hypertension leading to hypotension, premature ventricular complexes, prolonged PR interval and QRS on electrocardiogram, and cardiovascular collapse
      (a) Most common with bupivicaine, then etidocaine
      (b) Treatment = Prevention: frequent aspiration; inject slowly with divided doses—every dose is a test dose.
      (c) Treat hypotension with ephedrine and bradycardia with atropine

c. Neural damage
   (1) Spinal cord/roots most prone
   (2) Transient radicular irritation (TRI)
      (a) Pain in buttock, lower back, posterior thighs
      (b) Onset: 24 hours
      (c) Duration: 1 week
      (d) Associated with lidocaine
   (3) Cauda equina syndrome (CES):
      (a) Injury to lumbosacral plexus; sensory parasthesias, bowel and bladder dysfunction, paraplegia
      (b) Associated with microcatheters in spinal administration: lidocaine + tetracaine > bupivacaine > ropivacaine

C. Esters
   1. Cocaine
      a. First ester class drug used for clinical local anesthesia in 1884
      b. Excellent topical anesthetic
      c. Used for anesthesia and vasoconstriction in nasal mucosa before nasotracheal intubation and during nasal operations
      d. Sympathomimetic properties
         (1) Causes accumulation of synaptic norepinephrine
         (2) Inhibits reuptake of norepinephrine released from adrenergic nerve endings
         (3) Increased synaptic norepinephrine thus facilitates sympathomimetic responses.
         (4) Warning: cocaine can cause severe increases in heart rate and blood pressure and coronary artery vasoconstriction.
      e. CNS stimulant, especially cerebral cortex, because of accumulating synaptic norepinephrine
      f. Pyrogenic activity: potential side effect
      g. Administration route and dosage
         (1) Topical use as 4% to 10% solution for mucous membrane anesthesia, especially nasopharynx
         (2) No other uses because of side effects and toxicities
      h. Pharmacokinetics
         (1) Well absorbed from all routes
         (2) Hydrolyzed by plasma cholinesterases
      i. Drug interaction: causes myocardium to be more responsive and sensitive to catecholamines
      j. Nursing considerations
         (1) Potential for toxicity
         (2) High potential for abuse: powerful cortical stimulant
      k. Signs and symptoms of cocaine toxicity
         (1) Hypertension
         (2) Tachycardia
         (3) Coronary artery vasoconstriction
         (4) Cerebral vascular accidents
         (5) Hyperthermia
         (6) Seizures
         (7) Decreased uterine blood flow—fetal hypoxemia
   2. Procaine (Novocaine)
      a. First synthetic ester class local anesthetic (1904)
      b. Administration route
         (1) Local infiltration
         (2) Peripheral nerve block
         (3) Spinal anesthesia
      c. Pharmacokinetics
         (1) Absorption

(a) Vasoconstrictors prolong local anesthetic action: slower absorption diminishes chance for systemic toxicity.

(2) Metabolized by plasma cholinesterases, which include pseudocholinesterase (PChE)

3. Chloroprocaine (Nesacaine)
   a. Rapid onset, short duration, little systemic toxicity ester class drug
   b. Thrombophlebitis frequent side effect
   c. Notoriety of causing spinal neuropathy has limited its use.
      (1) Toxicity traced to bisulfite preservative and acidic pH of its solution.
      (2) Toxic combination of preservative and acidic solution is now removed.
   d. Administration route
      (1) Local infiltration
      (2) Peripheral nerve block
      (3) Epidural anesthesia (lumbar and caudal routes)
   e. Pharmacokinetics: metabolized by plasma cholinesterases (including PChE)
   f. Pharmacodynamics: blocks sensory more than motor nerves
4. Tetracaine (Pontocaine)
   a. Slow onset of analgesia, long duration, ester class drug synthesized in 1931
   b. Ten times more potent and toxic than procaine
   c. Causes extensive motor and sympathetic blockade
   d. Administration route
      (1) Topical anesthesia
         (a) Corneal
         (b) Endotracheal topical anesthesia
      (2) Spinal anesthesia
         (a) Isobaric solutions: 2 to 3 hours spinal anesthesia
         (b) Add epinephrine: 4 to 6 hours duration
   e. Pharmacokinetics
      (1) Readily absorbed from all routes
      (2) Metabolized by plasma cholinesterases (including PChE)
   f. Pharmacodynamics
      (1) Blocks sensory and motor nerves equally well

D. Amino-amides
   1. Prilocaine (Citanest)
      a. Intermediate potency amino-amide class drug
      b. Duration: 60 minutes
      c. Less vasodilation than lidocaine
      d. Uses
         (1) Local
         (2) Peripheral nerve block
         (3) IV
         (4) Epidural
         (5) Subarachnoid
      e. Metabolism
         (1) Prilocaine releases orthotoluidine, which converts hemoglobin to methemoglobin.
         (2) Prilocaine, 10 mg/kg, yields 3 to 5 g of methemoglobin.
         (3) Treat with methylene blue, 1 to 2 mg/kg (may repeat).
         (4) Symptoms of methemoglobinemia
            (a) Brown-grey cyanosis
            (b) Tachypnea
            (c) Metabolic acidosis
            (d) Hypoxia
            (e) Headache

      (f) Irritability

      (g) Chocolate-colored blood

  2. Lidocaine

    a. Medium-acting local anesthetic of amide class

    b. Quick, potent, and longer lasting than procaine

    c. High incidence of sleepiness and dizziness

    d. IV lidocaine depresses laryngeal and tracheal reflexes.

    e. Notable antidysrhythmic properties on the myocardium

    f. When infiltrated as a local anesthetic, its vasodilator activity facilitates its rate of absorption.

      (1) Epinephrine (coadministered with lidocaine) decreases this vasodilation and absorption, thus prolonging duration of block.

      (2) Mepivacaine does not have this vasodilator effect and thus can be a substitute for lidocaine with epinephrine when epinephrine's use is not desirable.

    g. Administration route and dosage

      (1) Local infiltration: 0.5% to 2% (with or without epinephrine)

      (2) Peripheral nerve block: 1% to 2% solutions (with or without epinephrine)

      (3) Epidural anesthesia: 1.5% to 2% solutions

        (a) Average dose: 15 to 20 mL of 1.5% to 2% solutions

        (b) Duration: 0.75 to 1.5 hours

      (4) Spinal anesthesia, hyperbaric: 1.5% or 5% solutions (with or without dextrose)

        (a) Average dose: 50 to 80 mg (1-1.6 mL)

        (b) Duration: 0.75 to 1.5 hours

        (c) Note: because of possible association with TRI, now recommended that 5% lidocaine solution be diluted with cerebrospinal fluid (CSF) to final concentration of 2% before injection

      (5) Topical anesthesia: 2% jelly or 4% solution

      (6) IV (Bier) block: 40 to 50 mL of 0.5% solution

    h. Pharmacokinetics: metabolized by hepatic microsomal enzymes

    i. Pharmacodynamics: blocks sensory and motor nerves equally well

    j. Nursing considerations

      (1) Lidocaine (topical or IV) useful in anesthetizing trachea before intubation

      (2) Topical or IV lidocaine will depress laryngeal and tracheal reflexes.

  3. Mepivacaine (Carbocaine)

    a. Medium-acting local anesthetic of amide class

    b. Longer duration of action than lidocaine

    c. Does not cause vasodilation as does lidocaine

    d. Moderate potency and toxicity

    e. Administration route and dosage

      (1) Local infiltration: 1% to 2% solutions

      (2) Peripheral nerve block: 1% to 2% solutions

      (3) Epidural anesthesia (lumbar and caudal routes): 1% to 2% solutions

        (a) Average dose: up to 25 mL of 2% solution

        (b) Duration: 1 to 2 hours

      (4) Not for use in spinal anesthesia

    f. Pharmacokinetics: longer acting than lidocaine

    g. Pharmacodynamics: similar to lidocaine (and other amide local anesthetics) except it does not cause vasodilation (alternative to lidocaine with epinephrine)

  4. Bupivacaine (Marcaine, Sensorcaine)

    a. High potency amino-amide

    b. Long duration of action: 3 to 10 hours

    c. Residual analgesia outlasts anesthetic effects.

    d. Cardiac toxicity warning: excessive dosing or accidental IV injection can cause ventricular dysrhythmias that are difficult to correct; do not exceed the maximally allowed dose.

    e. Administration route and dosage

        (1) Epidural or caudal anesthesia: 0.25% to 0.5% solutions

            (a) Average dose: 15 to 20 mL of 0.5% solution

            (b) Duration: 2 to 4 hours

        (2) Spinal anesthesia: 0.75% solution (with or without dextrose)

            (a) Average dose: 7.5 to 12 mg (1-1.6 mL)

            (b) Duration: 2 to 4 hours

    f. Pharmacokinetics: metabolized by hepatic microsomal enzymes

    g. Pharmacodynamics: blocks sensory more than motor nerves

    h. Uses

        (1) Local

        (2) Peripheral nerve block

        (3) Epidural

        (4) Subarachnoid

    i. Nursing considerations

        (1) Has a prolonged anesthetic and analgesic action

        (2) Frequently infiltrated during surgery as a postoperative analgesic for incision pain (analgesia lasts about 4-8 hours)

        (3) May cause ventricular dysrhythmias when local anesthetic doses become excessive or are injected IV by accident. Treatment must be with bretylium or amiodarone. Lidocaine will be ineffective or may worsen condition. Evidence in animal studies suggests Intralipid infusion offers some protection and has been suggested as immediately available in regional block areas.

5. Etidocaine (Duranest)

    a. High potency amino-amide of long duration

    b. Duration 5 to 10 hours

    c. Need high concentration for adequate sensory block

    d. Uses

        (1) Local

        (2) Peripheral nerve block

        (3) Epidural

6. Ropivacaine (Naropin)

    a. High potency amino-amide

    b. Chemically similar to bupivacaine

    c. Produces less motor blockage than bupivacaine

    d. Duration as long as 12 hours

        (1) Similar anesthetic properties to bupivacaine (i.e., both have more of an effect on sensory nerves than on motor nerves, although ropivacaine may have slightly less effect on motor nerves)

        (2) Appears to be somewhat less cardiotoxic than bupivacaine; however, cardiotoxicity may still be of concern with slightly larger doses.

        (3) Preliminary clinical experience suggests a dosing schedule similar to that of bupivacaine.

    e. Uses

        (1) Epidural

        (2) Safe for obstetric use

7. Levobupivacaine (Chirocaine)

    a. Amino-amide local infiltrate

    b. Similar pharmacokinetic profile as bupivacaine

    c. Fast onset, moderate duration

    d. Used for surgical anesthesia and pain management cases

    e. May be administered in combination with epidural fentanyl or clonidine

8. Preservative-free morphine

    a. Brand names: Duramorph, Astramorph, and others

      b. Used as an adjunct for neuraxial (NA) anesthesia

      c. Epidural administration provides pain relief for extended periods.

         (1) No loss of motor or sensory functions

         (2) Some dose-dependent decreases in sympathetic function may occur.

         (3) Respiratory depression always possible but not likely if conservative doses given

      d. Onset occurs 15 to 60 minutes after NA administration; analgesia may last 12 to 36 hours.

      e. Initial adult dose is 2 to 5 mg; duration 12 to 24 hours

      f. Delayed respiratory depression possible; patient should be monitored for 18 to 24 hours after administration, depending on dose given.

      g. Resuscitation equipment and naloxone should be available to counteract any potential respiratory depressant effects.

      h. Nausea and vomiting possible; need for antiemetics should be anticipated.

V. REGIONAL TECHNIQUES

  A. General facts

    1. Anesthetic injected into or around a nerve or nerve plexus

    2. Requires a knowledge of anatomy

    3. Absorption of excessive doses can lead to systemic toxicity.

    4. Epinephrine-containing solutions will delay systemic absorption and thus decrease systemic toxicity.

  B. Topical

    1. Anesthetic is applied directly to:

      a. Skin

      b. Mucous membrane

      c. Urethra

      d. Nose

      e. Pharynx

    2. Systemic absorption occurs after application to mucous membranes.

      a. Increases risk of toxicity if excessive doses applied (especially true of vascular tracheobronchial tree)

  C. IV (Bier blocks)

    1. Produces anesthesia of arm or leg

    2. Injection of large volumes of local anesthetic IV while circulation to the extremity is occluded by a tourniquet

    3. Onset rapid, muscle relaxation profound

    4. Duration depends on tourniquet time inflation.

    5. Risk of toxicity when tourniquet released

    6. No analgesia after circulation restored

    7. Bupivacaine contraindicated in bier blocks because of cardiovascular toxicity

  D. Local infiltration and field blocks

    1. Anesthetic injected directly into tissue

    2. Field block: anesthetic injected into surrounding tissue

      a. Blocks transmission of sensory impulses

      b. Warning: epinephrine-containing solutions should not be infiltrated into confined areas (fingers, toes, ears, nose, penis); gangrene may develop.

    3. Peripheral nerve block: specific site to block conduction

      a. Complications common to nerve blocks

         (1) Reaction to local anesthetic

         (2) Nerve damage

         (3) Failed block

         (4) Hematoma

      b. Infiltration—inject into tissue

      c. Field block—inject into surrounding tissues

      d. Cervical plexus block

         (1) Formed by first four cervical nerves

         (2) Common use for carotid endarterectomy

      e. Brachial plexus block (BPB)

   (1) Formed by anterior rami of C5-C8 and T1, which divide into three trunks to supply shoulders and upper extremity
   (2) Three approaches
    (a) Interscalene used for shoulder surgery
    (b) Supraclavicular anesthetizes entire plexus.
     (i) Risk of pneumothorax
    (c) Axillary
     (i) Most popular
     (ii) Easy and safe
     (iii) Surgery procedures distal to elbow
   (3) Complications
    (a) Horner's syndrome: secondary to stellate ganglion block
    (b) Phrenic nerve block: dyspnea
    (c) Recurrent laryngeal nerve block: hoarseness and weak voice
   (4) Disadvantages
    (a) Ulnar nerve frequently missed
    (b) Musculocutaneous nerve is most often missed with BPB (especially axillary); it is the most proximal branch of brachial plexus.
  f. Distal nerve block of upper extremity
   (1) Can block median, ulnar, and radial nerves
   (2) May be used for isolated finger or toe procedures
  g. Intercostal blocks
   (1) Twelve pair of intercostal nerves supply the ribs and abdominal wall skin and skeletal muscles.
   (2) Used for postoperative pain after thoracic or abdominal surgery
   (3) Used for pain of rib fractures
   (4) Risk of pneumothorax and intravascular injection
   (5) May need to sedate patient for procedure
  h. Lower extremity block
   (1) Supplied by widely separated nerves
   (2) To block entire lower extremity requires blocks of lumbar and sacral plexuses.
   (3) Unpopular because of multiple injections
   (4) Nerves blocked include:
    (a) Sciatic
    (b) Femoral
    (c) Lateral femoral cutaneous
    (d) Obturator
    (e) Saphenous
   (5) Ankle blocks require five nerves around the circumference to be injected.
 E. Sympathetic
  1. Stellate ganglion
  a. Used for diagnosis and treatment of reflex sympathetic dystrophies
  b. Used for management of circulatory insufficiency in upper extremity
  c. Signs of a successful block
   (1) Horner's syndrome
    (a) Ptosis
    (b) Miosis
    (c) Anhydrosis
   (2) Ipsilateral nasal congestion
   (3) Flushing of conjunctiva and skin
   (4) Temperature increase in ipsilateral arm and hand
  d. Common side effects
   (1) Sensation of "lump in the throat"
   (2) Temporary hoarseness and dysphasia because of recurrent laryngeal block

(3) Unpleasant effects of Horner's syndrome

(4) Hematoma

2. Celiac plexus block

a. Used for relief of severe visceral pain (i.e., pancreatic cancer)

b. Complicated technique

c. May see:

(1) Orthostatic hypotension

(2) Increased gastrointestinal motility with possible diarrhea

(3) Vascular injury because of close proximity to aorta

(4) Spinal block

3. Lumbar sympathetic block

a. Used for diagnostic, prognostic, and therapeutic purposes

b. Used for chronic pain syndromes by injecting phenol

c. Complications include:

(1) Neuritis of genitofemoral nerve

(2) Kidney perforation

(3) Subcapsular hematoma

(4) Horner's syndrome

(5) Somatic nerve damage

(6) Subarachnoid injection

(7) Intravascular injection

(8) Perforation of disk

(9) Stricture of ureter

(10) Infection

(11) Ejaculatory failure

(12) Chronic back pain

F. Spinal anesthesia (intrathecal or subarachnoid block)

1. Anesthetic solution injected into intrathecal space

a. Nerve roots and part of spinal cord anesthetized

b. Warning: spinal cord usually ends at L1-L2 interspace; agent should be injected below this level to avoid possible cord trauma.

2. Spinal—block nerve conduction in extremity or region of the body

3. Systemic toxicity: rare because of small doses given

4. Baricity (Table 22-3)

a. Addition of 5% to 10% glucose makes solution heavier than CSF.

b. Solution tends to "sink" within CSF according to pull of gravity.

c. Level of anesthesia influenced by body's position

d. Trendelenburg position will hasten cephalad spread of local anesthetic.

G. Epidural anesthesia

1. Specific facts

a. Anesthetic solutions can be administered into epidural space by:

(1) Single injection

■ TABLE 22-3
■ ■ **Baricity of Solution**

Type	Specific Gravity	Diluent	Uses
Hypobaric	<1.003	Distilled water	Perineal, rectal, and total hip arthroplasty procedures
Isobaric	1.003-1.009	Cerebrospinal fluid	Used when anesthesia required at a specific level (i.e., lower extremity surgery, fractured hips)
Hyperbaric	>1.009	Dextrose 10%	Most frequent use because solution settles to most dependent aspect of subarachnoid space

          (2) Repetitive bolus injections (by catheter)

          (3) Continuous infusion (by catheter)

    b. Produces nerve root, spinal cord, and paravertebral nerve anesthesia

    c. Produces less sympathetic blockade than intrathecal (spinal) block

    d. Higher chance for systemic toxicity than spinal block

          (1) Greater amount of drug needs to be administered for epidural anesthesia (in contrast to spinal anesthesia).

          (2) Greater amount of drug administered is systemically absorbed.

    e. Epidural—agents into thoracic or lumbar epidural space

    f. Because of procedural use of a larger needle, an increased risk for a more pronounced headache is present if inadvertent dural puncture occurs.

  2. Indications

    a. Procedures on abdomen

    b. Procedures on lower extremity

    c. Treatment of chronic pain

    d. Labor analgesia

H. Caudal—injection into sacral canal below dural sac

  1. Used in children and during labor

  2. Single shot for surgery below diaphragm

  3. Continuous block for pain relief

I. NA anesthesia

  1. Common properties for spinal and epidural blocks (i.e., anesthetics)

    a. Typically used for surgical cases involving abdomen, perineum, and lower extremities

    b. Dermatomes

          (1) Used in assessment of evolution and extent of an NA anesthetic

          (2) Nerve roots exiting spinal cord innervate skin in contiguous sensory bands or stripes (1-2 inches wide); these bands arise posteriorly (from spinal column) and typically radiate away laterally, anteriorly, or caudally (looking like zebra stripes, if they could actually be seen).

          (3) Each sensory stripe (dermatome) corresponds to a specific nerve root.

          (4) Each sensory stripe (dermatome) has been investigated, mapped, and standardized in such a manner as to portray the idealized person.

          (5) Anatomic relationships of representative dermatomes (Figure 22-1)

             (a) Neck: C3

             (b) Clavicles: C5

             (c) Nipples: T4

             (d) Xiphoid: T6

             (e) Navel: T10

             (f) Groin: L1

             (g) Knees: L4

             (h) Dorsum of foot: L5

             (i) Lateral ankles: S1

    c. Dermatomes are a guide to determining surgical anesthetic needs (Tables 22-4 and 22-5).

  2. Evolution of an NA anesthetic

    a. Evolution of an NA anesthetic influenced by a number of factors

          (1) Amount of agent given (dose), especially with spinal

          (2) Volume of solution, especially with epidural

          (3) Position of patient after injection (i.e., sitting, supine, Trendelenburg, reverse Trendelenburg)

          (4) Baricity of solution (spinal blocks)

          (5) Anatomic and physiologic considerations

             (a) Height

             (b) Hormonal influences

             (c) Obesity

             (d) Coincident pregnancy

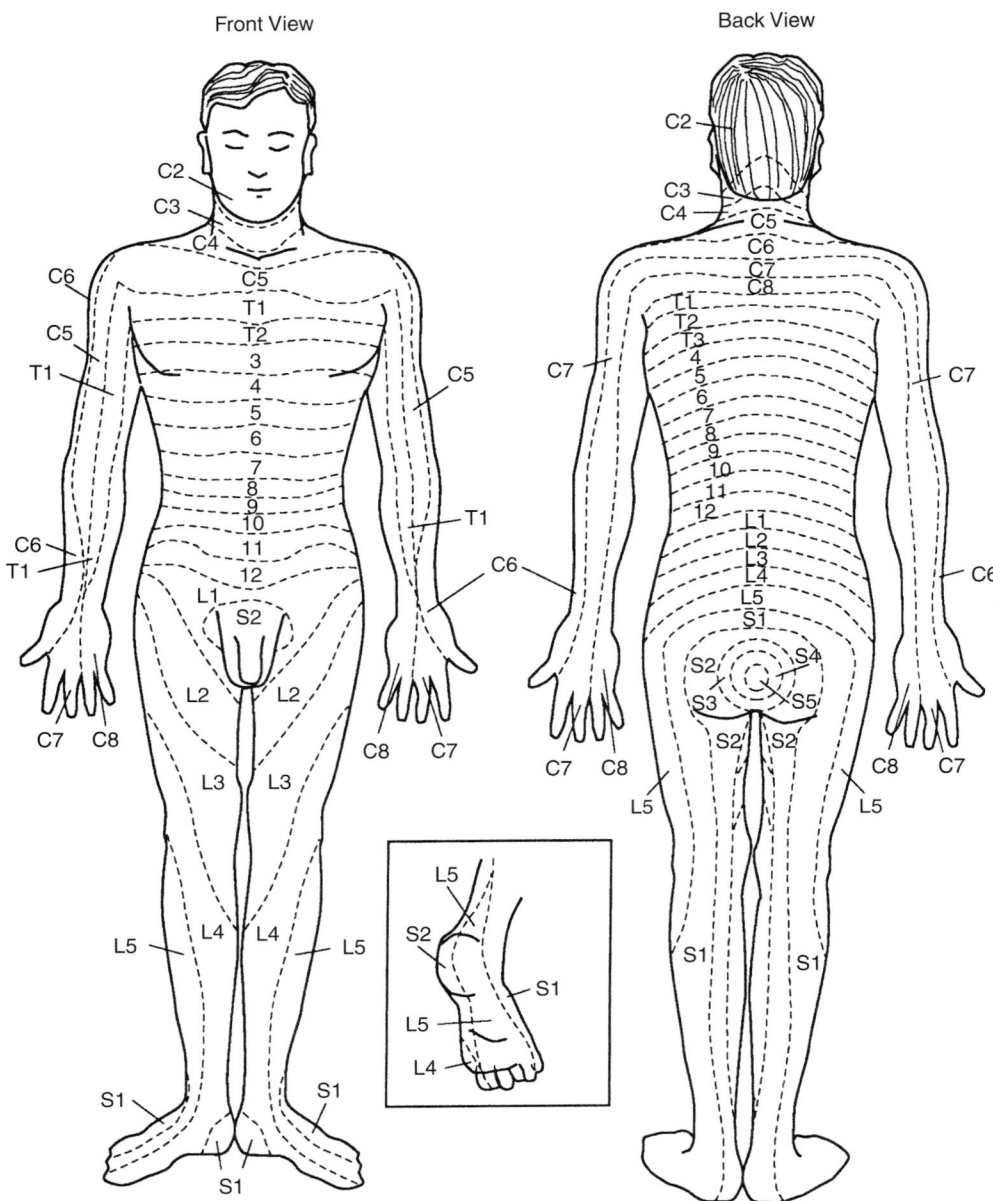

FIGURE 22-1 ■ Dermatomes. (From Cardona VD, Hurn PD, Mason PJB, et al: *Trauma nursing from resuscitation through rehabilitation*, ed 2, Philadelphia, 1994, WB Saunders, p. 444.)

    b. After NA injection, evolution of anesthetic block is monitored closely (as it moves cephalad) by assessing loss of sensation along previously mentioned dermatomal levels (Box 22-2).

    c. Assess loss of temperature sensation as first indication of sensory block (alcohol wipe).

    d. Assess loss of sensation to "sharp" (point of sterile needle) or "dull" (blunt hub of sterile needle).

    e. NA anesthetic noted to first take effect in feet and then move cephalad (degree of cephalad movement being influenced by factors mentioned previously)

  3. Side effects

■ TABLE 22-4
■ ■ **Dermatomes in Relation to Surgical Need and Significance**

Cutaneous Level	Segmental Level	Significance
Pinky digit	C8	Knocked out T1-4
		Cardioaccelerator fibers
Inner arm	T1-2	Some cardioaccelerator fibers blocked
Apex of axilla	T3	Good landmark
Nipple	T4/5	Possible cardioaccelerator fiber block
Xiphoid tip	T7	Splanchnic (T5-L1) may be blocked
Umbilicus	T10	SNS legs (vasodilate)
Inguinal ligament	T12	No SNS block of legs
Outer foot	S1	Most difficult nerve root to anesthetize

SNS, Sympathetic nervous system.

■ TABLE 22-5
■ ■ **Dermatomes Related to Common Surgical Procedures**

Sensory Level	Type of Surgery
T4	Cesarean section, upper abdomen, uterine surgery
T6/7	Lower abdomen, appendectomy, hernia repair
T10	Hip surgery, transurethral resection of prostate, vaginal delivery
T7/8	Tourniquet pain
L1	Lower extremity surgeries, knee surgeries
L2/3	Foot surgery
S2/5	Hemorrhoidectomy, genitalia/buttocks

■ BOX 22-2
■ **SEQUENCE OF SPINAL RESOLUTION**

Order of Loss of Function
1. Autonomic or sympathetic functions (vasomotor, bladder control)
2. Sense of temperature
3. Pain
4. Touch
5. Movement
6. Proprioception (sense of body location)

Example: "Phantom response" is a response in which patients may ask you to straighten their legs when they are already straight. The last position the patients were in before the regional medications taking effect is that position they believe they are still in.

Order of Return of Function
1. Proprioception
2. Movement
3. Touch
4. Pain
5. Sense of temperature
6. Autonomic or sympathetic functions (vasomotor, bladder control)
   Last blocked is first to recover.

    a. Sympathetic blockade more likely to be caused by a spinal rather than an epidural block

    b. Hypotension more likely with an NA block higher than T6 (but less than T3) because such blocks tend to impair sympathetic vasoconstrictor outflow from spinal cord (T6 to L2) to blood vessels of mesentery and lower extremities; this effect can lead to:

      (1) Reduction in venous tone

      (2) Reduction in venous return to heart

      (3) Decrease in cardiac filling and cardiac output

      (4) Decrease in arterial blood pressure

      (5) Reflex increase in heart rate

      (6) Potential for a decrease in coronary blood flow

      (7) Probable increase in myocardial O_2 consumption

    c. Bradycardia more likely with a block higher than T3 because such blocks tend to impair sympathetic cardioaccelerator outflow (T1 to T4) to sinoatrial (SA) and atrioventricular (AV) nodes of myocardium; this effect leaves cardiodecelerator effects of vagus nerve (cranial nerve X) unrestrained.

      (1) Treat with atropine as needed.

      (2) Precautionary treatments that may be considered before potential development of hypotension from sympathetic blockade include:

        (a) Preblock fluid loading: use 20 to 25 mL/kg of normal saline or lactated Ringer's solution.

        (b) Prophylactic administration of intramuscular (IM) ephedrine, 25 to 50 mg

        (c) Not using excessive amounts of NA anesthetics

      (3) Treatment options for hypotension after there has been an excessive NA sympathetic block

        (a) Elevation of patient's legs (this does not necessarily mean placing patient in Trendelenburg position; under some circumstances, Trendelenburg position, if initiated too early, can worsen a high NA block)

        (b) IV fluid boluses as needed to fill dilated venous capacitance vessels

        (c) Vasopressors to support poor vascular tone (i.e., hypotension) until block resolves, such as phenylephrine bolus or infusion

          (i) Consider IV phenylephrine if tachycardia present (incremental IV doses of 20 to 100 mcg). Caution: phenylephrine may cause reflex bradycardia.

          (ii) Consider IV atropine if bradycardia present; incremental IV doses of 0.5 to 1 mg per advanced cardiac life support protocol.

          (iii) Do not hesitate to use incremental doses of IV epinephrine or ephedrine if cardiovascular collapse appears imminent.

          (iv) Consider infusion if cardiovascular depression has occurred.

          (v) Consider placement of arterial line for blood pressure monitoring if needed.

      (4) "High" sensory block equates to neurogenic shock.

        (a) Block higher than T1 may cause severe cardiopulmonary collapse.

        (b) Hydration, vasopressors and vagolytics, intubation, and cardiopulmonary resuscitation may be needed as NA blockade moves closer toward brainstem.

  4. Neurological complications

    a. Postdural puncture headache (PDPH)

      (1) Incidence

(a) Directly related to size of hole made in dura by spinal or epidural needle used: larger needles make larger holes.
(b) Inversely related to age of patient: older patients less likely to experience PDPHs
(c) With regard to spinal anesthesia, blunt (spreading tip) needles less likely than sharp (cutting tip) needles to produce headaches; Whitacre, Sprotte, and Gertie-Marx needles are examples of "blunt tip" category; Quincke needles are an example of the "cutting tip" type.
(2) Symptoms of PDPH
(a) Headache typically felt in frontal or occipital location or both (worsened by sitting or standing up); onset usually after 24 to 72 hours
(b) Associated symptoms: neck ache or stiffness (57%), backache (35%), and nausea (22%)
(c) Less commonly associated symptoms: shoulder pain, blurred vision, vomiting, tinnitus, auditory difficulties, and diplopia (i.e., cross-eyed, from a bilateral abducens nerve palsy)
(d) Severity of PDPH may be relieved by pressure on jugular veins or worsened by pressure on carotid arteries.
(3) Symptomatic treatment includes hydration, analgesics, and caffeinated beverages.
(4) Definitive treatment, if symptoms persist, includes an epidural blood patch that may be given 24 hours after PDPH develops.
  b. Adhesive arachnoiditis
(1) Caused by introduction of foreign materials into intrathecal space
(2) Results in chronic inflammation of arachnoid
(3) Progressive weakness and sensory loss of perineum or lower limbs
(4) May advance to paraplegia
  c. Cauda equina syndrome
(1) May be caused by adhesive arachnoiditis
(2) Persistent paresis of legs
(3) Sensory loss in perineum
(4) Bowel and bladder dysfunction
(5) Effects usually permanent and may slowly deteriorate
(6) In some cases, slow regression of symptoms occurs over months.
  d. Peripheral nerve palsy usually temporary but can be permanent from nerve root damage
  e. Septic meningitis
(1) Symptoms appear within 24 hours of intrathecal contamination.
(a) Fever
(b) Headache
(c) Neck rigidity
(d) Kernig's sign: with patient in supine position, thigh is flexed to a right angle with the trunk; Kernig's sign present if same-sided leg cannot be extended completely because of severe neck pain
(2) Good outcome if diagnosed early; must be treated immediately with antibiotics
5. Respiratory effects
  a. Effects on ventilatory system increase as NA block moves in cephalad direction.
  b. First, ability to cough is weakened from paralysis of abdominal muscles; inability to cough can impair patient's capacity to clear airway secretions.
  c. Next, progressive cephalad anesthesia of intercostal nerves increasingly becomes impaired.
(1) Intercostal sensory nerves and patient's ability to perceive that he or she is breathing by usual sensory cues from the skin (i.e., that the chest wall is moving normally with each breath)

(2) Intercostal motor nerves and patient's ability to take deep breaths (patient's inspiratory capacity also progressively lost)

(3) Note: some deprivation of chest wall sensation can be unavoidable under ordinary circumstances; reassurance helpful in allaying patient's anxiety

(4) Warning: with complete loss of chest wall sensation and patient's complaints of increasing difficulty breathing, possibility of an NA block progressing toward complete phrenic nerve paralysis (C3 to C5) should be suspected: emergent intubation of trachea may be immediately necessary!

    d. Finally, a high enough NA block to cause paralysis of phrenic nerve (C3 to C5) is rarely seen if reasonable attention to technique is provided; however, if apnea does occur, patient will require assisted ventilation and possibly intubation to protect airway from secretions or aspiration of possible gastric contents.

J. Nursing interventions

  1. Hypotension is a common side effect.

  2. Have respiratory support equipment available.

  3. Assess residual block.

    a. Motor block can outlast some sensory blocks.

    b. Be careful standing patients.

    c. Motor assessment

      (1) Dorsiflexion/plantar flexion (push down on gas pedal)

      (2) Invert and evert movement (windshield wiper movement of foot)

      (3) Extension

  4. Some resolution of block before discharge from PACU

  5. Appropriate discharge instructions should be given.

    a. Do not get up without assistance first few times.

    b. Patient may have long-acting local anesthetic drug on board so may not have return of complete sensation and motor ability.

  6. Contraindications

    a. Absolute contraindications

      (1) Patient refusal

      (2) Coagulation deficiencies

      (3) Infection at block site

    b. Relative contraindications

      (1) Patient age (i.e., older uncooperative children, Alzheimer's)

      (2) Lack of cooperation or inability to follow directions or consent

      (3) Chronic neurological disorders

      (4) Allergy to local anesthetics

      (5) Specific cardiac problems

        (a) Locals intensify Mobitz I, II, and third-degree AV blocks.

        (b) Aortic stenosis or idiopathic hypertrophic subaortic stenosis with subarachnoid block (SAB): do not tolerate vasodilation

  7. Additive opioids to epidural NAs

    a. Morphine: 3 to 10 mg; duration 12 to 24 hours

    b. Demerol: usually epidurally—early respiratory depression

    c. Fentanyl: 20 to 100 mcg; duration 2 to 3 hours

    d. Sufentanil: 40 to 50 mcg—early respiratory depression

VI. IV ANESTHETIC INDUCTION AGENTS

  A. Common properties

    1. General facts

      a. IV administration

      b. Good patient acceptance

      c. Quick onset

      d. Very brief duration

      e. Quick offset because of redistribution

    f. IV administration quickly and reversibly induces anesthesia.
      (1) CNS depression occurs.
      (2) Spontaneous ventilation arrested
      (3) Laryngeal reflexes lost
      (4) Increased risk for aspiration can occur.
    g. Patients generally recover within 5 to 10 minutes after a single dose.
    h. Specific agents have variable side effects, depending on circumstances.
  2. Elimination
    a. Amount of anesthetic agent distributed to each region of body is directly proportional to amount of blood each region receives; those regions receiving greatest amounts of blood will be anesthetized first.
      (1) Highly perfused regions
        (a) Brain
        (b) Heart
        (c) Kidney
        (d) Liver
      (2) Moderately perfused regions
        (a) Muscle
        (b) Skin
      (3) Mildly perfused regions
        (a) Fat
        (b) Bone marrow
      (4) Poorly perfused regions
        (a) Tendons
        (b) Ligaments
        (c) Bone
    b. Although metabolism does occur for most of these drugs, plasma levels are initially reduced, primarily by redistribution.
    c. Redistribution occurs very quickly with IV induction agents.
      (1) On IV injection (single dose), injected drug is diluted into primary vascular space (i.e., central compartment—concentration of drug in blood now at its maximum).
      (2) Next (and very quickly), central compartment distributes drug first to those organs richly supplied by the vasculature.
        (a) Because brain and heart are small, only minor amounts of drug distributed here
        (b) At this time, concentration of drug in central compartment still near its peak level
        (c) Note that drug's effects on CNS and cardiovascular system are now maximal.
      (3) As time proceeds, drug in central compartment is redistributed into larger organs and tissue less richly supplied by vasculature (i.e., muscle, skin, fat, and bone marrow).
        (a) If monitored, concentration of drug in vascular space would now appear to decline.
        (b) Clinically, effects of drug on CNS and cardiovascular system begin to wane.
  3. Respiratory effects
    a. Respiratory, laryngeal, and pharyngeal reflexes blunted
    b. Upper airway obstruction can be caused by relaxation of surrounding soft tissue muscle tone.
    c. Ventilatory depression usually guaranteed
  4. Immune response effect
    a. Initial studies suggest that T-lymphocyte proliferations inhibited by most of the induction agents (thiopental more than methohexital and etomidate, which have equal effect) except propofol
    b. Propofol may be one of the least T lymphocyte–inhibiting drugs to use for immunocompromised patients.

    5. Nursing considerations
      a. Ventilation will need to be supported until effects of these agents wear off.
      b. If gastric contents present, airway and lungs will need to be protected until protective airway reflexes return.
        (1) Be vigilant.
        (2) Maintain proper positioning of airway.
        (3) Be prepared for immediate suctioning of airway if vomiting occurs.

B. Thiopental
  1. General facts
    a. Brand name: Sodium Pentothal and others
    b. Used as anesthetic IV induction agent
      (1) Generally rapid
      (2) Pleasant
    c. Used for:
      (1) Cardioversion
      (2) Brain protection (cardiopulmonary arrest)
    d. Dose-dependent depression of CNS function: effects range from sedation through coma
  2. Administration route and dosage
    a. Individuals with adequate cardiovascular stability
      (1) 2.5 to 5 mg/kg, titrated to effect
    b. Individuals without adequate cardiovascular stability (slower administration recommended)
      (1) Induction dosage of thiopental must be reduced.
      (2) Consider alternate IV agents: etomidate or ketamine.
      (3) Lowers blood pressure 25% to 30%
    c. Respiratory impact
      (1) Decreased tidal volume
      (2) Apnea may occur.
      (3) Garlic taste
  3. Pharmacokinetics
    a. Onset: less than 30 seconds
    b. Duration: 5 to 10 minutes
    c. Metabolism
      (1) Hepatic microsomal enzymes (slow metabolism; toxic accumulation can occur)
      (2) Chronic use causes predictable enzyme induction.
    d. Elimination
      (1) Termination of action primarily by redistribution
      (2) Multiple dosing saturates this process and will delay clinical recovery.
      (3) Thiopental largely eliminated in urine as water-soluble metabolites
      (4) Elimination half-life 12 hours (large volume of distribution); hangover effect
  4. Pharmacodynamics
    a. Dose-dependent depression of CNS function
      (1) Depresses polysynaptic responses
      (2) Thought to potentiate effect of inhibitory neurotransmitter (gamma-aminobutyric acid [GABA])
      (3) Important locus of depression is reticular activating system (required for wakefulness).
    b. Hyperalgesic effect at low blood levels; patient may perceive more pain.
  5. Hepatic effects
    a. With liver disease, metabolism impaired, drowsiness prolonged, and ventilation depressed
  6. Nursing considerations

    a. Reconstituted solution very alkaline (pH >10) and incompatible with acidic solutions

        (1) Infiltrated injections may need special attention: apply warm compresses.

    b. Patient may display yawning, hiccoughing, and possible laryngospasm.

    c. Contraindicated with sulfa allergy

    d. Contraindicated with history of porphyria

    e. Causes histamine release (cautious use with asthma)

    f. Intra-arterial thiopental—arterial spasm, thrombosis, and distal limb ischemia—gangrene and necrosis (dilute then vasodilate)

        (1) Stop injection but leave needle in artery.

        (2) Arterial injection of lidocaine (10 mL of 1%) provides analgesia and vasodilatation.

        (3) Brachial plexus block will have same action for a more prolonged period.

        (4) Papaverine (40-80 mg in 20 mL saline) is an effective vasodilator.

        (5) Anticoagulate with a heparin.

C. Methohexital

  1. General facts

    a. Brand name: Brevital and others

    b. Used as anesthetic induction agent

    c. Electroconvulsive therapy

    d. Dose-dependent depression of CNS function: effects range from sedation through coma.

    e. Potency: twice that of thiopental

    f. Action: similar to thiopental at equianesthetic doses but has less effect on respiratory depression

  2. Administration route and dosage

    a. IV induction: 1 to 2 mg/kg

    b. Rectal doses

        (1) 20 to 30 mg/kg

        (2) Used in pediatric patients

        (3) Onset in about 7 minutes

        (4) Recovery usually begins in about 45 minutes.

  3. Pharmacokinetics (see section VI.B.3)

  4. Pharmacodynamics (see section VI.B.4)

  5. Nursing considerations

    a. Several side effects on injection: pain, myoclonus, hiccoughs

D. Etomidate

  1. General facts

    a. Brand name: Amidate

    b. Used as anesthetic induction agent

    c. Agent of choice in patients with cardiovascular disease

    d. Excellent cardiovascular stability

        (1) Less likely to cause hypotension than thiopental

        (2) Heart rate and cardiac output tend to remain constant; negative inotropic effects are minimal.

        (3) Slight decrease in blood pressure possible because of slight peripheral vascular relaxation

    e. Dose-dependent suppression of adrenal steroidogenesis

        (1) Up to 24 hours after one induction dose

        (2) Also occurs after prolonged infusions

            (a) Use contraindicated in critically ill patients

            (b) May cause reversible adrenal insufficiency

    f. Dissolved in propylene glycol: pain and venoirritation may occur on injection.

  2. Administration route and dosage

    a. IV induction: 0.2 to 0.4 mg/kg

3. Pharmacokinetics
   a. Onset: 15 to 45 seconds
   b. Duration: 3 to 12 minutes
   c. Metabolism: hepatic microsomal enzymes and plasma esterases; hydrolysis of this drug nearly complete
   d. Elimination
      (1) Action terminated primarily by redistribution
      (2) Rapid metabolism also contributes to prompt awakening.
      (3) Overall, clearance five times faster than with thiopental
4. Pharmacodynamics
   a. Hypnotic without analgesic effect
   b. Unconsciousness in 1 minute or less
5. Cardiovascular effects: see General Facts, section VI.D.1.
6. Respiratory effects
   a. Dose-dependent hypoventilation and apnea
   b. Rapid return of spontaneous ventilation
7. Skeletal muscle effects
   a. Myoclonus occasionally seen on induction
   b. Premedication with narcotic or benzodiazepine diminishes myoclonus.
8. Nursing considerations
   a. Several side effects on injection
      (1) Dose-dependent suppression of adrenal function
         (a) Etomidate inhibits cortisol synthesis.
         (b) Circulating levels of cortisol are depressed.
         (c) Circulating levels of ACTH are increased.
         (d) Effects may last up to 24 hours after a single dose.
      (2) Myoclonus
      (3) Pain when rapidly injected into small vein
      (4) Nausea or vomiting common
   b. Use of etomidate infusions in intensive care units (ICUs) leads to adrenocortical suppression with increased morbidity and mortality.
      (1) Adrenal insufficiency possible
      (2) Use contraindicated in critically ill patients

E. Ketamine
   1. General facts
      a. Brand name: Ketalar
      b. Used as anesthetic induction agent
      c. Used in MAC procedures
      d. Intense analgesic properties
      e. Useful in minor surgical procedures
         (1) Burn debridement
         (2) Oral surgery where intense analgesia is necessary
      f. Related to phencyclidine (PCP) and lysergic acid diethylamide (LSD); vivid hallucinations possible during and after surgery
   2. Administration route and dosage
      a. IV doses
         (1) Induction: 1 to 2 mg/kg
            (a) Rapid onset
            (b) Recovery usually begins in about 5 to 10 minutes.
         (2) Maintenance: 0.5 to 1 mg/kg every 5 to 30 minutes
         (3) Infusion: 1 mg/kg per hour (may have fewer aftereffects)
      b. IM dose: 5 to 10 mg/kg
         (1) Onset within 3 to 5 minutes
         (2) Recovery usually begins in about 10 to 20 minutes.
      c. Sedation or MAC
         (1) 0.2 to 0.8 mg/kg over 2 to 3 minutes
         (2) 2 to 4 mg/kg IM
      d. Preemptive analgesia (prevention of chronic pain)
         (1) 0.15 to 0.25 mg/kg IV

e. Combined with propofol for MAC sedation (less respiratory depression than with propofol alone)
   (1) Loading: 1 to 3 mg/kg IV; infusion: 5 to 20 mcg/kg per minute
   (2) Run propofol at normal MAC dosing
3. Pharmacokinetics
   a. Onset: 15 to 45 seconds
   b. Duration: 3 to 12 minutes
   c. Metabolism: occurs extensively by hepatic microsomal enzymes
   d. Elimination
      (1) Action terminated primarily by redistribution
      (2) Largely eliminated in urine
4. Pharmacodynamics
   a. Depresses neocortex
   b. Produces excellent analgesia
   c. Stimulates limbic system
   d. Does not depress reticular activating system
   e. Produces dissociation of thalamoneocortical and limbic systems
   f. Produces dissociative anesthesia
      (1) No recollection of surgery
      (2) Patient appears to be awake.
      (3) Minimal respiratory depression
5. CNS effects
   a. Increases cerebral blood flow; has been reported to increase intracranial pressure
   b. Emergence from anesthesia can be associated with delirium.
      (1) Alterations in mood and body image
      (2) Vivid dreams, sometimes progressing to hallucinations
      (3) Out-of-body experiences or psychomotor activity
   c. Recurrent illusions or flashbacks (may occur up to several weeks after anesthesia)
   d. Strategies to reduce or eliminate "emergence" phenomena
      (1) Use diazepam or barbiturate as premedicant.
      (2) Preoperatively mention possibility of dreams.
      (3) Recovery in dark, quiet environment has no beneficial effect.
6. Cardiovascular effects
   a. Increases heart rate, blood pressure, and cardiac output
7. Respiratory effects
   a. Respiratory, laryngeal, and pharyngeal reflexes remain nearly normal although not considered protective.
   b. Spontaneous ventilation tends to be maintained.
   c. Ventilatory depression and obstruction indicate overdosage or rapid administration.
   d. Potential for increased salivary gland secretion may require patient premedication with an antisialagogue such as glycopyrrolate.
   e. Note: in acutely hypovolemic patients, ketamine acts as a myocardial depressant with depletion of endogenous catecholamines
8. Skeletal muscle effects
   a. Usually causes increase in muscle tone
9. Contraindications
   a. Hypertension
   b. Previous stroke
   c. Psychiatric disorders
   d. Elevated intracranial pressure
   e. Pulmonary hypertension
10. Nursing considerations
   a. Can produce vivid hallucinations in PACU; patient may need to be restrained or require benzodiazepine sedation.
   b. Incidence of delirium

(1) Greater in adults than in children
(2) Fifty percent of adults older than 30 years experience excitement and delirium.
  c. Preanesthetic visit should mention potential for dreamlike effects that may be experienced on emergence and during first day after ketamine exposure.
  d. Can produce irritability and compromise suck in infants
F. Propofol
  1. General facts
    a. Brand name: Diprivan
    b. Used as anesthetic induction agent
    c. Used in MAC sedation
    d. ICU sedation
    e. Formulated in a milky white emulsion of glycerin, lecithin (from egg yolks), and soybean oil
      (1) Avoid in patients with allergy to eggs and soybean.
    f. May cause hypotension if injected too rapidly; more pronounced in hypovolemic patients
    g. Mechanism of action
      (1) Decreases rate of dissociation of GABA from GABA-A receptor
      (2) GABA-mimetic
    h. No analgesic effects
    i. Rapid and alert emergence
    j. High incidence of pain on IV injection
      (1) Distal veins: 40%
      (2) Larger veins: 10%
      (3) IV lidocaine used to decrease this pain (usually 2% lidocaine used)
    k. No preservatives: cannot be stored after opening ampules (opened ampules can support vigorous growth of microorganisms)
      (1) Continuous IV infusions with bottle reservoirs must be discarded after 12 hours.
  2. Administration route and dosage
    a. Reduce dosage in elderly, premedicated, and hypovolemic patients.
    b. Induction: 1.5 to 2.5 mg/kg
    c. Maintenance: vary infusion from 50 to 150 mcg/kg per minute.
      (1) Propofol can be used as primary anesthetic.
      (2) Narcotics and nitrous oxide (N_2O) may be added as adjuncts.
      (3) Infusion discontinued 10 to 15 minutes before case ends
  3. Pharmacokinetics
    a. Onset: 15 to 45 seconds
    b. Duration: 5 to 10 minutes
    c. Metabolism: extremely rapid
    d. Elimination
      (1) Action terminated primarily by redistribution; prolonged administration, however, can saturate this process.
      (2) Largely eliminated in urine
      (3) Clearance 5 to 10 times faster than with thiopental
      (4) Clearance significantly greater than liver blood flow
      (5) Pulmonary uptake extensive
  4. Nursing considerations
    a. Lower incidence of postoperative side effects
      (1) Less hangover
      (2) Less nausea and vomiting
      (3) Less psychomotor impairment
    b. Earlier ambulation and discharge after outpatient surgery
      (1) Recovery time decreased
      (2) Outpatients ready to go home earlier
      (3) Patients resume day-to-day activities earlier.

           (4) Patients more alert and drink fluids and eat earlier

           (5) Patients often more responsive and in elevated mood

      c. Rapid emergence from anesthesia may hasten pain awareness.

           (1) Propofol does not provide any residual postanesthetic analgesic effect.

           (2) Intraoperative or postoperative analgesics may need to be administered.

      d. Allergic reactions

           (1) Rarely, clinical features of anaphylaxis have occurred shortly after administration of propofol.

G. Benzodiazepines (see section VIII.C)

  1. Diazepam (Valium)

  2. Midazolam (Versed)

  3. Lorazepam (Ativan)

VII. IV OPIOID ANESTHETICS

  A. Common properties

    1. General facts

      a. Synthetic opioids

      b. Used as analgesic or anesthetic induction agents

      c. Also used as premedicant: sedative, analgesic, or anesthetic adjunct

      d. Intraoperative use will decrease requirement for general anesthesia.

    2. Pharmacokinetics

      a. Onset: rapid

      b. Duration of analgesia: 30 minutes

      c. Redistribution half-life: 15 minutes

      d. Metabolized by liver

      e. Elimination

           (1) Lower doses: termination of action primarily by redistribution; multiple doses or large doses will saturate this process (see section VI.A.2.c)

           (2) Higher doses: primarily by metabolism; various half-lives

              (a) Remifentanil: 0.25 to 0.33 hours

              (b) Alfentanil: 1.5 hours

              (c) Sufentanil: 2.5 hours

              (d) Fentanyl: 3.5 to 4 hours

              (e) Morphine: 3 to 4 hours

              (f) Meperidine: 3 to 4 hours

              (g) Hydromorphone (Dilaudid): 2 to 3 hours

    3. Pharmacodynamics

      a. Appears to modulate intracellular production of cyclic adenosine monophosphate

      b. May inhibit transmembrane calcium currents

           (1) Effect appears to be potentiated by calcium channel blockers.

           (2) Effect at presynaptic neurons may decrease release of neurotransmitters.

      c. Overall, opioids inhibit pain by modulating synaptic impulse transmission.

      d. Opioids decrease perception of and response to pain by:

           (1) Effects at level of dorsal horn cells of spine

           (2) Activation of descending inhibitory pathways from brainstem

           (3) Altering emotional response to pain in limbic cortex

           (4) Opioids relieve continuous "dull" pain better than intermittent sharp pain.

    4. Side effects

      a. Miosis: stimulation of oculomotor nerve; reversed by naloxone, atropine, or glycopyrrolate

      b. Bradycardia: stimulation of vagus nerve treatable with atropine or glycopyrrolate

      c. Muscle rigidity: alfentanil worst offender; more pronounced when injected rapidly
      d. Nausea and vomiting: use antiemetics.
      e. Hypotension
        (1) May be caused by bradycardia and/or a decrease in sympathetic tone
        (2) Exaggerated in patients who are anxious, hypovolemic, or in pain
      f. Delayed awakening
      g. Respiratory depression: background partial pressure of carbon dioxide in arterial blood ($Paco_2$) required to stimulate normal ventilation is increased.
   5. Nursing considerations
      a. Observe for respiratory depression in PACU.
        (1) Assess need for ventilatory support.
        (2) Naloxone should be readily available.
      b. Reduce doses in elderly and hypovolemic patients.
      c. Respiratory depression can outlast analgesic effect.
 B. Morphine
   1. General facts
      a. Prototype and other narcotics compared with it
      b. Use preservative-free for epidural and intrathecal doses.
      c. Mu receptor agonist
   2. Administration route and dosage
      a. Guidelines for IV loading dose (titrated to effect)
        (1) Perioperative analgesia: 2 to 15 mg
          (a) Onset: 1 to 5 minutes
          (b) Peak analgesia at 20 minutes
          (c) Duration: 4 hours
        (2) Epidural anesthesia: 2- to 5-mg bolus
        (3) Intrathecal: 0.2 to 1.0 mg
        (4) Often used in patient-controlled analgesia pumps postoperatively
      b. Histamine release resulting in:
        (1) Hypotension
        (2) Pruritis
        (3) Wheezing
        (4) Red-streaking along IV route
        (5) Skin wheal formation
   3. Active metabolite may accumulate in renal-impaired patients.
   4. Useful in treatment of angina in acute coronary syndromes (decreases preload and pain associated)
   5. Spasm biliary smooth muscle (incidence 3%)
 C. Meperidine
   1. General facts
      a. Brand name: Demerol
      b. Synthetic narcotic analgesic
      c. Structurally similar to atropine
        (1) Mydriasis, tachycardia, and dry mouth secondary to anticholinergic effects (like atropine)
      d. One tenth as potent as morphine
   2. Administration route and dosage
      a. Guidelines for IV loading dose (titrated to effect)
        (1) Perioperative: used for shivering
        (2) Thought to act through a potassium receptor mechanism
        (3) Use 12.5 to 25 mg for postoperative shivering.
        (4) Contraindicated in patients receiving monoamine oxidase inhibitors
   3. Contraindicated in seizure disorders
      a. Normeperidine is primary metabolite.

(1) One half as active as meperidine in regards to analgesia
(2) Toxicity manifests as myoclonus and seizures.

D. Hydromorphone
  1. General facts
    a. Brand name: Dilaudid
    b. Synthetic narcotic analgesic
  2. Administration route and dosage
    a. Guidelines for IV loading dose (titrated to effect)
      (1) Perioperative analgesia: 0.5 to 2.0 mg
        (a) Onset: less than 1 minute
        (b) Duration: 2 to 4 hours
    b. Six times more potent than morphine

E. Alfentanil
  1. General facts
    a. Brand name: Alfenta
    b. Used as analgesic and anesthetic adjuvant
    c. Synthetic narcotic analgesic
      (1) One tenth as potent as fentanyl
      (2) Ten times more potent than morphine
    d. Metabolized in liver (not for patients with liver failure)
      (1) Note: Emycins, cimetidine, calcium channel blockers, and antifungals inhibit liver metabolism; may see increased effects
  2. Administration route and dosage
    a. Guidelines for IV loading dose (titrated to effect)
      (1) Perioperative analgesia: 10 to 25 mcg/kg
      (2) Balanced anesthesia: 50 to 150 mcg/kg
    b. Guidelines for continuous IV infusion (titrated to effect)
      (1) Perioperative analgesia: 0.25 to 1 mcg/kg per minute
      (2) Balanced anesthesia: 0.5 to 3 mcg/kg per minute

F. Fentanyl
  1. General facts
    a. Brand name: Sublimaze
    b. Used as analgesic and anesthetic adjuvant
    c. Synthetic narcotic analgesic: 100 times more potent than morphine
    d. Duration of analgesia: 30 to 60 minutes
    e. Mu receptor agonist
    f. Pharmacokinetics
      (1) Lungs are a large, inactive storage site.
      (2) Up to 75% of first doses goes through first pass effect in lungs.
  2. Administration route and dosage
    a. Guidelines for IV loading dose (titrated to effect)
      (1) Perioperative analgesia: 1 to 3 mcg/kg
      (2) Balanced anesthesia: 5 to 15 mcg/kg
    b. Guidelines for continuous IV infusion (titrated to effect)
      (1) Perioperative analgesia: 0.01 to 0.03 mcg/kg per minute
      (2) Balanced anesthesia: 0.03 to 0.1 mcg/kg per minute

G. Remifentanil
  1. General facts
    a. Brand name: Ultiva
    b. Used as analgesic and anesthetic adjuvant
    c. Synthetic narcotic with extremely short half-life
    d. After initial loading dose, effects of this drug must be continued by continuous infusion.
    e. Abrupt discontinuation of infusions of this drug can cause sudden onset of extreme pain and related adverse effects.
    f. Because remifentanil by itself cannot ensure unconsciousness, its exclusive use in general anesthesia not recommended

       g. Spinal or epidural use not recommended because of motor dysfunctions that might occur from its glycine vehicle (glycine is a spinal cord neurotransmitter)

  2. Administration route and dosage

      a. Guidelines for IV loading dose (titrated to effect)

         (1) Balanced anesthesia: 0.5 to 2 mcg/kg

      b. Guidelines for continuous IV infusion (titrated to effect)

         (1) Balanced anesthesia: 0.25 to 0.5 mcg/kg per minute

  3. Nursing considerations

      a. Sudden discontinuation of infusions of this drug after surgery may bring on sudden onset of intense pain; supplemental use of longer-lasting analgesics must be anticipated and administered without delay.

      b. Because of its high potency, remifentanil not administered by nursing personnel

      c. Rapid onset of remifentanil may be associated with life-threatening rigidity if large doses administered by bolus or rapid infusion.

H. Sufentanil

  1. General facts

      a. Brand name: Sufenta

      b. Used as analgesic and anesthetic adjuvant

      c. Mu receptor agonist

      d. Synthetic narcotic analgesic

         (1) Is 500 to 1000 times more potent than morphine

         (2) Is 5 to 10 times more potent than fentanyl

      e. Used in balanced general anesthesia

         (1) For induction and maintenance

         (2) In major surgical procedures

  2. Administration route and dosage

      a. Guidelines for IV loading dose (titrated to effect)

         (1) Balanced anesthesia: 1 to 3 mcg/kg

      b. Guidelines for continuous IV infusion (titrated to effect)

         (1) Balanced anesthesia: 0.01 to 0.05 mcg/kg per hour

         (2) Discontinue infusion 30 to 45 minutes before wake-up.

I. Opioid antagonist: naloxone (Narcan)

  1. General facts

      a. Nonselective competitive antagonist at all opioid receptors

         (1) Administer slowly to avoid side effects: pulmonary edema, hypertension, dysrhythmias, and pain.

      b. Short duration of action: 30 to 45 minutes

      c. Monitor for returned respiratory depression.

  2. Administration route and dosage

      a. Dose of 0.2 to 0.4 mg reverses opioid-induced respiratory depression; titrate 0.04 mg to avoid acute reversal of analgesia.

      b. Plasma half-life: 1 to 1.5 hours; shorter than most opioids

      c. Clinical effects last 30 to 90 minutes.

      d. Narcan infusion: 5 mcg/kg per hour

VIII. IV ANESTHETIC ADJUNCTS

  A. Droperidol

    1. General facts

        a. Brand name: Inapsine

        b. Because of its antiemetic properties, this antipsychotic agent widely used in anesthesia

        c. Moderate antiemetic effects; dose: 0.0625 to 0.125 mg IV

        d. Neuroleptic anesthesia (Innovar)

           (1) Combines properties of droperidol with those of fentanyl in a 50:1 mixture

           (2) Primary effects

              (a) Ataraxia

          (b) Some amnesia

          (c) Reduced motor movement

          (d) Patient arousable and responsive but indifferent

      e. Additional effects

          (1) Alpha-adrenergic blocking activity produces vasodilation and mild to moderate hypotension.

          (2) Elevates threshold for myocardial dysrhythmias but may also prolong QT interval

          (3) Anticonvulsant action

          (4) Slight respiratory depression

  2. Pharmacokinetics: metabolized by liver

  3. Pharmacodynamics: works within CNS as dopamine antagonist

  4. Side effects

      a. Dystonic reaction: muscle spasm of face, neck, tongue, or upper back

          (1) Occurs in about 1% of patient population

          (2) May also be caused by metoclopramide

          (3) Treatment: diphenhydramine (Benadryl), 25 to 50 mg by slow IV

          (4) Alternate treatment: benztropine (Cogentin), 1 to 2 mg IV

      b. Postanesthetic dysphoria (internalized overwhelming fear)

          (1) May occur when droperidol (a psychotropic drug) is given alone without beneficial effect of narcotics such as fentanyl

          (2) May occur if beneficial effect of a coadministered narcotic wanes

          (3) Effect of droperidol usually persists longer than that of narcotics.

          (4) Patients and their families may require some reassurance if dysphoric effect occurs.

      c. Contraindicated in Parkinson's

      d. Black box warning: QT-interval prolongation, torsade de pointes, cardiac arrest, and ventricular tachycardia have been reported in patients; should have electrocardiogram monitoring when administering IV

B. Anticholinergics

  1. Atropine

      a. Dose: 0.5 to 1 mg IM or IV

      b. Inhibits salivary and respiratory tract secretions

      c. Causes bronchodilation

      d. Counteracts bradycardia and related dysrhythmias

      e. Given with antiacetylcholinesterase (anti-AChE) agents at end of general anesthesia

      f. Crosses blood-brain barrier, causes CNS stimulation

      g. Can produce central anticholinergic syndrome

          (1) Restlessness, irritability, disorientation, delirium

          (2) Can be major cause of postoperative dysphoria

          (3) Central effects can be reversed by physostigmine.

  2. Scopolamine

      a. Same preoperative use as atropine

      b. Dose: 0.3 to 0.6 mg IM or IV

          (1) Dose transdermal: 5 mcg/h

      c. Causes CNS depression, drowsiness, amnesia, euphoria, fatigue

      d. May cause paradoxical excitation

      e. Less effective at preventing bradycardia

      f. Higher incidence of postoperative dysphoria and delirium

      g. May cause short-term amnesia when given with morphine

  3. Glycopyrrolate (Robinul)

      a. Longer acting than atropine

      b. More potent antisialagogue than atropine

      c. Dose: 0.1 to 0.2 mg IM or IV

      d. More potent inhibitor of gastric acid secretion than atropine

      e. Does not cross blood-brain barrier

      f. Does not produce sedation

      g. Does not produce central anticholinergic syndrome

      h. More rapid postoperative awakening than with atropine

      i. Prevents bradycardia and less likely to cause tachycardia than atropine

C. Benzodiazepines

  1. General facts

     a. Administered by oral, IM, or IV routes

     b. Absorbed from gastrointestinal tract

     c. Metabolized by hepatic oxidative microsomal enzymes; inactive metabolites excreted in urine

     d. Lack of analgesic properties

     e. Dose-related depression of ventilation

     f. Warning: ventilatory rate must be monitored closely after IV sedation; use pulse oximetry to confirm patient's return to normalcy.

     g. Exhibits amnestic, anxiolytic, hypnotic, sedative properties

     h. Also exhibits anticonvulsant and muscle relaxant properties

     i. Bind to modulating sites on GABA receptors in CNS

     j. Leads to hyperpolarization of postsynaptic membranes; highest density of benzodiazepine receptors is in cerebral cortex, where there is an inhibitory effect on excitation of neurons.

       (1) Mild cardiovascular depressant effects: mild vasodilation

       (2) Minor direct myocardial depression

       (3) Greater effects from midazolam than from diazepam and lorazepam

     k. Skeletal muscle relaxation reflects action on spinal internuncial neurons.

       (1) Skeletal muscle tone reduced

       (2) Benzodiazepines do not reduce surgical requirements for muscle relaxants.

     l. Recovery of fine motor skills

       (1) More rapid with midazolam than with diazepam or lorazepam

     m. Can markedly attenuate cardiostimulatory effects of ketamine; also minimizes emergence sequelae of ketamine

     n. Smoking, consumption of alcohol, increased age, and use of antacids and cimetidine all decrease clearance of benzodiazepines

  2. Diazepam

     a. Brand name: Valium and others

     b. Used as a sedative and anesthetic adjunct

     c. Insoluble in water

     d. Parenteral formulation contains propylene glycol; injection may be associated with venous irritation and pain.

     e. Dosing schedule

       (1) Sedation

         (a) IV: 2.5 to 5 mg

         (b) Orally (PO): 5 to 10 mg

       (2) Induction of general anesthesia: 0.25 to 0.5 mg/kg IV

       (3) Treatment of seizures: 0.10 mg/kg IV and titrate to effect

     f. Onset

       (1) IV: rapid

       (2) PO: 30 to 60 minutes

     g. Duration: IV, 15 minutes to 3 hours

     h. Low hepatic clearance rates: elimination half-life, 20 to 40 hours

     i. Metabolism

       (1) Desmethyldiazepam active metabolite

       (2) Onset may cause resedation in 4 to 6 hours

       (3) 48 to 96 hours for desmethyldiazepam before elimination

  3. Lorazepam

     a. Brand name: Ativan

     b. Used as sedative and anesthetic adjunct

     c. IV sedation during regional anesthesia

        d. Use as an anticonvulsant

        e. More potent than Valium or Versed

        f. Insoluble in water

            (1) Parenteral formulation contains propylene glycol; injection may be associated with pain and venous irritation.

        g. Dosing schedule for sedation

            (1) IV: 1 to 2 mg

            (2) PO: premedicant, 0.05 mg/kg (not to exceed 4 mg)

        h. Onset

            (1) May be slow and somewhat unpredictable

                (a) May be marked lag between peak blood concentration and clinical effect

                (b) Clinical effect may be difficult to titrate.

            (2) IV: 5 to 20 minutes

            (3) IM: 0.5 to 2 hours

            (4) PO: 1 to 2 hours

        i. Duration

            (1) IV: 4 to 6 hours

            (2) IM: 8 hours

            (3) PO: 8 hours

        j. Elimination half-life: 10 to 20 hours

    4. Midazolam

        a. Brand name: Versed

        b. Used as sedative and anesthetic adjunct

        c. Water-soluble formulation

        d. Minimal local irritation on injection

        e. Midazolam has a steep dose-response curve; careful titration very important

        f. Dosing schedule

            (1) Sedation

                 (a) IV: 1 to 4 mg

                 (b) IM: 0.05 to 0.1 mg/kg

            (2) Induction of general anesthesia: 0.1 to 0.2 mg/kg IV

        g. Onset

            (1) IV: 15 minutes

            (2) IM: 10 to 30 minutes

         h. Duration

            (1) IV: 2 to 6 hours (induction dose)

            (2) IM: 1 to 2 hours

         i. Rapid and extensive hepatic metabolism and renal excretion; elimination half-life, 2 to 4 hours

D. Benzodiazepine competitive antagonist

    1. Flumazenil

        a. Brand name: Romazicon

        b. Only drug available in this class

        c. Specific benzodiazepine receptor antagonist

        d. Blocks CNS effects of benzodiazepines

        e. Dosing schedule: IV doses of 0.1-mg increments to maximum of 1 mg

        f. Onset (IV): within 1 minute

        g. Duration: 1 to 2 hours

        h. Hepatic metabolism and renal excretion

            (1) Redistribution half-life: about 5 minutes

            (2) Elimination half-life: about 60 minutes

        i. Nursing considerations

            (1) Must monitor for resedation because duration of action less than all benzodiazepines' duration of action

            (2) Contraindicated for chronic benzodiazepine users (precipitates seizures)

    E. Alpha$_2$-agonists
      1. Alpha$_2$-receptors
        a. Majority are in presynaptic nerve terminals.
        b. Activation inhibits adenylate cyclase activity, which limits norepinephrine release from storage vesicles.
        c. Major physiological effect (negative feedback mechanism)
          (1) Vascular smooth muscle: postsynaptic alpha$_2$ receptors produce vasoconstriction.
          (2) CNS postsynaptic alpha$_2$ receptor agonism causes sedation and peripheral vasodilation, resulting in decreased blood pressure.
      2. Clonidine: prototypical drug
        a. Premedication dosing: 0.1 to 0.3 mg (typical adult dose)
        b. Side effects: dry mouth, sedation, bradycardia, and contact dermatitis
        c. Decreased minimum alveolar concentration of inhaled and decreased IV drug requirements
        d. Used for prevention/treatment of emergence delirium in children
        e. Analgesic activity: epidural/SAB administration produces analgesia.
        f. Withdrawal symptoms: rebound hypertension
        g. Useful in preemptive analgesia (prevention of chronic pain)
        h. Useful in treatment of chronic pain in combination with clonazepam
      3. Dexmeditomidine (Precedex)
        a. Produces cooperative sedation, pain relief, anxiety reduction, stable respiratory rates, and predictable cardiovascular response
        b. Uses
          (1) MAC sedation
          (2) ICU sedation
          (3) Adjunct to general or regional anesthesia
        c. Dosage and administration
          (1) Used only as a continuous infusion lasting less than 24 hours
          (2) Loading dose: 1 mcg/kg over 10 minutes
          (3) Maintenance: 0.2 to 0.7 mcg/kg per hour
          (4) Cautions: may potentiate effects of opioids, sedatives/hypnotics, anesthetics, and other vasoactive agents
  IX. VOLATILE INHALATIONAL ANESTHETICS
    A. Common properties
      1. General facts
        a. Exist as liquids that evaporate at room temperature
        b. Amount of liquid evaporated controlled by a device called a vaporizer
        c. Concentration of vapor administered determines patient's depth of anesthesia.
        d. The term minimum alveolar concentration defines the concentration (vol%) of anesthetic vapor (at 1 atmosphere of pressure) that prevents skeletal muscle movement in 50% of patients given a painful stimulus (surgical skin incision). Minimum alveolar concentration is determined only after anesthetic has had time to equilibrate throughout body.
      2. Administration route and dosage
        a. "Simple" inhalational anesthesia
          (1) Volatile agent used by itself with no adjuncts
          (2) Either halothane or sevoflurane used because they are pleasant smelling; these two agents recommended for mask inductions and maintenance anesthesia
          (3) Enflurane, isoflurane, and desflurane used only for maintenance anesthesia because they are too irritating to inhale for mask inductions; with these agents, general anesthesia commenced with a short-acting IV induction agent
        b. "Balanced" inhalational anesthesia
          (1) IV adjuncts (narcotics, N_2O, muscle relaxants) added to enhance effects of volatile agents, thus reducing doses of inhalational agents required

3. Pharmacokinetics
   a. Uptake into capillary blood (from alveoli) directly proportional to lipid solubility of anesthetic vapor
   b. Amount of anesthetic agent distributed to each region of body directly proportional to amount of blood each region receives; those regions receiving greatest amounts of blood will be anesthetized first.
      (1) Highly perfused regions
          (a) Brain
          (b) Heart
          (c) Kidney
          (d) Liver
      (2) Moderately perfused regions
          (a) Muscle
          (b) Skin
      (3) Mildly perfused regions
          (a) Fat
          (b) Bone marrow
      (4) Poorly perfused regions
          (a) Tendons
          (b) Ligaments
          (c) Bone
   c. Vapor elimination from various regions of body (back to lungs) also determined by regional rates of blood flow; elimination slowest from regions with poorest blood supply
      (1) Poorly perfused regions serve as storage sites for volatile anesthetics— the extent of this "storage" being a function of the time allowed these regions to absorb anesthetic agent and their size (i.e., obese patients have a larger capacity to store volatile anesthetics than slender patients).
4. Pharmacodynamics
   a. Dose-dependent CNS depression
   b. Several sites and mechanisms of action are under consideration; all of these are not completely understood.
   c. Overall, it can be stated simply that general anesthetics "anesthetize" by impairing CNS synaptic transmission.
5. CNS effects
   a. Impairs CNS synaptic transmission
   b. Decreases cerebral metabolism
   c. Increases cerebral blood flow (CBF)
      (1) Effect occurs within minutes.
      (2) CBF variably increased by each agent
      (3) Intracranial pressure (ICP) also variably increased
      (4) Increases in intracranial swelling and ICP are serious concerns in cases involving head trauma; note that the above deleterious effects of volatile agents can be attenuated by intentionally hyperventilating the patient to achieve hypocarbia.
6. Cardiovascular effects
   a. Sensitization of myocardium to dysrhythmogenic actions of catecholamines
      (1) Halothane > isoflurane = enflurane
      (2) Ventricular ectopy, tachycardia, or fibrillation all possible
7. Respiratory (ventilatory) system
   a. Dose-dependent depression of spontaneous ventilation
   b. Dulls ventilatory responsiveness to hypoxemia and hypercarbia
   c. Obtunds laryngeal and pharyngeal reflexes
      (1) Some of the agents can be used to facilitate intubation (i.e., halothane and sevoflurane).
      (2) Depressed laryngeal reflexes increase risk for aspiration (if gastric contents are present).
   d. Bronchodilation

(1) Direct relaxing effect on bronchial smooth muscles

(2) All the volatile agents can be useful in unconscious patients, but only halothane and sevoflurane are useful in initiating anesthesia by mask (the others are too irritating to inhale by awake patients).

8. Renal effects

   a. Dose-dependent decreases in renal blood flow, glomerular filtration, and urine output can be offset by adequate prehydration.

9. Hepatic effects

   a. Dose-dependent reductions in total hepatic blood flow can lead to impaired hepatocyte oxygenation and a self-limiting form of hepatic dysfunction (can be more significant with halothane).

   b. Although all volatile anesthetics can cause a rare form of severe hepatitis, certain adults exposed to halothane appear to be at greater risk (see section IX.B.7.c).

10. Gastrointestinal effects

    a. Relaxes smooth muscle and motility

11. Uterine effects

    a. Dose-dependent relaxation of uterine smooth muscle

       (1) Greater degrees of relaxation may cause greater amounts of uterine bleeding during cesarean sections.

       (2) A safe rule of thumb is to administer volatile anesthetics at a dose equal to 0.5 minimum alveolar concentration (a dose that should only inhibit uterine contractility by about 80%); supplemental analgesia can be provided by coadministration of N_2O with O_2 in a 50:50 mixture.

12. Drug interactions that potentiate effects of volatile anesthetics (some of these drugs can also introduce some of their own unique problems)

    a. Acute ethanol intoxication

    b. Ketamine

       (1) May enhance occurrence of dreams and hallucinations

       (2) When used in patients with asthma receiving aminophylline, may induce seizures (i.e., combinations of ketamine and aminophylline can lower seizure threshold)

    c. N_2O (see section X)

    d. Narcotics (morphine, fentanyl, sufentanil)

       (1) Cause a dose-dependent desensitization in normal ventilatory response to increases in plasma CO_2; narcotics upwardly reset concentration of plasma CO_2 that is considered to be "normal" by medullary chemoreceptors.

       (2) Higher-than-normal concentrations of plasma CO_2 eventually will restore "normal" spontaneous tidal volumes, but this assumes that ventilation is sufficient in the meantime to maintain an adequate supply of O_2.

       (3) As a consequence of this dose-dependent narcotic-induced hypercapnia, CO_2 levels will continue to rise until catecholamines released trigger cardiac dysrhythmias or until hypercapnia becomes so severe that CNS becomes progressively depressed.

       (4) Patients who have received narcotics must be monitored closely to ensure that their ventilatory patterns are sufficient to maintain adequate oxygenation and exhalation of CO_2; supplemental O_2 and ventilatory equipment must be available.

       (5) Patients with stiff chest or wooden chest syndrome can be associated with supranormal dosages of IV potent narcotics.

    e. Sedatives (benzodiazepines and barbiturates)

       (1) As with narcotics, sedatives decrease chemoreceptor sensitivities to plasma CO_2, but unlike narcotics, sedatives also depress the maximal response that can be achieved to increase ventilation (i.e., no increase

in plasma CO_2 will ever be sufficient to stimulate chemoreceptors enough to restore normal tidal volumes); thus excessive use of sedatives (more so than narcotics) threatens a patient with irreconcilable hypercapnia.

    (2) Patients must also be monitored closely to ensure adequate oxygenation and exhalation of CO_2; supplemental O_2 and ventilatory equipment must be supplied as needed.

  f. Acute tetrahydrocannabinol (marijuana) intoxication

13. Drug interactions that antagonize effects of volatile anesthetics (increase amount of volatile anesthetics required)
- **a.** Amphetamines
- **b.** Cocaine
- **c.** Chronic ethanol intoxication
- **d.** Naloxone
- **e.** Chronic tetrahydrocannabinol (marijuana) intoxication

14. Toxicities
- **a.** Respiratory depression
- **b.** Respiratory arrest (apnea)
- **c.** Cardiovascular depression
- **d.** Postobstructive pulmonary edema
- **e.** Malignant hyperthermia

15. Nursing considerations
- **a.** Impairment of spontaneous ventilation
  - (1) CNS response to hypercapnia may be depressed.
  - (2) CNS response to hypoxemia may be depressed.
- **b.** Depression of laryngeal and pharyngeal reflexes
  - (1) Aspiration risks are increased. Warning: be vigilant!
- **c.** Volatile anesthetics have dysrhythmogenic effects (to varying degrees); these effects are worsened by concomitant use of epinephrine (in mixture with local anesthetics).
- **d.** Volatile anesthetics offer no residual analgesic effect.
  - (1) When general anesthesia is discontinued, patients will awaken into an awareness of the pain of their surgery (unless IV analgesics, regional anesthetics, or local anesthetics are used before patient's emergence from general anesthesia).
  - (2) Rapidity with which patients awaken into pain is determined in part by how fast their anesthetic wears off.
- **e.** Be vigilant for malignant hyperthermia (see Chapter 24); its onset is sometimes delayed and may first be recognized in PACU.
- **f.** Monitoring vital signs will trace waning residual effects of anesthesia.
- **g.** Monitoring urine output will assess patient's volume status, renal blood flow, glomerular filtration rate, and overall health of kidneys.
- **h.** Hypothermia
  - (1) Results from marked intraoperative heat loss
  - (2) May lead to marked peripheral vasoconstriction
    - (a) If skin appears blanched, suspect vasoconstriction.
    - (b) If skin appears hyperemic, vasoconstriction less likely
  - (3) Temperature of patient must be normalized.
    - (a) Administer warmed IV fluids.
    - (b) Use active rewarming methods (warmed blankets or air).
  - (4) May lead to profound shivering
    - (a) Increases O_2 consumption (important in anemic patients or in patients with poor pulmonary or cardiac reserve)

B. Halothane
- **1.** General facts
  - **a.** Brand name: various manufacturers
  - **b.** Oldest agent currently in use; commonly used in pediatric anesthesia
  - **c.** Its vapor is pleasant smelling and nonirritating.

      d. Commonly used for mask inductions

      e. Not likely to cause coughing and laryngospasm

      f. Can be used for maintenance anesthesia

  2. Administration route

      a. Inhalation only

  3. Pharmacokinetics

      a. Metabolism: by hepatic microsomal enzymes

      b. Elimination

          (1) Unmetabolized drug: lungs (80%)

          (2) Metabolized drug: kidneys (20%)

  4. CNS effects

      a. Cerebral vasodilation

          (1) Greatest with halothane

          (2) Can induce increase in ICP

          (3) Hypocapnia, if induced before exposure, will blunt increase in ICP.

  5. Cardiovascular effects

      a. Myocardial depression: decreased heart rate, contractility, stroke volume, and cardiac output

      b. Systemic vasodilation: decreased systemic vascular resistance (SVR) by direct relaxant effect on vascular tone

      c. Impairs normal function of AV node

          (1) Bradycardia

          (2) Nodal rhythms

          (3) Wandering pacemaker

      d. Dysrhythmias

          (1) Sensitization of myocardium (by volatile anesthetics) to exogenously administered epinephrine is highest seen (i.e., greater in halothane than in isoflurane and desflurane, which are equal in effect but greater than enflurane).

             (a) Dose of exogenously administered epinephrine (e.g., found in some local anesthetics) should be kept to less than 2 mcg/kg body weight.

             (b) Above sensitization to epinephrine can be lessened by coadministration of lidocaine.

  6. Renal effects

      a. Decreased renal blood flow and glomerular filtration may be offset by adequate prehydration.

  7. Hepatic effects

      a. Reversible reduction in hepatic blood flow is possible.

      b. Reversible decrease in hepatic function and self-limited hepatotoxicity is possible.

      c. Halothane hepatitis

          (1) Rare (1:20,000 to 1:200,000); less likely in children

          (2) Can lead to massive hepatic necrosis and death

          (3) Occurs 5 to 6 days after exposure

          (4) Risk factors may include enzyme induction, female gender, genetic predisposition, hypoxemia, hypermetabolic states, multiple exposures, middle age, and obesity.

          (5) Appears to be caused by covalent binding of oxidative metabolites to liver parenchyma

             (a) Binding of these metabolites to the liver deranges its molecular architecture in such a way that the body does not recognize the liver as "self" anymore (thus, neoantigens are formed), and the immune system begins to attack the "nonself" liver with antibodies.

          (6) Disease presents with marked increases in serum alanine aminotransferase (ALT), aspartate aminotransferase (AST), and bilirubin; other findings include hepatomegaly, hepatic encephalopathy, fever, jaundice, malaise, and nonspecific gastrointestinal symptoms.

8. Sympathetic nervous system effects
   a. Sensitizes heart to dysrhythmogenic action of catecholamines
9. Skeletal muscle effects
   a. Causes mild relaxation
   b. Can augment overall effect of muscle relaxants
10. Toxicities (by two different mechanisms)
    a. Self-limited mild hepatotoxicity (related to decreased blood flow) with presenting symptoms and signs of low-grade fever, nausea, lethargy, and mild transient elevations of liver aminotransferase enzymes (ALT, AST)
    b. "Halothane hepatitis" is a much rarer but more severe toxicity (see section IX.B.7).
11. Drug interactions
    a. Adrenergic blockers: hypotension as a result of decrease in heart rate and contractility

C. Enflurane
1. General facts
   a. Brand name: Ethrane
      (1) Older agent used with decreasing popularity, in part because of its slow onset and offset of anesthetic action
   b. Volatile liquid with pungent and irritating odor
      (1) Not useful for mask inductions; may cause breath-holding, coughing, and laryngospasm
      (2) Used only for maintenance anesthesia after general anesthesia has been initiated with IV induction agents
   c. In an unwanted reaction, enflurane can be degraded into carbon monoxide as it passes through the CO_2 absorbent of the anesthesia machine. Normally, enflurane passes through the anesthesia machine unchanged and does not interact with soda lime or Baralyme of CO_2^- absorbing canisters. However, if enflurane is exposed to excessively dry soda lime or Baralyme, it can be chemically degraded and released as carbon monoxide gas.
2. Administration route
   a. Inhalation only
3. Pharmacokinetics
   a. More resistant to metabolism than halothane
   b. Some liver metabolism (2%)
   c. Metabolites excreted by kidneys
   d. Primarily eliminated as unchanged exhaled vapor (80%-95%)
4. CNS effects
   a. Motor hyperactivity in 2% of patients
      (1) May see electroencephalographic seizure patterns (contraindicated in patients with seizure disorders)
      (2) May progress to tonic-clonic seizures
5. Cardiovascular effects
   a. Hypotension possible
      (1) Mild depression of cardiac output
      (2) Mild relaxation of vascular resistance
   b. Dysrhythmias
      (1) Stable heart rate
      (2) Sensitization of myocardium (by volatile anesthetics) to exogenously administered epinephrine is minimal (i.e., greater with halothane than with isoflurane and desflurane, which are equal but greater than enflurane).
      (3) Dose of exogenously administered epinephrine (e.g., found in some local anesthetics) should be kept to less than 11 mcg/kg body weight.
6. Respiratory effects (see section IX.A.7)
7. Hepatic effects
   a. Less likely when compared with halothane but still may cause syndrome such as "halothane hepatitis" (see section IX.B.7.c)

8. Skeletal muscle effects
    a. Promotes and potentiates neuromuscular blockade, although it is not a true nondepolarizing or depolarizing muscle relaxant
9. Drug interactions (see section IX.A.12)
10. Nursing considerations
    a. May enhance seizure activity
    b. Patients more hemodynamically stable than with halothane
    c. Enflurane, which is slowly eliminated, most likely of all volatile anesthetics to produce a lingering CNS depressant effect in PACU
    d. Caution: increased risk of fluoride toxicity leading to acute renal failure if hepatic enzyme induced or taking isoniazid

D. Isoflurane
  1. General facts
    a. Brand name: Forane
    b. Clinically useful anesthetic for maintenance of general anesthesia
    c. Volatile liquid with strongly pungent and irritating odor
    d. Not useful for mask inductions; may cause breath-holding, coughing, and laryngospasm
    e. Used only for maintenance anesthesia after general anesthesia has been initiated with IV induction agents
    f. In an unwanted reaction, isoflurane can be degraded into carbon monoxide as it passes through the CO_2 absorbent of the anesthesia machine (see carbon monoxide discussion, section IX.C.1.c).
  2. Administration route and dosage
    a. Inhalation only
  3. Pharmacokinetics
    a. More resistant to metabolism than enflurane and halothane
    b. Eliminated primarily by exhalation as an intact molecule
    c. Some metabolism (0.2%) by liver
    d. Metabolites excreted by kidneys
  4. CNS effects (see section IX.A.5)
  5. Cardiovascular effects
    a. Myocardial function only slightly affected
      (1) Weak negative inotrope
      (2) Increases coronary blood flow; may promote "coronary steal" phenomenon
    b. Peripheral vasodilation
    c. Dysrhythmias
      (1) No bradycardia
      (2) Possible tachycardia
      (3) Sensitization of myocardium (by volatile anesthetics) to exogenously administered epinephrine is less than that seen with halothane (i.e., greater effect with halothane than with isoflurane and desflurane, which are equal in effect but greater than enflurane).
      (4) Dose of exogenously administered epinephrine should be kept to less than 7 mcg/kg body weight.
  6. Respiratory effects (see section IX.A.7)
  7. Hepatic effects
    a. Historically, a possible carcinogenic effect reported
      (1) Original study and results not reproducible
      (2) Clinical use now widely accepted
  8. Skeletal muscle effects
    a. Promotes and potentiates neuromuscular blockade
  9. Toxicity: rare
  10. Drug interactions (see section IX.A.12)
  11. Nursing considerations
    a. Commonly used inhalational agent
    b. Postoperative shivering may be caused by increased heat loss from intraoperative vasodilation.

E. Desflurane
   1. General facts
      a. Brand name: Suprane
      b. Newest clinically useful anesthetic for maintenance of general anesthesia
      c. Volatile liquid with pungent and irritating odor
      d. Not useful for mask inductions; may cause breath-holding, coughing, and laryngospasm
      e. Used only for maintenance anesthesia after general anesthesia has been initiated with IV induction agents
      f. In an unwanted reaction, desflurane can be degraded into carbon monoxide as it passes through the CO_2 absorbent of the anesthesia machine (see carbon monoxide discussion, section IX.C.1.c).
      g. Solubility in blood extremely low and similar to N_2O
      h. Allows for very fast onset and offset of CNS effects
   2. Administration route and dosage
      a. Inhalation only
   3. Pharmacokinetics
      a. Extremely resistant to metabolism (only 0.02% metabolized)
      b. Most chemically inert of all volatile anesthetic agents
      c. Eliminated primarily by exhalation as an intact molecule
   4. Cardiovascular effects
      a. May have coronary arteriolar vasodilator effects that promote "coronary steal" and myocardial ischemia; this concern is controversial clinically but should not be a problem perioperatively as long as O_2 supply to myocardium is maintained and its O_2 demand is minimized.
      b. During sudden increases in inspired gas concentrations, desflurane stimulates a transient, sympathetically mediated increase in heart rate and blood pressure (to a lesser extent this is also observed with isoflurane); this response can be blunted by preadministration of narcotics such as fentanyl.
      c. Dysrhythmias
         (1) Sensitization of myocardium (by volatile anesthetics) to exogenously administered epinephrine is comparable to that seen with isoflurane (i.e., greater effect with halothane than with isoflurane and desflurane, which are equal in effect but greater than enflurane).
         (2) Dose of exogenously administered epinephrine should be kept to less than 7 mcg/kg body weight.
   5. Respiratory effects (see section IX.A.7)
   6. Hepatic and renal systems
      a. Hepatic and renal blood flow appear to be well preserved.
   7. Skeletal muscle effects
      a. Promotes and potentiates neuromuscular blockade
   8. CNS effects
      a. Remarkably fast onset and offset of anesthesia
      b. Solubility in blood very low (as with N_2O)
      c. Preliminary evidence suggests that desflurane at 1 minimum alveolar concentration significantly increases CSF pressure more so than 1 minimum alveolar concentration isoflurane.
   9. Nursing considerations
      a. Commonly used for maintenance anesthesia in adults and in ambulatory surgery settings
      b. Extremely rapid onset and offset of CNS effects; rapid offset leaves no lingering analgesia; requirement for supplemental analgesia must be anticipated.
F. Sevoflurane
   1. General facts
      a. Brand name: Ultane
      b. Because of chemical configuration, it cannot be broken down into carbon monoxide even if it does pass through dry CO_2 absorbents (see section IX.C.1.c).

      c. Sevoflurane can, however, be converted into other toxic products, including compounds A and B (see section IX.F.10).

      d. Its vapor is pleasant smelling and nonirritating.

         (1) Very useful for mask inductions

         (2) Also useful for maintenance anesthesia as long as certain criteria are followed (see section IX.F.10)

  2. Administration route

      a. Inhalation only

  3. Pharmacokinetics

      a. Up to 5% of administered dose metabolized by liver

  4. Cardiovascular effects

      a. Has less potent coronary arteriolar vasodilator effects and does not appear to cause "coronary steal"

      b. During sudden increases in inspired gas concentrations, it does not result in transient, sympathetically mediated increases in heart rate and blood pressure (i.e., unlike desflurane and to a lesser extent isoflurane).

      c. Dysrhythmias

         (1) Unlike other volatile agents, sevoflurane does not appear to sensitize myocardium to dysrhythmogenic effects of exogenously administered catecholamines.

  5. Respiratory effects

      a. Dose-dependent depression of ventilation

      b. Pleasant smelling and nonirritating; of all the volatile agents, least likely to cause coughing, breath-holding, excessive salivation, or laryngospasm

  6. Hepatic and renal systems

      a. Hepatic and renal blood flow appear to be well preserved.

      b. Hexafluoroisopropanol, one of the metabolites, is conjugated in liver with glucuronic acid and excreted by kidneys into urine.

      c. Fluoride ion, the other metabolite, may be associated with renal impairment if allowed to accumulate (see section IX.F.10).

  7. Skeletal muscle effects

      a. Promotes and potentiates neuromuscular blockade

  8. CNS effects

      a. Solubility in blood very low (as with desflurane and N_2O)

         (1) Allows for fast onset and offset of CNS effects

         (2) Speed of onset and offset slightly slower than desflurane and N_2O

      b. Not associated with convulsive or epileptic activity (unlike enflurane)

      c. Causes minimal increases in ICP over the 0.5 to 1 minimum alveolar concentration range

  9. Toxicity of metabolites

      a. Fluoride ion can be nephrotoxic if levels allowed to rise high enough.

         (1) Peak concentration of fluoride ion appears to be similar to that after enflurane use.

         (2) No clinical demonstration of nephrotoxicity has yet been described, even though moderately elevated plasma levels of fluoride ion have been seen.

         (3) Caution is advised in using sevoflurane in patients with known renal impairment.

      b. Hexafluoroisopropanol is potentially hepatotoxic if not eliminated rapidly by glucuronidation (beware in patients with hepatic disease); glucuronide metabolite is excreted by kidneys (be wary in patients with renal impairment).

  10. Breakdown product

      a. Sevoflurane can be broken down by exposure to Baralyme or soda lime; rate of this breakdown is increased by certain conditions.

      b. Several breakdown products can be formed.

         (1) Compounds A, B, C, D, and E

(2) Note: only compound A (and to a lesser extent compound B) is likely to be clinically relevant.

(3) Compound A causes renal, hepatic, and cerebral damage in animal studies.

    (a) This has led to recommendation that sevoflurane fresh gas flow rate not be titrated below 2 L/min for greater than 2 minimum alveolar concentration hours.

11. Nursing considerations
    a. Pediatric use becoming more common and competing with halothane usage
    b. Adult use in ambulatory surgery settings becoming more common
    c. Least irritating of all the volatile agents used
    d. Extremely rapid onset and offset of CNS effects; rapid offset leaves no lingering analgesia; requirement for supplemental analgesia must be anticipated.
    e. May not be useful in patients with hepatic or renal insufficiency

X. GASEOUS INHALATIONAL ANESTHETIC (N_2O)
A. General facts
    1. Exists as an inorganic gas at atmospheric pressure
    2. Brand name: various manufacturers
    3. Odorless to sweet-smelling inorganic gas
    4. Nonflammable but will support combustion
    5. Prominent analgesic effects
        a. Reduces amount of volatile agents required
        b. Analgesic effect further enhanced by narcotics
    6. Weak anesthetic effects
        a. Not potent enough to provide anesthesia
        b. Minimal muscle relaxant properties
B. Administration route
    1. Administered by inhalation
    2. Clinically useful doses range between 50% and 70% fraction of inspired gases
        a. Use of greater concentrations may cause hypoxia.
        b. Clinical doses at 50% to 70% provide limited analgesic effects.
        c. The limited analgesia provided may be enhanced by co-administration of opioids.
C. Pharmacokinetics
    1. Quick onset of effects occurs over minutes.
        a. Quick onset related to its very low solubility in blood
        b. Quick onset also related to high concentrations used
    2. Metabolism negligible
    3. Offset of effects
        a. Five to 10 minutes (assuming adequate ventilations)
        b. Related to its very low solubility in blood
        c. Assumes adequate ventilation of fresh O_2 into lungs
    4. Diffusion hypoxia and anoxia
        a. When an N_2O-O_2 blend is being delivered into patients' lungs, N_2O cannot accumulate in alveoli more than the 50% to 70% being given; however, when external delivery of N_2O is stopped, the entire amount of N_2O that accumulated within the patient can diffuse back into alveoli at a concentration approaching 100% if the patient is poorly ventilated.
        b. Back diffusion of N_2O dilutes alveolar O_2 and ultimately causes hypoxemia.
        c. Accumulating alveolar N_2O must be ventilated out of lungs and replaced with a fresh supply of 100% O_2.
D. CNS effects
    1. Mild amnesia (incomplete CNS depression)
    2. Very good analgesic effects
    3. May increase CBF and ICP

  E. Cardiovascular system
     1. May initially increase heart rate, SVR, and cardiac contractility indirectly by evoking release of catecholamines
     2. However, ultimately decreases heart rate, SVR, and cardiac contractility by a direct depressant effect
        a. Depressant effect seen when catecholamine stores in sympathetic nerve endings depleted because of prolonged hypovolemia, cardiac failure, shock, or trauma
  F. Pulmonary and ventilatory system
     1. Chemoreceptor response to hypercapnia decreased
     2. High inhaled concentrations (50%-70%) required for analgesia
        a. Must mix this agent with 100% O_2, not air (21% O_2)
        b. Must be vigilant for possible development of hypoxemia
  G. Uterine effects
     1. Does not alter contractility in doses used for analgesia
  H. Untoward effects
     1. Diffusion hypoxia (see section X.C.4)
     2. Nausea may be related to diffusion of N_2O into middle ear.
     3. Undesirable expansion by N_2O of closed gaseous spaces (within body) filled with nitrogen
        a. Room air approximately 80% nitrogen
        b. When N_2O introduced into lungs, it (as do all gases) will begin to evenly distribute itself (through bloodstream) throughout body's fluid space, and also into any collections of air or nitrogen.
        c. As it moves down its concentration gradient into the blood and any collections of air, it will be met by the opposite movement of nitrogen down its concentration gradient (from the collections of air) toward the lungs full of N_2O (and O_2) but very little nitrogen.
        d. Given enough time, these two gases will equilibrate down their gradients.
        e. Because N_2O is 34 times more soluble in blood than nitrogen, N_2O equilibrates first and thus tends to expand any pockets of air trapped within the body until the nitrogen eventually equilibrates "out."
        f. In the interim (while nitrogen is trying to leave), there can be a tremendous increase in the volume and pressure of these pockets of gases, which leads to the undesirable gaseous expansions.
        g. Examples of trapped air that can expand (with consequent dilemmas) include middle ear (nausea, a ruptured tympanic membrane), small air pneumothoraces (tension pneumothorax), air emboli in blood (myocardial infarction, stroke), and air emboli in CSF (tension pneumoencephaly).
     4. Undesirable collapse of closed gaseous spaces (within body) filled with N_2O
        a. Exact opposite of the preceding can occur after a patient has been under general anesthesia with N_2O for a long period; in this case, an eardrum can be severely retracted until room air nitrogen equilibrates back into the gaseous vacuum left behind in the middle ear space after the N_2O equilibrated "out."
  I. Drug interactions
     1. Narcotics enhance analgesia and may enhance circulatory depression (see sections X.A.5 and X.E.2).
  J. Nursing considerations
     1. Be wary of diffusion hypoxemia in patients who have received intraoperative N_2O; on their initial arrival in the PACU, patients may have some degree of diffusion hypoxia if N_2O was not adequately eliminated from their bodies before their departure from the operating room (OR).
     2. Be wary of potential for increased nausea.
     3. Be wary of potential for expanded or retracted pockets of air.

XI. NONDEPOLARIZING MUSCLE RELAXANTS (NDMRs)
   A. Common properties
      1. Physiology of neuromuscular junction (NMJ) (Figure 22-2)
         a. Anatomy and physiology
            (1) Presynaptic nerve terminal
               (a) Releases "packets" of neurotransmitter
            (2) Neurotransmitter
               (a) Acetylcholine (ACh)
               (b) Transmits a chemical signal across the synaptic cleft
            (3) Synapse (synaptic cleft)
               (a) Extremely narrow, extracellular interconnection point between a nerve ending and a muscle cell
            (4) Postsynaptic ACh receptors (on muscle cells)
         b. Presynaptic activity
            (1) Impulse conducted down presynaptic neuron
            (2) Presynaptic nerve ending depolarized.
            (3) Nerve ending releases ACh into synapse.
         c. Synaptic activity
            (1) Released ACh diffuses across synapse to postsynaptic receptors on muscle cell.
         d. Postsynaptic activity
            (1) ACh binds to receptors on muscle cell.
            (2) Postsynaptic membrane of muscle cell is depolarized.
            (3) Membrane depolarization triggers a mechanism within muscle cell that leads to contraction.
         e. Termination of skeletal muscle contraction
            (1) Impulses no longer conducted down presynaptic neuron
            (2) Presynaptic nerve ending repolarizes.
            (3) ACh release into synapse reduced
            (4) Cholinesterase in synapse hydrolyzes previously released ACh.
            (5) Insufficient ACh remains in synapse to continue depolarization of postsynaptic side of NMJ.
            (6) Muscle cells return to noncontracted state.
      2. Pharmacokinetics
         a. Absorption
            (1) Poorly absorbed from gastrointestinal tract
            (2) Typically given by IV injection
            (3) Onset of paralysis by IV injection: 1 to 2 minutes
         b. Elimination
            (1) First, redistribution occurs.
            (2) Next, hepatic or renal excretion or both

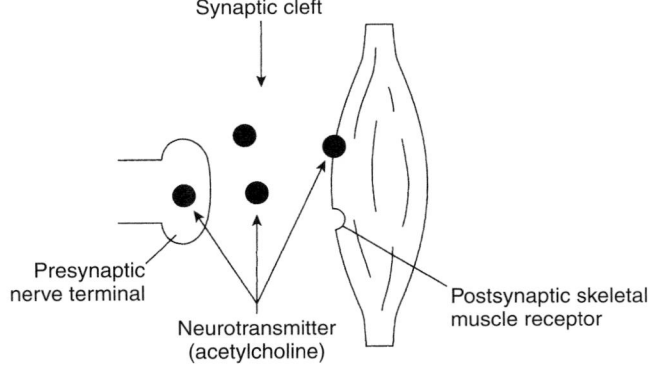

FIGURE 22-2 ■ Neuromuscular junction.

3. Pharmacodynamics
   a. NDMRs block binding of ACh to postsynaptic receptors of skeletal muscle, impairing skeletal muscle contraction (Figure 22-3).
      (1) NDMRs bind to postsynaptic receptors.
      (2) ACh still released from presynaptic terminals
      (3) However, NDMRs compete with ACh for postsynaptic receptor sites.
      (4) Degree of competition (i.e., extent of muscle paralysis) depends on dose of NDMR given.
   b. Sequence of paralysis
      (1) Advances from fine to gross motor impairment (eyes → jaw → hands → limbs and neck → intercostal muscles → diaphragm)
   c. Sequence of recovery in reverse order of sequence of paralysis
   d. Reversal of NDMR effects
      (1) Various mechanisms lead to "natural decay" in concentration of NDMR within synapse (thus restoring ability of "naturally" released ACh to reach postsynaptic muscle receptors).
         (a) Redistribution
         (b) Metabolism
         (c) Renal excretion
         (d) Biliary excretion
      (2) Reversal can be enhanced or expedited by "pharmacologic intervention" to exaggerate amount of ACh "naturally" found within synapse during blocked neuromuscular transmission; increased amounts of ACh can compete more easily with NDMRs for postsynaptic muscle receptors (see section XIII).
4. CNS effects
   a. NDMRs do not cross blood-brain barrier.
      (1) No CNS effects
      (2) Patient can be paralyzed and not speaking but be fully awake and alert!
      (3) No analgesic properties
5. Toxicity
   a. Ventilatory paralysis requires ventilatory support.
   b. Recurarization (i.e., reblockade) occurs when some condition or factor invigorates a previously attenuated neuromuscular blockade (this effect requires presence of "subtherapeutic" amounts of NDMR that would not normally cause skeletal muscle paralysis).

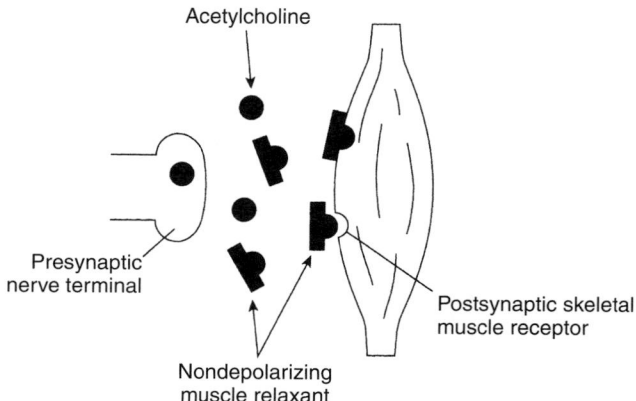

FIGURE 22-3 ■ Nondepolarizing muscle relaxants compete with acetylcholine for skeletal muscle receptor site.

(1) Can be induced when respiratory acidosis occurs because of injudicious use of narcotic analgesics

(2) Can occur when long-acting NDMRs are "reversed" with short-acting NDMR reversal agents (see section XIII)

6. Interactions

   a. NDMR paralysis can be enhanced by drugs.

      (1) Aminoglycosides

      (2) Calcium channel blockers

      (3) Clindamycin

      (4) Lithium

      (5) Magnesium

      (6) Tetracyclines

      (7) Volatile anesthetics

      (8) Cyclosporine

   b. NDMR paralysis can be enhanced by physiological imbalances.

      (1) Respiratory acidosis

      (2) Dehydration

      (3) Hypercapnia

      (4) Hypokalemia

      (5) Hyponatremia

      (6) Hypermagnesemia

      (7) Hypothermia

   c. NDMR paralysis can be antagonized by drugs.

      (1) NDMR reversal agents (increase synaptic ACh)

      (2) Caffeine

      (3) Epinephrine

      (4) Norepinephrine

      (5) Theophylline

   d. NDMR paralysis can be antagonized by physiological imbalances.

      (1) Hypocapnia

      (2) Hyperkalemia

      (3) Hypernatremia

      (4) Respiratory alkalosis

7. Nursing considerations

   a. CNS

      (1) Never assume a paralyzed patient asleep

      (2) Paralyzed patient may be fully awake and feeling pain.

   b. Paralysis may be potentiated by many drugs or conditions (see section XI.A.6).

   c. Hypothermia

      (1) Can prolong recovery from a neuromuscular block

   d. Warning: watch for "reparalysis" in patients who may be inadequately reversed or may still have unacceptably high residual amounts of long-acting NDMRs.

      (1) Need to clinically assess each patient's muscle strength

      (2) Inquire as to if, how much, and when a long-acting NDMR was given.

      (3) Note: be familiar with long-acting NDMRs by name: doxacurium, pancuronium, pipecuronium, and tubocurarine.

B. Atracurium

   1. General facts

      a. Brand name: Tracrium

      b. Classified as intermediate-acting NDMR

      c. Commonly used

      d. Drug spontaneously "self-destructs" systemically by a process known as Hoffman elimination.

         (1) No enzyme systems required

(2) Occurs only in mildly alkaline solutions or blood at its normal pH of 7.4

(3) Process can still occur when hepatorenal systems impaired.

(4) Hoffman elimination slower and paralysis lasts longer if blood acidotic

   e. Drug can also be degraded by ester hydrolysis in an otherwise healthy patient.

  2. Administration route and dosage

   a. IV doses: 0.4 to 0.5 mg/kg for intubation

  3. Pharmacokinetics

   a. Onset: 3 to 5 minutes

   b. Duration: 20 to 35 minutes

   c. Elimination

    (1) Hoffman elimination normally eliminates 33% of a given dose with production of two metabolites: laudanosine and a monoacrylate compound.

     (a) Laudanosine does not have NDMR properties, but in high concentrations has been shown to cause vasodilation, cerebral excitation, and seizure activity in animals.

     (b) Laudanosine principally eliminated by kidneys; theoretically, may accumulate in patients with renal failure

    (2) Under normal conditions, spontaneous recovery from paralysis can occur in 40 to 60 minutes.

    (3) Even with hepatic or renal system failure, complete recovery can still occur (albeit slower) by way of Hoffman elimination.

  4. Cardiovascular effects

   a. Histamine release may cause hypotension and tachycardia.

    (1) Depends on dose and rate of IV injection

    (2) More likely to occur if dose injected rapidly

    (3) More likely to occur if dose exceeds 0.4 to 0.5 mg/kg

  5. Effect of physiochemical extremes on elimination

   a. Hypothermia, hypercarbia, and acidemia may lengthen time of paralysis by slowing Hoffman degradation.

   b. Hyperthermia and alkalemia may shorten time of paralysis by hastening Hoffman degradation.

  6. Nursing considerations

   a. Eliminated by nonrenal and nonhepatic pathways

   b. Hypothermia, hypercarbia, and acidemia prolong paralysis and weakness.

   c. Residual paralysis or weakness easily reversed with NDMR reversal agents

C. Cisatracurium

  1. General facts

   a. Brand name: Nimbex

   b. Classified as intermediate-acting NDMR

   c. Is 1 of 10 stereoisomers of atracurium

   d. Three times more potent than atracurium

   e. In contrast to atracurium, primarily eliminated (80%) by process known as Hoffman elimination

   f. In sharp contrast to atracurium, not significantly degraded by nonspecific plasma esterases

   g. Clinically, less laudanosine generated

   h. Overall, may offer advantages over atracurium when used during very long operations or in ICU for patients requiring long-term mechanical ventilation (especially those with renal failure)

  2. Administration route and dosage

   a. IV doses: 0.15 to 0.2 mg/kg for intubation

  3. Pharmacokinetics

   a. Onset: 1.5 to 2 minutes

   b. Duration: 50 to 60 minutes

      c. Elimination
          (1) Hoffman elimination: 80% of a given dose
          (2) Plasma esterase hydrolysis: not significant
          (3) Renal and hepatic excretion: 20% of a given dose
          (4) Even with hepatic or renal system failure, complete recovery can still occur by way of Hoffman elimination.
  4. Cardiovascular effects
      a. Histamine release less of a concern than with atracurium
  5. Effect of physicochemical extremes on elimination
      a. Hypothermia, hypercarbia, and acidemia may lengthen time of paralysis by slowing Hoffman degradation.
      b. Hyperthermia and alkalemia may shorten time of paralysis by hastening Hoffman degradation.
  6. Nursing considerations
      a. May be considered an improved form of atracurium
      b. Greater use for long OR cases or mechanically ventilated ICU patients

D. Curare (d-tubocurarine)
  1. General facts
      a. Brand name: various manufacturers
      b. Classified as long-acting NDMR
      c. Oldest NDMR in clinical use
      d. Not commonly used clinically anymore as a primary NDMR
      e. Has greatest potential of all NDMRs to release histamine
      f. Some preparations contain sulfite preservatives.
          (1) Ascertain sulfite presence in brand to be used.
          (2) Allergic reactions may occur in susceptible patients.
      g. Reversal of blockade should not be attempted unless some spontaneous recovery has begun (this point applies to all NDMRs, especially long-acting NDMRs).
  2. Administration route and dosage
      a. IV dose: 0.6 mg/kg for intubation
  3. Pharmacokinetics
      a. Onset: 3 to 5 minutes
      b. Duration: 60 to 90 minutes
      c. Hepatic metabolism: not significant
      d. Biliary excretion (unchanged drug): 10% to 40%
      e. Renal excretion (unchanged drug): 45%
      f. Uptake: some drugs may be taken up into inactive tissue sites for a prolonged period (>24 hours).
  4. Cardiovascular effects
      a. Hypotension
          (1) Caused by release of histamine from mast cells
          (2) Amount of histamine released depends on curare dose and rate of injection.
          (3) Can be caused by blockade of autonomic ganglia if predominant autonomic tone is sympathetic
          (4) More pronounced in presence of hypovolemia
      b. Bradycardia and decreased contractility
          (1) Can be caused by blockade of autonomic ganglia if predominant autonomic tone is sympathetic
      c. Tachycardia
          (1) Can be caused by blockade of autonomic ganglia if predominant autonomic tone is parasympathetic
          (2) May be potentiated by a reflex response secondary to previously mentioned hypotension
  5. Gastrointestinal effects
      a. Impaired peristaltic activity can be caused by blockade of autonomic ganglia if predominant tone is parasympathetic (peristaltic).

     6. Side effects

       a. Secondary to histamine release

         (1) Wheals

         (2) Pruritus

         (3) Erythema

         (4) Hypotension

         (5) Bronchospasm

         (6) Bronchial and salivary secretions

         (7) Decreased coagulability caused by concomitant release of heparin from mast cells

       b. Secondary to ganglionic blockade

         (1) Affects many systems but is usually incomplete (see preceding)

     7. Toxic effects

       a. Cardiovascular collapse

         (1) Excessive histamine release

         (2) Ganglionic blockade of a dominant sympathetic tone

       b. Some preparations contain benzyl alcohol preservatives.

         (1) Toxicity may occur in neonates.

     8. Nursing considerations

       a. Hypotension

         (1) More profound in presence of hypovolemia

         (2) Rehydrate and support blood pressure as needed.

       b. History of allergies, asthma, and/or anaphylactic reactions

         (1) Avoid curare.

       c. Use not recommended in patients with renal disease

         (1) Decreased renal elimination causes slower recovery from paralysis.

  E. Doxacurium

     1. General facts

       a. Brand name: Nuromax

       b. Classified as long-acting NDMR

       c. Most potent NDMR currently available: 2.5 to 3 times more potent than pancuronium

       d. Recommended for use during long surgical cases

       e. Useful in cases requiring cardiovascular stability (minimal drug-related changes in blood pressure and heart rate)

       f. Reversal of blockade should not be attempted unless some spontaneous recovery has begun (this point applies to all NDMRs, especially long-acting NDMRs).

     2. Administration route and dosage

       a. IV dose: 0.04 to 0.08 mg/kg for intubation

     3. Pharmacokinetics

       a. Onset: 4 to 6 minutes

       b. Duration: 60 to 90 minutes

       c. Hepatic metabolism: unknown

       d. Biliary excretion (unchanged drug): unknown

       e. Renal excretion (unchanged drug): 70%

     4. Cardiovascular effects

       a. Does not cause clinically significant hemodynamic effects; slight decrease in heart rate, central venous pressure, or pulmonary artery pressure possible

     5. Side effects uncommon but can include:

       a. Flushing

       b. Urticaria

       c. Hypotension

       d. Bronchospasm

     6. Nursing considerations

       a. Very long-acting NDMR

       b. Elimination depends on renal and biliary excretion.

       c. Renal and hepatic disease slows recovery from paralysis.

          d. Requires adequate reversal or long, spontaneous recovery period

              (1) Warning: be watchful for a downward trend in minute ventilation in PACU.

              (2) Return of paralysis can be caused by administration of inadequate amounts or inappropriate selections of NDMR reversal agents.

              (3) Return of paralysis can also be caused by administration of excessive amounts of this long-acting NDMR given too close toward end of surgery.

              (4) Note: additional reversal agent may be required in PACU.

F. Gallamine

   1. General facts

      a. Brand name: various manufacturers

      b. Classified as long-acting NDMR

      c. Not commonly used clinically

      d. Substantial "vagolytic" (antimuscarinic) effect

         (1) May cause tachycardia

      e. Histamine release only with excessive doses

   2. Administration route and dosage

      a. IV dose: 3 to 4 mg/kg for intubation

      b. Not suitable for prolonged surgery because of its solubility in fat

         (1) Repetitive dosing may lead to accumulation of drug in fat tissue.

         (2) Weakness or paralysis may be prolonged in obese patients.

   3. Pharmacokinetics

      a. Onset: 3 to 5 minutes

      b. Duration: 60 to 90 minutes

      c. Hepatic metabolism: not significant

      d. Biliary excretion (unchanged drug): ~0%

      e. Renal excretion (unchanged drug): ~100%

   4. Drug interactions: same as with curare

   5. Nursing considerations

      a. Excreted entirely by kidneys

      b. Useful in patients with hepatic impairment

      c. Not useful in patients with renal impairment

      d. Moderate solubility in fat

         (1) Warning: reparalysis or prolonged weakness may occur in obese patients.

G. Metocurine

   1. General facts

      a. Brand name: various manufacturers

      b. Classified as long-acting NDMR

      c. Not commonly used anymore

      d. Small amount of histamine release (dose dependent)

   2. Administration route and dosage

      a. IV dose: 0.3 to 0.4 mg/kg for intubation

   3. Pharmacokinetics

      a. Onset: 3 to 5 minutes

      b. Duration: 60 to 90 minutes

      c. Hepatic metabolism: not significant

      d. Biliary excretion (unchanged drug): 1% to 2%

      e. Renal excretion (unchanged drug): ~43%

      f. Uptake: some drug may be taken up into inactive tissue sites for a prolonged period.

   4. Cardiovascular effects: negligible

   5. Drug interactions: same as with curare

   6. Nursing considerations: same as with curare

H. Pancuronium

   1. General facts

      a. Brand name: Pavulon and others

      b. Classified as long-acting NDMR

        c. Commonly used

        d. Potential histamine release with excessive doses

        e. Reversal of blockade should not be attempted unless some spontaneous recovery has begun (this point applies to all NDMRs, especially long-acting NDMRs).

    2. Administration route and dosage

        a. Dose: 0.08 to 0.10 mg/kg for intubation

    3. Pharmacokinetics

        a. Onset: 3 to 5 minutes

        b. Duration: 60 to 90 minutes

        c. Hepatic metabolism: 10% to 40%

        d. Biliary excretion (unchanged drug): 5% to 10%

        e. Renal excretion (unchanged drug): 80%

    4. Cardiovascular effects

        a. Anticholinergic and vagolytic action may cause tachycardia.

        b. Sympathomimetic actions

            (1) Enhances release of norepinephrine from adrenergic nerve endings

            (2) Inhibits reuptake of norepinephrine from adrenergic nerve endings

            (3) Overall sympathetic effect may increase heart rate and blood pressure.

    5. Nursing considerations

        a. Requires adequate reversal or long, spontaneous recovery period

            (1) Warning: be watchful for a downward trend in minute ventilation in PACU.

            (2) Return of paralysis can be caused by administration of inadequate amounts or inappropriate selections of NDMR reversal agents.

            (3) Return of paralysis can also be caused by administration of excessive amounts of this long-acting NDMR given too close toward end of surgery.

            (4) Note: additional NDMR reversal agent may be required in PACU.

I. Pipecuronium

    1. General facts

        a. Brand name: Arduan

        b. Classified as long-acting NDMR

        c. Recommended for use during prolonged surgery

        d. Recommended for cases requiring cardiovascular stability

        e. Reversal of blockade should not be attempted unless some spontaneous recovery has begun (this point applies to all NDMRs, especially long-acting NDMRs).

    2. Administration route and dosage

        a. IV dose: 0.07 to 0.085 mg/kg for intubation

        b. Recovery: usually begins in 45 minutes

    3. Pharmacokinetics

        a. Onset: 3 to 5 minutes

        b. Duration: 60 to 90 minutes

        c. Hepatic metabolism: 10%

        d. Biliary excretion (unchanged drug): 20%

        e. Renal excretion (unchanged drug): 70%

    4. Cardiovascular effects

        a. Does not cause clinically significant hemodynamic effects

    5. Side effects

        a. Rash and urticaria: possibly related to histamine release

        b. Hypoventilation and apnea: caused by effects of residual NDMR

    6. Nursing considerations

        a. Long-acting NDMR

        b. Elimination depends on renal excretion; dose should be reduced in patients with renal impairment.

        c. Requires adequate reversal or long, spontaneous recovery period

            (1) Warning: inadequate reversal may have been given in OR.

(2) Warning: watch for downward trend in minute ventilation.

(3) Paralysis may recur once effect of reversal agent has worn off; additional reversal may be required in PACU.

J. Rocuronium
  1. General facts
      a. Brand name: Zemuron
      b. Classified as short-acting NDMR
      c. No histamine release
      d. Appears devoid of cardiovascular effects
      e. Very fast onset of muscle relaxation
      f. However, in certain situations, succinylcholine may still be best choice for emergency intubations.
  2. Administration route and dosage
      a. IV dose: 0.5 mg/kg for intubation
  3. Pharmacokinetics
      a. Onset: 1 minute
      b. Duration: 15 to 20 minutes
      c. Metabolism: does not appear to be significant
      d. Elimination: unchanged by liver and kidney
  4. Nursing considerations
      a. Similar to vecuronium (see section XI.K.4)

K. Vecuronium
  1. General facts
      a. Brand name: Norcuron
      b. Classified as intermediate-acting NDMR
      c. No histamine release (even at high doses)
      d. Generally speaking, no cardiovascular effects
          (1) Minimal, if any, effects on blood pressure and heart rate
          (2) Occasional reports of histamine-like reactions
  2. Administration route and dosage
      a. IV dose: 0.08 to 0.1 mg/kg for intubation
  3. Pharmacokinetics
      a. Onset: 3 to 5 minutes
      b. Duration: 20 to 35 minutes
      c. Hepatic deacetylation: 20% to 30%
      d. Biliary excretion (unchanged drug): 40% to 75%
      e. Elimination can be prolonged with severe liver disease.
      f. Renal excretion (unchanged drug): 15% to 25%
  4. Nursing considerations
      a. Lack of cardiovascular effects; useful in cardiac surgery
      b. Hepatobiliary excretion: prolonged effect with severe liver disease

XII. DEPOLARIZING MUSCLE RELAXANTS (SUCCINYLCHOLINE)
  A. General facts
      1. Succinylcholine (SCh) only drug of this class in United States
      2. Brand names: Anectine, Quelicin, and Sucostrin
      3. Classified as ultrashort-acting depolarizing muscle relaxant (DMR)
      4. Very rapid onset and offset
      5. Frequently used when intubating conditions needed rapidly
      6. Warning: Use in children controversial and potentially dangerous
          a. Use may be appropriate if benefits of promptly intubating the trachea are greater than risks of using SCh.
          b. Be wary of cardiac standstill due to SCh-induced release of intracellular skeletal muscle potassium causing
              (1) Hyperkalemic crisis
              (2) Depolarization of contractile tissue of the heart
          c. Treatment of SCh-induced cardiac standstill
              (1) Basic Life Support

        (2) Titrate doses of calcium chloride
           (a) Stabilizes and repolarizes resting membrane potential of cardiac cells
        (3) Titrate insulin, glucose and bicarbonate
           (a) Helps pump extracellular potassium back into skeletal muscle cells

    7. Warning: contraindicated in patients after acute phase (after 2-4 days) of certain types of neuromuscular injury (because of potential for release of life-threatening amounts of intracellular potassium from denervated skeletal muscle subsequently exposed to SCh)
      a. Major burns
      b. Multiple trauma
      c. Upper motor neuron injury
      d. Lower motor neuron injury
      e. Cerebrovascular accidents
      f. Extensive denervation of skeletal muscle

    8. Warning: may also be contraindicated in patients with chronic illnesses (after several days) because of an excessive release of intracellular potassium from skeletal muscle that has been in a state of chronic disuse
      a. Disuse atrophy
      b. Critical illness
      c. Severe infection
      d. Prolonged immobilization
      e. Recent discontinuation of prolonged NDMR use in a critical care setting

    9. Warning: use in children with muscular dystrophies or myotonias particularly ill-advised; these children may be more likely to develop a life-threatening type of prolonged skeletal muscle spasm, or malignant hyperthermia (see Chapter 24).

  B. Administration route and dosage
    1. Usually as single IV bolus
      a. About 1 to 1.5 mg/kg for intubation
      b. Infusion "titrated to effect" may be used to prolong relaxation.
    2. Phase I block (occurs after a brief single-dose exposure to SCh)
      a. Type of neuromuscular paralysis typically associated with DMRs
        (1) Caused by single doses of SCh not exceeding 3 mg/kg
        (2) Relaxant effect wears off quickly (usually within minutes) after SCh is rapidly metabolized and NMJ completely repolarizes (see exceptions involving atypical PChE, sections XII.D.6 and XII.D.7).
        (3) If nerve stimulator is used minutes after administration of SCh
           (a) Brief sustained (titanic) stimulation to the nerve of a muscle will produce a contraction of low but sustained amplitude.
           (b) As effects of the DMR block wear off, each subsequent titanic stimulation will produce sustained amplitudes of contraction with increasing amplitudes overall.
        (4) If an anticholinesterase drug is given during the drug recovery period
           (a) Augmentation of the DMR block
           (b) Return of neuromuscular paralysis
           (c) Brief titanic stimulation produces a sustained contraction of decreased or no amplitude.
    3. Phase II block (acts more as an NDMR block)
      a. Type of neuromuscular paralysis similar to that caused by NDMR
        (1) Occurs after a single bolus dose of >3 mg/kg or after a continuous infusion (total dose) of >7 mg/kg
        (2) Postsynaptic ACh receptor appears to change with interaction with SCh.
           (a) SCh binds to ACh receptor, but depolarization no longer occurs.
           (b) With chronic exposure to SCh, ACh receptor protects itself by responding as if SCh were a NDMR.
           (c) General anesthetics may facilitate this phenomenon.

(3) Note that phase II relaxant effect of SCh does not wear off quickly and completely; thus prolonged apnea, slow recovery from paralysis, and prolonged intubation and mechanical ventilation may be observed.

(4) Brief tetanic stimulation to the nerve of a muscle recovering from a phase II block will produce contractions of low and unsustained amplitude. As effects of the NDMR block wear off, each subsequent tetanic stimulation (allowing for rest periods in between) continues to produce unsustained amplitudes of contraction (within each tetanic period) but with ever-increasing amplitudes overall. As effects of phase II block completely resolve, the unsustained amplitudes (seen during a tetanic stimulation) ultimately become sustainable.

(5) If an anticholinesterase drug is given during the drug recovery period, there will be a beneficial antagonism of the phase II block and a return of neuromuscular function; edrophonium, 0.1 mg/kg IV, may be used to briefly test whether a phase II–type block exists (effects of this small dose are short-lived if a phase I–type block is actually present).

C. Pharmacokinetics
  1. Absorption
    a. Must be given by IV or IM injection
    b. Onset of paralysis after IV injection occurs in about 1 minute.
  2. Duration
    a. Generally short (about 5 minutes), after a single intubating dose
    b. Complete recovery normally occurs in about 15 minutes.
  3. Metabolism
    a. Normally hydrolyzed by PChE
    b. Not hydrolyzed by AChE
    c. Decreases in quantity (concentration) or quality (i.e., molecular defects) of PChE will prolong effects of an administered dose of SCh.
    d. See following information on plasma cholinesterase (section XII.D).
  4. Renal excretion (unchanged drug): 10%
D. Plasma cholinesterase (PChE)
  1. Also called pseudocholinesterase
  2. Produced by liver
  3. Serum albumin and PChE levels
    a. Tend to be directly related
    b. Hypoalbuminemic patients tend to have PChE deficiency.
  4. Role of PChE
    a. No clearly understood physiological role
    b. Responsible for metabolism of SCh, local anesthetics (esters), and trimethaphan (an antihypertensive medication)
  5. Typical homozygous PChE
    a. Majority of population has this genetic variant.
    b. SCh metabolized with rapid rate of ester hydrolysis
  6. Atypical heterozygous PChE
    a. 4% of population
    b. SCh metabolized with mildly reduced rate of hydrolysis
    c. Mild prolongation of intraoperative apnea possible if SCh given
  7. Atypical homozygous PChE
    a. 0.03% of population
    b. SCh metabolized with severely reduced rate of hydrolysis
    c. Severe prolongation of postoperative apnea possible if SCh given
E. Acquired changes in PChE activity
  1. Decreased activity (decreased quantity of active enzyme molecules)
    a. Advanced age
    b. Renal failure
    c. Malnutrition

   d. Severe anemia

   e. Severe hepatic disease

   f. Bronchogenic carcinoma

   g. Prolonged cardiopulmonary bypass

   h. Postpartum period (levels lowest on third postpartum day)

   i. Inquire as to recent administration of NDMR reversal agents (i.e., neostigmine and pyridostigmine).

  2. Increased activity (increased quantity)

   a. Obese have more activity than nonobese patients.

   b. Whole blood, packed red blood cells, and fresh frozen plasma are an exogenous source of PChE.

 F. Pharmacodynamics

  1. SCh depolarizes NMJ of skeletal muscle as endogenous ACh does (Figure 22-4).

   a. Normally, ACh binds to nicotinic receptors of NMJ, but this binding is short-lived because ACh is rapidly hydrolyzed by presence of AChE.

   b. SCh also binds to nicotinic receptors of NMJ and, notably, does so more effectively; binding and depolarization of NMJ by SCh lasts longer than that caused by ACh.

  2. Sequence of SCh-induced paralysis

   a. Advances from fine to gross motor impairment

   b. Eyes, jaw, and hands → limbs and neck → intercostal muscles → diaphragm

  3. Initial depolarization causes transient fasciculations.

   a. May or may not cause postoperative myalgia

   b. Myalgia can be reduced by pretreatment with small dose of NDMR.

   c. May transiently increase intraocular pressure (IOP) (possibly involves transient contraction or fasciculation of extraocular muscles)

   d. Use of SCh may cause extrusion of eye contents in "open globe" cases.

 G. CNS effects

  1. Does not cross blood-brain barrier

   a. No CNS effects

   b. Patient can be paralyzed (and not speaking) but be fully awake and alert!

 H. Cardiovascular effects

  1. Stimulation of vagal nuclei and nerve (vagus nerve innervates atria and SA/AV nodes) leads to:

   a. Bradycardia and supraventricular dysrhythmias

   b. "Digitalized patients" may manifest exaggerated bradycardia.

  2. Stimulation of sympathetic ganglia

   a. Hypertension and tachycardia may follow usual doses because of initial (phase I) effects of SCh on ganglionic nicotinic receptors.

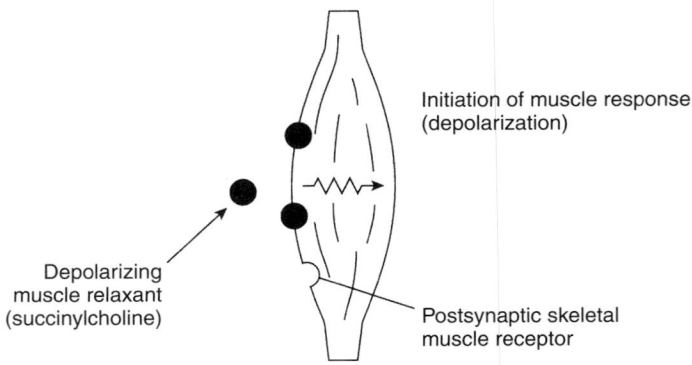

FIGURE 22-4 ■ Paralysis with succinylcholine: initiation of skeletal muscle response. First, depolarization initiates uncontrolled random contractions (fasciculations); then during the next several minutes, persisting receptor depolarization leads to muscle paralysis/relaxation.

  3. Inhibition of sympathetic ganglia
    a. Hypotension and bradycardia may subsequently follow extremely high doses of SCh because of its phase II blockade of ganglionic nicotinic receptors.
I. Respiratory effect
  1. Ventilation must be artificially supported during muscle paralysis.
J. Gastrointestinal effects
  1. Increases intragastric and intra-abdominal pressure
  2. But also increases lower esophageal sphincter pressure
    a. Therefore risk of regurgitation lower than expected
    b. Aspiration precautions should still be maintained.
K. Hepatic effects (none)
L. Renal effects
  1. Direct: not likely
  2. Indirect: excessive fasciculations may cause myoglobinuria; however, myoglobinuria most likely seen in children or adults in whom malignant hyperthermia develops (see Chapter 24)
M. Histamine release
  1. Occasionally causes mild reaction: rash on arms and upper chest
N. Eye effect (transiently raises IOP)
  1. Contracts extraocular muscles
  2. Contraindicated in patients with eye injuries (i.e., open globe) because eye contents may be extruded during initial SCh-induced fasciculations of extraocular muscles
O. Induced hyperkalemia
  1. Depolarization of skeletal muscle causes release of intracellular potassium into extracellular fluid (ECF).
    a. Normally amounts to about 0.5 mEq/L
    b. Effect peaks in 5 minutes; normalizes in 10 to 15 minutes
    c. Excessive increases in serum potassium can cause cardiac arrest.
  2. As mentioned above, SCh-induced depolarization of denervated skeletal muscle causes a copious release of potassium into ECF (effect observed initially 2 to 4 days after denervation and is maximal after 14 days); this unusual release of potassium occurs because denervated skeletal muscle increases its population of nicotinic receptors in the hope of reestablishing contact with its formerly attached and functioning nerve endings.
  3. Conditions that can lead to some form of skeletal muscle denervation
    a. Severe burns
    b. Denervation injuries
    c. Massive muscle or soft tissue trauma
    d. Spinal cord injury (up to 6 months after initial insult)
    e. Upper motor neuron lesions: stroke, encephalitis
  4. Muscle fasciculations
    a. Related to wholesale depolarization of skeletal muscles throughout human body
    b. Very small and judicious doses of NDMRs (administered before use of SCh) used by some clinicians to reduce these fasciculations
P. Concurrent hyperkalemia
  1. As stated previously, SCh releases potassium into ECF.
  2. Use of SCh may be inadvisable with some conditions.
    a. Renal disease
    b. Severe intra-abdominal infections
    c. Patients experiencing congestive heart failure or receiving digoxin
Q. Toxic effects
  1. Prolonged apnea
  2. Cardiac arrest
  3. Malignant hyperthermia (see Chapter 24)

 R. Interactions

  1. Enhancement of DMR effects by drugs

   a. Calcium channel blockers

   b. NDMR reversal agents inhibit PChE.

   c. Note: if SCh administered in PACU, a patient who has been given the NDMR reversal agent neostigmine or pyridostigmine (not edrophonium) can have an unanticipated period of prolonged muscle paralysis (see section XIII).

  2. Drugs that inhibit PChE can prolong effects of SCh.

   a. Trimethaphan

   b. Local anesthetic esters (procaine, chloroprocaine, and tetracaine)

  3. DMR paralysis can be enhanced by physiological imbalances.

   a. Respiratory alkalosis

   b. Hyperkalemia

   c. Hypermagnesemia

   d. Hypothermia

   e. Decreased renal function

   f. Dehydration

   g. Lithium pharmacotherapy

   h. Low quantity or abnormal quality of PChE

  4. DMR paralysis can be antagonized by physiological imbalances.

   a. Respiratory acidosis

   b. Hypokalemia

   c. Decreased peripheral perfusion

 S. Nursing considerations

  1. SCh has no effect on mentation; thus never assume that a paralyzed patient is asleep or pain free.

  2. Malignant hyperthermia

   a. May or may not occur during anesthesia

   b. May first manifest itself in PACU

  3. Postoperative myalgia

   a. Caused by SCh-induced fasciculations

   b. Can be lessened by a very small dose of NDMR before SCh

  4. If a slow recovery occurs from SCh-induced paralysis:

   a. Check serum albumin level; if low, PChE level may also be low.

  5. Treatment of phase II block

   a. Careful clinical correlation required

   b. Reversal of paralysis attempted with an anticholinesterase drug

  6. SCh use after patient has received an anticholinesterase drug

   a. Acceptable if SCh used to treat postoperative laryngospasm

   b. Acceptable if SCh used to reintubate patient in PACU

   c. Remember that relaxation of skeletal muscle will be prolonged if PChE inhibited.

   d. Note: neostigmine and pyridostigmine will inhibit PChE as well as AChE.

   e. Note: edrophonium inhibits AChE but not PChE.

XIII. NDMR REVERSAL AGENTS (ANTICHOLINESTERASES)

 A. Common properties

  1. Physiology

   a. Physiology of NMJ (see section XI.A.1)

   b. Released ACh depolarizes skeletal muscle by binding to postsynaptic nicotinic receptors at the NMJ.

    (1) Contraction of skeletal muscle initiated in this manner

    (2) Contraction ceases when neural release of ACh ends and when residual ACh in synapse destroyed: such destruction of ACh performed rapidly by the synaptic enzyme AChE

   c. NDMRs prevent released ACh from reaching nicotinic receptors of skeletal muscle.

    (1) Molecules of NDMRs bind to and block these receptors.

    (2) Voluntary control of skeletal muscle contraction thereby weakened or lost

2. Pharmacodynamics
    a. NDMR reversal agents provide a means of overpowering the effects of NDMRs.
        (1) This is done by inhibiting synaptic AChE and thus increasing synaptic levels of ACh.
        (2) Greater amounts of NDMR displaced from nicotinic receptors as synaptic concentration of ACh exceeds that of NDMR.
        (3) Return of neuromuscular control can be hastened as synaptic concentration of ACh is artificially increased concurrent with the progressive reduction in concentration of NDMR (by breakdown, metabolism, excretion, and discontinuing its administration).
    b. NDMR reversal agents exert a desired effect by increasing synaptic levels of ACh at nicotinic receptors of skeletal muscle.
    c. However, NDMR reversal agents exert an undesired effect by increasing synaptic levels of ACh at muscarinic receptors in the following organs:
        (1) Eyes: miosis
        (2) Heart: bradycardia
        (3) Lungs: bronchospasm
        (4) Gastrointestinal tract: enhanced peristalsis
        (5) Secretory glands: enhanced secretions
    d. Undesired effects of NDMR reversal agents can be minimized by coadministration of antimuscarinic agents (atropine or glycopyrrolate).
    e. If excessive doses of NDMR reversal agents are administered, an excessive increase in synaptic ACh will occur; this will result in synaptic depolarization (by ACh) and resulting skeletal muscle weakness.
3. CNS effects
    a. NDMR reversal agents have no direct effects (they do not cross blood-brain barrier).
4. Toxicities
    a. Minimal if dosed properly and combined with appropriate antimuscarinic drug
B. Neostigmine
    1. General facts
        a. Brand name: various manufacturers
        b. Commonly used reversal agent for NDMRs
        c. Binds to synaptic AChE
            (1) Prevents AChE from breaking down ACh
                (a) Half-life of neostigmine-AChE binding: 30 minutes
                (b) Half-life of ACh-AChE binding: 42 microseconds
            (2) Synaptic levels of ACh accumulate.
                (a) Competitive antagonism between ACh and NDMR occurs.
            (3) Bound neostigmine eventually hydrolyzes spontaneously.
                (a) Thereafter, AChE available to bind more ACh
        d. Inhibits PChE and will prolong effects of other drugs metabolized by PChE
            (1) SCh
            (2) Mivacurium
            (3) Trimethaphan
            (4) Local anesthetic esters (i.e., procaine, chloroprocaine, and tetracaine)
    2. Administration route and dosage
        a. IV dose: 0.05 mg/kg
            (1) Must be given concurrently with IV glycopyrrolate (0.01 mg/kg)
            (2) Should not be given unless some spontaneous recovery of NMJ evident (assess motor strength before dosing)
    3. Pharmacokinetics
        a. Onset (IV injection)
            (1) 50% of peak activity within 3.5 minutes
            (2) 100% of peak activity within 7 minutes

        b. Duration: 60 minutes
        c. Metabolism: ester hydrolysis by AChE and PChE
        d. Excretion: renal (50%)
        e. Elimination: primarily renal (75%)
            (1) Metabolites from hydrolysis
            (2) Unchanged drug, small amount
    4. Pharmacodynamics
        a. Reversibly inhibits synaptic AChE
            (1) Dose-dependent increase in synaptic ACh
            (2) ACh competitively antagonizes presence of NDMRs.
        b. Alert: neostigmine also reversibly inhibits PChE.
            (1) Effect may last up to 4 hours.
            (2) This will prolong effects of drugs metabolized by PChE.
                (a) SCh
                (b) Mivacurium
                (c) Trimethaphan
                (d) Local anesthetics, esters
        c. Note: excessive neostigmine can actually cause neuromuscular paralysis.
            (1) Depolarization block can occur (as with SCh).
            (2) Caused by effects of excessive doses (>0.075 mg/kg)
                (a) Direct effects: in excessive doses, neostigmine can directly depolarize nicotinic receptors.
                (b) Indirect effects: maximally increased levels of ACh in synapse may also cause a depolarization block of NMJ.
    5. Cardiovascular effects
        a. Bradycardia
            (1) Caused by increased ACh at sites of vagal innervation: SA and AV nodes
            (2) Can profoundly lower heart rate and cardiac output
        b. Peripheral vasodilation may cause hypotension.
            (1) Caused by activation of vascular muscarinic receptors
    6. Drug combinations
        a. Neostigmine with atropine
            (1) Not a preferred combination
            (2) Onset and effect of atropine precede that of neostigmine.
                (a) More tachycardia
                (b) More dysrhythmias
        b. Neostigmine with glycopyrrolate
            (1) Preferred combination for neostigmine
            (2) Onset time of glycopyrrolate better matches that of neostigmine.
                (a) Less tachycardia
                (b) Fewer dysrhythmias
            (3) In addition, neither drug crosses blood-brain barrier; therefore CNS effects are minimal.
    7. Nursing considerations
        a. Commonly used reversal agent for NDMRs
        b. Monitor vital signs and pulse oximetry (Spo_2) when reversal agents given.
C. Edrophonium
    1. General facts
        a. Brand name: Enlon
        b. Frequently used anticholinesterase for NDMRs
        c. Alert: onset of effects is rapid; a profound increase in vagal tone (muscarinic tone) on the heart will occur if atropine is not coadministered; severe bradycardia, or even asystole, may result.
        d. Good reversal agent if used correctly (atropine must be coadministered with edrophonium)
        e. Does not inhibit PChE (neostigmine and pyridostigmine will)

2. Administration route and dosage
   a. IV: 0.5 to 1 mg/kg
      (1) Not given unless some spontaneous recovery evident
      (2) Given in combination with IV atropine (7-14 mcg/kg)
3. Pharmacokinetics
   a. Onset (IV injection)
      (1) 50% of peak activity within 0.5 minutes
      (2) 100% of peak activity within 1 minute
   b. Duration: 60 minutes
   c. Metabolism: conjugation to glucuronide
   d. Elimination: primarily renal (75%)
      (1) Tubular secretion
      (2) Metabolites from hydrolysis
      (3) Small amount of unchanged drug
4. Drug combinations
   a. Edrophonium with atropine
      (1) Preferred combination for edrophonium
      (2) Onset time of atropine matches that of edrophonium.
         (a) Less bradycardia
         (b) Fewer dysrhythmias
         (c) Much less likely to see asystole
      (3) Atropine does cross blood-brain barrier.
   b. Edrophonium with glycopyrrolate
      (1) Potentially dangerous combination
      (2) Onset time of glycopyrrolate lags behind that of edrophonium: severe bradycardia, asystole, cardiovascular collapse can occur.
5. Nursing considerations
   a. Formerly was not a popular reversal agent because not regarded as being very potent
      (1) This was true historically; however, inadequate doses were given.
      (2) Dose should be 0.5 to 1 mg/kg (in combination with atropine).
   b. Currently is used more
      (1) Edrophonium available in solution by itself (Enlon); use atropine concurrently.
      (2) Edrophonium also comes premixed with atropine (Enlon Plus).
   c. Alert: edrophonium still not recommended for reversing a dense block; neostigmine (in combination with glycopyrrolate) will be more effective.
D. Pyridostigmine
   1. General facts
      a. Brand name: various manufacturers
      b. Less commonly used reversal agent for NDMRs
      c. Less potent reversal agent than neostigmine; only 20% of reversal activity of neostigmine
      d. Duration of action (4-5 hours): 40% longer than that of neostigmine
      e. Fewer muscarinic effects
      f. Profound depression of PChE
         (1) Longer lasting than neostigmine
         (2) Will prolong effects of drugs metabolized by PChE
            (a) SCh
            (b) Mivacurium
            (c) Trimethaphan
            (d) Local anesthetics, esters
   2. Administration route and dosage
      a. IV dose: 0.25 mg/kg
         (1) Not given unless some spontaneous recovery evident
         (2) Given in combination with IV glycopyrrolate (0.01 mg/kg); administer slowly to diminish side effects.

3. Pharmacokinetics
   a. Onset (IV injection)
      (1) 50% of peak activity in 4 minutes
      (2) 100% of peak activity in 12 minutes
   b. Duration: about 90 minutes
   c. Metabolism: hydrolysis by AChE and PChE
   d. Elimination: primarily renal (75%)
4. Drug combinations
   a. Pyridostigmine with atropine
      (1) Not a preferred combination
      (2) Onset time of atropine precedes that of pyridostigmine.
         (a) More tachycardia
         (b) More dysrhythmias
   b. Pyridostigmine with glycopyrrolate
      (1) Preferred combination for pyridostigmine
      (2) Onset time of glycopyrrolate better matches that of pyridostigmine.
         (a) Less tachycardia
         (b) Fewer dysrhythmias
         (c) Neither crosses blood-brain barrier.
5. Cardiovascular effects
   a. Fewer autonomic side effects
   b. Fewer dysrhythmias in elderly
6. Nursing considerations
   a. Less commonly used NDMR reversal agent
   b. Longer onset time than edrophonium or neostigmine

BIBLIOGRAPHY

1. Abram S: *Pain medicine: The requisites in anesthesiology*, St Louis, 2006, Mosby.
2. Atlee J: *Complications in anesthesia*, Philadelphia, 2007, Saunders.
3. Barash P, Cullen B, Stoelting R, eds: *Clinical anesthesia*, ed 6, Philadelphia, 2009, Lippincott Williams & Wilkins.
4. Burden N, DeFazio Quinn D, O'Brien D, et al: *Ambulatory surgical nursing*, ed 2, Philadelphia, 2000, Saunders.
5. Cole D, Schlunt M: *Adult perioperative anesthesia: Requisites in anesthesiology*, St Louis, 2004, Mosby.
6. Drain C, Odom Forren J: *Perianesthesia nursing: A critical care approach*, ed 5, Philadelphia, 2009, Saunders.
7. Faust R: *Anesthesiology review*, ed 3, New York, 2002, Churchill Livingstone.
8. Godden B, ed: *Competency based orientation and credentialing program for the registered nurses in the perianesthesia setting*, Cherry Hill, NJ, 2009, American Society of PeriAnesthesia Nurses.
9. Karlet M: *Nurse anesthesia secrets*, St Louis, 2005, Mosby.
10. Leung J: *Cardiac and vascular anesthesia: The requisites in anesthesiology*, St Louis, 2004, Mosby.
11. Miller R, ed: *Anesthesia*, ed 6, New York, 2004, Churchill Livingstone.
12. Nagelhout J, Zaglaniczny K: *Nurse anesthesia* ed 3, St Louis, 2005, Saunders.
13. Rathmell J, Neal J, Viscomi C: *Regional anesthesia: The requisites in anesthesiology*, St Louis, 2004, Mosby.
14. Roisen M, Fleisher L: *Essence of anesthesia practice*, ed 2, Philadelphia, 2002, Saunders.
15. Springman S: *Ambulatory anesthesia: The requisites in anesthesiology*, St Louis, 2006, Mosby.
16. Stoelting R: *Pharmacology and physiology in anesthetic practice*, ed 3, Philadelphia, 2000, Lippincott-Raven.
17. Stoelting R, Miller R: *Basics of anesthesia*, ed 5, New York, 2004, Churchill Livingstone.
18. Zaglaniczny K, Aker J: *Clinical guide to pediatric anesthesia*, Philadelphia, 1999, Saunders.

23 Moderate Sedation/ Analgesia

JAN ODOM-FORREN

OBJECTIVES

At the conclusion of this chapter, the reader will be able to:

1. Define moderate sedation, deep sedation, and general anesthesia.
2. Identify the statutory, regulatory, practice guidelines, and promulgated professional standards of care for nurses administering moderate sedation and analgesia.
3. State the components of presedation patient assessment.
4. List sedative and analgesic medications, dosing guidelines, and nursing considerations associated with their administration.
5. Identify required monitoring parameters for the patient receiving moderate sedation and analgesia.
6. State postsedation monitoring requirements for the patient receiving sedation.
7. Identify risk management strategies used to reduce the incidence of complications associated with the delivery of sedative and analgesic medications.

I. SEDATION
  A. Definitions
    1. Minimal sedation (anxiolysis)
      a. Respond normally to verbal commands.
      b. Cognitive function and coordination may be impaired.
      c. Ventilatory and cardiovascular functions are unaffected.
    2. Moderate sedation and analgesia (formerly referred to as "conscious sedation")
      a. A drug-induced depression of consciousness
      b. Patients respond purposefully to verbal commands either alone or accompanied by light tactile stimulation.
      c. No interventions required to maintain a patent airway
      d. Spontaneous ventilation adequate
      e. Cardiovascular function usually maintained
    3. Deep sedation and analgesia
      a. A drug-induced depression of consciousness
      b. Patients cannot be easily aroused.
      c. Respond purposefully after repeated or painful stimulation.
      d. Independent ability to maintain ventilatory function may be impaired.
      e. May require assistance in maintaining a patent airway
      f. Spontaneous ventilation may be inadequate.
      g. Cardiovascular function usually maintained
    4. Anesthesia
      a. Consists of general anesthesia and spinal or major regional anesthesia
      b. Does not include local anesthesia
      c. General anesthesia is a drug-induced loss of consciousness.
        (1) Patients not arousable, even with painful stimulation
        (2) Ability to independently maintain ventilatory function often impaired

      d. Often require assistance in maintaining a patent airway

      e. Positive pressure ventilation may be required because of:

         (1) Depressed spontaneous ventilation

         (2) Drug-induced depression of neuromuscular function

      f. Cardiovascular function may be impaired.

  5. Goals and objectives of moderate sedation and analgesia

      a. Maintain adequate sedation with minimal risk.

      b. Relieve anxiety.

      c. Produce amnesia.

      d. Provide relief from pain and other noxious stimuli.

      e. Overall goal: to allay patient fear and anxiety with a minimum of medication

      f. Altered mood

      g. Enhanced patient cooperation

      h. Elevation of pain threshold

      i. Stable vital signs

      j. Intact protective reflexes

      k. Rapid recovery

      l. Unconsciousness and unresponsiveness are not goals of moderate sedation and analgesia.

  6. Indications for moderate sedation and analgesia

      a. Diagnostic and therapeutic procedures that require anxiolysis and/or analgesia, widely used throughout health care facilities and physician offices, including, but not limited to:

         (1) Burn unit dressing changes

         (2) Cardiology, heart station, cardiac catheterization and electrophysiology laboratories

         (3) Cosmetic surgery

         (4) Gastroenterology

         (5) General surgery procedures

         (6) Gynecology

         (7) Ophthalmology

         (8) Oral surgery

         (9) Orthopedic procedures

         (10) Pulmonary biopsy and bronchoscopy

         (11) Radiology, interventional radiology

         (12) Urology

         (13) Emergency department procedures

B. Legal scope of practice issues

  1. Requires:

      a. An understanding of definition and levels of sedation

      b. Adherence to clinical criteria outlined

  2. Nurses required to comply with legal scope of practice issues in many jurisdictions

      a. Legal scope of practice issues related to nursing delegated and administered through state boards of nursing

      b. Nurses engaged in administration of sedation must ascertain their state board of nursing's formal position or policy statement delineating their role and responsibility in the delivery of sedation and analgesia.

      c. Most states have adopted guidelines, but some states have not taken formal action on the issue or lack statutory authority to enact such legislation.

C. The Joint Commission (TJC)

  1. TJC has taken an active role in the development of policies, standards, and intents related to operative or other high-risk procedures and/or the administration of moderate or deep sedation or anesthesia.

      a. The standards apply when patients receive in any setting:

         (1) Moderate or deep sedation

         (2) General anesthesia

        (3) Spinal anesthesia

        (4) Other major regional anesthesia

  2. It is the obligation of each institution to develop institution-wide appropriate protocols for patients receiving sedation.

  3. TJC states:

    a. Moderate or deep sedation and anesthesia are provided by qualified individuals.

    b. Sufficient numbers of qualified personnel are present during procedures using moderate or deep sedation and anesthesia.

    c. Presedation and preanesthesia assessment is performed for each patient before beginning:

        (1) Moderate or deep sedation

        (2) Anesthesia induction

    d. Moderate or deep sedation and anesthesia care are planned.

    e. Patient's physiological status is monitored during sedation or anesthesia administration.

    f. Patient's postprocedure status is assessed on admission to and before discharge from the postsedation or postanesthesia recovery area.

D. Professional organizations

  1. In July 1991, the Nursing Organizations Liaison Forum in Washington, D.C., endorsed a position statement for the management of patients receiving intravenous sedation for short-term therapeutic, diagnostic, or surgical procedures.

    a. This position statement has been adopted by many professional nursing organizations.

  2. Professional organizations have developed specialty guidelines for use.

  3. Participating professional organizations

    a. American Society of PeriAnesthesia Nurses

    b. Association of periOperative Registered Nurses

    c. American Society of Anesthesiologists

    d. American Association of Nurse Anesthetists

    e. Society of Gastroenterology Nurses and Associates

    f. American Society for Gastrointestinal Endoscopy

  4. Professional organization guidelines, TJC standards, and statutory regulations require policy development that prepares the nurse participating in the delivery of sedation to demonstrate:

    a. Knowledge of anatomy, physiology, cardiac dysrhythmias, and complications related to the administration of sedative agents

    b. Knowledge of pharmacokinetic and pharmacodynamic principles associated with moderate sedation medications

    c. Presedation assessment and monitoring of physiologic parameters including:

        (1) Respiratory rate and ventilatory function

        (2) Oxygen saturation

        (3) Blood pressure

        (4) Cardiac rate and rhythm

        (5) Level of consciousness

    d. Understanding of principles of oxygen delivery and the ability to use oxygen delivery devices

    e. Ability to rapidly assess, diagnose, and intervene in the event of an untoward reaction associated with administration of moderate sedation

    f. Proven skill in airway management

    g. Accurate documentation of the procedure and medications administered

    h. Competency validation for training and education conducted on a regular basis

II. PRESEDATION ASSESSMENT
  A. Presedation assessment goals
    1. Identify preexisting pathophysiological disease.
    2. Obtain baseline patient information.
    3. Take history and perform physical examination.
    4. Reduce patient anxiety through education and communication.
    5. Prepare a plan for the procedure.
    6. Obtain informed consent.
  B. Components of presedation assessment
    1. General health
      a. Height and weight
      b. Obesity or recent weight loss
      c. Current medications or herbal use
      d. Baseline vital signs and temperature
      e. History of tobacco or alcohol use
      f. Physical handicaps and level of mobility
      g. Pain assessment
    2. Medical history
      a. Cardiac
        (1) Angina
        (2) Coronary artery disease
        (3) Dysrhythmias
        (4) Exercise tolerance
        (5) Hypertension
        (6) Myocardial infarction
        (7) Presence of a pacemaker or implantable cardioverter defibrillator
      b. Pulmonary
        (1) Asthma
        (2) Bronchitis, tuberculosis, pneumonia
        (3) Dyspnea
        (4) Exercise tolerance
        (5) Cigarette smoking
        (6) Recent cold or flu
        (7) Airway assessment
          (a) Mallampati assessment or other assessment such as having patient open mouth, stick out tongue, and flex neck (see Figure 23-1)
          (b) Craniofacial abnormalities
        (8) Sleep apnea
      c. Hepatic
        (1) Ascites
        (2) Cirrhosis
        (3) Hepatitis
      d. Renal
        (1) Dialysis
        (2) Renal failure
        (3) Renal insufficiency
      e. Neurological
        (1) Convulsive disorders
        (2) Headaches
        (3) Level of consciousness
        (4) Stroke
        (5) Syncope
        (6) Cerebrovascular insufficiency
        (7) Preexisting neurological deficit
      f. Endocrine
        (1) Adrenal disease
        (2) Diabetes
        (3) Thyroid disease

(a) Hyperthyroidism
(b) Hypothyroidism
g. Gastrointestinal
(1) Hiatal hernia
(2) Predisposition to nausea and vomiting
(3) Chronic diarrhea or constipation
h. Hematology
(1) Anemia
(2) Aspirin, nonsteroidal anti-inflammatory drug use
(3) Excessive bleeding
i. Musculoskeletal
(1) Arthritis
(2) Back pain
(3) Joint pain
3. Nothing by mouth (NPO) status
a. *Guidelines for Preoperative Fasting* (American Society of Anesthesiologists) include:

Ingested Materials	Minimum Fasting Period[†] (h)
Clear liquids[‡]	2
Breast milk	4
Infant formula	6
Nonhuman milk[§]	6
Light meal[¶]	6

These recommendations apply to healthy patients who are undergoing elective procedures. They are not intended for women in labor. Following the guidelines does not guarantee a complete gastric emptying has occurred.
[†]The fasting periods apply to all ages.
[‡]Examples of clear liquids include water, fruit juices without pulp, carbonated beverages, clear tea, and black coffee.
[§]Since nonhuman milk is similar to solids in gastric emptying time, the amount ingested must be considered when determining an appropriate fasting period.
[¶]A light meal typically consists of toast and clear liquids. Meals that include fried or fatty foods or meat may prolong gastric emptying time. Both the amount and type of foods must be considered when determining an appropriate fasting period.

b. Emergent procedures require consideration of:
(1) NPO status
(2) Risk of gastric acid aspiration
c. Histamine-blocking and gastrokinetic agents may be used to decrease gastric acidity and decrease gastric volume.
III. PROCEDURAL CARE
A. Monitoring
1. Monitoring process during the procedure includes:
a. Observation and vigilance
b. Interpretation of data
c. Initiation of corrective action when required
2. Electrocardiogram (ECG)
a. ECG monitoring during sedation procedures is required to detect:
(1) Dysrhythmias
(2) Myocardial ischemia
(3) Electrolyte disturbance
(4) Pacemaker function

    b. Cardiac rhythm and dysrhythmias that may be encountered include:

      (1) Sinus tachycardia

      (2) Sinus bradycardia

      (3) Sinus arrhythmia

      (4) Premature atrial contractions

      (5) Supraventricular tachycardia

      (6) Atrial flutter

      (7) Atrial fibrillation

      (8) Junctional rhythm

      (9) Premature ventricular contractions

      (10) Ventricular tachycardia

      (11) Ventricular fibrillation

    c. See Chapter 32 for description, ECG criteria, and treatment protocol for specific dysrhythmias.

3. Noninvasive blood pressure

    a. Hypotension

      (1) A decrease in systolic arterial blood pressure of 20% to 30% and may be caused by a variety of factors including:

        (a) Hypovolemia

        (b) Myocardial ischemia

        (c) Pharmacological agents

        (d) Acidosis

        (e) Parasympathetic stimulation (pain, vagal stimulation)

      (2) Treatment

        (a) Administer oxygen.

        (b) Administer a fluid challenge (300-500 mL crystalloid).

        (c) Correct acidosis or hypoxemia.

        (d) Relieve myocardial ischemia.

          (i) Nitrates

          (ii) Oxygen

          (iii) Analgesia

        (e) Titrate sympathomimetic medications.

        (f) Titrate inotropic agents.

    b. Hypertension

      (1) Normal blood pressure should be less than 120/80 mm Hg for an adult.

    c. Blood pressure that stays between 120/80 mm Hg and 139/89 mm Hg considered prehypertension

    d. Systolic blood pressure greater than 140 mm Hg or a diastolic blood pressure greater than 90 mm Hg considered hypertension

      (1) Increases bleeding

      (2) Predisposes patient to hemorrhage

      (3) May lead to cardiac dysrhythmias

      (4) Increases systemic vascular resistance

      (5) Increases myocardial oxygen consumption

      (6) Treatment

        (a) Diuresis for fluid overload

        (b) Noxious stimuli require analgesia or discontinuation of stimuli.

        (c) Sympathetic nervous stimulation may require alpha and beta blockade.

        (d) Myocardial ischemia requires nitrates and analgesia.

4. Ventilatory function

    a. Assessed using auscultation and having patients take deep breaths

    b. Pulse oximetry

      (1) Required with sedation to monitor oxygenation status of patient

      (2) Provides a noninvasive, continuous monitoring parameter to assess the percentage of hemoglobin combined with oxygen

      (3) Pulse oximetry technology allows two light-emitting diodes to measure the intensity of transmitted light across the vascular bed.

      (4) Early indication of developing hypoxemia

    c. Capnography
       (1) Consider using to monitor ventilatory status (end-tidal carbon dioxide levels)
       (2) Provides a graphic representation of exhaled carbon dioxide levels with a tracing (capnogram)
       (3) Best monitor for measuring adequacy of ventilation
       (4) Must use to monitor ventilatory function during deep sedation
  5. Level of sedation scoring system
    a. Ramsey Sedation Scale (Table 23-1)
    b. Modified Observer's Assessment of Alertness/Sedation Scale (Table 23-2)
    c. Sedation Visual Analogue Scale (0-100 mm)
    d. Sedation Scale by M. McCaffery and C. Pasero (Box 23-1)

■ TABLE 23-1
■ ■ **Ramsay Sedation Scale**

Score	Responsiveness
1	Patient is anxious and agitated or restless, or both.
2	Patient is cooperative, oriented, and tranquil.
3	Patient responds to commands only.
4	Patient exhibits brisk response to light glabellar tap or loud auditory stimulus.
5	Patient exhibits a sluggish response to light glabellar tap or loud auditory stimulus.
6	Patient exhibits no response.

From Ramsay MA, Savege TM, Simpson BR, et al: Controlled sedation with alphaxalone-alphadolone. *Br Med J* 2:656–659, 1974.

■ TABLE 23-2
■ ■ **Modified Observer's Assessment of Alertness/Sedation Scale**

Responsiveness	Score
Agitated	6
Responds readily to name spoken in normal tone (alert)	5
Lethargic response to name spoken in normal tone	4
Responds only after name is called loudly and/or repeatedly	3
Responds only after mild prodding or shaking	2
Does not respond to mild prodding or shaking	1
Does not respond to deep stimulus	0

From Cohen LB, DeLegge MH, Aisenberg J, et al: AGA Institute review of endoscopic sedation. *Gastroenterology* 133:675–701, 2007.

■ BOX 23-1
■ **SEDATION SCALE**

S = Sleep, easy to arouse
1 = Awake and alert
2 = Slightly drowsy, easily aroused
3 = Frequently drowsy, arousable, drifts off to sleep during conversation
4 = Somnolent, minimal or no response to physical stimulation

From McCaffery M, Pasero C: *Pain: Clinical manual*, ed 2, St Louis, 1999, Mosby.

B. Procedural considerations
   1. All syringes labeled
   2. Emergency medications and equipment immediately available
   3. Adequate intravenous access established before the procedure
   4. "Time out" immediately before procedure
   5. Turn alarms on and keep them on.
   6. Documentation of care every 5 minutes during procedure and at least every 15 minutes during phase I recovery
      a. Vital signs
      b. Oxygen saturation
      c. Level of sedation
IV. AIRWAY MANAGEMENT AND MANAGEMENT OF RESPIRATORY COMPLICATIONS
   A. Evaluation of airway
      1. Oral cavity inspection
         a. Loose, chipped, capped teeth
         b. Dental anomalies
            (1) Crowns
            (2) Bridges
            (3) Dentures
         c. Obstruction to airflow
            (1) Tumors
            (2) Edema
            (3) Inflammatory processes
      2. Temporomandibular joint examination
         a. Conducted with patient's mouth opened wide
            (1) Normal distance between upper and lower central incisors is 4 to 6 cm.
         b. Indications of reduced temporomandibular joint mobility
            (1) Clicking sound when mouth opened
            (2) Pain associated with opening mouth
            (3) Reduced ability to open mouth
      3. Physical characteristics
         a. The following physical characteristics may indicate potential for difficult airway management:
            (1) Recessed jaw
            (2) Protruding jaw (hypognathous)
            (3) Deviated trachea
            (4) Large tongue
            (5) Short, thick neck
            (6) Protruding teeth
            (7) High, arched palate
      4. Mallampati airway classification system (Figure 23-1)
         a. Initially described in 1983
         b. Offers clinician a grading system for anticipation of difficult intubation
         c. Examination conducted while patient's head is maintained in a neutral position and mouth is opened 50 to 60 mm.
         d. Classes I to IV are based on anatomic areas visualized.
            (1) Class I: uvula, tonsillar pillars, soft and hard palate visualized
            (2) Class II: uvula, hard and soft palate visualized
            (3) Class III: portion of uvula and hard palate visualized
            (4) Class IV: portion of hard palate visualized
      5. Anesthesia provider should be consulted for any patient determined at risk for airway management.
   B. Complications
      1. Potent synergistic effect when following medications used together
         a. Sedative
         b. Hypnotic
         c. Analgesic

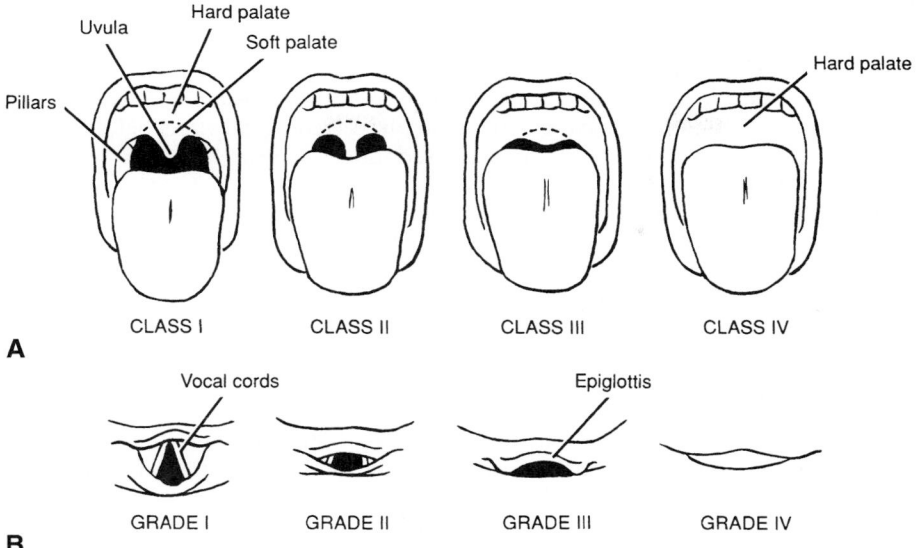

FIGURE 23-1 ■ Mallampati airway classification. (From Mallampati SR: Clinical signs to predict difficult tracheal intubation [hypothesis]. *Can Anaesth Soc J* 30:316, 1983.)

   2. Decreased oropharyngeal muscle tone predisposes patient to airway obstruction, leading to apnea and hypoxemia.
   3. Steps for restoration of airflow
      a. Lateral head tilt
      b. Chin lift
      c. Jaw thrust
      d. Nasal airway insertion
      e. Oropharyngeal airway insertion
      f. Endotracheal tube insertion
   4. Oxygen delivery devices: because of respiratory depressant effects associated with administration of sedative, hypnotic, or opioid medications, it is strongly recommended that supplemental oxygen be administered to all patients receiving sedation and analgesia (see Chapter 31).
 V. PHARMACOLOGICAL AGENTS
   A. Sedation and analgesia medications
      1. Benzodiazepines (see Chapter 22 for general facts, pharmacokinetics, and pharmacodynamics)
         a. Midazolam (Versed) sedation
            (1) Dosing guidelines are individualized and titrated to effect.
            (2) Do not administer by rapid injection.
            (3) Titration to effect means administration of drug until:
               (a) Somnolence
               (b) Nystagmus
               (c) Slurred speech
            (4) Healthy patients: before the procedure
               (a) Small increments (0.5 mg) of midazolam are administered over 2 minutes.
               (b) Initial intravenous dose should not exceed 2.5 mg.
               (c) Some patients may respond to as little as 0.5 to 1 mg.
            (5) Adults 60 years or older: elderly, debilitated, chronically ill patients or patients with reduced pulmonary reserve

(a) Require small, incremental (0.25-0.5 mg) doses administered over 2 minutes

(b) Initial dose should not exceed 1.5 mg.

(c) If additional sedation is required, it is imperative to wait 2-3 minutes to evaluate the pharmacological effect before administering additional sedation.

b. Diazepam sedation

(1) Dosing guidelines: individualized and titrated to effect

(2) Before the planned procedure, 1 to 2 mg of intravenous diazepam is titrated over a minute.

(3) Additional 1-mg increments may be administered over several minutes during the procedure.

(4) Additional time must be allowed to evaluate pharmacological effect in geriatric or debilitated patients or patients with decreased cardiac output.

(5) Do not administer by rapid or single-bolus injection.

(6) Extreme care must be exercised when administering diazepam concurrently with opioids.

c. Benzodiazepine antagonist: flumazenil (Romazicon)

(1) Specific benzodiazepine antagonist

(2) Reverses central nervous system effects of benzodiazepines through competitive inhibition of benzodiazepine receptor sites on the γ-aminobutyric acid (GABA) benzodiazepine receptor complex

(3) Duration and degree of reversal related to total dose administered and plasma benzodiazepine concentration

(4) Dose: 0.2 mg administered intravenously over 15 seconds.

(5) If desired level of consciousness not obtained after waiting an additional 45 seconds, a further dose of 0.2 mg can be injected.

(6) May be repeated at 60-second intervals when necessary (up to a maximum of four additional times) to a maximum total dose of 1 mg

(7) Dosage should be individualized based on patient's response, with most patients responding to doses of 0.6 to 1 mg.

(8) Onset: 1 to 2 minutes; an 80% response will be achieved within 3 minutes of administration.

(9) Duration: 40 to 80 minutes; monitor (up to 120 minutes) for resedation.

2. Opioids

a. Opioids bind to specific opiate receptor subtypes located within central nervous system.

(1) Mu

(2) Kappa

(3) Delta

(4) Sigma

b. See Chapter 22 for general facts, pharmacokinetics, and pharmacodynamics.

c. Dosing guidelines

(1) Fentanyl: 1 to 2 mcg/kg titrated in 25-mcg increments

(2) Meperidine: 0.5 to 1 mg/kg titrated in 25-mg increments

(3) Morphine: 0.05 to 0.2 mg/kg titrated in 1- to 2-mg increments

3. Sedatives, hypnotics, and dissociative anesthetic agents

a. Sedative, hypnotic, and dissociative medications are added to deepen levels of sedation.

(1) Administration of these medications by registered nurses depends on statutory, regulatory, and recommended standards of care.

(2) Manufacturer recommendations generally advise that these agents be administered by anesthesia providers.

(3) Nurse-administered propofol sedation varies with state board of nursing.

(a) Advantages of using propofol for nurse administration of sedation
  (i) Short action of medication
  (ii) Rapid recovery
  (iii) Lower incidence of postoperative/postprocedure nausea and vomiting
  (iv) Faster discharge of patients
(b) Disadvantages of using propofol for nurse administration of sedation
  (i) Unpredictability of action
  (ii) Demanding airway requirements
  (iii) No known reversal
  (iv) Package insert with propofol states that it is to be used by individuals trained in administering general anesthesia
(c) Perianesthesia nurses should check the scope of practice in the state employed.
(d) See Box 23-2 for safe use of propofol.
  b. See Chapter 22 for general facts, pharmacokinetics, and pharmacodynamics.
B. Techniques of administration
  1. Single-dose injection technique uses individual medications titrated slowly to effect.
    a. To establish an analgesic base, often opioids are administered before benzodiazepines.
    b. Two to three minutes before the procedure, intravenous opioids may be slowly administered to establish analgesia.
    c. Benzodiazepines are then added and titrated to patient effect.
      (1) Combining medications (opioids, benzodiazepines, and hypnotics)
        (a) Reduces total dosage through synergistic action
        (b) Assists clinician in maintenance of sedation and analgesia parameters
        (c) Provides rapid patient recovery

■ BOX 23-2
■ **SAFE USE OF PROPOFOL**

Responsible physician:
- Must have education and training to manage complications
- Must be proficient in airway management
- Have ACLS training
- Must understand pharmacology of drugs

Practitioner administering propofol:
- Must have education and training to identify and mange airway and cardiovascular changes of patient who enters state of general anesthesia
- Must have ability to assist in management of complications
- Must be present throughout procedure with no other responsibilities other than monitoring patient
- Must monitor patient, assessing level of consciousness, ventilation, oxygen saturation, heart rate, blood pressure with monitoring of exhaled carbon dioxide when possible
- Must identify early signs of hypotension, bradycardia, apnea, airway obstruction, oxygen desaturation
- Must have age-appropriate equipment immediately available
- Must not be involved in conduct of surgical/diagnostic procedure

---

ACLS, Advanced cardiac life support.
From Odom-Forren J: The evolution of nurse-monitored sedation. *J Perianesth Nurs* 20:395, 2005.

      d. Despite the speed with which a desired plasma concentration can be achieved, risks associated with a bolus technique outweigh potential benefits.

      e. Small incremental doses allow therapeutic plasma levels to be reached slowly and produce the desired pharmacological effect with a minimum of medication.

  2. Continuous infusion techniques produce a constant medication plasma level.

      a. Avoids fluctuations in medication plasma levels associated with bolus technique

      b. Popular sedative technique in critical care units for mechanically ventilated or agitated patients

      c. Additional benefits of continuous infusion techniques

         (1) Shorter recovery time

         (2) Reduced medication requirement

         (3) Minimized side effects

      d. Careful titration based on predetermined clinical endpoints (nystagmus, slurred speech, sedation) allows a rapid return to an alert state after infusion is discontinued at conclusion of procedure.

      e. Continuous infusion techniques are extremely difficult to master as a clinician, particularly in establishing a baseline level of sedation.

         (1) When establishing baseline sedation levels, patients are predisposed to oversedation as the clinician is attempting to establish a desired level of sedation.

         (2) This frequently results in patient's entering a state of deep sedation or general anesthesia.

VI. POSTSEDATION RECOVERY

  A. Monitoring

    1. Purpose

      a. Ensure return of physiological function.

      b. Assess patient.

      c. Assess readiness for discharge.

      d. Treat complications.

    2. Monitoring and discharge policies

      a. Required by accrediting bodies

      b. Recommended by professional organizations

    3. Dependent on:

      a. Diagnostic or surgical procedure performed

      b. Length of procedure

      c. Preprocedure physiological status

      d. Intraprocedural complications

      e. Medications administered

      f. Quantities of medications administered

    4. Documentation of recovery parameters

      a. Use of a postprocedure objective scoring tool (e.g., Aldrete scoring system) to determine readiness to move from phase I to phase II level of care

      b. Objective parameters must assess:

         (1) Activity

         (2) Respiration

         (3) Circulation

         (4) Level of consciousness

         (5) Oxygenation

      c. Upon completion of the procedure, all patients must be monitored until all institution-approved discharge criteria are met.

         (1) These discharge criteria must be developed in conjunction with statutory, regulatory, and professional organization standards (see Chapter 30 for more discharge criteria).

(2) One of the following objective scoring tools for outpatient "street fitness" may be used to assess for discharge readiness.
  (a) Chung's Postanesthesia Discharge Scoring System
  (b) Modified Postanesthesia Discharge Scoring System
  (c) Aldrete's Modified Postanesthesia Recovery Score (see Box 23-3)

■ BOX 23-3
■ **DISCHARGE CRITERIA SCORING**

Modified Aldrete Scoring System*

Category	Score = 2	Score = 1	Score = 0
Respirations	Breathes and coughs freely	Dyspnea	Apnea
O_2 Saturation	$SpO_2 > 92\%$ on R/A	Supplemental O_2	$SpO_2 < 92\%$ on O_2
Circulation	BP +/− 20 mmHg pre-op value	BP +/− 20-50 mmHg pre-op value	BP +/− 50 mmHg pre-op value
LOC	Awake and oriented	Wakens with stimulation	Non-responsive
Movement	Moves 4 limbs spontaneously	Moves 2 limbs spontaneously	Moves 0 limbs spontaneously

Postanesthesia Discharge Scoring System (PADSS)
1. Vital signs
   2 = Within 20% of preoperative value
   1 = 20-40% of preoperative value
   0 = 40% of preoperative value
2. Ambulation and mental status
   2 = Oriented ×3 and has a steady gait
   1 = Oriented ×3 or has a steady gait
   0 = Neither
3. Pain or nausea/vomiting
   2 = Minimal
   1 = Moderate
   0 = Severe
4. Surgical bleeding
   2 = Minimal
   1 = Moderate
   0 = Severe
5. Intake and output
   2 = Has had PO fluids and voided
   1 = Has had PO fluids or voided
   0 = Neither
The total score is 10, with patients scoring ≥9 fit for discharge home.

MODIFIED Postanesthetic Discharge Scoring System (MPADSS)
1. Vital Signs
   2 = Within 20% of preoperative value
   1 = 20-40% of preoperative value
   0 = 40% of preoperative value
2. Ambulation
   2 = Steady gait/no dizziness
   1 = With assistance
   0 = None/dizziness

Continued

■ BOX 23-3
■ **DISCHARGE CRITERIA SCORING—cont'd**

> **3.** Nausea/vomiting
> 2 = Minimal
> 1 = Moderate
> 0 = Severe
> **4.** Pain
> 2 = Minimal
> 1 = Moderate
> 0 = Severe
> **5.** Surgical bleeding
> 2 = Minimal
> 1 = Moderate
> 0 = Severe
> The total score is 10, with patients scoring ≥9 fit for discharge home.

*A minimum score of 9/10 (and/or return to similar preop status) is achieved prior to transferring the patient to a Phase II recovery area.
From Chung F: Discharge criteria – a new trend. *Can J Anaesth* 42(11):1056-1058, 1995.

B. Postsedation
  1. Instruction
    a. Conduct in presence of a responsible adult assuming care of patient on discharge
    b. Written discharge instructions addressing medications, diet, and procedure-specific information must be reviewed with each patient.
    c. To protect patient, sedation and analgesia discharge instructions identify:
      (1) Medication used
      (2) Side effects
      (3) Specific postprocedural guidelines
  2. Patient criteria for discharge
    a. Patients should be alert and oriented or return to baseline status.
    b. Parents should be informed that pediatric patients are at risk for airway obstruction if head falls forward while child is secured in a car seat.
    c. Vital signs should be stable and within acceptable limits.
    d. Outpatients should be discharged in presence of a responsible adults who will accompany them home. (This includes all patients who have received sedation, whether minimal, moderate, or deep.)
  3. Sedation and analgesia postsedation follow-up
    a. A mechanism to ascertain postprocedure status is recommended for patients discharged on day of procedure.
    b. Inpatient information may be gathered by the moderate sedation practitioner after the procedure.
    c. Methods of gathering data include the following:
      (1) Patient questionnaire
      (2) Telephone interview
      (3) Satisfaction survey
    d. Purpose of postsedation assessment is to evaluate the following:
      (1) Incidence of complications related to administration of moderate sedation
      (2) Delayed recovery
      (3) Procedural complication rate
      (4) Return to function

VII. SEDATION RISK MANAGEMENT
   A. Strategies
      1. Quality: defined as the comprehensive positive outcome of a product
         a. Achievement of excellence in health care requires quality care and service evaluation.
      2. Quality of sedation services based on:
         a. Compliance with prescribed standards
         b. Recommended practice guidelines
      3. Implementation of a successful moderate sedation program based on:
         a. Delivery of highly technical aspects of care
         b. Positive outcomes
      4. Unexpected events and complications may occur as a result of:
         a. Human error
         b. Periods of reduced observation
         c. Environmental factors
         d. Poor communication
         e. Haste
         f. Poor patient selection
         g. Lack of preparation
      5. To prevent or reduce the number of adverse events:
         a. Implement a risk reduction strategy for all units and personnel engaged in administration of moderate sedation.
         b. Individual injury prevention strategies include the following:
            (1) Development of a complete sedation plan
            (2) Presedation preparation and patient assessment
            (3) Application and use of required monitoring equipment
            (4) Selection of appropriate pharmacological medications and techniques
            (5) Preparation and presence of emergency resuscitation equipment and personnel
            (6) Preparation for specific procedures and locations
            (7) Postsedation monitoring and discharge planning
      6. Management of risks and liability for the moderate sedation practitioner
         a. Practice issues: know the state board of nursing's position on the practice.
         b. Policies and procedures: must know sedation policy and procedure for facility and adhere to practices.
         c. Education and competence: must be educated in all aspects of practice of sedation and analgesia and show competence in delivery of care.
         d. Preprocedure care: assessment is important risk tool to determine whether patient is appropriate for nurse-monitored sedation.
         e. Medication administration: know sedation continuum and titrate to moderate sedation.
         f. Documentation: all nursing care should be documented to give accurate picture of patient's care.
         g. Wrong-site surgery: implement in all settings to decrease risks of wrong person or wrong procedure.
         h. Administration of anesthetic agents: know state board of nursing's position, organizational statements, support or lack of support from the institution, and personal education and competence to deliver the care.
      7. Ideally, individual risk reduction strategies prevent injury before an adverse incident or event takes place.

   a. Application of a risk management program
     (1) Department or institution basis
     (2) Development and implementation of mechanisms aimed at:
       (a) Risk
       (b) Identification
       (c) Analysis
       (d) Control
   b. Creation of a moderate sedation database program, as depicted in Figure 23-2, is essential.
   c. Coordinator guides input into moderate sedation database.
   d. Once database has been instituted, strategies to implement changes are used.

Conscious Sedation: Clinical Indicator Form

Patient Identification #_____   Age:_____   Date of Service:_____/ _____/_____

Attending Physician: _____   Procedure:_____

CS Nurse: _____   Location:_____

MONITORING INDICATORS

A. Continuous ECG monitoring?   ☐ Yes   ☐ No
B. Continuous respiratory monitoring?   ☐ Yes   ☐ No
C. Continuous blood pressure monitoring?   ☐ Yes   ☐ No
D. Continuous pulse oximetry monitoring?   ☐ Yes   ☐ No
E. Continuous level of consciousness monitoring?   ☐ Yes   ☐ No
F. Continuous patient monitoring by nurse?   ☐ Yes   ☐ No

PREPROCEDURE INDICATORS

☐ Preprocedure assessment complete
☐ Incomplete informed consent/no signature
☐ Incomplete patient chart
☐ Incomplete labwork
☐ Medical consult requires
☐ Noncompliance; NPO status
☐ Noncompliance; preprocedure medication instructions

PROCEDURE INDICATORS

☐ Respiratory depression
☐ Respiratory complication: stridor/laryngospasm/arrest
☐ Cardiovascular complications: cardiac arrest/ischemia/CHF/pulmonary edema
☐ Cardiovascular complications: hypotension/hypertension/dysrhythmias
☐ Level of consciousness: unresponsive/obtunded reflexes/agitation
☐ Medication: allergic reaction/wrong medication administered
☐ All medications administered as per facility policy
☐ Reversal agents administered (Flumazenil/Naloxone)

POSTPROCEDURE INDICATORS

☐ Prolonged somnolence
☐ Unexpected admission secondary to sedation
☐ Additional reversal agents administered (Flumazenil/Naloxone)
☐ Nausea/Vomiting: _____ times post discharge, current status:_____
☐ Evidence of postprocedure monitoring
☐ Documentation of discharge criteria
☐ Evidence of patient/family dissatisfaction
☐ Postprocedure follow-up complete

FIGURE 23-2 ■ Conscious sedation database program. (From Kost M: *Manual of conscious sedation,* Philadelphia, 1998, WB Saunders. Copyright 1996, Specialty Health Consultants.)

BIBLIOGRAPHY

1. Aldrete J: Postanesthesia recovery score revisited. *J Clin Anesth* 7:84, 1995.
2. American Heart Association: *About high blood pressure*. Available at: www.american-heart.org. Accessed November 3, 2008.
3. American Nurses Association: *Nursing liaison forum: Policy statement on conscious sedation*, Washington, DC, 1991, American Nurses Association.
4. American Society of Anesthesiologists: *Practice guidelines for management of the difficult airway*. Available at: www.asahq.org/publica tionsAndServices/Difficult%20Airway. pdf. Accessed August 13, 2008.
5. American Society of Anesthesiologists Task Force on Sedation and Analgesia by Non-anesthesiologists: Practice guidelines for sedation and analgesia by non-anesthesiologists. *Anesthesiology* 96(4):1004-1017, 2002.
6. Association of periOperating Registered Nurses: Standards, recommended practices and guidelines. *AORN J* 75:642-652, 2002.
7. Cohen LB, DeLegge MH, Aisenberg J, et al: AGA Institute review of endoscopic sedation. *Gastroenterology* 133:675-701, 2007.
8. Foster F: *Conscious sedation…coming to a unit near you*, Springhouse, PA, 2001, Springhouse Corp, SpringNet.
9. Kost M: *Manual of conscious sedation*, Philadelphia, 1998, WB Saunders.
10. Kost M: *Moderate sedation/analgesia: Core competences for practice*, ed 2, Philadelphia, 2004, Saunders.
11. Kost M, Brown D, DeZayas B: The administration of conscious sedation by non-anesthesia personnel. *Anesth Today* 11(2):11-15, 2000.
12. Lightdale JR, Goldman DA, Feldman HA, et al: Microstream capnography improves patient monitoring during moderate sedation: A randomized, controlled trial. *Pediatrics* 117(6):e1170-e1178, 2006.
13. Meltzer B: RNs pushing propofol. *Outpatient Surgery* 4(7):24-37, 2003.
14. Moos DD, Cuddeford JD: Implications of obstructive sleep apnea syndrome for the perianesthesia nurse. *J Perianesth Nurs* 21(2):103-115, 2006.
15. Odom-Forren J: The evolution of nurse monitored sedation. *J Perianesth Nurs* 20(6):385-398, 2005.
16. Odom-Forren J: The propofol debate continues. *J Perianesth Nurs* 21(2):77-78, 2006.
17. Odom-Forren J: Perioperative patient safety and procedural sedation. *Perioperative Nursing Clinics* 3(4):355-366, 2008.
18. Odom-Forren J, Watson D: *Practical guide to moderate sedation/analgesia*, Philadelphia, 2005, Saunders.
19. Ramsay MA, Savege TM, Simpson BR, et al: Controlled sedation with alphaxalone-alphadolone. *Br Med J* 2:656-659, 1974.
20. The Joint Commission: *Hospital accreditation standards*, Oakbrook Terrace, IL, 2008, The Joint Commission.
21. Vargo JJ: Minimizing complications: Sedation and monitoring. *Gastrointest Endosc Clin N Am* 17(1):11-28, v-vi, 2007.

Thermoregulation

VALLIRE D. HOOPER

OBJECTIVES

At the conclusion of this chapter, the reader will be able to:

1. Describe the physiology of thermoregulation.

2. Identify two complications of altered thermoregulation in the perianesthesia/perioperative setting.

3. Define unplanned perioperative hypothermia.

4. List three common causes of perioperative hypothermia.

5. Identify four adverse outcomes related to perioperative hypothermia.

6. Describe phase-specific recommendations for the management of perioperative hypothermia.

7. Define the pathophysiology of malignant hyperthermia (MH).

8. Identify the signs and symptoms of MH.

9. Describe the treatment of MH.

I. BASIC TERMS AND DEFINITIONS
   A. Thermal compartments
      1. Core thermal compartment
         a. Well-perfused tissues with temperature remaining relatively uniform
         b. Consists of organs of:
            (1) Trunk
            (2) Head
         c. Comprises 50% to 60% of body mass
      2. Peripheral thermal compartment
         a. Consists of arms and legs
         b. Temperature nonhomogeneous and varies over time
            (1) Temperature usually 2° C to 4° C lower than core temperature
            (2) Difference can be larger in more extreme thermal and/or physiological circumstances.
               (a) Lower core-to-peripheral gradients
                  (i) Warm environment
                  (ii) Vasodilation in response to an increased metabolic heat (generated in the core)
               (b) Higher core-to-peripheral gradients
                  (i) Cold environment
                  (ii) Vasoconstriction in an attempt to shift metabolic heat to the core
   B. Temperature
      1. Core temperature
         a. Temperature of core thermal compartment
         b. Most accurate core temperature measurement sites
            (1) Pulmonary artery (PA)
               (a) Obtained using a PA catheter
               (b) Most accurate because the artery brings blood directly from the core and its surroundings

          (c) Affected by:
              (i)   Large, rapid infusions of warmed or cold fluids
              (ii) Respiratory cycles
              (iii) Lower limb pneumatic compression devices
      (2) Distal esophagus
          (a) Best alternative to PA site
          (b) Affected by:
              (i)   Active cooling phase of cardiopulmonary bypass
              (ii) Surgery involving an open thorax or exposure of the
                    diaphragm
      (3) Nasopharynx
          (a) Used to monitor brain temperature
          (b) Not recommended with:
              (i)   Substantial anticoagulation
              (ii) Manipulation of nasal mucosa
      (4) Oral
          (a) Temperature readings vary dependent on placement in oral cavity
              (Figure 24-1).
          (b) Accurate reflection of core temperature when taken in left or right
              posterior sublingual (buccal) pocket
          (c) Site is dependable even in presence of:
              (i)   Oxygen therapy
              (ii) Warmed and cooled inspired gases
              (iii) Varied respiratory rates
          (d) Do not use in patients who are:
              (i)   Disoriented
              (ii) Shivering
              (iii) Having seizures
  c. Other temperature measurement sites used in the perianesthesia
     setting
     (1) Tympanic membrane (Figure 24-2)
         (a) Accuracy of reading dependent on:
             (i)   Operator technique
             (ii) Patient anatomy

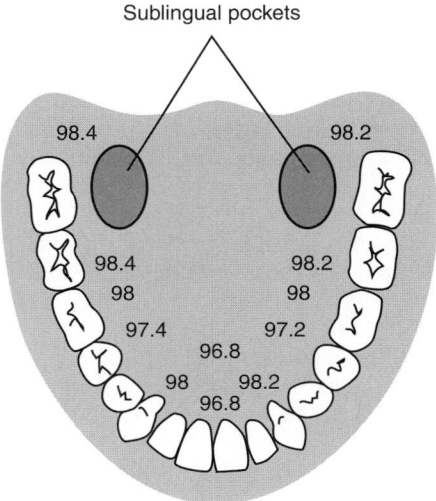

Sublingual pockets

98.4   98.2

98.4   98.2
98   98
97.4   97.2
        96.8
98   98.2
        96.8

FIGURE 24-1 ■ Temperature variations in the oral cavity. (From Nicoll LH: Heat in motion: Evaluating and managing temperature. *Nursing* 32:s1-s12, 2002.)

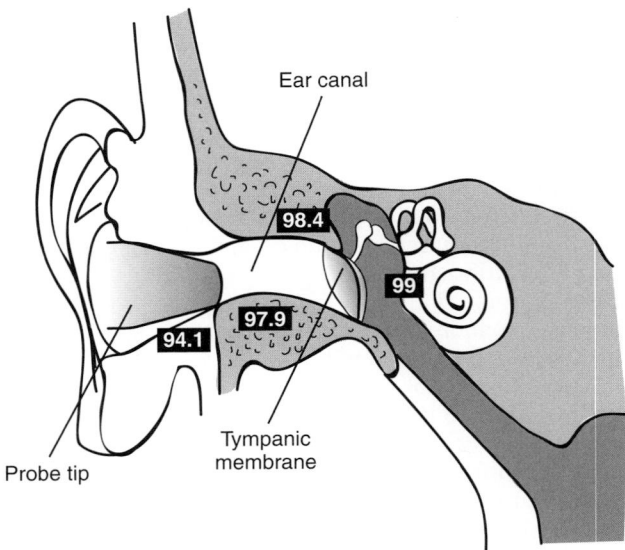

Ear canal

98.4

99

97.9

94.1

Tympanic membrane

Probe tip

FIGURE 24-2 ■ Tympanic temperature monitoring. (From Nicoll LH: Heat in motion: Evaluating and managing temperature. *Nursing* 32:s1-s12, 2002.)

         (iii) Accurate calibration
         (iv) Inherent instrument error of instrument used
      (b) Shown to be inaccurate to true core temperature measurements
    (2) Temporal artery
      (a) Favorably compares to tympanic and rectal measurements in children
      (b) Less reliable in adults
      (c) Lack of evidence to support accuracy to core temperature measurements in adults
    (3) Axillary
    (4) Bladder
      (a) Subject to thermal lag in unsteady thermal states
      (b) Continuous urinary drainage required
      (c) Useful indicator of total body warming
    (5) Rectum
      (a) Subject to thermal lag in unsteady thermal states
      (b) Potential for probe to be inserted into stool
    (6) Skin
  2. Normothermia: core temperature of 36° C to 38° C (96.8° F to 100.4° F)
  3. Hypothermia: core temperature less than 36° C (96.8° F)
  4. Hyperthermia: core temperature greater than 38° C (100.4° F)
C. Unplanned perioperative hypothermia
  1. Active warming measures
    a. Forced air convective warming
    b. Circulating mattresses
    c. Resistive heating blankets
    d. Radiant warmers
    e. Negative-pressure warming systems
    f. Warmed humidified inspired oxygen
  2. Passive thermal care measures
    a. Warmed cotton blankets
    b. Reflective blankets

   c. Circulating water mattress
   d. Socks
   e. Head covering
   f. Limited skin exposure
  3. Prewarming
   a. Warming of peripheral tissues or surface skin before anesthesia induction
  4. Risk factor
   a. Independent predictor, not an associated factor of an untoward event
  5. Thermal comfort
   a. Patient perception that they are neither too warm or too cold
 D. MH
  1. Hereditary abnormality of muscle metabolism
   a. Caused by certain triggering agents
   b. Results in a life-threatening pharmacogenetic disorder
  2. Must have specific genes for MH to occur
   a. Relatives of patient who has had an MH crisis are at risk.
    (1) Siblings
    (2) Parents
    (3) Children
   b. Inheritance by autosomal dominant pathway
    (1) Risk diminishes as relationship becomes further removed.
  3. Characterized by muscular hypercatabolic reactions
   a. Level of intracellular calcium reuptake is impaired producing:
    (1) Muscle tetany
    (2) Increased production of:
     (a) Heat
     (b) Carbon dioxide
     (c) Lactate
II. THERMOREGULATION PHYSIOLOGY
 A. Most of body's heat provided by basal metabolic rate
  1. Core body temperature remains fairly constant.
  2. Skin and extremity temperatures may vary with:
   a. Environmental changes
   b. Thermoregulatory responses
 B. Temperature regulation in conscious adults mediated by the hypothalamus
  (Figure 24-3) through a combination of behavioral and physiological responses
  1. Hypothalamus

Hypothalamic "Thermostat"

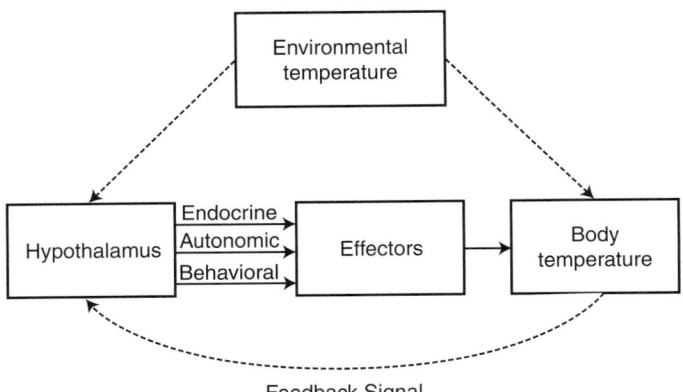

FIGURE 24-3 ■ The hypothalamic thermostat. (From Pressley TA: *Temperature regulation, 2000.* Available at: http://phy025.lubb.ttuhsc.edu/Pressley/Course/Temp-Reg.htm. Accessed March 2003.)

    a. Nestled at base of the brain
    b. Primary temperature control center
        (1) Maintains normothermia by regulating heat loss with heat production
        (2) Receives input via spinal cord from thermoreceptors located in:
            (a) Skin
            (b) Nose
            (c) Oral cavity
            (d) Thoracic viscera
            (e) Spinal cord
    c. Generates conscious and unconscious responses to maintain normothermia
  2. Mechanisms of temperature regulation
    a. Behavior
        (1) Adding or removing clothing or covering
        (2) Changing location
        (3) Adjusting temperature of dietary intake
        (4) Adjusting environmental temperature
    b. Endocrine
        (1) Hormones released in response to hypothalamic stimulation
        (2) Initiates organ and tissue responses in all systems
    c. Autonomic
        (1) Changes in peripheral circulation
        (2) Peripheral shell expands or contracts in response to peripheral and core temperature changes (Figure 24-4).
C. Mechanisms of heat production and loss
  1. Mechanisms of heat production
    a. Body tissues produce heat in proportion to their metabolic rates.
        (1) Metabolism is the only natural internal source of heat.
        (2) Brain and major organs (core thermal compartment)
            (a) Most metabolically active
            (b) Generate more metabolic heat than skeletal muscle at rest

Relative Size of Insulating Shell

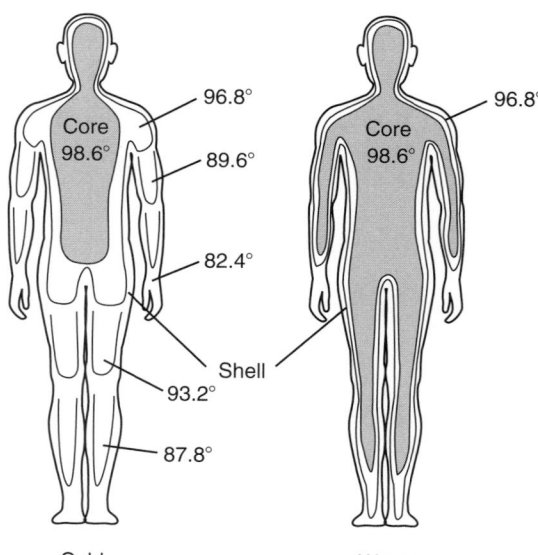

FIGURE 24-4 ■ Relative size of the insulating shell in response to temperature changes. (From Pressley TA: *Temperature regulation, 2000.* Available at: http://phy025.lubb.ttuhsc.edu/Pressley/Course/Temp-Reg.htm. Accessed March 2003.)

(3) Skeletal muscle can briefly exceed the basal metabolic rate by a factor of 10.

b. Increased metabolism related to work or physical exercise

c. Thermogenesis

(1) Accomplished by shivering and nonshivering means

(2) Nonshivering

(a) Limited physiologic response of newborn infant to hypothermia

(b) Involves catabolism of brown fat, which is not coupled with adenosine triphosphate formation

(c) Releases energy in the form of heat

(3) Shivering

(a) Can increase heat production by up to 500%

(b) Accompanied by increased:

(i) Metabolic rate

(ii) Oxygen demand

2. Mechanisms of heat loss

a. Processes controlling heat transfer (Figure 24-5)

(1) Radiation

(a) Loss of energy through radiant electromagnetic waves in the infrared spectrum

(b) Involves no direct contact between the objects involved

(i) Energy (or heat) radiates from warmer object to cooler one.

(ii) Uncovered skin in operative patient will radiate energy away from patient, reducing the body temperature.

(c) Accounts for 40% to 60% of all heat loss

(d) Accentuated in the elderly and neonates

(2) Convection

(a) Loss of body heat by means of transfer to surrounding cooler air

(b) Need a temperature gradient between the body and surrounding air

(c) Heat transfer may occur in two ways

(i) Passive movement

[a] Warm air rises.

[b] Loss of body heat as a result of basic skin exposure

(ii) Active movement

[a] Fan or wind blowing across the body surface

[b] Facilitated by laminar flow systems in operating room (OR)

(d) Accounts for 25% to 35% of heat lost and 10 kilocalories/hour (kcal/h)

(3) Conduction

(a) Transfer of heat energy through direct contact between objects

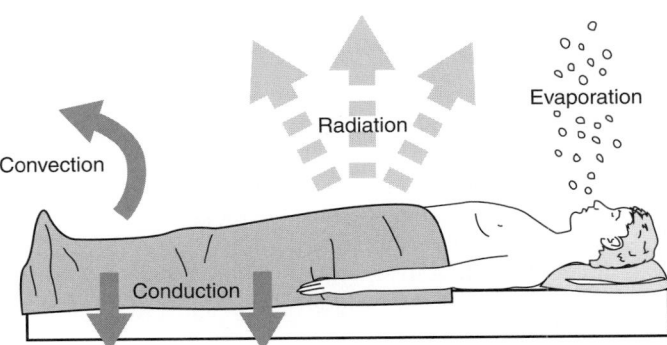

FIGURE 24-5 ■ Mechanisms of heat loss. (From Sessler DI: Perioperative heat balance. *Anesthesiology* 92:583, 2000.)

        (b) Heat loss occurs with contact with any of the following:
            (i)   Cold OR table
            (ii) Skin preparation solutions
            (iii) Intravenous (IV) fluids
            (iv) Irrigants
            (v) Cold sheets and drapes
        (c) Causes core body heat to move out to cooler periphery
        (d) Accounts for up to 10% of heat loss
            (i)   With IV fluid infusion, 16 kcal/h loss
            (ii) With blood infusion, 30 kcal/h loss
    (4) Evaporation
        (a) Transfer of heat that occurs when a liquid changed into a gas
        (b) Routes of heat loss
            (i)   Perspiration (12-16 kcal/h)
            (ii) Evaporation (12-16 kcal/h)
            (iii) Exposed viscera during surgery or trauma
                [a] The larger the wound, the greater the heat loss
                [b] Can result in a 400 kcal/h loss
        (c) May account for up to 25% of heat loss
  b. Other routes of heat loss in perioperative setting
    (1) Infusion of IV fluids that are cooler than body temperature
        (a) A mass is added to the body that is cooler than current body temperature.
        (b) Average body temperature falls.
        (c) Fluid exits the body as urine or blood after being warmed to body temperature.
        (d) Net loss of heat energy occurs.
    (2) Ventilation with dry gas
        (a) Gas is cooler than body temperature.
        (b) Warmed, heated, and humidified in tracheobronchial tree
        (c) Warmed and saturated with water vapor, the gas is exhaled at body temperature.
        (d) Significant heat energy loss may occur over time.
D. Physiological responses to changes in environmental temperature
  1. Cold environment
    a. Physiological goal is to minimize heat loss while maximizing heat production.
    b. Sympathetic stimulation
      (1) Increases thickness of insulating shell through vasoconstriction
      (2) Stimulates nonshivering thermogenesis
      (3) Initiates piloerection
    c. Shivering thermogenesis initiated
    d. Long-term exposure also results in release of thyrotropin-releasing hormone from the hypothalamus.
  2. Hot environment
    a. Physiological goal is to maximize heat loss.
    b. Vasodilation shrinks insulating shell.
    c. Sudomotor response (stimulation of sweat glands)
      (1) Regulates sensible evaporative heat loss
      (2) Increases activity of cholinergic pathways
      (3) Critical for cooling in an environment that is hotter than the body
      (4) May also promote vasodilation
    d. Decreased heat production
    e. Long-term exposure
      (1) Increase in sweating capacity of sweat glands
      (2) Aldosterone-mediated increase in sodium retention

III. PERIOPERATIVE THERMOREGULATION
  A. Unless actively warmed, patients receiving an anesthetic become hypothermic.
    1. Usual temperature drop is 1° C to 3° C.
    2. Temperature loss depends on:
      a. Type and dose of anesthetic
      b. Amount of surgical exposure
      c. Ambient temperature
    3. Normal physiological responses used to regulate the core temperature impaired by anesthetic agents
      a. Patient tends to become poikilothermic.
      b. Body takes on temperature of environment.
  B. Redistribution hypothermia occurs.
    1. Mechanisms of redistribution
      a. General anesthesia reduces the vasoconstriction threshold.
        (1) Threshold drops well below normal core temperature.
        (2) Centrally mediated thermoregulatory constriction is inhibited.
      b. General and regional anesthesia also cause peripheral vasodilation.
        (1) Blood flow to skin increased
        (2) Core heat lost through peripheral tissues
    2. Both mechanisms result in a core-to-peripheral redistribution of body heat (Figure 24-6).
  C. Typical patterns of heat loss during a surgical case (Figure 24-7)
    1. Core temperature drop of 1° C to 1.5° C occurs during first hour of surgery.
      a. Caused by core-to-peripheral redistribution
      b. Affected by other factors
        (1) Initial body heat content
        (2) Body morphology
        (3) Amount of systemic heat loss
    2. Initial heat loss followed by 2 to 3 hours of a slower, more linear drop
      a. Metabolic rate drops 15% to 40% with administration of general anesthesia.
      b. Heat loss exceeds metabolic heat production.
      c. Heat loss mediated by the four fundamental mechanisms of heat loss (Figure 24-6)

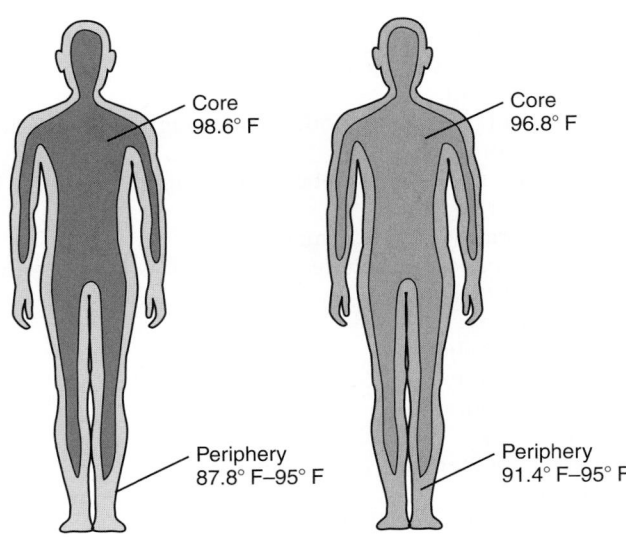

Core
98.6° F

Core
96.8° F

Periphery
87.8° F–95° F

Periphery
91.4° F–95° F

Vasoconstricted — Anesthesia → Vasodilated

FIGURE 24-6 ■ Core-to-peripheral redistribution after the administration of anesthesia. (From Sessler DI: Perioperative heat balance. *Anesthesiology* 92:581, 2000.)

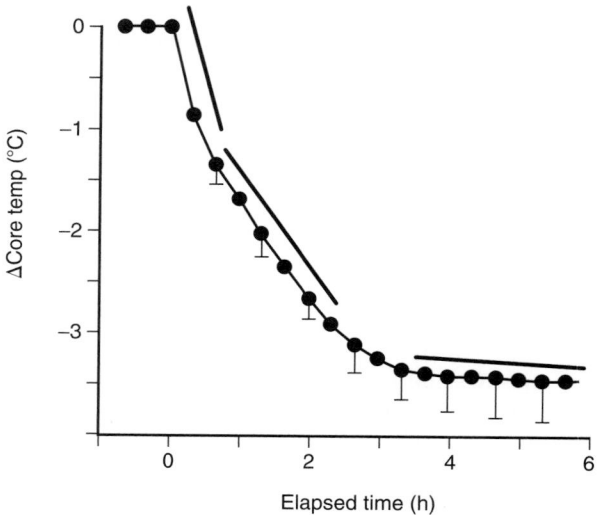

FIGURE 24-7 ■ Perioperative heat loss over time. (From Sessler DI: Perioperative heat balance. *Anesthesiology* 92:580, 2000.)

           (1) Radiation
           (2) Convection
           (3) Conduction
           (4) Evaporation
    3. Patient enters a plateau phase where the core temperature stabilizes.
       a. Usually develops 2 to 4 hours into surgery
       b. Characterized by a constant core temperature
       c. May be passively or actively maintained
          (1) Passive plateau
             (a) Metabolic heat production equals heat loss without activating thermoregulatory defenses.
             (b) Commonly seen in small operations in which patients are well covered with effective insulators
          (2) Active plateau
             (a) Patient becomes hypothermic enough to trigger thermoregulatory vasoconstriction.
             (b) To occur with anesthetics, core temperature drops to 34° C to 35° C (93.2° F to 95° F)
  D. Postoperative return to normothermia
    1. Brain anesthetic concentration decreases to allow for triggering of normal thermoregulatory responses.
    2. Can be impaired by:
       a. Residual anesthetics
       b. Postoperative opioids
    3. May take 2 to 5 hours
    4. Can be affected by:
       a. Degree of hypothermia
       b. Age of patient
IV. PLANNED PERIOPERATIVE HYPOTHERMIA
  A. Hypothermia may be intentionally induced in some surgical cases to prevent intraoperative complications.
    1. Cardiac ischemia
    2. Cerebral ischemia

    B. Most common cases include:
       1. Cardiac surgery requiring cardiopulmonary bypass
         a. Decreases amount of oxygen required by myocardial cells
         b. Slows metabolic demands
       2. Neurosurgical procedures
         a. Decreases intracranial pressure
         b. Decreases amount of bleeding
    C. Intentionally induced hypothermia has been shown to be effective in:
       1. Acute stroke
       2. Perinatal asphyxia
       3. Neurological outcome after cardiac arrest
       4. Severe head injury
V. UNPLANNED PERIOPERATIVE HYPOTHERMIA (UPH)
    A. Unexpected core temperature decrease to less than 36° C (96.8° F) as a result of surgery or other procedure.
    B. May be present regardless of patient's temperature if:
       1. Patient complains of feeling cold.
       2. Patient presents with common signs and symptoms.
         a. Shivering
         b. Peripheral vasoconstriction
         c. Piloerection
    C. Risk factors
       1. Every patient undergoing surgery
       2. Risk factors supported by weak evidence:
         a. Age
         b. Female gender
         c. Systolic blood pressure
         d. Level of spinal block
       3. Risk factors supported by insufficient (mixed) evidence
         a. Body Mass Index (BMI) below normal
         b. Normal BMI
         c. Procedure duration
         d. Body surface/wound area uncovered
         e. Anesthesia duration
         f. History of diabetes with autonomic dysfunction
    D. Negative effects associated with UPH
       1. Patient discomfort related to:
         a. Shivering
         b. Unpleasant sensation of being cold
       2. Adrenergic stimulation resulting in an increase in serum catecholamine levels
       3. Untoward cardiac events
         a. Increased catecholamines may cause myocardial ischemia.
         b. Cardiac function directly impaired at temperatures less than 33° C (91.4° F)
         c. Threshold for dysrhythmias around 31° C (87.8° F)
         d. Ventricular fibrillation likely at 30° C (86° F)
       4. Coagulopathy
         a. Platelet function reduced
         b. Clotting cascade slowed
         c. Blood loss increased
       5. Altered drug metabolism
         a. Elimination of injectable drugs prolonged
         b. Duration of anesthetic agents prolonged
       6. Impaired wound healing/surgical site infection
         a. Tissue oxygenation decreased
         b. Immunity and collagen production impaired
         c. Infection rates increased
           (1) 19% in a hypothermic patient
           (2) 6% in a normothermic patient

    7. Increased hospital costs
       a. Hypothermia of 1.5° C below normal results in a $2500 to $7000 increase.
       b. Elevated costs related to:
          (1) Increased length of stay in:
             (a) Post anesthesia care unit (PACU)
             (b) Intensive care unit (ICU)
             (c) Hospital
          (2) Increased use of:
             (a) Red blood cells
             (b) Plasma
             (c) Platelets
          (3) Increased need for mechanical ventilation
          (4) Management of adverse cardiac events
  E. Perioperative patient management
    1. Preoperative (Figures 24-8 and 24-9)
       a. Assessment
          (1) Identify patient's risk factors for UPH.
          (2) Measure patient's temperature.
          (3) Determine patient's thermal comfort level.
          (4) Assess for other signs and symptoms of hypothermia.
          (5) Document and communicate all risk factor assessment findings to all members of the anesthesia/surgical team
       b. Interventions
          (1) Implement passive thermal care measures.
          (2) Maintain ambient room temperature at or above 24° C (75° F).
          (3) Institute active warming for hypothermic patients.
          (4) Consider preoperative warming to reduce the risk of intra/postoperative hypothermia.
             (a) Minimum of 30 minutes of prewarming may reduce the risk of subsequent hypothermia.
       c. Outcome
          (1) Patient will express thermal comfort.
          (2) Nonemergent patients will be normothermic before going to the OR/procedure area.

Thermal Management Flow Chart

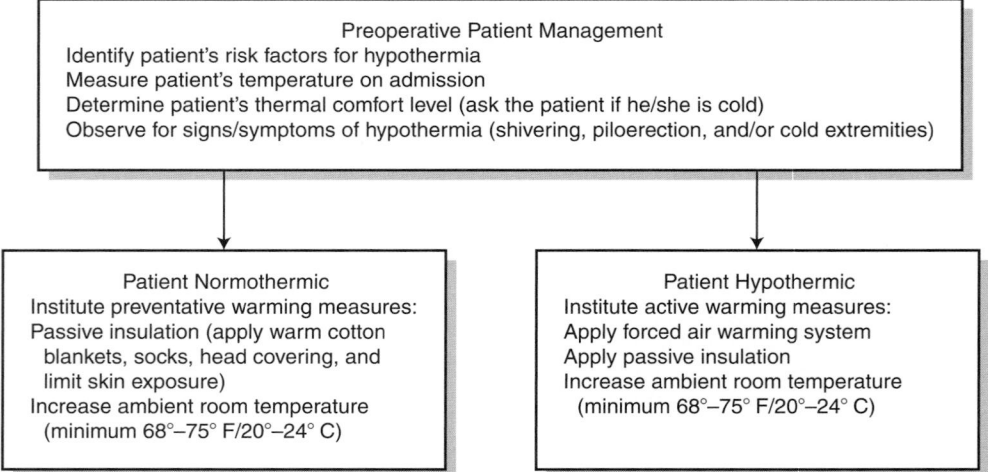

FIGURE 24-8 ■ Preoperative patient management. (From American Society of PeriAnesthesia Nurses: Clinical guideline for the prevention of unplanned perioperative hypothermia. In *2008-2010 Standards of perianesthesia nursing practice,* Cherry Hill, NJ, 2008, American Society of PeriAnesthesia Nurses, p 24.)

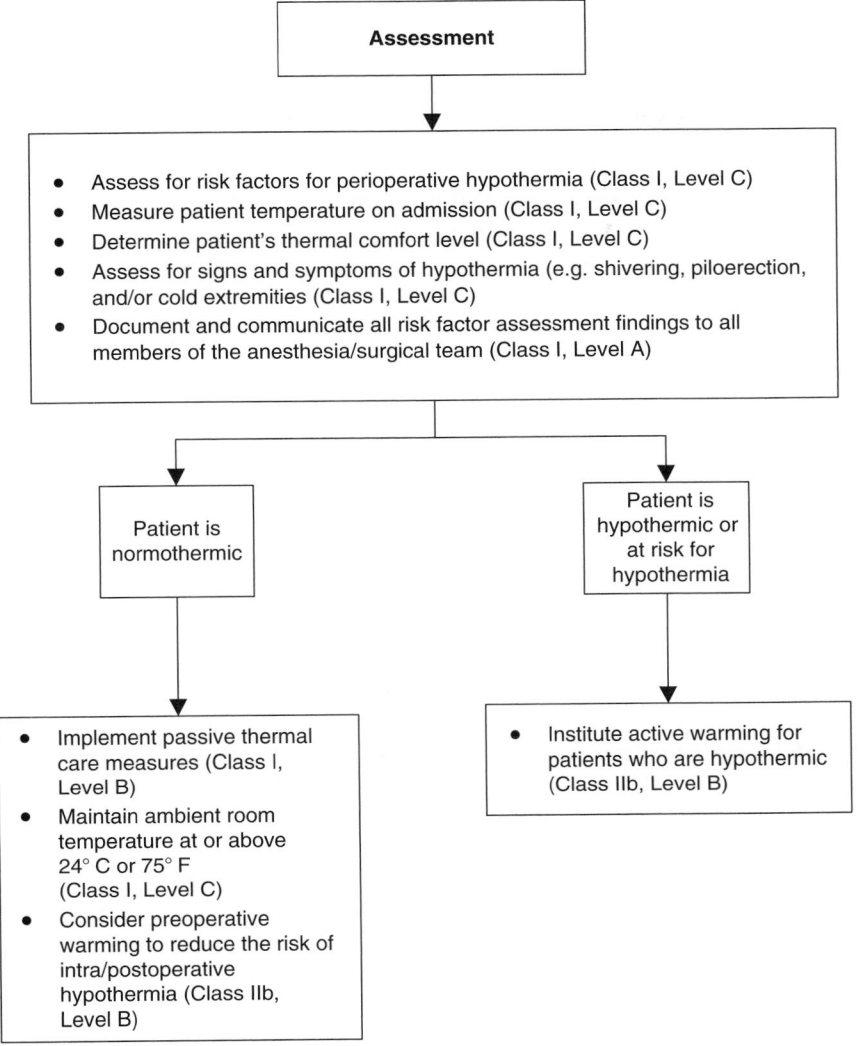

FIGURE 24-9 ■ Preadmission/Preoperative recommendations. (From American Society of PeriAnesthesia Nurses: Preadmission/preoperative recommendations. *Journal of PeriAnesthesia Nursing,* in Press.)

2. Intraoperative (Figures 24-10 and 24-11)
   a. Assessment
      (1) Identify patient's risk factors for UPH.
      (2) Consider frequent temperature monitoring in all cases.
      (3) Determine patient's thermal comfort level.
      (4) Assess for signs and symptoms of hypothermia.
      (5) Document and communicate all risk factor assessment findings to all members of the anesthesia/surgical/nursing team.
   b. Interventions
      (1) All patients
         (a) Passive warming measures
         (b) Maintain ambient room temperature as per Association of periOperative Registered Nurses (AORN) and architectural recommendations.
         (c) Limit skin exposure.
      (2) Procedures longer than 30 minutes
         (a) Forced air warming

Intraoperative Patient Management

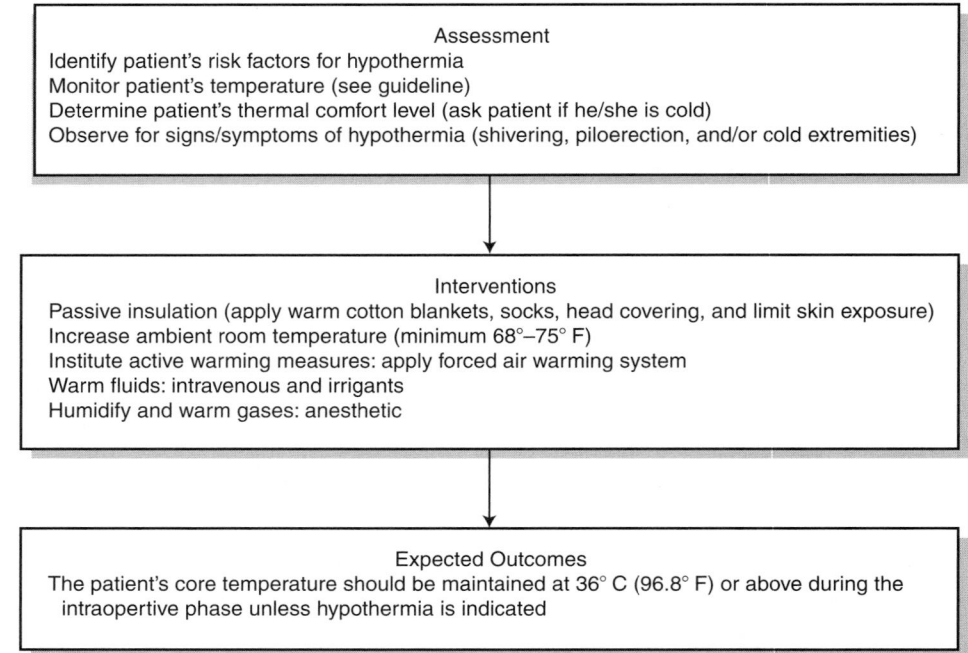

Assessment
Identify patient's risk factors for hypothermia
Monitor patient's temperature (see guideline)
Determine patient's thermal comfort level (ask patient if he/she is cold)
Observe for signs/symptoms of hypothermia (shivering, piloerection, and/or cold extremities)

Interventions
Passive insulation (apply warm cotton blankets, socks, head covering, and limit skin exposure)
Increase ambient room temperature (minimum 68°–75° F)
Institute active warming measures: apply forced air warming system
Warm fluids: intravenous and irrigants
Humidify and warm gases: anesthetic

Expected Outcomes
The patient's core temperature should be maintained at 36° C (96.8° F) or above during the
intraopertive phase unless hypothermia is indicated

FIGURE 24-10 ■ Intraoperative patient management. (From American Society of PeriAnesthesia Nurses: Clinical guideline for the prevention of unplanned perioperative hypothermia. In *2008-2010 Standards of perianesthesia nursing practice,* Cherry Hill, NJ, 2008, American Society of PeriAnesthesia Nurses, p 24.)

       (3) Alternative warming measures that may be used alone or in combination with forced air
         (a) Warmed IV fluids
         (b) Warmed irrigation fluids
         (c) Circulating water garments
         (d) Circulating water mattress
         (e) Radiant heat
         (f) Gel pad (Artic Sun©) surface warming
         (g) Resistive heating
    c. Patient will be normothermic on discharge from the OR/procedure area
  3. Postoperative patient management: phase I PACU (Figures 24-12 and 24-13)
    a. Assessment
      (1) Identify patient's risk factors for UPH.
      (2) Assess temperature on admission to phase I PACU.
         (a) If hypothermic:
            (i)   Monitor serial temperatures at least every 15 minutes.
            (ii) Monitor until normothermia reached.
         (b) If normothermic, assess temperature:
            (i)   At least hourly
            (ii) Before discharge
            (iii) As ordered or indicated
      (3) Determine patient's thermal comfort level.
      (4) Assess for signs and symptoms of hypothermia.
    b. Interventions
      (1) If normothermic:
         (a) Institute thermal comfort measures.
         (b) Maintain ambient room temperature at or above 24° C (75° F).

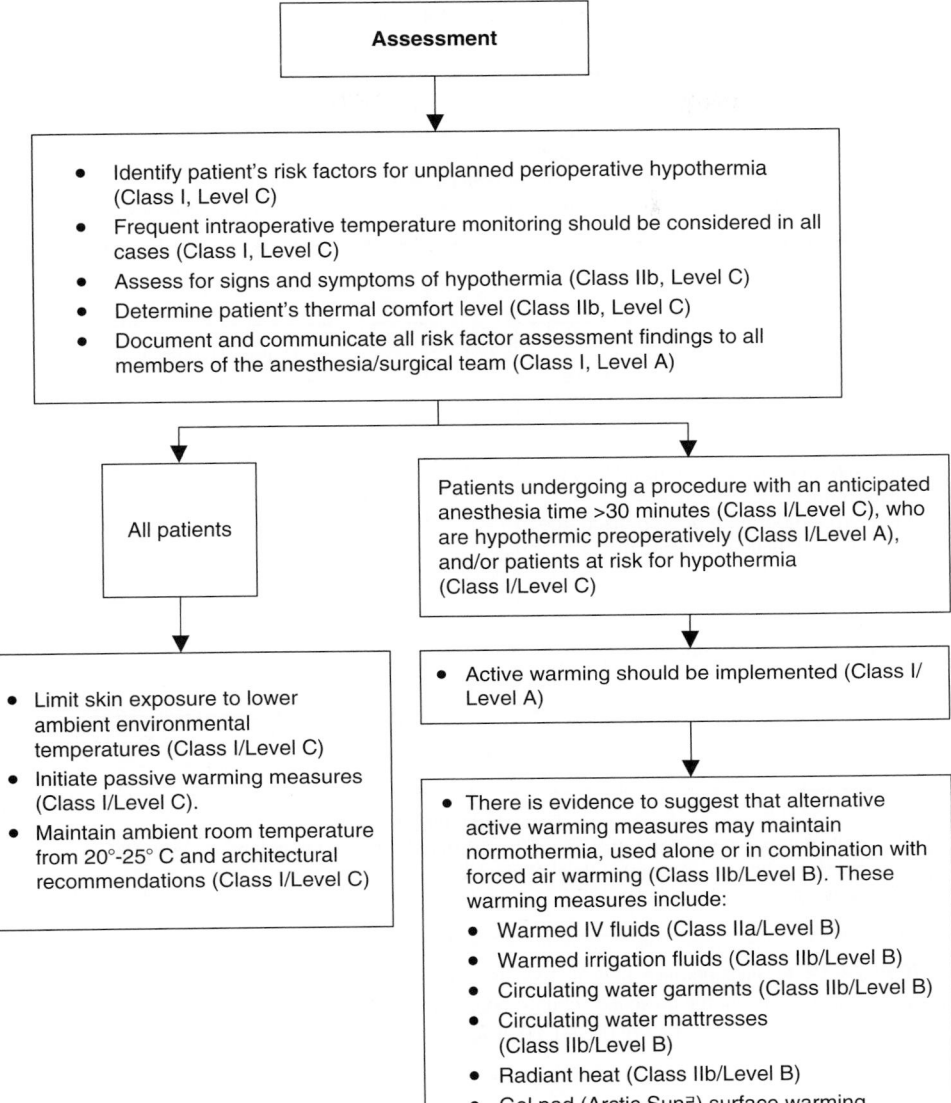

FIGURE 24-11 ■ Intraoperative recommendations. (From American Society of PeriAnesthesia Nurses: Preadmission/preoperative recommendations. *Journal of PeriAnesthesia Nursing,* in Press.)

    (c) Assess patient's thermal comfort level.
        (i) On admission
        (ii) Discharge
        (iii) As indicated
    (d) Observe for signs and symptoms of hypothermia.
    (e) Reassess temperature:
        (i) If patient's thermal comfort level decreases
        (ii) If patient shows signs or symptoms of hypothermia
    (f) Measure patient's temperature before discharge.
  (2) If hypothermic:
    (a) Initiate active warming measures.
    (b) Consider adjuvant measures.

Postoperative Patient Management: Phase I PACU

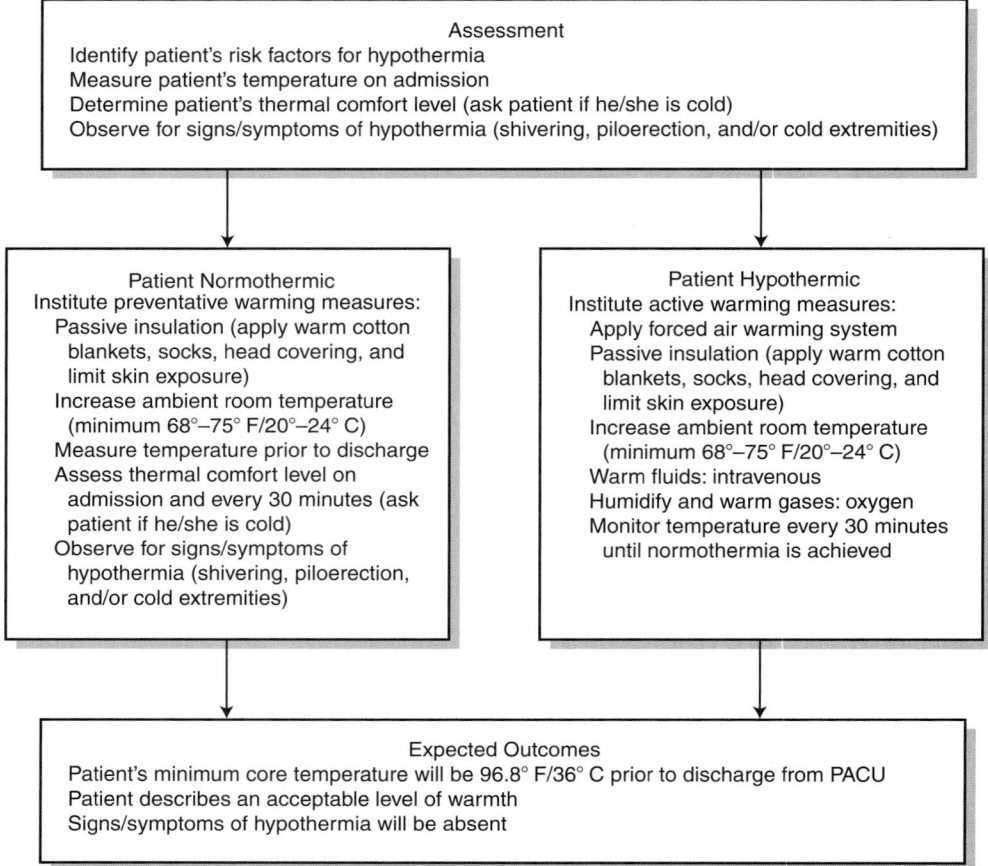

Assessment
Identify patient's risk factors for hypothermia
Measure patient's temperature on admission
Determine patient's thermal comfort level (ask patient if he/she is cold)
Observe for signs/symptoms of hypothermia (shivering, piloerection, and/or cold extremities)

Patient Normothermic
Institute preventative warming measures:
  Passive insulation (apply warm cotton
    blankets, socks, head covering, and
    limit skin exposure)
  Increase ambient room temperature
    (minimum 68°–75° F/20°–24° C)
  Measure temperature prior to discharge
  Assess thermal comfort level on
    admission and every 30 minutes (ask
    patient if he/she is cold)
  Observe for signs/symptoms of
    hypothermia (shivering, piloerection,
    and/or cold extremities)

Patient Hypothermic
Institute active warming measures:
  Apply forced air warming system
  Passive insulation (apply warm cotton
    blankets, socks, head covering, and
    limit skin exposure)
  Increase ambient room temperature
    (minimum 68°–75° F/20°–24° C)
  Warm fluids: intravenous
  Humidify and warm gases: oxygen
  Monitor temperature every 30 minutes
    until normothermia is achieved

Expected Outcomes
Patient's minimum core temperature will be 96.8° F/36° C prior to discharge from PACU
Patient describes an acceptable level of warmth
Signs/symptoms of hypothermia will be absent

FIGURE 24-12 ■ Postoperative patient management: PACU. (From American Society of PeriAnesthesia Nurses: Clinical guideline for the prevention of unplanned perioperative hypothermia. In *2008-2010 Standards of perianesthesia nursing practice,* Cherry Hill, NJ, 2008, American Society of PeriAnesthesia Nurses, p 25.)

        (i) Warm IV fluids.
        (ii) Humidify and warm oxygen.
     (c) Assess every 15 minutes until normothermia reached.
        (i) Temperature
        (ii) Thermal comfort level
   (3) Discharge teaching (Figure 24-14)
     (a) Instruct patient and responsible adult in methods to maintain
       normothermia after discharge
        (i) consumption of warm liquids
        (ii) application of blankets, socks, and other warm clothing
        (iii) increased room temperature
VI. MALIGNANT HYPERTHERMIA
  A. Incidence of MH
    1. More common in children
      a. Children: 1:15,000 anesthetics administered
      b. Adults: 1:20,000 to 1:50,000 anesthetics administered
    2. Many cases undetected
      a. Never anesthetized
      b. Short anesthetic period

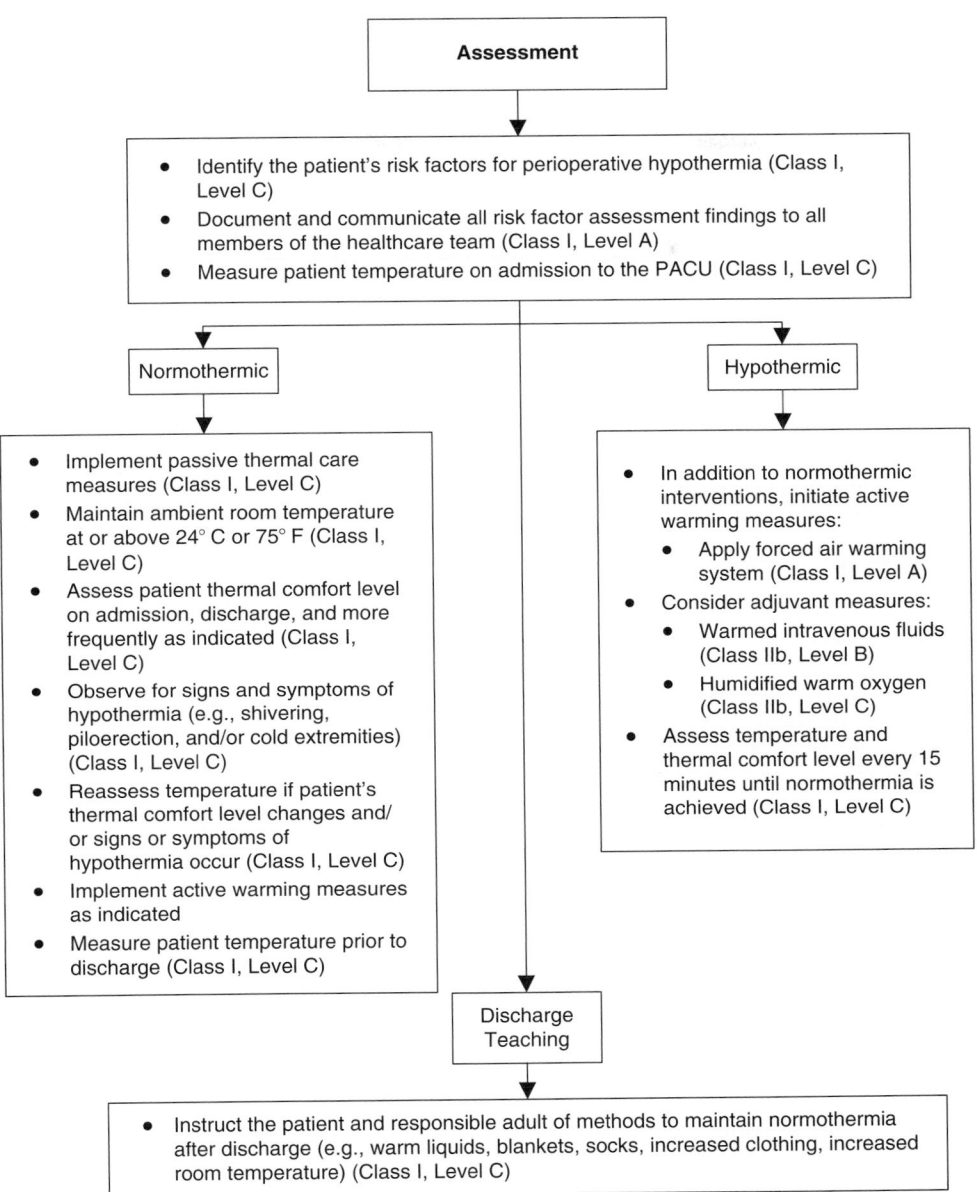

FIGURE 24-13 ■ Phase I/II PACU postoperative patient management recommendations. (From American Society of PeriAnesthesia Nurses: Preadmission/preoperative recommendations. *Journal of PeriAnesthesia Nursing,* in Press.)

    c. Effects of triggering agent may be modified by preceding with use of nontriggering agents.
        (1) Thiobarbiturates
        (2) Nondepolarizing muscle relaxants
        (3) Hypothermia
    d. Many cases mild, not diagnosed
  B. Mortality significantly reduced since availability of dantrolene in late 1970s
    1. Before 1970: 70%
    2. 1976: 28%
    3. Has remained 6% to 7% since the late 1980s
    4. Most deaths still occur in otherwise healthy children and adults.
  C. Triggering agents

Postoperative Patient Management: Phase II PACU (ASU)

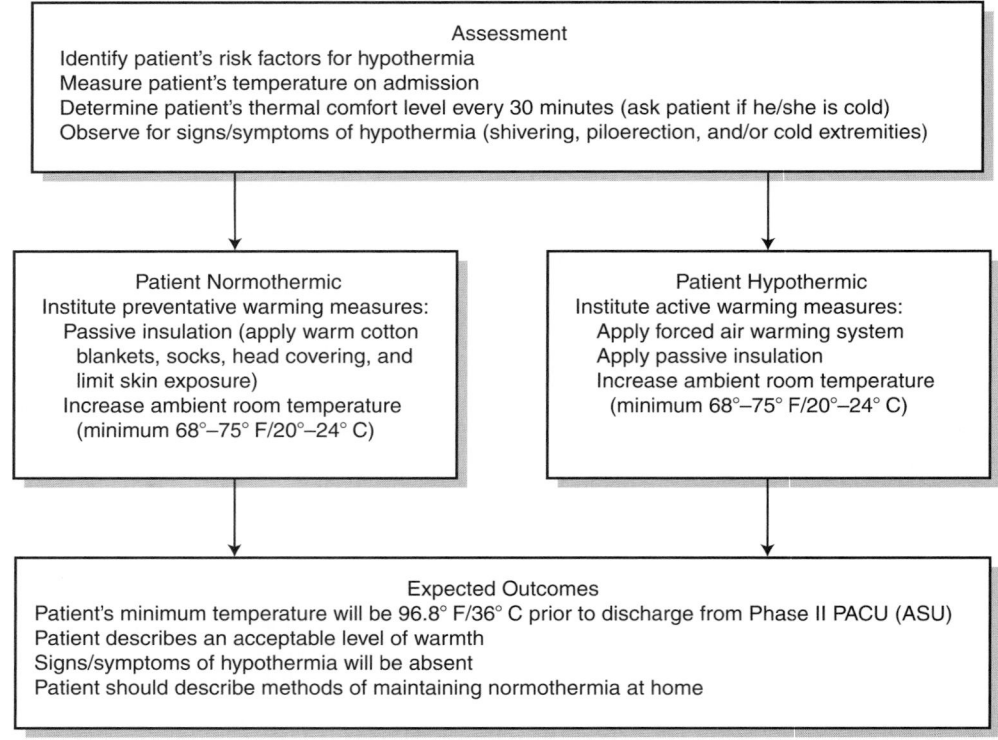

FIGURE 24-14 ■ Postoperative patient management: Phase II PACU. (From American Society of PeriAnesthesia Nurses: Clinical guideline for the prevention of unplanned perioperative hypothermia. In *2008-2010 Standards of perianesthesia nursing practice,* Cherry Hill, NJ, 2008, American Society of PeriAnesthesia Nurses, p 26.)

  1. Pharmacological
     a. Succinylcholine
     b. All volatile inhalation agents
        (1) Halothane
        (2) Enflurane
        (3) Isoflurane
        (4) Sevoflurane
        (5) Desflurane
        (6) Chloroform (trichloromethane, methyltrichloride)
        (7) Trichloroethylene
        (8) Xenon (rarely used)
 D. Safe anesthetic agents (Table 24-1)
 E. Preoperative detection
    1. History
       a. Patient with previous MH episode
       b. Fifty percent with MH have had previous anesthesia without a problem.
       c. Family member with MH who has had crisis provides warning.
       d. History of family member who died during surgery and anesthesia
    2. Examination
       a. Usually reveals nothing
       b. Muscle weakness and myopathies associated with MH-like syndromes
          (1) Duchenne muscular dystrophy
          (2) Central core disease
          (3) Myotonia
          (4) Other unusual myopathies

■ TABLE 24-1
■ ■ **Drugs That Are Considered Safe to Administer to a Patient with MHS**

Barbiturates/Intravenous Anesthetics	Opioids	Anxiety-Relieving Medications
Diazepam	Alfentanil (Alfenta)	Ativan (Lorazepam)
Etomidate (Amidate)	Anileridine	Centrax
Hexobarbital	Codeine (Methyl Morphine)	Dalmane (Flurazepam)
Ketamine (Ketalar)	Diamorphine	Halcion (Triazolam)
Methohexital (Brevital)	Fentanyl (Sublimaze)	Klonopin
Midazolam	Hydromorphone (Dilaudid)	Librax
Narcobarbital	Meperidine (Demerol)	Librium (Chlordiazepoxide)
Propofol (Diprivan)	Methadone	Versed (Midazolam)
Thiopental	Morphine	Paxipam (Halazepam)
	Naloxone	Restoril (Temazepam)
	Oxycodone	Serax (Oxazepam)
	Phenoperidine	Tranxene (Clorazepate)
	Remifentanil	Valium (Diazepam)
	Sufentanil (Sufenta)	
INHALED NONVOLATILE GENERAL ANESTHETIC	**SAFE MUSCLE RELAXANTS**	**LOCAL ANESTHETICS**
Nitrous oxide	Arduan (Pipecuronium)	Amethocaine
	Curare (active ingredient is Tubocurarine)	Articaine
		Bupivacaine
	Gallamine	Dibucaine
	Metocurine	Etidocaine
	Mivacron (Mivacurium)	Eucaine
	Neuromax (Doxacurium)	Lidocaine (Xylocaine)
	Nimbex (Cisatracurium)	Levobupivacaine
	Norcuron (Vecuronium)	Mepivacaine (Carbocaine)
	Pavulon (Pancuronium)	Procaine (Novocain)
	Tracrium (Atracurium)	Prilocaine (Citanest)
	Zemuron (Rocuronium)	Ropivacaine
		Stovaine

MHS, Malignant hyperthermia syndrome.
From Drain C, Odom-Forren J: *Perianesthesia nursing: A critical care approach*, ed 5, Philadelphia, 2009, Saunders.

     3. Laboratory tests
       a. Caffeine-halothane contracture test
         (1) Most reliable test for preoperative diagnosis
         (2) Few hospitals (about eight) in United States and Canada can perform this test.
         (3) Requires muscle biopsy
            (a) Must be performed at one of the testing hospitals
            (b) Cannot be mailed to testing center
         (4) Costly
       b. Molecular genetic testing
         (1) Detects 30% to 50% of patients at risk for MH
         (2) Can be obtained with a simple blood sample
   F. Signs and symptoms of MH
     1. Increasing end-tidal carbon dioxide
     2. Muscle rigidity
       a. Masseter muscle spasm after administration of succinylcholine
       b. Generalized trunk or total body rigidity

     3. Tachycardia/tachypnea

     4. Mixed respiratory and metabolic acidosis

     5. Temperature elevation (often a late sign)

     6. Myoglobinuria

  G. Treatment (Box 24-1)

     1. Immediate treatment

       a. Discontinue anesthesia and surgery immediately.

       b. Administer 100% oxygen.

       c. Halt procedure as soon as possible.

     2. Administer dantrolene (Dantrium) 2.5 mg/kg rapidly through a large-bore IV.

       a. Dantrolene supplied in 20-mg vials

         (1) Reconstitute with 60 mL of preservative-free sterile water.

         (2) Shake vigorously.

         (3) Warming bottle of solution may hasten mixing.

       b. Side effects of dantrolene

         (1) Difficulty in walking

         (2) Fatigue

         (3) Muscle weakness

■ BOX 24-1

■ **SUGGESTED EQUIPMENT AND DRUGS TO BE USED IN TREATMENT OF ACUTE MALIGNANT HYPERTHERMIA**

Equipment Needed
Intravenous lines with assorted cannula gauges
Central venous pressure sets (2)
Transducer kits for arterial and central venous cannulation
Esophageal or other core temperature probes
Pulmonary artery catheter
Laboratory test tubes for blood chemistry analysis
Syringes (60 mL x 5) to dilute dantrolene
Crystalloid solution (ten 1000-mL bottles), labeled *for hyperthermia only* and stored in PACU refrigerator
Bucket of cracked ice, labeled *for hyperthermia only* and stored in freezer of PACU refrigerator
Cooling blanket
Nasogastric tubes
Urine meter (1)
Irrigation tray with piston syringe
Fan
Large, clear plastic bags for ice

Drugs Needed
Sodium bicarbonate (8.4%): 50 mL x 5
Furosemide: 40 mg/amp x 4 ampules
Calcium chloride (10%): 10-mL vial x 2
Glucose (2 bottles of 50% strength)
Iced intravenous saline solution (ten 1000-mL bottles in refrigerator)
Lidocaine for injection: 100 mg/5 mL or 100 mg/10 mL in preloaded syringes (3)
Amiodarone is also acceptable (ACLS protocol for treatment of cardiac dysrhythmias)
Regular insulin (1 ampule of 100 units; refrigerated)
Dantrolene (Dantrium) intravenous: 36 vials of lyophilized powder with at least 2200 mL of sterile water for injection, USP (without a bacteriostatic agent), to reconstitute dantrolene

ACLS, Advanced cardiac life support; *PACU,* post anesthesia care unit; *USP,* United States Pharmacopeia.
From Drain C, Odom-Forren J: *Perianesthesia nursing: A critical care approach,* ed 5, Philadelphia, 2009, Saunders.

        (4) Dizziness

        (5) Blurred vision

        (6) Nausea

        (7) Thrombophlebitis (late problem)

  3. Bicarbonate for metabolic acidosis

  4. Initiate patient cooling.

    a. IV infusion of iced sodium chloride (NaCl)

    b. Surface cooling for all patients

      (1) Ice packs to groin, axillae, head

      (2) Cooling blankets

      (3) Immersion in container of ice

    c. Lavage stomach, bladder, and rectum with cold saline

    d. Lavage with cold saline if peritoneal cavity open

    e. Extracorporeal cooling by heart-lung machine in exceptional cases

    f. Discontinue cooling interventions when temperature decreases to 38° C (100.4° F).

    g. Effective treatment in most situations includes:

      (1) Treatment with dantrolene

      (2) Discontinuation of anesthetic

      (3) Lavage of:

        (a) Stomach

        (b) Bladder

      (4) Cover exposed surfaces.

        (a) Iced cold towels

        (b) Cooling blankets

  5. Maintain fluid and electrolyte balance.

    a. Monitor arterial blood gases frequently.

    b. To guide fluid therapy, monitor:

      (1) Central venous pressure

      (2) PA catheter

    c. Use indwelling urinary catheter to monitor urine output.

    d. Administer IV fluids as ordered.

    e. Administer furosemide and mannitol as ordered.

    f. For hyperkalemia, administer:

      (1) Glucose (or dextrose)

      (2) Insulin

      (3) Calcium

  6. Monitor cardiac output.

    a. Maintain continuous cardiac monitoring.

    b. Treat ventricular dysrhythmias.

      (1) Procainamide

      (2) Lidocaine

      (3) Do NOT use calcium channel blockers.

H. Follow-up after initial treatment

  1. Repeat IV or oral dantrolene every 4 to 6 hours for up to 48 hours.

  2. Monitor for recurrence for 24 to 48 hours postoperatively in ICU.

  3. Monitor for development of disseminated intravascular coagulation.

  4. Follow serum creatine kinase levels for several days until normalized.

I. Miscellaneous issues

  1. MH-susceptible ambulatory patients

    a. May be discharged after 4 hours in PACU

    b. Uneventful surgery

  2. For inpatients

    a. Label patients' charts as "MH risk—do not use succinylcholine."

    b. MH patients who have required resuscitation have been given succinylcholine.

J. Preparing for an MH crisis
  1. Maintain MH cart.
    a. Drugs and fluids required to treat acute MH episode
    b. May share with OR
  2. Keep clear instructions with MH cart at all times.
  3. Post MH treatment protocol in highly visible place.
  4. Develop a detailed MH crisis response plan.
    a. Specify the roles of each staff member.
    b. Monitor and update education of all staff.
    c. Provide updates at least annually.
    d. Conduct mock MH crisis drills.
  5. Have dantrolene immediately available.
    a. At least 36 vials
    b. Not in locked cabinet or stored in pharmacy
  6. Have arterial blood gas laboratory immediately available.
  7. Information sources
    a. Malignant Hyperthermia Association of the United States (MHAUS)
      (1) PO Box 1069, 1139 East State St., Sherburne, NY 13460-1069
      (2) Phone
        (a) 1-607-674-7901
        (b) 1-800-98-MHAUS
        (c) 1-800-MH-HYPER (MH hotline)
      (3) www.mhaus.org
    b. North American Malignant Hyperthermia Registry
      (1) 1-888-274-7899
      (2) http://naregistry.mhaus.org

BIBLIOGRAPHY

1. AANA: *Scope and standards for nurse anesthesia practice*, 2007. Available at: www.aana.com/uploadedFiles/Resources/Practice_Documents/scope_stds_nap07_2007.pdf. Accessed September 11, 2008.
2. ASA: *Standards for basic anesthetic monitoring*, 2005. Available at: www.asahq.org/publicationsAndServices/standards/02.pdf. Accessed September 11, 2008.
3. ASPAN: *Clinical guideline for the prevention of unplanned perioperative hypothermia*, 2001. Available at: www.aspan.org/PDFfiles/HYPOTHERMIA_GUIDELINE10–02.pdf. Accessed March 5, 2007.
4. Dybwik K, Nielsen EW: Infrared temporal thermometry. *Tidsskr Nor Laegeforen* 6(21):3025–3026, 2003.
5. Girard T, Treves S, Voronkov E, et al: Molecular genetic testing for malignant hyperthermia susceptibility. *Anesthesiology* 100(5):1076–1080, 2004.
6. Good KK, Verble JA, Secrest J, et al: Postoperative hypothermia: The chilling consequences. *AORN J* 83(5):1054–1066, 2006.
7. Greenes DS, Fleisher GR: Accuracy of a noninvasive temporal artery thermometer for use in infants. *Arch Pediatr Adolesc Med* 155(3):376–381, 2001.
8. Holtzclaw BJ: Circadian rhythmicity and homeostatic stability in thermoregulation. *Biol Res Nurs* 2(4):221–235, 2001.
9. Hooper VD: *Unplanned perioperative hypothermia: The state of the science*. Presented at the ASPAN 27th National Conference, Grapevine, Texas, May 6, 2008.
10. Hooper VD, Andrews JO: Accuracy of noninvasive core temperature measurement in acutely ill adults: The state of the science. *Biol Res Nurs* 8(1):24–34, 2006.
11. Mahoney C, Odom J: Maintaining intraoperative normothermia: A meta-analysis of outcomes with costs. *AANA J* 67(2):155–163, 1999.
12. Malignant Hypothermia Association of the United States: Available at: www.mhaus.org. Accessed December 3, 2008.
13. Moran DS, Mendal L: Core temperature measurement: Methods and current insights. *Sports Med* 32(14):879–885, 2002.
14. Naecsu A: Malignant hyperthermia. *Nurs Stand* 20(28):51–57, 2006.
15. Nicoll LH: Heat in motion: Evaluating and managing temperature. *Nursing* 32:s1–s12, 2002.
16. Ostrowsky B, Ober J, Wenzel R, et al: The case of the cold thermometers. *Am J Infect Control* 31(1):57–59, 2003.

17. Rosenburg H: *Malignant hyperthermia syndrome*, 2006. Available at: www.mhaus.org/NonFB/Slideshow_eng/SlideShow_ENG_files/frame.htm. Accessed March 15, 2007.
18. Rupp ME, Heermann J, Uphoff ME: Need for a reliable system to measure body temperature. *Am J Infect Control* 32(3):184, 2004.
19. Sessler DI: Perioperative heat balance. *Anesthesiology* 92(2):578–596, 2000.
20. Sessler DI: Complications and treatment of mild hypothermia. *Anesthesiology* 95(2):531–543, 2001.
21. Suleman MI, Doufas AG, Akca O, et al: Insufficiency in a new temporal-artery thermometer for adult and pediatric patients. *Anesth Analg* 95(1):67–71, 2002.
22. Wagner DV: Unplanned perioperative hypothermia. *AORN J* 83(2):470, 473–476 2006.
23. Welch TC: AANA journal course. *AANA J* 70(3):227–231, 2002.

25 Postoperative Nausea and Vomiting

SUSAN JANE FETZER

OBJECTIVES

At the conclusion of this chapter, the reader will be able to:

1. Differentiate nausea, vomiting, and retching.
2. Describe the phases of perianesthesia-related nausea and vomiting.
3. Determine a patient's risk of experiencing postoperative nausea and vomiting (PONV).
4. Describe the difference between prophylactic and rescue therapy for PONV.
5. List five categories of PONV drugs that work on the chemoreceptor zone.
6. List five nursing interventions in the care of the patient at high risk for PONV or postdischarge nausea and vomiting (PDNV).
7. Describe the importance of risk-adjusted multimodal therapy for PONV.

I. DEFINITIONS
   A. Nausea
      1. Subjective sensation in back of throat or epigastrium
      2. Conscious cortical activity
      3. Conscious awareness of the need to vomit
      4. No expulsive muscular movements
      5. May not culminate in vomiting
      6. Synonyms: sick to my stomach, upset stomach, butterflies, queasy
   B. Vomiting
      1. Objective forceful evacuation of gastric contents through oral or nasal cavity
      2. Autonomic reflex directed by brainstem
      3. May or may not be preceded by nausea
      4. Coordinated muscular movements
      5. Associated with physiological changes
         a. Increased heart rate
         b. Increased respiratory rate
         c. Sweating
      6. Synonyms
         a. Pitching
         b. Barfing
         c. Ralphing
         d. Upchucking
         e. Puking
   C. Retching
      1. An attempt to vomit
      2. Nonproductive
      3. Synonyms
         a. Dry heaves
         b. Gagging

D. Vomiting and retching also termed emetic episodes
E. PONV
    1. Defined as nausea, vomiting, and retching separately or combined
    2. Occurs within first 24 hours after inpatient surgery
    3. Early PONV: First 2 to 6 hours after surgery
    4. Late PONV: After transfer to the postoperative unit, 6 to 24 hours after surgery
F. PDNV
    1. Occurs after discharge from health care facility
G. Delayed PDNV
    1. Occurs 24 hours after surgery
II. CONSEQUENCES OF PONV
  A. Physiological
    1. Surgical site disruption
    2. Esophageal tears
    3. Gastric herniation
    4. Fatigue
    5. Dehydration
    6. Electrolyte imbalance
    7. Airway compromise with aspiration
    8. Increased intracranial pressure
    9. Increased ocular pressure
  B. Delay of oral nutrition and drug therapy
    1. Poor pain management
    2. Interference with diabetic and antihypertensive drug regimens
    3. Potential for dehydration
  C. Increased costs
    1. Each vomiting episode delays discharge from post anesthesia care unit by an average of 20 minutes.
    2. Cost of treating vomiting is three times greater than cost of treating nausea.
    3. Readmission
    4. Increased length of stay
    5. Increased cost of complications
    6. Delay in resuming activities of daily living
    7. Increased nursing time
  D. Patient satisfaction
    1. PONV is among top 10 most undesirable outcomes after surgery.
III. ETIOLOGY OF PONV
  A. Nature of PONV is multifactorial.
  B. Vomiting center (VC)
    1. Located in the lateral reticular formation, medulla (mid brainstem) of the brain
    2. Composed of three major nuclei
      a. Nucleus tractus solitarius
      b. Dorsal motor nucleus of the vagus nerve
      c. Nucleus ambiguous involved with coordination of motor activity during vomiting
    3. Stimulated by multiple afferent sensory inputs
      a. Chemoreceptor triggering zone (CTZ)
      b. Pharyngeal nerve input
        (1) Stimulated by mechanical irritation
        (2) Gagging can result in retching and vomiting.
      c. Vagus mucosal pathways from gastrointestinal system
        (1) Mechanical receptors in stomach sensitive to distention and contraction
        (2) Chemoreceptors in duodenum and stomach sensitive to noxious substances
        (3) Vagal afferents also located in eye and oropharynx

(a) Manipulation of the eye can result in VC stimulation.
(b) Oropharyngeal suctioning can result in VC stimulation.
   d. Midbrain afferent pathways
      (1) Stimulated by increased intracranial pressure
   e. Neuronal pathways from vestibular apparatus
      (1) Direct stimulation from cranial nerve VIII
   f. Reflex afferent pathways from the cerebral cortex
      (1) Learned response of anticipatory nausea and vomiting
      (2) Cortical afferent stimulation
         (a) Emotional: stress, anxiety, fear
         (b) Sights and sounds of surgical suite
4. Chemoreceptors located in VC
   a. Cholinergic
   b. Histaminic
   c. Opioid (mu)
   d. Neurokinin 1 (NK1)
5. Response of VC to multiple inputs is activation of efferent motor pathways of vomiting reflex.
   a. Gastric efferent response
   b. Respiratory efferent response
C. CTZ
   1. Located in area postrema on floor of fourth ventricle of brain
   2. Adjacent to VC
   3. Very vascular, making it sensitive to decreased blood flow (e.g., hypotension)
   4. Outside the blood-brain barrier, making it responsive to emetogenic substances in blood or spinal fluid such as:
      a. Uremia, hypercalcemia
      b. Antineoplastic drugs
      c. Blood sugar fluctuations
      d. Hormonal influences
      e. Serum narcotic level
      f. Inhalation anesthetics
      g. Levels of dopamine and serotonin
   5. Sensitive to intracerebral pressure
   6. Contains chemoreceptors
      a. Serotonin type 3 (5-hydroxytryptamine, 5-HT$_3$)
      b. Dopamine type 2 (D$_2$)
      c. Histamine type 1 (H$_1$)
      d. Muscarinic cholinergic type 1 (M$_1$)
      e. Mu opioid
      f. Stimulation of CTZ chemoreceptors results in stimulation of VC
   7. Point of entry of vagal afferent nerve pathways
      a. Receives vagal stimulation resulting from noxious substances in gut and stomach
      b. Vagal stimulation triggers serotonin receptors.
      c. Stimulation of vagal afferents during perianesthesia period creates PONV through CTZ.
         (1) Opioids delay gastric emptying, promoting distention and vagal stimulation.
         (2) Handling abdominal contents during surgery promotes vagal stimulation.
         (3) Pneumoperitoneum secondary to laparoscopic procedures results in vagal stimulation.
         (4) Intestinal ischemia creates vagal stimulation.
         (5) Vagal stimulation results in serotonin release in GI tract.

8. Point of entry for vestibular afferent pathways
    a. Changes in motion and pressure increase vestibular activity.
    b. Vestibular apparatus of inner ear triggers histamine receptors.
        (1) Mechanism that creates motion sickness
        (2) Mechanism that results in PONV during rapid position changes
    c. Believed mechanism initiated by nitrous oxide
9. Point of entry for cortical afferent pathways
    a. Cortical emotional input = stress, anxiety, depression, fear, cognitive overload
    b. Physiological = hypoxia, pain, hypotension, intracranial pressure
    c. Sensory input = sight, sound, smell
    d. Nucleus tractus solitarius (NTS)
10. Physical proximity to CTZ
11. Major site of vagal afferents from vestibular apparatus
12. Contains chemoreceptors
    a. D_2
    b. $5\text{-}HT_3$
    c. H_1
    d. M_1
    e. Vomiting reflex
13. Efferent output of VC
14. Vomiting occurs in three phases.
    a. Preejection phase
        (1) Increase in salivation and swallowing
        (2) Decrease in gastric tone
        (3) Pallor, diaphoresis
        (4) Tachycardia
        (5) Regurgitation of small intestine content into stomach
        (6) Mediated by vagus nerve and acetylcholine
    b. Ejection phase
        (1) Respiratory inhibition
        (2) Closure of glottis to prevent aspiration
        (3) Elevation of soft palate
    c. Postejection phase
        (1) Associated with relief of nausea
IV. INCIDENCE OF PONV
    A. PONV occurs in one third of all patients undergoing surgery with anesthesia.
    B. Up to 80% incidence among patients with predetermined risk factors
    C. Incidence of PDNV up to 50%
    D. Patients with PONV are four times more likely to have PDNV.
    E. More than one third of patients with PDNV will not have PONV.
V. RISK FACTORS FOR PONV
    A. Independent risk factors
        1. Independent predictors of PONV
        2. Gender
            a. Females at two to four times higher risk starting at puberty
            b. No gender difference before puberty
            c. Unknown relationship of PONV to progesterone, estrogen, and gonadotropin hormonal levels
            d. Hormonal fluctuation in menstrual cycle may be responsible for PONV differences among women.
            e. Research has disapproved increased susceptibility during first week of menstrual cycle.
        3. Positive history of motion sickness or previous PONV
            a. Riding in car, plane flight, boat travel
            b. History of PONV in parent or sibling may be a risk factor.
            c. Patients with motion sickness appear to have a well-developed vestibular reflex arc.
            d. Increases risk of PONV two to three times

    4. Smoking status

      a. Nonsmokers at 1.5 to 2.5 times higher risk

      b. Chemical composition of cigarettes believed to increase hepatic enzyme activity to increase metabolism of anesthesia.

    5. Use of postoperative opioids

      a. Long-acting opioids appear to increase risk.

      b. Morphine associated with more PONV than fentanyl

B. Associated patient risk factors

    1. Factors that are not strong enough to predict PONV but are associated with an increased risk

    2. Age

      a. Risk of vomiting in children up to 42%

      b. Risk increases in children older than 2 years.

      c. Higher risk in school-age children aged 6 to 16 years, up to 51%

      d. Female gender adds greater risk after puberty.

      e. Risk stabilizes in adulthood and is decreased after age 70.

    3. Presence of delayed gastric emptying/increased gastric volume

      a. Pregnancy

      b. Neurological disease

      c. Diabetes

      d. Measurement of delayed emptying is unavailable.

      e. Degree of PONV risk is not known.

      f. Obesity (body mass index) has been disproved as a PONV risk factor.

    4. American Society of Anesthesiologists (ASA) status

      a. Healthier patients appear to be at higher risk.

      b. ASA 1 greater risk than ASA 3

    5. Anxiety

      a. Preoperative anxiety is a weak predictor of PONV.

      b. Increased circulating levels of catecholamines may stimulate receptors.

      c. Air swallowing increases gastric volume and decreases gastric motility.

      d. Anxiety has not been shown to be a risk factor for children.

    6. Pain

      a. Excessive pain increases the risk of PONV.

      b. Use of nonsteroidal anti-inflammatory agents to reduce need for opioids can lower risk of PONV.

      c. History of migraine is a possible risk for postoperative nausea.

    7. Preoperative fasting

      a. More liberal criteria for clear liquids appear to reduce incidence of PONV.

      b. Positive relationship exists between length of liquid fast and incidence of PONV.

      c. ASA recommendations allowing healthy adults to drink clear liquids as little as 2 hours before surgery are beneficial in PONV.

      d. A 35% reduction in systolic blood pressure during anesthesia induction is associated with an increased incidence of PONV.

C. Associated surgical risk factors

    1. Factors not strong enough to predict PONV but associated with an increased risk

    2. Surgery duration

      a. Longer duration of surgery increases the risk.

      b. Each 30-minute increase in outpatient surgical time increases baseline risk by 60%.

    3. Type of surgery

      a. Controversial risk factor

      b. Type of surgery may be related to pain experience, opioid use, length of surgery, and surgical manipulation of emetogenic stimuli.

      c. Ear, nose, and throat: middle ear surgery stimulates vestibular afferents.

      d. Adenotonsillectomy: introduces blood into stomach as emetogenic irritant, pharyngeal afferent stimulation

      e. Ophthalmic strabismus: stimulates vestibular afferents

      f. Gynecological and breast: gender-related risk

      g. Laparoscopy: increases gastric volume as vagal afferent stimulant

      h. Abdominal: decreases gastric emptying as vagal afferent stimulant

      i. Plastic and reconstructive: surgery duration, risk of hypovolemia

      j. Shoulder: pain afferent stimulation

      k. Craniotomy: intracranial pressure stimulation

    4. Hypovolemia

      a. Results in prolonged hypotension that can stimulate CTZ

      b. Results in postural hypotension

D. Associated anesthetic risk factors

    1. Factors not strong enough to predict PONV but associated with an increased risk

    2. Use of volatile anesthetics or nitrous oxide

      a. Increases risk by 20%

      b. Risk of early PONV within 2 hours of surgery

      c. Effect depends on duration of exposure.

      d. Omitting nitrous oxide is known antiemetic prophylactic measure.

      e. No relationship to delayed PONV

    3. Propofol

      a. Appears to have a protective effect in reducing PONV when used for maintenance

      b. No antiemetic effect when used for induction only

      c. Antiemetic effect lasts only 6 hours after surgery.

    4. Gastric distention

      a. Laryngeal mask airway may create air in stomach.

      b. Rapid sequence induction with cricoid pressure may reduce air in stomach.

    5. Perioperative opioid administration

      a. Direct action on the CTZ receptors

      b. Decreases gastric emptying times

      c. Slows gastric motility

    6. Type of approach

      a. General anesthesia has higher rate of PONV than regional approaches.

      b. Induction agents associated with higher incidence of PONV

        (1) Ketamine

        (2) Etomidate

      c. Inhalation agents have higher rate of PONV than intravenous agents.

      d. Selection of reversal agents: neostigmine and physostigmine may increase PONV.

E. Associated postoperative risk factors

    1. Pain

    2. Movement

    3. Hypotension

    4. Blood in stomach

      a. Oropharyngeal bleeding

        (1) Nasal surgery

        (2) Adenotonsillectomy

        (3) Dental extraction

        (4) Pharyngeal procedures

      b. Gastrointestinal procedures

F. Differences in PONV

    1. Research suggests that risk factors for nausea are different than risk factors for vomiting.

VI. ASSESSMENT OF PONV
   A. Preoperative assessment
      1. Risk scoring tools group independent risk factors to predict PONV.
      2. Simplified tools treat each risk factor equally.
         a. Apfel et al. risk assessment (1 point for each of four findings)
            (1) Risk assessment
               (a) Female
               (b) History of motion sickness or PONV
               (c) Nonsmoker
               (d) Anticipated use of postoperative opioids
            (2) Scores range from 0 to 4 points.
            (3) Risk of PONV by score
               (a) 0 = 10%
               (b) 1 = 21%
               (c) 2 = 39%
               (d) 3 = 61%
               (e) 4 = 79%
         b. Koivuranta et al. risk assessment (1 point for each of five findings)
            (1) Risk assessment
               (a) Female
               (b) History of PONV
               (c) History of motion sickness
               (d) Nonsmoker
               (e) Surgery over 60 minutes
            (2) Scores range from 0 to 5 points.
            (3) Risk of postoperative nausea and postoperative vomiting by score
               (a) 0 = 17% and 7%, respectively
               (b) 1 = 18% and 7%, respectively
               (c) 2 = 42% and 17%, respectively
               (d) 3 = 54% and 25%, respectively
               (e) 4 = 47% and 38%, respectively
               (f) 5 = 87% and 61%, respectively
         c. Eberhart et al. risk assessment (1 point for each of four findings)
            (1) Risk assessment
               (a) History of postoperative vomiting in child, parent, or sibling
               (b) Duration of surgery over 30 minutes
               (c) Age older than 3 years
               (d) Strabismus surgery
            (2) System developed for risk assessment of vomiting in children
            (3) Scores range from 0 to 4 points.
            (4) Risk of postoperative vomiting by score
               (a) 0 = 9%
               (b) 1 = 10%
               (c) 2 = 30%
               (d) 3 = 55%
               (e) 4 = 70%
         d. Scoring systems have 55% to 80% accuracy in predicting PONV.
         e. Score offers method to plan prophylactic antiemetic interventions.
      3. Carefully assess for motion sickness history.
         a. Nausea or vomiting when riding in a car, boat, plane, bus
         b. Avoidance of amusement park rides
      4. Carefully assess preoperative hydration status.
         a. Length and extent of "nothing by mouth" period
         b. Use of diuretics
         c. Administration of bowel preparation regimens

  B. Postoperative assessment
    1. Knowledge of patient PONV risk factors and risk score
    2. Knowledge of prophylactic antiemetics administered
      a. Receptor targeted
      b. Timing of administration
    3. Knowledge of patient fluid volume status
    4. Assess patient routinely for PONV.
      a. Only one third of patients communicate nausea to health care providers.
      b. Direct specific questioning captures a higher percentage of actual PONV incidence.
  C. PONV assessment
    1. Timing (early vs late)
    2. Duration
    3. Nausea
      a. Rated on scale of 0 to 10; 10 is worst it can get
      b. Continuous versus intermittent
      c. Precipitating events
        (1) Occurring with motion
        (2) Concurrent pain
        (3) Smells, sounds, visual stimuli
        (4) After eating/drinking
        (5) Hypotension
        (6) Medications
    4. Vomiting
      a. Amount of vomitus
      b. Frequency of episodes
      c. Color, consistency, presence of blood
      d. Precipitating events
VII. **PONV PLAN**
  A. Nursing diagnosis
    1. Calculate risk of PONV for each patient.
    2. Communicate risk to anesthesia provider.
  B. Multimodal therapy based on risk assessment.
    1. Prophylactic interventions (Table 25-1)
      a. Hydration
      b. Risk reduction interventions
      c. Pharmacological combination therapy
      d. Complementary therapy
    2. Rescue interventions
VIII. **PROPHYLACTIC INTERVENTIONS**
  A. Hydration
    1. Preoperative 20 mL/kg (1-1.5 L) isotonic fluid bolus has been shown to decrease incidence of PONV.
    2. Forced postoperative (predischarge) fluid consumption increases PONV by 60%.
  B. Intraoperative anesthetics
    1. Total intravenous anesthesia (TIVA) with propofol and oxygen decreases risk equivalent to one pharmacological receptor blocking agent.
  C. Risk factor score determines pharmacological prophylaxis.
    1. Low risk
      a. Chance of PONV 10% to 20%
      b. Interventions needed—none
    2. Moderate risk
      a. Chance of PONV 40%
      b. Interventions needed—one
    3. Severe risk
      a. Chance of PONV 60%
      b. Interventions needed—two

■ TABLE 25-1
■ **Prophylactic and Rescue Antiemetics**

Agent	Trade Name	Receptors Affected	Use	Route	Dosage	Notes
Aprepitant	Emend	NK_1	P	PO	40 mg	Best effect when given 1-3 hours prior to induction
Dexamethasone	Decadron	Unknown	P, R	IV	4 mg	Administer before anesthesia induction. Used in combination with other antiemetics; vaginal/anal itching side effects
Dimenhydrinate	Dramamine	H_1, M_1	P, R	IV, IM	50-100 mg	Anticholinergic effects include dry mouth, urinary retention
Dolastron	Anzemet	$5-HT_3$	P, R	IV	12.5 mg	
Droperidol	Inapsine	D_2	P, R	IV	.625-1.25 mg	Best effect when given at end of surgery; little anti-vomiting effect; dose dependent side effects; requires 3 hours of EKG monitoring after dosing
Granisetron	Kytril	$5-HT_3$	P, R	IV	5 mcg/kg-1mg	Increases GI motility; not used for gastric surgery; recommended dosage does not offer effective prophylaxis
Metoclopramide	Reglan	D_2	R	IV	10 mg	
Ondansetron	Zofran	$5-HT_3$	P, R	IV Sublingual	4 mg	Best effect when given 15-30 minutes prior to end of surgery; headache is common side effect
Prochloperazine	Compazine	D_2	R	IV, IM PR	5-10 mg 25 mg	Extrapyramidal symptoms possible; sedative; anticholinergic effects include dry mouth, urinary retention
Promethazine	Phenergan	D_2, H_1, M_1	R	IV IM, PR	6.25-12.5 mg 12.5-25 mg	
Scopolamine	Transderm Scop	H_1, M_1	P, R	Transdermal	1.5 mg patch	Apply 4 hours prior to end of surgery; interferes with vestibular impulse transmission; anticholinergic effects; not used for patients with narrow angle glaucoma include dry mouth, urinary retention

D_2, Dopamine receptor blocker; $5-HT_3$, serotonin receptor blocker; H_1, histamine receptor blocker; M_1, muscarinic receptor blocker; NK_1, NK receptor blocker; P, prophlaxis; R, rescue.

4. Very severe risk
    a. Chance of PONV 80%
    b. Interventions needed—three or more
5. Medical consequences
    a. Regardless of risk score, prophylaxis is indicated if medical consequences of vomiting are high (e.g., wired jaw).
D. Pharmacological interventions
    1. Efficacy based on number needed to treat (NNT)
        a. Number of patients needed to receive the intervention to prevent one emetic event that would have occurred if the intervention was not used
        b. Quantitative method to compare efficacy of interventions
        c. NNT translates into risk reduction for event (e.g., NNT of 5 equals a 20% risk reduction).
    2. Depending on risk score, consideration is given to the number of VC receptors to be blocked (i.e., D_2, M_1, H_1, 5-HT_3, NK1).
    3. Serotonin receptor antagonists
        a. Ondansetron (Zofran)
            (1) First marketed and most widely studied 5-HT3 antagonist
            (2) Appears to have better antivomiting effect than antinausea effect
            (3) Highly selective with a greater affinity for 5-HT3 receptor than any other receptor
            (4) Works by binding to the CTZ and vagal afferent 5-HT3 receptors
            (5) Administer 15 to 30 minutes before end of surgery.
            (6) Appears effective in PDNV
            (7) No value of additional dose if maximal dose of 4 mg has been administered in 24 hours
            (8) Oral form (oral disintegrating tablet [ODT]) can be used in PDNV.
            (9) NNT = 5 to 6
        b. Granisetron (Kytril)
        c. Dolasetron (Anzemet)
            (1) Administer 30 minutes before end of surgery to permit required conversion to hydrodolasetron.
            (2) Timing of administration for prophylaxis has little effect on efficacy.
            (3) Known to increase QT interval
        d. Palonosetron
            (1) Currently approved for chemotherapy-induced nausea and vomiting only
            (2) No apparent antinausea effect
            (3) High incidence of headache
        e. Overall, 5-HT_3 agents most effective when given at the end of surgery
        f. Little evidence supporting superiority in PONV of any one 5-HT_3 compound
        g. Fewer side effects than other antiemetics: headache, constipation
        h. Can be used in pediatrics
        i. Fewer side effects improve suitability for ambulatory surgery.
        j. NNT = 5 to 8
    4. Antidopaminergics = D_2 antagonists
        a. Butryophenone
            (1) Droperidol (Inapsine)
                (a) Appears to have a better antinausea effect than antivomiting effect
                (b) Better when administered at the end of surgery
                (c) NNT = 3 to 5 if given with patient controlled analgesia PCA opiates over 24 hours
                (d) Larger doses needed for vomiting
                (e) Side effects of sedation and dizziness, which are dose dependent
                (f) Decreases risk of hypotension, which can generate PONV
                (g) Extrapyramidal reactions including anxiety, agitation, restlessness
                (h) Food and Drug Administration Black Box warning (2001)

> > > (i) ECG monitoring required for 2 to 3 hours after dose
> > > (ii) Possible QT prolongation resulting in arrhythmias
> > > (iii) Restricted to use as second-line therapy
> > (2) Haloperidol (Haldol)
> b. Benzamide
> > (1) Metoclopramide (Reglan)
> > > (a) Blocks D_2 receptors in CTZ and VC
> > > (b) At higher doses blocks 5-HT3 receptors in CTZ
> > > (c) Weak effect
> > > (d) Only better than placebo in 50% of cases for nausea
> > > (e) Short half-life
> > > (f) Most common administered dose (10 mg IV) when given alone not effective for prophylaxis
> > > (g) Because of increased gastric emptying not recommended for gastric surgery
> > > (h) Unpleasant side effects even at normal dosages: restlessness, agitation, weakness, drowsiness

5. Phenothiazines
   a. Promethazine (Phenergan)
   b. Prochlorperazine (Compazine)
   c. Blocks D_2 receptors in CTZ
   d. Blocks H_1 receptors in CTZ
   e. Blocks M_1 receptors in vestibular apparatus
   f. Need to monitor patients for sedation, hypotension, and extrapyramidal symptoms
6. NK1 receptor agonists
   a. Aprepitant (Emend)
   b. Neuropeptide substance P receptors found in NTS and CTZ
   c. NK1 receptors also located in peripheral nervous system
7. Antihistamines
   a. Diphenhydramine, dimenhydrinate
   b. Block H_1 receptors in CTZ
   c. Act directly on VC
   d. Block M_1 receptors in vestibular apparatus
   e. Good for treatment of vertigo and motion sickness
   f. Side effects: drowsiness, blurred vision, and urinary retention
   g. NNT = 5 to 8
8. Anticholinergics
   a. Blocks M_1 receptors
   b. Scopolamine
      (1) Belladonna alkaloid
      (2) Also blocks H_1 receptors in VC
      (3) Suppresses the noradrenergic system leading to reduced vestibular sensitivity
      (4) Transdermal patch application behind ear
      (5) Applied 4 hours before anticipated end of surgery
      (6) May be applied preoperatively for short surgeries
      (7) Contraindicated for patients with narrow-angle glaucoma because of increase in intraocular pressure
      (8) Side effects: inhibits salivation (dry mouth), dizziness, increases heart rate, dilates pupils, drowsiness, urinary retention
      (9) Slow release system delivers dose over 3 days if left on.
      (10) Effective in PDNV
         (a) Patients sent home require education for side effects.
         (b) Patients sent home require education on proper use and removal of the patch.
      (11) Not appropriate for children
      (12) Use cautiously in elders, lactating mothers.
      (13) NNT = 4

9. Glucocorticoids
   a. Dexamethasone (Decadron), methylprednisolone (Solu-Medrol)
   b. Precise method of action unknown
   c. More effective when administered before anesthesia induction
   d. Minimal adverse effects
   e. Low cost
   f. Additive effect when used with other agents, especially 5-HT_3 blockers
   g. Effective for early and late PONV
   h. Appears effective for PDNV
   i. NNT late postoperative nausea = 4
   j. NNT late postoperative vomiting = 7
10. Gastroprokinetics
    a. Increases gastric motility, which decreases stomach distention
    b. Small quantities of clear fluids can result in gastroprokinesis.
    c. Metoclopramide (Reglan)
       (1) Enhances gastric emptying
       (2) Increases upper motility
       (3) Weak 5-HT_3 activity only in high doses
       (4) Short half-life
       (5) Not effective for prevention of PONV alone
       (6) May be effective when used in combination with dexamethasone
       (7) Side effects include hypotension, increased heart rate, sedation.
11. Mucosal blocking agents
    a. Vomiting is stimulated by gastric mucosa release of neuroactive agents:
       (1) 5-HT_3
       (2) Cholecystokinin
    b. Serotonin (5-HT_3) blockers inhibit 5-HT release.
    c. Different effect of agents related to individual genetic metabolism
    d. Greater effect on reducing vomiting than nausea
    e. Best effect for abdominal and pelvic surgeries
12. Cortical depressants
    a. Cannabinoids
    b. Benzodiazepines
    c. Scant research on effectiveness in PONV/PDNV
13. Multimodal therapy
    a. No antiemetic is entirely effective.
    b. Multimodal therapy refers to a combination of interventions that is more effective than a single strategy to increase antiemetic efficacy.
    c. Combining two or more antiemetics has demonstrated improved prophylaxis.
E. Reduce risk by maintaining cardiorespiratory stability.
   1. Treat hypotension aggressively.
   2. A 35% drop in blood pressure will change intestinal perfusion and increase PONV.
   3. Supplemental oxygen
F. Universal prophylaxis
   1. Likely PONV incidence of 10% to 20% despite any or all therapy
   2. Prophylaxis for everyone without regard for risk not cost-effective
   3. Universal prophylaxis increases risks of adverse drug effects.
IX. RESCUE INTERVENTIONS
   A. Despite prophylaxis, PONV occurs.
   B. Before using additional modalities, other causes of PONV should be ruled out.
   C. Rescuing the patient with PONV requires a different treatment approach than prophylaxis.
   D. A drug used for prophylaxis should not be used for rescue in the immediate postoperative period.
   E. Select agent with a different receptor blocking ability.

    F. Late PONV patients can be treated with any of the prophylactic agents except dexamethasone or scopolamine.

    G. Nurse must be aware of antiemetic drugs and their mechanisms of action.

    H. Aggressive fluid therapy if tolerated may be helpful.

    I. Delayed PDNV

        1. Ondansetron dissolving tablets (Zofran ODT)

        2. Promethazine suppository or tablet

        3. Prochlorperazine oral tablet or suppository

        4. Scopolamine patch

X. COMPLEMENTARY THERAPIES

    A. Ginger

        1. Possible antiemetic effect, although exact mechanism unknown

            a. Antiserotonin effects

            b. 5-HT$_3$ receptor antagonist

            c. Antispasmodic to reduce gastric motility

        2. Central nervous system and GI systems effects

        3. Dose is not clear, but evidence points to 1 gram or more.

        4. Active ingredients in ginger preparations have not been standardized.

        5. Research meta-analysis indicates better effect than placebo.

        6. Should not be recommended for patients taking warfarin

    B. Aromatherapy

        1. Essential oils including ginger, cardamom, and tarragon

        2. Peppermint oil

            a. Traditional cure for vomiting

            b. Some success with nausea in obstetrics and gynecology

        3. Isopropyl alcohol inhalation

            a. Risk free

            b. Low cost

            c. Efficacy has not been established through research.

    C. P6 stimulation

        1. Includes acupressure, acupuncture, transcutaneous electrical stimulation

        2. Better than placebo with NNT = 4 to 5

        3. May reduce nausea

        4. No effect shown in children

        5. Little impact on vomiting

    D. Supplemental oxygen

        1. Appears to affect GI tract, which has high metabolic demands and intolerance to ischemia

        2. Evidence is conflicting.

        3. Majority of research indicates that oxygen is of limited or no benefit.

        4. Reduces PONV by 50% in colorectal surgery

        5. Inexpensive and risk free

        6. Administered dose for 2 hours postoperatively

    E. Untested modalities

        1. Cool washcloths to forehead

        2. Deep breathing

        3. Repositioning

XI. PEDIATRIC PONV THERAPY CONSIDERATIONS

    A. Use of propofol increases risk of bradycardia during strabismus surgery.

    B. Droperidol causes more extrapyramidal reactions in children.

    C. Should not force oral fluids before discharge

    D. Nonpharmacological techniques have not shown effectiveness in children.

XII. NURSING INTERVENTIONS

    A. Knowledge of patient risk score

    B. Awareness of antiemetic prophylaxis plan of care

    C. Prepare environment to reduce emetic stimulation.

        1. Sights, smells, conversation
  D. Ensure adequate preoperative and postoperative hydration.
  E. Provide adequate analgesia.
        1. Appropriate opioids
        2. Appropriate nonsteroidal anti-inflammatory drugs
  F. Move and ambulate patients slowly postoperatively.
  G. Patient education
        1. Knowledge of risk factors
        2. Awareness of future risk
        3. Management of PDNV
           a. How to manage fluids and food
           b. How to manage medications with known gastric irritation
           c. When to contact health care provider
XIII. DOCUMENTATION
  A. Document each symptom: nausea, vomiting, retching.
  B. Nausea
        1. Timing
           a. Intermittent
           b. Continuous
           c. Preceding vomiting
        2. Preceding events
           a. Transport (motion induced)
           b. Medication (opioid induced)
           c. Food/fluids (gastric motility)
        3. Rank on severity scale
           a. Verbal descriptive scale
           b. Visual analog scale
  C. Vomiting
        1. Frequency
        2. Volume
        3. Characteristics of emesis
           a. Content
               (1) Undigested food
               (2) Hematemesis
               (3) Coffee ground
               (4) Bilious
               (5) Feculent
           b. Color
  D. Retching
        1. Frequency
        2. Precipitating events
  E. Efficacy of interventions for PONV
        1. Response to rescue pharmacology
        2. Response to complementary interventions

BIBLIOGRAPHY

1. American Society of PeriAnesthesia Nurses: ASPAN's evidence-based clinical practice guideline for the prevention and/or management of PONV/PDNV. *J Perianesth Nurs* 21(4):230–250, 2006.
2. Couture DJ, Maye JP, O'Brien D, et al: Therapeutic modalities for the prophylactic management of postoperative nausea and vomiting. *J Perianesth Nurs* 21(6):398–403, 2006.
3. Gan TJ: Risk factors of postoperative nausea and vomiting. *Anesth Analg* 102(6): 1884–1898, 2006.
4. Golembiewski JA, O'Brien D: A systematic approach to the management of postoperative nausea and vomiting. *J Perianesth Nurs* 17(6):364–376, 2002.
5. Golembiewski JA, Tokumaru S: Pharmacological prophylaxis and management of adult

postoperative/discharge nausea and vomiting. *J Perianesth Nurs* 21(6):385–397, 2006.

6. Habib AS, Gan TJ: Evidence-based management of postoperative nausea and vomiting: A review. *Can J Anaesth* 51(4):326–341, 2004.

7. Murphy MJ, Hooper VD, Sulivan E, et al: Identification of risk factors for postoperative nausea and vomiting in the perianesthesia adult patient. *J Perianesth Nurs* 21(6):377–384, 2006.

8. Odom-Forren J, Fetzer SJ, Moser DK: Evidence-based interventions for post discharge nausea and vomiting: A review of the literature. *J Perianesth Nurs* 21(6):411–430, 2006.

Pain and Comfort Management

LINDA WILSON, H. LYNN KANE, KATHLEEN FALKENSTEIN

OBJECTIVES

At the conclusion of this chapter, the reader will be able to:

1. Define pain, commonly used terms, and types of pain.

2. Describe nociception: basic process of normal pain transmission.

3. Describe harmful effects of unrelieved pain.

4. Identify pain and comfort management in the perianesthesia settings, including special considerations and key concepts in analgesic therapy.

5. Identify pharmacological and non-pharmacological interventions, including those for children and management of opioid complications.

6. Define comfort.

7. Identify the contexts in which comfort occurs.

I. PAIN
  A. Definition of pain
    1. Pain is whatever the experiencing person says it is, existing whenever he or she says it does.
    2. Pain is unpleasant sensory and emotional experience associated with actual or potential tissue damage.
  B. Types of pain
    1. Nociceptive pain—normal processing of stimuli that damages normal tissue or has the potential to do so if prolonged; usually responsive to nonopioids and/or opioids
      a. Somatic pain—usually aching or throbbing in quality and is well localized
        (1) Arises from:
          (a) Bone
          (b) Joint
          (c) Muscle
          (d) Skin
          (e) Connective tissue
      b. Visceral pain—arises from visceral tissue, such as the gastrointestinal (GI) tract and pancreas
    2. Neuropathic pain—abnormal processing of sensory input by the peripheral nervous system or central nervous system (CNS)
      a. Treatment usually includes adjuvant analgesics.
      b. Centrally generated pain
        (1) Deafferentation pain—injury to either the peripheral nervous system or CNS
        (2) Sympathetically maintained pain—associated with dysregulation of the autonomic nervous system

      c. Peripherally generated pain
        (1) Painful polyneuropathies—pain felt along the distribution of many peripheral nerves
        (2) Painful mononeuropathies—usually associated with a known peripheral nerve injury, and pain felt at least partly along the distribution of the damaged nerve

C. Definition of commonly used pain terms
1. Acute pain—usually elicited by the injury of body tissues and activation of nociceptive transducers at the site of local tissue damage; pain that extends until period of healing
2. Chronic pain—usually elicited by an injury but may be perpetuated by factors that are both pathogenetically and physically remote from originating cause: pain that extends beyond the expected period of healing (3-6 months since the initiation of pain)
3. Recurrent pain—episodic or intermittent occurrences of pain with each episode lasting for a relatively short period but recurring across an extended period
4. Transient pain—elicited by activation of nociceptors in the absence of any significant local tissue damage; this type of pain ceases as soon as the stimulus is removed (e.g., venipuncture).
5. Addiction—a behavioral pattern of psychoactive substance abuse; addiction is characterized by overwhelming involvement with the use of a medication, the securing of its supply, and a high tendency to relapse.
6. Adjuvant analgesia—a medication that is analgesic in some painful conditions, but that medication's primary indication is something other than analgesia
7. Allodynia pain—caused by stimulus that does not normally provoke pain
8. Analgesia—absence of the spontaneous report of pain or pain behaviors in response to stimulation that would normally be painful
9. Anxiolytic—a medication used primarily to treat episodes of anxiety
10. Central pain—initiated or caused by primary lesion or dysfunction in the CNS
11. Dysesthesia—an unpleasant, abnormal sensation, whether spontaneous or evoked
12. Hyperalgesia—an increased response to a stimulus that is normally painful
13. Hypoalgesia—diminished pain in response to a normally painful stimulus
14. Hypochondriasis—an excessive preoccupation that bodily sensations and fears represent serious disease despite reassurance to the contrary
15. Malingering—a conscious and willful feigning or exaggeration of a disease or effect of an injury to obtain a specific external gain
16. Neuralgia—pain in the distribution of a nerve or nerves
17. Neurogenic pain—initiated or caused by a primary lesion, dysfunction, or transitory perturbation in the peripheral nervous system or CNS
18. Neuropathic pain—initiated or caused by a primary lesion or dysfunction in the nervous system
19. NMDA—*N*-methyl-D-aspartate; an example of an NMDA receptor blocker is ketamine.
20. Noxious stimulus—a stimulus that is capable of activating receptors for tissue damage
21. Pain behavior—verbal or nonverbal actions understood by observers to indicate that a person may be experiencing pain and suffering
22. Pain relief—report of reduced pain after a treatment
23. Pain threshold—the least level of stimulus intensity perceived as painful
24. Pain tolerance level—the greatest level of noxious stimulation that an individual is willing to tolerate
25. Paresthesia—an abnormal sensation, whether spontaneous or evoked
26. Physical dependence—a pharmacologic property of a medication (e.g., opioid) characterized by the occurrence of an abstinence syndrome after abrupt discontinuation of the substance or administration of an antagonist; this does not imply addiction

27. Psychogenic pain—report of pain attributed primarily to psychological factors, usually in the absence of an objective physical pathology that could account for pain
28. Suffering—reaction to the physical or emotional components of pain with a feeling of uncontrollability, helplessness, hopelessness, intolerability, and interminableness
29. Tolerance—a physiological state in which a person requires an increased dosage of a drug to sustain a desired effect
D. Nociception: basic process of normal pain transmission
   1. Transduction—conversion of one energy from another
      a. Process occurs in the periphery when a noxious stimulus causes tissue damage.
      b. Damaged cells release substances that activate or sensitize nociceptors.
      c. This activation leads to the generation of an action potential.
      d. Sensitizing substances released by damaged cells
         (1) Prostaglandins
         (2) Bradykinin
         (3) Serotonin (5-hydroxytryptamine)
         (4) Substance P
         (5) Histamine
      e. An action potential results from:
         (1) Release of the preceding sensitizing substances (nociceptive pain)
         (2) A change in the charge along the neuronal membrane
         (3) Abnormal processing of stimuli by the nervous system neuropathic pain
         (4) A change in the charge along the neural membrane
            (a) Change in charge occurs when sodium ion (Na^+) moves into the cell and other ion transfers occur.
   2. Transmission—the action potential continues from the site of damage to the spinal cord and ascends to higher centers; transmission may be considered in three phases.
      a. Injury site to spinal cord
         (1) Nociceptors terminate in the spinal cord.
      b. Spinal cord to brainstem and thalamus
         (1) Release of substance P and other neurotransmitters continues the impulse across the synaptic cleft between the nociceptors and the dorsal horn neurons.
         (2) From the dorsal horn of the spinal cord, neurons such as the spinothalamic tract ascend to the thalamus.
         (3) Other tracts carry the message to different centers in the brain.
      c. Thalamus to cortex
         (1) Thalamus acts as a relay station sending the impulse to central structures for processing.
   3. Perception of pain—conscious experience of pain
   4. Modulation—inhibitor nociceptive impulses
      a. Neurons originating in the brain stem descend to the spinal cord.
      b. Released substances inhibit the transmission of nociceptive impulses.
         (1) Endogenous opioid
         (2) Serotonin
         (3) Norepinephrine (Figure 26-1)
E. Harmful effects of unrelieved pain
   1. Endocrine
      a. Increase in the following:
         (1) Corticotropin (Adrenocorticotropic hormone—ACTH)
         (2) Cortisol
         (3) Antidiuretic hormone
         (4) Catecholamines
            (a) Epinephrine
            (b) Norepinephrine

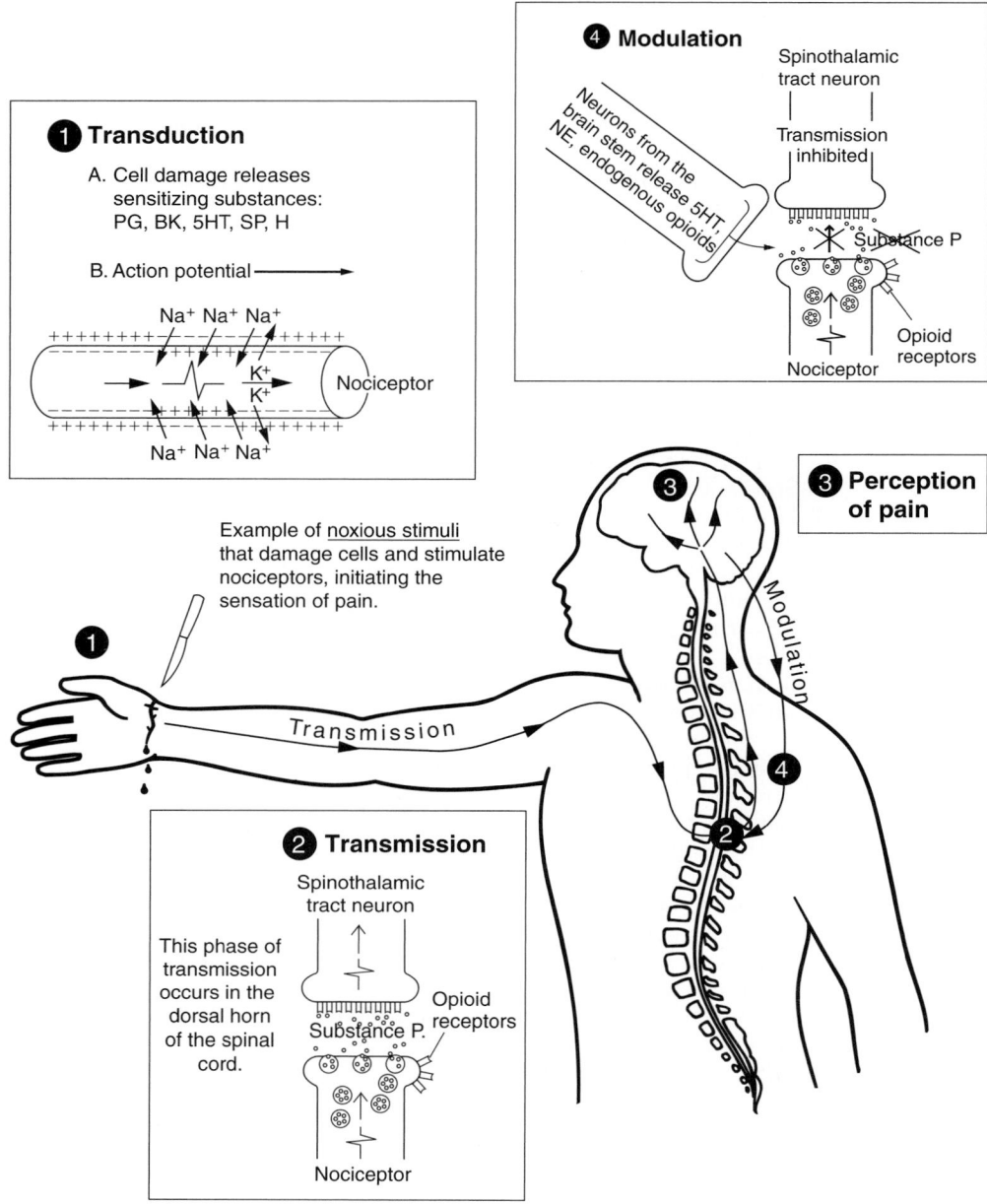

FIGURE 26-1 ■ Pain transmission. *BK*, Bradykinin; *H*, histamine; *5HT*, 5-hydroxytryptamine (serotonin); *NE*, norepinephrine; *PG*, prostaglandins; *SP*, substance P. (From McCaffery M, Pasero C: *Pain: Clinical manual,* St Louis, 1999, Mosby.)

        (5) Growth hormone
        (6) Renin
        (7) Angiotensin II
        (8) Aldosterone
        (9) Glucagons
        (10) Interleukin-1
   b. Decrease in:
        (1) Insulin
        (2) Testosterone

   2. Metabolic
     a. Gluconeogenesis
     b. Hepatic glycogenolysis
     c. Hyperglycemia
     d. Glucose intolerance
     e. Insulin resistance
     f. Muscle protein catabolism
     g. Increased lipolysis
   3. Cardiovascular
     a. Increase in the following
       (1) Heart rate
       (2) Cardiac output
       (3) Peripheral vascular resistance
       (4) Systemic vascular resistance
       (5) Hypertension
       (6) Coronary vascular resistance
       (7) Myocardial oxygen consumption
       (8) Hypercoagulation
       (9) Deep vein thrombosis
   4. Respiratory
     a. Decreased flows and volumes
     b. Atelectasis
     c. Shunting
     d. Hypoxemia
     e. Decreased cough
     f. Sputum retention
     g. Infection
   5. Genitourinary
     a. Decreased urinary output
     b. Urinary retention
     c. Fluid overload
     d. Hypokalemia
     e. Hyperkalemia
   6. Gastrointestinal (GI)
     a. Decreased gastric motility
     b. Decreased bowel motility
   7. Musculoskeletal
     a. Muscle spasm
     b. Impaired muscle function
     c. Fatigue
     d. Immobility
   8. Cognitive
     a. Reduction in cognitive function
     b. Mental confusion
   9. Immune response
     a. Depression
  10. Developmental
     a. Increased behavioral and physiological response to pain
     b. Altered temperaments
     c. Higher somatization
     d. Infant distress behavior
     e. Possible altered development of the pain system
     f. Increased vulnerability to stress disorders
     g. Addictive behavior
     h. Anxiety states
     i. Cultural considerations
  11. Debilitating chronic pain syndromes
     a. Postmastectomy pain
     b. Postthoracotomy pain

        c. Phantom pain

        d. Postherpetic neuralgia

   12. Quality of life

        a. Sleeplessness

        b. Anxiety

        c. Fear

        d. Hopelessness

        e. Increase thoughts of suicide

F. Special considerations

   1. Key principle: all patients deserve the best possible pain relief and comfort measures that can be safely provided.

   2. The following emphasizes some important key elements of care in patients with special needs.

        a. Elderly patients

           (1) Same pain assessment tools may be used in both cognitively intact elderly and younger patients.

           (2) Report of pain may be altered.

              (a) Physiological

              (b) Psychological

              (c) Cultural differences

           (3) Often have acute and chronic painful diseases

              (a) More than 80% have various forms of arthritis.

              (b) Most will have acute pain at some time.

           (4) Have multiple diseases

           (5) Take many medications

           (6) Prevalence of pain two-fold higher in those older than 60

           (7) Increased sensitivity to therapeutic and toxic effects of analgesics

              (a) Influenced by age-induced changes

                  (i) Drug absorption

                  (ii) Distribution

                  (iii) Metabolism

                  (iv) Elimination

           (8) Prone to constipation when given opioid analgesic

           (9) All nonsteroidal anti-inflammatory medications (NSAIDs) must be used with caution because of increased risk.

              (a) GI problems

              (b) Renal insufficiency

              (c) Platelet dysfunction

          (10) More sensitive to analgesic effects of opioid medications

              (a) May experience a higher peak effect

              (b) Longer duration of pain relief

              (c) Reduce initial dose by 25% to 50%.

              (d) Careful dose titration

              (e) Close monitoring of patient's responses

        b. Patients with known or suspected chemical dependency or history of such

           (1) Usually experience traumatic injuries

           (2) Experience a variety of health problems

           (3) Possible withdrawal caused by opioid absence may stimulate sympathetic nervous system.

              (a) Restlessness

              (b) Tachycardia

              (c) Sleeplessness

           (4) Focus on managing pain or discomfort, not detoxification.

           (5) There is no evidence that:

              (a) Withholding analgesics will increase the likelihood of recovery from addiction

              (b) Providing analgesics will worsen addiction

(6) Higher loading and maintenance doses of opioids may be required to reduce intensity of pain.

(7) Provide nonpharmacological interventions concomitantly with pharmacological interventions.

(8) May refer to an addiction specialist for ongoing care and rehabilitation after the acute pain period

(9) Patients with chronic alcoholism who are actively drinking

    (a) Maintain on benzodiazepines or alcohol throughout the intraoperative and postoperative periods to prevent withdrawal reaction or delirium tremens.

    (b) Dosage based upon individual evaluation

c. Concurrent medical conditions

(1) Involving either hepatic or renal impairment: result is medication accumulation

    (a) Elimination decreased in patient with renal failure

    (b) Doses must be lowered or given less frequently.

(2) Observe patient with respiratory insufficiency and chronic obstructive disease.

(3) Observe patient taking anxiolytics or other psychoactive medications for interaction with pain medications.

d. Patients with shock, trauma, or burns

(1) Observe for cardiorespiratory instability in the first hour of injury.

    (a) Carefully titrate opioid dosage.

    (b) Monitor closely.

(2) Peripheral nerve damage may result in neuropathic pain requiring adjuvant analgesics.

    (a) Tricyclic antidepressants

    (b) Anticonvulsants

    (c) Opioids

    (d) Nonopioids

e. Patients having procedures outside the operating room

(1) Analgesia may be withheld for a painful procedure when:

    (a) Immediate treatment of cardiorespiratory instability required

    (b) A competent patient declines treatment.

(2) Clinicians giving anesthetic or analgesic agents must understand:

    (a) Proper technique of administration

    (b) Dosage

    (c) Contraindications

    (d) Side effects

    (e) Treatment of overdose

(3) Monitor closely according to institutional policy when analgesic or adjuvant given.

f. Patients with chronic pain in perianesthesia setting

(1) Require special consideration and planning for pain management

(2) May request consultations with an acute pain management service and/or anesthesiologist familiar with chronic pain management

(3) Individualized detailed pain management plan communicated through all phases of perioperative care

g. Pediatric patients

(1) Provide adequate and unhurried preparation of the child and family.

    (a) Parental prediction of the child's response highly correlates with the actual degree of distress.

(2) Optimally manage preexisting pain.

(3) Requires frequent assessment and reassessment

    (a) Presence

    (b) Amount

    (c) Quality

    (d) Location of pain

(4) Emotional distress accentuates the experience of pain.
    (a) Focus on prevention.
    (b) Reduce anticipated pain.
(5) Inclusion of parents or caregiver essential to pain assessment
(6) Tailor assessment strategies to the development level and personality of the child.
(7) Physiological indicators may vary among children who are experiencing pain.
(8) Interpretation of physiological indicators crucial
    (a) In the context of the clinical condition
    (b) In conjunction with other assessment methods
(9) Effective interaction key to effective pain management
(10) Preferences of the child and family warrant respect and careful consideration.
(11) Primary obligation to ensure safe and competent care
(12) Environmental factors such as cold or crowded rooms and alarms on machines can intensify distress.

  h. Obstetric patients
    (1) During pregnancy
      (a) Analgesic considerations
        (i) May increase vascular resistance or decrease placental flow
        (ii) May cause transient or permanent harm to the fetus or infant
      (b) Encourage the use of nonpharmacological pain-relieving measures and caution against the use of analgesics.
      (c) Analgesics
        (i) Acetaminophen: safe for use in therapeutic doses
        (ii) NSAIDs: generally not recommended
        (iii) Opioid analgesics: a long history of safely relieving perinatal pain
          [a] Mu-agonists are recommended.
            [1] Morphine
            [2] Hydromorphone
            [3] Fentanyl
            [4] Oxycodone
            [5] Hydrocodone
            [6] Meperidine: not recommended as first-line opioid
        (iv) Adjuvant analgesics are used to treat pain of neuropathic origin.
          [a] Local anesthetics
          [b] Antidepressants
          [c] Anticonvulsants
          [d] Corticosteroids
          [e] Benzodiazepines
        (v) Types of pain related to pregnancy
          [a] Round ligament pain (sides of the uterus)
          [b] Headache
          [c] Back pain
          [d] Pyrosis (heartburn)
          [e] Braxton Hicks contractions
    (2) During childbirth
      (a) Labor pain considered the most agonizing of pain syndromes
      (b) Factors contributing to suffering
        (i) Lack of appropriate analgesics
        (ii) Lack of support person
        (iii) Hunger
        (iv) Fatigue
        (v) Low self-confidence

      (c) Alternate pain management methods
          (i)   Relaxation
          (ii)   Distraction
          (iii) Imagery
          (iv)   Effleurage
          (v)   Water heat
          (vi)   Acupuncture
      (d) Analgesics
          (i)   Mu-opioid agonists commonly used
          (ii)   Meperidine not recommended
          (iii) Local anesthetic bupivacaine used most often for epidural analgesia and anesthesia
          (iv)   Benzodiazepines recommended for muscle spasm only, and their use for childbirth not recommended
      (e) Regional techniques used
          (i)   Intrathecal analgesia
          (ii)   Epidural analgesia and anesthesia
          (iii) Combined spinal-epidural analgesia
  3. During postpartum
      a. Effective pain management very important postpartum
          (1) Clotting factors elevated
          (2) Increased risk for thrombophlebitis
          (3) Pain relief should be aimed at maximizing patient's mobility.
      b. Bonding with baby encouraged
      c. Types of pain
          (1) Uterine contractions
          (2) Episiotomy
          (3) Breast
          (4) Nipple
          (5) Post Cesarean section
  4. During breast-feeding
      a. Secretion of medications into breast milk: considerations
          (1) High lipid solubility
          (2) Low molecular weights
          (3) Nonionized state
  5. Neonates may receive 1% to 2% of the maternal dose of a medication.
      a. Medicating right before or right after breast-feeding may minimize medication transfer.
      b. Acetaminophen safe
      c. NSAIDs generally not recommended
      d. Opioid analgesics
          (1) Codeine
          (2) Fentanyl
          (3) Methadone
          (4) Morphine
      e. Adjuvant analgesic for neuropathic pain
G. Key concepts in analgesic therapy
  1. Balanced analgesia
      a. Continuous multimodal approach in treating pain
      b. Considered as the ideal by experts
      c. Use combined analgesic regimen.
          (1) Reduces the likelihood of significant side effects from a single agent or method
      d. Opioids commonly used in the balanced analgesia approach
          (1) Administered preemptively as well as after the noxious event occurs
  2. Preemptive analgesia
      a. Intervention implemented before noxious stimuli are experienced
      b. Designed to reduce the CNS impact of these stimuli

    c. NSAIDs reduce activation and centralization of nociceptors.

    d. Local anesthetics used to block sensory inflows

    e. Opioids act centrally to control pain.

    f. Local anesthetics provide effective preemptive analgesia.

       (1) Long-acting regional blocks indicated before painful procedures

       (2) Indicated whenever pain management expected to be difficult

3. Around-the-clock (ATC) dosing

    a. Two basic principles of providing effective pain management

       (1) Preventing pain

       (2) Maintaining a pain rating that is satisfactory to patient

    b. Indicated whenever pain is predicted to be present for at least 12 to 24 hours

    c. ATC dosing should be accompanied by provision of additional analgesic doses to relieve:

       (1) Breakthrough pain

       (2) Ongoing extreme pain

    d. Short-acting mu-agonist opioid analgesics used in breakthrough pain

       (1) Recommend that rescue doses are the same route and opioid as the ATC.

    e. Pain can have a sudden or gradual onset, and it can be brief or prolonged.

4. As needed (PRN) dosing

    a. Ordinarily, the patient requests analgesia.

    b. Effective PRN dosing requires active participation of patient.

       (1) Prompt patient to ask for medication before the pain is severe or out of control.

    c. Opioid analgesic is appropriate.

    d. ATC can be replaced with PRN dosing when acute pain is resolved.

5. Patient-controlled analgesia (PCA)

    a. An interactive method that permits patients to treat their pain by self-administering doses of analgesics.

    b. Initiating PCA in the post anesthesia care unit (PACU) is recommended.

       (1) Allows evaluation of patient's response to the therapy early in postoperative course

       (2) Prevents delays in analgesia on the nursing unit

    c. Types

       (1) Subcutaneous infusions

          (a) Rarely used for acute pain management

            (i) Slow onset

            (ii) When there is limited intravenous (IV) access

            (iii) Oral opioids not tolerated

            (iv) Intermittent bolusing for children

          (b) Hydromorphone and morphine most commonly used

          (c) Methadone causes irritation to the site.

          (d) Absorption and distribution dependent on needle placement and the patient's adipose tissue

          (e) Opioid concentrations high because infusion volumes must be limited

            (i) Most patients can absorb 2 or 3 mL/h.

            (ii) Some can absorb 5 mL/h.

            (iii) Infusion pump must be able to deliver in tenths of milliliter (0.1 mL/h).

          (f) Primary site of infusion

            (i) Left or right subclavicular anterior chest wall

            (ii) Left, right, or center abdomen

            (iii) Upper arms

            (iv) Thighs

            (v) Buttocks

(2) IV PCA
  (a) Used for immediate analgesic effect for acute, severe escalating pain
    (i) Includes bolus
    (ii) Continuous infusion
  (b) A steady state maintained better with continuous infusion
  (c) Duration of analgesia by bolus administration is dose dependent; the higher the dose, usually the longer the duration.
  d. Special considerations for pediatric IV PCA
    (1) Safe and effective use in children older than 5 years
    (2) Instruct parents and caregivers that only the designated child's pain manager should press the PCA.
    (3) Adult and pediatric selection guidelines are the same in the use of PCA.
    (4) Principles of starting dose estimates and titration for adults apply also to children.
6. Intraspinal analgesics (neuraxial)
  a. Epidural—needle inserted in epidural space
  b. Intrathecal—needle inserted in subarachnoid space
  c. Catheters removed after 2 to 4 days
  d. Long-term epidural and intrathecal catheters can be placed surgically.
    (1) Tunneled subcutaneously to an implanted pump
    (2) Subcutaneous pocket in the abdomen for pump
    (3) Implanted catheters easier to maintain
    (4) Risk of infection less
  e. Contraindications for intraspinal use
    (1) Patient refusal
    (2) Untreated sepsis, which could involve the site of injection
    (3) Shock
    (4) Hypovolemia
    (5) Coagulopathies
  f. Contraindications to use of opioid analgesia
    (1) Contraindications to epidural catheter insertion
    (2) History of adverse reactions to opioid medications
    (3) Central sleep apnea
    (4) Lack of familiarity of technique by patient caretakers
  g. Potential complications
    (1) Total or high spinal blockade
    (2) IV injection
    (3) Dural puncture resulting in a dural puncture headache
    (4) Bleeding resulting in an epidural hematoma
    (5) Catheter problems including:
      (a) Migration of epidural catheter
      (b) Breakage of catheter
      (c) Infection
  h. Analgesics and local anesthetics commonly used
    (1) Fentanyl
    (2) Sufentanil
    (3) Morphine
    (4) Hydromorphone
    (5) Ropivacaine
    (6) Bupivacaine
7. Transdermal
  a. Check for transdermal fentanyl patch placed by the patient for chronic pain.
  b. Fentanyl patches deliver the synthetic opioid passively.
  c. Consider fentanyl patch dose in the total opioid patient receives.
H. Site-specific surgery
  1. Dental surgery
    a. Patient's anxiety frequently disproportionate to the safety of the procedure
    b. May benefit from behavioral or pharmacological anxiolytic therapy

c. Manage mild pain associated with uncomplicated dental care with NSAIDs
   (1) Given preprocedure, shown to delay onset of postoperative pain and lessen its severity
d. Preoperative treatment can delay onset of pain postoperatively on more traumatic and intense procedure.
   (1) Ibuprofen
   (2) Application of long-acting local anesthetic
e. May require an opioid added to pain regimen
   (1) Codeine
   (2) Oxycodone

2. Radical head and neck
   a. Alternate routes for pain therapy may be required.
      (1) Gastrostomy
      (2) Jejunostomy
   b. Presence of tracheostomy may limit ability to describe pain or response to analgesic.
   c. Positioning of head and neck is critical.
   d. Positioning and padding
      (1) Minimize muscle spasm.
      (2) Minimize pressure point ulcer breakdown.
   e. Painful swallowing may require modification of diet.
      (1) Liquids and soft foods
      (2) Occasional use of topical anesthetics such as viscous lidocaine

3. Neurosurgery
   a. Opioid analgesics may affect abnormal neurological signs and symptoms that may be present.
      (1) Pupillary reflexes
      (2) Level of consciousness
   b. Balance analgesia to provide appropriate neurological monitoring.
   c. NSAIDs may be considered.
      (1) No effect on level of consciousness or pupillary reflexes
      (2) Risk of coagulopathy or hemorrhage

4. Thoracic surgery
   a. Preexisting disease, such as chronic obstructive pulmonary disease, common
   b. May have had prior medical treatment such as chemotherapy
   c. Epidural analgesia or neural blockade with local anesthetics improves pulmonary functions.
   d. Local epidural infusion provides dermatome bands of pain relief above and below epidural insertion site (T4 to T10).
   e. For patient experiencing pain above T4, ketorolac IV may provide excellent analgesia.
      (1) The potential risks of bleeding must be evaluated before a first dose.
      (2) Ketorolac IV might be used for 24 hours after surgery.
      (3) Use of opioids to reduce postoperative pain after thoracotomy is well documented.
   f. Use of PCA has:
      (1) Incrementally improved analgesia
      (2) Increased patient satisfaction
      (3) Improved pulmonary function
      (4) Contributed to early recovery and discharge

5. Cardiac surgery
   a. Close observation is essential to distinguish postoperative pain (chest wall and pleura) from cardiac pain (may be related to myocardial ischemia).
   b. Median sternotomy incision may require anesthetic induction of high dose of opioids.

      c. As techniques of less invasive surgical approaches progress and gain in popularity, anesthesia induction requirements may decrease.

   6. Upper abdominal surgery

      a. In preparation for surgery, review pain management choices and care plans with the patient.

         (1) Treatment for inadequate pain relief

         (2) Treatments for side effects

         (3) Scheduled postoperative opioid medication may be withheld in the event of respiratory depression, nausea, and vomiting.

   7. Lower abdominal surgery

      a. Pain management based on same principle as that for upper abdominal surgery

      b. Pain management during active labor requires special expertise and caution because side effects may impair fetal well-being.

      c. Epidural local anesthesia beneficial in suppressing pain and surgical stress responses

      d. Pain after procedures on the anus can be severe and require adjunctive measures.

         (1) Stool softeners

         (2) Dietary manipulation

         (3) Local anesthetic suppositories

   8. Back surgery

      a. Patient may experience chronic pain.

         (1) May be depressed, anxious, and irritable

         (2) Have a tolerance level to opioid medications

      b. Some procedures may limit use of epidural and spinal delivery of pain medications.

      c. Patient can experience paraspinal muscle spasm—appropriate to add muscle relaxant to supplement conventional opioid therapy.

      d. Require careful monitoring of neurological functions

   9. Surgery on extremities

      a. High degree of morbidity related to venous thromboembolic complications must be considered.

      b. Pain control postoperatively should allow early ambulation and movement in postoperative period.

      c. Pain therapy should not interfere with monitoring patient's neurologic functions.

      d. Epidural analgesia allows early mobility and minimizes complications from thromboemboli.

  10. Soft tissue surgery

      a. Local soft tissue resections: patient usually obtains pain control with oral opioids.

      b. Patient anxious about potential biopsy results may need adjuvant medication or nonpharmacological therapy.

I. Pharmacologic treatment of pain

   1. Equianalgesic dose chart (Table 26-1)

   2. Starting IV PCA prescription ranges for opioid-naïve adults (Table 26-2)

   3. Pediatric IV PCA dosing (Table 26-3)

   4. Managing opioid-induced side effects

      a. Constipation

         (1) Stool softener

         (2) Rectal exam to rule out impaction

         (3) Disimpaction—administer rescue analgesia or tranquilizer before procedure.

      b. Nausea and vomiting

         (1) Titrate opioid doses slowly and steadily.

         (2) Add or increase nonopioid or adjuvant for additional pain relief.

         (3) Antiemetic

         (4) Support use of relaxation techniques.

TABLE 26-1
Equianalgesic Dose Chart

Opioid	Parenteral (IM/SC/IV) (over ~4 h)	Oral (PO) (over ~4 h)	Onset (min)	Peak (min)	Duration* (h)	Half-life (h)
MU AGONISTS						
Morphine	10 mg	30 mg	30-60 (PO) 30-60 (CR)† 30-60 (R) 5-10 (IV) 10-20 (SC) 10-20 (IM)	60-90 (PO) 90-180 (CR)† 60-90 (R) 15-30 (IV) 30-60 (SC) 30-60 (IM)	3-6 (PO) 8-12 (CR)† 4-5 (R) 3-4 (IV)*‡ 3-4 (SC) 3-4 (IM)	2-4
Codeine	130 mg	200 mg NR	30-60 (PO) 10-20 (SC) 10-20 (IM)	60-90 (PO) UK (SC) 30-60 (IM)	3-4 (PO) 3-4 (SC) 3-4 (IM)	2-4
Fentanyl	100 mcg/h parenterally and transdermally ≈4 mg/h morphine parenterally; 1 mcg/h transdermally ≈ morphine 2 mg/24 h orally	—	5 (OT) 1-5 (IV) 7-15 (IM) 12-16 h (TD)	15 (OT) 3-5 (IV) 10-20 (IM) 24 h (TD)	2-5 (OT) 0.5-4 (IV)*‡ 0.5-4 (IM) 48-72 (TD)	3-4§ 13-24 (TD)
Hydrocodone (as in Vicodin, Lortab)	—	30 mg‖ NR	30-60 (PO)	60-90 (PO)	4-6 (PO)	4
Hydromorphone (Dilaudid)	1.5 mg¶	7.5 mg	15-30 (PO) 15-30 (R) 5 (IV) 10-20 (SC) 10-20 (IM)	30-90 (PO) 30-90 (R) 10-20 (IV) 30-90 (SC) 30-90 (IM)	3-4 (PO) 3-4 (R) 3-4 (IV)*‡ 3-4 (SC) 3-4 (IM)	2-3

Drug						
Levorphanol (Levo-Dromoran)	2 mg	4 mg	30-60 (PO) 10 (IV) 10-20 (SC) 10-20 (IM)	60-90 (PO) 15-30 (IV) 60-90 (SC) 60-90 (IM)	4-6 (PO) 4-6 (IV)*‡ 4-6 (SC) 4-6 (IM)	12-15
Meperidine (Demerol)	75 mg	300 mg NR	30-60 (PO) 5-10 (IV) 10-20 (SC) 10-20 (IM)	60-90 (PO) 10-15 (IV) 15-30 (SC) 15-30 (IM)	2-4 (PO) 2-4 (IV)*‡ 2-4 (SC) 2-4 (IM)	2-3
Methadone (Dolophine)	10 mg#	20 mg**	30-60 (PO) UK (SL) 10 (IV) 10-20 (SC) 10-20 (IM)	60-120 (PO) 10 (SL) UK (IV) 60-120 (SC) 60-120 (IM)	4-8 (PO) UK (SL) 4-8 (IV)*‡ 4-8 (SC) 4-8 (IM)	12-190
Oxycodone (as in Percocet, Tylox)	—	20 mg	30-60 (PO) 30-60 (CR)†† 30-60 (R)	60-90 (PO) 90-180 (CR)†† 30-60 (R)	3-4 (PO) 8-12 (CR)†† 3-6 (R)	2-3 4.5 (CR)
Oxymorphone (Numorphan)	1 mg	(10 mg R)	15-30 (R) 5-10 (IV) 10-20 (SC) 10-20 (IM)	120 (R) 15-30 (IV) UK (SC) 30-90 (PO)	3-6 (R) 3-4 (IV)*‡ 3-6 (SC) 3-6 IM	2-3
Propoxyphene (Darvon)		—	30-60 (PO)	60-90 (PO)	4-6 (PO)	6-12
Buprenorphine§§ (Buprenex)	0.4 mg	—	5 (SL) 5 (IV) 10-20 (IM)	30-60 (SL) 10-20 (IV) 30-60 (IM)	UK (SL) 3-4 (IV)*‡ 3-6 (IM)	2-3
Butorphanol§§ (Stadol)	2 mg	—	5-15 (NS)‖‖ 5 (IV) 10-20 (IM)	60-90 (NS) 10-20 (IV) 30-60 (IM)	3-4 (NS) 3-4 (IV)*‡ 3-4 (IM)	3-4
Dezocine (Dalgan)	10 mg	—	5 (IV) 10-20 (IM)	UK (IV) 30-60 (IM)	3-4 (IV)*‡ 3-4 (IM)	2-3

Continued

TABLE 26-1 ■ Equianalgesic Dose Chart—cont'd

MU AGONISTS—cont'd

Drug						
Nalbuphine§§ (Nubain)	10 mg	—	5 (IV) <15 (SC) <15 (IM)	10-20 (IV) UK (SC) 30-60 (IM)	3-4 (IV)*‡ 3-4 (SC) 3-4 (IM)	5
Pentazocine§§ (Talwin)	60 mg	180 mg	15-30 (PO) 5 (IV) 15-20 (SC) 15-20 (IM)	60-180 (PO) 15 (IV) 60 (SC) 60 (IM)	3-4 (PO) 3-4 (IV)*‡ 3-4(SC) 3-4 (IM)	2-3

*Duration of analgesia is dose dependent; the higher the dose, usually the longer the duration.

†As in, for example, MS Contin.

‡IV boluses may be used to produce analgesia that lasts approximately as long as IM or SC doses. However, of all routes of administration, IV produces the highest peak concentration of the medication, and the peak concentration is associated with the highest level of toxicity (e.g., sedation). To decrease the peak effect and lower the level of toxicity, IV boluses may be administered more slowly (e.g., 10 mg of morphine over a 15-minute period), or smaller doses may be administered more often (e.g., 5 mg of morphine every 1-1.5 hours).

§At steady state, slow release of fentanyl from storage in tissues can result in a prolonged half-life up to 12 hours.

‖Equianalgesic data not available.

¶The recommendation that 1.5 mg of parenteral hydromorphone is approximately equal to 10 mg of parenteral morphine is based on single-dose studies. With repeated dosing of hydromorphone (e.g., PCA), it is more likely that 2 to 3 mg of parenteral hydromorphone is equal to 10 mg of parenteral morphine.

#In opioid-tolerant patient converted from continuous IV hydromorphone to continuous IV methadone, start with 10% to 25% of the equianalgesic dose.

**In opioid-tolerant patient converted to methadone, start PO dosing PRN with 10% to 25% of equianalgesic dose.

††As in, for example, Oxycontin

‡‡65 to 130 mg = approximately one sixth of all doses listed in this chart.

§§Used in combination with mu agonists, may reverse analgesia and precipitate withdrawal in opioid-dependent patient.

‖‖In opioid-naive patient who is taking occasional mu agonists, such as codeine or oxycodone, the addition of butorphanol nasal spray may provide additive analgesia. However, in an opioid-tolerant patient, such as one receiving ATC morphine, the addition of butorphanol nasal spray should be avoided because it may reverse analgesia and precipitate withdrawal.

ATC, Around-the-clock; CR, oral controlled-release; IM, intramuscular; IV, intravenous; NR, not recommended; NS, nasal spray; OT, oral transmucosal; PO, oral; R, rectal; SC, subcutaneous; SL, sublingual; TD, transdermal; UK, unknown.

From McCaffery M, Pasero C: *Pain: Clinical manual*, ed 2, St Louis, 1999, Mosby.

■ TABLE 26-2
■ ■ **Starting IV PCA Prescription Ranges for Opioid-Naïve Adults***

Drug	Typical Concentration	Loading Dose	PCA Dose	Delay	Basal Rate	Hour Limit
Morphine	1 mg/mL	2.5 mg, repeat PRN	0.6-2.0 mg	5-10 min	0-1.25 mg/h	7.5-12.5 mg/h
Hydromorphone	0.2 mg/mL	0.4 mg, repeat PRN	0.1-0.3 mg	5-10 min	0-0.2 mg/h	1.2-2.0 mg/h
Fentanyl	10 mcg/mL	25 mcg, repeat PRN	5-20 mcg	4-8 min	0-10 mcg/h	75-125 mcg/h
Meperidine†	10 mg/mL	20 mg, repeat PRN	5-20 mg	5-10 min	0-10 mg/h‡ NR	50-100 mg/h

*To save time and prevent errors, tables with PCA prescription ranges commonly used for opioid-naïve patients with severe, moderate, and mild pain can be developed in advance. This table is an example for severe pain. Ranges for moderate pain are 50% of those for severe pain, for mild pain 25%.

†Should be used for very brief course, in patients who are allergic to the other opioids listed in this chart.

‡Accumulation of normeperidine can cause toxic CNS effects and is more likely to occur when meperidine is administered by continuous infusion.

IV, Intravenous; *NR*, not recommended; *PCA*, patient-controlled analgesia; *PRN*, as needed.

From McCaffery M, Pasero C: *Pain: Clinical manual*, ed 2, St Louis, 1999, Mosby. Data from American Pain Society (APS): *Principles of analgesic use in the treatment of acute and cancer pain*, ed 3, Glenview, IL, 1992, APS; and Hunt RF, Abbott Laboratories, Hospital Products Division: Letter communication to Malcolm Cohen, MD, Mt. Sinai Medical Center, Miami Beach, FL, July 11, 1989.

■ TABLE 26-3
■ ■ **Pediatric IV PCA Dosing**

Opioid Analgesic	PCA Dose	Delay (Lock-Out)	Basal Rate
Morphine	10-30 mcg/kg/dose	6-10 min	0-30 mcg/kg/h
Fentanyl	0.5-1.0 mcg/kg/dose	6-10 min	0-1.0 mcg/kg/h
Hydromorphone (Dilaudid)	3-5 mcg/kg/dose	6-10 min	0-5 mcg/kg/h

IV, Intravenous; *PCA*, patient-controlled analgesia.

From McCaffery M, Pasero C: *Pain: Clinical manual*, ed 2, St Louis, 1999, Mosby. Data from Houck CS: The management of acute pain in the child. In Ashburn MA, Rice LF, eds: *The management of pain*, ed 3, New York, 1998, Churchill Livingstone; and Yaster M, Krane EJ, Kaplan RF, et al (eds): *Pediatric pain management and sedation handbook: Formulary*, St Louis, 1997, Mosby.

    c. Pruritus
        (1) Reduce opioid by 25% if analgesia satisfactory.
        (2) Add or increase nonopioid or nonsedating adjuvant for additional pain relief.
        (3) Benadryl
        (4) Naloxone as a last resource
    d. Mental confusion
        (1) Evaluate underlying cause.
        (2) Eliminate nonessential CNS-acting medications (e.g., steroids).
        (3) Reduce opioid by 25% if analgesia satisfactory.
        (4) Reevaluate and treat underlying process.
        (5) If delirium persists:
            (a) Switch to another opioid.
            (b) Switch to intraspinal route.
        (6) Avoid naloxone.
    e. Sedation
        (1) Evaluate if related to sedation from opioid.
        (2) Eliminate nonessential CNS depressant medications.

(3) Reduce opioid by 1% to 25% if analgesia satisfactory.

(4) Add or increase nonopioid or nonsedating adjuvant for additional pain relief.

(5) Add stimulus during the day (e.g., caffeine).

f. Respiratory depression

(1) Monitor sedation level and respiratory rate.

(2) Add or increase nonopioid or nonsedating adjuvants.

(3) Decrease opioid by 25% if analgesia satisfactory.

(4) Stop opioid if patient minimally responsive.

J. Nonpharmacological and integrative therapies

1. Cutaneous stimulation

a. Definition: stimulation of skin by such methods

(1) Heat

(2) Cold

(3) Vibration

b. Potential benefits: range from making pain more tolerable to actual reduction of pain

c. A simple touch can be experienced as a therapeutic gesture of caring.

d. Touch modalities gaining popularity among patients who choose integrative therapies

2. Types

a. Cold therapy

(1) Cold tends to relieve pain faster and longer.

(2) It decreases bleeding and edema.

(3) Apply to site using:

(a) Waterproof bag with ice

(b) Conventional cold pack

(c) Commercial cold therapy device

(d) Effective for:

(i) Surgical incisions

(ii) Headache

(iii) Muscle spasms

(iv) Low back pain

(4) Avoid tissue damage by providing appropriate protective covering.

(5) Inspect skin to assess for potential tissue damage.

b. Heat therapy

(1) Heat therapy may be useful in the following types of pain:

(a) Muscle aches

(b) Spasms

(c) Low back pain

(2) Avoid tissue damage by providing appropriate protective covering.

(3) Inspect skin for potential tissue damage.

c. Vibration

(1) A form of an electric massage

(2) Has a soothing effect

(3) Vibration with moderate pressure may relieve pain by causing:

(a) Numbness

(b) Paresthesia

(c) Anesthesia

(4) May change character of sensation from sharp to dull

(5) Handheld and stationary vibrators can be used.

d. Touch modalities

(1) Reiki techniques

(a) Originated nearly 3000 years ago and is believed to balance energy and bring harmony to:

(i) Body

(ii) Mind

(iii) Soul

    (b) Usually performed by a trained Reiki master
    (c) Technique involves light touch over clothing.
      (i) Begin with the head.
      (ii) Work down the body front and back.
    (d) Helpful in reducing stress and anxiety
    (e) Promotes relaxation
   (2) Therapeutic touch
    (a) Introduced in 1979
      (i) Unlike laying-on of hands
      (ii) Does not require physical touch
      (iii) Name can be misleading
    (b) Practitioners believe:
      (i) Human beings are open energy systems.
      (ii) Flow of energy between people is a natural and continuous event.
    (c) Practitioner uses self to facilitate healing that occurs during the treatment.
    (d) Provides:
      (i) Calming response
      (ii) Decreased anxiety
      (iii) Promotes sleep when used alone or with sedatives
    (e) Since physical touch not necessary when doing therapeutic touch, it can ideally be used in patients for whom touch would be painful.
 3. Relaxation techniques
  a. Definition: relaxation is a state of relative freedom from both anxiety and skeletal muscle tension.
  b. Benefits
   (1) Not a substitute for appropriate pain management
   (2) May reduce anxiety
   (3) Decrease muscle tension
   (4) Promote the ability to sleep
  c. More beneficial when patient:
   (1) Receives preoperative instructions to practice relaxation techniques
   (2) Coached to use during postoperative phase
  d. Researchers suggest a 20-minute technique be used three times a day for maximum stress-reducing response.
  e. Types
   (1) Slow deep breathing
    (a) Clench fists.
    (b) Breathe in deeply.
    (c) Hold breath a moment.
    (d) Breathe out.
    (e) Let oneself go limp.
    (f) Start yawning.
   (2) Imagery: effective approach to relaxation that reduces pain intensity
    (a) Involves closing one's eyes to recall:
      (i) Pleasant or peaceful experiences
      (ii) Calming places or events
   (3) Superficial massage
    (a) Handholding
    (b) Rubbing a shoulder
    (c) Rhythmic application of pressure to skin and muscles
    (d) Techniques may:
      (i) Decrease pain
      (ii) Relax muscles
      (iii) Facilitate sleep
    (e) Must obtain patient's permission to be touched

(f) Common areas for massage include:
  (i) Back and shoulders
  (ii) Hand
  (iii) Feet
(g) Can communicate care and concern when verbal interactions are limited
(4) Music therapy
  (a) Learn to use music for:
    (i) Distraction
    (ii) Relaxation
  (b) Researchers found that patients who listen to music may have more satisfying hospital experiences.
  (c) Use soothing background music in preoperative area.
  (d) Small, portable tape players with headsets help block out extraneous noises and promote relaxation.
  (e) Establish a tape library with available music selections and relaxation tapes.
  (f) Encourage patient to request personal preferences.

4. Distraction
  a. Definition: sometimes referred to as cognitive refocusing; attention and concentration directed at stimuli other than pain
  b. Benefits: although the effects as a method of pain management are unpredictable, it may:
    (1) Decrease intensity of pain.
    (2) Increase pain tolerance.
    (3) Make more acceptable pain sensation.
    (4) Improve positive mood.
  c. Often beneficial in mild to moderate pain associated with a procedure
    (1) Peripheral IV insertion
    (2) Repositioning
  d. Distraction used more effectively before pain actually begins
    (1) Types
      (a) Music
      (b) Video games
      (c) Imagery
      (d) Prayer
      (e) Aromatherapy
      (f) Hypnotherapy
      (g) Humor

5. Nonpharmacological approaches to pain management for children
  a. Distraction
    (1) Involve parent and child in identifying strong distractions.
    (2) Involve child in play by:
      (a) Using radio
      (b) Tape recorder
      (c) Record player
      (d) Having child sing
      (e) Using rhythmic breathing
    (3) Have child take a deep breath and blow it out until told to stop.
    (4) Have child blow bubbles to "blow the hurt away."
    (5) Have child concentrate on yelling or saying "ouch" by focusing on "yelling loud or soft as you feel it hurt; that way I know what's happening."
    (6) Have child look through kaleidoscope and concentrate on the different designs.
    (7) Use humor: watch cartoons, tell jokes or funny stories, or act silly.
    (8) Have child read, play games, or visit with friends.

        b. Relaxation
           (1) Hold in a comfortable, well-supported position, such as vertical against chest and shoulder.
           (2) Rock in a chair.
           (3) Repeat one or two words softly: "Mommy's here."
           (4) Ask child to take a deep breath and go limp like a rag doll.
           (5) Suggest child float like a balloon.
        c. Imagery for distraction or relaxation
           (1) Have child identify some highly pleasurable stories or pretend experiences.
           (2) Have child describe details of the events.
           (3) Have child write down or record script.
           (4) Encourage child to concentrate on pleasurable events during painful time.
        d. Cutaneous stimulation
           (1) Rhythmic rubbing
           (2) Pressure
           (3) Electric vibrator
           (4) Massage with hand lotion.
           (5) Powder or menthol cream
           (6) Application of heat and cold on site before giving injection
           (7) Application of ice to site opposite painful area

II. COMFORT
    A. Definition: the immediate experience of being strengthened by having a need for relief, ease, and transcendence met in four contexts
        1. Physical
        2. Psychospiritual
        3. Sociocultural
        4. Environmental
    B. Context of comfort
        1. Physical—pertaining to bodily sensations and homeostatic mechanisms that may or may not be related to specific diagnoses
        2. Psychospiritual—whatever gave life meaning for an individual and entailed:
           a. Self-esteem
           b. Self-concept
           c. Sexuality
           d. Relationship to a higher order or being
        3. Sociocultural—pertaining to interpersonal, family, and societal relationships including:
           a. Finances
           b. Education
           c. Support
             (1) Family histories
             (2) Traditions
             (3) Language
             (4) Clothes
             (5) Customs
        4. Environmental—pertaining to external surroundings, conditions, and influences
    C. Methods for pain and comfort assessment
        1. Pain scales (Figures 26-2 and 26-3)
        2. FLACC Scale (Face, Legs, Activity, Cry, Consolability) (Figure 26-4)
        3. PACU Behavioral Pain Rating Scale (Figures 26-5 and 26-6)

III. PAIN AND COMFORT MANAGEMENT
    A. Preoperative phase—assessment
        1. Vital signs including pain and comfort goals (e.g., 0-10 scale)
        2. Medical history
           a. Neurological status
           b. Cardiac and respiratory instability
           c. Allergy to medication, food, and objects
           d. Use of herbs

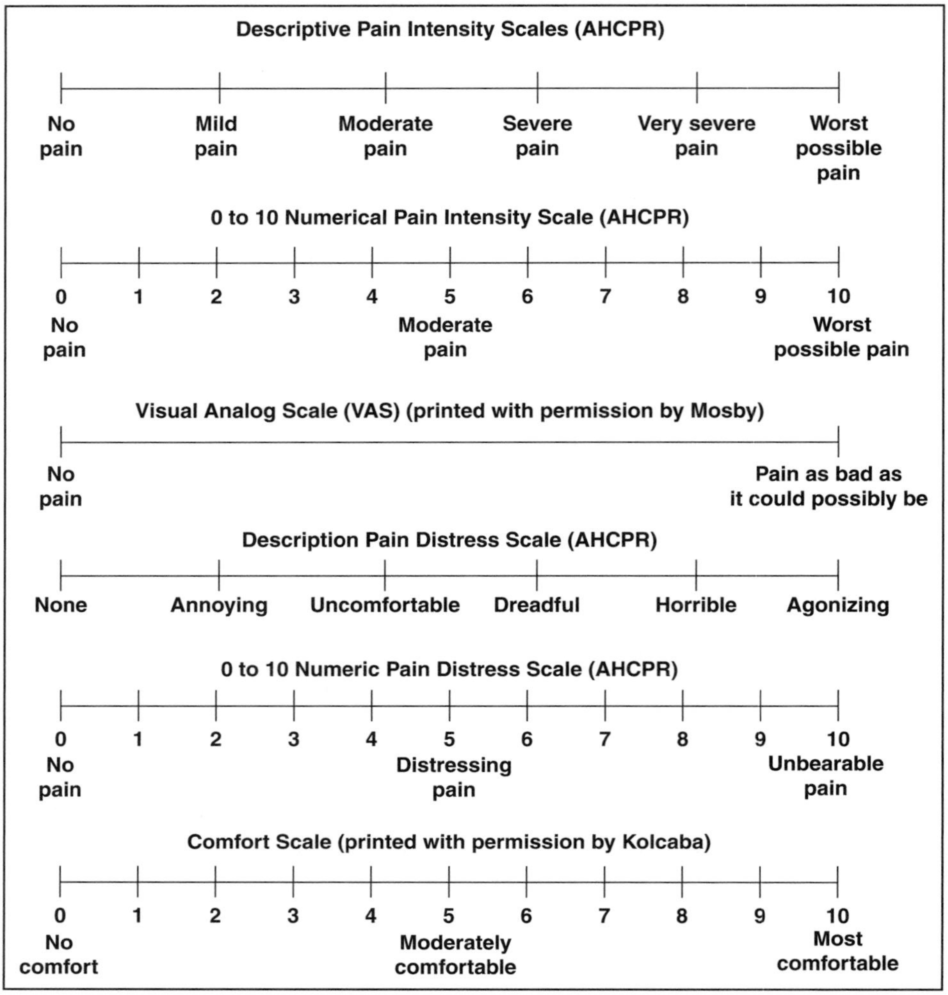

Descriptive Pain Intensity Scales (AHCPR)

| No pain | Mild pain | Moderate pain | Severe pain | Very severe pain | Worst possible pain |

0 to 10 Numerical Pain Intensity Scale (AHCPR)

| 0 | 1 | 2 | 3 | 4 | 5 | 6 | 7 | 8 | 9 | 10 |

No pain — Moderate pain — Worst possible pain

Visual Analog Scale (VAS) (printed with permission by Mosby)

No pain — Pain as bad as it could possibly be

Description Pain Distress Scale (AHCPR)

| None | Annoying | Uncomfortable | Dreadful | Horrible | Agonizing |

0 to 10 Numeric Pain Distress Scale (AHCPR)

| 0 | 1 | 2 | 3 | 4 | 5 | 6 | 7 | 8 | 9 | 10 |

No pain — Distressing pain — Unbearable pain

Comfort Scale (printed with permission by Kolcaba)

| 0 | 1 | 2 | 3 | 4 | 5 | 6 | 7 | 8 | 9 | 10 |

No comfort — Moderately comfortable — Most comfortable

FIGURE 26-2 ■ Pain scales.

    e. Motion sickness
    f. Sickle cell
    g. Fibromyalgia
    h. Use of caffeine, substance abuse
    i. Fear and anxiety
  3. Pain history
    a. Preexisting pain
    b. Acute, chronic pain level
    c. Pattern

FACES Scale

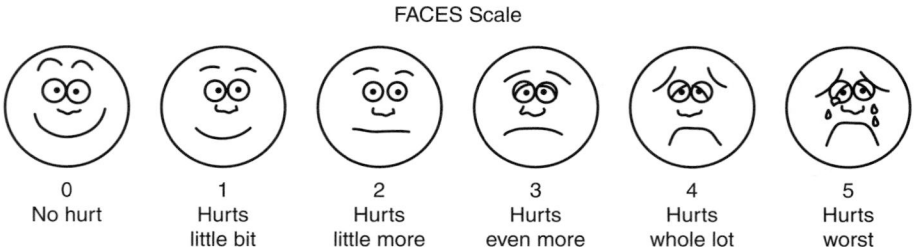

| 0 | 1 | 2 | 3 | 4 | 5 |
| No hurt | Hurts little bit | Hurts little more | Hurts even more | Hurts whole lot | Hurts worst |

FIGURE 26-3 ■ FACES scale. (From Wong DL, Hockenberry M, Wilson D, et al: *Whaley and Wong's nursing care of infants and children*, ed 7, St Louis, 2003, Mosby. Printed with permission by Elsevier.)

FLACC

	0	1	2
Face	No particular expression or smile	Occasional grimace or frown, withdrawn, disinterested	Frequent to constant frown, clenched jaw, quivering chin
Legs	Normal position or relaxed	Uneasy, restless, tense	Kicking or legs drawn up
Activity	Lying quietly, normal position, moves easily	Squirming, shifting back and forth, tense	Arched, rigid or jerking
Cry	No cry (awake, or asleep)	Moans or whimpers, occasional complaint	Crying steadily, screams or sobs, frequent complaints
Consolability	Content, relaxed	Reassured by touching, hugging, talking	Difficult to console or comfort

FLACC Behavioral Pain Scale

0 = Relaxed
1–3 = Mile discomfort
4–6 = Moderate pain
7–10 = Severe discomfort

When using this scale also use Self-report
Watch awake patients 2–5 minutes
Watch sleeping patients 5 minutes

FIGURE 26-4 ■ FLACC Pain Assessment Tool. (From Merkel S, Voepel-Lewis T, Shayevitz J, et al: The FLACC: A behavioral scale for scoring postoperative pain in young children. *Pediatr Nurs* 23(3):293-297, 1997. With permission of Jannetti Publications, Inc.)

    d. Quality
    e. Type of source
    f. Intensity
    g. Location
    h. Duration and time
    i. Course
    j. Pain affect
    k. Effects on personal life
4. Pain behaviors and expressions or history
    a. Grimacing
    b. Frowning
    c. Crying
    d. Restlessness
    e. Tension and discomfort behaviors
        (1) Shivering
        (2) Nausea
        (3) Vomiting
    f. Note that physical appearance may not necessarily indicate pain and discomfort or their absence.
5. Analgesic history
    a. Type
        (1) Opioid
        (2) Nonopioid
        (3) Adjuvant analgesics
    b. Dose
    c. Frequency
    d. Effectiveness
    e. Adverse effects
    f. Other medications that may influence choice of analgesics
        (1) Anticoagulants
        (2) Antihypertensives
        (3) Muscle relaxants

Instructions:

Ask the patient to self report pain. If unable, may use Pain Behavioral Pain Reporting Scale (PBPRS). If PBPRS is used:

1. Identify which behavior(s) are being demonstrated. Patient may demonstrate 1 or more pain behaviors with different intensities.
2. Identify the behavior that indicates the highest intensity of pain, for example, sounds 3 (severe-cries out or sobs). This correlates to self report of pain (Scale 1–10: 1–3 = mild, 4–6 = moderate, and 7–10 = severe).
3. Note: Pain behaviors are highly individual and the absence of any specific behavior (e.g., facial expression, body movement) does not mean the absence of pain.

Pain Behaviors	Definition
Restless: 0 = Relaxed 1 = Slightly .... 2 = Moderately .... 3 = Very	 Head turns to side Movements of upper/lower extremities (raising hands or lifting legs) Change of position >2× within 10 minutes, flapping extremities (1 or 2 legs or feet), pulling all covers (blanket), *or* attempts to get out of bed
Frowning/Grimacing: 0 = None 1 = Slight .... 2 = Moderate .... 3 = Severe	 Tightening of skin around the eyes Lowering and raising the eyebrows or closing eyes tightly Raising the upper lip, wrinkling the nose, stretching the lips horizontally, *or* opening of the mouth
Sounds: 0 = None 1 = Mild .... 2 = Moderate .... 3 = Severe	 Groans, moans softly Groans and moans loudly Cries or sobs
Muscle Tension: 0 = Relaxed 1 = Slight .... 2 = Moderate .... 3 = Severe	 Bracing (side rails and bed) or making closed fist Guarding hands, interlocking or pressing together, hyperextention of legs or pantar flexion (stationary), *or* rubbing abdomen (more than 2×/10 minutes) Bending knee (stationary)

FIGURE 26-5 ■ PACU Pain Behavioral Pain Scale. (Printed with permission by Johns Hopkins Hospital.)

6. Patient's preferences for pain relief and comfort measures
   a. Expectations
   b. Concerns
   c. Aggravating and alleviating factors
   d. Clarification of misconceptions
7. Pain and comfort acceptable levels
   a. Patient and family (as indicated) agree on plan of treatment and interventions postoperatively.
8. Comfort history
   a. Physical
      (1) Warming measures
      (2) Positioning
   b. Sociocultural
   c. Psychospiritual
      (1) Spiritual beliefs and symbols
   d. Environment

Form 3.1 **Initial Pain Assessment Tool**

Date _____

Patient's Name _____ Age _____ Room _____

Diagnosis_____ Physician _____

Nurse_____

1. LOCATION: Patient or nurse mark drawing.

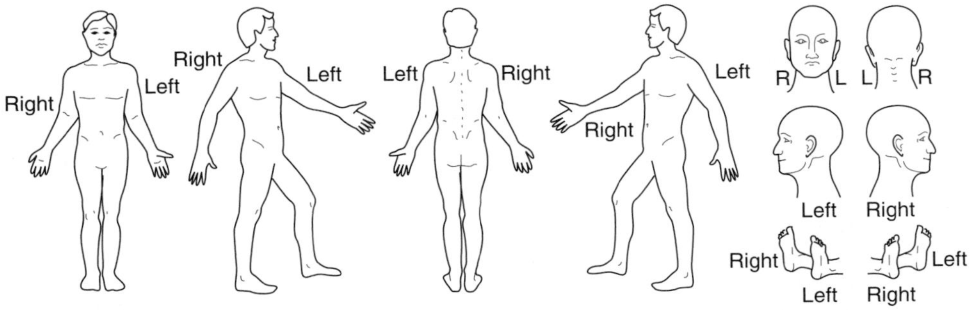

2. INTENSITY: Patient rates the pain. Scale used _____
   Present:_____
   Worst pain gets:_____
   Best pain gets:_____
   Acceptable level of pain: _____
3. QUALITY: (Use patient's own words, e.g., prick, ache, burn, throb, pull, sharp) _____
   _____
4. ONSET, DURATION, VARIATIONS, RHYTHMS: _____
   _____
5. MANNER OF EXPRESSING PAIN: _____
   _____
   _____
6. WHAT RELIEVES THE PAIN? _____
   _____
   _____
7. WHAT CAUSES OR INCREASES THE PAIN? _____
   _____
   _____
8. EFFECTS OF PAIN: (Note decreased function, decreased quality of life.)
   Accompanying symptoms (e.g., nausea)_____
   Sleep _____
   Appetite _____
   Physical activity_____
   Relationship with others (e.g., irritability) _____
   Emotions (e.g., anger, suicidal, crying) _____
   Concentration_____
   Other_____
9. OTHER COMMENTS: _____
   _____
10. PLAN: _____
   _____
   _____

FIGURE 26-6 ■ Initial Pain Assessment Tool. (From McCaffery M, Pasero C: *Pain: Clinical manual*, St Louis, 1999, Mosby.)

      (1) Music
      (2) Comfort objects
      (3) Privacy
      (4) Factors related to nausea and vomiting
   9. Educational needs
     a. Consider age or level of education.
     b. Cognitive
     c. Language appropriateness
     d. Barriers to learning

      10. Cultural language preference, identification of personal beliefs, and resulting restrictions
      11. Pertinent laboratory results in patient with epidural catheter
        a. Prolonged prothrombin time (PT)
        b. Prolonged partial thromboplastin time (PTT)
        c. Abnormal international normalized ratio (INR)
        d. Platelet count

B. Preoperative phase—interventions
    1. Identify patient.
    2. Validate physician's order and procedure.
      a. Correct name of drug, dose, amount, route, and time
      b. Validate type of surgery and correct surgical site as applicable.
    3. Discuss pain and comfort assessment.
      a. Presence
      b. Location
      c. Quality
      d. Intensity
      e. Age
      f. Language
      g. Condition
      h. Cognitive appropriate pain rating scale (assessment method must be the same for consistency)
        (1) 0 to 10 (see Figure 26-1)
        (2) Comfort Scale (see Figure 26-2)
        (3) FACES Scale (see Figure 26-3)
    4. Discuss with patient and family information about reporting pain intensity using numerical or FACES rating scales and available pain relief and comfort measures.
      a. Include discussion of patient's preference for pain and comfort measures.
    5. Implement comfort measures as indicated by patient.
      a. Physiological
      b. Sociocultural
      c. Spiritual
      d. Environmental support
    6. Discuss and dispel misconceptions about pain and pain management.
    7. Encourage patient to take a preventive approach to pain and discomfort by asking for relief measures before pain and discomfort are severe or out of control.
    8. Educate on purpose of IV or epidural PCA as indicated.
    9. Educate about use of nonpharmacological methods.
      a. Cold therapy
      b. Relaxation breathing
      c. Music
    10. Discuss potential outcomes of pain and discomfort treatment approaches.
    11. Establish pain relief and comfort goals with the patient.
      a. A pain rating of less than 4 (scale 0–10) to make it easy to:
        (1) Cough
        (2) Deep breathe
        (3) Turn
    12. Premedicate patient for sedation, pain relief, comfort.
      a. Nonopioid
      b. Opioid
      c. Antiemetics
      d. Consider needs of patient with chronic pain.
    13. Arrange interpreter throughout the continuum of care as indicated.
    14. Use interventions for sensory-impaired patients.
      a. Device to amplify sound
      b. Sign language
      c. Interpreters

15. Report abnormal findings including laboratory values for patient with epidural catheter.
    a. Prolonged PT (>12.5 seconds)
    b. PTT (>35 seconds)
    c. INR (>5)
    d. Platelet (<150,000/mm^3)
16. Arrange for parents to be present for children.

C. Preoperative phase—expected outcomes
    1. Patient states understanding of care plan and priority of individualized needs.
    2. Patient states understanding of pain intensity scale, comfort scale, and pain relief and comfort goals.
    3. Patient establishes realistic and achievable pain relief and comfort goals.
       a. A pain rating of less than 4 (scale 0–10) to make it easy to:
          (1) Cough
          (2) Deep breathe
          (3) Repositioning
    4. Patient states understanding or demonstrates correct use of PCA equipment as indicated.
    5. Patient verbalizes understanding of importance of using other nonpharmacological methods of alleviating pain and discomfort.
       a. Cold therapy
       b. Relaxation breathing
       c. Music

D. Postanesthesia phase I—assessment
    1. Refer to preoperative phase assessment, interventions, and outcomes data.
    2. Type of surgery and anesthesia technique, anesthetic agents, reversal agents
    3. Analgesics
       a. Nonopioid
       b. Opioid
       c. Adjuvants given before and during surgery
       d. Last dose time and amount
       e. Regional (e.g., spinal and epidural)
    4. Pain and comfort levels on admission and until transfer to receiving unit or discharge to home
       a. Reassess frequently until pain or discomfort is controlled.
       b. Assess continuously during sedation procedure.
    5. Assessment parameters
       a. Functional level and ability to relax
       b. Pain
          (1) Type
          (2) Location
          (3) Intensity
          (4) Use self-report pain rating scale whenever possible.
             (a) Age
             (b) Language
             (c) Condition
             (d) Cognitively appropriate tools
                (i) Quality
                (ii) Frequency (continuous or intermittent)
                (iii) Sedation level
       c. Patient's method of assessment and reporting needs to be the same during the postoperative continuum of care for consistency.
       d. Self-report of comfort level using numerical scale (scale 0–10) or other institutional approved instruments
       e. Physical appearance

(1) Pain and discomfort behaviors

(2) Note: pain behaviors are highly individual and the absence of any specific behavior (e.g., facial expression, body movement) does not mean the absence of pain.

    f. Other sources of discomfort

      (1) Position

      (2) Nausea and vomiting

      (3) Shivering

      (4) Environment

        (a) Noise

        (b) Noxious smell

6. Achievement of pain relief and comfort treatment goals

7. Age, cognitive ability, and cognitive learning method

8. Status and vital signs

    a. Airway patency

    b. Respiratory status

    c. Breath sounds

    d. Level of consciousness

    e. Pupil size as indicated

    f. Other symptoms related to effects of medications

    g. Blood pressure

    h. Pulse and cardiac monitor rhythm

    i. Oxygen saturation

    j. Motor and sensory functions after regional anesthesia technique

E. Postanesthesia phase I—interventions

  1. Identify patient correctly.

  2. Validate physician's order.

  3. Implement correct name of drug, dose, amount, route, and time.

  4. Include type of surgery and surgical site as applicable.

  5. Consider multimodal therapy.

  6. Pharmacological (as ordered)

    a. Mild to moderate pain—use nonopioids.

      (1) Acetaminophen

      (2) NSAIDs

      (3) Cox-2 inhibitors

      (4) All the patient's regular nonopioid prescription medications should be made available unless contraindicated.

      (5) May consider opioid

    b. Moderate to severe pain

      (1) Combine nonopioid and opioid.

    c. Use the three analgesic groups appropriately.

      (1) Nonopioids

        (a) Aspirin

        (b) Acetaminophen

        (c) NSAIDs

          (i) Ketorolac

          (ii) Ibuprofen

        (d) Cox-2 inhibitors

      (2) Mu-agonist opioids

        (a) Morphine

        (b) Hydromorphone

        (c) Fentanyl

      (3) Adjuvants

        (a) Multipurpose for chronic pain

          (i) Anticonvulsants

          (ii) Tricyclic antidepressants

          (iii) Corticosteroids

          (iv) Antianxiety medication

(b) Multipurpose for moderate to severe acute pain
  (i)   Local anesthetics
  (ii) Ketamine, an NMDA receptor blocker (patient education should include telling the patient to expect dreamlike feelings during administration)
(c) Continuous neuropathic pain
  (i)   Antidepressants
  (ii) Tricyclic antidepressants
  (iii) Oral or local anesthetic
(d) Lancinating (stabbing, knifelike pain) neuropathic pain
  (i)   Anticonvulsant
  (ii) Baclofen
(e) Malignant bone pain
  (i)   Corticosteroids
  (ii) Calcitonin
(f) Postorthopedic surgery
  (i)   Consider muscle relaxants if patient experiences muscle spasm.
(4) Initiate and adjust regional infusions (PCA) as indicated and ordered, based on hemodynamics status.
  (a) Refer to institutional permissive procedure.
(5) Nonpharmacological interventions—use to complement, not replace, pharmacological interventions.
  7. Administer comfort measures as needed.
    a. Physical
      (1) Positioning
      (2) Pillow
      (3) Heat and cold therapies
      (4) Sensory aids
        (a) Dentures
        (b) Eye glasses
        (c) Hearing aids
      (5) Use meperidine (Demerol) for shivering as ordered.
    b. Sociocultural
      (1) Family and caregiver
      (2) Interpreter visit
    c. Psychospiritual
      (1) Chaplain or cleric of choice
      (2) Religious objects and symbols
    d. Environmental
      (1) Confidentiality
      (2) Privacy
      (3) Reasonably quiet room
    e. Cognitive behavioral
      (1) Education and instruction
      (2) Relaxation
      (3) Imagery
      (4) Music
      (5) Distraction
      (6) Biofeedback
F. Postanesthesia phase I—expected outcomes
  1. Patient maintains hemodynamic stability including respiratory and cardiac status and level of consciousness.
  2. Patient states achievement of pain relief and comfort treatments goals (e.g., acceptable pain relief with mobility at time of transfer or discharge).
  3. Patient feels safe and secure.
  4. Patient demonstrates effective use of at least one nonpharmacological method.
    a. Breathing relaxation techniques

    5. Patient demonstrates effective use of PCA as indicated, and discusses expected results of regional techniques.

    6. Patient verbalizes evidence of receding pain level and increased comfort with pharmacological and nonpharmacological interventions.

G. Postanesthesia phase II and extended observation—assessment

    1. Refer to preoperative phase and phase I assessments, interventions, and outcomes data.

    2. Achievement of pain and comfort treatment goals and level of satisfaction with pain relief and comfort management

    3. Pain relief and comfort management plan for discharge and patient agreement

    4. Educational and resource needs, considering age, language, condition, and cognitive appropriateness

H. Postanesthesia phase II and extended observation—interventions

    1. Identify patient correctly.

    2. Validate physician's order.

    3. Implement correct name of medication, dose, amount, route, and time.

    4. Pharmacological interventions (as ordered)

        a. Nonopioid

            (1) Acetaminophen

            (2) NSAIDs

            (3) Cox-2 inhibitors

        b. Mu-agonist opioids

            (1) Morphine

            (2) Hydromorphone

            (3) Fentanyl

        c. Adjuvant analgesics

            (1) Local anesthetics

    5. Continue and/or initiate nonpharmacological measures from phase I.

    6. Educate patient, family, and caregiver.

        a. Pain and comfort measures

        b. Untoward symptoms to observe

        c. Regional or local anesthetic effects dissipating after discharge

            (1) Numbness

            (2) Motor weakness

            (3) Inadequate relief

    7. Discuss misconceptions and expectations, and implement plan of action satisfactory to patient.

    8. Address nausea with pharmacological interventions or other techniques and discuss expectations.

I. Postanesthesia phase II and extended observation—expected outcomes

    1. Patient states acceptable level of pain relief and comfort with movement or activity at time of transfer or discharge to home.

    2. Patient verbalizes understanding of discharge instruction plans.

        a. Specific medication to be taken

        b. Frequency of medication administration

        c. Potential side effects of medication

        d. Potential adjustments as applicable

        e. Potential medication interactions

        f. Specific precaution to follow when taking medication

            (1) Physical limitation

            (2) Dietary restrictions

        g. Name and telephone number of physician or resource to notify about pain, problems, and other concerns

    3. Patient states understanding or demonstrates effective use of nonpharmacological methods.

        a. Cold and heat therapy

        b. Relaxation breathing

    c. Imagery
    d. Music
  4. Patient states achievement of pain and comfort treatment goals and level of satisfaction with pain relief and comfort management in perianesthesia setting.

BIBLIOGRAPHY

1. American Society for Pain Management Nursing: *Pain management nursing: Scope and standards of practice,* Silver Spring, MD, 2005, Nursesbooks.
2. American Society of PeriAnesthesia Nurses: *Standards of perianesthesia nursing practice 2008–2010,* Cherry Hill, NJ, 2008, ASPAN.
3. Ballantyne J: *The Massachusetts General Hospital handbook of pain management,* Philadelphia, 2006, Lippincott, Williams & Wilkins.
4. Bayley E, Turcke S: *A comprehensive curriculum for trauma nursing,* Park Ridge, IL, 1998, Roadrunner Press.
5. Burden N, Quinn D, O'Brien D, et al: *Ambulatory surgical nursing,* ed 2, Philadelphia, 2000, Saunders.
6. Cole D, Schlunt M: *Adult perioperative anesthesia,* St Louis, 2004, Mosby.
7. Drain C, Odom-Forren J: *Perianesthesia nursing: A critical care approach,* ed 5, Philadelphia, 2009, Saunders.
8. Dunwoody C, Krenzischek D, Pasero C, et al: Assessment, physiological monitoring and consequences of inadequately treated acute pain. *J Perianesth Nurs* 23(Suppl 1):S15–S27, 2008.
9. Kolcaba K: *Comfort theory and practice: A vision for holistic health care and research,* Philadelphia, 2003, Springer.
10. Kolcaba KY: A taxonomic structure for the concept of comfort. *Image J Nurs Sch* 23(4):237–240, 1991.
11. Kolcaba KY: Holistic comfort: Operationalizing the construct as a nurse sensitive outcome. *ANS Adv Nurs Sci* 15(1):1–10, 1992.
12. Kolcaba KY: A theory of holistic comfort for nursing. *J Adv Nurs* 19(6):1178–1184, 1994.
13. Kolcaba KY: *The comfort line website.* Available at: www.thecomfortline.com/index.html. Accessed August 25, 2008.
14. Kolcaba K, DiMarco M: Comfort theory and its application to pediatric nursing. *Pediatr Nurs* 31(3):187–194, 2005.
15. Kolcaba K, Dowd, Steiner R: Development of an instrument to measure holistic client comfort as an outcome of healing touch. *Holist Nurs Pract* 20:122–129, 2006.
16. Kolcaba K, Schirm V, Steiner R: Effects of hand massage on comfort of nursing home residents. *Geriatr Nurs* 27(2):85–91, 2006.
17. Kolcaba K, Tilton C, Drouin C: Comfort theory: A unifying framework to enhance the practice environment. *J Nurs Adm* 36(11):538–544, 2006.
18. Kolcaba K, Wilson L: Comfort care: A framework for perianesthesia nursing. *J Perianesth Nurs* 17(2):102–111; quiz 111–113, 2002.
19. Krenzischek D, Wilson L: An introduction to the ASPAN pain and comfort clinical guideline. *J Perianesth Nurs* 18(4):228–236, 2003.
20. Loeser J: *Bonica's management of pain,* ed 3, Philadelphia, 2001, Lippincott, Williams & Wilkins.
21. McCaffery M, Pasero C: *Pain: Clinical manual,* St Louis, 1999, Mosby.
22. Merkel S, Shobha M: Pediatric pain: Tools and assessment. *J Perianesth Nurs* 15(6):408–414, 2000.
23. Merkel S, Voepel-Lewis T, Shayevitz J, et al: The FLACC: A behavioral scale for scoring postoperative pain in young children. *Pediatr Nurs* 23(3):293–297, 1997.
24. Pasero C: Fentanyl for acute pain management. *J Perianesth Nurs* 20(4):279–284, 2005.
25. Pasero C: Procedure specific pain management: PROSPECT. *J Perianesth Nurs* 22(5):335–340, 2007.
26. Pasero C: The registered nurse's role in the management of analgesia by catheter technique. *J Perianesth Nurs* 23(1):53–56, 2008.
27. Pasero C, McCaffery M: Orthopaedic postoperative pain management. *J Perianesth Nurs* 22(3):160–172; quiz 172–173, 2007.
28. Sibell D, Kirsch J: *The 5 minute pain management consult,* Philadelphia, 2006, Lippincott, Williams & Wilkins.
29. Wardwell DW, Engebretson J: Biological correlates of Reiki touch healing. *J Adv Nurs* 33(4):439–445, 2001.
30. Wilson L, Kolcaba K: Practical application of comfort theory in the perianesthesia setting. *J Perianesth Nurs* 19(3):164–173, 2004.

Hemodynamic Monitoring

MAUREEN MCLAUGHLIN

OBJECTIVES

At the conclusion of this chapter, the reader will be able to:

1. Identify surgical patients who may benefit from hemodynamic monitoring based on their risk of oxygen supply and demand imbalance.
2. Define the physiological variables affecting cardiac function and link their interactions.
3. Describe the principles of pressure monitoring and strategies to optimize accuracy.
4. Determine the indications, risks, complications, and perioperative considerations for specific hemodynamic monitoring, including arterial pressure, central venous pressure, and pulmonary artery pressure (PAP).
5. Identify normal waveform configurations for the preceding catheters.
6. List the various ports of the pulmonary artery (PA) catheter, and list their functions.
7. Identify normal and calculated hemodynamic pressures, and link the clinical significance of alterations in surgical patients.
8. Compare and contrast the bolus and continuous cardiac output techniques for thermodilution cardiac output, and determine the significance of altered cardiac output states in surgical patients.
9. Define the function of mixed venous oxygen saturation (Svo_2) and identify causes for variances.

I. GOALS OF HEMODYNAMIC MONITORING
   A. Aid in the diagnosis of critically ill patients
   B. Evaluate therapies such as vasoactive medications, fluid boluses, mechanical ventilation, etc.
   C. Assess and optimize the balance between oxygen supply and demand.
II. INDICATIONS
   A. Benefit and patient acuity must outweigh cost and potential for complications.
   B. High risk and/or hemodynamically unstable surgical patients
III. PHYSIOLOGICAL VARIABLES AFFECTING CARDIAC FUNCTION
   A. Cardiac output (CO)
      1. Definition: amount of blood ejected from the ventricles measured in liters per minute
      2. CO = Stroke volume (SV) × Heart rate (HR)
      3. Influences on CO
         a. HR
         b. SV
            (1) CO definition: amount of blood ejected from the ventricle with each beat
            (2) Influences on SV
               (a) Preload (right and left)
                   (i) Definition: amount of end-diastolic stretch on myocardial muscle fibers; determined by volume of blood filling the ventricle at the end of diastole
                   (ii) Right-sided preload: central venous pressure (CVP) or right atrial pressure (RAP)
                   (iii) Left-sided preload

[a] Left atrial pressure (LAP)
[b] Pulmonary artery diastolic (PAD) pressure
[c] Pulmonary artery occlusion (wedge) pressure (PAOP)
[d] Pulmonary capillary wedge pressure (PCWP)
(iv) Influences on preload
[a] Any condition that increases blood return to the heart or decreases ejection of blood from the heart. Examples:
[1] Pulmonary hypertension decreases the ability of the right ventricle (RV) to pump, thereby decreasing the ejection of blood from the RV and increasing RV preload.
[2] Fluid infusions increase circulating blood volume, thereby increasing right-sided and left-sided preload.
(b) Afterload (right and left)
(i) Definition: resistance, impedance, or pressure the ventricle must overcome to eject blood
(ii) Affected by:
[a] Volume and viscosity of the blood
[b] Size and thickness of the ventricle
[c] Tone of the vascular beds
(iii) Right-sided afterload: pulmonary vascular resistance
(iv) Left-sided afterload: systemic vascular resistance
(v) Influences on afterload: any condition that increases or decreases the pressure required for the ventricle to eject volume; conditions that would affect afterload include:
[a] Vascular resistance
[b] Valve function
[c] Increased blood viscosity
[d] Examples:
[1] Aortic stenosis would result in a narrowed outflow tract, increasing the pressure required for the left ventricle (LV) to eject blood and therefore increasing left-sided afterload.
[2] Use of a vasodilator would relax the vessel beds and increase the diameter of the vessels, decreasing the pressure required for the ventricles to eject blood and therefore decreasing afterload.
(c) Contractility
(i) Definition: inherent ability of myocardial muscle fibers to shorten and contract regardless of preload or afterload
(ii) Indirectly assessed through a calculated stroke work index
c. Atrioventricular (AV) synchrony
(1) Definition: coordinated contraction pattern between atria and ventricles
(2) Influences on AV synchrony
(a) Ischemia
(b) Infarction
(c) Conduction deficits
(d) Dysrhythmia
(3) Loss of synchrony
(a) Decreases CO
(b) Decreases blood pressure (BP)
(c) Decreases SV
(d) Increases LAP
IV. HEMODYNAMIC EVALUATION OF CARDIAC FUNCTION
A. Hemodynamic normal values (Table 27-1)
B. Hemodynamic calculations (Table 27-2)

■ TABLE 27-1
■ ■ **Hemodynamic Normal Values (Adult)**

Pressure	Value	Range
Right atrial pressure (RAP)	Mean	2-6 mm Hg
Central venous pressure (CVP)	Mean	3-8 cm H_2O
Right ventricular pressure (RVP)	Systolic	15-30 mm Hg
	Diastolic	0-8 mm Hg
Pulmonary artery pressure (PAP)	Systolic	15-30 mm Hg
	Diastolic	5-15 mm Hg
	Mean	10-20 mm Hg
Left atrial pressure (LAP)	Mean	8-12 mm Hg
Pulmonary artery occlusion pressure (PAOP)	Mean	8-12 mm Hg
Pulmonary capillary wedge pressure (PCWP)	Mean	8-12 mm Hg
Left ventricular end-diastolic pressure (LVEDP)	Mean	4-12 mm Hg

From Dennison R: *Pass CCRN!*, ed 3, St Louis, 2007, Mosby.

■ TABLE 27-2
■ ■ **Hemodynamic Calculations (Adult)**

Pressure	Formula	Value
Mean arterial pressure	Systole + (2 × Diastole) / 3	70-105 mm Hg
Cardiac output	HR × SV	4-8 L/min
Cardiac index	CO/BSA	2.5-4.0 L/min/m²
Stroke volume	(CO/HR) × 1000	60-100 mL
Stroke index	SV/BSA *or* CI/HR	30-65 mL/beat/m²
Left ventricular stroke work index	[1.36 × SI × (MAP − PAOP)] / 100	45-65 g-m/beat/m²
Right ventricular stroke work index	[1.36 × SI × (MPAP − RAP)] / 100	5-12 g-m/beat/m²
Systemic vascular resistance	[(MAP − RAP) × 80] / CO *or* [(MAP − CVP) × 80] / CO	900-1400 dynes/sec/cm⁻⁵
Pulmonary vascular resistance	{[RAP − (PAOP × MPAP)] × 80} / CO	<250 dynes/sec/cm⁻⁵
Ejection fraction	(SV/EDV) × 100	55%-75% (left ventricle)

BP, Blood pressure; *BSA,* body surface area; *CI,* cardiac index; *CO,* cardiac output; *CVP,* central venous pressure; *EDV,* end-diastolic volume; *HR,* heart rate; *MAP,* mean arterial pressure; *MPAP,* mean pulmonary artery pressure; *PAOP,* pulmonary artery occlusion pressure; *RAP,* right atrial pressure; *SI,* stroke index; *SV,* stroke volume.
From Dennison R: *Pass CCRN!*, ed 3, St Louis, 2007, Mosby.

V. LIMITATIONS OF HEMODYNAMIC MONITORING
    A. Presumptions and assumptions
        1. Major presumption: Pressure = Volume
            a. RAP = Right ventricular end-diastolic volume = RV preload
            b. PA diastolic pressure = LAP = PCWP = Left ventricular end-diastolic volume = LV preload

  2. Reality

    a. Relationship between pressure and volume is curvilinear.

    b. Influenced by compliance or ease of distensibility of the ventricle

VI. PRINCIPLES OF PRESSURE MONITORING

  A. Uses a fluid-filled tubing system with a pressure transducer

  B. Mechanical impulse transmitted from tip of catheter through the fluid to the transducer chip

    1. Impulse converted from a mechanical signal to an electronic signal

    2. Signal sent to the monitor through the transducer cable to be displayed as an electronic waveform on the monitor screen

  C. Optimizing accuracy of pressures

    1. Remove bubbles from tubing when priming.

    2. Use a continuous flush system with 300 mm Hg pressure to infusion bag.

    3. Eliminate tubing extensions if possible (use only nondistensible extension tubing).

    4. Level and zero transducer when indicated.

      a. Position patient in 0° to 45° supine position (position of tolerance).

      b. Place air and fluid interface at the phlebostatic axis (fourth intercostal space, midchest) and open to air while activating the zero function on your bedside monitor (Figure 27-1).

      c. Transducer must be leveled and zeroed to atmospheric pressure initially and whenever the tubing is disconnected or changed.

        (1) Standards of care for the leveling and zeroing of pressure lines vary per institution.

        (2) Common practice is to level and zero the transducer:

          (a) At change of shift

          (b) After a change in patient's position

          (c) Whenever there is a significant change in filling pressures

      d. Allow 5 minutes after position changes before measuring pressures.

      e. Maintain as much consistency in patient's position as possible for measurement.

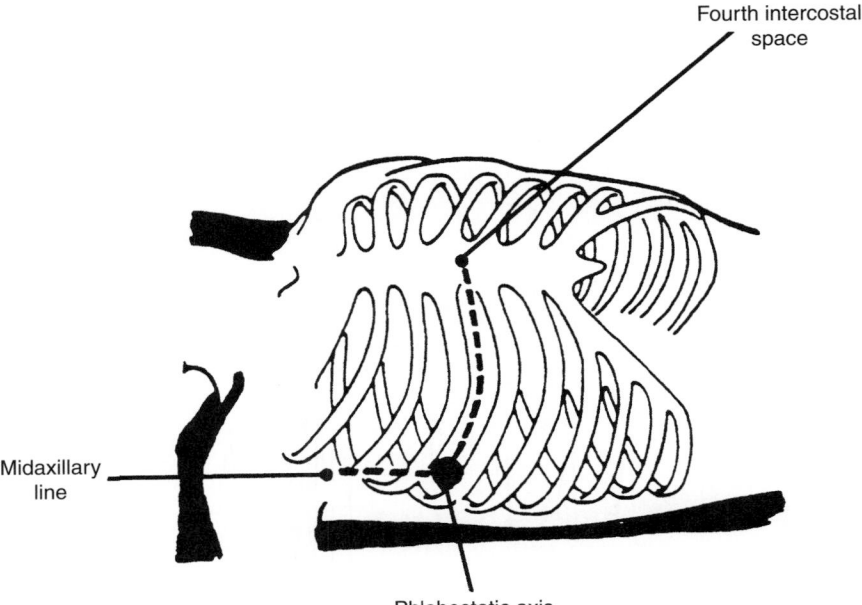

FIGURE 27-1 ■ Phlebostatic axis is an approximation of right atrium and is used for leveling air interface port of pressure monitoring system. (Adapted from Dresden DG: *Core curriculum for perianesthesia nursing practice*, ed 4, Philadelphia, 1999, Saunders.)

5. Square wave test: evaluates dynamic response of pressure monitoring system (Figure 27-2)
   a. Perform by:
      (1) Activate the fast flush device for 1 to 2 seconds.
      (2) Immediately evaluate configuration on the monitor.
      (3) Waveform will be replaced with a square wave.
   b. Analyze waveform.
      (1) Optimally damped waveform
         (a) One to two oscillations
         (b) No peaks >1 mm apart
         (c) Straight vertical downstroke back to baseline
      (2) Overly damped system
         (a) Slurred upstroke with downstroke
         (b) No oscillations after the square wave
         (c) Treat
            (i) Check for occlusion.
            (ii) Ensure nonpliable tubing being used.
            (iii) Make sure all components securely connected.

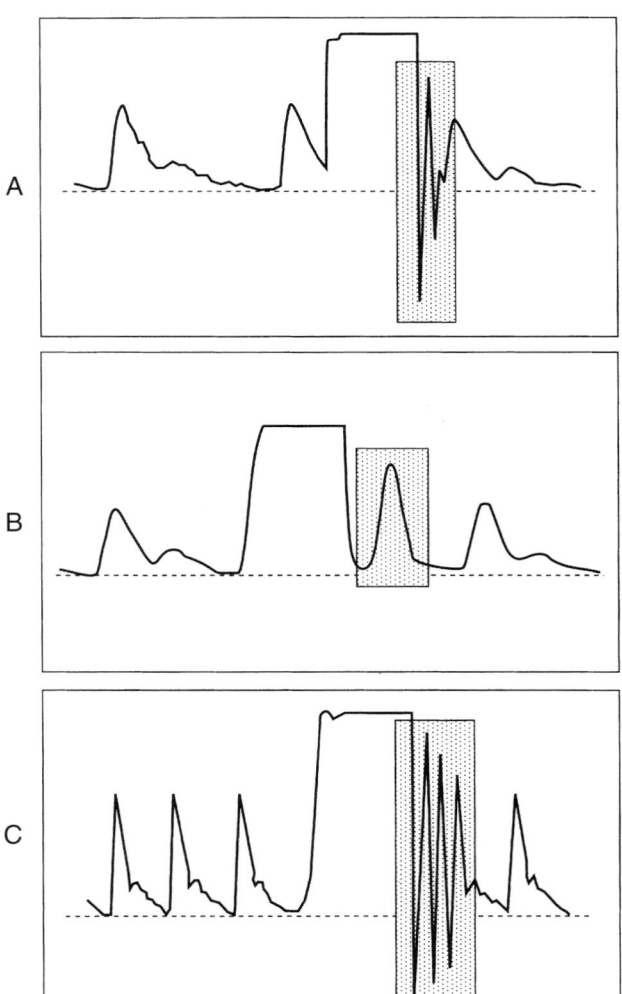

FIGURE 27-2 ■ Square wave test using the fast-flush valve. **A,** Normal test and accurate waveform. **B,** Overdamped. **C,** Underdamped. (From Dennison RD: *Pass CCRN!,* ed 3, St Louis, 2007, Mosby.)

(3) Underdamped
    (a) Numerous oscillations above and below baseline after activation
        of flush
    (b) Overestimation of systolic pressure
    (c) Underestimation of diastolic pressure
    (d) Treatment
        (i) Restrict catheter and tubing length to 4 feet.
        (ii) Remove all air bubbles.
VII. DIRECT INTRA-ARTERIAL PRESSURE MONITORING (ARTERIAL LINE)
   A. Allows for continuous observation of the patient's systemic BP with calculation
      of the mean arterial pressure
   B. Provides more accuracy than use of a sphygmomanometer during low CO states
   C. Under optimal conditions, an indirect BP, such as an auscultated BP or one
      obtained via an automated BP cuff, will underestimate the systolic pressure and
      overestimate the diastolic pressure by about 5 mm Hg.
   D. Indications
      1. Cardiopulmonary bypass
      2. Procedures with potential for wide variation in BP intraoperatively or
         postoperatively, such as:
         a. Carotid endarterectomy
         b. Aortic aneurysm resection
         c. Craniotomies
      3. Need for strict BP control
      4. Multiple arterial blood gases or laboratory tests
      5. Titration of vasoactive medications (particularly those with an extremely
         short half-life, e.g., nitroprusside)
   E. Placement
      1. Site needs to be accessible and easily compressible in case of bleeding.
      2. Radial artery (most common)
         a. Allen test should be performed before insertion to assess for collateral
            ulnar flow.
            (1) Procedure
                (a) Compress both ulnar and radial arteries on one extremity while
                    the patient repeatedly makes a tight fist to squeeze blood out of
                    the hand.
                (b) Release compression of the ulnar artery to observe for reperfusion
                    indicated by a blush of color.
                (c) Color should return within 5 to 10 seconds or radial artery should
                    not be cannulated.
                (d) Test can be repeated on radial artery for evidence of brisk
                    perfusion.
      3. Femoral
         a. Most commonly seen with patients undergoing cardiac catheterization
            laboratory procedures
      4. Other sites may include axillary, brachial, or pedal artery (uncommon).
   F. Arterial pressure waveform; two components (Figure 27-3)
      1. Anacrotic limb: a sharp uprise in the tracing that reflects the outflow of
         blood from the ventricle and into the arterial system
      2. Dicrotic limb: descending of the pressure tracing that reflects the decrease
         in pressure during diastole. Beginning of diastole is seen as a small notch on
         the descending limb of the tracing caused by the closing of the aortic valve
         and is commonly called the dicrotic notch.
   G. Risks and complications
      1. Vascular compromise (e.g., thrombus, spasm)
      2. Disconnection: hemorrhage
      3. Accidental injection of drugs or air
      4. Infection
      5. Nerve damage

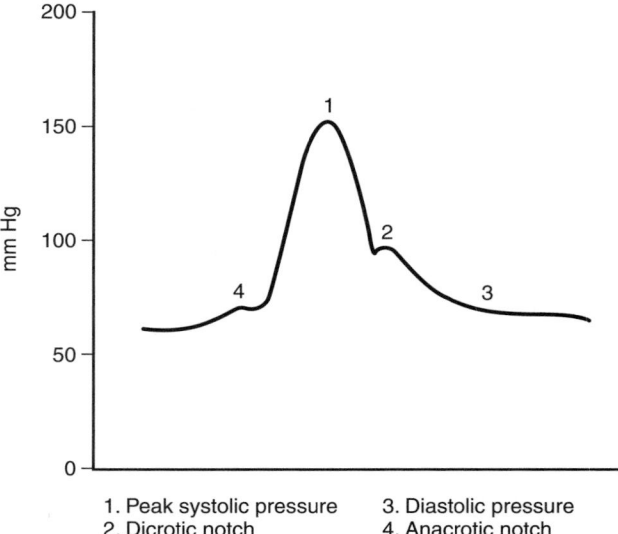

Components of Arterial Pulse

1. Peak systolic pressure   3. Diastolic pressure
2. Dicrotic notch   4. Anacrotic notch

FIGURE 27-3 ■ Arterial pressure waveform. (From Headley JM: *Invasive hemodynamic monitoring: Physiological principles and clinical applications,* Irvine, CA, 1996, Edwards Lifesciences.)

    H. Preoperative considerations
        1. Patient teaching
            a. Potential for extremity immobilization
            b. Instructed to inform nurse if experience coldness, numbness, pain, or tingling
            c. May require arterial line postoperatively
  I. Intraoperative and postoperative considerations
        1. Maintain aseptic technique.
            a. Keep dead-end caps on stopcock ports.
            b. Occlusive dressing
            c. Sterile technique maintained during insertion
        2. Monitor pressures continuously (an arterial line should always be connected to the transducer cable and waveform displayed on the monitor).
        3. Assess and document appearance of site, immobilization, capillary refill of extremity, temperature and color of extremity.
        4. Document a monitor strip of the waveform in the chart to display waveform appearance.
        5. Always use luerlock connections.
        6. Level and zero transducer per standard of care or institutional policy.
        7. Troubleshoot variances in the patient waveform.
            a. Always assess patient first when troubleshooting a dampened waveform (Figure 27-4).
VIII. CVP MONITORING
    A. Indications
        1. Rapid infusion of fluid or blood
        2. Inability to cannulate peripheral veins
        3. Administration of vesicants or drugs that may cause peripheral sclerosis
            a. Potassium
            b. Epinephrine
            c. Norepinephrine
            d. Chemotherapeutic agents
            e. Aminoglycosides

Troubleshooting/Nursing Interventions

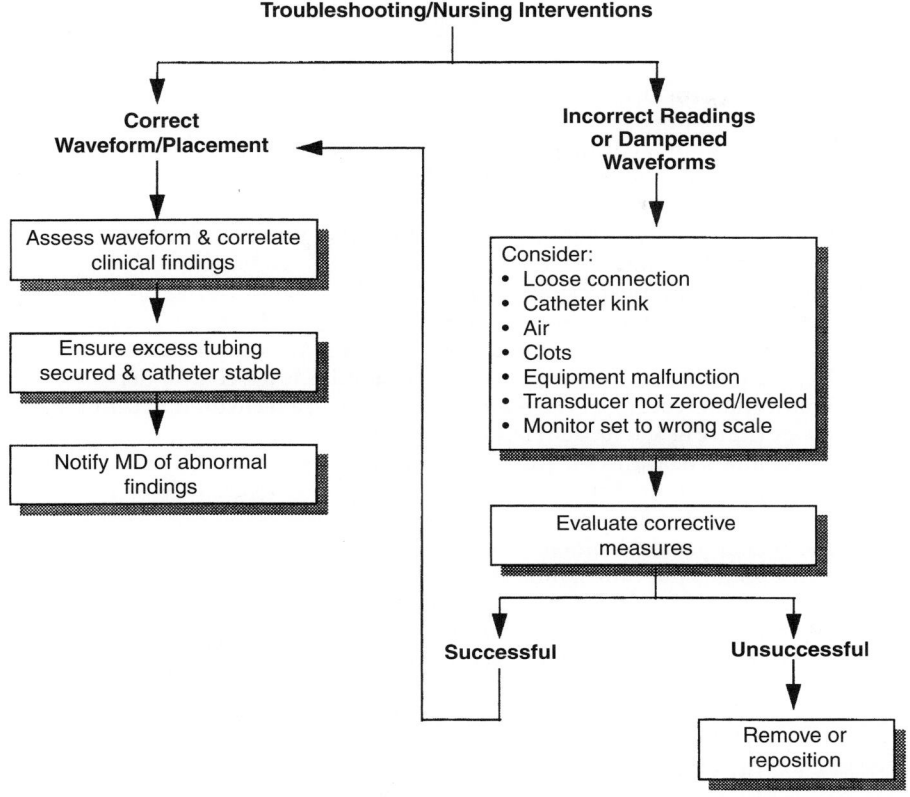

FIGURE 27-4 ■ Arterial pressure monitoring: Troubleshooting and nursing interventions. (From Dresden DG: *Core curriculum for perianesthesia nursing practice*, ed 4, Philadelphia, 1999, Saunders.)

    4. Administration of hyperalimentation
    5. Access site for temporary transvenous pacing.
    6. Assessment of fluid status
    7. Assess right-sided heart function.
    8. Aspiration of air emboli in neurosurgical patients who are positioned
       intraoperatively in the upright position and thus at risk for an air embolism
  B. Placement
    1. Single-lumen or multilumen catheter placed in a major vein leading to
       superior vena cava
       a. Subclavian
       b. Internal jugular
       c. Femoral
       d. Brachial
    2. Side port of PA catheter introducer and proximal port of PA catheter can also
       be used as a central venous access.
       a. Chest x-ray should always be performed:
          (1) To confirm correct placement
          (2) To rule out complications such as a pneumothorax
  C. Risks and complications
    1. Carotid artery puncture with insertion (internal jugular approach)
    2. Infection
    3. Thrombus or embolic event
    4. Air embolism
    5. Pneumothorax from insertion (increased risk with subclavian approach)
    6. Hematoma formation

       7. Arrhythmias

       8. Vascular erosion

       9. Improper placement, including heart chamber

    D. Preoperative considerations

       1. Patient teaching

         a. Information regarding catheter insertion should be:

           (1) Included in preoperative teaching

           (2) Part of informed consent

         b. Differentiate whether lines will be placed in preoperative holding or after induction of anesthesia.

    E. Intraoperative and postoperative considerations

       a. Obtain an order for a postinsertion chest x-ray to verify line placement and rule out complications, such as a pneumothorax, malposition.

       b. Maintain a sterile dressing per hospital standards for central lines.

       c. Intermittent readings via a water manometer are measured in centimeters of water (mm Hg x 1.36 = cm H_2O) (2-8 cm H_2O).

       d. Continuous readings via pressure transducer are measured in millimeters of mercury (2-6 mm Hg).

       e. Must be leveled and zeroed to phlebostatic axis

       f. Assessment and documentation

         (1) Pressures per unit standard

         (2) Location of catheter and appearance of site if visualized

         (3) Strip recording of waveform in chart (Figure 27-5)

           (a) Record waveform on two-channel recorder concurrently with electrocardiogram to identify individual waves of waveform to ensure accuracy with increased respiratory artifact.

             (i) Zero reference point is the phlebostatic axis.

             (ii) CVP values should not be recorded when patient is in a lateral position.

           (b) CVP waveform reflects the respiratory variation.

             (i) Record pressure at mean of the "a" wave at end-exhalation (see Figure 27-8).

           (c) Mean CVP value may be falsely elevated when the patient is receiving positive end-expiratory pressure (PEEP) during mechanical ventilation.

           (d) CVP values should be examined for trends and incorporated into other assessment data such as:

             (i) Urine output

             (ii) Heart rate

             (iii) BP

       g. Troubleshooting and nursing interventions (Figure 27-6)

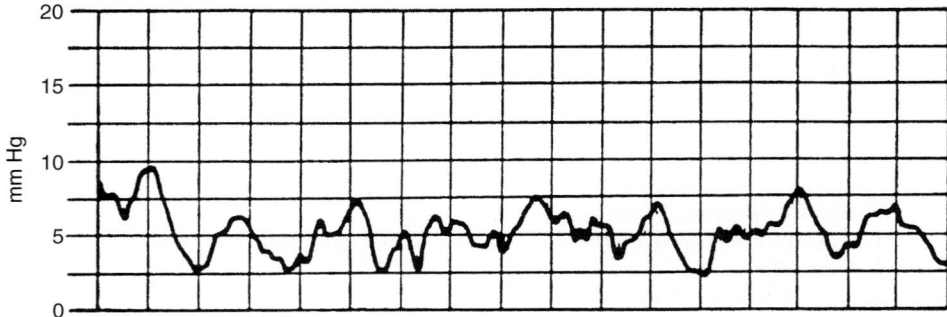

FIGURE 27-5 ■ Central venous pressure monitoring: Waveform. (From Dresden DG: *Core curriculum for perianesthesia nursing practice*, ed 4, Philadelphia, 1999, Saunders.)

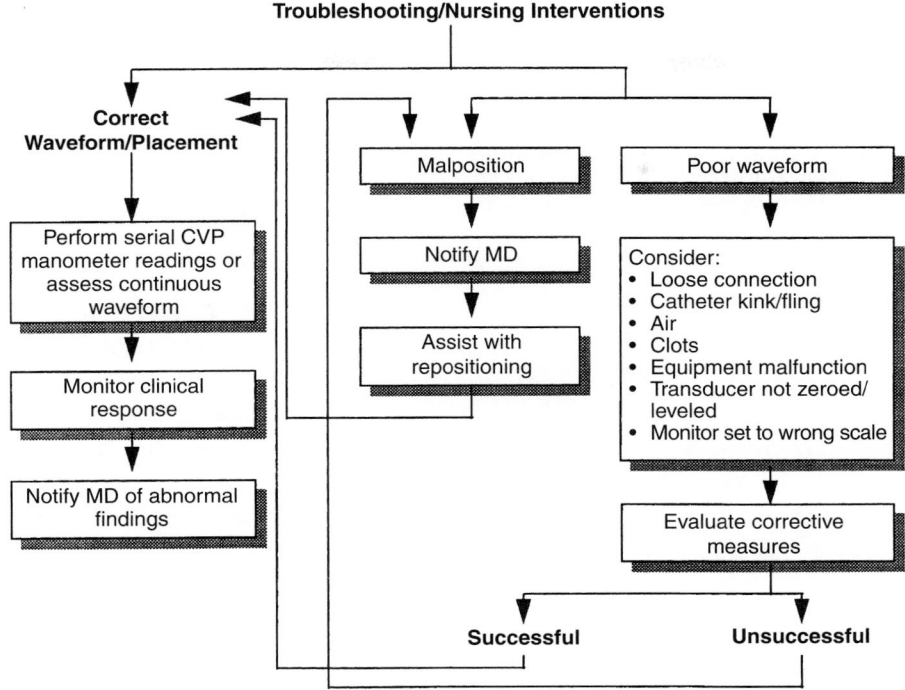

FIGURE 27-6 ■ Central venous pressure monitoring: Troubleshooting and nursing interventions. (From Dresden DG: *Core curriculum for perianesthesia nursing practice*, ed 4, Philadelphia, 1999, Saunders.)

IX. PAP MONITORING (PA CATHETER)
   A. Indications
   1. Intraoperative patient risk that exceeds the cost and risk of complications of insertion of the catheter
      a. Perioperative monitoring of surgical patients with major preexisting systems dysfunction undergoing extensive operative procedures
         (1) Thoracic or abdominal aortic aneurysms
         (2) Coronary artery bypass and valvular replacement
         (3) Extensive intra-abdominal resections
         (4) Prolonged orthopedic procedures
         (5) Thoracic or abdominal aortic aneurysms
         (6) Patients with a history of congestive heart failure, cardiomyopathy
      2. Shock of severe or prolonged duration or unknown etiology
      3. Assessment of cardiovascular function and response to therapy in patients with complicated, unstable cardiovascular disease unresponsive to conventional therapy
      4. Use of mechanical assist devices (i.e., intra-aortic balloon pump, ventricular assist device)
      5. Titration of cardioactive and vasoactive drugs
   B. Placement
      1. Internal jugular and subclavian veins are preferred, but may also be placed in the brachial or femoral vein.
   C. Catheter types: all catheters are flow-directed thermal dilutional PA catheters.
      1. Most common type of PA catheter contains several ports (detailed below) that allow for measurement of PAP, PAOP (PCWP), and CVP or RAP. The catheter allows for bolus injection of solutions for measuring CO and contains a thermistor port that measures core body temperature.
      2. Most PA catheters also contain an additional "VIP" port that can be used for the infusion of medications and intravenous fluids.

3. Paceport—has an RV port for insertion of a ventricular pacing wire
4. Svo_2—has a fiberoptic tip that measures continuous mixed venous oxygen saturation in the PA
5. Continuous cardiac output (CCO)—measures CCO by emitting random thermal energy impulses (Edwards Lifesciences)
6. CCOmbo—measures continuous CO plus Svo_2 (Edwards Lifesciences) (Figure 27-7)
7. CCOmbo V—measures RV end-diastolic volume and RV ejection fraction as well as CCO and Svo_2 (Edwards Lifesciences)

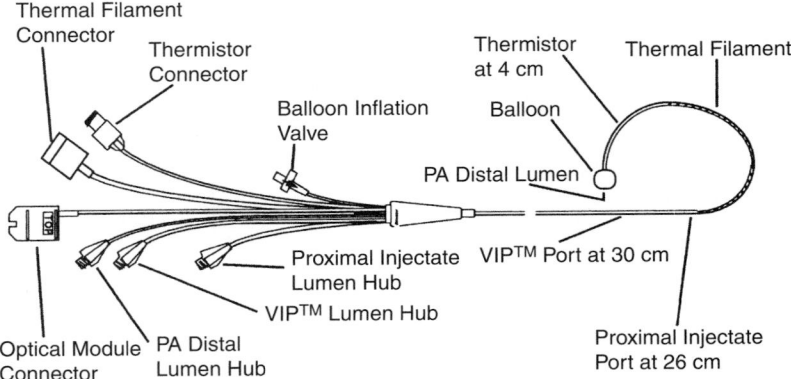

FIGURE 27-7 ■ Swan-Ganz CCO/Svo_2/VIP TD catheter. *CCO*, Continuous cardiac output; *Svo_2*, mixed venous oxygen saturation; *VIP*, venous infusion port; *TD*, thermodilution. (Reprinted with permission from Edwards Lifesciences, Irvine, CA.)

D. Ports and measurements
   1. Distal port
      a. Exits at tip of catheter in PA
      b. Measures PAP (systolic/diastolic/mean), PAOP (PCWP), Svo_2 (see Table 27-1)
         (1) PAP systolic: 15 to 30 mm Hg
         (2) Diastolic: 5 to 15 mm Hg
         (3) Mean: 10 to 20 mm Hg
         (4) PAOP (PCWP) : 8 to 12 mm Hg
         (5) Svo_2: 60% to 80%
      c. Infuse only pressurized saline or heparinized saline at 300 mm Hg.
         (1) Refer to institutional policy regarding the use of heparin-containing products as a flush solution.
      d. Indirectly reflects right-sided (systolic) and left-sided (diastolic) heart pressures in the absence of lung or valvular disease
      e. May be used to sample mixed venous blood
   2. Proximal port
      a. Exits in RA usually at 26- to 30-cm mark
      b. Measures RAP (CVP) and used for infusion of injectate with bolus CO
      c. RAP: 2-6 mm Hg
      d. May be used for infusion, although blood products and vasoactive drugs are discouraged
      e. Aspirate blood before performing bolus CO if using for infusion of medications (to prevent bolus of drugs).
   3. Balloon port or gate valve
      a. To obtain PAOP (PCWP), inflate balloon with up to 1.5 mL of air for the 7.0- to 8.0-French catheters. (Generally, balloon volume printed on hub of catheter)
      b. Balloon should wedge with 1.25 to 1.5 mL of air. Allow syringe to passively refill, then lock gate valve when not in use.
      c. Do not inflate for more than 15 seconds or two respiratory cycles.

      d. Read pressure at end-expiration.

      e. PAOP (PCWP) should be within 2 to 5 mm Hg of PAD pressure.

      f. Indirectly reflects LAP and left ventricular end-diastolic pressure

   E. Waveforms (Figures 27-8 to 27-12)

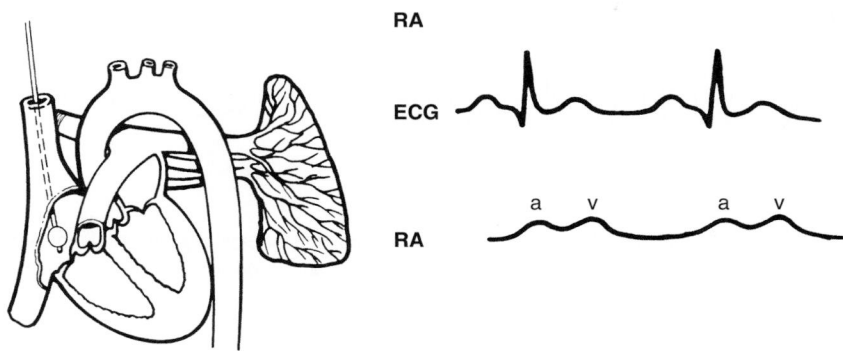

FIGURE 27-8 ■ Pulmonary artery waveforms: Right atrial waveform. (From Headley JM: *Invasive hemodynamic monitoring: Physiological principles and clinical applications,* Irvine, CA, 1996, Edwards Lifesciences.)

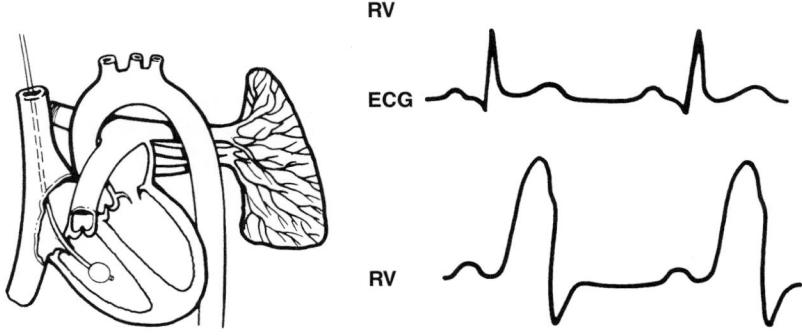

FIGURE 27-9 ■ Pulmonary artery waveforms: Right ventricular waveform. (From Headley JM: *Invasive hemodynamic monitoring: Physiological principles and clinical applications,* Irvine, CA, 1996, Edwards Lifesciences.)

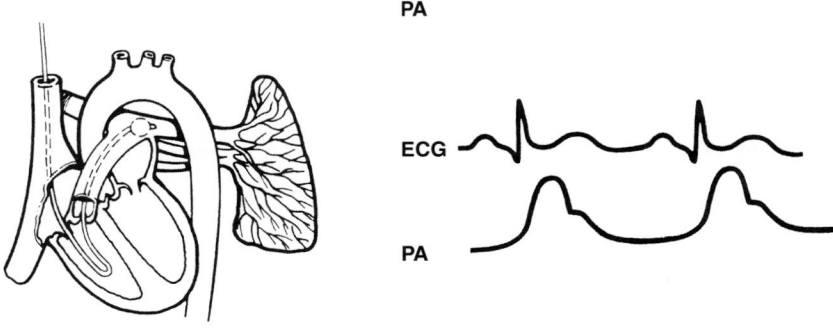

FIGURE 27-10 ■ Pulmonary artery catheter waveforms: Pulmonary artery. (From Headley JM: *Invasive hemodynamic monitoring: Physiological principles and clinical applications,* Irvine, CA, 1996, Edwards Lifesciences.)

Pulmonary Artery Wedge Waveform

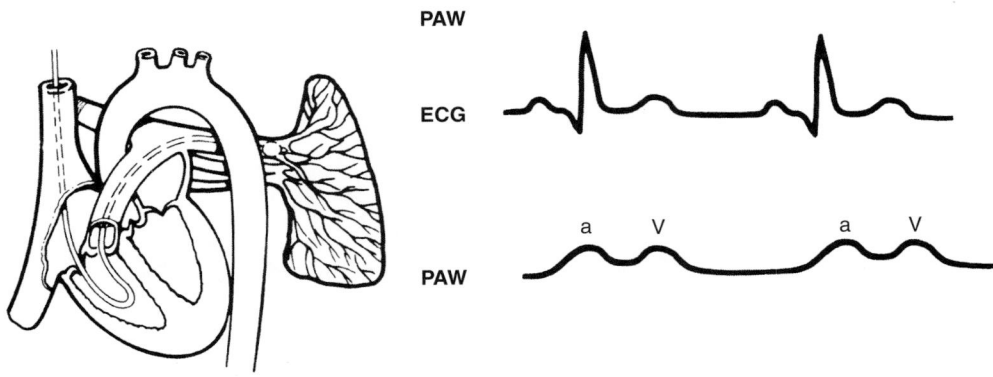

FIGURE 27-11 ■ Pulmonary artery catheter waveforms: Pulmonary capillary wedge. (From Headley JM: *Invasive hemodynamic monitoring: Physiological principles and clinical applications,* Irvine, CA, 1996, Edwards Lifesciences.)

Normal Insertion Tracings

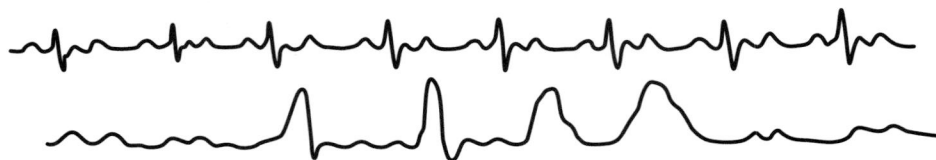

FIGURE 27-12 ■ Pulmonary artery catheter waveforms: Normal insertion tracings. (From Headley JM: *Invasive hemodynamic monitoring: Physiological principles and clinical applications,* Irvine, CA, 1996, Edwards Lifesciences.)

 F. Risks and complications
  1. Carries the same risks and complications of an arterial line and central venous line plus some unique to the PA catheter
   a. Pulmonary artery rupture
   b. Perforation of RV
   c. Dysrhythmias
   d. Electrical microshocks
   e. Catheter migration backward to RV or forward to wedged position
   f. Catheter knotting or kinking
   g. Balloon rupture
   h. Overwedging or failure to unwedge, resulting in pulmonary necrosis or infarction
 G. Preoperative considerations
  1. Must have informed consent involving explanation of risks, alternatives, and benefits
  2. Patient teaching
   a. Important to stress this is a diagnostic aid and does not assist the heart or lungs
   b. Generally inserted after initiation of anesthesia
 H. Intraoperative and postoperative considerations
  1. Ensure accuracy of measurements.
   a. Visualize waveform for normal configuration.
   b. Pressure readings
    (1) Measure all readings at end-expiration.
    (2) PCWP readings reflect respiratory variations and should be based on the mean of the "a" wave (see Figures 27-8 to 27-12).

      c. Level air-water interface stopcock to the phlebostatic axis and zero transducer to atmospheric pressure initially and if tubing is opened to air or changed.

      d. Read pressures with the patient in the same position for consistency.

        (1) Most accurate is supine position with head of bed less than 45° upright.

      e. Maintain catheter in position where balloon wedges with 1.25 to 1.5 mL of air, and document placement (depth) to ensure consistency.

      f. Remove all air bubbles from tubing and maintain distal infusion fluids at 300 mm Hg.

      g. Discourage use of extra extension tubing.

  2. Assessment and documentation

      a. Measure and document hemodynamic parameters including calculated parameters upon insertion and per standard (initiation of vasoactive therapy or change in patient condition).

      b. Assess site for bleeding or hematoma. Mark and document size of hematoma in centimeters.

      c. Note and document centimeter markings at hub of catheter. (Thin markings are 10 cm, and thick markings are 50 cm.)

  3. Apply sterile central line dressing per hospital standard.

      a. Avoid taping across sheath covering external catheter.

  4. Maintain aseptic technique: cover stopcock ports with sterile dead-ender caps.

I. PA catheter insertion in post anesthesia care unit

  1. Assemble all equipment (e.g., insertion supplies, catheter, monitor cables).

  2. Obtain consent if required.

  3. Instruct patient.

  4. Assess need for sedation.

  5. Prime or flush transducer tubing to expel all air bubbles (must be done before insertion).

  6. Maintain sterile technique.

  7. Monitor patient during procedure (BP, oxygen saturation as measured by pulse oximetry [Spo_2], rhythm).

  8. Be prepared to inflate balloon.

  9. Cover site and obtain hemodynamic parameters quickly postinsertion.

  10. Obtain chest x-ray after insertion to verify placement and rule out complications.

  11. Document pressures and waveform strips in chart.

J. Clinical significance of alterations in hemodynamic pressures in surgical patients

  1. Elevated PAP (systolic) may be caused by any condition that directly or indirectly increases pressure and/or volume in the lungs or RV.

      a. Pulmonary hypertension

      b. LV failure and mitral stenosis

      c. Constrictive pericarditis

      d. Cardiac tamponade

      e. Congestive heart failure

      f. Atrial or ventricular septal defects

  2. Elevated PAP (diastolic) may be caused by any condition that directly or indirectly increases pressure and/or volume in the lungs or LV.

      a. LV failure

      b. Mitral stenosis

      c. Pulmonary hypertension

      d. Left-to-right shunts

  3. Elevated PAOP(PCWP) may be caused by any condition that increases pressure and/or volume in LV.

      a. Constrictive pericarditis

      b. LV failure

      c. Mitral valve dysfunction

      d. Aortic insufficiency

      e. Fluid overload

      f. Ischemia

      4. Decreased PAP and PAOP (PCWP) may be caused by any condition or situation that decreases volume and/or pressure in the LV or decreases the pressure the LV must generate to open the aortic valve.

        a. Hypotension

        b. Hypovolemia

        c. Vasodilating drugs causing decreased afterload

X. THERMODILUTION CO

  A. Method that applies indicator dilution principles, using temperature change as the indicator

  B. Direct measurement that indirectly reflects myocardial performance

    1. Bolus method

      a. Known amount of saline (generally 5 or 10 mL) injected into RA via proximal port

      b. This cooler solution mixes with and cools surrounding blood, and temperature is measured in PA by a thermistor bead on tip of catheter.

      c. Computer plots change in temperature on a time-temperature curve.

    2. CCO

      a. Special PA catheter contains a thermal filament between 14 and 25 cm from distal tip.

      b. This filament emits a random thermal signal, resulting in a minute elevation in blood temperature downstream.

      c. Computer continuously cross-correlates the input signal with the temperature change to produce a thermodilution washout curve.

      d. Computer continuously updates CO data.

    3. Continuous-wave Doppler probe

      a. Noninvasively measures thoracic electrical impedance via external electrodes placed on neck and chest wall

  C. CO is 4 to 8 L/min; cardiac index (CI) is 2.5 to 4 L/min/m^2.

  D. Indications

    1. Used for determination of calculated hemodynamic variables

    2. Perioperative fluid management

    3. Assessment of intra-aortic balloon pump therapy and PEEP

    4. Evaluation of effects of cardioactive drugs

    5. Indication for myocardial ischemia and infarction

  E. Techniques for accurate assessment

    1. Use accurately measured injectate volume (generally 10 mL for adults and 5 mL for children).

    2. Iced or room temperature (19° C to 24° C) injectate can be used.

    3. Room temperature saline may be used for most patients.

    4. In patients with either a high or low CO, use of cold injectate may improve results.

    5. Ice-cold saline for injection if hyperthermic or in a high-flow state

    6. Use correct computation constant (packaged with catheter and based on catheter size and amount and temperature of injectate).

    7. Inject rapidly and smoothly within 4 seconds; wait 60 seconds between injections.

    8. Average three to five injections, preferably with results within 10% of each other.

    9. Perform injection during the same time in the respiratory cycle (end-expiration).

    10. Visibly inspect CO curve for technique and accuracy (Figures 27-13 and 27-14).

  F. Significance of CO and CI in surgical patients

    1. Low CO states

      a. Decreased or increased preload

        (1) Hypovolemia or hypervolemia

        (2) Hemorrhage

        (3) Tamponade

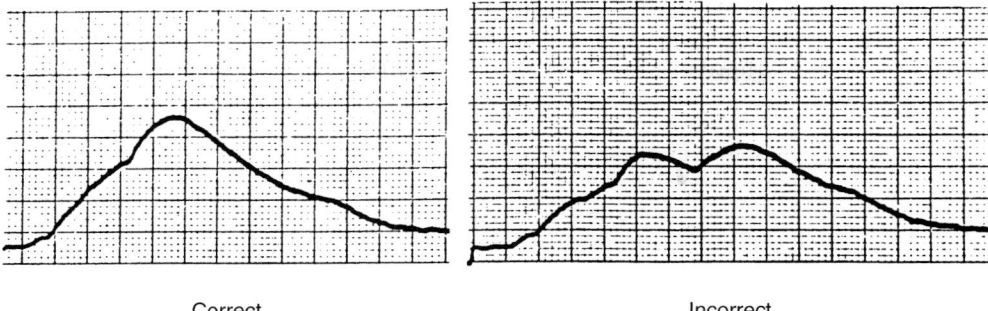

Correct   Incorrect

FIGURE 27-13 ■ Bolus cardiac output waveform. (From Dresden DG: *Core curriculum for perianesthesia nursing practice*, ed 4, Philadelphia, 1999, Saunders.)

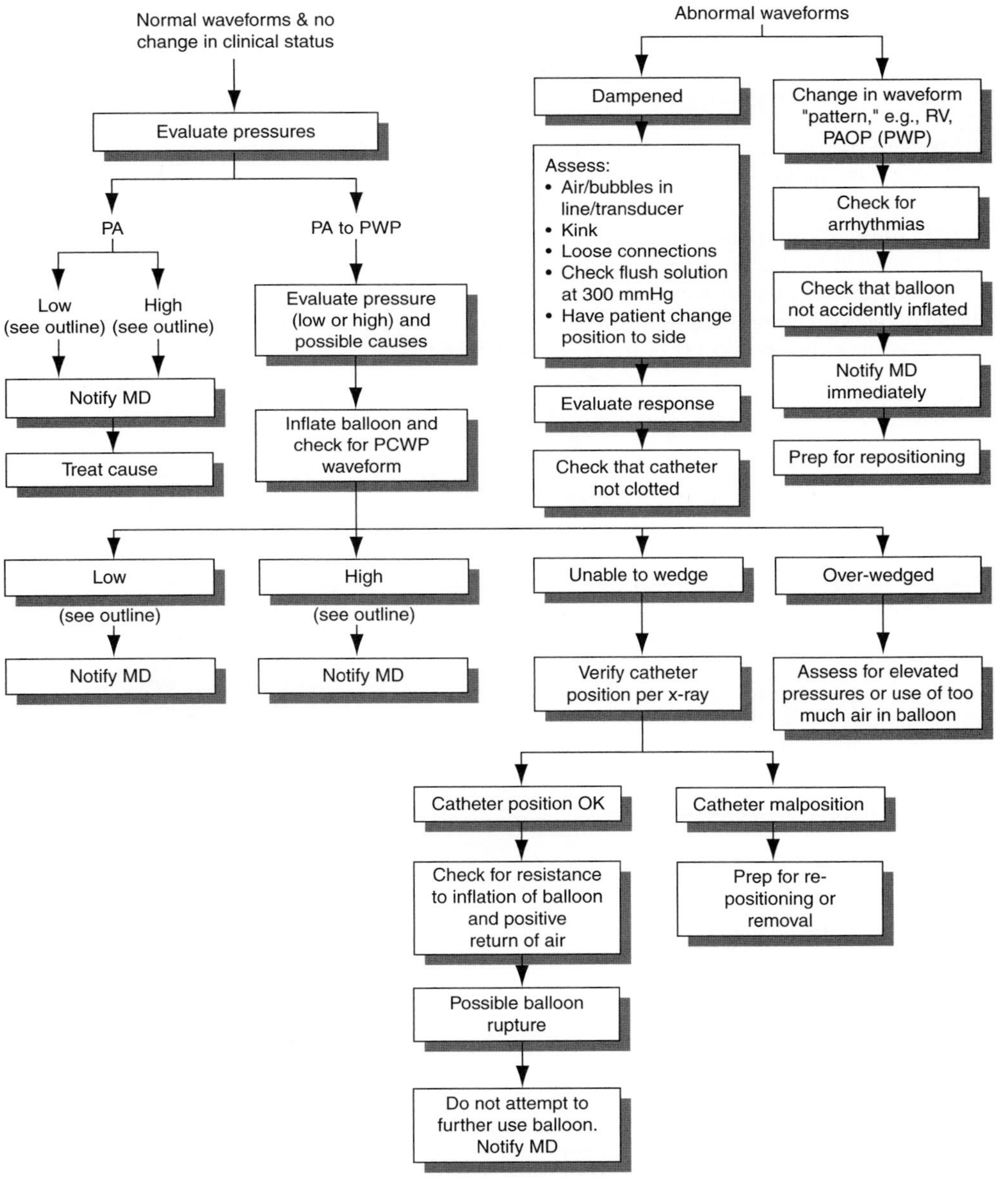

Normal waveforms & no
change in clinical status

↓

Evaluate pressures

↓

PA   PA to PWP

Low   High
(see outline) (see outline)

↓   ↓

Notify MD

↓

Treat cause

Evaluate pressure
(low or high) and
possible causes

↓

Inflate balloon and
check for PCWP
waveform

Abnormal waveforms

Dampened   Change in waveform
                  "pattern," e.g., RV,
                  PAOP (PWP)

Assess:
• Air/bubbles in
  line/transducer
• Kink
• Loose connections
• Check flush solution
  at 300 mmHg
• Have patient change
  position to side

Check for
arrhythmias

↓

Check that balloon
not accidently inflated

↓

Notify MD
immediately

↓

Prep for repositioning

Evaluate response

↓

Check that catheter
not clotted

Low   High   Unable to wedge   Over-wedged
(see outline)   (see outline)

↓   ↓   ↓   ↓

Notify MD   Notify MD   Verify catheter   Assess for elevated
                                   position per x-ray   pressures or use of too
                                                           much air in balloon

Catheter position OK   Catheter malposition

↓   ↓

Check for resistance   Prep for re-
to inflation of balloon   positioning or
and positive   removal
return of air

↓

Possible balloon
rupture

↓

Do not attempt to
further use balloon.
Notify MD

FIGURE 27-14 ■ Troubleshooting and nursing interventions in thermodilution cardiac output.

          b. Decreased myocardial contractility

            (1) Drugs

            (2) Myocardial infarction

            (3) LV failure

            (4) Dysrhythmias

          c. Decreased or increased afterload

            (1) Body temperature

            (2) Valvular dysfunction

            (3) Vasoconstriction or dilation

            (4) Vasoactive drugs

            (5) Loss of vascular neural control—spinal anesthesia

      2. High CO states

        a. Hypervolemia

        b. Decreased afterload

          (1) Vasodilatation

          (2) Sepsis

        c. High metabolic states

          (1) Hyperthyroid states

          (2) Pregnancy

XI. Svo_2

    A. Global measures of end result of both oxygen delivery and consumption at the tissue level

    B. Oxygen leftovers (hemoglobin [Hb] saturation) measured via a fiberoptic filament on distal tip of PA catheter by using reflective spectrophotometry

    C. Sensitive, early indicator of oxygenation imbalances but not specific as to whether cause associated with an oxygen supply or demand problem

    D. Necessary measurement for calculation of oxygen delivery (Dao_2) and oxygen consumption (Vo_2) (Figure 27-15 and Table 27-3)

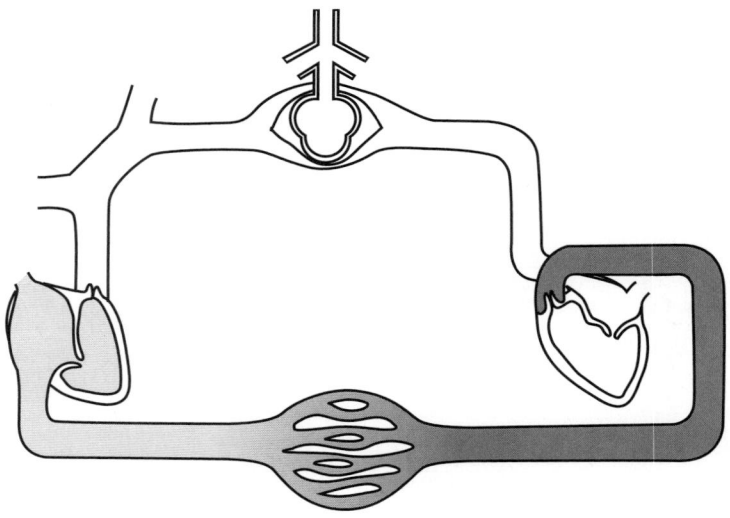

Mixed Venous
$C_VO_2 = 15.5$ vol%
$P_VO_2 = 35\text{-}45$ mm Hg
$S_VO_2 = 60\%\text{-}80\%$
$DO_2 = 75$ mL O_2/min

Arterial
$CaO_2 = 20.1$ vol%
$PaO_2 = 80\text{-}100$ mm Hg
$SaO_2 = 95\%\text{-}98\%$
$DO_2 = 1005$ mL O_2/min

$$\dot{V}O_2 = CO \times Hb \times 13.8 \times (SaO_2 - S_VO_2)$$
$$= 230 - 250 \text{ mL } O_2/\text{min}$$
$$\text{Extraction} = 250/1000 \text{ mL } O_2 = 25\%$$

FIGURE 27-15 ■ Normal oxygenation values. (From *Understanding continuous mixed venous oxygen saturation [Svo₂]: Monitoring with the Swan-Ganz® Oximetry TD System*, ed 2, Irvine, CA, 1996, Edwards Lifesciences.)

■ TABLE 27-3
■ ■ **Oxygenation Parameters (Adult)**

Parameters	Equations	Normal Range
Partial pressure of arterial oxygen (Pao_2)		80-100 mm Hg
Partial pressure of arterial CO_2 ($Paco_2$)		35-45 mm Hg
Bicarbonate (HCO_3)		22-26mEq/L
pH		7.35-7.45
Arterial oxygen saturation (Sao_2)		>95%
Mixed venous saturation (Svo_2)		60%-80%
Arterial oxygen content (Cao_2)	$(0.0138 \times Hgb \times Sao_2) + (0.0031 \times Pao_2)$	17-20 mL/dL
Venous oxygen content (Cvo_2)	$(0.0138 \times Hgb \times Svo_2) + (0.0031 \times Pvo_2)$	12-15 mL/dL
A-V oxygen content difference ($C[a-v]o_2$)	$Cao_2 - Cvo_2$	4-6 mL/dL
Oxygen delivery (Dao_2)	$Cao_2 \times CO \times 10$	900-1100 mL/min
Oxygen delivery index (Dao_{2i})	$Cao_2 \times CI \times 10$	550-650 mL/min/m²
Oxygen consumption (Vo_2)	$(C[a-v]o_2) \times CO \times 10$	200-300 mL/min
Oxygen consumption index (Vo_2I)	$(C[a-v]o_2) \times CI \times 10$	110-160 mL/min/m²
Oxygen extraction ratio (o_2ER)	$([Cao_2 - Cvo_2]/Cao_2) \times 100$	22%-30%
Oxygen extraction index (o_2EI)	$(Sao_2 - Svo_2)/Sao_2 \times 100$	20%-275%

A-V, Arteriovenous; *CI,* cardiac index; *CO,* cardiac output; *CO_2,* carbon dioxide; *Hgb,* hemoglobin; *Pvo_2,* partial oxygen pressure in mixed venous blood.
Data from Dennison RD: *Pass CCRN!,* ed 3, St Louis, 2007, Mosby.

1. Dao_2 definition: amount of oxygen delivered to tissues measured in milliliters per minute (normal ≈1000 mL/min)
2. Vo_2 definition: amount of oxygen consumed by tissues measured in milliliters per minute (normal ≈250 mL/min)
3. Oxygen demand definition: amount of oxygen necessary to maintain aerobic metabolism
   a. A dynamic variable dependent on the process of metabolism
   b. Impossible to measure
   c. We can indirectly support oxygen demand by assessing and optimizing Dao_2 and Vo_2.
E. Normal Svo_2 is 60% to 80%.
F. Decreased Svo_2 (<60%) a result of:
   1. Decreased oxygen delivered
      a. Lowered CO, lowered Hb level, or lowered Sao_2
   2. Increased oxygen consumption
      a. Increased cellular oxygen demand
         (1) Fever
         (2) Pain
         (3) Shivering
         (4) Seizing
         (5) Injury
         (6) Increased intracranial pressure
G. Increased Svo_2 (>80%) a result of:
   1. Increased oxygen delivery
      a. Increased CO
         (1) Hyperthyroidism
         (2) Pregnancy

(3) Sepsis
(4) Vasodilatation
    2. Decreased oxygen consumption
      a. Hypothermia,
      b. Anesthesia
      c. Neuromuscular paralysis
    3. Faulty calibration of equipment
  H. Techniques for ensuring accuracy
    1. Calibrate PA catheter
      a. Before insertion (in vitro)
      b. After insertion (in vivo)
      c. Daily
      d. With major changes in Hb (2 g or more)
    2. Withdraw blood sample for in vivo calibration from distal port very slowly (over 1-2 minutes) after discarding waste.
    3. Maintain PA catheter position that requires 1.25 to 1.5 mL of air to wedge balloon.
    4. Maintain PA catheter position for a signal quality index of 1 to 2.
  I. Clinical application of Svo_2
    1. Assess for causes of a 5% change in Svo_2 that does not return to baseline within 5 minutes.
    2. Differentiate between alterations in oxygen supply versus demand.

BIBLIOGRAPHY

1. Chulay M, Gawlinski A, ed: *Protocols for practice: Hemodynamic monitoring*, Aliso Viejo, CA, 2001, American Association of Critical-Care Nurses.
2. Darovic G: *Hemodynamic monitoring: Invasive and noninvasive clinical application*, ed 3, Philadelphia, 2002, WB Saunders.
3. Dennison R: *Pass CCRN!*, ed 3, St Louis, 2007, Mosby.
4. Druding MC: Integrating hemodynamic monitoring and physical assessment. *Dimens Crit Care Nurs* 19(4):25–30, 2000.
5. Lichtenthal PR: *Quick guide to cardiopulmonary care*, Irvine, CA, 1998, Edwards Lifesciences.
6. McMillen P: Calculating medication dosages. *Crit Care Nurse* 20(6):17–19, 2000.
7. Nagelhout J, Plaus K: *Nurse anesthesia*, ed 4, St Louis, 2010, Saunders.
8. Rice WP, Fernandez EG, Jrog D, et al: A comparison of hydrostatic leveling methods in invasive pressure monitoring. *Crit Care Nurse* 20(6):20–30, 2000.
9. Springhouse: *Critical care nursing made incredibly easy*, Philadelphia, 2004, Lippincott Williams & Wilkins.
10. Springhouse: *Hemodynamic monitoring made incredibly visual*, Philadelphia, 2007, Lippincott Williams & Wilkins.

28 Perianesthesia Complications

LOIS SCHICK

OBJECTIVES

At the conclusion of this chapter, the reader will be able to:

1. List three potential airway complications that may occur in the immediate postanesthesia period.

2. Describe the signs and symptoms associated with pulmonary edema.

3. Describe the signs, symptoms, and treatment of a patient with suspected pseudocholinesterase deficiency.

4. Identify two common causes of hypovolemia in the immediate postoperative setting.

5. Identify three risk factors that predispose a patient to postoperative nausea and vomiting (PONV).

I. PERIANESTHESIA SETTING
   A. Patient complications can occur at any time
   B. Critical communication
      1. Safe transfer of care (Table 28-1)
         a. Anesthesia provider, either an anesthesiologist or a Certified Registered Nurse Anesthetist
         b. Special procedure unit reports to PACU nurse.
         c. Surgery nurse conveys report to the PACU nurse.
      2. Written or computerized record
         a. Convey patient's stable progressive transition from sedation to wakefulness.
         b. Inform all caregivers of:
            (1) Events
            (2) Complications
            (3) Consultations
            (4) Interventions
         c. Complete, accurate, legible
   C. PACU nurses
      1. Assess continually the patient's status.
      2. Identify potential complications.
      3. Treat untoward reactions.
II. CRITICAL POSTANESTHESIA ASSESSMENTS
   A. Assessment priorities
      1. Simultaneous overview of organ systems and responses during admission
         a. Respiratory effort, oxygen saturation: artificial airway, intubated
         b. Cardiac rate, rhythm, and vital signs: hypotensive, hypertensive, abnormal rhythm
         c. Awareness, level of consciousness, and ability to move: arousable
         d. Pain severity and anxiety: agitated or calm, implement pain scale
         e. Residual effect of local anesthetic blocks, regional anesthetics
            (1) Motor and sensory dermatome levels after spinal or epidural block

■ TABLE 28-1
■ ■ **Admission to Phase I: Content of Report**

Expected communications PACU nurse receives on patient admission

COMMUNICATE	**ASSESS**
Patient's name and age	Airway patency
Preoperative medical history	Breathing quality
Anesthetic technique and duration	Cardiovascular stability
INTRAOPERATIVE MEDICATIONS, TIMES, DOSES	**DETERMINE AND MANAGE**
Sedatives, narcotics, relaxants	Consciousness
Reversal medications	Pain
Antibiotics, steroids, adjunctives	Muscle strength
Fluid balance	Wounds and drains
	Critical procedural events

PACU, Post anesthesia care unit.

      (2) Regional block renders extremity numb and difficult to control.
         (a) Block effect provides wonderful pain management.
         (b) Safety concern: protect from flailing, floppy extremity.
   f. Thermoregulation: temperature and comfort
 2. Determine need for 1:1 nursing care according to American Society of PeriAnesthesia Nurses (ASPAN) standards.
 3. Repeat assessment at regular intervals according to standards and policies.
B. Surgery-specific observations
 1. Integrity of dressings or visible suture lines, any drainage
 2. Position, patency, and function of every monitoring line and wound drain
 3. Abdominal girth, distention, nausea
 4. Neurological and neurovascular status
  a. Consciousness, respiratory effort, pupil size and equality, seizures, posturing, and movement after intracranial surgeries
   (1) Stimulus required to elicit response
     (a) Spontaneous?
     (b) Touch or voice?
     (c) Sternal rub?
   (2) Degree and quality of response
   (3) Improvement or decline during PACU observation
  b. Capillary refill, sensation, motion, strength after spinal, orthopedic, peripheral vascular procedures
   (1) Pulses, color, motion, sensation, temperature
     (a) Shoulders to fingertips
     (b) Hips to toes
   (2) Doppler assessment if circulation or pulse quality questionable
     (a) Cool or vasoconstricted extremity
     (b) May be normally diminished if peripheral vascular disease
   (3) Is any deficit new or present preprocedure worse or improved?
  c. Impairment related to surgical position or events
   (1) Vision impairment reported after hypotensive episodes
   (2) Skin damage at pressure points: redness, blisters, breaks
   (3) Peroneal nerve compression after legs in stirrups
     (a) Numbness or tingling after urological, gynecological procedures
   (4) Ulnar nerve stretch while areas extended and muscle relaxed
     (a) Numbness
     (b) Tingling
     (c) Weakness

    d. Impairment related to procedure

        (1) Circulation distal to line site with:

            (a) Intravenous (IV) infiltration

            (b) Medication extravasation

            (c) Arterial monitoring lines

        (2) Edema or bleeding in surgical extremity can impair circulation.

        (3) Tight casts, splints, and wraps can restrict venous return.

        (4) Compartment syndrome

            (a) Increased pressure in extremity's fascial compartments

            (b) Perfusion impaired: muscle and nerve ischemia result.

            (c) Prompt pressure released lest tissue necrosis result.

                (i) Surgical fasciotomy

                (ii) Remove or split cast.

                (iii) Monitor for hyperkalemia after muscle destroyed.

            (d) Report immediately:

                (i) Extreme pain unrelieved by narcotics

                (ii) Paresthesia or paralysis

                (iii) Pallor

                (iv) Pulselessness of limb

  5. Genitourinary status

    a. Bladder distention: urge to void? Verify time of last void.

    b. Catheter patency, urine color, clarity, volume, clots

    c. Titrate flow of bladder irrigation systems.

    d. Bladder ultrasound to assess bladder volumes

    e. Determine necessity of urination before discharge.

        (1) Consider increasing IV fluid rate to promote bladder volume.

        (2) Instruct to strain urine for particles after lithotripsy.

  6. Obtain, report, and review necessary x-rays, laboratory assessments.

    a. Chest x-ray to verify placement of new central lines, endotracheal (ET) tube

    b. Spinal or extremity x-rays per surgeon orders

    c. Arterial blood gases if patient intubated and mechanically ventilated

    d. Serum glucose in diabetics

    e. Hemoglobin if significant blood loss during procedure

    f. Electrolytes if extended surgery with multiple transfusions, extensive muscle destruction

C. Clearly document all assessments and events according to facility style and policy.

  1. Observed deficits, physician consultations, orders

  2. Outcomes of interventions

  3. Times of each assessment, intervention

    a. Increase frequency of assessments when deficit or compromise.

    b. Every change in clinical status, improvement or decline

    c. Airway removal, monitoring line insertion, laboratory and x-ray results

III. AIRWAY INTEGRITY (Box 28-1)

A. Complications heralded by:

  1. Hypoxia: oxygen desaturation, decreasing partial pressure of oxygen (Pao_2)—insufficient delivery

    a. Arterial oxygen saturation (Sao_2) of 90% corresponds with partial pressure of oxygen in arterial blood (Pao_2) of 60 mm Hg.

    b. Monitored oxyhemoglobin saturation <90%

    c. Reduced respiratory rate, depth, effort

    d. Oversedation: limited consciousness reduces stimulus to breathe.

    e. Restlessness: still anesthetized patient may actually be disoriented, "air hunger."

        (1) May indicate return of narcotic or muscle relaxant effect

        (2) Always ensure adequate oxygenation and ventilation before sedating.

        (3) Only provide judicious, sparing analgesia until patient alert.

■ BOX 28-1
■ **RESPIRATORY ASSESSMENT**

Assessments and Perianesthesia Nurse Competencies Related to Respiratory Evaluation

Critical Nursing Behaviors

Never leaves patient unattended
Lists signs and symptoms of respiratory depression
Stimulates wakefulness, movement, and deep breathing
Assesses ventilation
■ Monitors oxygen saturation
■ Auscultates lungs and observes chest movement
■ Provides supplemental oxygen as appropriate
Positions patient for effective respiratory effort and chest expansion
■ Slight head and chest elevation, particularly if patient is obese
■ Ensures adequate blood pressure and patent airway
Plans interventions for airway obstruction
■ Demonstrates mandibular lift (jaw support) for airway patency
■ Suctions airway with proper technique before extubation and as needed
■ Inserts oral or nasal airway when appropriate
■ States indications for endotracheal reintubation
■ Secures endotracheal tube and demonstrates use of bag-valve-mask device
■ Describes criteria for extubation readiness
Describes physiology and interventions for renarcotization, recurarization, pseudocholinesterase deficiency, and pulmonary edema
■ Monitors and provides oxygen
■ Obtains and prepares appropriate medications and emergency equipment
■ Remains within sight near the patient's head
■ Uses touch and soft, reassuring words
Prepares equipment for positive pressure airway support or mechanical ventilation
Consults anesthesiologist and communicates airway status
Documents events and interventions

    f. Cardiovascular status varies: hypertension to hypotension, dysrhythmias.
    g. "High" spinal blockade
  2. Hypercarbia: respiratory acidosis, increasing partial pressure of carbon dioxide ($Paco_2$)
  3. Factors that may increase airway risk
    a. Anatomy: limit chest expansion, diaphragm, respiratory muscle movement.
      (1) Obesity or pregnancy
      (2) Neck: large and/or short neck
      (3) Receding chin, "no" jaw
      (4) Upper abdominal surgery
      (5) History of obstructive sleep apnea
    b. Poor muscle tone
      (1) Medication effects
        (a) Narcotics
        (b) Muscle relaxants
      (2) Neuromuscular diseases
        (a) Myasthenia gravis
        (b) Quadriplegia
    c. Facial, throat swelling
      (1) Anaphylaxis
      (2) Surgical manipulation
      (3) Edema

B. Obstruction: interrupted patency—an emergency in any PACU
   1. Common when patient very sedated: airway reflexes blunted
      a. Soft tissue obstruction: oropharynx blocked to air entry
         (1) Slippage of tongue
         (2) Foreign body (i.e., loose teeth)
      b. Partial airway obstruction: snoring signals
         (1) Reposition or elevate head.
         (2) Turn patient to side-lying position.
         (3) Jaw support
         (4) Insert oral or nasal airway.
      c. Total obstruction: rocking, asynchronous chest movements indicates:
         (1) No chest expansion, no air entry audible with auscultation
         (2) Flaring nostrils, tracheal tug, abdominal, accessory muscles
         (3) Muscle relaxation or reintubation if jaw support ineffective
   2. Risk
      a. Hypoventilation or even apnea
      b. Vomiting and aspiration
         (1) Peptic ulcer
         (2) Hiatal hernia
         (3) Obesity
   3. Nursing responsibility
      a. Never leave the bedside of the sedated, inadequately breathing patient.
      b. Be prepared.
         (1) Sudden, silent vomiting
         (2) Airway obstruction
         (3) Apnea
         (4) Wild disorientation
      c. Ask a colleague to contact help or obtain supplies, medications.
      d. Open airway.
         (1) Turn patient to side.
         (2) Mandibular extension or jaw thrust
         (3) Insert artificial nasal or oral airway.
         (4) Backward tilt of head
         (5) Towel roll under shoulders
C. Laryngospasm and airway edema
   1. Spasm of laryngeal muscles with partial or complete closure
      a. Stridor: high-pitched, crowing respirations indicates partial obstruction.
      b. Absent breath sounds indicates total obstruction.
   2. Airway spasm precipitated by irritants or allergy
      a. Blood, vomitus, mucus on vocal cord
         (1) Suction well before extubation.
         (2) Reduce stimulation of extubation.
            (a) Remove ET tube or laryngeal mask airway (LMA) while deeply anesthetized.
            (b) Wait until fully awake.
      b. Smoking
      c. Chronic obstructive pulmonary disease (COPD)
      d. Airway irritability
      e. History of asthma (bronchospasm)
      f. Airway trauma
         (1) Procedure: long or difficult intubation or LMA
         (2) Never remove LMA while patient deeply sedated, unresponsive.
         (3) Premature extubation or LMA removal predisposes patient to:
            (a) Airway spasm plus aspiration
            (b) Coughing
            (c) Retching
            (d) Obstruction

        (4) Procedures
           (a) Frequent suctioning
           (b) Laryngoscopy
           (c) Difficult intubation
    g. Postintubation croup common among children
    h. Coughing, upper respiratory infection
  3. May be able to speak, indicating partial closure
    a. Auscultate lungs for wheezes, air entry; monitor oximetry.
    b. Constant nurse presence and assessment
    c. Coach calmness, slow breathing; perhaps hyperextend head.
        (1) Elevate head; provide humidified oxygen.
        (2) Racemic epinephrine inhalations reduce swelling.
        (3) Lidocaine to reduce irritability
        (4) Decadron to reduce inflammation
        (5) Edema symptoms may recur: observe several hours later.
    d. Consult anesthesia provider, immediately if total obstruction.
        (1) Provide 100% oxygen by positive pressure ventilation.
        (2) Low (subparalytic) dose of succinylcholine to relax laryngeal muscles, then reintubate per anesthesia provider.
        (3) Corticosteroids and/or lidocaine may be ordered to reduce airway irritation and swelling.
D. Bronchospasm
  1. Event
    a. Constriction of bronchial smooth muscle
    b. Closure of small pulmonary airways
        (1) Edema
        (2) Increased secretions
    c. Reaction caused by stimulating airway irritants
        (1) Allergic response: airway and vascular response
           (a) Occurs within 3 minutes after IV injection
           (b) Sensitivity to:
               (i) Medications
               (ii) Chemicals
               (iii) Latex
        (2) Aspiration
        (3) Intubation or endotracheal suctioning
    d. Response more likely if preexisting COPD, asthma
  2. Symptoms
    a. Wheezing, often shallow, "noisy" respiration
    b. Decreased oxygen saturation
    c. Dyspnea
    d. Intercostal retractions
    e. Increased respiratory rate
  3. Intervention
    a. Increase oxygen delivery; consider humidified source.
    b. Remove the irritant.
    c. Therapy with inhaled aerosol of bronchodilator like albuterol or patient's personal inhaler
    d. Relax airway passages in severe responses.
        (1) Muscle relaxants
        (2) Lidocaine
        (3) Epinephrine
        (4) Hydrocortisone
E. Pulmonary edema: pink frothy sputum, dyspnea, wheezing, rales, hypoxia
  1. Fluid accumulation in the alveoli causes:
    a. Increase in hydrostatic pressure
        (1) Fluid overload
        (2) Left ventricular failure

(3) Mitral valve dysfunction
(4) Ischemic heart disease
b. Decrease in interstitial pressure
(1) Prolonged airway obstruction
c. Increase in capillary permeability
(1) Sepsis
(2) Aspiration
(3) Transfusion reaction
(4) Trauma
(5) Anaphylaxis
(6) Shock
(7) Disseminated intravascular coagulation
2. Noncardiac origin: sudden onset in young, healthy patients
a. Etiology: upper airway obstruction, rapid naloxone injection
(1) A strong patient's effort to breathe against closed glottis
(2) Negative pressure increases within chest cavity.
(3) Sharp increase in hydrostatic pressure pulls water to lungs.
b. Symptoms
(1) Decreased lung compliance
(2) Chest x-ray findings
(a) Normal heart size
(b) No congestive heart failure
3. Cardiac origins: maximized cardiac compliance
a. Etiology
(1) Fluid overload
(2) Ischemic heart disease, cardiomyopathy
(3) Ventricular failure and/or cardiac valve dysfunction
(4) Increase in pulmonary capillary permeability
(a) Sepsis
(b) Critical multisystem illness
(c) Debilitation: cancer, liver failure
(5) Anaphylaxis or transfusion reaction
b. Symptoms
(1) Tachycardia
(2) Dyspnea
(3) Tachypnea
(4) Confusion
(5) Wheezing
(a) Rales
(b) Crackles
(6) Decreased blood pressure
(7) Paroxysmal nocturnal dyspnea
4. Intervention: treat cause.
a. Evaluate chest x-ray: pulmonary infiltrates
(1) Reintubation
(2) Mechanical ventilation to maintain oxygen
b. Morphine relaxes patient and pulmonary vasculature.
c. Diuretics if cardiac origin—not deemed useful if noncardiac
d. Monitor hemodynamics.
e. Reduce hypoxemia.
f. Upright sitting position
g. Oxygen administration
F. Pulmonary embolus: blood flow obstruction in pulmonary vessels
1. Likely causative factors in perianesthesia period
a. Thrombus as a result of perioperative venous stasis and immobility
b. Fat embolism after pelvic or long-bone fracture and/or surgery
c. Hypercoagulability conditions, dehydration, or damaged vessels

    2. Symptoms and assessment
       a. Acute onset of pleuritic chest pain
       b. Tachypnea
       c. Tachycardia
       d. Agitation
       e. Apprehension
       f. Hemoptysis
       g. Hypoxia
       h. Hypotension likely
    3. Intervention
       a. Correct hypoxia, cardiovascular instability.
       b. Prompt anticoagulation, initially with heparin
       c. Prophylactic prevention
          (1) Elastic hose
          (2) Sequential compression sleeves/devices
             (a) Foot
             (b) Calf
G. Aspiration pneumonitis: prevention most prudent therapy
    1. Always a potential, albeit rare complication among the sedated or anesthetized
    2. Inhalation of gastric contents as a result of:
       a. Full stomach: residual gastric volume, especially if particulate
       b. Acidic gastric contents
       c. Inability to protect airway: inhibited airway reflexes
       d. Obesity
       e. Pregnancy
       f. Hiatal hernia
       g. Diabetic: gastroparesis
       h. Upper abdominal surgery. Laryngeal mask airway (LMA)
          (1) Aspiration: an underreported complication
          (2) If malpositioned, coughing, straining on LMA, risk is increased.
          (3) Potential greater when placed by the inexperienced provider
       i. Trauma patients
    3. Inhalation of blood or foreign body
       a. Loose teeth
       b. Trauma during oropharyngeal manipulation or surgery
    4. Assessment
       a. Coughing, wheezing, hypoxia, hypercarbia, tachypnea
       b. Bronchospasm or atelectasis, particularly if foreign body
       c. Heart rate changes, dysrhythmias, hypotension
    5. Interventions
       a. Prevent by reducing risk.
          (1) Ensure nothing by mouth (NPO) status of recommended duration.
          (2) Side-lying position for sedated or obtunded patients
          (3) Rapid sequence induction for at-risk patients
       b. Chest x-ray to document infiltrates
       c. Ensure airway patency; turn sedated patient to side.
       d. Provide humidified oxygen; intubate if necessary.
       e. Constant observation: never step away from bedside.
       f. Count minute respiratory rate; observe depth.
       g. Stimulate patient toward consciousness, deep breathing.
       h. Frequently assess vital signs and act to maintain stability.
       i. Continuously monitor oxygen saturation, even after PACU discharge.
       j. Bronchoscopy if foreign body, large particles
       k. Steroids controversial; antibiotic use only if indicated
       l. Histamine antagonists
          (1) Antacids
          (2) Antiemetic therapy

        (3) H$_2$ receptor blockers
           (a) Cimetidine
           (b) Ranitidine
           (c) Famotidine

H. Hypoventilation: ineffective respiratory effort
   1. Results in:
      a. Decreased oxygen saturation (Po$_2$), which may be first sign
      b. Subdued respiratory rate, depth, effort
      c. Obliterated airway protective gag and cough reflexes
      d. Increased risk of pulmonary aspiration
      e. Decreased level of consciousness: minimal responsiveness
      f. Hypercarbia: increasing Pco$_2$
         (1) Compounds unresponsiveness
         (2) Respiratory acidosis; if unresolved:
           (a) Less responsiveness
           (b) Cardiac dysrhythmia
           (c) Unstable blood pressure
   2. Contributing origins
      a. Associated conditions
         (1) Obesity
         (2) Pregnancy
         (3) Lengthy or upper abdominal surgeries/procedures
         (4) Prolonged exposure to:
           (a) Muscle relaxants
           (b) Narcotic doses
      b. Hemoglobin loss
         (1) Reduces hemoglobin available to transport oxygen
         (2) Consider low hemoglobin.
           (a) Patient pale
           (b) Oxygen saturation low
           (c) Tachycardia
      c. Renarcotization: residual narcotic or sedative effect
         (1) Recurrence of extreme somnolence, poor ventilation
         (2) Caused by gradual migration of narcotics and sedatives from tissues back into bloodstream
         (3) Consider titrating a narcotic or benzodiazepine antagonist.
           (a) Dramatically reverses narcotic effect
           (b) Expect quick wakefulness, pain, agitation, tachycardia.
           (c) Extend observation period at least 30 minutes.
           (d) Opioid half-life is longer than single dose of antagonist.
      d. Reparalysis or recurarization: protracted muscle weakness
         (1) Neuromuscular blockade recreated
         (2) Residual nondepolarizing muscle relaxants in tissue "outlive" effects of anticholinesterase (reversal) medications.
         (3) Migrate into bloodstream and recreate weakness
         (4) Muscles uncoordinated, weak, "floppy"
         (5) Respirations shallow, gaspy; chest expansion minimal
         (6) Awake patients panicked, anxious, restless
         (7) Often pain despite weakness: no analgesia in muscle relaxants
         (8) May need additional reversal doses, respiratory support, even temporary intubation
      e. Pseudocholinesterase deficiency: genetic absence or lack
         (1) Insufficient amount of the intrinsic enzyme needed to hydrolyze succinylcholine, the depolarizing muscle relaxant
           (a) Normally breaks down within 3 to 5 minutes
           (b) Affects 1 in 2500 to 1 in 2800 individuals
           (c) Patient may be unaware of genetic predisposition until after receiving succinylcholine.

    (2) Prolonged duration of succinylcholine effect in patients with abnormal or low levels of plasma cholinesterase
      (a) Liver disease
      (b) Malnutrition
      (c) Severe anemia
      (d) Pregnancy
      (e) End-stage renal disease
      (f) Acidosis
    (3) Irreversible muscle weakness ("floppy") and apnea
    (4) Requires mechanical ventilation to support respiration
      (a) Necessary until muscle strength gradually returns
      (b) Psychological support, information, sedation
    (5) Constant vigilance: patient alert, fearful, feels pain
    (6) Educate patient and family to reveal before next anesthetic.
    (7) Physician may recommend laboratory measure of dibucaine levels.

  f. Pneumothorax: air entry into pleural space
    (1) Acute chest pain, dyspnea, reduced or absent breath sounds in affected area from deflation of lung, lobe, or pleural bleb
    (2) Caused by:
      (a) Alveolar rupture from mechanical ventilation
      (b) Surgical chest procedures that invade pleura
      (c) Central line placement
      (d) Complication of nerve blocks
        (i) Interscalene
        (ii) Intercostals
        (iii) Brachial plexus
    (3) Tension pneumothorax: after air entry into chest, intrapleural pressure increases and lung deflates; heart and great vessels pulled toward the intact lung.
      (a) Hypoxia and inability to ventilate
      (b) Decreased venous return
      (c) Hypotension
      (d) Tachycardia
    (4) Monitor oxygenation.
    (5) Elevate head of bed.
    (6) Serial chest x-rays
      (a) If <20% deflation, observe.
      (b) If >20% or patient symptomatic, insert chest tube.

 3. Care of intubated, perhaps ventilated patient
  a. Verify effective placement of ET tube.
    (1) Auscultate breath sounds.
      (a) Bilateral air entry all lobes
      (b) Clear sounds without rhonchi
      (c) Chest x-ray as indicated
    (2) Continuous monitoring of oxygen saturation with pulse oximetry
    (3) Sample arterial blood gases.
      (a) Basis to assess adequacy of ventilator settings
      (b) Determine acidosis.
  b. Periodically suction via ET tube to clear secretions using sterile technique.
  c. Sedate, relax to minimize stress of awareness while intubated.
    (1) Propofol infusion: sedation, quick consciousness within minutes
    (2) Precedex infusion: short-term sedation without respiratory depression. Use sanctioned for up to 24 hours only
    (3) Paralytics: muscle relaxants used to prevent activity, gagging on ET tube
    (4) Narcotics, analgesics must be given.
      (a) Sedatives, muscle relaxants offer no pain reduction.
      (b) Torture for patient to be responsive with light sedative but in pain and unable to indicate by movement or communication

    d. Be aware of sedation goals.
        (1) Deep sedation if intubated for days
        (2) Light sedation allows for regular, brief wake-up intervals to assess neurological status.
    e. Stir up regimen
        (1) Every 10 to 15 minutes
            (a) Deep breathe.
            (b) Cough.
            (c) Move extremities.
            (d) Turn from side to side.
    f. Extubation criteria
        (1) Return of muscle strength after muscle relaxants
            (a) Equal hand grasps
            (b) Able to initiate head lift from bed and sustain at least 5 seconds
        (2) Respiratory parameters
            (a) Tidal volume at least 5 mL/kg
            (b) Vital capacity at least 15 to 20 mL/kg
            (c) Negative inspiratory force of 20 to 25 cm water pressure
        (3) Patient should respond appropriately to questions.
            (a) "Yes" or "no" head movements
            (b) Other forms of communication
                (i) Sign or picture board
                (ii) Writing
            (c) Protrude the tongue.
            (d) Open eyes widely.
        (4) Swallow and cough reflexes present.
        (5) Regular respiratory pattern >10 breaths per minute
        (6) After extubation, close observation for hypoventilation
            (a) Presence of ET tube may have stimulated patient to remain awake and breathing adequately.
IV. CARDIOVASCULAR STABILITY (Box 28-2)
  A. Hypotension: consider an array of possible causes to plan interventions.
    1. Evidence: clinical signs of hypoperfusion
      a. Measured blood pressure 20% to 30% below baseline
      b. Mean arterial pressure (MAP) <65 mm Hg
      c. Initially, compensates with peripheral vasoconstriction unless sepsis

---

■ BOX 28-2
■ **CARDIOVASCULAR ASSESSMENT**

> **Assessments and Perianesthesia Nurse Competencies Related to Cardiovascular Evaluation**
> **Critical Nursing Behaviors**
> Assesses cardiac and breath sounds and documents peripheral pulses
> Discusses causes, physiological responses, and interventions for hypotension
> - Increases frequency of blood pressure monitoring
> - Identifies factors that alter vasoconstrictive reflexes and heart rate
> - Infuses a small bolus (up to 250 mL) of crystalloid
> - Observes for significant or ongoing blood loss
> - Consults with anesthesiologist and surgeon
> Describes causes, physiological responses, and interventions for hypertension
> - Increases frequency of blood pressure monitoring
> - Identifies patients at risk and procedural or anesthesia-related causes
> - States actions and effects of pharmacological interventions (nifedipine, labetalol, esmolol, hydralazine, nitroprusside, nitroglycerin)
> Identifies causes and interventions for common cardiac rhythms

          (1) Pale, cool, clammy skin ("cold" shock)
          (2) Warm extremities and hypotension suggest sepsis ("warm" shock).
          (3) Tachycardia: may precede blood pressure decrease
      d. Perfusion deficits as cardiac output continues to fall: act quickly to restore.
          (1) Nausea, sometimes vomiting
          (2) Dizziness
          (3) Confusion or even loss of consciousness if extreme
          (4) Chest pain, dysrhythmias if susceptible or preexisting cardiac disease
          (5) Oliguria and metabolic acidosis if hypotension uncorrected
      e. Consider causes.
          (1) Hypoxia
          (2) Hypoglycemia
          (3) Electrolyte imbalances alter contractile strength of cardiac muscle.
             (a) Hypomagnesemia
             (b) Hypocalcemia
             (c) Acidosis exacerbates electrolyte disturbance (Table 28-2).
      f. Consider allergic response: accompanied by angioedema, urticaria.
      g. Prompt, aggressive fluid resuscitation: multiple methods to calculate need
          (1) Improve cardiac output and therefore contractility first.
          (2) Calculate overall fluid replacement by "3 in 1" rule (Table 28-3).
             (a) Replace 300 mL isotonic fluid rapidly for every 100 mL shed blood.
          (3) Infusion of 500 mL saline bolus; then assess, repeat.
          (4) Vasopressin infusion may augment response to vasopressor medications; improves survival outcomes in critically ill.
  2. Colloid versus crystalloid controversy
      a. No studies clearly indicate improved outcomes with either therapy.
      b. To restore circulating volume and improve blood pressure, most perianesthesia patients need only boluses of isotonic fluid.
      c. Measure hemoglobin: does patient need blood transfusion?
      d. Critically or chronically ill may respond to colloid to increase osmotic effect in vascular system (extracellular fluid).

■ TABLE 28-2
■ ■ **Severe Metabolic Acidosis**

Quickly intervene when hypotension and hypoxia occur in critically ill patients; inadequately treated hypoperfusion and hypoxia contribute to worsening metabolic acidosis.

	Normal Values	Severe Acidosis
pH	7.35-7.45	<7.20
HCO_3	22-26 mEq/L (ABG)	<22 mEq/L
Total CO_2	24-32 mEq/L (chemistry panel)*	
Anion gap	8-12 mEq/L†	>13 mEq/L as HCO_3^- ions are depleted when used to buffer acids

Acidotic Conditions	Clinical Signs	Interventions
Lactic acidosis	Hyperkalemia	Correct cause
Ketoacidosis	Cardiac contractility decreases	Perfusion
Diabetic	Pulmonary resistance increases (edema)	Oxygenation
Uremic	Poor catecholamine response	Monitor ABG
Starvation	Ventricular fibrillation more likely	Titrate $NaHCO_3$
Aspirin intoxication	Hyperventilation	Controversial in therapy; few
	Decreased muscle energy	studies report improved outcomes, though usually ordered
	Weakens respiratory strength	

*Total Carbon Dioxide (CO_2) = Bicarbonate (HCO_3^-) +Dissolved CO_2+ Carbonic Acid (H_2CO_3). Total CO_2 should nearly equal HCO_3^-.
†Anion gap is a guide to acidosis severity. It is calculated by subtracting primary anions from primary cations: (Na^+) − (Cl^- + HCO_3^-).
ABG, Arterial blood gas; *NaHCO_3*, sodium bicarbonate.

■ TABLE 28-3
■ ■ **Treating Hypotension: Fluid Replacement**

Guide to approximate fluid replacement requirements

Goal	Action	Outcome

Increase preload
Also increases contractile force
	Volume replacement: Rapidly!
	Rate guide: 300 mL for each
	    100 mL of fluid loss*
		First priority
		Mean arterial pressure
		    >65 mm Hg[†]
		Lower heart rate

Restore hemoglobin	Laboratory measure if persistent hypotension	

Clinical shock if 20% loss of
    circulating volume*
	Transfuse according to physician
	    orders.
	Review patient history and clinical
	    status.
	Increase oxygen-carrying capacity.
	Initiate vasopressors.
		Improve O_2 delivery.
		Less hypoxia
		Less acidosis
		pH toward 7.4
		
		Only after fluid volume replaced!

Deliver oxygen	Find most effective method.	Raise oxygen saturation.

If	Then Replace

1. Blood loss ~800 mL
   Heart rate <100 beats/min
   BP normal
	Up to 2400 mL
	Isotonic crystalloid

2. Blood loss ~1500 mL
   Heart rate >100 beats/min
   BP normal
	About 4500 mL
	Isotonic crystalloid

3. Blood loss >2000 mL
   Heart rate >140 beats/min
   Hypotensive
   Tachypneic, oliguric
	About 6000 mL
	Crystalloid + transfuse

*Fluid replacement examples.
[†]Calculation: Diastolic BP + $\frac{1}{3}$(systolic BP – diastolic BP).
BP, Blood pressure.

        (1) Albumin
        (2) Hetastarch
        (3) Needed blood components
   3. Often transient, mild, but must plan response to profound low blood pressure
     a. Orthostatic (postural) hypotension
        (1) In ambulatory surgery or procedural areas, may not be evident until patient sits or stands
        (2) Peripheral vessels incompetent: remain vasodilated from effect of anesthetic medications
        (3) Monitor blood pressure as patient changes position, walks.
     b. Continued effect of spinal or epidural (regional) anesthetic
        (1) Remaining vasodilation from sympathetic block
           (a) Increases relative size of vascular compartment
           (b) Peripheral pooling of blood
        (2) Most likely after high residual motor and sensory block
           (a) Respiratory compromise above level T4
           (b) Symptoms persist until blockade recedes.
              (i) Hypotension
              (ii) Heat loss
        (3) Nursing intervention: remain at stretcher side.
           (a) Generous fluid volumes to fill expanded vascular space

        (b) Reclining, foot-elevated position

        (c) Consult anesthesia provider.

        (d) Explain situation.

        (e) Support emotionally.

        (f) Observe constantly.

     (4) Give vasopressors.

        (a) Epinephrine

        (b) Neosynephrine

     (5) Monitor oxygen saturations; observe respiratory quality.

        (a) Recognize hypoventilation.

        (b) Intubate, mechanically ventilate if hypoventilation persists.

  c. Hypothermia: rewarm slowly, cautiously.

     (1) Initially, vasoconstrictive responses caused by cold temperature

        (a) Masks inadequate circulating fluid volumes

     (2) Peripheral vessels dilate as temperature normalizes.

        (a) Relative vascular space increases.

        (b) Blood pressure plummets.

  d. Sepsis

     (1) Consider rewarming if hypotension does not resolve after fluid.

     (2) More likely after:

        (a) Urological procedure

        (b) Preexisting infection

        (c) Intra-abdominal leaks

        (d) Gastrointestinal necrosis

        (e) Trauma

     (3) Massive peripheral vasodilation

        (a) Low vascular resistance

        (b) Maintains large vascular space

     (4) Provide copious fluid volumes, antibiotics, vasopressors.

     (5) Act quickly to normalize blood pressure, electrolytes.

     (6) Close, even 1:1 observation in PACU, then consider intensive care unit admission

  e. Cardiogenic causes

     (1) New-onset periprocedural myocardial infarction

     (2) Cardiac tamponade

     (3) Embolism

     (4) Inability to respond with tachycardia, vasoconstriction

        (a) Medication effects: negative inotropics and chronotropics

4. Hypovolemia: intravascular volume deficit

  a. Most common cause of hypotension, particularly in perianesthesia areas

     (1) Procedure-related bleeding

     (2) Insufficient replacement of fluid volume, considering:

        (a) Intraoperative blood loss

        (b) NPO duration

        (c) Insensible losses

  b. Assessment indicators

     (1) Hypotension: always ask, "Is patient hypovolemic?"

     (2) Compensatory tachycardia

     (3) Significant bleeding: check

        (a) Wound drains

        (b) On or under dressings, splints, casts

        (c) Increasing abdominal girth after abdominal procedures

        (d) Hematuria or blood in emesis

        (e) Vascular integrity after orthopedic surgery

     (4) Cumulative losses from sampling for laboratory measures

     (5) Coagulopathy

        (a) Preprocedural condition

   (b) Aspirin, anticoagulants, and herbals not stopped preoperatively
   (c) After multiple transfusions
   (d) May require treatment with:
     (i) Vitamin K
     (ii) Platelets
     (iii) Cryoprecipitate
     (iv) Fresh frozen plasma
     (v) Desmopressin (DDAVP)
     (vi) Amicar
  c. Intervention: treat underlying cause.
   (1) Assess fluid volume status in all perianesthesia phases.
    (a) Transfuse with packed red cells if hemoglobin <7 to 9 g/dL.
    (b) Individual patient with cardiac disease may need transfusion at higher hemoglobin level.
    (c) Autologous: predonated by patient
    (d) Donated to patient by another of same blood type
    (e) Banked blood: donated by unknown
   (2) Always provide oxygen if patient hypotensive and/or bleeding.
   (3) Fluid, blood product replacement according to calculated need
   (4) Early treatment of acidosis particularly if large blood loss
   (5) Return to operating room for reexploration of surgical site.
   (6) Elevate legs to increase venous return (preload).
B. Hypertension
 1. At least 20% increase above baseline or greater than 140/90 mm Hg can cause:
  a. Surgical bleeding
  b. Cardiac ischemia or failure
 2. Causes in perianesthesia units
  a. Preexisting high blood pressure: most common postprocedural cause
   (1) Encourage patient to take antihypertensive medications before procedure.
  b. Inadequately treated pain, anxiety, or delirium
  c. Full, distended bladder
  d. After vascular surgeries: carotid endarterectomy, cardiac surgery
  e. Fluid overload
  f. Preeclampsia among pregnant patients
  g. Hypothermia and shivering
 3. Treat by alleviating cause.
  a. Antihypertensives
   (1) Beta-blockers
    (a) Peripheral vasodilation
    (b) Heart rate reduction
   (2) Nitroprusside
    (a) Peripheral vasodilation
    (b) Reduces afterload
   (3) Hydralazine: relaxes arterioles
  b. Diuresis, bladder emptying
  c. Rewarming: promotes vasodilation
  d. Manage pain, anxiety.
 4. Autonomic dysreflexia: sudden, dramatic blood pressure elevations
  a. Unimpeded discharge of sympathetic neurons
  b. Paraplegic or quadriplegic patients
  c. Prompted by stimulation
   (1) "Oscopy" procedures
   (2) Surgical manipulation
   (3) Full bladder: verify catheter patency.
   (4) Distended colon
   (5) Increased muscle spasm

        d. Symptoms

          (1) Severe, vessel-rupturing hypertension to 250/150 mm Hg

            (a) Seizures or stroke

            (b) Cardiac arrest

            (c) Surgical bleeding

          (2) Above level of spinal cord injury

            (a) Profuse sweating, flushed skin

            (b) Throbbing headache

          (3) Below spinal cord injury level

            (a) Pale skin

            (b) Gooseflesh

        e. Quick interventions

          (1) Empty bladder.

            (a) Void or catheterize.

            (b) Straighten tubing kinks.

          (2) Treat pain.

            (a) Markedly relaxes patient

            (b) Dilates peripheral vasculature

          (3) Vasodilating medications: nitroprusside, labetalol

          (4) Elevate head of bed.

C. Cardiac dysrhythmias (see Chapter 32)

    1. Sinus bradycardia: common, usually benign

        a. Heart rate less than 60 beats/min

          (1) Especially among young, healthy athletes

          (2) Sleepy, understimulated patients

          (3) Expected response when using beta-blocking medications

          (4) Response to anesthetic medications: sinus and junctional

        b. No treatment unless:

          (1) Dangerously low blood pressure

          (2) Progressive heart block

            (a) New or chronic cardiac disease

            (b) Atropine increases sinus firing and atrioventricular conduction.

            (c) Pacemaker for persistent, symptomatic blocks

        c. Vagal nerve stimulation: profound bradycardia, even asystole

          (1) Normally sustains heart rate balance; opposes acceleration tendencies

          (2) Undeterred stimulation as a result of:

            (a) Valsalva: straining at stool or urination

            (b) Vomiting and retching

          (3) Likely results in:

            (a) Nausea

            (b) Profound hypotension

            (c) Dizziness

            (d) Lethargy

            (e) Unconsciousness

          (4) Intervene with:

            (a) Recumbent flat position

            (b) Close monitoring of vital signs, cardiac rhythm, alertness

            (c) Medications as indicated per anesthesia provider or protocols

            (d) Defer transfer from PACU.

               (i) May occur when moving about in phase II; consider return to phase I care.

    2. Atrial fibrillation or flutter

        a. Often a chronic condition, especially among elderly surgical patients

        b. Report to physician.

          (1) New onset could reflect:

            (a) Fluid overload in cardiac-sensitive patient

            (b) Perianesthesia cardiac concern

          (2) Rapid, uncontrolled ventricular response

(3) Physical decompensation
    (a) Associated with significant hypotension or hypertension
    (b) Chest pain
    (c) Respiratory changes: dyspnea, pulmonary congestion

3. Premature ventricular contractions may:
  a. Be benign, normally occurring
  b. Reflect hypokalemia, acidosis, hypercapnia: assess labs
  c. Indicate hypoxia: supplement oxygen, stimulate groggy patient
  d. Suggest cardiac ischemia

4. Supraventricular tachycardia: common, usually self-limiting
  a. Heart rate 100 to 140 beats/min often a normal compensatory response to:
    (1) Surgical stress response
    (2) Pain and/or anxiety
    (3) Bladder distention
    (4) Hypovolemia or low hemoglobin (anemia)
    (5) Fever
    (6) Reflexive response to medications
      (a) Muscle relaxant reversal: glycopyrrolate
      (b) Vasoactive medications: nitroprusside, dopamine
  b. Malignant hyperthermia
    (1) Unexplained, ultrarapid tachycardia
    (2) Every PACU staff must be prepared with a protocol, supplies, personnel education to respond promptly to this anesthesia crisis.

D. Chest pain: presume cardiac cause until excluded!
  1. At-risk patients
    a. Preexisting cardiac disease
    b. Obesity
    c. Diabetes
    d. Debilitation
  2. Assess subjective description.
    a. Pleural versus angina
    b. Sharp versus pressure
    c. Location
      (1) Jaw
      (2) Chest
      (3) Left arm
      (4) Radiation to neck
      (5) Back
      (6) Indigestion
    d. Notice accompanying diaphoresis, nausea, dyspnea.
    e. Associated cardiac arrhythmias or blood pressure instability
  3. Differentiate
    a. Gas, especially after laparoscopy, colon surgery
    b. Referred surgical pain
    c. Pleural causes: pneumothorax, pleural effusion, pneumonia
    d. Gastrointestinal (GI) causes
      (1) Reflux esophagitis
      (2) Ulcer, pancreatitis
  4. Interventions
    a. Monitor rate and rhythm.
      (1) Obtain 12-lead electrocardiogram (ECG).
      (2) Compare with preoperative ECG.
    b. Decrease myocardial work and manage complications.
      (1) Relieve pain and consider morphine for vasodilating benefits.
      (2) Antianginal (nitroglycerin)
      (3) Dysrhythmia treatment
      (4) Blood pressure therapies
      (5) Adequate oxygenation
      (6) Hydration

      c. Laboratory tests
        (1) Serial troponins
        (2) Cardiac enzymes
      d. Peripheral vascular integrity
      e. Reposition patient
      f. Offer antacids, which may relieve noncardiac pain

V. GASTROINTESTINAL (GI) ISSUES
  A. Nausea and vomiting
    1. All too common, miserable, resistant anesthesia outcome
      a. Alters patient reports of satisfaction with procedure
      b. Sedation increases aspiration risk.
      c. Persistent retching
      d. Recurrent emesis increases pain.
      e. Dehydration
      f. May result in unplanned hospital admission after procedures, ambulatory surgery
    2. Physiology: narcotics, sedatives can trigger brain's emetic center.
      a. Retching controlled by vomiting center in medulla
      b. Vomiting center receives input from:
        (1) Cerebral cortex: olfactory, visual, emotional stimuli
        (2) GI tract
        (3) Vestibular system
        (4) Chemoreceptor trigger zone
    3. Risk factors for developing PONV (see Chapter 25)
      a. Predisposing factors
        (1) Patient specific
          (a) Female gender
          (b) Nonsmoking status
          (c) History of PONV
          (d) History of motion sickness or vestibular problems
          (e) Delayed gastric emptying or pressure
            (i)   Morbid obesity
            (ii) Pregnancy (early stage)
            (iii) Gastroparesis
               [a] Neurological diseases
               [b] Diabetes
          (f) Increased gastric volume
            (i)   Full stomach, insufficient duration of the nothing by mouth (NPO) status
            (ii) Anxiety
          (g) Hypotension, bradycardia: sudden unexpected emesis
          (h) Severe pain
          (i) Dehydration including NPO duration in fluid replacement calculations
        (2) Anesthetic related
          (a) Use of volatile anesthetics
          (b) Nitrous oxide
          (c) IV medications: ketamine, etomidate
          (d) Postoperative use of opioids
            (i)   Meperidine
            (ii) Morphine
          (e) Duration of anesthesia
        (3) Surgery related
          (a) Duration of surgery
          (b) Type of surgery
            (i)   Laparoscopic procedures particularly gynecologic
            (ii) Strabismus surgery primarily in children
            (iii) Middle ear procedures

    b. Intervention: no panacea, "wonder" therapy
      (1) Prevention most effective treatment
        (a) Assess risk indicators.
        (b) Hydration: generous IV fluid replacement
        (c) Avoid brisk head movement, restlessness.
        (d) Provide adequate analgesia; position for comfort.
        (e) Encourage deep breathing, relaxation.
      (2) Avoid gastric distention.
        (a) Restrict oral fluids until nausea passes.
        (b) Oral hygiene: many complain of anesthetic "taste."
        (c) Ensure patent nasogastric tube.
      (3) Medicate: preemptive combinations, particularly if high risk or history of PONV
        (a) Anticholinergics: scopolamine patch behind ear
        (b) Serotonins: ondansetron (Zofran) or cousin dolasetron (Anzemet)
        (c) Butyrophenones: droperidol (Inapsine). Consider the black box warning.
          (i) Only limited use; recommended for outpatients because of unpleasant extrapyramidal effects, also drowsiness
        (d) Corticosteroids: dexamethasone (Decadron)
        (e) Sedatives: propofol (Diprivan) has antiemetic properties.
        (f) Phenothiazines
          (i) Prochlorperazine (Compazine): per rectal suppository, particularly if outpatient with resistant nausea
          (ii) Chlorpromazine (Thorazine)
        (g) Antihistamines
          (i) Hydroxyzine (Vistaril, Atarax)
          (ii) Diphenhydramine (Benadryl)
        (h) Benzamide
          (i) Metoclopramide (Reglan)
      (4) Adjunctive complementary modalities to reduce dizziness, nausea
        (a) Acupressure antiemetic wrist bands
        (b) Power of suggestion
        (c) Hydration: up to 2000 mL for even minor procedures
        (d) Aromatherapy
        (e) Music
      (5) May vomit after discharge despite interventions
        (a) Persist up to 48 hours after discharge from phase I PACU
        (b) Oral fluids and food too soon actually increase likelihood.
        (c) For patients discharged home, advise:
          (i) Rest
          (ii) Nonnarcotic medications if possible
          (iii) Gradual increases in fluid intake: "treat yourself as though you had the flu."
          (iv) Contact physician for unrelenting vomiting.
B. GI perfusion: remember the gut!
  1. Potential for GI ischemia an overlooked consideration for critically ill patients
    a. Mesentery not directly visible for assessment
      (1) Absent bowel sounds may mean dead or poorly perfused gut.
      (2) Involve gastroenterology assessment quickly in sepsis.
    b. Crucial concern when evaluating sepsis, especially if:
      (1) Unresolving hypotension, progressive acidosis
      (2) Trauma, pancreatitis, burns: potential for GI dysfunction high
    c. No specific, convenient measure to assess viability of GI tissue
      (1) GI symptoms often not treated until symptomatic—perhaps too late
        (a) Outcome worse the longer patient with sepsis is hypotensive with low MAP
        (b) Alcoholism history increases risk of GI ischemia.

(i) Poorly functioning liver

(ii) Immunosuppressed

(2) Kupffer cells: critical to protecting "gut"

(a) Immune (phagocytic) cells in liver kill bacteria released from "gut."

(b) If unhealthy gut, more endotoxins circulate through liver, then seed other organs.

(c) Impaired Kupffer cells predispose to sepsis, pulmonary failure (acute respiratory distress syndrome)

(d) Liver function tests only reflect injury, not systemic function: enzyme levels rise only if cell death.

(3) Tonometry studies cumbersome at bedside but recommend:

(a) Improve oxygen delivery, cardiac output before acidosis

(b) Survival from sepsis increased if maintain oxygenation

2. Prevent multisystem organ failure (MSOF) or dysfunction(MSOD).

a. Per tonometry studies, prevent MSOF if perfuse gut.

b. Recommend postpyloric tube feedings to maintain viability and structural integrity of microvilli in small bowel cell walls.

(1) If not stimulated, microvilli flatten.

(2) Can occur even if NPO for 4 days

(3) Bypass stomach when inserting feeding tube.

(4) Infuse high glutamine solution, even in small amount.

VI. NEUROLOGICAL CONCERNS AND ANESTHESIA

A. Delayed emergence: slow to arouse, failure to return to preanesthetic baseline

1. Consider multiple possible reasons and treat the cause (Box 28-3).

a. Understimulated patient: actively stimulate at regular intervals.

(1) Touch, shake, and call to patient.

(2) Remain at stretcher side; do not leave unresponsive patient unattended.

(3) Know patient's neurological baseline, medical history, laboratory results.

b. Assess adequate ventilation and oxygenation.

(1) Poor ventilation will only extend arousal period.

(2) Hyperventilation

(a) May be normal response: effort to exhale volatile (gas) anesthetics—observe, may rouse soon.

(b) If diabetic, consider superelevated hyperglycemia and acidosis.

(3) Hypercarbia (increased Pco_2) impairs consciousness, extends sedation.

(4) Hypoxia (decreased Po_2) deprives tissues of oxygen, produces acidosis.

(5) Monitor oxygen saturation, deliver oxygen.

(6) Consult anesthesiologist.

(7) Extended unresponsiveness: draw arterial blood gases.

c. Hypothermia

(1) Cold body temperatures delay metabolism of medications.

(2) Gradually rewarm while monitoring vital signs: prevent hypotension.

d. Prolonged action of anesthesia medications: most likely cause

(1) Ongoing neuromuscular blockade: is patient awake but unable to move?

(2) Observe pupils: pinpoint constriction suggests continued narcotic effect.

(3) Has sufficient time elapsed for medication metabolism and elimination?

(4) Consider reversing narcotics, benzodiazepines, muscle relaxants.

e. Metabolic causes: correct imbalances.

(1) Hypoglycemia or hyperglycemia: measure blood glucose.

(2) Electrolyte imbalance

(3) Preexisting reasons: hepatic, renal, Cushing's disease, hypothyroidism

f. Organic dysfunction

(1) Perioperative myocardial infarction. Assess 12-lead ECG.

(2) Cerebrovascular issues: stroke, seizure, intracerebral hemorrhage

(3) Air embolism related to surgical procedure
    (a) Cardiopulmonary bypass during heart surgery
    (b) Sitting position during cervical (neck) surgery
(4) Craniotomy: new hematoma

B. Emergence delirium: "Waking up wild!" (see Box 28-3)
  1. Suspect hypoxia first!
    a. Ensure adequate ventilation, oxygenation before giving any sedation.
    b. Patient may move but remain anesthetized, disoriented, air hungry.
      (1) Residual muscle relaxants: unable to "get enough air"
      (2) Narcotics, sedatives: hypercarbia from ineffective respiratory effort
      (3) Electrolyte or acid-base imbalance, hemoglobin deficiency
    c. Agitation may signal cerebral hypoxia.
    d. Consider severe anemia: is patient bleeding actively?
      (1) Consider procedural blood loss according to preanesthetic hemoglobin.
      (2) Measure hemoglobin: adequate to transport oxygen to tissues?
  2. Transient restless, agitated, confused, or dysphoric arousal
    a. Squirmy, crying, strongly pushing away caregiver common in children, teens
    b. Normal response to pain, urgent call of a full bladder when not fully awake!
    c. Untoward response: fewer than 10% of all surgical patients

■ BOX 28-3
■ **SAFE EMERGENCE: DELIRIUM AND DELAYED RESPONSE**

Assessments and Perianesthesia Nurse Competencies Related to Emergence Delirium and Delayed Arousal After Anesthesia

Critical Nursing Behaviors

Discern hidden causes of agitation, especially hypoxia, undetected internal hemorrhage, or acidosis
Identify physiological possibilities for delayed emergence from anesthesia and appropriate nursing and medical interventions
Explain physiological influence of medications used to calm the restless patient or to stir the slow-to-respond patient

- Medicate only when oxygenation is adequate
- Phyostigmine, an anticholinesterase medication, penetrates the blood-brain barrier to increase neuromuscular acetylcholine: quickly transforms agitation to calm
- Titrate midazolam, lorazepam, narcotics prn
- Narcotic or benzodiazepine antagonists to reverse sedation
- Medications to correct physiologic imbalance
- Quickly transforms agitation to calm

Describe rationale to ensure the agitated patient's safety while restless

- Remain with the patient and frequently assesses oxygenation
- Loosely apply limb restraints; aware that limiting movement may increase fear, disorientation, and agitation
- Protect sensitive corneas from abrasion by flailing hands that rub eyes
- Involve family members
- Parents calm a wild child.
- A familiar voice might help reorient a patient with visual, hearing, intellectual, or emotional impairment.

Describe rationale to ensure safety of a patient with delayed arousal

- Always remain with the patient
- Closely monitor oxygenation, airway patency, and respiratory quality
- Frequently attempt to arouse patient
- Consult physician as appropriate when sedation persists
- Rewarm a hypothermic patient; consider other medical possibilities

(1) History may indicate prior occurrence with anesthetic exposure.
(2) Confluence of multiple medications
    (a) Dreams, hallucinations when adults receive ketamine
    (b) Extrapyramidal effects caused by droperidol
    (c) Anesthetics and medications to treat organic brain syndrome
(3) Continuation of preprocedural anxiety about life or procedure
  d. Signals chronic alcoholism: consult physician.
    (1) Drinkers often underestimate consumption.
    (2) When was the last drink? Is patient also tachycardic?
    (3) Consider delirium tremens.
      (a) Arrange for close observation after PACU discharge.
      (b) Initiate sedation protocol, often with lorazepam (Ativan), per physician order.
  e. Signals substance abuse, either legal or illicit
3. Consider systemic causes.
  a. Acute dilutional hyponatremia: measure serum sodium.
    (1) May absorb intraoperative irrigant after transurethral resection of prostate (TURP), also known as "TURP syndrome"
    (2) Women after hysteroscopy
  b. Hypotension: inadequate oxygen delivery
  c. Sepsis
  d. Hypothermia: unable to express feeling cold and slows medication elimination
4. Safety: irrational, agitated, thrashing patient is usually extremely strong.
  a. Constant presence of nurse required to ensure safe passage through this stage
  b. Multiple personnel needed at bedside to:
    (1) Restrain patient.
    (2) Keep patient on stretcher.
    (3) Avoid bodily injury to patient and nurse.
  c. Remain calm, speak softly to connect with and reorient patient.
    (1) Encourage, guide patient toward stillness.
    (2) When you can interact with patient, ask questions to assess.
      (a) Breathing: "getting enough air?"
      (b) Pain: presence and severity
      (c) Awareness of situation
        (i) Does patient recall having procedure?
        (ii) Know who he or she is?
        (iii) Where he or she is?
      (d) Feeling cold?
    (3) Although tempting, overwhelming patient with forceful restraint and loud commands serves only to further agitate.
    (4) Carefully apply limb restraints according to facility protocol.
    (5) Maintain quiet environment.
    (6) Prevent injury.
      (a) Fall from stretcher
      (b) Scratched corneas with random movements
  d. Protracted delirium may resolve with physostigmine; consult anesthesia provider.
  e. Judiciously treat pain: chemical restraint
    (1) Prevent sudden somnolence.
    (2) Pain may be severe in patients who chronically use oral narcotics.
      (a) Did patient take scheduled narcotics preprocedure?
      (b) If not, likely reacting incoherently to severe pain
C. Recall of intraoperative or procedural events
  1. Rare and haunting occurrence for patient and anesthesia provider
    a. Alert, oriented patient, perhaps ready for discharge, relates details of intraoperative events.

(1) Specifics of conversations, comments, or an occurrence
   (a) Pain and being "unable to tell anyone"
   (b) Interprets conversations he or she overheard to be about self, even if they were not
(2) Most associated with "light" general anesthetic for:
   (a) Cesarean section
   (b) Bypass cardiac surgery
  b. Allow to talk.
   (1) May feel scared, angry, sad, confused
   (2) Listen closely; document all communication.
   (3) Acknowledge that awareness does occur.
   (4) Consult and inform anesthesia provider, who should visit patient.
  D. Local anesthetic toxicity
   1. Central nervous system effects: cross blood-brain barrier
    a. Tinnitus
    b. Light-headedness and/or confusion
    c. Circumoral numbness
    d. Unresponsiveness
    e. Seizures
   2. Cardiovascular and respiratory effects
    a. Peripheral vasodilatation: relaxation of vascular smooth muscle
    b. Hypotension, circulatory collapse at extremely high doses
    c. Dysrhythmias
     (1) Bradycardia
     (2) Atrioventricular block
     (3) Intraventricular conduction delay
    d. Respiratory arrest
   3. Cause: large intravascular bolus of local anesthetic
    a. Sudden release or failure of tourniquet during Bier Block
    b. Inadvertent injection when placing regional blocks
    c. Improperly set infusion rate of IV lidocaine
   4. Intervention: largely supportive to resuscitate
    a. Oxygenation, airway maintenance
    b. Generous IV fluid volume
    c. Symptomatic treatment of:
     (1) Seizures
     (2) Hypotension
     (3) Apnea
VII. THERMOREGULATION (see Chapter 24)
  A. Hypothermia: iatrogenic complication
   1. Perianesthesia origins
    a. Vasodilating anesthetic medications and techniques
     (1) General anesthetics: alter thermoregulation at the hypothalamus
      (a) Patient cools to temperature of room (poikilothermia).
     (2) Spinal blockade: lose heat through dilated peripheral vessels
      (a) Heat loss continues until spinal resolved, even in PACU.
    b. Open body cavities, room temperature tissue irrigants during procedure
    c. Cold room temperatures in procedure rooms
   2. Heat loss physics
    a. Radiation: heat transfer between two surfaces of different temperatures
    b. Convection: surface loss of heat when fluid flows across at a lower temperature
    c. Conduction: heat transfer between two touching objects of different temperatures as when warm human body in direct contact with cooler surgical table
    d. Evaporation: heat loss through insensible water loss from skin, the respiratory tract, open incisions, and wet drapes

3. Potential consequences: vary with significance of heat loss
   a. Increased oxygen consumption as a result of shivering
      (1) Normal autonomic response to generate heat
      (2) Heat production by muscular contractions
      (3) Potential cardiac or pulmonary failure for compromised patient
         (a) Oxygen consumption increases 400% to 500%.
         (b) Tachycardia and hypertension
         (c) Pain and thermal discomfort: feels cold
            (i) Temperature may actually meet discharge criteria.
            (ii) Patients describe as "thought I'd freeze to death."
   b. Wound infection: studies indicate hypothermia delays wound healing.
   c. Cardiac disturbance: marked increase in cardiac output, breathing
   d. Delayed emergence from anesthesia: prolonged medication effect and delayed elimination, especially if temperature below 95° F (35° C)
   e. Coagulopathy
   f. Assessment interference
      (1) Vasoconstriction and shivering movements impede measurement of oxygen saturation.
4. Interventions: preventing unplanned heat loss recommended
   a. Rewarming measures: gradual to prevent sudden hypotension
      (1) Active methods for warmth and comfort
         (a) Forced-air warming system: billowy blankets filled with warmed air
      (2) Passive insulation
         (a) Warmed cotton blankets
         (b) Thermal drapes
         (c) Fluid and blood warmers
         (d) Heated humidifiers for oxygen delivery
         (e) Infrared lights
      (3) Increasing the thermostat to warm the procedure area
   b. Supplemental oxygen, particularly if shivering
   c. Regularly measure temperature, every 30 minutes if hypothermic.
      (1) Discharge only after attaining facility's discharge temperature.
      (2) Discharge criteria per ASPAN discharge criteria: 96.8° F (36° C)
      (3) ASPAN clinical practice guideline, established at a multispecialty consensus conference on hypothermia
         (a) Defines normothermia as 96.8° F to 100.4° F (36° C to 38° C)
   d. Meperidine, as little as 10 mg IV, effectively suppresses shivering.
B. Hyperthermia
   1. Fever: normal physiological response to infection
      a. May arrive for surgery, perhaps for wound debridement or appendectomy: less febrile postoperatively
      b. May be indication for surgery cancellation of elective spine, joint replacement involving implanted hardware
         (1) Evaluate for pulmonary infection.
         (2) Urinary tract infection
      c. Prelude to sepsis
         (1) Heighten vigilance and assessment.
         (2) Anticipate hypotension, hypoxia.
   2. Malignant hyperthermia: a true anesthesia crisis
      a. Causes
         (1) Rare, genetically determined skeletal muscle response
            (a) Calcium prevented from reentering cell
         (2) Specific triggers
            (a) Succinylcholine
            (b) Volatile inhalation agents, including desflurane, isoflurane, enflurane, halothane, and sevoflurane
         (3) Most likely in the young and healthy

  b. Goal: prevention
    (1) Identify susceptibility: ask all preoperative patients if there is a personal or family history of:
      (a) Anesthetic-related death
      (b) Muscle disorder
      (c) Developing a fever or dark urine after previous surgery
  c. Observations
    (1) Sudden unexplained tachycardia may be initial signal.
    (2) Unexpected surge of end-tidal CO_2 in anesthetized patient
    (3) Profound muscle rigidity: often first noted at masseter muscle
    (4) Extreme metabolic acidosis
    (5) Respiratory acidosis
    (6) Cyanosis
    (7) Tachypnea
    (8) Hemodynamic instability
    (9) Fever a late sign
  d. Interventions: aggressive, intensive to ward off terminal acidosis
    (1) Immediate cooling: pack in ice, chilled IV fluids
    (2) Massive doses of dantrolene sodium (Dantrium), a skeletal muscle relaxant
    (3) Find personnel help: a crisis with multiple tasks
    (4) Oxygenate: hyperventilate at 100%.
    (5) Work to correct severe metabolic acidosis.
    (6) Monitor
      (a) Hemodynamics
      (b) Urine
      (c) Laboratory studies

BIBLIOGRAPHY

1. American Society of PeriAnesthesia Nursing: *Standards of perianesthesia nursing practice 2008-2010*, Cherry Hill, NJ, 2008, American Society of PeriAnesthesia Nursing.
2. Anthony D, Jasinski DM: Postoperative pain management: Morphine versus ketorolac. *J Perianesth Nurs* 17:30–42, 2002.
3. Barnes S, O'Brien D: Considering bypass of phase I PACU? *J Perianesth Nurs* 17:193–195, 2002.
4. Bennett J, Wren KR, Haas R: Opioid use during the perianesthesia period. *J Perianesth Nurs* 16:255–259, 2001.
5. Benumof JL: Obstructive sleep apnea in the adult obese patients: Implications for airway management. *Anesthesiol Clin N Am* 20:789–811, 2002.
6. Bogetz MS: Using the laryngeal mask airway to manage the difficult airway. *Anesthesiol Clin N Am* 20:863–870, 2002.
7. Burns SM: Revisiting hypothermia: A critical concept. *Crit Care Nurse* 21:83–86, 2001.
8. Burns SM: Safely caring for patients with a laryngeal mask airway. *Crit Care Nurse* 21:72–74, 2001.
9. Burns SM: Delirium during emergence from anesthesia: A case study. *Crit Care Nurse* 23:66–69, 2003.
10. Calswell JE: Rapid sequence intubation: Is rocuronium an alternative? *Semin Anesth Periop Med Pain* 21:99–103, 2002.
11. Childs SG: Tension pneumothorax: A pulmonary complication secondary to regional anesthesia from brachial plexus interscalene nerve block. *J Perianesth Nurs* 17:404–412, 2002.
12. Connor EL, Wren KR: Detrimental effects of hypothermia: A systems analysis. *J Perianesth Nurs* 15:151–155, 2000.
13. Cowling GE, Haas R: Hypotension in the PACU: An algorithmic approach. *J Perianesth Nurs* 17:159–163, 2002.
14. Drain C, Odom-Forren J: *Perianesthesia nursing: A critical care approach*, ed 5, Philadelphia, 2009, Saunders.
15. Erickson LI: Acquired neuromuscular disorders in the critically ill patient. *Semin Anesth Periop Med Pain* 21:135–139, 2002.
16. Floyd PT: Latex allergy update. *J Perianesth Nurs* 15:26–30, 2000.
17. Golembiewski JA, Obrien D: A systematic approach to the management of postoperative nausea and vomiting. *J Perianesth Nurs* 17:364–376, 2002.
18. Gray JR: *Steering clear of sepsis skid: Interventions in sepsis, organ, and renal failure.* Lecture on April 21, Robbinsdale, MN, 2003, North Memorial Center.
19. Irvin SM: Sensorineural hearing loss after select procedures. *J Perianesth Nurs* 17:89–101, 2002.

20. Kervin MW: Residual neuromuscular blockade in the immediate postoperative period. *J Perianesth Nurs* 17:152–158, 2002.

21. Knoerl DV, McNulty P., Estes C., et al: Evaluation of orthostatic blood pressure testing as a discharge criterion from PACU after spinal anesthesia. *J Perianesth Nurs* 16:11–18, 2001.

22. Learman JB: The challenging role of the perianesthesia nurse in the office-based surgical suite. *J Perianesth Nurs* 15:31–52, 2000.

23. Moline BM: Pain management in the ambulatory surgical population. *J Perianesth Nurs* 16:388–398, 2001.

24. Nagelhout J, Plaus K: *Nurse anesthesia*, ed 4, St. Louis, 2010, Saunders.

25. Nunnelee JD, Spaner DS: Assessment and nursing management of hypertension in the perioperative period. *J Perianesth Nurs* 15:163–168, 2000.

26. O'Brien D: Acute postoperative delirium: Definition, incidence, recognition and interventions. *J Perianesth Nurs* 17:384–392, 2002.

27. Prielipp RC, Young CC: Current drugs for sedation of critically ill patients. *Semin Anesth Periop Med Pain* 20:85–94, 2001.

28. Redmond MC: Malignant hyperthermia: Perianesthesia recognition, treatment, and care. *J Perianesth Nurs* 16:259–269, 2001.

29. Rose JB, Watcha MF: Postoperative nausea and vomiting. In Benumof JL, Saidman LJ, editors: *Anesthesia and perioperative complications*, ed 2, St Louis, 1999, Mosby.

30. Sandlin D: Transderm scopolamine: A painless, noninvasive option for control of postoperative nausea and vomiting. *J Perianesth Nurs* 17:427–429, 2001.

31. Sommers MS: The cellular basis of septic shock. *Crit Care Nurs Clin North Am* 15:13–26, 2003.

32. Spitellie PH, Holmes MA, Domino KB: Awareness during anesthesia. *Anesthesiol Clin N Am* 20:317–332, 2002.

33. Watche MF: Postoperative nausea and emesis. *Anesthesiol Clin N Am* 20:471–484, 2002.

34. Watkins AC, White PF: Fast-tracking after ambulatory surgery. *J Perianesth Nurs* 16:379–387, 2001.

35. Watson CB: Respiratory complications associated with anesthesia. *Anesthesiol Clin N Am* 20:275–299, 2002.

36. Williams EL: Postoperative blindness. *Anesthesiol Clin N Am* 20:367–384, 2002.

37. Wilson M: Giving postanesthesia care in the critical care unit. *Dimens Crit Care Nurs* 19:38–43, 2000.

29 Hematological Care

WANDA RODRIGUEZ

OBJECTIVES

At the conclusion of this chapter, the reader will be able to:

1. Describe normal and abnormal laboratory values and initiate appropriate nursing interventions as needed.

2. Describe the nursing care of a patient with a hematological disorder.

3. Describe the nursing interventions for a patient with a disorder in hemostasis.

4. Describe nursing responsibilities associated with blood and blood component transfusions.

5. Identify the types of transfusion reactions and the appropriate nursing interventions.

I. OVERVIEW
    A. Common blood dyscrasias in the following areas:
        1. Hematology
        2. Hemostasis
    B. Chapter broadly presents:
        1. Clinical signs
        2. Laboratory results
        3. Nursing interventions
II. PERIANESTHESIA ISSUES RELATE TO HEMATOLOGY
    A. Preoperative clinical assessment with laboratory tests
        1. Alterations affect outcomes, especially oxygenation and hemostasis.
            a. Critically assess potential for:
                (1) Anemia
                (2) Coagulopathy
            b. Review clinical indications and medical history.
            c. No established minimum value for presurgical hemoglobin (Hgb)
            d. Routine laboratory screening is neither required nor recommended for every preoperative patient.
                (1) When preoperative Hgb low, continue with surgery as planned depending on:
                    (a) Acuity of anemia
                    (b) Patient's cardiopulmonary response
                    (c) Surgical urgency
            e. Preoperative hemoglobin selectively recommended for:
                (1) Neonates to detect physiological anemia
                (2) Elderly patients
                (3) Menstruating women
                (4) Bone marrow suppression
                (5) Malignancy
                (6) Genetically determined anemic conditions
            f. Preanesthetic screening may uncover unrecognized coagulopathy.
                (1) Documented coagulation disorder seldom appropriate for surgery in the nonacute ambulatory setting.
        2. American Society of Anesthesiologists (ASA) "Practice Guidelines for Perioperative Blood Transfusion and Adjuvant Therapies"
            a. Preoperative intervention recommendations

(1) Discontinue anticoagulation in advance of surgery.
(2) Delay surgery in elective cases until drug effects (e.g., warfarin, clopidogrel, aspirin) dissipate.

B. Transfusion is not innocuous; there are potential risks.

   1. Complications cannot be overlooked or minimized.

     a. Hemolytic reactions (Refer to section V, subsection C.)

     b. Transfusion-related acute lung injury

       (1) Occurs usually within 2 hours of beginning of transfusion or appears within 6 hours

       (2) Food and Drug Administration (FDA) reporting indicates leading cause of transfusion-related fatality

       (3) In-hospital mortality rate: 5% to 10%

       (4) Causes

         (a) Antibodies in plasma against human white blood cell antigen lead to immune-mediated response.

         (b) Lipid inflammatory agents mediate granulocyte antigens.

       (5) Signs and symptoms

         (a) Acute dyspnea

         (b) Noncardiogenic pulmonary edema

         (c) Frothy sputum

         (d) Diffuse bilateral infiltrates

         (e) Crackles

         (f) Fever

         (g) Tachycardia

         (h) Hypotension

       (6) Treatment

         (a) Stop transfusion.

         (b) Administer oxygen.

         (c) Intubate.

         (d) Place on mechanical ventilation.

         (e) Hypotension not responding to fluids, administer vasopressors.

         (f) Involves noncardiogenic pulmonary edema

         (g) No diuretics as can worsen the situation

         (h) Nonsteroidal anti-inflammatory drugs (NSAIDs)

         (i) Prostaglandins

     c. Transfusion transmitted

       (1) Human immunodeficiency virus (HIV)

       (2) Cytomegalovirus (CMV)

         (a) Carried by 70% of donors

       (3) Viral infections such as hepatitis

         (a) Hepatitis not detected by donor testing: long "seronegative" period; most (>90%) transmitted hepatitis is hepatitis C.

       (4) Especially threatening to the immunosuppressed

         (a) Occurs 3 to 6 weeks post transfusion of large amounts of fresh blood

       (5) Bacterial contamination: in blood bank

         (a) Stored units can cause severe septicemia.

         (b) Mortality nearly 60% because of endotoxins producing gram-negative organisms

         (c) FDA reporting indicates third most common cause of transfusion-related fatality

     d. Transfusion-related immunomodulation

       (1) Immunosuppression occurs after transfusion.

       (2) May cause reactivation of latent viruses such as CMV

       (3) Causal relationship not proven but linked in recurrence of:

         (a) Resected malignancies (especially colorectal cancer)

         (b) Inflammatory bowel disease

(c) Spontaneous abortions

    (4) Associated in development of postoperative infections

    (5) Leukocyte-depleted transfusions suggested as an alternative

2. Weigh against serious anemia risk: oxygen deficit, decreased perfusion

    a. If mild:

        (1) Palpitations

        (2) Tachycardia

        (3) New ejection murmur

    b. If severe:

        (1) Stroke

        (2) Myocardial infarction

    c. ASA "Practice Guidelines for Perioperative Blood Transfusion and Adjuvant Therapies"

        (1) Intraoperative and postoperative management recommendations

            (a) "Red blood cells should usually be administered when the hemoglobin level is low (e.g., less than 6 g/dL in a young healthy patient), especially when anemia is acute."

            (b) "Red blood cells are usually unnecessary when the level is more than 10 g/dL."

            (c) "These conclusions may be altered in the presence of:

                (i) Anticipated blood loss.

                (ii) Active critical (i.e., myocardium, central nervous system, or renal) organ ischemia."

        (2) "The determination of whether intermediate Hgb concentrations (i.e., 6-10 g/dL) justify or require red blood cell transfusion should be based on:

            (a) Any ongoing indication of organ ischemia

            (b) Potential or actual ongoing bleeding (rate and magnitude)

            (c) The patient's intravascular volume status

            (d) The patient's risk factors for complications of inadequate oxygenation."

        (3) "These risk factors include a:

            (a) Low cardiopulmonary reserve

            (b) High oxygen consumption."

3. Metabolic effects of stored blood: a 35- to 42-day "shelf life"

    a. Toxic enzymes from dead white blood cells (WBCs) and platelets "significant" after 14 days of storage

    b. Hypocalcemia: ionized calcium binds with citrate used to preserve stored blood.

    c. Aging blood results in:

        (1) Hyperkalemia: potassium released from cell lysis

        (2) Acidosis

        (3) Independent risk factors for multiple organ failure

    d. Postoperative infection and immunosuppression risk

        (1) May not be evident for months posttransfusion

        (2) After spinal fusion, joint replacement, transfusion associated with iatrogenic wound infection, longer hospital stay, and more days of fever, antibiotic therapy

        (3) Tumor recurrence linked to transfusion, unproven

C. Autologous transfusion: alternative to allogenic transfusion

    1. Preoperative autologous donation. Patient predonates units of own blood.

        a. Patients may be ineligible for presurgical donation because of:

            (1) Weight

            (2) Age

            (3) Restrictions

            (4) Anemia

            (5) Cardiac conditions

       b. Advantages
          (1) Prevention of disease transmission
          (2) Some adverse transfusion reactions
          (3) Reassurance about blood risks
       c. Disadvantages
          (1) Higher cost
          (2) Wastage of unused blood
          (3) Potential for clerical error
          (4) Likelihood of requiring transfusion due to risk of perioperative anemia
    2. Reinfusion of salvaged blood intraoperatively or postoperatively
       a. Recovered red blood cells (RBCs) have oxygen transport properties equivalent to allogenic transfusions.
       b. As long as the salvaged blood stays connected with the patient's circulation, intraoperative blood salvage is often acceptable to Jehovah's Witnesses.
    3. Acute normovolemic hemodilution
       a. Removal of patient's blood and restoring intravascular volume with:
          (1) Crystalloid
          (2) Colloid
       b. Done before start of the operative procedure after induction
       c. Dilution of patient's blood reduces RBC losses, when blood is lost during surgery.
       d. Reinfusion can occur at any time during or after surgery.
  D. Alternatives to allogenic transfusions
    1. Epoetin alfa (recombinant human erythropoietin)
       a. Stimulates erythropoiesis in the bone marrow
       b. Frequently used in:
          (1) Cancer-related anemia
          (2) Anemia with renal insufficiency
          (3) Anemia in the critically ill
       c. Products: Epogen or Procrit
    2. Antifibrinolytic agents
       a. Blood loss reduction after surgery, especially cardiac, and in trauma
       b. Products
          (1) Aprotinin (Trasylol)
          (2) Aminocaproic acid (Amicar)
          (3) Tranexamic acid (Cyklokapron)
       c. FDA issued a Public Health Advisory for aprotinin.
          (1) Adverse effects
             (a) Myocardial infarction
            (b) Stroke
            (c) Renal dysfunction
  E. Bloodless medicine programs
    1. Team approach in providing best medical care to all patients using alternative to allogenic transfusions
    2. Advocating for patients who do not accept transfusions (e.g., Jehovah's Witness)
III. HEMATOLOGY COMPONENTS: BLOOD CELLS AND CLOTTING FACTORS
  A. Hemoglobin: carried on RBCs
    1. RBC physiology (Box 29-1)
       a. Critical transporter of oxygen to tissues
          (1) Carried on hemoglobin molecule to tissues
          (2) Normally concave on both sides (biconcave)
          (3) Proportion (percentage) in total blood volume is hematocrit.
       b. Produced in bone marrow and removed by the spleen
       c. Production stimulated by erythropoietin, which is produced by the kidney

■ BOX 29-1
■ **HEMATOLOGY: NORMAL LABORATORY VALUES***

Red blood cells (RBCs)
- Male: 4.6-6.2 million per microliter
- Female: 4.2-5.4 million per microliter

Hemoglobin (Hgb)
- Male: 13-18 grams per deciliter (g/dL)
- Female: 12-16 g/dL

Hematocrit (HCT): proportion of RBCs in circulating blood volume
- Male: 40%-54%
- Female: 37%-47%

White blood cells (WBCs): 4500-11,000 per microliter

Differential:
- Segmented neutrophils: 54%-62%
- Band neutrophils: 3%-5%
- Lymphocytes: 25%-33%
- Monocytes: 3%-7%
- Eosinophils: 1%-3%
- Basophils: 0-1%

Platelets: 150,000-400,000 per microliter
Prothrombin time (PT): 12-14 seconds
Usually expressed as International Normalized Ratio (INR): 0.7-1.8
Activated partial thromboplastin time (APTT): 30-40 seconds
Partial Prothrombin time (PTT): 25-41 seconds
Fibrinogen level: 200-400 mg/100 mL
Thrombin time (TT): 14-16 seconds
Fibrin degradation (split) products: 2-10 mcg/mL
D-dimer <250 ng/mL

*Guidelines only: normal values vary with clinical laboratory.

    d. Life span approximately 120 days
  2. Anemia: hemoglobin or RBC deficit; hematocrit reduction
    a. Cardiovascular symptoms vary with hemoglobin level and acuity of cell loss: weakness and fatigue common.
    b. Assess and suspect acutely low hemoglobin if:
      (1) Low oxygen saturation as measured by pulse oximetry (Spo_2), particularly if intraoperative blood loss was significant
      (2) Hypotension, perhaps noted by orthostatic changes when head of bed raised or ambulatory surgery patient stands
      (3) Tachycardia, likely a compensatory way to sustain cardiac output and sustain normal blood pressure
        (a) A multipurpose indicator representing a response by sympathetic nerves of the autonomic system
        (b) Consider hypovolemia.
          (i)   With or without low hemoglobin
          (ii) Heart rate increases
        (c) Heart rate increased with:
          (i)   Stress
          (ii) Anxiety
          (iii) Fever
        (d) Patients who cannot respond with tachycardia
          (i)   Patients taking beta-blocker medications
          (ii) Patients with transplanted hearts, which are denervated and so lack autonomic responses

    c. Causes of hemoglobin deficit
      (1) Loss
        (a) Hemorrhagic: usually acute as in:
          (i) Trauma
          (ii) Surgical loss
          (iii) Gastrointestinal
          (iv) Uterine
          (v) Nasal
          (vi) Vascular
        (b) Hemodilution from fluid volume expansion
          (i) Normal during pregnancy
          (ii) Replacement with non-RBC colloid or crystalloids
        (c) Researchers implicate laboratory draws (phlebotomy) as source of accumulated blood loss, especially for intensive care unit patients: up to 40 to 70 mL daily.
      (2) Inadequate RBC production
        (a) Insufficient vitamin B_{12} (intrinsic factor) needed for erythropoiesis
          (i) Postgastrectomy: insufficient hydrochloric acid secretion along with atrophy of gastric parietal cells
          (ii) Pernicious anemia: autoimmune destruction and atrophy of the gastric parietal cells along with insufficient hydrochloric acid secretion
        (b) Endocrine factors: insufficient erythropoietin production, as in:
          (i) Chronic renal failure
          (ii) Addison's disease
          (iii) Thyroid diseases
        (c) Liver disease: drug or alcoholic induced
        (d) Aplasia: bone marrow suppression
          (i) Decreased
            [a] Hemoglobin
            [b] RBCs
            [c] WBCs
            [d] Platelet count
          (ii) Etiology
            [a] Malignancy: infiltration of marrow
            [b] Chemotherapy
            [c] Chemical or radiation exposure: dose dependent
            [d] Medications: phenytoin, chloramphenicol
        (e) Inflammatory conditions
          (i) Rheumatoid arthritis
          (ii) Autoimmune diseases such as lupus erythematosus
          (iii) About 15% of asymptomatic HIV-positive patients are anemic.
        (f) Genetic predisposition: mutation or recessive traits
          (i) Alters a link in the chain of hemoglobin formation
          (ii) Produces hemolytic anemias such as:
            [a] Sickle cell anemia (Box 29-2)
              [1] Affects 1% of African Americans
              [2] Hypoxia, fever, acidosis spur RBC change from biconcave to sickled.
              [3] Severe pain: joints, limbs, abdomen
              [4] Jaundice, ischemia, organ infarction
            [b] Thalassemia (Cooley's)
              [1] Major: early death, altered growth, transfusion dependency
              [2] Minor (trait): few symptoms, hemoglobin <12 g/dL
            [c] Spherocytosis
              [1] RBCs spherical rather than biconcave disks; survival reduced to 14 days

■ BOX 29-2
■ **SICKLE CELL ANEMIA: PREDISPOSED BY HEREDITY**

Genetic Characteristics
Most commonly, patients inherit the HbS trait from both parents.
Specific stimuli cause RBCs to alter shape and function.
Forms mutant HbS rather than normal HbA
Trait carried by 10% of African Americans
Fewer than 1% of African Americans develop disease.

Clinical Concerns
Abnormal HbS cell forms have decreased affinity for oxygen.
Oxygen deficit causes cells to change shape and sickle.
Sickled cells rupture or clog small vessels.
Sickling crisis stimulated by:
- Altered temperature: fever or cold
- Acidosis and hypoventilation
- Dehydration
- Changes in altitude

Clinical Outcomes
Chronic anemia one of the hallmark clinical signs and exacerbations
Sluggish peripheral circulation due to sludging or vaso-occlusion
- Thrombosis, organ infarction
- Cerebral changes, altered renal function, cardiopulmonary compromise
- Limb ulcerations, necrosis
Ischemic pain, especially at limbs, joints, bones, and abdomen
Infection susceptibility

Nursing Responsibility: Crisis Prevention and Anemia Management
Ensure oxygenation: Prevent hypoventilation, acidosis.
- Monitor respiratory quality, rate, and depth.
- Provide supplemental oxygen; titrate to oxygen saturation.
- Adequately reverse muscle relaxants.
- Position patient for effective lung expansion.
- Early mobility
Promote peripheral circulation: minimize vasoconstriction.
- Maintain normothermia.
- Ensure adequate hydration to reduce blood viscosity.
- Regularly assess limb, organ ischemia.
- Limit peripheral blood stagnation.
- Monitor renal labs, urine volume.
Reduce stress.
- Analgesia: manage pain.
- Antibiotics: prevent or control infection.
- Calming environment
Avoid if possible vasodilators—may cause hypotension
Avoid if possible vasoconstrictors—may cause circulatory stasis
Other therapies
- Transfusions
- Hydroxyurea
- Cytotoxic agent that can elevate HbF levels, decreasing HbS formation

HbA, Hemoglobin A (adult hemoglobin); *HbF*, hemoglobin F (fetal hemoglobin); *HbS*, hemoglobin S (sickle cell hemoglobin); *RBCs*, red blood cells.

(3) Destruction of RBCs: normal vitamin B_{12} levels
  (a) Pharmaceuticals, burns: destroys or impairs function
  (b) Excessive physical stress
  (c) Hemolysis: cell trauma, destruction, or consumption
    (i) Defective prosthetic heart valves or blood pumps
    (ii) Infection: bacterial or viral
(4) Inadequate intake of folic acid or iron
  (a) Malnutrition: dietary lack, alcoholism, chronic anorexia
  (b) Malabsorption as a result of ileal disease, surgical resection

d. Perianesthesia nursing interventions and evaluation related to anemia
  (1) Need sufficient RBC numbers and hemoglobin level to bind oxygen for delivery to tissues
  (2) No absolute minimum hemoglobin measure established, although acute loss may cause more hemodynamic instability than chronic deficit
    (a) Hemoglobin of 9 to 10 g/dL is desired.
    (b) Anesthesia may be safely administered to patients with hemoglobin of 6 to 7 g/dL, such as:
      (i) Patients with chronic renal failure whose erythropoietin is suppressed
      (ii) Acutely ill Jehovah's Witnesses who refuse blood on religious principles
    (c) Acute anemia is unlikely in ambulatory surgery setting.
  (3) Fully saturate circulating hemoglobin.
    (a) Monitor oxygen saturation, ensure adequate oxygenation, limit oxygen demand.
      (i) Stimulate the sedated patient.
      (ii) Position the patient for optimal lung expansion.
      (iii) Deliver supplemental oxygen by mask or nasal cannula, with or without humidity.
      (iv) Provide analgesia to promote deep breathing.
      (v) Reduce stress: provide anxiolytics if safe.
      (vi) Remember that hypoxia alters acid-base balance.
    (b) Measure hemoglobin.
      (i) Particularly if oxygen saturation decreases
      (ii) Monitor postoperative blood and volume losses from drains, dressings, suction.
      (iii) Prevent profound hypotension.
        [a] Increase preload (volume) and support cardiac output: hydrate with crystalloid, colloid if necessary.
        [b] Anticipate orthostatic effects: gradual position changes to upright, noting blood pressure and heart rate.
        [c] Transfuse if ordered by physician per facility protocol.

3. Polycythemia: exaggerated RBC, hemoglobin, hematocrit, WBC production
  a. Increased RBC production unrelated to erythropoietin level
    (1) Blood volume and viscosity profoundly increased: cause unknown
    (2) Hypertension, vein engorgement, cardiac arrhythmia, thrombosis, tissue hypoxia can result.
    (3) One form (polycythemia vera) occurs in adults older than 60 years, primarily men.
      (a) Erythropoietin level low
  b. Physiological response by bone marrow as:
    (1) Adaptive response to altitude: normal compensation to environment
    (2) Pharmaceutical response to parenteral erythropoietin given to patients with chronic renal failure
    (3) Compensatory response to "perceived" hypoxemia associated with chronic cardiopulmonary conditions
      (a) Valvular or structural cardiac anomalies impede cardiac outflow and therefore oxygen delivery to tissue.

        (b) Pulmonary obstructive diseases such as asthma, emphysema

        (c) Pulmonary hypertension, pheochromocytoma

    c. Assessment, intervention, evaluation

       (1) Laboratory tests: hemoglobin >18 g/dL, hematocrit >54%, RBCs, WBCs, platelet count elevated

       (2) Symptoms: ruddy complexion, headache, weakness, angina, palpitations, hypertension, splenomegaly, claudication, phlebitis

       (3) Treatment: chronic anticoagulation, splenectomy, phlebotomy

B. Leukocytes: WBCs

  1. Physiology: mediate immune response with assorted WBC cell types

    a. Primary functions

       (1) Neutrophils—phagocytosis

       (2) Lymphocytes—antibody production and cell-mediated immunity

       (3) Monocytes—phagocytosis and antibody production,

       (4) Eosinophils and basophils—allergic hypersensitivity reactions

  2. Leukocytosis: increased WBC production up to 100,000 per microliter and anemia

    a. Appropriate inflammatory response to "invasion" by foreign substances or infection

    b. Pathological response: bone marrow proliferation, elementary WBCs

       (1) Acute lymphocytic leukemia

         (a) More common in children, with:

           (i) Pain

           (ii) Fatigue

           (iii) Bleeding

           (iv) Enlarged lymph nodes

           (v) Enlarged liver

           (vi) Enlarged spleen

           (vii) History of fever with no apparent cause

         (b) Cure rate in children is 80%.

         (c) Treatment: eradicate leukemic cells from marrow, lymph tissue, and/or residual disease from central nervous system.

           (i) Chemotherapy

           (ii) Targeted drug therapy

           (iii) Radiation therapy

           (iv) Bone marrow–stem cell transplantation

       (2) Chronic lymphocytic leukemia

         (a) Affects men older than 50 years with enlarged spleen and neck lymph nodes

         (b) Symptoms may develop slowly due to the abnormal cells increasing at slower rate.

         (c) Treatment: alleviate symptoms and slow down progression.

           (i) Chemotherapy, stem cell transplantation, and/or radiation for palliative care

       (3) Acute myelocytic leukemia

         (a) Characterizes 80% of all adult leukemias

         (b) Produces fever, bruising, pallor, joint pain, fatigue, enlarged liver, spleen

         (c) Treatment: eradicate leukemic stem cell.

           (i) Chemotherapy, immunotherapy, bone marrow transplant, and/or radiation therapy

       (4) Hodgkin's disease (Hodgkin's lymphoma)

         (a) Originates with enlarged lymph nodes, starting at neck, axilla

         (b) Common in early adulthood between the ages of 20 and 40 years with fever, night sweats, weight loss, fatigue, liver and spleen enlargement

         (c) Symptoms will manifest anywhere in the body depending on the location.

         (d) Treatment: combined chemotherapy and radiotherapy

(5) Non-Hodgkin's lymphomas
    (a) Large group of cancers that originate in the lymphatic system
    (b) Two classifications
        (i) Indolent: grow slowly and fewer symptoms
            [a] Diffuse large B-cell lymphoma, follicular lymphoma
        (ii) Aggressive
            [a] Burkitt's lymphoma, diffuse small non–cleaved cell lymphoma
    (c) Swollen lymph nodes, neck, axilla, or groin, fever, night sweats, abdominal pain or swelling
    (d) Treatment: different therapies and approaches for indolent (low or high tumor burden) and aggressive
        (i) Indolent
            [a] Low tumor burden: radiotherapy and/or combined with chemotherapy
            [b] High tumor burden: biology-based therapies (e.g., monoclonal antibodies, interferon, or vaccines)
        (ii) Aggressive
            [a] Early: chemotherapy combined with radiotherapy
            [b] Recurrent: high-dose chemotherapy and bone marrow or stem cell transplantation
(6) Multiple myeloma
    (a) Malignancy of the plasma cell that produces immunoglobulin
    (b) Affects adults older than 70 years with bone pain, fractures, bleeding, and bruising
    (c) Common in men and in African Americans
    (d) Treatment: alleviate symptoms and slow down progression.
        (i) High-dose chemotherapy with stem cell transplantation
        (ii) Corticosteroids alone or with other drugs such as:
            [a] Thalidomide
            [b] Lenalidomide (Revlimid)
            [c] Bortezomib (Velcade)

c. Perianesthesia interventions and evaluation
  (1) Increase oxygen delivery with supplemental oxygen.
  (2) Prevent tissue damage, bruising.
    (a) Use soft-tipped suction catheters.
    (b) Position gently; pad stretcher siderails if indicated.
    (c) Apply pressure; monitor venous, arterial puncture sites.
  (3) Transfuse blood components as ordered.
  (4) Prevent infection: respect protective isolation precautions when WBC, platelets dangerously low.
    (a) Provide post anesthesia care unit (PACU) care in operating room or patient's room per hospital policy rather than PACU.

3. Leukopenia: production reduced to fewer than 5000 per microliter of blood
  a. Bone marrow suppression by:
    (1) Disease
    (2) Immunosuppression
    (3) Radiation
    (4) Toxins
    (5) Drugs
  b. Patient safety may require protective isolation to prevent exposure to iatrogenic infection.

4. Perianesthesia nursing assessments and interventions
  a. Report deviation from normal parameters.
    (1) Preadmission tests might be first recognition of infection or leukemia.
    (2) Leukopenia and unusual bruising may coexist with anemias and platelet dysfunction.

      b. Obtain accurate history: ask pointed preanesthetic questions.
        (1) Fevers, with or without chills?
        (2) Easy bruising or bleeding?
        (3) Increased fatigue?
        (4) Pain, especially in joints?
      c. Think "protection."
        (1) Avoid pressure to skin and joints, and provide soft surfaces against skin.
        (2) Prevent hematoma during venipuncture and suctioning.
        (3) Isolate as required: infectious versus protective.

IV. COAGULATION: A CHAIN OF EVENTS TO ENSURE HEMOSTASIS
    A. Physiology: clotting is an intricate balance that requires:
      1. Adequate liver function to produce a cascade of interrelated clotting factors that circulate until activated
      2. Functional platelets, normal calcium, and specific enzymes
        a. Platelets "plug" injury site.
        b. About 66% circulate for their 7- to 10-day life span, rest in spleen.
        c. Aspirin renders platelets less "sticky."
      3. Vascular integrity ensures a smooth, "healthy" endothelial wall for:
        a. Adherence of a platelet plug bound by a fibrin clot
        b. Appropriate local constriction to limit local blood flow
      4. Synergy among a host of clotting factors (proteins) along the coagulation pathway
        a. Coagulation factors (Box 29-3)
          (1) Vitamin K–dependent factors are factors II, VII, IX, and X.
          (2) Platelets affect factor XIII.
        b. Naturally occurring coagulation inhibitors include:
          (1) Alpha-1 antitrypsin
          (2) Protein C
          (3) Antithrombin 3
        c. Clotting pathways (Table 29-1)
          (1) Extrinsic pathway: triggered by tissue injury; thromboplastin released and a sequence of events leading to fibrin clot formation
          (2) Intrinsic pathway: occurs within blood; proenzyme (factor VII) activated, spurs a cascade of clotting factors
        d. Fibrin
          (1) Strands of structural support for platelet plug; formed when fibrinogen activated
          (2) Effect limited to injury site to prevent massive coagulation

■ BOX 29-3
■ **CLOTTING FACTORS***

Factor I	Fibrinogen
Factor II	Prothrombin
Factor III	Tissue thromboplastin
Factor IV	Calcium ions
Factor V	Proaccelerin
Factor VII	Prothrombin conversion accelerator
Factor VIII	Antihemophilic factor A/von Willebrand factor
Factor IX	Christmas factor (autoprothrombin II)
Factor X	Stuart factor (autoprothrombin I)
Factor XI	Plasma thromboplastin antecedent
Factor XII	Hageman factor (enzyme)
Factor XIII	Fibrin-stabilizing factor

*Activated in specific points in clotting sequence.

■ TABLE 29-1
■ ■ **Coagulation**

	Extrinsic	**Intrinsic**
Response	Tissue	Within blood
Activates	Thromboplastin (factor III)	Circulating clotting factors and platelets
Result	Prothrombin (made in liver) converted to thrombin via plasma proteins, enzymes, and clotting factors Fibrin forms from thrombin	Platelets aggregate, form plug
Laboratory tests	PT and INR	**PTT**

   B. Laboratory assessments of coagulation (see Box 29-1)
      1. Prothrombin time (PT): assesses conversion of prothrombin to thrombin and factors I, II, V, VII, and X
         a. Specific monitor for Warfarin (Coumadin), which affects the external coagulation pathway
         b. If prolonged: significant bleeding risk during surgery, trauma, or soft tissue injury and must correct preprocedure
            (1) Liver disease, vitamin K deficiency
            (2) Fibrinogen; prothrombin; clotting factors V, VII, X
         c. Clinical interventions to correct abnormal lab values
            (1) Vitamin K injections
            (2) Fresh frozen plasma
      2. International normalized ratio (INR): standardized method of reporting the PT
         a. Used to monitor Warfarin (Coumadin)
      3. Partial thromboplastin time (PTT): assesses intrinsic coagulation pathway
         a. Monitor if administering heparin.
         b. Detects alteration in clotting factors I, II, V, VIII, IX through XII
      4. Thrombin time (TT): assesses thrombin activity to stimulate fibrin creation at coagulation's final stage
         a. Prolonged by fibrinogen (factor I) deficiency
      5. Platelet count: number, shape, and size of circulating platelets
         a. Surgical bleeding is rare if numbers are 100,000 or greater.
         b. Anticipate spontaneous bleeding if platelet numbers <20,000.
         c. Aspirin alters function for the 7-day life of a platelet.
         d. NSAIDs alter platelet function, with recovery within 2 days.
   C. Coagulopathies: acquired or hereditary disorders of clotting sequence
      1. Idiopathic immune thrombocytopenic purpura (ITP): characterized by spontaneous bleeding
         a. Autoimmune disorder: active antiplatelet antibodies and profoundly reduced platelet numbers, causing epistaxis, petechiae, bruising
         b. Acutely affects young children after immunization or viral infection with chicken pox, mumps, or measles
         c. Chronic ITP affects adults, primarily women, younger than 50 years.
         d. Treatment: depends on severity
            (1) In children: no treatment; may go away on its own within 6 months
            (2) In adults: no treatment for mild to moderate with no bleeding
            (3) Modalities: corticosteroids, intravenous immunoglobin, or splenectomy
      2. Disseminated intravascular coagulopathy (DIC): clotting factor consumption in response to surgery, pregnancy toxemia, sepsis, cancer, trauma, or multiple transfusions

      a. Simultaneous active bleeding and intravascular (capillary) clotting

        (1) Prolonged

          (a) PT

          (b) PTT

          (c) INR

          (d) TT

        (2) Decreased

          (a) Platelets

          (b) Fibrinogen

        (3) Increased

          (a) Fibrin degradation (split) products (degree of fibrinolysis)

          (b) D-dimer (breakdown of fibrin)

      b. Reflects severe, overwhelming response to organ system crisis

      c. Treatment focus is replacing clotting factors and correcting imbalances.

        (1) Administer blood and coagulation factors as ordered.

        (2) Administer volume resuscitation and, if indicated for refractory shock, inotropes as ordered.

      d. Occurrence in ambulatory surgery setting is highly unlikely.

  3. Hereditary coagulopathies

      a. Hemophilia: sex-linked clotting factor deficiency affecting men

        (1) Hemophilia A: clotting factor VIII lacking

          (a) Significant bleeding into tissues and joints if active factor VIII is <5%

          (b) PTT prolonged and PT normal

        (2) Hemophilia B (Christmas disease): clotting factor IX lacking

          (a) Prevents formation of stable clots; regular infusions of cryoprecipitate or fresh frozen plasma (FFP) likely

          (b) Intraoperative FFP needed to support factor IX

          (c) PTT, PT, and TT all within normal limits

        (3) Drug approved for use of bleeding, prophylaxis: NovoSeven (recombinant factor VIIa product)

          (a) No human plasma used in its manufacture, nor stabilized with albumin

          (b) Risk of transmission of human virus essentially zero

      b. Von Willebrand's disease: common disorder affecting men and women with mucous membrane bleeding, epistaxis, mild bruising

        (1) Defective von Willebrand factor (vWF)

          (a) Reduced activity of factor VIII: PTT increased

          (b) Platelet "stickiness" impaired, numbers adequate

        (2) Preoperative therapies

          (a) Desmopressin (DDAVP) can increase vWF.

          (b) Cryoprecipitate (has factor VIII) in scheduled twice-daily doses

D. Perianesthesia nursing assessments and interventions

  1. Preanesthesia

      a. Identify at-risk patients: coagulation risk and bleeding history.

        (1) Risk of intraspinal or epidural hematoma increases if an anticoagulated patient receives regional anesthesia.

        (2) Undetected coagulopathy can underlie persistent postsurgical bleeding.

      b. Document date and time of most recent anticoagulant medication.

        (1) Coumadin, heparin, clopidogrel

        (2) Aspirin, NSAIDs

        (3) Chemotherapy agents that suppress bone marrow

      c. A patient with a significant bleeding disorder is an unlikely candidate for outpatient surgery with discharge home.

  2. Postanesthesia

      a. Observe often for insidious bleeding.

        (1) Always look under the patient as well as at the wound itself.

        (2) Increasing abdominal girth after laparoscopic procedures

(3) An obese patient can accumulate a lot of blood in the abdomen before distention or tenderness is evident.

(4) Oozing and bruising from incisions or venipuncture sites

b. Link vital signs and oxygenation changes with bleeding potential.

(1) Continuously monitor oxygen saturation, observe respiratory quality. Persistently low SpO_2 may indicate undetected hemoglobin loss.

(2) Measure hemoglobin: anemia often associated with coagulopathy.

(3) Support blood pressure with adequate fluid volume.

(a) Maintain IV patency and limit venipuncture.

(b) Consider central or arterial line for laboratory sampling.

(4) Transfuse selected blood components as indicated per physician order.

V. TRANSFUSION PHYSIOLOGY: BLOOD CELL COMPATIBILITY

A. Blood and blood components

1. Whole blood: 1 unit = 500 mL with hematocrit of approximately 35%

a. Used if profound bleeding or desired component unavailable

b. Contains RBCs, plasma, WBCs, and platelets

c. Must be ABO identical

d. Irradiated whole blood: donor leukocytes inactivated

(1) Reduce risk of graft-versus-host disease

2. Packed RBCs: 1 unit = 250 to 300 mL with hematocrit of approximately 60%

a. Most commonly transfused component: used to restore oxygen-carrying capacity

b. Contains

(1) RBCs

(2) Nonfunctional WBC

(3) Platelets

(4) Minimal plasma

c. Must be ABO compatible

d. In the average adult who is not bleeding or hemolyzing:

(1) Hemoglobin increases by 1 g/dL.

(2) Hct increases by 3% per 1 unit.

e. Leukocyte-reduced RBCs

(1) Indication

(a) History of multiple febrile nonhemolytic transfusion reactions

(b) Frequent transfusion candidates—risk for alloimmunization to leukocyte antigens

(c) Targeted populations—immunocompromised (prevent CMV infection)

f. Irradiated RBCs

(1) Leukocytes inactivated; reduce risk of graft-versus-host disease

(2) Highly immunocompromised (e.g., bone marrow or solid organ transplant)

3. Platelet concentrates:

a. One pack = 50 to 300 mL

b. One unit of platelets increases platelet count (5000-10,000 for average sized adult)

c. Restore clotting ability

d. Pooled platelets donor but some patients may require single platelet donor

4. Available depending on the indication, leukocyte-reduced or irradiated

a. Treats:

(1) Leukemia

(2) DIC

(3) Bleeding caused by thrombocytopenia

(4) Platelet suppression caused by chemotherapy or radiation

5. FFP: 1 unit = 125 to 260 mL

a. Unconcentrated plasma containing all coagulation factors except platelets

b. Must be ABO compatible; use within 24 hours after thawing.

    c. Treats:
       (1) Coagulation deficiencies secondary to liver disease
       (2) DIC
       (3) Antithrombin III deficiency
       (4) Dilutional coagulopathy after massive blood replacement
6. Cryoprecipitate antihemophilic factor (Cryo)
    a. ABO-compatible preferred
       (1) Rh type does not need to be considered.
    b. Concentrated factors derived from FFP, ABO compatibility preferred
       (1) Rh type need not be considered.
    c. Contains:
       (1) Fibrinogen
       (2) Factors
          (a) VIII
          (b) vWF
          (c) XIII
    d. Use within 4 hours after thawing to treat:
       (1) Hemophilia A
       (2) DIC
       (3) Von Willebrand's disease
       (4) Obstetric complications
       (5) Fibrinogen deficiency
7. Granulocytes
    a. Usage
       (1) Neutropenic patients with documented infections and do not respond to antibiotics
       (2) Hereditary neutrophil function defects
    b. Must be ABO compatible
    c. Irradiated: reduces risk of graft-versus-host disease
8. Serum albumin: 5% solution, up to 500 mL; 25% solution, up to 100 mL
    a. Sterile product contains:
       (1) 96% albumin
       (2) 4% globulin
       (3) Other proteins
    b. Obtained from pooled plasma, heat treated to inactivate hepatitis virus
    c. Widely used for its oncotic properties
    d. Treats:
       (1) Hypovolemia: expands plasma volume
       (2) Hypoproteinemia
9. Plasma protein fraction (Plasmanate, PPF) 1 unit = 50, 250, or 500 mL
    a. Contains:
       (1) 88% albumin
       (2) 12% globulins
       (3) No coagulation factors
    b. Obtained from pooled plasma, heat treated to inactivate hepatitis virus
    c. Treats:
       (1) Hypovolemia: a volume expander
       (2) Hypoproteinemia
B. Four major blood types: A, B, AB, O
  1. A or B antigens, or both, carried on surface of RBCs
  2. Form blood type A, B, or AB (Table 29-2)
    a. "Universal recipient"
       (1) Blood type AB
       (2) Produces no antibodies
    b. "Universal donor"
       (1) Blood type O
    c. Plasma carries naturally occurring antibodies to antigens not present on the red cell.

■ TABLE 29-2
■ ■ **Red Cell Blood Type and Compatibility**

Patient Blood Type	Compatible Donor	Antigen	Antibody
A	A or O	A	B
B	B or O	B	A
AB	AB, or A, B, O	AB	None
O	O only	None	AB

C. Rh type: determined primarily by the D antigen
   1. Positive or negative antigen carried on surface of RBCs
      a. Rh⁺ (positive for the D antigen) occurs in more than 80% of people.
      b. Rh⁻ (negative for the D antigen) occurs in less than 20%.
   2. Rh⁺, must receive Rh⁺ cells; and Rh⁻, must receive Rh⁻ cells.
   3. Detection crucial to prevent:
      a. Significant antibody stimulation from multiple transfusions: makes crossmatching for future transfusions difficult
      b. Hemolytic disease of newborn antibodies produced in Rh⁻ woman pregnant with Rh⁺ fetus
         (1) Give RhoGAM per physician order to Rh⁻ mother to prevent hemolysis of a future baby's blood whether after full-term birth, miscarriage, or abortion.

VI. ADMINISTERING BLOOD AND BLOOD PRODUCTS
   A. Why transfuse? Indications
      1. Restore circulating volume.
      2. Increase oxygen transport to tissues.
      3. Replace coagulation factors or correct bleeding.
      4. Replace granulocytes or treat sepsis.
   B. Accuracy required to ensure patient safety; for every blood component
      1. Check patient orders.
      2. Verify correct patient and blood component: follow facility policy.
      3. Verify patient consent for transfusion.
      4. At patient's bedside, two (2) licensed staff simultaneously match information on patient, blood component, and blood bank compatibility label.
         a. Patient name and hospital identification number
         b. Donor number on blood product
         c. ABO and Rh type
         d. Expiration date of component
      5. Report any identification discrepancy to blood bank immediately and delay transfusion.
      6. Prepare to transfuse.
         a. Prime blood tubing with normal saline; cover filter in drip chamber.
            (1) D₅W (5% dextrose in water) is hypotonic and causes hemolysis.
            (2) Ringer's lactate contains calcium, can initiate coagulation.
            (3) Change blood tubing and filter after every 2 units: filter traps clots and coagulant debris.
            (4) Never add medications to a unit of blood or piggyback into tubing— this includes narcotic analgesics delivered by patient-controlled analgesia.
         b. Gently mix contents and examine unit carefully for bubbles, plasma discoloration.
         c. Explain procedure and transfusion need to patient.
         d. Verify:
            (1) IV patent
            (2) Nonreddened site
            (3) An 18- or 19-gauge catheter

e. Before starting transfusion, measure and document patient's temperature, blood pressure, vital signs, and heart rate.

f. Keep patient warm for comfort.

    (1) Use blood warmer, particularly if transfusing multiple units.

    (2) Apply warm blankets, active rewarming device.

    (3) Note transfusion reaction signals:

        (a) New-onset of chills

        (b) Shivering

        (c) Immediately stop blood transfusion.

g. Start infusion slowly, and remain with patient for initial 15 to 20 minutes of infusion: document vital signs and observe for transfusion reaction.

h. Frequently monitor infusion and patient response.

    (1) Rate: 30 minutes to 4 hours according to acuity, patient tolerance

        (a) Apply pressure bag to rapidly administer cells or volume.

        (b) FDA regulations require a transfusion to be completed within 4 hours.

    (2) Document vital signs if clinical change and after infusion.

i. Should a transfusion reaction occur, notify:

    (1) Blood bank

    (2) Surgeon

    (3) Anesthesiologist

    (4) Follow established protocols of institution.

C. Transfusion complications

  1. Hemolytic reaction is a severe reaction caused by:

    a. ABO incompatibility: immediate hemolysis of RBCs after infusion of the first few milliliters of blood

    b. Human clerical error: patient or blood component not properly identified and matched; usual cause of hemolytic reactions

    c. Assessment and observations

        (1) Burning sensation along vein receiving transfusion

        (2) Sudden fever (temperature >104° F [40° C]) and chills

        (3) Hypotension, hematuria, and hemolysis with:

            (a) Hematuria, flank pain, and renal failure

            (b) Dyspnea, tachypnea, tachycardia, palpitations, substernal pain

        (4) Abnormal bleeding or DIC

    d. Be especially vigilant with the anesthetized or sedated patient.

        (1) Immediately report unexplained, significant oozing.

        (2) Patient cannot report pain, anxiety.

        (3) Difficult to distinguish hypotension caused by transfusion reaction from hypotension caused by hypovolemic shock

        (4) Muscle relaxant may limit shivering response.

    e. Intervention and evaluation

        (1) Discontinue transfusion immediately!

        (2) Assess and document patient's clinical condition.

        (3) Infuse normal saline (use new tubing) and inform physician.

        (4) Complete transfusion reaction profile and return.

            (a) Facility's investigation form to blood bank

            (b) Intact set of blood component unit, tubing, and accompanying IV fluid to blood bank

            (c) Blood samples as indicated by facility

            (d) Urine sample for urine hemoglobin to laboratory

        (5) Simultaneously treat patient per physician orders.

            (a) Acetaminophen for fever

            (b) Diphenhydramine (Benadryl) for itching

            (c) Cautious fluid management

            (d) Furosemide if needed for diuresis

            (e) Frequently monitor and document patient's response.

  2. Delayed hemolytic transfusion reaction

    a. Usually occurs several days after transfusion: transfused cells have antigen to which recipient has been previously sensitized

        b. Causative antibodies: Anti-E, Anti-C, Kidd system

        c. Assessment

            (1) Unexplained fever

            (2) Definite hemoglobin decrease 2 to 10 days posttransfusion

            (3) Positive direct Coombs' test, elevated bilirubin

  3. Pyrogenic (febrile) transfusion reaction

        a. Not hemolytic: onset 1 hour into transfusion, may last 8 to 10 hours

        b. Causes

            (1) WBC or platelet antibodies

            (2) Contaminating pyrogenic bacteria

            (3) Pregnancy or previous transfusion

        c. Assessment and intervention

            (1) New-onset chills with fever, temperature increase 2° F.

            (2) Flushed skin, headache, tachycardia

            (3) Hemolysis: bacteria replicate quickly even when refrigerated—symptoms after infusion of first 50 mL of blood.

            (4) Severe hypotension, abdominal and extremity pain

            (5) Hematuria, DIC, and renal failure

        d. Intervention and evaluation

            (1) Discontinue transfusion! Early signs parallel early hemolytic reaction.

            (2) Begin transfusion reaction investigation.

            (3) Antipyretics (acetaminophen) and antihistamine for itching (diphenhydramine)

            (4) Fluids to support blood pressure and urine volume; monitor airway.

  4. Allergic transfusion reaction

        a. Hypersensitivity response: accounts for 1% to 3% of transfusion reactions

        b. Occurs as a result of antibodies to donor blood foreign proteins, often in a patient with significant allergy history

        c. Develop urticaria with hives, itching

        d. Assessment and intervention

            (1) Stop transfusion! Reaction may progress unpredictably.

            (2) Assess for glottal edema.

            (3) Give IV antihistamine (Diphenhydramine/Benadryl).

BIBLIOGRAPHY

1. American Red Cross: *Practice guidleines for blood transfusion, a compilation from recent peer-reviewed literature*, ed 2, 2007.
2. Adamson JD: New Blood, Old Blood, or No Blood? *N Engl J Med* 358:1295–1296, 2008.
3. Advancing Transfusion and Cellular Therapies Worldwide: *Circular of information for the use of human blood and blood components*, 2002.
4. ASA: Practice guidelines for perioperative blood transfusion and adjuvant therapies. *Anesthesiology* 105:198–208, 2006.
5. ASA: *Questions and answers about blood management*, ed 4, 2006–2007.
6. Dennison RD: *Pass CCRN*, ed 3, St Louis, 2007, Mosby.
7. Goodnough LT, Shander A: Blood management. *Arch Pathol Lab Med* 131:695–701, 2007.
8. Joyce JA: Toward reducing perioperative transfusions. *AANA J* 76:131–137, 2008.
9. Justice HM, Mason JD: Recognizing acquired thrombocytopenic coagulations. *Emerg Med* 39(7):7–13, 2007.
10. Lambing A: Bleeding disorders: Patient history key to diagnosis. *Nurse Pract* 32:16–24, 2007.
11. Kam PCA: Anaesthetic management of a patient with thrombocytopenia. *Curr Opin Anaesthesiol* 21:369–374, 2008.
12. Klein H, Spahn D, Carson J: Red blood cell transfusion in clinical practice. *Lancet* 370:415–26, 2007.
13. Knippen MA: Transfusion-related acute lung injury. *AJN* 106:61–64, 2006.
14. Nagelhout J, Plaus K: *Nurse anesthesia*, ed 4, St Louis, 2010, Saunders.
15. Platt O: Hydroxyurea for the treatment of sickle cell anemia. *N Engl J Med* 358:1362–1369, 2008.
16. Rempher KJ: Assessment of red blood cell and coagulation laboratory data. *AACN Adv Crit Care* 15:622–637, 2004.
17. Roisen MF, Fleisher L: *Essence of anesthesia practice*, ed 2, Philadelphia, 2002, WB Saunders.

30 Phase I Discharge Criteria

SUSAN JANE FETZER

OBJECTIVES

At the conclusion of this chapter, the reader will be able to:

1. Define terminology describing discharge definitions.
2. Describe commonly used post anesthesia care unit (PACU) discharge criteria.
3. Describe the function of discharge criteria.

I. OVERVIEW
   A. Standard: PACU nurses must assess and evaluate the patient's readiness for discharge. Using a criteria-based scoring system ensures patients are adequately prepared for transfer to PACU phase II extended observation or a nursing unit.
   B. Definitions
      1. Discharge ready: a multifaceted concept that describes a patient's functional and cognitive state as sufficiently recovered from anesthesia and able to leave the PACU and be safely cared for in a less intensive nursing environment
      2. Discharge readiness: the state of being ready to leave the PACU and be cared for in a less intensive nursing environment
      3. Discharge criterion: a standard or test by which to judge or decide whether a PACU patient is discharge ready
      4. Discharge score: a quantitative measurement applied to one or more discharge criteria that have been assigned numerical values to categories of achievement; a discharge score is a summation of criteria ratings into a total score.
      5. Ready for transfer: a description of the patient who is discharge ready
      6. Fast-tracking: an action bypassing PACU phase I recovery when phase I criteria have been met before leaving the operating room (OR)
      7. Evidence of discharge readiness includes:
         a. An assessment by the attending anesthesia personnel
         b. Meeting established criterion or criteria
         c. Achieving an acceptable score on an established discharge scoring system
         d. Documentation of nursing assessment that reflects that the patient is:
            (1) Physiologically stable
            (2) Responsive to external stimuli
            (3) Free from anesthetic and surgical complications
            (4) Adequately recovered from the major effects of anesthesia
      8. Ready for transfer criteria may extend to include patient characteristics that are not included under discharge criteria but fall within the jurisdiction of nursing judgment such as:
         a. Attaining an acceptable level of pain
         b. Attaining an acceptable level of nausea
         c. Need for ongoing pharmacological or technological treatments
            (1) Completed blood transfusion
            (2) Chest x-ray
            (3) Respiratory treatment

        d. Need for ongoing collaboration with other health care providers
          (1) Respiratory therapy
          (2) Surgeon
    9. Ready-for-transfer criteria may extend to include institutional characteristics that affect the patient's ability to leave the PACU environment such as:
        a. Ability of receiving unit to accept transfer due to bed availability
        b. Ability of receiving unit to accept transfer due to personnel availability
 C. Function of discharge criteria
    1. Ensure standard of care is met for all patients.
    2. Guide practice decisions without dictating practice.
    3. Promote efficient use of fiscal and personnel resources.
        a. Use of discharge criteria shown to reduce PACU time by 24%.
        b. Use of discharge criteria shown to decrease discharge delays.
        c. Use of discharge criteria had no significant differences in adverse events.
    4. Allow nurses to act on behalf of anesthesia personnel.
        a. American Society of Anesthesiologists (ASA) states in their Standards for Postanesthesia Care that "in the absence of the physician responsible for the discharge, the PACU nurse shall determine that the patient meets the discharge criteria."
    5. Meet Joint Commission requirements.
        a. Relevant discharge criteria rigorously applied to determine the readiness of the patient for discharge
        b. Discharge criteria approved by the medical staff
    6. Meet American Society of PeriAnesthesia Nurses (ASPAN) Standards of Perianesthesia Nursing Practice 2008-2010.
    7. Nurse Practice Act: determining discharge readiness is a delegated act (refer to specific practice act of each state).
 D. Requirements for determining discharge readiness
    1. ASA *Standards for Postanesthesia Care*
        a. Standard V: Physician is responsible for the discharge of the patient from the post anesthesia care unit.
        b. Standard V.1. When discharge criteria are used, they must be approved by the Department of Anesthesiology and the medical staff. They may vary depending upon whether the patient is discharged to a hospital room, to the intensive care unit (ICU), to a short stay unit, or home.
    2. Discharge criteria must be applied consistently.
    3. Discharge criteria must be enforced.
    4. Compliance to discharge criteria must be monitored.
 E. Application of discharge criteria
    1. Applied when patient is about to leave the OR to determine eligibility for fast-tracking
    2. Applied when patient is admitted to PACU as part of nursing assessment
    3. Applied routinely (every 15 or 30 minutes depending on institutional policy) as part of a nursing assessment
    4. Used to monitor intraoperative and postanesthesia interventions for effectiveness during quality assurance activities
    5. Used in nursing research to monitor the effect of interventions on patient outcomes
    6. Supports physician and nursing critical judgment of discharge readiness
 F. Variations of discharge readiness
    1. PACU to ICU
        a. Achievement of discharge criteria reflects need for ongoing critical care nursing to monitor and intervene.
        b. All discharge criteria may not be met.
        c. Discharge score defining discharge readiness may not be achieved.
        d. Physician evaluation is used in place of discharge criteria or discharge score.
        e. Discharge readiness and ready to transfer should occur concurrently.

  2. PACU to acute care
     a. Discharge criteria met with one or two exceptions.
     b. Discharge score attained within acceptable range set by policy.
     c. Reasons for exceptions included in nursing documentation.
     d. Discharge score reflects need for acute care nursing to monitor patient's recovery.
     e. Institutional policies identify exceptions that must be reported to the physician before transfer.
     f. Discharge readiness may be attained before ready to transfer.
  3. PACU to phase II/extended observation
     a. Achievement of most discharge criteria with the likelihood that all discharge criteria will be attained shortly after discharge to phase II
     b. Discharge criteria are met, but occasionally other patient characteristics (e.g., pain control, nausea) may restrict the patient from phase II discharge to home.
     c. Discharge score attained within acceptable range set by institutional policy.
     d. Discharge readiness may be attained before ready to transfer.
  4. PACU to home
     a. Achievement of all PACU discharge criteria and all phase II discharge criteria met
     b. Any discharge criteria exceptions documented and reported to the physician
     c. Order to discharge home documented
     d. Appropriate for patients receiving monitored anesthesia care
II. STANDARDS FOR DISCHARGE CRITERIA
  A. Discharge criteria are:
    1. Objective
    2. Measurable
    3. Understandable
    4. Able to be applied by knowledgeable health care providers
  B. Discharge criteria are valid.
    1. Criterion reflects the concept being measured (e.g., arterial oxygen saturation [Sao_2] is a more valid measurement of oxygenation than patient color).
    2. Criterion acknowledged as appropriate by content experts
    3. Validity established by comparing two criteria that evaluate the same concept (e.g., level of sensory block and extremity movement)
    4. Reflect the ability of the criterion to be sensitive to changes in patient status and able to measure change in patient status appropriately
    5. Can be supported by testing the criterion against future predictions
    6. Validity evaluated on a continuum
    7. A discharge criterion may be valid for one population of patients but not for another (e.g., discharge criterion of Sao_2 >92% is not valid for a patient with chronic obstructive pulmonary disease who has baseline Sao_2 of 89%).
  C. Discharge criteria are reliable.
    1. Criterion applied the same way regardless of health care provider (interrater reliability)
    2. Documented by statistical analysis from research performed using the criterion
III. COMMONLY USED DESCRIPTORS FOR PACU DISCHARGE CRITERIA
  A. Respiratory criteria
    1. Respiratory stability
     a. Able to breathe deeply
     b. Able to breathe deeply and cough freely
     c. Coughs on commands or cries
     d. Tachypnea with a good cough
     e. Maintains good airway
     f. Dyspnea or limited breathing
     g. Dyspnea, limited breathing, or tachypnea

      h. Dyspnea with a weak cough
      i. Apneic
      j. Apneic or on mechanical ventilator
      k. Requires airway maintenance
    2. Oxygen saturation
      a. Maintains value >92% on room air
      b. Needs O_2 inhalation to maintain saturation >90%
      c. Requires supplemental oxygen
      d. Saturation <92% with supplemental oxygen
      e. O_2 saturation <90% with supplemental oxygen
    3. Color
      a. Pink
      b. Pink and warm
      c. Pale, dusky, blotchy, jaundice, others
      d. Cyanotic
  B. Cardiovascular criteria: hemodynamic stability
    1. Blood pressure within 15%, 30%, 50% of preoperative baseline
    2. Blood pressure >90 mm systolic and within 30 mm Hg of preoperative baseline
    3. Blood pressure within 20%, 20% to 50%, 50% of preanesthetic level
    4. Blood pressure within 20%, 20% to 49%, 50% of preanesthetic level
    5. Exception: children who are crying
  C. Musculoskeletal criteria: physical activity
    1. Able to stand up and walk straight
    2. Able to move all extremities on command
    3. Able to move all extremities voluntarily or on command
    4. Active motion, voluntary or on command
    5. Head lift with closed mouth for 5 seconds
    6. Moving limbs purposefully
    7. Vertigo when erect
    8. Some weakness in movement of extremities
    9. Dizziness when supine
    10. Weak motion, voluntary or on command
    11. Able to move two extremities on command
    12. Able to move two extremities voluntarily or on command
    13. Nonpurposeful movements; unable to move extremities voluntarily
    14. Unable to move extremities voluntarily or on command
    15. No motion
  D. Neurological criteria: level of consciousness
    1. Fully awake
    2. Awake and oriented
    3. Fully awake or easily aroused when called
    4. Verbal response to spoken command
    5. Arousable with minimal stimulation
    6. Responding to stimuli
    7. Responds to stimuli and exhibits presence of protective reflexes
    8. Arousable on calling
    9. Responsive to only tactile stimulation
    10. Not responding
    11. No response or absence of protective reflexes
  E. Temperature
    1. Core temperature at least 36° C (96.8° F)
    2. Patient describes feeling acceptable level of warmth.
    3. No signs and symptoms of hypothermia
    4. Exception: can be discharged to critical care with temperature less than 36° C
  F. Presence of pain
    1. Pain free
    2. No pain or mild pain

      3. Moderate to severe, controlled with analgesics
      4. Mild pain handled by oral medication
      5. Persistent severe pain
      6. Severe pain requiring parenteral medication
      7. Comfortable with regard to pain

G. Additional criteria considered concurrently with discharge criteria
    1. Emetic symptoms
      a. Able to drink fluids
      b. None or mild nausea with no vomiting
      c. Nauseated
      d. Transient vomiting or retching
      e. Nausea and vomiting
      f. Persistent moderate or severe nausea and vomiting
    2. Urinary symptoms
      a. Has voided
      b. Unable to void but comfortable
      c. Unable to void and uncomfortable
      d. Bladder ultrasound less than 400 mL
    3. Surgical site
      a. Dry and clean
      b. Wet but stationary or marked
      c. Growing area of wetness

H. Additional regional anesthesia (epidural/spinal) discharge criteria
    1. Orthostatic blood pressure challenges
      a. Intervals of 30 minutes
      b. Less than 10% decrease in mean arterial pressure
    2. Sensory level
      a. Less than or equal to T10
    3. Block has started and continues to recede.
    4. Two segment regression of sensory block
    5. Receding block to L1 or lower

I. Additional regional anesthesia (shoulder/ankle) discharge criteria
    1. No sensory or motor criteria required for discharge from PACU

J. Minimum mandatory stay as a discharge requirement
    1. Insufficient research literature to support minimum 1-hour stay in PACU
    2. Length of stay should be determined on case-by-case basis.

K. Sources of discharge criteria descriptors as noted in preceding sections
    1. Postanesthesia Recovery Score (PARS)—Aldrete and Kroulik (1970)
    2. Steward (1975)
    3. Thomas and Davis (1984)
    4. Soliman et al (1988)
    5. Alexander et al (1989)
    6. Postanesthesia Recovery Score for Ambulatory Patients (PARSAP)—modified Aldrete (1995)
    7. Marley and Moline (1996)
    8. White (1999)
    9. Cohen et al (1998)
    10. ASPAN (2008)

IV. OVERVIEW OF DISCHARGE SCORING MEASURES
  A. Quantitatively summarizes clinical observations and judgments
  B. Composed of discharge criteria that best reflect the patient's overall status
  C. Discharge criteria used for discharge score may be patient specific
    1. Criteria and scoring system for general anesthesia patient
    2. Criteria and scoring system for obstetric patient
    3. Criteria and scoring system for regional anesthesia patient
  D. Each criteria has two or more levels on which patient can be described.
    1. Point for each level of criterion attained

    2. Greater total score reflects:
      a. Increased patient stability
      b. Lower risk of complications upon transfer
      c. Progress toward discharge readiness
  E. Requirements for discharge scoring measures
    1. Simple to administer
    2. Easy to remember
    3. Applicable to all situations
    4. Able to discriminate among patients at different levels of recovery (validity)
    5. Able to be scored similarly by two different providers simultaneously (reliability)
V. EXAMPLES OF DISCHARGE CRITERIA SCORING SYSTEMS
  A. Aldrete (also known as PARS)
    1. Developed in 1970
    2. Five criteria rated from 0 to 2
      a. Activity
      b. Respiration
      c. Circulation
      d. Consciousness
      e. Color
    3. Maximum score of 10
    4. Scores 8 and 9 reflect discharge readiness.
    5. Scores less than 7 are dangerous.
    6. Recommended assessment every 30 minutes
    7. Evidence of validity and reliability
      a. Aldrete (1970)
        (1) Studied 352 patients undergoing general anesthesia
        (2) Seventy-eight percent of patients scored 8 or higher upon PACU admission.
      b. Figueroa (1972)
        (1) Studied 500 cases with 89% having general anesthesia
        (2) Fifty-six percent of patients scored lower than 7 upon PACU admission.
        (3) Eleven percent of patients scored 10 upon PACU admission.
        (4) Age, sex and surgical procedure did not influence scores.
      c. Holzgrafe (1972)
        (1) Studied 456 patients
        (2) Twenty-four percent of patients scored 8 or higher upon PACU admission.
        (3) Circulation criteria were likely to have higher score on admission.
        (4) Level of consciousness and activity had lowest scores on admission to PACU.
      d. Soliman et al. (1988)
        (1) Studied 81 children undergoing general anesthesia
        (2) Used PARS with additional oxygen saturation criterion
        (3) No significant association with PARS score and oxygen saturation was identified.
        (4) Twelve children had PARS scores higher than 8 with Sao_2 less than 95%.
  B. Steward
    1. Proposed in 1975
    2. Three criteria rated from 0 to 2
      a. Consciousness
      b. Airway
      c. Movement
    3. Maximum score of 6
    4. Excluded color because deemed color was not objective and difficult to interpret

5. Excluded blood pressure because of little constant relation to recovery from general anesthesia
6. Minimum score for discharge not recommended
7. Evidence of validity and reliability not published

C. Thomas and Davis
  1. Proposed in 1984
  2. Five criteria rated either 0 or 1
     a. Systolic blood pressure above 90 mm Hg, but not 30 mm Hg above or below the preoperative reading
     b. Pink and warm
     c. Verbal response to spoken command
     d. Head lift with closed mouth for 5 seconds
     e. Comfortable with regard to pain
  3. Minimum score of 5 required for discharge
  4. Evidence of validity and reliability not published

D. Modified Aldrete (also known as PARSAP)
  1. Reported in 1995 in response to trends in ambulatory surgery for ambulatory surgery patients
  2. Modified one criterion of original PARS by replacing color index with Sao_2
  3. Ten criteria rated from 0 to 2
     a. Activity
     b. Respiration
     c. Circulation
     d. Consciousness
     e. Oxygenation
     f. Dressing
     g. Pain
     h. Ambulation
     i. Fast feeding
     j. Urine output
  4. Maximum score of 20
     a. PACU phase I discharge requires minimum score of 8 to 10 using original PARS criteria.
     b. Home discharge requires minimum score of 18.
  5. Addition of five criteria to original PARS when determining discharge from phase II
     a. Dressing appearance
     b. Pain severity
     c. Ability to ambulate
     d. Tolerance of oral fluids
     e. Ability to urinate
  6. Useful for combined PACU phase I and phase II units
  7. Evidence of validity and reliability
     a. Aldrete (1998)
        (1) Studied 740 adult patients
        (2) Sixty-two percent of patients scored 18 and higher within an hour of arrival in PACU.

E. White
  1. Developed in 1999
  2. Used for fast-tracking
  3. More sensitive and selective than Modified Aldrete Scale
  4. Seven criteria rated from 0 to 2
     a. Level of consciousness
     b. Physical activity
     c. Hemodynamic stability
     d. Respiratory stability
     e. Oxygen saturation status

      f. Postoperative pain assessment

      g. Postoperative emetic symptoms

    5. Maximum score of 14

    6. Requirements for discharge to phase II

      a. Minimum score of 12

      b. All criteria with scores of 1 or above

    7. Evidence for validity and reliability not published

  F. Cohen et al.

    1. Reported in 1998

    2. Proposed specific PACU discharge criteria for obstetric patients after regional anesthesia

    3. Criteria

      a. Stable cardiorespiratory status

      b. Block started to recede

      c. Block continuing to recede

    4. Evidence for validity and reliability

      a. Retrospective review of 6-month data from 358 patients

      b. All patients kept 1 hour in PACU and monitored for events.

      c. Patients who received epidurals were discharged sooner than those who received spinals.

BIBLIOGRAPHY

1. Aldrete JA: The post anesthesia recovery score revisited. *J Clin Anesth* 7(1):89–91, 1995.

2. Aldrete JA: Modifications to the postanesthesia score for use in ambulatory surgery. *J Perianesth Nurs* 13(3):148–155, 1998.

3. Aldrete JA, Kroulik D: A postanesthetic recovery score. *Anesth Analg* 49(6):924–934, 1970.

4. Alexander CM, Teller LE, Gross JB, et al: New discharge criteria decrease recovery room time after subarachnoid block. *Anesthesiology* 70(4):640–643, 1989.

5. American Society of Anesthesiologists: *Standards for postanesthesia care*, Park Ridge, IL, 2004, American Society of Anesthesiologists.

6. American Society of PeriAnesthesia Nurses: Clinical guidelines for the prevention of unplanned perioperative hypothermia. *J Perianesth Nurs* 16:305–314, 2001.

7. American Society of PeriAnesthesia Nurses: *Standards of perianesthesia nursing practice 2008–2010*, Cherry Hill, NJ, 2008, ASPAN.

8. Brown I, Jellish WS, Kleinman B, et al: Use of postanesthesia discharge criteria to reduce discharge delays for inpatients in the postanesthesia care unit. *J Clin Anesth* 20(3):175–179, 2008.

9. Cohen SE, Hamilton CL, Riley ET, et al: Obstetric postanesthesia care unit stays. *Anesthesiology* 89(6):1559–1565, 1998.

10. Fetzer S: Factors used to determine discharge readiness. *J Perianesth Nurs* 13(6):337–339, 1998.

11. Figueroa M Jr: The postanesthesia recovery score: A second look. *South Med J* 65(7):791–795, 1972.

12. Holzgrafe RE: A postanesthesia recovery score. *Wis Med J* 71(11):239–241, 1972.

13. Kuc JA, Pietro J: Safe discharge from the PACU and ambulatory care setting. *J Nurs Law* 6(2):7–14, 1999.

14. Marley RA, Moline BM: Patient discharge from the ambulatory setting. *J Post Anesth Nurs* 11(1):39–49, 1996.

15. Mulroy MF, Salinas FV, Larkin KL, et al: Ambulatory surgery patients may be discharged before voiding after short-acting spinal and epidural anesthesia. *Anesthesiology* 97(2):315–319, 2002.

16. Soliman IE, Patel RI, Ehrenpreis MB, et al: Recovery scores do not correlate with postoperative hypoxemia in children. *Anesth Analg* 67(1):53–56, 1988.

17. Steward DJ: A simplified scoring system for the post-operative recovery room. *Can Anaesth Soc J* 22(1):111–113, 1975.

18. Thomas D, Davis AC: A post-anesthetic scoring system. *Anaesth Intensive Care* 12(2):125–126, 1984.

19. Wetchler BV: Perianesthesia scoring system: Discharging ambulatory surgery patients. *AORN J* 41(2):382–384, 1985.

20. White PF: Criteria for fast-tracking outpatients after ambulatory surgery. *J Clin Anesth* 11(1):78–79, 1999.

21. White PF, Rawal S, Nguyen J et al: PACU fast-tracking: An alternative to "bypassing" the PACU for facilitating the recovery process after ambulatory surgery. *J Perianesth Nurs* 18(4):247–253, 2003.

22. White PF, Song D: New criteria for fast-tracking after outpatient anesthesia: A comparison with the modified Aldrete scoring system. *Anesth Analg* 88(5):1069–1072, 1999.

SURGICAL SPECIALTIES

31 Respiratory Care

REX A. MARLEY
BECKI L. HOYLE

■ ■ ■

OBJECTIVES

At the conclusion of this chapter, the reader will be able to:

1. Describe the anatomy and physiology relevant to the care of the pulmonary surgical patient.
2. Describe signs and symptoms of specific pulmonary pathological conditions.
3. Describe components of preoperative assessment in the evaluation of a patient presenting for pulmonary surgery.
4. Explain surgical procedures used in the diagnosis and treatment of the pulmonary patient.
5. State the major complications seen postoperatively in the patient undergoing thoracic surgery.
6. Describe the key nursing assessments and interventions in the immediate postoperative phase of the patient undergoing thoracic surgery.
7. Describe risk factors for the development of postoperative hypoxemia.
8. List the indications and applications of various airway management devices.
9. Differentiate between the advantages and disadvantages of synchronized intermittent mandatory, volume and pressure assist control, and pressure support ventilation.
10. Identify extubation criteria for the post anesthesia care unit (PACU) patient.
11. Explain the application of pulse oximetry and capnography.
12. Describe commonly encountered adverse perianesthesia respiratory events.

I. RESPIRATORY ANATOMY AND PHYSIOLOGY
   A. Gross anatomy of the respiratory system
      1. Nose: serves to humidify, filter, and heat or cool the inspired air better than oral breathing.
         a. The olfactory region senses whether the inspired gas has noxious qualities.
         b. If the inspired air is sufficiently noxious, a sneeze may result in an attempt to cleanse the nose of the noxious gas.
      2. Pharynx: stems from Greek word meaning "throat"
         a. Nasopharynx: pharynx above the soft palate
            (1) Lymphatic tissue, known as the pharyngeal tonsils, located here
               (a) When tonsils hypertrophy, known as adenoids
            (2) Eustachian tubes allow for equalization of air pressure between the middle ear and the atmosphere.
         b. Oropharynx: region below the nasopharynx, above the laryngopharynx and posterior to the oral cavity
            (1) Palatine tonsils, located in the posterior oropharyngeal wall
               (a) Similar to the pharyngeal tonsils
               (b) Located to neutralize pathogens taken into pharynx
            (2) Tongue: posterior portion of tongue located in the oropharynx
               (a) Highly innervated muscular organ that accounts for the strong gag reflex when stimulated
         c. Laryngopharynx: airway below base of tongue to larynx

3. Larynx: complex series of cartilages connected to bones by muscles; serves as the distinction between the upper and lower airways
   a. Functions include:
      (1) Gas conduction
      (2) Prevention of food entry into the lower respiratory tract
      (3) Facilitation of cough and phonation
   b. Consists of:
      (1) Three paired cartilages
         (a) Arytenoids
         (b) Corniculate
         (c) Cuneiform
      (2) Epiglottis: chief guardian of the laryngeal opening; closes during swallowing to prevent pulmonary aspiration
      (3) Vocal cords: altering positions of the vocal cords allows for phonation and the basis for speech.
      (4) Glottic opening (glottis)
         (a) Opening between vocal cords
         (b) Entrance to trachea
         (c) Narrowest portion of adult's airway when factoring endotracheal tube size
      (5) Thyroid cartilage: largest of all laryngeal cartilages; Adam's apple is anterior prominence of thyroid cartilage.
      (6) Cricoid cartilage: located immediately caudal to thyroid cartilage
         (a) Only completely ringed cartilage surrounding the trachea
         (b) Narrowest portion of child's airway, until approximately 10 years of age, when factoring endotracheal tube size
      (7) Cricothyroid membrane: small space separating the thyroid and cricoid cartilages anteriorly
         (a) Cricothyroidotomy: small incision through the cricothyroid membrane to establish an emergency airway into the trachea
4. Trachea: the lower airway starts at the trachea and includes the tracheobronchial tree and parenchyma of the lungs (Figure 31-1).
   a. Composed of 16 to 20 horseshoe-shaped cartilages with the posterior wall composed of nonstriated trachealis muscle
      (1) Differences between infants and adults (Table 31-1)
   b. Carina: bifurcation point of trachea into right and left primary bronchi
      (1) Important marker in endotracheal tube placement. Proper endotracheal tube positioning is routinely proximal to the carina.
      (2) Anatomic landmark is the angle of Louis (angle formed at the junction of the manubrium and body of the sternum).
5. Lungs
   a. Primary bronchi
      (1) Right bronchus is slightly larger in diameter than the left.
      (2) Left bronchus angles more sharply (45°-55° from midline) toward its lung than the right bronchus (20°-30° from midline).
      (3) Most common site of pulmonary aspiration is the right lung because the right primary bronchus is wider and has a straighter angle than the left bronchus.
   b. Each primary bronchus further divides at least 20 times (the first 16 generations of airways, to the level of the terminal bronchioles, do not participate in gas exchange) forming:
      (1) Bronchi: lobar > segmental > subsegmental > small
      (2) Bronchioles: primary > secondary > terminal > respiratory. The first site of gas exchange occurs in the respiratory bronchioles.
      (3) Alveolar ducts: thin-walled tubes that lead into alveolar sacs
      (4) Alveoli: cluster of thin-walled sacs where primary gas diffusion occurs; 200 to 600 million in healthy lungs

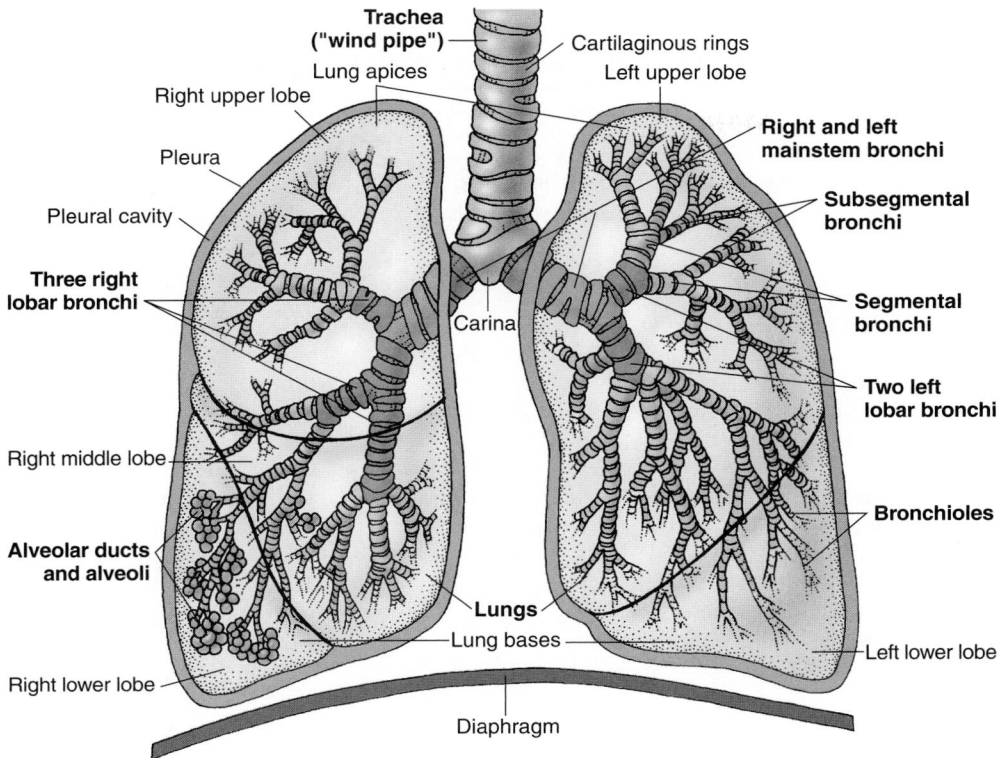

FIGURE 31-1 ■ Anatomy of lower respiratory tract. (From Ignatavicius DD, Bayne V: *Medical-surgical nursing: A nursing process approach,* ed 4, Philadelphia, 2002, WB Saunders.)

6. Thoracic cavity: cone shaped; composed of bone and cartilage to protect the vital organs
    a. Bony structures
        (1) Sternum (breastbone), which is composed of three parts
            (a) Manubrium (uppermost)
            (b) Body
            (c) Xiphoid process (lower end)
        (2) Ribs: typically 12 pairs form the rib cage.
        (3) Clavicle
        (4) Vertebrae: 7 cervical, 12 thoracic, 5 lumbar, 5 sacral, coccyx 4 fused segments
        (5) Scapulae
    b. Muscles of breathing: the muscles of respiration (Box 31-1)
        (1) Inspiration (active phase)
            (a) Diaphragm: dome-shaped skeletal muscle separating the thoracic and abdominal cavities
                (i) Major muscle of inspiration
                (ii) Only inspiratory muscle active during quiet ventilation
                (iii) Innervation by the phrenic nerve from the cervical plexus (C3-C5)
            (b) Accessory muscles silent during normal breathing
                (i) Patients with advanced chronic obstructive pulmonary disease (COPD) use to:
                    [a] Assist the flattened diaphragm
                    [b] Help relieve their increased work of breathing
        (2) Expiration
            (a) Normally proceeds passively to functional residual capacity
            (b) Expiratory muscles

■ TABLE 31-1
■ ■ **Comparative Mean Values for Normal Infant and Adult Airway Parameters**

Parameter	Infant	Adult
ANATOMIC DIFFERENCES		
Narrowest portion of airway	Cricoid ring	Glottis
Epiglottis	Narrow, short, U-shaped	Broad
Tongue	Large	—
Glottis location	C3-4	C5-6
Tracheal length (mm)	57	120
Tracheal diameter (mm)	4	16
LUNG VOLUMES		
Tidal volume (V_T; mL/kg)	7	7
Anatomic dead space (V_D; mL/kg)	2-2.5	2.2
V_D/V_T ratio	0.3	0.3
Residual volume (mL/kg)	19	16
Closing volume (mL/kg)	12	7
Closing capacity (mL/kg)	35	23
Functional residual capacity (mL/kg)	27-30	34
Vital capacity (mL/kg)	35	70
Total lung capacity (mL/kg)	70	80
RESPIRATION		
Frequency (breaths/min)	30-50	12-16
Alveolar ventilation (mL/kg/min)	100-150	60
Airway resistance (cm H_2O/L/s)	18-29	2-3
Oxygen consumption (mL/kg/min)	7-9	3

From Aker J, Marley RA, Manningham RJ: Anesthesia for pediatric patients with respiratory diseases. In Zaglaniczny K, Aker J, eds: *Clinical guide to pediatric anesthesia*, Philadelphia, 1999, WB Saunders.

      (i) Become active when minute volume exceeds 40 L/min
      (ii) When airway obstruction occurs
  c. Pleura: two layers that normally slide easily over each other during ventilation
    (1) Visceral
      (a) Lines the lung surface
      (b) No sensory innervation
    (2) Parietal

■ BOX 31-1
■ **MUSCLES OF RESPIRATION**

Inspiratory Muscles	Expiratory Muscles
Diaphragm	Internal intercostals
Accessory muscles of respiration	Abdominals
External intercostals	External & internal obliques
Scalenes	Transverse abdominis
Sternocleidomastoids	Rectus abdominis
	Glottic muscles (narrow glottis during expiration)
	Diaphragm (early expiratory contraction acts as a "brake")

From Grippi MA, Litzky LA, Manaker S, eds: *Pulmonary science and medicine: A review of fundamental principles*, Baltimore, 2001, Lippincott Williams & Wilkins.

               (a) Lines the chest wall

               (b) Sensory innervation

          (3) Pleural space

               (a) Formed by the apposition of the parietal pleura and the visceral pleura

               (b) Potential space containing a thin film of fluid, usually 10 mL, to provide lubrication for the sliding of the visceral pleura on the parietal pleura with each breath

               (c) Pressure within normally subatmospheric (-4 to -5 cm H_2O)

   d. Mediastinum: located between the two lungs; contains the major airways and great vessels, including portions of or all of:

       (1) Aortic arch and branches

       (2) Thymus

       (3) Innominate veins

       (4) Pulmonary artery and veins

       (5) Vena cava

       (6) Heart and pericardium

       (7) Lymphatic tissue and thoracic ducts

       (8) Trachea

       (9) Hilum of each lung

      (10) Azygos and hemizygous venous system

      (11) Esophagus

      (12) Vagus, cardiac, and phrenic nerves

      (13) Sympathetic nerve chains

   e. Lungs

       (1) Right lung

          (a) Shorter and wider than the left

          (b) Enjoys slightly greater ventilation than the left lung

          (c) Consists of three lobes

              (i) Upper

             (ii) Middle

             (iii) Lower

       (2) Left consists of two lobes.

          (a) Upper

          (b) Lower

       (3) Apex of the lung extends upward into the base of the neck, about 4 cm above the midpoint of the clavicle.

       (4) Lung bases are concave, with the right lung base higher than the left.

       (5) Hilum is the root portion of each lung, located medially; contains:

          (a) Pulmonary artery

          (b) Two pulmonary veins

          (c) Primary bronchus

          (d) Bronchial vessels

          (e) Lymphatics

          (f) Lymph nodes

          (g) Nerves

7. Pulmonary circulation

   a. Purpose: to deliver deoxygenated blood to pulmonary capillaries where gas exchange occurs at the alveolar-capillary membrane

       (1) Oxygen taken on

       (2) Carbon dioxide removed

   b. Pulmonary circulation acts as reservoir for left side of heart.

       (1) Approximately 30% of pulmonary vessels perfused at any given time

   c. High volume, low-pressure (one sixth of systemic arterial pressure), low-resistance system

   d. Distribution of pulmonary ventilation and perfusion

       (1) Distribution of blood flow affected by posture (gravitational influence)

          (a) In upright position, blood flow increases linearly from apex to base.

          (b) In supine position, blood flow is greater to posterior (dependent) regions.

(2) Lung zone I (upper): ventilation exceeds perfusion.

(3) Lung zone II (middle): ventilation equals perfusion.

(4) Lung zone III (lower): perfusion exceeds ventilation.

8. Neural control of ventilation

   a. Respiratory center

     (1) Responsible for generating the rhythmic pattern of inspiration and expiration

     (2) Receives input from:

       (a) Chemoreceptors

       (b) Lung and other receptors

       (c) Cortex

       (d) Major output to the phrenic nerves

     (3) Medulla

       (a) Inspiratory area: responsible for basic ventilatory rhythm

       (b) Expiratory area

         (i) Passive at rest

         (ii) Responsible for active expiration during forceful breathing

           [a] Exercise

     (4) Pons

       (a) Pneumotaxic center

         (i) Located in upper pons

         (ii) Controls the "switch-off" point of inspiration

         (iii) Controls inspiratory time

       (b) Apneustic center

         (i) Located in lower pons

         (ii) Prolongs inspiration if stimulated

   b. Chemical feedback mechanisms

     (1) Central chemoreceptors

       (a) Located on anterolateral surface of medulla

       (b) Influenced by pH of cerebrospinal fluid

         (i) Increase in hydrogen ion concentration stimulates ventilation to increase in depth and rate.

       (c) Responsible for normal control of ventilation

       (d) In chronic situations of hypercapnia:

         (i) Chemoreceptors become less sensitive to changes in carbon dioxide levels as reflected in hydrogen ion concentration.

     (2) Peripheral chemoreceptors

       (a) Located in the aortic arch and carotid bodies close to the bifurcation of the common carotid arteries

       (b) Have high metabolic rates so are sensitive to changes in oxygen supply

       (c) A decrease in partial pressure of oxygen in arterial blood ($Pao_2 < 60$ mm Hg) causes stimulation of the medulla's respiratory center, resulting in:

         (i) Increase in rate and depth of respiration, thus an increase in minute ventilation

         (ii) Tachycardia and hypertension, thus an increase in cardiac output

         (iii) Increase in pulmonary resistance

   c. Nerves

     (1) Autonomic

       (a) Parasympathetic

         (i) Main neural influence over airways in normal conditions

         (ii) Causes smooth muscle contraction

       (b) Sympathetic: causes smooth muscle dilation

     (2) Phrenic: motor innervation for diaphragm

(3) Intercostals—motor innervation for:
- (a) Intercostal muscles
- (b) Muscles
- (c) Skin of anterolateral thorax

d. Receptors
- (1) Pulmonary stretch receptors (Hering-Breuer reflex)
  - (a) Located predominantly in the airways rather than in the alveoli
  - (b) When lung inflation stretches these receptors:
    - (i) Send inhibitory impulses to the medulla stopping further inspiration
    - (ii) Activated only at large tidal volumes (>800–1000 mL)
  - (c) May be important in infants by regulating the work of breathing
    - (i) Immaturity of this reflex, such as in the preterm infant, shortens inspiratory effort.
    - (ii) May lead to central apnea
  - (d) Minimal functional significance in healthy adult individuals
- (2) Irritant receptors located between airway epithelial cells
  - (a) Sensitive to noxious stimuli
    - (i) Cigarette smoke
    - (ii) Inhaled dusts
    - (iii) Cold air
  - (b) Stimulation causes:
    - (i) Reflex cough
    - (ii) Bronchoconstriction
    - (iii) Sneezing
    - (iv) Tachypnea
    - (v) Narrowing of the glottis
- (3) Juxtacapillary (J) receptors: located in alveolar walls adjacent to capillaries when stimulated by the following result in rapid, shallow breathing and dyspnea
  - (a) Alveolar inflammatory processes (i.e., pneumonia)
  - (b) Pulmonary vascular congestion (i.e., congestive heart failure)
  - (c) Pulmonary edema
- (4) Extrapulmonary receptors
  - (a) Nose and upper airway: respond to mechanical and chemical stimuli
  - (b) Joint and muscle: increase ventilation during exercise
  - (c) Chest wall: probably instrumental in sensation of dyspnea

B. Components of gas exchange
1. Ventilation: movement of gas between atmosphere and alveoli
   a. Pressure changes during ventilation
   - (1) Airflow moves from an area of higher pressure to lower pressure.
   - (2) At rest, intrapulmonic pressure equals atmospheric pressure.
   - (3) During normal inspiration, the diaphragm and intercostal muscles contract, pulling the lungs outwards with the chest wall.
   - (4) The intrapulmonic pressure becomes negative relative to atmospheric pressure, usually 2 to 3 cm H_2O, and air moves into the lungs.
   b. Volumes (Figure 31-2, Table 31-1).
   - (1) Tidal volume: volume of air inspired or expired during each respiratory cycle
   - (2) Minute ventilation: product of the tidal volume and respiratory frequency per minute; adult at rest approximately 6 L/min
   - (3) Vital capacity: maximum volume of air that can be expelled from the lungs after a maximal inspiration
   - (4) Functional residual capacity: volume of air present in the lungs after a normal expiration
   - (5) Alveolar ventilation: portion of ventilation that takes part in gas exchange

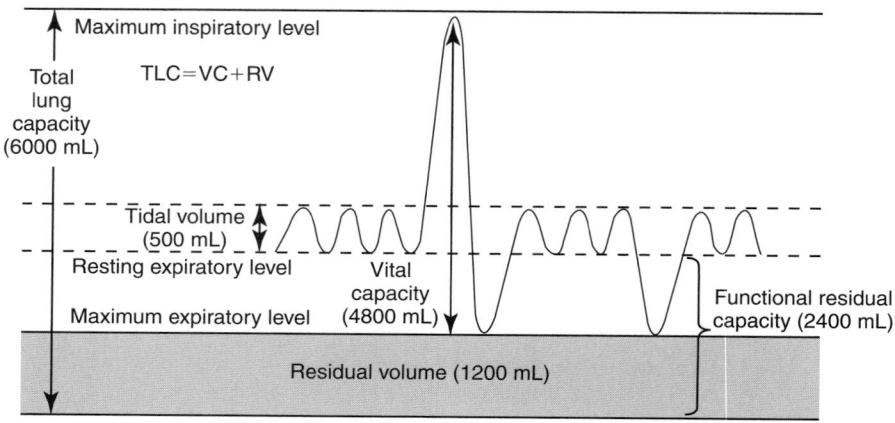

FIGURE 31-2 ■ Basic lung volumes and capacities of a normal adult male spirogram. (From Kersten LD: *Comprehensive respiratory nursing: A decision making approach,* Philadelphia, 1989, WB Saunders.)

    (6) Dead space ventilation: portion of ventilation that is not involved in gas exchange; two main components:
        (a) Anatomic dead space
           (i)   Nose
           (ii) Mouth
           (iii) Pharynx
           (iv) Larynx
           (v)   Trachea
           (vi) Bronchi
           (vii) Bronchioles
        (b) Alveolar dead space (e.g., ventilated but not perfused alveoli)
  c. Gravity determines where ventilation goes in the lungs.
    (1) Dependent regions of lungs ventilate better than uppermost regions.
  d. Work of breathing
    (1) Normally under basal conditions, the muscles of respiration account for less than 5% of the body's total oxygen consumption.
    (2) Energy required for ventilation can be divided into three components:
        (a) Compliance work: energy required to overcome elastic forces of lung
        (b) Tissue resistance work: energy required to overcome tissue friction of lung and thoracic cage during inspiration and expiration
        (c) Airway resistance work: energy required to overcome resistance to air movement in and out of lungs
  e. Elastic recoil: tendency of the lung to return to its resting position after being stretched; tendency of chest wall to spring out
  f. Critical closing volume: volume of alveolar distention at which force of recoil becomes greater than force of distention; below this volume, alveolus collapses
  g. Pulmonary compliance
    (1) Measurement of distensibility of chest wall and lung parenchyma
    (2) How easily the elastic forces in the lung accept a volume of air
    (3) The volume change per unit of pressure change
    (4) Conditions that increase compliance
        (a) COPD
        (b) Aging process
    (5) Conditions that decrease compliance (reduced compliance requires that patient does more muscular work to achieve same minute ventilation)
        (a) Acute respiratory distress syndrome (ARDS)
        (b) Bronchospasm

    (c) Pulmonary edema
    (d) Pulmonary fibrosis
    (e) Deformities of chest wall
    (f) Obesity, pregnancy, abdominal distention
    (g) Postoperative splinting, atelectasis, or pneumonia

  h. Airway resistance: impedance that air encounters as it moves through the airways

    (1) Factors affecting airway resistance
      (a) Airway diameter: the smaller the airway radius, the greater the resistance
      (b) Airway length: the greater the length, the greater the resistance
      (c) Airflow rate: if flow rate is increased, airway pressure increases and therefore resistance increases.

    (2) Major sites of resistance to gas flow are the nose, mouth, and large airways (typically turbulent flow) (80%), while the airways less than 2 mm in diameter (typically laminar flow) account for the remaining 20%.

    (3) Conditions that can increase resistance (increased resistance requires that patient does more muscular work to achieve same minute volume)
      (a) Edema of airways
      (b) Bronchospasm
      (c) Obstruction
        (i) Secretions
        (ii) Mucous plugs
        (iii) Tumor
      (d) COPD: loss of tissue elasticity results in a decrease in airway diameter and thus an increase in airway resistance (not reversible with a bronchodilator).
      (e) Endotracheal or tracheostomy tubes

2. Diffusion: movement of gas across alveolocapillary membrane from an area of high concentration to a region of lower concentration

  a. Factors affecting diffusion
    (1) Available surface area of alveoli and capillaries
      (a) Decrease in lung tissue (i.e., postpneumonectomy)
      (b) COPD
    (2) Integrity of alveolocapillary wall; thickness of alveolocapillary membrane
      (a) Interstitial disease
      (b) Pulmonary edema
    (3) Hemoglobin level
    (4) Difference of partial pressure of gas in alveolus versus blood
      (a) High altitude conditions decrease the gradient for diffusion.
    (5) Solubility of gas
      (a) Carbon dioxide diffuses more readily across the alveolocapillary membrane than oxygen; therefore, factors that affect diffusion are much more likely to affect oxygen than carbon dioxide.

  b. Oxygen transport: oxygen transported either dissolved in plasma (3%) or bound to hemoglobin (97%)
    (1) Assessment of the basic blood gas measurements reflecting oxygenation involves interpreting data that identify:
      (a) Partial pressure of oxygen in the plasma (Pao_2)
      (b) Amount of oxygen bound to hemoglobin (Sao_2)
      (c) Total content of oxygen in the arterial blood (Cao_2)
    (2) Oxyhemoglobin dissociation curve graphically represents relationship of Pao_2 to percentage of oxygen saturation of hemoglobin (Figure 31-3).
      (a) Upper flat curve indicates a relatively unchanged hemoglobin affinity at Pao_2 levels greater than 70 mm Hg.

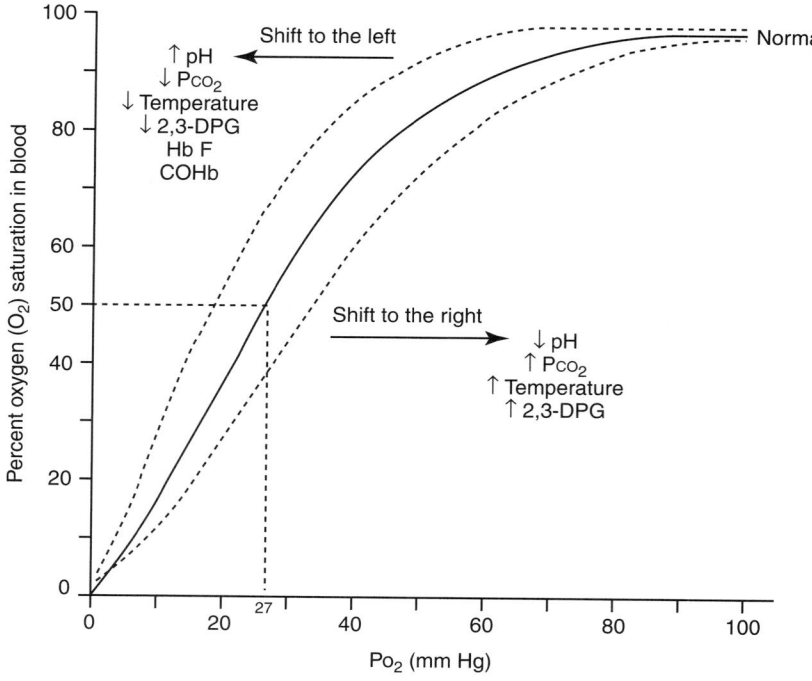

FIGURE 31-3 ■ Oxyhemoglobin dissociation curve.

    (b) Steep slope of curve ($Pao_2 < 60$ mm Hg) indicates:
        (i) Small decreases in Pao_2 result in a lessening affinity of oxygen for the hemoglobin molecule.
        (ii) Release of large amounts of oxygen to the tissues
        (iii) At a normal pH of 7.4, oxygen saturation as measured by pulse oximetry (Spo_2) of 96% = Pao_2 of 90 mm Hg.
    (c) Factors that promote the release of oxygen from hemoglobin (shift to right); more oxygen available to the tissues
        (i) Acidosis
        (ii) Hypercapnia
        (iii) Hyperthermia
        (iv) Increased levels of 2,3-diphosphoglycerate (2,3-DPG)
    (d) Factors that decrease the release of oxygen from hemoglobin (shift to left); less oxygen available to the tissues
        (i) Alkalosis
        (ii) Hypocapnia
        (iii) Hypothermia
        (iv) Decreased levels of 2,3-DPG
(3) Cao_2: a function of the amount of oxygen bound to hemoglobin and dissolved in the plasma
    (a) In whole blood, each gram of normal hemoglobin (Hb) can carry approximately 1.34 mL of oxygen.
    (b) The amount of dissolved oxygen in the blood is calculated as:
        (i) Dissolved oxygen (mL/dL) = $Pao_2 \times 0.003$
        (ii) Thus the $Cao_2 = (Hb \times 1.34$ mL $\times Sao_2) + (Pao_2 \times 0.003)$
(4) Oxygen transport: $Cao_2 \times 10 \times$ cardiac output (CO)
(5) Causes of hypoxemia
    (a) Low inspired oxygen concentration
    (b) Alveolar hypoventilation
    (c) Diffusion abnormalities

        (d) Ventilation-perfusion (V/Q) abnormalities
           (i)   Decreased cardiac output
           (ii) Shunting
        (e) Increased oxygen consumption
    c. Carbon dioxide transport
      (1) Dissolved in plasma
      (2) Carbaminohemoglobin
      (3) Bicarbonate ion
  3. Perfusion: movement of oxygenated blood to tissues
    a. Control of pulmonary circulation: hypoxic vasoconstriction
    b. V/Q ratios and abnormalities
      (1) Average-sized adult alveolar ventilation equals 4 L/min with a cardiac output of 5 L/min.
      (2) Normal V/Q ratio therefore approximates 0.8 to 0.85.
        (a) Regional variations in V/Q are mainly caused by gravity, thus are most evident in the upright position.
        (b) Changes in lung ventilation or pulmonary blood flow alter relationships; this results in abnormalities of gas exchange.
    c. Alveolar shunts: venous blood enters into the lung in areas without alveolar ventilation—thus cannot pick up oxygen or unload carbon dioxide and returns to the left side of the heart unchanged.

II. RESPIRATORY ASSESSMENT
  A. Medical history
    1. Goal of preprocedure preparation is to:
      a. Properly evaluate and optimize the patient's condition.
      b. Decrease postanesthesia complications that may further compromise patient's status.
    2. The best evaluation of the patient's respiratory function comes from a comprehensive medical history of the patient's quality of life.
    3. Four main objectives of the patient interview
      a. Collect information.
      b. Develop rapport.
      c. Respond to concerns.
      d. Educate the patient.
    4. Chief complaint and present illness
    5. Current health status
    6. Significant medical history
      a. Respiratory disease
      b. Acquired immune disease
      c. Cardiovascular disease
      d. Neuromuscular disease
      e. Musculoskeletal disease
      f. Hematological disease
      g. Diabetes
      h. Renal or hepatic dysfunction
      i. Smoking history: smoking exposure is crudely derived by the number of "pack years" smoked, which is the number of years smoked multiplied by the number of packs per day smoked.
      j. Family history—for example:
        (1) Household exposure to tuberculosis
        (2) Inherited diseases
          (a) Cystic fibrosis
          (b) $Alpha_1$-antitrypsin deficiency
          (c) Hereditary hemorrhagic telangiectasia
          (d) Immotile cilia syndrome
        (3) Familial intrinsic asthma
        (4) Passive smoke exposure
      k. Occupational or environmental exposure
        (1) Occupational asthma

   (2) Asbestosis
   (3) Silicosis
   (4) Irritant inhalant injury
   (5) High-altitude pulmonary edema
   (6) Berylliosis
   (7) Spanish toxic oil syndrome
   (8) Occupational bronchitis
   (9) Paraquat injury
   (10) Acute silicosis
   (11) Chronic cadmium exposure
   (12) Hard metal disease
   (13) Uranium mining
   (14) Coke oven work

7. Major pulmonary symptoms
 a. Cough: the most common symptom for which patients seek medical care and the second most common reason for a general medical examination
  (1) Two main reasons for coughing are:
   (a) To prevent pulmonary aspiration of foreign material
   (b) To clear foreign material and excessive secretions from the lower respiratory tract
  (2) Acute (<3 weeks) or chronic (≥3 weeks) cough
   (a) Acute: most common causes are viral or bacterial upper respiratory tract infection.
    (i) Common cold
    (ii) Acute bacterial sinusitis
    (iii) Pertussis
    (iv) Exacerbations of COPD
    (v) Allergic rhinitis
    (vi) Environmental irritant rhinitis
    (vii) Potentially life-threatening conditions that may also cause acute coughing
     [a] Asthma
     [b] Congestive heart failure
     [c] Pneumonia
     [d] Pulmonary embolism
     [e] Pulmonary aspiration
   (b) Chronic—most common causes are:
    (i) Postnasal drip syndrome secondary to rhinosinus conditions
    (ii) Asthma
    (iii) Gastroesophageal reflux disease
    (iv) Chronic bronchitis
    (v) Bronchiectasis
 b. Sputum production
  (1) Foul-smelling: indicative of anaerobic infection; for example, lung abscesses or necrotizing pneumonia
  (2) Plentiful frothy saliva-like: rare symptom of bronchoalveolar carcinoma
  (3) Pink-tinged foamy: pulmonary edema
  (4) Rust-colored or prune juice colored: pneumococcal pneumonia
  (5) Copious purulent with intermittent blood streaking: bronchiectasis
 c. Dyspnea
  (1) Key areas to elicit
   (a) Persistence or variability of dyspnea
   (b) Intermittent dyspnea probably caused by reversible events
    (i) Bronchoconstriction
    (ii) Congestive heart failure
    (iii) Pleural effusion
    (iv) Acute pulmonary emboli
    (v) Hyperventilation syndrome

(c) Continual or progressive dyspnea more characteristic of chronic circumstances
  (i)   COPD
  (ii) Interstitial fibrosis
  (iii) Chronic pulmonary emboli
  (iv) Dysfunction of the diaphragm or chest wall
(d) Aggravating or precipitating factors
  (i)   Activity: during exertion or at rest
  (ii) Timing: paroxysmal nocturnal dyspnea
  (iii) Position: orthopnea
  (iv) Exposures
      [a] Cigarettes
      [b] Allergens
  (v)   Eating
(e) Measures (e.g., positioning or medications helpful in lessening dyspnea)
(2) Physiological conditions contributing to dyspnea
  (a) Mechanical interference with ventilation
    (i)   Obstruction to airflow
    (ii) Resistance to expansion of the lungs
    (iii) Resistance to expansion of the chest wall or diaphragm
  (b) Weakness of the respiratory pump
    (i)   Absolute
        [a] Poliomyelitis
        [b] Neuromuscular disease
    (ii) Relative
        [a] Hyperinflation
        [b] Pleural effusion
        [c] Pneumothorax
  (c) Increased respiratory drive
    (i)   Hypoxemia
    (ii) Metabolic acidosis
    (iii) Stimulation of intrapulmonary receptors
  (d) Wasted ventilation
    (i)   Capillary destruction
        [a] Emphysema
        [b] Interstitial lung disease
    (ii) Large-vessel obstruction
  (e) Pulmonary emboli
  (f) Pulmonary vasculitis
  (g) Psychological dysfunction
    (i)   Bodily preoccupation
    (ii) Anxiety
    (iii) Depression
    (iv) Litigation
  (h) Cardiac abnormalities resulting in inefficient pumping of the left ventricle
d. Wheezing: expiratory sound produced by turbulent gas flow through narrowed airways; be aware of the adage that "all that wheezes is not bronchospasm."
e. Hemoptysis: expectoration of any blood is indicative of hemoptysis.
  (1) Any newfound or substantial hemoptysis merits a complete diagnostic evaluation.
  (2) Common causes
    (a) Chronic bronchitis
    (b) Bronchiectasis
    (c) Neoplasm
    (d) Tuberculosis becoming less important

    f. Chest pain: sources, types, and most common causes include:
      (1) Pleuropulmonary disorders
        (a) Pleuritic pain
        (b) Pain of pulmonary hypertension
        (c) Tracheobronchial pain
      (2) Musculoskeletal disorders
        (a) Costochondral pain
        (b) Neuritis-radiculitis
        (c) Shoulder–upper extremity pain
        (d) Chest wall pain
      (3) Cardiovascular disorders
        (a) Myocardial ischemia
        (b) Pericardial pain
        (c) Substernal and back pain
      (4) Gastrointestinal disorders
        (a) Esophageal pain
        (b) Epigastric-substernal pain
      (5) Psychiatric disorders (e.g., atypical anginal pain)
      (6) Others (e.g., substernal pain)
    g. Voice changes or hoarseness may indicate
      (1) Recurrent laryngeal nerve damage
      (2) Compression associated with tumor
    h. Dysphagia may indicate
      (1) Esophageal involvement
      (2) Acute epiglottitis
    i. Constitutional signs
      (1) Weakness or decreased exercise tolerance
      (2) Weight loss, anorexia
      (3) Night sweats
      (4) Fever
    j. Abnormal chest radiograph
    k. Superior vena cava syndrome
      (1) Dyspnea
      (2) Cough
      (3) Dilation of veins on head, neck, and arms
      (4) Edema of face, arms, and upper body associated with compression
        of vena cava
B. Physical examination
  1. Inspection: visual skill used to gather patient information during the patient interview
    a. General appearance (e.g., sex, age, size, posture)
    b. State of sensorium
    c. Temperature, turgor, moisture of skin
    d. Skin color
      (1) Peripheral cyanosis
      (2) Central cyanosis
    e. Nutritional status
    f. Speech
    g. Chest configuration
      (1) Pectus excavatum
      (2) Pectus carinatum
      (3) Lordosis
      (4) Kyphoscoliosis
      (5) Scoliosis
      (6) Ankylosing spondylitis

    h. Ventilatory effort (e.g., rate, rhythm, depth of respirations)

    i. Breathing abnormalities

       (1) Tachypnea: rapid shallow breathing

       (2) Kussmaul's breathing: rapid, deep breathing (air hunger); may be secondary to metabolic acidosis

       (3) Cheyne-Stokes breathing: rhythmic waxing and waning of the depth of breathing with regularly recurring periods of apnea; may be secondary to diseases of central nervous system, congestive heart failure

       (4) Biot's breathing: irregular breaths interspersed with variable periods of apnea, sometimes prolonged; may be secondary to stroke, trauma, increased intracranial pressure, or uncal or tentorial herniation

       (5) Cough

       (6) Stridor

       (7) Wheezing

       (8) Prolonged expiratory time (i.e., with COPD, bronchospasm)

    j. Chest wall movement

       (1) Excursion

       (2) Symmetry

    k. Fingers for clubbing or nicotine stains

    l. Use of accessory muscles of ventilation

    m. Dependent edema

2. Palpation: placing the palms of the hands on the chest to assess the degree of chest movement; least productive and thus not routinely performed by many

    a. Chest excursion and symmetry

    b. Tracheal position in the suprasternal notch may detect shifts of the mediastinum.

    c. Subcutaneous air

    d. Vocal fremitus: patient speaks "one, two, three" while examiner positions both palms horizontally from top to bottom on each side.

       (1) Increased fremitus in areas of increased sound transmission (e.g., pneumonia)

       (2) Decreased fremitus in areas of impaired sound transmission (e.g., pleural effusion)

3. Percussion: tissue vibrations will produce different sounds with varying tissue density.

    a. Dullness: percussion note heard and felt over areas of lung consolidation or fluid accumulation

    b. Tympany: percussion note heard and felt in regions of increased air in the lung

4. Auscultation: process of listening for sounds produced in the body

    a. Vesicular breath sounds: soft, low-pitched sounds heard over most of the normal chest

       (1) Sound may originate in the periphery of the lung at the area of the terminal respiratory units.

       (2) Inspiratory phase longer than expiratory phase and inspirations often softer (or inaudible) compared with expirations

    b. Adventitious breath sounds: abnormal lung sounds produced by movement of air in the lungs

    c. Bronchial breath sounds: loud, high-pitched sounds usually of a "tubular" quality

       (1) Normal sound if heard over the manubrium

       (2) Pathological if heard over the periphery

    d. Crackles: discontinuous adventitious lung sounds (e.g., rale-type sounds heard primarily on inspiration produced by fluid, heard in the peripheral fields)

       (1) Atelectasis

       (2) Airway fluid

    e. Wheezes: high-pitched, continuous, musical adventitious lung sounds

       (1) May be heard on inspiration and expiration

       (2) Most commonly associated with a combination of bronchoconstriction and retained secretions

    f. Rub

      (1) Grating or scraping sound of inflamed parietal visceral surfaces as they approximate at end of inspiration

      (2) Normal sound postthoracotomy

    g. Voice sounds: amplified transmission of voice through thorax as a result of increased lung density of areas of atelectasis

      (1) Bronchophony: increased transmission of spoken words "ninety nine"

      (2) Egophony: spoken "ee" is auscultated "aa."

      (3) Whispered pectoriloquy: auscultation of whispered voice is enhanced.

C. Diagnostic testing

  1. Laboratory

    a. Standard hematologic: routine laboratory screening not cost-effective or predictive of complications

      (1) Various tests will be ordered based on the presenting symptoms and the likelihood that these symptoms will yield abnormal laboratory test results.

    b. Arterial blood gas (ABG) analysis: cornerstone in the diagnosis and management of clinical oxygenation and acid-base disturbances.

      (1) There is an increased postoperative risk with:

        (a) Pao_2 <50 mm Hg (breathing room air)

        (b) $Paco_2$ >45 mm Hg

    c. Cultures and serologic testing: laboratory diagnosis of lower respiratory tract infection includes obtaining specimens for microbiologic examination.

    d. Laboratory testing for the respiratory surgical patient may be expected to include:

      (1) Complete blood count

      (2) Coagulation studies

        (a) International normalized ratio (INR)

        (b) Prothrombin time

        (c) Partial thromboplastin time

      (3) Electrolytes

      (4) Blood urea nitrogen

      (5) Creatinine

  2. Radiographic techniques: play an essential role in the detection, diagnosis, and follow-up care of patients with pulmonary disease

    a. Chest radiography: provides instant and inexpensive imaging of the cardiopulmonary system; plays a primary role in screening, emergency medicine, and intensive care setting

      (1) Routine examination consists of posteroanterior view and sometimes a left lateral projection with suspected chest disease.

    b. Pulmonary angiography: primarily used for the detection or exclusion of pulmonary embolism

    c. Computed tomography (CT)

      (1) Has become the major imaging modality of choice for the evaluation of patients with lung carcinoma and entities such as:

        (a) Arteriovenous fistulas

        (b) Rounded atelectasis

        (c) Fungus balls

        (d) Mucoid impaction

        (e) Infarcts

      (2) CT is useful for:

        (a) Staging

        (b) As a guide to surgical management

        (c) Determination of appropriate methods for surgical staging

    d. Magnetic resonance imaging (MRI) techniques: valuable for specific problem solving of issues in the thorax, which include evaluation of:

      (1) Mediastinal masses

      (2) Superior sulcus tumors

      (3) Thoracic aorta

e. Positron emission tomography (PET) imaging in the thorax: powerful diagnostic nuclear medicine tool that produces a three-dimensional image; used to determine the presence and severity of:
  (1) Cancers
  (2) Cardiovascular disease
  (3) Neurological conditions

3. Cardiac: certain electrocardiogram (ECG) changes might occur under various presenting pulmonary conditions.
  a. Severe asthma
    (1) Sinus tachycardia
    (2) Right axis deviation
    (3) Clockwise rotation
    (4) Partial right bundle branch
    (5) ST-T abnormalities
    (6) P-pulmonale (associated with hypercapnia and acidemia)
    (7) Right ventricular strain
  b. COPD: 75% of these patients have abnormal ECGs.
    (1) Multifocal atrial tachycardia
    (2) Right axis deviation
    (3) Clockwise rotation
    (4) Diminished QRS amplitude
    (5) Incomplete to complete right bundle branch block
  c. Pulmonary embolism
    (1) Sinus tachycardia
    (2) T-wave inversion
    (3) ST-segment depression
    (4) Low voltage in frontal plane
    (5) Left axis deviation
    (6) ST-segment elevation
    (7) Right bundle branch block
    (8) Premature ventricular contractions

4. Pulmonary function tests
  a. Designed to evaluate lung function; these tests may evaluate:
    (1) Airway function
    (2) Lung volumes and ventilation
    (3) Diffusing capacity
    (4) Metabolic requirements
  b. Appropriate testing in patients scheduled for major lung resection or inpatients who have severe pulmonary dysfunction may include:
    (1) Spirometry, including:
      (a) Forced vital capacity (FVC)
      (b) Forced expiratory volume in the first second (FEV_1)
      (c) Maximum breathing capacity (MBC)
      (d) Increased postoperative risk with
        (i) FVC <50% of predicted, FEV_1 <50% of FVC
        (ii) 1.5 L for lobectomy and 2 L for pneumonectomy
        (iii) MBC <50% of predicted or 50 L/min
      (e) Residual volume and total lung volume: increased postoperative risk with residual volume/total lung volume >50%
    (2) Diffusion capacity: increased postoperative risk with diffusion capacity ≤55% of predicted
    (3) Xenon scanning: to assess lung ventilation and perfusion patterns
    (4) Pulmonary artery pressure with unilateral balloon occlusion (if pulmonary resection or pneumonectomy considered)
      (a) Increased postoperative risk if pulmonary artery pressure during unilateral occlusion >30 mm Hg

(b) An indicator of oxygen consumption ($Vo_{2\,MAX}$) of:

(i) <10 mL/kg/min (<40% of predicted)—indicates the patient is unsuitable for any pulmonary resection

(ii) <15 mL/kg/min—high risk for postoperative cardiorespiratory complication after lung resection

(iii) >20 mL/kg/min (>75% of predicted)—indicates pneumonectomy may be reasonable

(5) Exercise testing: oxygen consumption during maximal exercise

5. Certain measures can be implemented before the patient's surgery in an attempt to optimize his or her condition (Box 31-2).

III. RESPIRATORY PATHOPHYSIOLOGY

A. Obstructive diseases

1. Chronic diseases characterized by:

a. Obstruction to airflow in lung parenchyma or airways

b. Commonly seen as secondary medical conditions in patients undergoing thoracic surgery

c. Includes patients with:

(1) Chronic airflow obstruction (bronchitis and emphysema)

(2) Destruction of alveolar tissue (emphysema)

(3) Potentially reversible airway disease (asthma)

2. COPD

a. Distinguished by the progressive development of airflow obstruction that is not fully reversible

b. Primary diseases of COPD

(1) Emphysema

(a) Condition of the lung characterized by abnormal permanent enlargement of the air spaces distal to the terminal bronchioles accompanied by destruction of their walls and without obvious fibrosis

---

■ BOX 31-2

■ **RISK REDUCTION STRATEGIES TO DECREASE THE INCIDENCE OF POSTOPERATIVE COMPLICATIONS IN PATIENTS WITH COPD**

Preoperative

- Encourage cessation of smoking for at least 8 weeks.
- Treat evidence of expiratory airflow obstruction, e.g., bronchodilator therapy.
- Treat respiratory infection with appropriate antibiotics.
- Initiate patient education regarding lung volume expansion maneuvers.

Intraoperative

- Use minimally invasive surgical (laparoscopic) techniques when possible.
- Consider use of regional anesthesia.
- Avoid use of long-acting neuromuscular blocking drugs.
- Avoid surgical procedures >3 hours.

Postoperative

- Continue tracheal intubation and mechanical ventilation (likely after abdominal or intrathoracic surgery and a preoperative $Paco_2$ >50 mm Hg and FEV_1/FVC <0.5; maintain Pao_2 at 60–100 mm Hg and $Paco_2$ in a range that maintains the pH at 7.35–7.45).
- Institute lung-volume expansion maneuvers (voluntary deep breathing, incentive spirometry, continuous positive airway pressure).
- Chest physiotherapy
- Maximize analgesia (neuraxial opioids, intercostal nerve blocks, patient-controlled analgesia).

COPD, Chronic obstructive pulmonary disease; FEV_1, forced expiratory volume in 1 second; *FVC*, forced vital capacity; $Paco_2$, partial pressure of carbon dioxide in arterial blood; Pao_2, partial pressure of oxygen in arterial blood.

From Stoelting RK, Dierdoff SF: *Handbook for anesthesia and co-existing disease,* ed 2, New York, 2002, Churchill Livingstone. Adapted from Smetana GW: Preoperative pulmonary evaluation. *N Engl J Med* 340:937-944, 1999.

          (b) Loss of elastic recoil allows collapse of distal, poorly supported airways, leading to premature airway closure and chronic air trapping.

          (c) This leads to increased compliance and impairment of gas exchange.

          (d) Frequently found in association with chronic bronchitis

       (2) Chronic bronchitis: chronic inflammation results in hypertrophy and hyperplasia of mucus-secreting glands resulting in:

          (a) Increased sputum production

          (b) Narrowing of bronchioles and small bronchi by edema and mucous gland enlargement, and chronic cough

          (c) Definition: presence of chronic productive cough for 3 or more months in each of 2 successive years in the absence of persistent cough-producing disorders that have been ruled out

             (i) Tuberculosis

             (ii) Neoplasm

             (iii) Bronchiectasis

             (iv) Cystic fibrosis

             (v) Chronic congestive heart failure

  c. Etiology of COPD: chronic exposure to tobacco smoke is the major predisposing factor leading to the development of COPD.

  d. Clinical manifestations of COPD

       (1) Chronic productive cough: most common symptom

       (2) Dyspnea: reason for seeking medical attention

       (3) Sputum production: mucoid but purulent during infections; greater in smokers

       (4) Hemoptysis: chronic bronchitis most common cause

       (5) Barrel-shaped chest, increased anteroposterior diameter of chest

       (6) Tachypnea

       (7) Prolonged expiratory time, indicative of significant obstruction when it exceeds 4 seconds

       (8) Pursed lip breathing

       (9) Decreased excursion

      (10) Crackles (inspiratory) and wheezing (not consistent finding)

      (11) Diminished breath sounds

      (12) Emaciation

  e. Laboratory findings

       (1) Chest radiograph and CT

          (a) Chronic bronchitis: "dirty chest" appearance, including increased bronchial wall thickness and prominent lung markings

          (b) Emphysema

             (i) Hyperlucency of the lungs secondary to arterial vascular deficiency (oligemia), attenuation of pulmonary vascular shadows

             (ii) Hyperinflation: flattening of the diaphragm, increase in the width of the retrosternal air space

             (iii) Bullae

  f. Pulmonary function tests

       (1) Decreased forced expiratory flow tests

          (a) FEV_1 (volume expired in the first second)

          (b) FEV_1/FVC ratio

          (c) FEF_{0-25} (average flow over the first quarter of forced expiration) ratio

          (d) PEF (peak expiratory flow)

          (e) Typically minimal improvement in these tests in response to a bronchodilator

       (2) Lung volumes in emphysema

          (a) Increased total lung capacity

          (b) Increased residual volume

(c) Increased functional residual capacity

(d) Decreased vital capacity secondary to the increased residual volume

(3) Diffusing capacity: single-breath diffusing capacity is decreased with severe emphysema.

g. ABG analysis

    (1) Early-stage COPD: mild to moderate hypoxemia without hypercapnia

    (2) Later-stage COPD

        (a) Moderate to severe hypoxemia with hypercapnia

        (b) Increased serum bicarbonate levels

h. Complications

    (1) Pneumothorax

    (2) Cor pulmonale

    (3) Pneumonia

    (4) Sleep abnormalities

i. Treatment

    (1) Influenza and pneumococcal vaccinations

    (2) Smoking cessation

    (3) Improve airway clearance of secretions.

    (4) Chest physiotherapy

    (5) Adequate hydration; diuresis if cor pulmonale present

    (6) Mucolytic or expectorant medications

    (7) Oxygen therapy—assess ABG for:

        (a) Pao_2 <55 mm Hg

        (b) Hematocrit >55%

        (c) Keep Pao_2 at 60 to 80 mm Hg.

    (8) Minimize airflow obstruction with $beta_2$-agonists or anticholinergics (most effective in COPD).

    (9) Reduce inflammation.

        (a) Corticosteroids

        (b) Antibiotics if infection present

        (c) Avoidance of smoking and other irritants

    (10) Noninvasive nasal mask ventilation during acute exacerbations

    (11) Lung volume reduction surgery in select emphysematous patients

    (12) Emotional support

3. Obstructive sleep apnea (OSA)

a. Breathing disorder distinguished by pattern of repeated collapse of the upper airway during sleep with cessation of breathing, leading to:

    (1) Intermittent patient arousal

    (2) Restored muscle tone

    (3) Airway becoming patent again

    (4) Pattern is often repeated during course of sleep.

    (5) Almost all patients with OSA have history of snoring.

b. Predisposing factors

    (1) Anatomic

        (a) Obesity

        (b) Increased neck circumference

        (c) Adenotonsillar hypertrophy

        (d) Craniofacial abnormalities or conditions

            (i) Retrognathia

            (ii) Micrognathia

    (2) Neuromuscular abnormalities

        (a) Cerebral palsy

        (b) Down syndrome

c. Clinical manifestations

    (1) Snoring

    (2) Sleep apnea (repeated episodes of complete cessation of airflow for ≥10 seconds)

   (3) Paradoxical movement of abdomen and rib cage
   (4) Fragmented sleep may lead to:
    (a) Daytime somnolence
    (b) Fatigue
    (c) Morning headaches
    (d) Diaphoresis
    (e) Nocturnal enuresis
    (f) Decreased cognition
    (g) Decreased intellectual function
    (h) Personality and behavioral changes
   (5) Cardiovascular manifestations may include:
    (a) Pulmonary and systemic hypertension
    (b) Right and left ventricular hypertrophy
    (c) Increased incidence of dysrhythmias
    (d) Myocardial infarction
    (e) Congestive heart failure
    (f) Stroke
  d. Diagnostic indicators and laboratory findings
   (1) Polysomnography to confirm sleep apnea diagnosis
   (2) Drop in oxygen saturation of >4%.
   (3) ABG analysis
    (a) Hypoxemia
    (b) Chronic hypercarbia
  e. Treatment
   (1) Behavioral
    (a) Weight loss in overweight patients
    (b) Avoidance of:
     (i) Alcohol
     (ii) Sedatives
     (iii) Hypnotics
    (c) Sleep in lateral position
   (2) Medical: Nasally applied continuous positive airway pressure (N-CPAP)
    (a) Most consistently effective treatment
    (b) Includes bilevel positive airway pressure (BiPAP) and auto-titrating CPAP
    (c) Should be available in immediate postoperative setting, when appropriate
   (3) Surgical
    (a) Tonsillectomy and adenoidectomy
    (b) Laser-assisted uvulopalatoplasty
    (c) Uvulopalatopharyngoplasty
    (d) Radiofrequency volumetric tissue reduction of the palate
    (e) Nasal septal reconstruction
    (f) Uvulopalatopharyngoglossoplasty
    (g) Laser midline glossectomy
    (h) Lingualplasty
    (i) Inferior sagittal mandibular osteotomy
    (j) Genioglossal advancement, with hyoid myotomy and suspension
    (k) Maxillomandibular osteotomy
    (l) Permanent tracheostomy
 4. Asthma
  a. Chronic disease characterized by chronic airway inflammation, airway hyperresponsiveness, and at least partially reversible airflow obstruction
  b. Etiology (Box 31-3)

■ BOX 31-3

■ **ETIOLOGIC FORMS OF ASTHMA ALLERGEN-INDUCED (IMMUNOLOGIC ASTHMA, MOST COMMON FORM OF REVERSIBLE EXPIRATORY AIRFLOW OBSTRUCTION)**

- Exercise-induced asthma
- Nocturnal asthma
- Aspirin-induced asthma (includes nonsteroidal anti-inflammatory drugs; patients with asthma may be sensitive to bisulfite and food processing and certain drugs)
- Occupational asthma (latex sensitivity in health care personnel may manifest as increasing expiratory obstruction to airflow during the normal workday in the operating room)
- Infectious asthma

From Stoelting RK, Dierdoff SF: *Handbook for anesthesia and co-existing disease,* ed 2, New York, 2002, Churchill Livingstone.

    c. Clinical manifestations: recurrent episodes occur predominantly at nighttime or in the early morning and consist of:
        (1) Wheezing
        (2) Dyspnea
        (3) Chest tightness
        (4) Coughing
    d. Laboratory findings
        (1) Chest radiograph: lung hyperinflation with flattened diaphragm
        (2) Pulmonary function testing
            (a) Asthmatics are bronchodilator responsive, such that the airway obstruction is reversible.
            (b) FEV_1 and maximum midexpiratory flow rates are diminished; during an asthmatic attack they may be <35% and <20% of normal, respectively.
            (c) Periodic peak inspiratory flow measurements should be performed to evaluate the effectiveness of inhaled pharmacological agents.
        (3) ECG: during an acute asthmatic attack, acute right-sided heart failure and ventricular irritability may be present.
        (4) ABG analysis
            (a) With mild asthma, Pao_2 and $Paco_2$ values typically are normal.
            (b) With severe asthma, as the patient fatigues:
                (i) FEV_1 <25% of predicted
                (ii)   Arterial hypoxemia
                (iii) Increasing $Paco_2$
    e. Treatment
        (1) Prevent and control bronchial inflammation with corticosteroids as a first line of therapy.
            (a) Cromolyn, a mast cell stabilizer, is effective in reducing inflammation and may be part of the treatment protocol.
        (2) Beta$_2$-agonist bronchodilators are recommended for symptomatic relief of acute occurrences whenever corticosteroids are inadequate and for the prevention of exercise-induced asthma.
        (3) Control environmental factors (i.e., cigarette smoke, dust) to minimize acute exacerbations.
        (4) Therapeutic protocol for the treatment of intermittent and persistent asthma (Table 31-2)
  5. Bronchiectasis
    a. Localized, irreversible dilatation of proximal bronchi (>2 mm in diameter) caused primarily by chronic bacterial infections; inflammatory response may erode arteries, leading to hemoptysis.
    b. Clinical manifestations
        (1) Cough: chronic, productive
        (2) Large quantities of purulent sputum production

■ TABLE 31-2
■ ■ **Stepwise Approach to Asthma Management***

Step 1 Mild, Intermittent	Step 2 Mild, Persistent	Step 3 Moderate, Persistent	Step 4 Severe, Persistent
Quick relief Short-acting inhaled B_2-agonist as needed for symptoms Long-term control Daily medications not necessary	Short-acting inhaled B_2-agonist as needed for symptoms Daily medications: Low-dose ICS or Cromolyn, nedocromil or Theophylline or Leukotriene inhibitors	Short-acting inhaled B_2-agonist as needed for symptoms Daily medications: Low- to medium-dose ICS + LABA or Medium-dose ICS or Low- to medium-dose ICS + sustained-release theophylline or Low- to medium-dose ICS + leukotriene modifier	Short-acting inhaled B_2-agonist as needed for symptoms Daily medications: High-dose ICS + LABA Plus, if needed: systemic corticosteroids Addition of a third controller medication has not been adequately studied

*Preferred therapies are shown in boldface type.
ICS, Inhaled corticosteroid; *LABA*, long-acting beta-agonist.
From Boushey HA, Corry DB, Fahy JV, et al: Asthma. In Mason RJ, Broaddus VC, Murray JF, et al (eds): *Murray and Nadel's textbook of respiratory medicine*, ed 4, Philadelphia, 2005, Saunders.

      (3) Hemoptysis
      (4) Signs of recurrent infection
  c. Treatment
      (1) Antibiotics as dictated by sputum or bronchoalveolar lavage fluid culture for aerobes, anaerobes, and mycobacteria
      (2) Chest physical therapy, including chest percussion and vibration along with postural drainage
      (3) Mucolytics and methods to increase mucociliary clearance
      (4) Surgical resection may be considered in patients with localized disease that has not responded to medical management.
 6. Cystic fibrosis
  a. Inherited autosomal recessive disorder characterized by chronic airway obstruction and infection and by exocrine pancreatic insufficiency
  b. Clinical manifestations
      (1) Very salty-tasting skin
      (2) Persistent coughing
      (3) Wheezing or pneumonia
      (4) Excessive appetite but poor weight gain
      (5) Bulky stools
  c. Laboratory findings
      (1) The sweat test is the accepted diagnostic examination for cystic fibrosis by measuring the amount of salt in the sweat.
      (2) A high salt level indicates that a person has cystic fibrosis.
  d. Treatment
      (1) Similar to that of bronchiectasis
         (a) Infection control
         (b) Airway clearance
      (2) Correction of organ dysfunction
         (a) Pancreatic enzyme replacement
      (3) Bronchodilator therapy if the patient exhibits bronchial hyperreactivity

    B. Restrictive diseases
        1. Pulmonary disorders
            a. Result in impaired respiratory function characterized by decreases in total lung capacity
            b. Principally an intrinsic process that alters the elastic properties of the lungs, causing the lungs to stiffen
            c. As compared with obstructive lung diseases, in restrictive diseases the expiratory flow rates remain normal.
        2. Acute intrinsic restrictive lung disease
            a. Typically presenting clinical symptoms of pulmonary edema (i.e., intravascular fluid leakage into the lung interstitium and alveoli)
            b. Acute hypoxemic respiratory failure: arises from collapse or filling of alveoli leading to adverse consequences on gas exchange; interstitial and alveolar fluid accumulation causes an increase in lung stiffness.
            c. Aspiration pneumonitis: secondary to pulmonary aspiration of acidic gastric contents
            d. Neurogenic pulmonary edema: develops secondary to acute brain injury; secondary massive expression of sympathetic nervous system impulses leads to widespread vasoconstriction and a shift of blood volume into the pulmonary circulation.
            e. Drug-induced pulmonary edema: principally heroin and cocaine
                (1) Cocaine usage can lead to pulmonary edema because of:
                    (a) Myocardial ischemia and infarction
                    (b) Pulmonary vasoconstriction
                    (c) Pulmonary capillary membrane injury
            f. High-altitude pulmonary edema: secondary to hypoxic pulmonary vasoconstriction and increased pulmonary vascular pressure that leads to high-permeability pulmonary edema
            g. Reexpansion of collapsed lung: unilateral pulmonary edema may occur in patients whose lung has been rapidly reinflated after a varied period of collapse.
            h. Postobstructive pulmonary edema: sudden onset of pulmonary edema of varying severity after vigorous inspiratory efforts against an obstructed upper airway, leading to increased pulmonary venous pressure and leakage of fluid and blood into the alveoli.
            i. Congestive heart failure
        3. Chronic intrinsic restrictive lung disease
            a. Attributable to inflammatory response and diffuse scarring of alveolar walls, leading to pulmonary fibrosis
            b. Sarcoidosis: systemic granulomatous disease resulting in inflammation, scarring, and occasionally hypercalcemia that interferes with organ function
            c. Hypersensitivity pneumonitis
                (1) Diffuse granulomatous response to the breathing of dust containing fungi, spores, or animal or vegetable material
                (2) Recurring period of hypersensitivity pneumonitis leads to pulmonary fibrosis.
            d. Eosinophilic granuloma
            e. Alveolar proteinosis: deposition of lipid-rich proteinaceous material in the alveoli
            f. Lymphangiomyomatosis
                (1) Proliferation of smooth muscle in:
                    (a) Abdominal and thoracic lymphatics
                    (b) Veins
                    (c) Bronchioles
                (2) May present with:
                    (a) Interstitial lung thickening
                    (b) Chylous effusion
                    (c) Pneumothorax

(3) Occurs in females of reproductive age
   g. Drug-induced pulmonary fibrosis
4. Chronic extrinsic lung disease
   a. Secondary to disorders affecting the thoracic cage that interfere with lung expansion
   b. Obesity
   c. Ascites
   d. Pregnancy
   e. Deformities of the chest wall
     (1) Kyphoscoliosis
     (2) Ankylosing spondylitis
   f. Deformities of the sternum
   g. Chest trauma
     (1) Flail chest: multiple rib fractures (typically double fractures of three or more contiguous ribs or combined sternal and rib fractures) produce a segment of the rib cage that is disconnected from the rest of the chest wall and deforms markedly with breathing (paradoxical).
     (2) Pulmonary contusion: blunt injury to lung parenchyma, airways, and alveoli, which may result in ventilation and perfusion mismatches
   h. Neuromuscular disorders
     (1) Spinal cord transection
     (2) Guillain-Barré syndrome
     (3) Myasthenia gravis
     (4) Eaton-Lambert syndrome
     (5) Muscular dystrophies
5. Disorders of the pleura and mediastinum
   a. Pleural thickening
   b. Pleural effusion
     (1) Fluid in pleural space; may be exudative (high-protein content) or transudative (low-protein content)
     (2) Etiology
       (a) Infection
       (b) Tumor
       (c) Congestive heart failure
       (d) Hepatic cirrhosis
       (e) Pancreatic abscess
     (3) Signs and symptoms
       (a) Hypoxemia
       (b) Tachypnea, dyspnea
       (c) Dullness to percussion
       (d) Decreased or absent fremitus
       (e) Diminished breath sounds
     (4) Treatment
       (a) Thoracentesis
       (b) Chest tube with water seal drainage
   c. Empyema
     (1) Pus in pleural space; may be acute or chronic
     (2) Etiology
       (a) Pneumonia
       (b) After thoracic surgery
     (3) Signs and symptoms
       (a) Malaise
       (b) Fever
       (c) Pleuritic pain
       (d) Leukocytosis
     (4) Diagnosis: lateral chest radiograph

      (5) Treatment
- (a) Appropriate antibiotic therapy based on pleural fluid cultures
- (b) Thoracentesis; consider closed or open drainage.
- (c) Thoracoscopy with decortication

  d. Pneumothorax
- (1) Air in pleural space as result of traumatic, iatrogenic, or spontaneous causes
- (2) Etiology: trauma, surgical procedure or central venous line insertion, nerve block (i.e., intercostal, supraclavicular, interscalene), positive-pressure ventilation, spontaneous subpleural emphysematous bleb rupture
- (3) Diagnosis: suggested by the clinical history and physical examination; chest radiograph (demonstrating a pleural line) or chest CT
- (4) Signs and symptoms
  - (a) Depends on size of pneumothorax
  - (b) Dyspnea
  - (c) Tachypnea
  - (d) Chest pain
  - (e) Increased work of breathing
  - (f) Decreased fremitus
  - (g) Decreased excursion
  - (h) Tracheal deviation to contralateral side
  - (i) Decreased or absent breath sounds
- (5) Treatment
  - (a) Supplemental oxygen therapy: increases rate of pleural absorption
  - (b) If pneumothorax >20%, re-expand lung with chest tube to water seal drainage.

  e. Tension pneumothorax
- (1) Life-threatening disorder in which air enters pleural space but cannot escape; as intrapleural volume of air increases, lungs and mediastinal structures are compressed and shifted to contralateral side, impairing respiratory and cardiac function.

  f. Hemothorax
- (1) Presence of blood in pleural space
- (2) Etiology: trauma, surgical procedure, neoplasm, pulmonary infarction
- (3) Treatment: depends on rate and volume of bleeding, thoracostomy and tube drainage, thoracoscopy or thoracotomy and exploration

  g. Mediastinal mass

  h. Pneumomediastinum

C. Vascular diseases

  1. Pulmonary edema

    a. A pathological state of abnormal accumulation of extravascular liquid in the lungs

    b. Acute pulmonary edema may be caused by:
- (1) Increased capillary pressure edema
  - (a) Hydrostatic
  - (b) Cardiogenic
- (2) Increased capillary permeability

    c. Signs and symptoms
- (1) Dyspnea, cough, and tachypnea are early signs.
- (2) Increased pressure edema; may complain of:
  - (a) Vague fatigue
  - (b) Mild pedal edema during the day
  - (c) Exertional or paroxysmal nocturnal dyspnea
  - (d) With severe alveolar edema, cough with frothy, pink sputum may be a presenting symptom.
- (3) Increased permeability edema
  - (a) Do not have symptoms of underlying cardiac disease

           (b) May offer history of exposure
               (i)   Toxic gases or chemicals
               (ii) Near drowning
               (iii) Drug ingestion
               (iv) Trauma

d. Risk factors
   (1) Sepsis
   (2) Pancreatitis
   (3) Pneumonia
   (4) Emesis
   (5) Seizures
   (6) Burns
   (7) High altitude

e. Treatment
   (1) Increased pressure edema (usually caused by cardiac failure): goal is to reduce the hydrostatic pressure.
   (2) Treatment measures may include:
      (a) Upright (high Fowler's) position
      (b) Antianxiety (morphine, a vasodilator)
      (c) Maintenance of satisfactory oxygenation
         (i)   Supplemental oxygen therapy
         (ii) CPAP and positive end-expiratory pressure (PEEP)
      (d) Decrease venous return (vasodilators).
      (e) Improve cardiac output (positive inotropics).
      (f) Diuresis
   (3) Increased permeability edema
      (a) Decrease edema accumulation.
         (i)   Ensure lowest possible pulmonary microvascular pressure.
         (ii) Reduce vascular volume.
      (b) Identify infection and treat.
      (c) Supportive therapy
         (i)   Administer oxygen.
         (ii) Lung protection ventilation strategy
         (iii) Optimize blood pressure and cardiac output.
      (d) Avoid:
         (i)   Hypotension
         (ii) Volume overload
         (iii) Infection

2. Pulmonary thromboembolism
  a. An obstruction of the pulmonary artery or one of its branches
  b. May be secondary to:
    (1) Amniotic fluid
    (2) Long bone fractures
    (3) More commonly a result of venous thrombosis
  c. Signs and symptoms
    (1) Isolated dyspnea—sudden onset
    (2) Unexplained tachypnea (respiratory rate >20 breaths/min)
    (3) Reflex bronchoconstriction
    (4) Pulmonary edema
    (5) Pleuritic pain
    (6) Hemoptysis
    (7) Right ventricular dysfunction
       (a) Bulging neck veins
       (b) Increased central venous pressure
       (c) Right ventricular hypokinesis
       (d) Accentuated pulmonic component of the second heart sound
    (8) Circulatory collapse

    d. Diagnostic tests
      (1) D-dimer test
      (2) Ultrasound
      (3) CT
      (4) V/Q scans
      (5) Pulmonary angiography
    e. Treatment
      (1) Heparin: administered initially via continuous infusion to maintain a target activated partial thromboplastin time ratio of 2.0 to 3
      (2) Inotropes (e.g., dopamine, dobutamine) to manage low–cardiac output states
      (3) Supplemental oxygen therapy to alleviate the hypoxic pulmonary vasoconstriction
      (4) Endotracheal intubation and mechanical ventilation with PEEP as needed for oxygenation
      (5) Analgesics may be required to treat pleuritic pain.
      (6) Inferior vena cava filters
      (7) Emergent pulmonary artery embolectomy with cardiopulmonary bypass for massive emboli may be required.

D. Malignant diseases
  1. Ninety percent of cases are symptomatic and advanced when diagnosed.
  2. Obstruction or compression of structures such as bronchi, blood vessels, and nerves are responsible for symptoms.
  3. Symptoms include:
    a. Cough
    b. Hoarseness
    c. Chest pain
    d. Dyspnea
  4. Systemic symptoms are:
    a. Fatigue
    b. Fever
    c. Anorexia
    d. Weight loss
    e. Malaise
  5. Lung cancer
    a. Leading cause of cancer death worldwide (28% of all cancer deaths)
    b. Cigarette smoking is the primary cause of lung cancer (90% of total deaths).
    c. Squamous cell carcinoma
      (1) Approximately 30% of all lung cancers
      (2) Characteristic development is centrally in major segmental bronchi with extension to lobar and mainstem bronchus.
      (3) Associated with the most favorable prognosis since this tumor is more amenable to resection
      (4) Lymph nodes should be examined, either by mediastinoscopy or by dissecting and sampling during the operation, to stage the disease.
      (5) Lobectomy or pneumonectomy are recommended whenever possible.
      (6) Limited lung resection may be more appropriate in the patient with compromised pulmonary status.
    d. Adenocarcinoma
      (1) Approximately 35% of all lung cancers
      (2) Characteristic development in peripheral parenchyma and is asymptomatic until mass becomes large; frequently metastasizes before becoming apparent.
      (3) Lymph nodes should be examined, either by mediastinoscopy or by dissecting and sampling during the operation, to stage the disease.
      (4) Lobectomy or pneumonectomy are recommended whenever possible.
      (5) Limited lung resection may be more appropriate in the patient with compromised pulmonary status.

  e. Large cell carcinoma
   (1) Accounts for 9% of all lung carcinomas
   (2) Characteristic rapid growth in lung periphery
   (3) Lymph nodes should be examined, either by mediastinoscopy
       or by dissecting and sampling during the operation, to stage the
       disease.
   (4) Lobectomy or pneumonectomy are recommended whenever possible.
   (5) Limited lung resection may be more appropriate in the patient with
       compromised pulmonary status.
  f. Small cell lung carcinoma (SCLC)
   (1) Twenty percent of all lung cancers; incidence would be reduced 80% if
       exposure to tobacco smoke were eliminated.
   (2) Characteristic endobronchial lesion in chronic cigarette smokers with
       hilar enlargement and disseminated disease
   (3) Two recognized subtypes
       (a) Pure SCLC: accounts for 90% of SCLC cases
       (b) Combined SCLS, with a mixture of any non–small cell type; occurs
           in fewer than 10% of cases
   (4) Often metastases to brain, liver, bone, bone marrow, and adrenal gland
       at diagnosis
   (5) Rarely amenable to surgical resection since typically widely
       disseminated at the time of presentation; early-stage solitary tumors
       without metastases may be treated with surgical resection.
  g. Bronchial carcinoid tumor
   (1) One to 2% of all invasive lung malignancies; frequently is invasive and
       metastasizes.
   (2) Characteristic central tracheobronchial tree location
   (3) Treatment is surgical resection. Typical carcinoid has excellent
       prognosis, with the 5-year survival between 60% and 80%.
  h. Metastatic tumor
   (1) Malignant tumors with pulmonary metastases are common and occur
       in 30% to 40% of patients with cancer.
   (2) The majority of adults presenting with pulmonary metastases do not
       have curable cancers, and palliative therapy is suitable.
   (3) Medical management for selected cancers may consist of:
       (a) Chemotherapy
       (b) Radiation therapy
       (c) Hormonal therapy
       (d) Immunological therapies
   (4) Surgical resection of the pulmonary metastases may be indicated if:
       (a) The tumor's primary site has been controlled.
       (b) The patient's physical status is such that he or she can tolerate the
           surgery.
       (c) No metastases to other sites
       (d) No radiological proof that the tumor is unresectable
6. Pleural tumors
  a. Main primary tumors involving the pleura are malignant
     mesotheliomas.
  b. Asbestos exposure accounts for most cases of malignant
     mesothelioma.
  c. Primary attempts at curing malignant mesothelioma involve surgery
     (extrapleural pneumonectomy) along with chemotherapy and
     radiotherapy.
7. Esophageal tumors
  a. Squamous cell
  b. Adenocarcinoma

8. Mediastinal tumors
   a. Common nonthoracic cancers that metastasize to the mediastinum include tumors arising from the skin (malignant melanoma), breast, genitourinary tract, and the head and neck.
   b. Tissue sampling techniques may include:
      (1) Transbronchial needle aspiration
      (2) Suprasternal mediastinoscopy
      (3) Anterior mediastinotomy
   c. The majority of mediastinal tumors must be surgically removed whether they are benign or malignant.
   d. Neurogenic tumors (20% of adults; 40% of children) are mostly benign and asymptomatic in adults, but in children, most are malignant and symptomatic.
   e. Thymoma: the most common mediastinal neoplasm is managed by surgical resection. Up to 50% of all thymomas are associated with myasthenia gravis.
   f. Germ cell tumors account for 10% to 12% of mediastinal tumors and are classified as either:
      (1) Teratoma and teratocarcinoma
      (2) Seminoma
      (3) Embryonal cell carcinoma
      (4) Choriocarcinoma
   g. Lymphoma: 10% to 20% of mediastinal masses are lymphomas occurring from:
      (1) Hodgkin's disease
      (2) Non-Hodgkin's lymphoma
      (3) Human immunodeficiency virus–infected patients
      (4) Anterior thoracotomy or mediastinoscopy are indicted to make the diagnosis, but surgical resection is typically not part of the therapy.

IV. PULMONARY DIAGNOSTIC AND SURGICAL PROCEDURES
   A. Patient management
      1. Premedication
         a. Sedation: given as needed to allay anxiety
            (1) Diazepam, 5 mg orally in the adult, may be supplemented with incremental intravenous midazolam.
            (2) Opioids are typically avoided because they may impair ventilatory reflexes and spontaneous deep breathing.
         b. Antisialagogue: glycopyrrolate, 0.2 mg intravenously, adult dose; may be given to decrease oral secretions
      2. Intraprocedural/intraoperative care
         a. Monitoring
            (1) Circulatory
               (a) ECG to monitor heart rate, rhythm, and ischemia, using simultaneous leads II and V_5.
               (b) Blood pressure cuff
               (c) Arterial line, if frequent determinations of ABGs, one-lung ventilation, or serious cardiac problems are anticipated.
               (d) Central venous pressure monitoring, only when there is documented:
                  (i)   Left ventricular dysfunction
                  (ii) Severe pulmonary hypertension
                  (iii) Cor pulmonale
               (e) Intake and output
               (f) Capillary refill
            (2) Respiratory
               (a) Esophageal stethoscope or precordial stethoscope over the dependant lung
               (b) Inspired oxygen concentration
               (c) End-tidal CO_2

  (d) ABG analysis, when indicated
  (e) Peak airway pressure
  (f) Pulse oximetry
  (3) Temperature: esophageal temperature probes inaccurate when the chest is open
  (4) Urine output: to evaluate circulatory and renal function
  (5) Neuromuscular blockade by peripheral nerve stimulator
b. Anesthesia: general anesthesia in combination with epidural anesthesia is the preferred technique for major thoracic surgery.
c. Airway adjuncts and management
  (1) Oropharyngeal airways
    (a) Indications
      (i) To treat supraglottic soft-tissue airway obstruction (e.g., relaxation of the soft palate, pharyngeal walls, or tongue) in patients without a patent gag reflex
      (ii) To prevent the patient from biting down and obstructing an endotracheal tube or laryngeal mask airway (LMA)
    (b) Contraindications
      (i) In the semiconscious patient, coughing, gagging, vomiting, or laryngospasm may be triggered from the oropharyngeal airway.
      (ii) Caution should be exercised in patients with extremely poor dentition or friable oropharyngeal tissue.
    (c) Technique of insertion
      (i) Sizing: an external landmark for estimating the proper length includes placing the airway along the cheek and measuring the distance from the corner of the mouth to the tragus of the ear.
      (ii) Insert right side up (consider using a tongue blade to assist with displacing the tongue) or upside down and then rotate 180° into the proper position.
      (iii) Avoid trauma to the teeth, and confirm the tongue or lips are not sandwiched between the airway and teeth.
      (iv) Ensure that the tongue is not displaced back into the pharynx to contribute to further obstruction.
  (2) Nasopharyngeal airways
    (a) Indications
      (i) A temporary method to treat supraglottic soft-tissue airway obstruction (e.g., relaxation of the soft palate, pharyngeal walls, or tongue)
      (ii) Appropriate in the patient with upper airway obstruction who exhibits a clenched jaw, mouth trauma, tongue abnormality, or tooth pathology
      (iii) A nasopharyngeal airway is less stimulating and better tolerated in the semiconscious patient than the oropharyngeal airway.
      (iv) In patients with persistent upper airway obstruction, consider using both oropharyngeal and nasopharyngeal airways together.
    (b) Contraindications
      (i) Avoid the nasopharyngeal airway after tonsillectomy, adenoidectomy, or cleft palate repair.
      (ii) Insertion of the airway into the cranial vault may occur after basilar skull fracture.
      (iii) Use with caution in patients with coagulopathy or nasal deformities because nasal hemorrhage may result.
    (c) Technique of insertion
      (i) Use the larger nostril for airway insertion.
      (ii) Sizing: distal tip of the nasopharyngeal airway should rest just above the open epiglottis.

[a] An external landmark for estimating the proper length includes having the proximal end positioned at the nares and the distal tip placed at the tragus of the ear.

(iii) Consider spraying a nasal vasoconstrictive agent (e.g., oxymetazoline) if appropriate.

[a] Laryngospasm may be a possibility should the liquid stimulate the vocal cords in the semiconscious patient.

(iv) Lubricate the airway with a water-soluble lubricant (i.e., lidocaine gel) if the patient is awake.

(v) When inserting, point the bevel medially to prevent trauma to the turbinates.

(vi) Advance the airway posteriorly (not upward toward the cribriform plate), parallel to the hard palate and beneath the inferior turbinate.

(vii) If significant resistance is encountered, withdraw, rotate 90°, and readvance with gentle, steady pressure.

(viii) Ease difficult passage by using a soft-suction catheter as an introducer.

[a] A flared proximal end or adjustable disk may be used to limit insertion depth.

(3) LMA

(a) Indications

(i) Substitute for face mask or endotracheal tube during elective anesthesia in the spontaneously breathing patient. The LMA is effective and safe for positive pressure ventilation in patients with normal compliance and airway resistance using normal tidal volumes.

(ii) Difficult ventilation: to improve a difficult airway seal without endotracheal intubation as with the bearded or edentulous patient

(iii) Difficult laryngoscopy: as an aide to endotracheal intubation (i.e., with the intubating LMA [LMA-Fastrach])

(iv) Emergency ventilation when cannot-intubate, cannot-ventilate scenario presents

(b) Contraindications

(i) Patients with pharyngeal pathology interfering with its placement

(ii) Patients with glottic or subglottic airway obstruction

(iii) Extremely limited mouth opening (<1.5 mm) or neck extension

(iv) When access to the airway is compromised (e.g., prone surgery)

(v) With low pulmonary compliance or high airway resistance (if peak airway pressures >20 cm H_2O)

(vi) Presence of increased risk of regurgitation

[a] Morbid obesity

[b] Pregnancy

[c] Insufficient fasting interval

[d] Hiatal hernia

[e] Intestinal obstruction

(c) Technique of insertion

(i) Use the largest size that will comfortably fit in the oral cavity.

[a] For adult female: #3 or #4

[b] For adult male: #4 or #5

(ii) LMA insertion (Figure 31-4)

(iii) After placement, the LMA cuff should be inflated with the minimal volume of air required to achieve an adequate seal. Most practitioners commonly inflate the cuff with more volume.

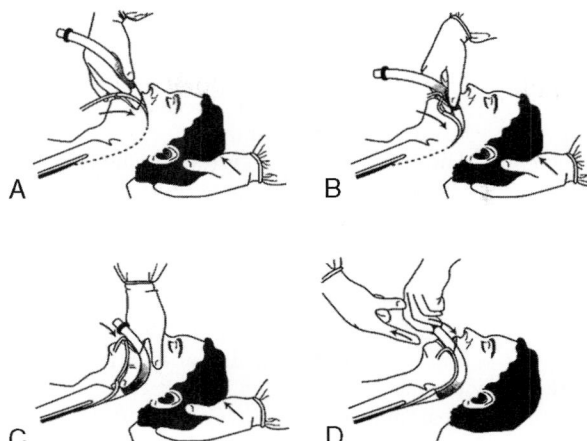

A

B

C

D

FIGURE 31-4 ■ Insertion technique for the laryngeal mask airway (LMA). **A,** With the head extended and the neck flexed, carefully flatten the LMA tip against the hard palate. To facilitate LMA introduction into the oral cavity, gently press the middle finger down on the jaw. **B,** The index finger pushes the LMA in a cranial direction following the contours of the hard and soft palates. **C,** Maintaining pressure with the finger on the tube in the cranial direction, advance the mask until definite resistance is felt at the base of the hypopharynx. Note the flexion of the wrist. **D,** Gently maintain cranial pressure with the nondominant hand while removing the index finger. (From LMA North America Inc, San Diego, CA.)

      [a] 20 mL for #3
      [b] 30 mL for #4
      [c] 40 mL for #5
  (d) Removal of the LMA
      (i)   LMA should be removed in the supine or lateral position, with the patient deeply anesthetized or awake, but not at a halfway stage. Consideration should be given to removing the LMA with the patient awake in cases where difficult mask ventilation is anticipated.
      (ii)   If suction is required around the oral cavity or down the airway tube, it should be carried out before recovery of reflexes. Suctioning and physical stimulation may provoke laryngeal spasm if anesthesia is light.
      (iii) Leave the patient undisturbed until reflexes are restored, except to administer oxygen and perform monitoring procedures.
      (iv) Watch for signs of swallowing. It is usually safe and convenient to remove adhesive tape when swallowing begins.
      (v)   Deflate (or partially deflate the cuff to assist with secretion removal that accumulated above the device) the cuff and simultaneously remove the device only when the patient can open the mouth on command. If the cuff is deflated before the return of effective swallowing and cough reflexes, secretions in the upper pharynx may enter the larynx, provoking coughing or laryngeal spasm. Verify airway patency and respiratory depth.
  (4) Support of the nonintubated airway. Airway maneuvers may be required to open an obstructed upper airway in the spontaneously breathing patient or to assist with ventilation in the patient not maintaining adequate minute ventilation.
    (a) Manual maneuver to open the airway: the goal is to lift the tongue away from the back wall of the pharynx, thus opening an obstructed airway.

    (i)   Head tilt–chin lift
        [a] Tilt the head back on the atlanto-occipital joint while keeping the teeth approximated by placing the edge of one hand on the patient's forehead and two fingers of the other hand under the chin.
        [b] The chin is lifted up while the head is tilted backward. Pressure on the submandibular soft tissue should be avoided because it can cause airway obstruction.
        [c] Consider placing the adult patient in the "sniffing" position by elevating the head 1 to 4 inches above the level of the shoulders.
        [d] Avoid the head tilt in patients with suspected neck injury and in patients with Down syndrome.

    (ii) Jaw thrust
        [a] Designed to open the airway while maintaining a neutral position in patients with suspected neck injury
        [b] The teeth will have to be slightly opened to allow the mandibular teeth freedom to slide over the maxillary teeth as the mandible subluxes forward.
        [c] The mandible is grasped bilaterally with the fingertips and lifted forward.

(b) Two-handed mask ventilation: assisted ventilation will be required in the patient unable to maintain sufficient gas exchange.
    (i)   Effective two-person mask technique allows the most skilled provider to perform a two-handed mask seal with jaw thrust, while the second rescuer uses one hand to enhance mask seal and the second hand to squeeze the bag.
    (ii) Select the appropriate size mask covering from above the nose to below the lower lip that allows a good seal between the mask and the patient's face; apply pressure to the mask sides with the thumb sides of the palms of both hands.
    (iii) Use the head tilt–chin lift or jaw thrust to open the airway; insert an oropharyngeal or nasopharyngeal airway as indicated; keep the mouth open if an airway is not used.
    (iv) Interface the mask with a self-inflating bag connected with an oxygen source; a second rescuer should initiate manual ventilation with a tidal volume approximating 10 to 15 mL/kg over 1 to 2 seconds.
    (v) Cricoid pressure should be applied in the patient at risk for pulmonary aspiration of gastric contents.

(5) Endotracheal intubation
  (a) Indications
    (i)   Ensure an unobstructed airway.
    (ii) Protect patient's airway from pulmonary aspiration of gastric contents.
    (iii) To facilitate mechanical ventilation
    (iv) To enable suctioning of pulmonary secretions
    (v) Provide conduit for medication delivery.
    (vi) If it is feared that ventilation and intubation may later become impossible (i.e., acute epiglottitis)
    (vii) Airway adjunct for general anesthesia
        [a] Thoracoabdominal surgery
        [b] Remote access to the head
        [c] Airway surgery in which secretions or blood might contaminate the trachea
  (b) Complications
    (i)   Suture lines may be disrupted if the patient coughs or strains on the tube.

(ii) Postextubation laryngeal edema

(iii) Postobstructive pulmonary edema

(iv) Tachycardia, hypertension

(v) Bronchospasm in susceptible patients

(vi) Hoarseness, pharyngitis

(c) Technique of insertion

    (i) Equipment for laryngoscopy

        [a] Oxygen source and self-inflating bag

        [b] Pharmacological agents for induction of anesthesia and muscle relaxation as necessary (i.e., hypnotic agent and muscle relaxant)

        [c] Face mask in various sizes

        [d] Oropharyngeal and nasopharyngeal airways in various sizes along with tongue blades and lubricant

        [e] Endotracheal tubes (ETT) in various sizes

        [f] Endotracheal tube stylet

        [g] Intubating (Magill) forceps

        [h] Syringe (i.e., 10 mL) for endotracheal tube cuff inflation

        [i] Suction apparatus with tonsil tip suction catheter (i.e., Yankauer)

        [j] Two laryngoscope handles with fresh batteries

        [k] Laryngoscope blades in various sizes: common blades include the curved (Macintosh) and straight (Miller)

        [l] Pillow, towel, blanket, or foam pad for head positioning

        [m] Monitoring equipment: ECG, pulse oximeter, blood pressure, and stethoscope.

        [n] Means to detect exhaled carbon dioxide to confirm proper endotracheal tube placement in the trachea

    (ii) Procedure for direct laryngoscopy

        [a] Secure intravenous access.

        [b] Assess the airway to determine anticipated ease of intubation.

        [c] Position patient, as tolerated, in the "sniff" or rapid airway management position (RAMP) to aid with aligning the axis of the airway.

        [d] Preoxygenate and denitrogenate the patient by having the patient breathe 100% oxygen via a tight-fitting face mask before induction, as appropriate.

        [e] Administer hypnotic agent (i.e., propofol, etomidate) as appropriate.

        [f] Apply cricoid pressure if the patient is at risk for pulmonary aspiration of gastric contents.

        [g] Administer muscle relaxant (i.e., rocuronium, succinylcholine) as appropriate once patient loses consciousness. Confirm relaxed state with peripheral nerve stimulator.

        [h] Open mouth using fingers or head extension.

        [i] Insert laryngoscope blade and sweep tongue to the left side of mouth.

        [j] Position laryngoscope blade in appropriate position (curved blade in vallecula; straight blade under epiglottis) and lift up and away to expose glottic opening.

        [k] Consider laryngeal manipulation (i.e., optimal external laryngeal manipulation), by an assistant to improve the view.

        [l] Place the ETT through the glottic opening an appropriate distance (i.e., 3–4 cm in the adult) into the trachea.

        [m] Inflate the ETT cuff.

[n] Connect the self-inflating bag and initiate ventilation.

[o] Confirm proper tube positioning by presence of exhaled carbon dioxide, visually observing the chest rise, and bilateral breath sounds confirmed via auscultation in the midaxillary region.

(6) Double-lumen ETT/bronchial blocker considerations

(a) During thoracic surgery, use either a double-lumen ETT or a bronchial blocker (a single-lumen tube with a built-in advanceable balloon to occlude the operative side main bronchus). At the appropriate time, the operative lung is separated from the nonoperative lung, and the nonoperative lung continues to be ventilated while the surgical lung is not.

(b) After surgery, the double-lumen ETT is exchanged, when possible, for a conventional single-lumen tube if the patient is to remain intubated. A single-lumen tube is preferred, as the double-lumen ETT causes more laryngeal trauma the longer it remains in place, and weaning is more difficult.

(7) The difficult airway

(a) Difficulty in endotracheal intubation is encountered in 1% to 4% of attempts, depending on the skill of the intubator.

(b) Failed intubation is encountered approximately 0.05% to 0.35% of time.

(c) The "can't intubate and can't ventilate" rate is 0.0001% to 0.02%.

(d) Several algorithms have been designed to facilitate the management of the difficult airway to minimize adverse outcomes (Figures 31-5 through 31-8). Familiarization with details of how to proceed when faced with a difficult airway is best learned before the experience.

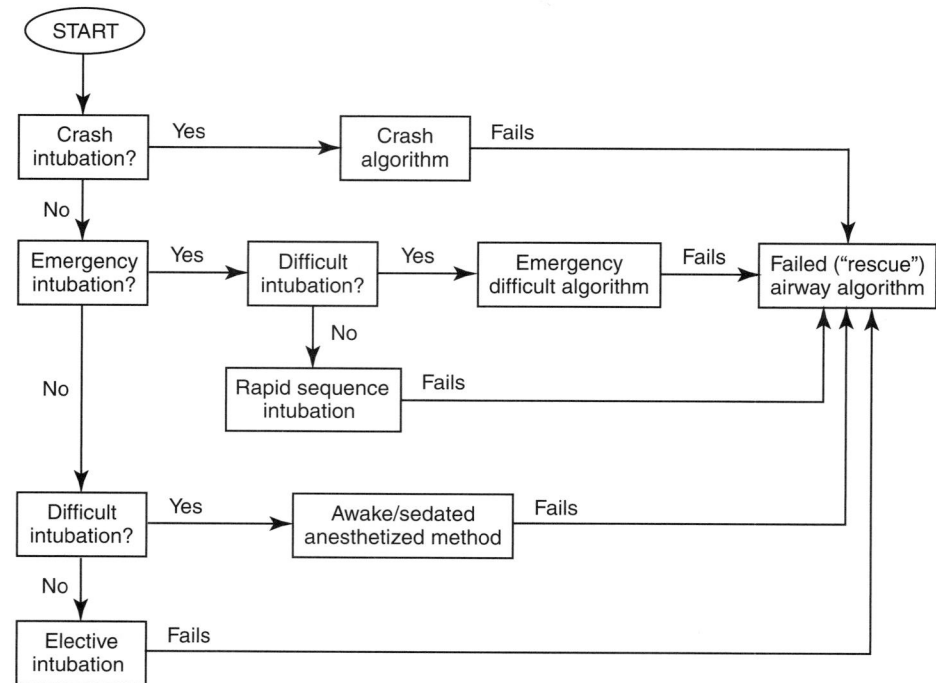

FIGURE 31-5 ■ Airway management overview. (From Murphy MF, Crosby ET: The algorithms. In Hung O, Murphy MF, eds: *Management of the difficult and failed airway,* New York, 2008, McGraw-Hill.)

    d. Positioning: supine for mediastinoscopy; typically lateral decubitus for thoracotomy or thoracoscopy

       (1) Circulatory effects of lateral decubitus

          (a) Pooling of blood can produce decreased venous return and fall in cardiac output.

          (b) Hyperabduction of the up-side arm, as might occur when the arm is suspended from the armrest, has resulted in peripheral gangrene.

       (2) Respiratory effects of lateral decubitus: mechanical interference with chest movement and thus limitation of lung expansion; most common long-term respiratory complication of lateral decubitus position is atelectasis.

       (3) Neurological effects of lateral decubitus: care must be exercised while positioning the patient to prevent injury to the brachial plexus and its peripheral branches, the long thoracic nerve, and nerves of the lower extremity (common peroneal nerve, sciatic nerve).

    e. One-lung ventilation: placement of a double-lumen endobronchial tube or bronchial blocker ETT is indicated for lung isolation.

       (1) Absolute indications for lung isolation

          (a) Isolate one lung from the other to avoid spillage or contamination (e.g., infection or massive hemorrhage).

          (b) Control the distribution of ventilation.

             (i) Bronchopleural fistula

             (ii) Bronchopleural cutaneous fistula

             (iii) Surgical opening of a major conducting airway

             (iv) Giant unilateral lung cyst or bulla

             (v) Tracheobronchial tree disruption

             (vi) Life-threatening hypoxemia related to unilateral lung disease

          (c) Unilateral bronchopulmonary lavage (pulmonary alveolar proteinosis)

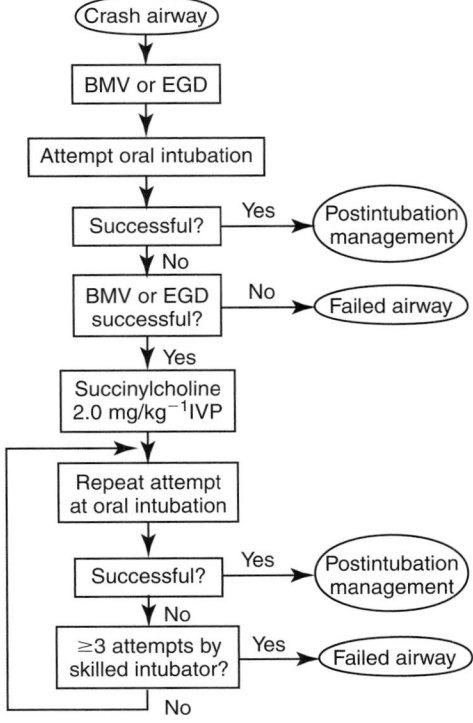

FIGURE 31-6 ■ Crash airway algorithm. *BMV*, Bag-mask ventilation; *EGD*, extraglottic device; *IVP*, intravenous push. (From Murphy MF, Crosby ET: The algorithms. In Hung O, Murphy MF, eds: *Management of the difficult and failed airway*, New York, 2008, McGraw-Hill.)

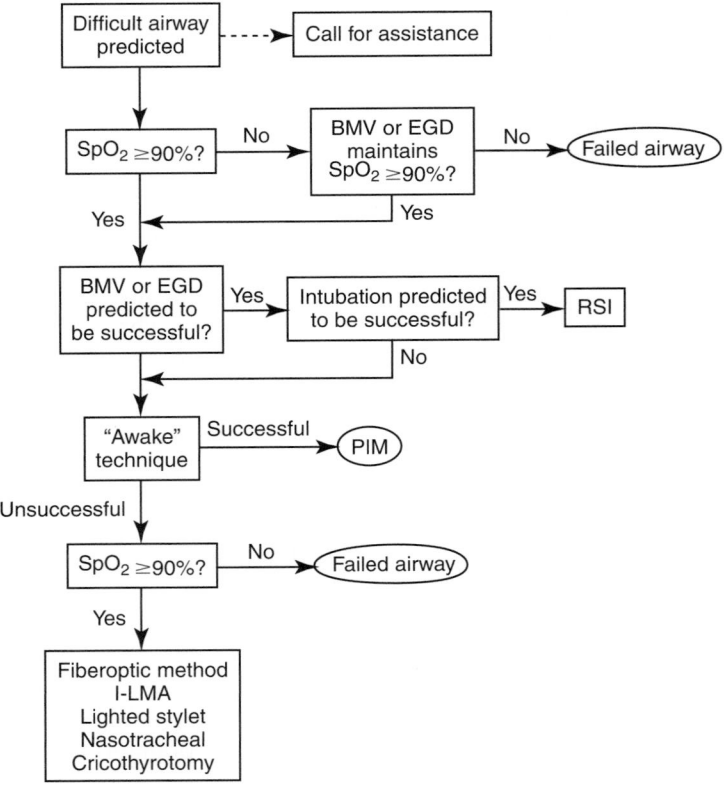

FIGURE 31-7 ■ The emergency difficult airway algorithm. *Spo₂*, Oxyhemoglobin saturation derived via pulse oximetry; *BMV*, bag-mask ventilation; *EGD*, extraglottic device; *RSI*, rapid sequence induction; *PIM*, postintubation management; *I-LMA*, intubating laryngeal mask airway. (From Murphy MF, Crosby ET: The algorithms. In Hung O, Murphy MF, eds: *Management of the difficult and failed airway,* New York, 2008, McGraw-Hill.)

(2) Relative indication for lung isolation
    (a) Facilitation of surgical exposure (high priority) for:
        (i) Thoracic aortic aneurysm
        (ii) Pneumonectomy
        (iii) Upper lobectomy
        (iv) Mediastinal exposure
        (v) Thoracoscopy
        (vi) Traumatic pulmonary hemorrhage
        (vii) Pulmonary resection via median sternotomy
    (b) Facilitation of surgical exposure (low priority) for:
        (i) Esophageal resection
        (ii) Middle and lower lobectomies
        (iii) Segmental resection
        (iv) Procedures on the thoracic spine
(3) Special considerations
    (a) Hypoxemia is a common occurrence when one-lung ventilation is used; thus patients are ventilated with 100% oxygen during this time.
    (b) If the patient cannot be extubated at the end of surgery, the double-lumen tube will be exchanged for a conventional ETT.
  f. Special intraoperative considerations
    (1) Blood loss is usually modest but can be substantial in situations of previous thoracotomy, chronic infection, and extrapleural pneumonectomy (for tuberculous disease and mesothelioma).

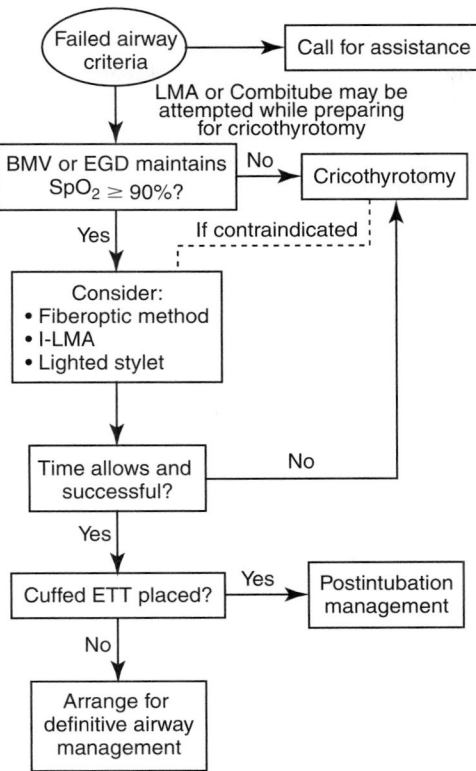

FIGURE 31-8 ■ Failed airway algorithm. *Spo₂*, Oxyhemoglobin saturation derived via pulse oximetry; *BMV*, bag-mask ventilation; *EGD*, extraglottic device; *I-LMA*, intubating laryngeal mask airway; *ETT*, endotracheal tube. (From Murphy MF, Crosby ET: The algorithms. In Hung O, Murphy MF, eds: *Management of the difficult and failed airway*, New York, 2008, McGraw-Hill.)

      (2) Chest cavity may be filled with saline while the suture site is subjected to a sustained positive airway pressure of 30 cm H_2O to check for air leak from the site of resection. This maneuver is also beneficial for reexpanding atelectatic regions.

      (3) Chest tube to water seal drainage (typically −20 cm H_2O suction) to drain the pleural cavity and promote lung expansion

      (4) Endotracheal extubation is the goal at the end of surgery.

B. Diagnostic

  1. Bronchoscopy

    a. Indications include:

      (1) Visualizing the airways

      (2) Assessing airway patency

      (3) Removing:

        (a) Abnormal tissue

        (b) Retained secretions

        (c) Mucus plugs

        (d) Foreign bodies

      (4) Evaluating lung lesions of unknown etiology by obtaining samples for:

        (a) Culture

        (b) Cytological study

        (c) Histological examination

      (5) Staging lung cancers

      (6) Bronchoalveolar lavage

      (7) Application of medication or radiopaque medium

      (8) Performance of difficult intubation

     b. Complications
       (1) Airway obstruction
         (a) Laryngospasm
         (b) Bronchospasm
         (c) Glottic or subglottic edema
       (2) Hypoxemia
       (3) Pneumothorax occurs in 5% to 10% of patients after transbronchial lung biopsies.
       (4) Hemorrhage: less than 50 mL blood loss considered normal
       (5) Local anesthetic toxicity
         (a) Numb tongue
         (b) Metallic taste
         (c) Tinnitus
         (d) Irritability
         (e) Confusion
         (f) Bradycardia
         (g) Agitation
         (h) Hypotension
         (i) Seizure activity
       (6) Hemodynamic alterations
         (a) Bradycardia
         (b) Tachycardia
         (c) Hypotension
         (d) Asystole
         (e) Atrial ectopy present in 40% of patients
  2. Mediastinoscopy
     a. Small transverse incision just above the suprasternal notch for visualization or biopsy of tumors or lymph nodes at tracheobronchial junction, subcarina, or upper lobe bronchi
     b. Complications
       (1) Hemorrhage
       (2) Venous air embolism
       (3) Airway, esophageal injury
         (a) Subcutaneous emphysema
         (b) Chest pain
         (c) Pneumothorax
       (4) Recurrent laryngeal nerve injury; hoarseness, vocal cord paralysis
  3. Laryngoscopy
     a. Visualization and/or biopsy of oropharynx, laryngopharynx, larynx, and proximal trachea
     b. Complications
       (1) Include trauma to:
         (a) Upper lip
         (b) Mucous membranes of oropharynx
         (c) Teeth
         (d) Eyes
       (2) Rupture of esophagus
       (3) Hypoxemia
       (4) Laryngospasm
  4. Thoracoscopy
     a. Visualization within pleural cavity to allow diagnosis of variety of pulmonary diseases and conditions
     b. Able to perform variety of procedures
       (1) Decortication of hemothorax and empyema
       (2) Blebectomy and bullectomy for spontaneous or secondary pneumothorax with persistent air leak
       (3) Lung volume reduction
       (4) Pleurectomy or pleurodesis

(5) Biopsy and excision of mediastinal lesions

(6) Pulmonary resection for bronchogenic carcinoma

(7) Drainage of pleural effusion and pericardial effusion

(8) Sympathectomies

(9) Vagotomies

(10) Thymectomies

  c. Advantage

    (1) Minimize incision pain.

    (2) Loss of muscle function

5. Percutaneous needle aspiration

  a. Used for the diagnosis of infectious and malignant diseases, often under the guidance of CT scanning or ultrasonography

  b. Complications

    (1) Tension pneumothorax

    (2) Endobronchial hemorrhage

    (3) Air embolism

6. Scalene node biopsy

  a. Positive biopsy indicates extramediastinal tumor involvement.

  b. Complications—injury to the:

    (1) Great vessels

      (a) Internal jugular

      (b) Subclavian veins

    (2) Phrenic nerve

    (3) Thoracic duct on left

    (4) Lymphatic structure on right

C. Therapeutic

1. Repair of pectus excavatum (funnel chest) or carinatum (pigeon breast): principally a cosmetic procedure to improve contour and body image of the sternum and lower costal cartilages

2. Chest wall reconstruction: removal of portions of the thoracic cage may be required, most commonly for lung cancer that has invaded the chest wall or radiation necrosis; wide skin flaps may be required to achieve adequate closure.

  a. Complication: flap ischemia—assessment of tissue perfusion every hour, including color, temperature, and flap turgor

3. Thoracoplasty: removal of several ribs or portions of ribs to obliterate an existing pleural space (i.e., empyema) or to collapse a portion of diseased lung

4. Decortication with pleurodesis

  a. Thoracoscopy is primarily performed to remove all fibrous tissue and pus from pleural space.

  b. Pleural sepsis is eliminated, and underlying lung is allowed to expand.

  c. This pleural thickening may develop secondary to empyema, blood, or fluid in pleural space.

5. Open window thoracostomy: surgical creation of an opening in the chest

  a. Involves resection of ribs to allow for drainage and irrigation of postpneumonectomy empyema

  b. Opening may be closed surgically at completion of empyema treatment.

6. Wedge resection of lung lesion: removal of a lung mass including 1-cm margins in a manner that does not remove an entire anatomic pulmonary segment

7. Segmentectomy: excision of individual bronchoalveolar segments of a lobe of lung; can be done if peripheral lesion is present without chest wall involvement

8. Lobectomy: excision of a lobe of the lung

9. Pneumonectomy: excision of either right or left lung

  a. Right pneumonectomy removes 55% of vascular bed and breathing capacity, so it is tolerated less well than left pneumonectomy.

    b. Chest tube may be clamped after surgery to allow serosanguineous effusion to fill hemithorax.
      (1) If bleeding is suspected, chest film is obtained to ascertain fluid level in chest.
      (2) Assess for tracheal deviation to ascertain excessive pressure in hemithorax.
    c. Volume overload: extremely sensitive to volume administration
      (1) Monitor for signs and symptoms of congestive heart failure.
        (a) Crackles
        (b) Tachypnea
        (c) Dyspnea
        (d) Hypoxemia
        (e) Increased filling pressure
    d. Phrenic nerve may be severed on operative side to elevate hemidiaphragm.
    e. Pericardium may be opened during procedure.
      (1) Ascertain whether pericardial closure was performed.
      (2) Check with surgeon regarding positioning restrictions.
      (3) Monitor for signs of cardiac herniation (acute cardiovascular compromise).
10. Sleeve resection: removal of tracheobronchial tree and associated lung segment or lobe and reattachment of remaining lung tissue; sleeve pneumonectomy may also be performed.
11. Lung volume reduction surgery
    a. Palliative surgery for patients with end-stage COPD involving removal of emphysematous lung tissue
    b. Procedure relieves pressure and increases expansion of functional lung tissue.
    c. Increases thoracic expansion and improves respiratory mechanics and gas exchange
    d. Unilateral or bilateral and usually requires multiple chest tubes
12. Lung transplant: removal of recipient lung and replacement with donor lung; most common reason for a single-lung transplant is end-stage emphysema.
13. Thymectomy: performed via a median sternotomy; treatment of choice for myasthenia gravis
    a. Preoperative pulmonary function testing may be done.
    b. Avoid or limit muscle relaxant during surgery. Patients with myasthenia gravis are usually:
      (1) Resistant to succinylcholine (larger intubating doses may be required)
      (2) Sensitive to nondepolarizing muscle relaxants (titrate with use of peripheral nerve stimulator)
    c. Avoid drugs or conditions that potentiate neuromuscular blockade.
      (1) Metabolic acidosis
      (2) Aminoglycoside antibiotics
      (3) Calcium channel blockers
      (4) Magnesium
      (5) Lithium
      (6) Hypothermia
      (7) Serum potassium disturbances
    d. Neurologist may help to determine time to restart anticholinesterase drugs.
    e. Complications
      (1) Ineffective breathing pattern
      (2) Ineffective airway clearance
      (3) Myasthenic, cholinergic crisis
      (4) Phrenic nerve injury
      (5) Bleeding: innominate, internal mammary artery

V. POSTANESTHESIA RESPIRATORY CARE

   A. PACU admission assessment (see Chapter 50)

      1. Before the PACU nurse accepts responsibility for the nursing care of the patient, the patient's condition will be reevaluated and a report will be given per the anesthesia care provider and OR circulating nurse.

      2. American Society of PeriAnesthesia Nurses (ASPAN) standards and guidelines for PACU admission will be followed (see Chapter 2).

      3. Initial report will include:

         a. Intraoperative vital sign trends

         b. Pertinent surgical and medical history

         c. Anesthetic medications and other medications administered intraoperatively

            (1) Beta-blockers

            (2) Insulin

            (3) Local anesthetics

            (4) Antibiotics

         d. Special intraoperative events

         e. Intraoperative intake and output

         f. Epidural/intrathecal dermatome anesthesia level: patients who have received a central neuraxial block with local anesthesia will be assessed bilaterally.

         g. Airway support measures

         h. Supplemental oxygen therapy requirements

         i. Vital signs, cardiac rhythm, continual pulse oximetry, ventilation assessment (e.g., end-tidal carbon dioxide).

         j. Location and type of dressings, tubes, and drains, including chest tube location (i.e., mediastinal or pleural)

         k. Intravenous infusions and invasive monitoring

         l. Chest radiograph to verify:

            (1) Chest tube positioning

            (2) Resolution of pneumothorax

            (3) Presence of hemothorax

            (4) Position of endotracheal tube or central intravenous line if present

         m. Intraoperative laboratory results

      4. Physical assessment

         a. Inspection

            (1) Airway patency and presence of artificial airways

            (2) General condition

               (a) Level of consciousness

               (b) Confusion, restlessness, or anxiety, consider:

                  (i)　Hypoxemia

                  (ii)　Hypercapnia

                  (iii)　Medication

                  (iv)　Hemodynamic stability

                  (v)　Pain

                  (vi)　Distended bladder

            (3) Respiratory rate

               (a) Tachypnea

                  (i)　Hypoxemia

                  (ii)　Hypercapnia

                  (iii)　Acidosis

                  (iv)　Fever

                  (v)　Pain

                  (vi)　Anxiety

               (b) Bradypnea

                  (i)　Hypercapnia

                  (ii)　Residual anesthetic effect

                  (iii)　Opioid effect

                  (iv)　Increased intracranial pressure

(4) Ventilatory rhythm and pattern
    (a) Regular
    (b) Cheyne-Stoke's
        (i) Periods of apnea alternating with rhythmic, shallow, progressively deeper and then shallower respirations
    (c) Biot's
        (i) Quick, shallow inspiration followed by regular or irregular periods of apnea
        (ii) May be secondary to stroke, trauma, or uncal or tentorial herniation
    (d) Ataxic respirations
        (i) Similar to Biot's but pattern of respiration and apnea completely irregular
        (ii) Usually progresses to complete apnea
    (e) Prolonged expiratory time (i.e., with COPD, bronchospasm)
(5) Depth
    (a) Hypoventilation (with respiratory acidosis) common in early postoperative phase
(6) Chest wall movement
    (a) Decreased: hypoventilation, pain
    (b) Asymmetric
        (i) Atelectasis
        (ii) Pleural effusion
        (iii) Diaphragmatic paralysis
        (iv) Mainstem bronchus endotracheal intubation
        (v) Splinting
        (vi) Hemothorax, pneumothorax
(7) Cyanosis: bluish color of skin and mucous membranes associated with deoxyhemoglobin
    (a) Causes
        (i) Inadequate circulation
        (ii) Pulmonary or cardiac disease or defect
        (iii) Poisoning (i.e., drugs, chemicals)
        (iv) Low-oxygen environment
    (b) Cyanosis is not a reliable sign of hypoxemia; thus if cyanosis is present, Pao_2 should be determined.
    (c) At least 5 g% of deoxyhemoglobin must be present in the blood before cyanosis will appear; therefore it may be:
        (i) Marked in patients with polycythemia
        (ii) Difficult to detect in the anemic patient
(8) Use of accessory muscles, which is indicative of increased work of breathing
    (a) Abdominals
    (b) Sternocleidomastoid
    (c) Scalene
    (d) Pectoralis major
    (e) Trapezius
(9) Nasal flaring: one of the first physiological compensations in infants with impaired oxygenation or ventilation; decreases airway resistance
(10) Retractions secondary to patient's effort to generate more negative pressure to improve ventilation; cardinal sign of respiratory distress in pediatric patient
(11) Grunting: increases end-expiratory pressure; in infants is indicative of respiratory distress
(12) Sputum production: note appearance and amount.
(13) Thoracoabdominal dyscoordination: retraction of abdomen during inspiration; indicates diaphragmatic fatigue and ventilatory failure
b. Palpation
    (1) Chest wall: observe for expansion.
    (2) Trachea

(a) Should be midline
(b) Deviates toward hemithorax with lowest intrathoracic pressure
    (i)   Atelectasis
    (ii) Phrenic nerve paralysis
    (iii) Pneumonia
    (iv) Pneumonectomy
(c) Deviates away from pathological, space-occupying disorders
    (i)   Tension pneumothorax
    (ii) Hemothorax
    (iii) Pleural effusion

(3) Subcutaneous emphysema
(a) Palpable crackling sensation that results from air that has escaped from disrupted alveoli or small bronchi through a breach in the pleura into subcutaneous tissue
(b) Excessive amounts of subcutaneous emphysema may lead to airway obstruction and respiratory compromise.
(c) If the condition appears to be worsening, placement of a chest drain (or an additional one if one is already present) should be considered.
(d) Sources of air leak contributing to subcutaneous emphysema postoperatively include:
    (i)   Pneumothorax
    (ii) Tracheostomy wound
    (iii) Alveolar rupture from barotrauma
    (iv) Tracheobronchial or esophageal injury

(4) Fremitus
(a) Vibratory tremors felt through chest wall
(b) Increased
    (i)   Consolidation
    (ii) Mucus in airways
(c) Decreased
    (i)   Atelectasis
    (ii) Pneumothorax
    (iii) Pneumonectomy
    (iv) COPD
    (v) Pleural effusion
    (vi) Space-occupying mass

c. Auscultation
(1) Potential causes of absent breath sounds
(a) Obstruction
    (i)   Upper airway (e.g., tongue or soft tissue)
    (ii) Kink in endotracheal tube
    (iii) Laryngospasm
    (iv) Foreign body
(b) Secretions
(c) Pneumonectomy
(d) Pleural effusion
(e) Pneumothorax
(f) Mainstem endobronchial intubation
(g) Atelectasis
(2) Diminished vesicular sounds from:
(a) Obesity
(b) Hypoventilation
(c) COPD
(d) Mainstem endobronchial intubation

B. Oxygenation: the patient's ability to normally oxygenate is impaired for several days after pulmonary surgery.
    1. Etiology of postoperative hypoxemia

    a. Alveolar hypoventilation as a result of impaired breathing or increased dead space

    b. Preexisting pulmonary dysfunction

    c. Pain with splinting can make the patient prone to atelectasis.

    d. Loss of lung parenchyma as a result of the surgery

    e. Atelectasis

    f. Decreased wall compliance secondary to surgery

    g. ARDS

    h. Mainstem endobronchial intubation

    i. Low cardiac output states

2. Risk factors for postoperative hypoxemia

    a. Patient age: younger than 1 year and older than 60 years

    b. Hypobaric conditions: high altitudes

    c. Obesity

      (1) Males >120 kg

      (2) Females >100 kg

      (3) High risk for obstructive sleep apnea

      (4) Incidence: middle-aged men (4%) and women (2%)

    d. Cardiopulmonary disease (e.g., preexisting COPD including asthma)

    e. Smoking: once smoking exceeds 8 to 10 pack years

    f. Duration of anesthesia: surgeries lasting more than 1 hour

    g. Type of anesthesia: general anesthesia higher risk than regional techniques

    h. Order of risk by operative site from highest to lowest

      (1) Thoracic

      (2) Upper abdomen

      (3) Lower abdomen

      (4) Neck, extremities, head

    i. Abdominal distention: contributes to atelectasis

    j. Pain: splinting secondary to uncontrolled pain

3. Monitoring oxygenation

    a. Clinical signs of acute hypoxemia

      (1) Respiratory

        (a) Shallow, rapid respirations or normal, infrequent respirations depending upon the etiology

        (b) Tachypnea from carotid body chemoreceptor stimulation and lactic acidosis

        (c) Dyspnea, increased work of breathing

        (d) Oxyhemoglobin saturation <90%

      (2) Neurological

        (a) Anxiety, restlessness, inattentiveness

        (b) Altered mental status, confusion

        (c) Dimmed peripheral vision

        (d) Seizures

        (e) Unconsciousness

      (3) Skin

        (a) Diaphoresis

        (b) Cyanosis

      (4) Cardiac

        (a) Early: tachycardia

          (i)   Increased cardiac output

          (ii) Increased stroke volume

          (iii) Increased blood pressure

        (b) Late: bradycardia, hypotension

        (c) Dysrhythmias

    b. Pulse oximetry

      (1) General principle of operation

(a) Sensor usually placed on distal portion of patient's finger, toe, bridge of nose, or earlobe; consists of light-emitting diodes (LEDs) and a photodetector

(b) LEDs emit two wavelengths of light, red and infrared, which are transmitted through the body part to the photodetector.

    (i) Photodetector determines amount of light absorbed as it passes through the body part.

    (ii) Red light is absorbed by deoxygenated hemoglobin.

    (iii) Infrared light is absorbed by oxyhemoglobin (dyshemoglobins, e.g., carboxyhemoglobin and methemoglobin, are not measured).

    (iv) Pulse oximeter then:

        [a] Calculates the ratio of saturated hemoglobin to total hemoglobin

        [b] Provides a digital readout

(c) Ratio of oxyhemoglobin to total hemoglobin is then expressed in a percent (Spo_2).

(d) Pao_2 can be estimated from the Spo_2 by referring to the oxyhemoglobin dissociation curve (see Figure 31-3).

(2) Indications

  (a) For the continual, noninvasive, and instantaneous Spo_2 determination

  (b) Routine perioperative evaluation of oxygenation

  (c) Evaluate efficacy of changes in supplemental oxygen therapy.

  (d) Monitor perfusion distal to a surgical or traumatic injury site.

(3) Factors influencing the accuracy of pulse oximetry

  (a) Fingernail polish (e.g., blue, green, and black interfere more than purple and red nail polish to produce falsely low readings)

    (i) Clear acrylic nails do not affect Spo_2.

  (b) Venous pulsation (e.g., secondary to tricuspid valve regurgitation or venous engorgement) may yield falsely low readings.

  (c) With deeply pigmented skin, falsely high readings may be recorded or unobtainable.

    (i) The finger probe will be more accurate than the ear probe.

  (d) Exogenous and endogenous dyes (methylene blue greater effect than indocyanine green, which is greater than indigo carmine) will produce falsely low readings.

  (e) Anemia (hematocrit <10%) yields falsely low readings at low oxyhemoglobin values.

  (f) Reduced pulsatile component yields inaccurate, unobtainable, or falsely low readings secondary to:

    (i) Hypotension

    (ii) Vasoconstriction

    (iii) Use of vasoconstrictors

    (iv) Raynaud's disease

    (v) Hypothermia

    (vi) Ear probe more accurate than finger probe in this instance

  (g) Hypoxemia (oxyhemoglobin saturations <75%) can give inaccurately low or high readings.

  (h) Carboxyhemoglobinemia yields falsely high readings.

  (i) Motion artifact yields falsely low readings.

  (j) Methemoglobinemia yields falsely high readings at high oxyhemoglobin saturations and variable readings at low oxyhemoglobin saturations.

  (k) Ambient light may yield falsely low readings.

  (l) Incorrectly fitting probes yield falsely low readings.

c. Arterial blood gas analysis (see Chapter 21)

4. Nursing interventions
   a. Continually monitor oxyhemoglobin saturation.
      (1) Adjust supplemental oxygen therapy to maintain sufficient oxyhemoglobin saturation.
      (2) ABGs as indicated
   b. Positioning: head of bed elevated 30° to 45° or, if needed, to an upright sitting position to facilitate diaphragmatic excursion
      (1) Postpneumonectomy, the patient will be positioned with head of bed elevated, supine, or with the operative side in the dependent position.
   c. Ensure sufficient alveolar ventilation.
      (1) Residual anesthetic agents
         (a) Depress ventilation
         (b) Make patient prone to hypoxemia
      (2) Judicious use of opioids and patient stimulation
   d. Periodic alveolar expansion and lung hyperinflation: measures designed to maintain terminal airway and alveolar patency to minimize the occurrence of microatelectasis
      (1) Encourage cooperative patient to take in a maximal breath and hold for several seconds.
         (a) Repeat four times consecutively.
         (b) Periodically repeat while in the PACU.
      (2) Incentive spirometry every hour
   e. Appropriate pain management to promote effective ventilation
   f. Chest physiotherapy is designed to improve the mobilization of secretions, thus improving the matching of ventilation and perfusion. Physiotherapy incorporates:
      (1) Postural drainage
      (2) Breathing exercises
      (3) Percussion
      (4) Chest compressions
      (5) Using pillow support to the appropriate rib cage location before coughing
   g. CPAP via nasal or full-face mask
      (1) May be considered in the patient with marginal oxygenation in whom reintubation is not desirable
      (2) Should be routinely available for the patient with obstructive sleep apnea who uses this therapy at home
   h. Encourage turning, coughing, and deep breathing (known as Stir-up regimen).
   i. Early ambulation as appropriate
   j. Provide postoperative supplemental oxygen therapy as appropriate; can be anticipated for several days after thoracic surgery.
5. Supplemental oxygen therapy
   a. Humidity and aerosol-generating devices
      (1) Indications
         (a) Humidity therapy involves adding water vapor and sometimes heat to the inspired gas.
         (b) Medical gases are anhydrous, which can:
            (i) Precipitate airway drying
            (ii) Lead to inspissated secretions and mucus plugging
      (2) Humidify dry medical gases.
      (3) Overcome the humidity deficit created when the upper airway is bypassed (i.e., in the intubated patient since the normal mechanism of humidifying inspired gas is bypassed).
      (4) Medication delivery
      (5) Maintain mucous blanket stability.
      (6) Warm humidified inspired gas.
         (a) Accelerates recovery from hypothermia

   (b) Therapeutic for upper airway inflammation
   (c) Blunts reactive airway response to cold inspired gas
   (d) Liquefies and mobilizes tenacious pulmonary secretions
(7) Types of humidifiers
   (a) Note: sterile water should be used to prevent nosocomial infection.
   (b) Bubble diffuser: humidifier diffuses an underwater gas stream into small bubbles to raise the water vapor content of the gas to ambient levels.
      (i) Provides approximately 25% relative humidity at body temperature
      (ii) Used with devices when oxygen flow rates exceed 4 L/min
         [a] Nasal cannula
         [b] Simple face mask
         [c] Partial rebreathing masks
         [d] Loses effectiveness at flow rates >10 L/min
   (c) Cascade: a passover humidifier where gas flows over the surface of a volume of water (usually heated)
      (i) Typically used with mechanical ventilators or CPAP masks
      (ii) Can provide up to 100% humidity
   (d) Room humidifier (cool mist): adds humidity to room air; can provide 100% humidity in a confined space
   (e) Heat and moisture exchanger: a passive humidifier, sometimes referred to as an artificial nose, for short-term use in the intubated patient whose normal mechanism for heating and humidifying inspired gases is bypassed
      (i) When placed close to the artificial airway, exhaled heat and moisture are collected on this humidifier and returned to the patient during the following inspiration.
      (ii) This device does not provide sufficient heat and humidity for long-term therapy.
(8) Types of aerosol generators
   (a) Jet: a small-volume nebulizer commonly used for the delivery of aerosolized medication
   (b) Babington: a popular large-volume nebulizer (e.g., Solosphere or Hydrosphere) capable of delivering a high-density mist with oxygen concentrations ranging from 21% to 100%
   (c) Ultrasonic nebulizers: converts radio waves into high-frequency mechanical vibrations that are transmitted to a liquid surface to create an aerosol. Home "cool" mist devices are an example of the ultrasonic nebulizer.
   b. Oxygen therapy devices
   (1) Appropriate device for individual patient use will depend on the supplemental oxygen requirements of the patient and how well he or she tolerates a particular device (Table 31-3).
   (2) For higher inspired oxygen therapy requirements, combination therapy (e.g., nasal cannula in conjunction with a nonrebreathing mask or a double oxygen flowmeter setup) may be required.
6. Guidelines for postoperative oxygen therapy
   a. Supplemental oxygen therapy will be provided to treat and prevent hypoxemia as needed.
   b. Monitor patients continually with pulse oximetry while in PACU.
   c. Pulse oximetry and supplemental oxygen therapy should be available for patient transport from the operating room to the PACU as required.
   d. Patients at high risk for hypoxemia may require supplemental oxygen therapy for an extended time after surgery.
   e. Patients requiring assurance of adequate oxygen delivery
   (1) Anemia
   (2) Low cardiac output

■ TABLE 31-3
■ ■ **Common Oxygen Therapy Devices**

Device	F_{IO_2}	O_2 Flow Rate	Comment
Nasal cannula	0.24–0.44	1–6 L/min	More comfortable, better tolerated; reservoir: nasopharynx; avoid O_2 flow rate >6 L/min since nasal irritation is likely and inspired oxygen increase is negligible.
Simple O_2 mask	0.40–0.60	5–10 L/min	Oxygen flow rate should be at least 5 L/min to prevent a buildup of carbon dioxide within the mask.
Partial rebreathing mask	0.40–0.70	Minimum of 10 L/min	Adjust oxygen flow rate to keep reservoir bag partially inflated at peak inspiration to avoid room air entrainment.
Nonrebreathing mask	0.60–0.80	>15 L/min (prevent bag collapse on inspiration)	Leaflet valves closing both exhalation ports are not recommended because of the risks of suffocation.
Air entrainment mask	0.24, 0.28, 0.35, 0.40, 0.50	4 L/min for 0.24; 6 L/min for 0.28; 8 L/min for 0.35; 12 L/min for 0.40; 12 L/min for 0.50	Total gas flow (oxygen and air) should be sufficient to meet the patient's peak inspiratory flow requirements. The higher the F_{IO_2}, the less room air is entrained, thus the need for higher oxygen flow rates.
Aerosol mask	0.28–0.98*	>8 L/min	When the F_{IO_2} exceeds 0.5, the total gas flow to the patient may be insufficient to prevent room air dilution.
Face tent	Variable; $\uparrow \rightarrow$ 70% with close fit and sufficient O_2 flow*	>8 L/min	When the F_{IO_2} exceeds 0.5, the total gas flow to the patient may be insufficient to prevent room air dilution; good for patients with facial deformities and burns; used when the F_{IO_2} is not crucial.
Tracheostomy collar	0.28–0.98*	>8 L/min	When the F_{IO_2} exceeds 0.5, the total gas flow to the patient may be insufficient to prevent room air dilution.
T-piece with reservoir	0.28–0.98*	Sufficient to have continuous mist exiting from the reservoir tube	When the F_{IO_2} exceeds 0.5, the total gas flow to the patient may be insufficient to prevent room air dilution.

*Can deliver F_{IO_2} of 0.21 if used with compressed air instead of oxygen.
F_{IO_2}, Fraction of inspired oxygen.

      (3) Posttrauma
      (4) Cardiovascular disease with dysrhythmias
      (5) Increased metabolic rate
         (a) Fever
         (b) Shivering
   C. Ventilatory care: early extubation is the goal to minimize air leak and barotrauma, which have a disruptive influence on fresh bronchial or pulmonary staple lines, and can lead to the development of bronchopleural fistulas.
     1. The most common causes of delayed extubation are:
       a. Concomitant pulmonary disease
       b. Cardiac dysfunction
       c. Multiorgan dysfunction
       d. Hemodynamic instability

2. Postoperative respiratory failure: condition in which postoperative exchange of oxygen and/or carbon dioxide between alveoli and pulmonary capillaries is inadequate
   a. Etiology: effective minute ventilation may be impacted by several factors occurring in the immediate postoperative phase.
      (1) Residual anesthetic effects
         (a) Potent inhalational agents and opioids decrease sensitivity of the respiratory center to carbon dioxide.
         (b) Residual neuromuscular relaxants leave the patient with inadequate respiratory muscular function.
      (2) Epidural anesthesia with high block may impair intercostal muscle function.
      (3) Preexisting pulmonary dysfunction
      (4) Pain with splinting
      (5) Obesity-related hypoventilation
   b. Signs and symptoms of respiratory failure
      (1) Shallow, rapid respirations secondary to:
         (a) Residual neuromuscular blockade
         (b) Bradypnea
         (c) Effects of opioids
         (d) Potent inhalational agents
      (2) Hypoventilation
      (3) Hypercapnia
      (4) Decreased breath sounds
   c. Nursing interventions
      (1) Assess level of consciousness, level of fatigue, work of breathing.
      (2) Monitor rate, quality, and depth of respiration.
      (3) Auscultate breath sounds.
      (4) Pulmonary stir-up regimen
      (5) Positioning: head of bed elevated 30° to 45° or, if needed, to an upright sitting position to facilitate diaphragmatic excursion
      (6) Appropriate pain management to promote effective ventilation
      (7) Pressure support ventilation and CPAP with nasal or full-face mask, if appropriate, as a temporizing measure to manage the lethargic patient with respiratory acidosis in the PACU
      (8) ABG analysis to monitor and trend $Paco_2$
      (9) If adequate ventilation and oxygenation cannot be achieved with noninvasive measures, prepare for reintubation.
3. Mechanical ventilation
   a. Objectives of mechanical ventilation
      (1) Physiological objectives
         (a) To support or manipulate pulmonary gas exchange to maintain:
            (i)   Normal ventilation
            (ii) Deliberate hyperventilation
            (iii) Oxygen delivery at or near normal
         (b) To increase lung volume:
            (i) To prevent or treat atelectasis with adequate end-inspiratory lung inflation
            (ii) To achieve and maintain an adequate functional residual capacity (FRC)
         (c) To reduce the patient's work of breathing
      (2) Clinical objectives
         (a) Reverse acute respiratory failure
         (b) Reverse respiratory distress
         (c) Reverse hypoxemia
         (d) Reverse atelectasis
         (e) Prevent barotrauma
         (f) Reverse ventilatory muscle fatigue

        (g) Permit sedation and/or paralysis

        (h) Reduce myocardial oxygen consumption

    b. Ventilation modes (Table 31-4)

    c. Expiratory phase maintenance

        (1) PEEP: a small amount of positive pressure (typically 1–20 cm H_2O) is kept in the airways upon exhalation.

■ TABLE 31-4
■ ■ **Characteristics of Basic Modes of Mechanical Ventilation**

Modes	Description	Advantages	Disadvantages
VOLUME MODES			
1. Volume Assist-Control	Delivers V_T that is machine or patient triggered, flow targeted, and at a frequency that at least equals the preset rate; each breath is terminated by a preset V_T (volume cycle-off).	Guaranteed V_E; often used as initial mode of mechanical ventilation	Not easy to monitor plateau pressure. May be uncomfortable in patients who require high inspiratory flow. Large inflation volumes may contribute to barotrauma.
2. Synchronized Intermittent Mandatory Ventilation (SIMV)	Delivers synchronized breaths at preset V_T that is machine triggered, flow or pressure targeted, and at a preset frequency; patients can breathe spontaneously with or without pressure support ventilation between machine breaths.	Guaranteed V_E; periods of spontaneous breathing help to prevent progressive lung hyperinflation and auto-PEEP. Weaning is accomplished by gradually lowering the set rate and allowing the patient to assume more ventilatory work.	Increased work of breathing. Less capable of changing V_E as patient's status changes. May prolong weaning
PRESSURE MODES			
1. Pressure Assist-Control	Delivers V_T that is machine or patient triggered, pressure targeted, and at a frequency that at least equals the preset rate; each breath is terminated by a preset T_i (time cycle-off).	Pressure limiting. Patient comfort. Used for limiting plateau pressures that can cause barotrauma; infant and adult respiratory distress syndrome	No guaranteed V_T or V_E
2. Pressure Support Ventilation (PSV)	Delivers V_T that is patient triggered and pressure targeted; each breath is terminated by preset inspiratory flow (flow cycle-off); V_T, T_i, and frequency are determined by the patient; can be used alone or with IMV; when used with IMV, machine breaths have a predetermined pressure.	Patient comfort. Better patient-ventilator synchrony. Used as a weaning mode	No guaranteed V_E. Monitor V_T changes that may indicate changes in compliance. Inadequate for patients with unreliable respiratory drive

IMV, Intermittent mandatory ventilation; *PEEP*, positive end-expiratory pressure; T_i, inspiratory time; V_E, minute ventilation; V_T, tidal volume.
Modified from Yuh-Chin T, Huang JS: Basic modes of mechanical ventilation. In Papadakos PJ, Lachmann B, eds: *Mechanical ventilation: Clinical applications and pathophysiology*, Philadelphia, 2008, Saunders.

(a) Helps maintain alveoli diameter (increases FRC) for improved oxygenation

(b) When used with spontaneous breathing (no set rate, volume, or pressure), this is called CPAP.

(c) Goal: to enhance tissue oxygenation and maintain Pao_2 >60 mm Hg, using an Fio_2 <0.4, while maintaining adequate cardiovascular function

(d) Complications

  (i) Decreased venous return and cardiac output (i.e., with hypovolemia)

  (ii) Hypotension

  (iii) Pneumothorax or tension pneumothorax

  (iv) Increased intracranial pressure

  (v) Decreased urine output

  (vi) Barotrauma: injury to the lungs as the result of a sustained increase in intramural airway pressure secondary to alveolar overdistention

4. Monitoring of ventilation

  a. ABG analysis with $Paco_2$ is the "gold standard"; however, this assessment is intermittent and invasive (see Chapter 21).

  b. Capnography

    (1) Represents the measurement of carbon dioxide partial pressure in exhaled gas ($PETco_2$).

    (2) A graphic waveform is incorporated to display the pattern of gas exhalation.

    (3) The most common methods of gas measurement are with infrared spectroscopy and mass spectroscopy.

    (4) Under stable conditions, $PETco_2$ approximates $Paco_2$ with the values differing less than 10 mm Hg.

    (5) Conditions of pulmonary hypoperfusion (e.g., pulmonary embolism, hypotension, hemorrhage, and cardiac arrest) will increase the gradient between arterial and end-tidal carbon dioxide values.

    (6) Indications for capnography

      (a) Monitoring adequacy of mechanical ventilation

      (b) Assessing intubation of trachea versus esophagus

      (c) Monitoring the integrity of the mechanical ventilatory circuit and artificial airway

      (d) Monitoring the adequacy of pulmonary and coronary blood flow (e.g., with cardiopulmonary resuscitation)

      (e) Monitoring carbon dioxide production

    (7) Capnography in the nonintubated patient

      (a) $PETco_2$ monitoring via devices (e.g., nasal cannula or masks) has been described in the nonintubated patient.

      (b) Knowledge of the limitation of these devices is required; at the least, they may serve as an apnea monitor.

5. Criteria for routine "awake" endotracheal extubation

  a. No indication to keep the patient intubated

  b. Subjective clinical criteria

    (1) Patient follows commands.

    (2) Clear oropharynx and hypopharynx (e.g., no active bleeding, cleared secretions).

    (3) Airway reflexes are recovered.

    (4) Muscle relaxant fully reversed (i.e., patient able to sustain a head lift for >5 seconds)

    (5) Adequate pain control

    (6) Minimal residual inhaled anesthetic agent

  c. Objective criteria

    (1) Patient hemodynamically stable

    (2) Tidal volume: >6 mL/kg

    (3) Vital capacity ≥10–15 mL/kg
    (4) Maximum inspiratory pressure ≤–20 cm H_2O
    (5) Sustained tetanic contraction >5 seconds with peripheral nerve stimulator
    (6) Respiratory rate <25 breaths/min in the adult

  6. Routine tracheal extubation
    a. Patient meets weaning criteria.
      (1) Appropriate return of consciousness
      (2) Spontaneous respiration
      (3) Resolution of neuromuscular block
      (4) Ability to follow simple commands (sustained head lift ≥5 sec)
    b. Personnel and equipment are available should reintubation become necessary.
    c. Pharynx is suctioned to remove secretions.
    d. Increase inspired oxygen concentration to 100% for several minutes to denitrogenate the lungs.
    e. Remove tape securing the endotracheal tube.
    f. Deflate the endotracheal tube cuff, if present.
    g. Apply positive airway pressure or have the cooperative patient take a deep breath, then remove the tube.
    h. Suction the oropharynx again if secretions are present and the patient is unable to adequately expectorate.

  7. Considerations for extubating the difficult airway
    a. Patient at high risk for glottic edema and/or stridor, such as the patient having prolonged surgery in the prone position. Before extubation, a cuff-leak test may be performed using one of two techniques:
      (1) Deflate cuff entirely and occlude the endotracheal tube. The patient is asked to inhale and exhale slowly as the endotracheal tube is occluded. Monitor for an audible leak around the tube. With no leak present, the patient is at high risk for postextubation obstruction.
      (2) Deflate cuff while continuing mechanical ventilation. The proportion of lost tidal volume to delivered tidal volume may be predictive. Volume loss to peritubular leakage should not exceed 15% of the delivered tidal volume.
    b. Patient who was difficult to intubate
      (1) Place a hollow tube exchanger into the trachea via the endotracheal tube before extubation.
        (a) Used to oxygenate and ventilate the patient if necessary
        (b) Should be left in place until concern for the airway is resolved
        (c) Reintubation, if required, can be facilitated with the hollow tube exchanger in place.

D. Administration of aerosolized medications
  1. Clinical indications for pharmacologically active aerosol therapy
    a. To relieve upper airway inflammation (i.e., glottic or subglottic edema or laryngotracheobronchitis)
    b. To provide topical anesthesia to the upper and/or central airway (i.e., for awake endotracheal intubation)
    c. To relieve vascular congestion before nasopharyngeal instrumentation
    d. To promote bronchodilation (i.e., treatment for reactive airway disease)
  2. Advantages of aerosol drug delivery
    a. Drug delivery targeted to the respiratory system for local pulmonary effect
    b. Smaller dosage necessary
    c. More effective drug response
    d. Rapid therapeutic onset of action
    e. Systemic side effects fewer and less severe than with oral or parenteral therapy
    f. Painless self-administration possible by the patient
  3. Disadvantages of aerosol drug delivery
    a. Failure to master the technique of aerosol drug delivery; insufficient knowledge of administration protocol

      b. Shorter duration of action in acute asthma

      c. Difficulty in dosage appraisal and reproducibility

  4. Technique of aerosol delivery

      a. Assemble necessary equipment.

      b. Explain procedure and rationale to the patient.

      c. Position patient in semi-Fowler or sitting position as tolerated.

      d. Perform baseline monitoring.

          (1) Heart rate

          (2) Breath sounds

          (3) Blood pressure

          (4) Oxyhemoglobin saturation with pulse oximetry

          (5) Respiratory rate

      e. Considerations for small-volume jet nebulizer

          (1) Select mask or mouthpiece delivery (nose clips may be needed with mouthpiece).

          (2) Add appropriate medication to the reservoir: standard amounts of normal saline to mix with the medication include 2 to 2.5 mL for children and 3 to 3.5 mL for adults if commercially prepared mixtures are unavailable.

          (3) Driving gas (typically oxygen) flow rates should range between 6 and 8 L/min. This promotes ideal aerosol particle size while keeping the treatment time to less than 10 minutes.

          (4) Use conserving system by aerosolizing medication only during inspiration, when permitted, to deliver more medication to the patient and less to the atmosphere.

          (5) Coach patient to breathe slowly through the mouth at normal tidal volume.

          (6) Periodically tap the sides of the nebulizer to return droplets back into the liquid reservoir. Once sputtering occurs, either the treatment is completed or additional medicated solution should be added to the nebulizer's liquid reservoir.

      f. Considerations for metered dose inhaler (MDI)

          (1) Warming MDI canister to body temperature will yield a particle size closer to ideal.

          (2) Remove protective cap and make sure no foreign objects are present in the mouthpiece.

          (3) Vigorously shake canister to mix canister contents, then prime the canister by discharging it (three or four puffs should be wasted) if the unit has not been used during the previous 24 hours.

          (4) Encourage patient to breathe out normally.

          (5) Instruct patient to maintain his or her neck in a neutral position.

          (6) MDI without a spacer: position the MDI approximately 4 cm from the patient's lips and aim the actuator mouthpiece at an open mouth and initiate inspiration after canister actuation.

          (7) MDI with a spacer

             (a) Position patient's lips around the spacer's mouthpiece.

             (b) Begin inspiration after canister actuation.

             (c) Timing is not as critical when a spacer is used.

          (8) Inspiration should continue slowly (may take 3–5 seconds) until maximal effort is achieved. Encourage patient to hold his or her breath for 10 seconds.

          (9) Exhalation should continue normally, and wait 1 minute or longer before repeating the next prescribed puff.

          (10) Replace protective cap on actuator mouthpiece after treatment completion to prevent foreign object contamination.

E. Select postanesthesia respiratory complications

  1. Bronchospasm

      a. Risk factors

(1) Endobronchial intubation
(2) Pulmonary edema
(3) Pulmonary embolus
(4) Pulmonary aspiration of gastric contents
(5) Pneumothorax
(6) Histamine release associated with medications
(7) Allergic or anaphylactic reactions to medications, latex, contrast media, or blood products
(8) Tobacco use
(9) History of bronchospasm
(10) Recent upper respiratory tract infection

b. Signs and symptoms
(1) Prolonged expiratory time
(2) Wheezing
(3) Spontaneously breathing patients
    (a) Accessory muscle recruitment
    (b) Labored ventilation
    (c) Increased work of breathing
(4) Mechanically ventilated patients: high peak inspiratory pressure

c. Management
(1) Determine the cause and treat (e.g., with endobronchial intubation, reposition the tube to terminate in the trachea).
(2) Remove source of laryngeal irritation if indicated.
(3) Implement beta$_2$-agonist therapy.
(4) If ventilation is still compromised and labored after albuterol therapy, consider aminophylline loading dose and maintenance infusion.
(5) Bronchospasm resistant to beta$_2$-agonist therapy may improve with an anticholinergic medication (e.g., ipratropium bromide).

2. Laryngospasm
  a. Definition
    (1) Exaggerated, prolonged protective closure reflex of the vocal folds
    (2) Hypoxia and hypercarbia will result if the condition goes untreated.
    (3) May occur secondary to stimulation from:
      (a) Foreign body in oropharyngeal or nasopharyngeal airway
      (b) Secretions such as vomitus on or around the vocal cords
    (4) May also be secondary to airway irritation; accounts for 23% of all critical postoperative respiratory events in adults

  b. Risk factors
    (1) Foreign body or secretion stimulation of the vocal folds in association with a light plane (i.e., associated with emergence) of anesthesia
    (2) Upper respiratory tract infection, especially in the pediatric population

  c. Signs and symptoms
    (1) Partial laryngospasm
      (a) High-pitched inspiratory stridor
      (b) Thoracoabdominal dyscoordination
      (c) Tracheal tug
      (d) Apprehension
    (2) Complete laryngospasm: as described for partial laryngospasm except absence of stridor or air exchange

  d. Management
    (1) Immediately remove source of irritation.
      (a) Gently suction pharynx.
      (b) Encourage the cooperative patient to cough.
      (c) Consider the lateral decubitus position to promote drainage.
    (2) Gentle, positive pressure ventilation with bag-valve-mask with 100% supplemental oxygen; consider esophageal opening pressure of 18 to 20 cm H_2O and the likelihood of gastric insufflation.

        (3) Anterior displacement of mandible

    e. If these measures unsuccessful:

        (a) Succinylcholine 0.1 to 0.2 mg/kg (10–20 mg, adult) intravenously

        (b) Be prepared to assist ventilation with bag-valve-mask with 100% supplemental oxygen for 5 to 10 minutes.

        (c) If the patient is aware, offer continual reassurance and sedation as appropriate.

      (1) Lidocaine 1.5 mg/kg, intravenously, may be effective in preventing or minimizing partial laryngospasm.

      (2) Consider endotracheal intubation.

        (a) If unable to maintain adequate respiration with bag-valve-mask

        (b) If ventilation required in patients at high risk of pulmonary aspiration of gastric contents.

        (c) With persistent, symptomatic partial laryngospasm

3. Postobstructive pulmonary edema

    a. Risk factors

      (1) Upper airway obstruction (e.g., laryngospasm, upper airway mass, strangulation) when the patient attempts vigorous inspiratory efforts

      (2) Sustained ventilatory efforts by the patient may generate high negative intrapleural pressures.

      (3) Creates acute and marked increases in left ventricular preload and afterload

    b. Signs and symptoms

      (1) Appearance of:

        (a) Pink, frothy fluid

        (b) Decreasing oxyhemoglobin saturation

        (c) Wheezing

        (d) Dyspnea

        (e) Increased respiratory rate

      (2) Chest radiograph: diffuse, usually bilateral interstitial pulmonary infiltrates

    c. Management

      (1) Supportive measures

        (a) Relief of the obstruction and maintenance of a patent airway

        (b) Supplemental oxygen

        (c) Diuretics may be indicated in select cases.

        (d) Recovery usually occurs rapidly within hours after surgery without intensive therapy.

      (2) Mechanical ventilation with PEEP, or CPAP, may be required in severe cases.

4. Oxygen-induced hypoventilation

    a. Risk factors—include patients with:

      (1) A history of oxygen-induced hypoventilation

      (2) End-stage COPD and chronic hypoventilation with presenting signs and symptoms of acute respiratory decompensation and deteriorating hypoxemia

      (3) The "blue bloater" appearance, with peripheral edema from decompensated right-sided heart failure (cor pulmonale) along with hypercapnia and hypoxemia, but minimal or no dyspnea

      (4) Sleep apnea syndrome, especially those with daytime hypoventilation and sleepiness ("Pickwickian" syndrome)

      (5) Acute hypoxemia and hypersomnolence not secondary to sedative medications

    b. Signs and symptoms

      (1) If undetected initially, worsening hypercapnia and acidosis when exposed to preceding ambient levels of oxygen

    c. Management

      (1) Avoidance of this problem is ideal.

(a) Identify high-risk patients in advance.
(b) Judiciously use supplemental oxygen therapy for this high-risk patient to maintain a target Pao_2 of 50 to 60 mm Hg with either nasal cannula or air entrainment mask.
(2) Nasal cannula
(a) Initiate supplemental oxygen therapy at 1 L/min oxygen flow rate.
(b) Increase the oxygen flow rate by 0.5-L/min increments until Pao_2 reaches at least 50 mm Hg.
(3) Air entrainment mask
(a) Set oxygen percentage at 24% or 28% initially at the manufacturer's recommended oxygen flow rate.
(b) Adjust inspired oxygen concentration until Pao_2 reaches at least 50 mm Hg.
(4) Tissue oxygenation is an overriding priority.
(a) Oxygen must never be withheld from exacerbated, hypoxemic patients with end-stage COPD for any reason.
(b) Be prepared to mechanically support ventilation if supplemental oxygen induces severe hypoventilation.
(5) Progressive hypercapnia and respiratory acidosis are rare with overzealous supplemental oxygen therapy.
(a) Patient assessment should include ABG analysis to monitor these conditions.
5. Postextubation laryngeal edema
a. Risk factors
(1) Patient age: especially younger than 4 years
(2) History of infectious or postextubation croup
(3) Anaphylactic reaction
(4) Inflammatory airway changes (e.g., upper respiratory tract infection)
(5) Surgery of head, neck, and oral cavity
(6) Surgery lasting longer than 1 hour
(7) Traumatic intubation or emergence
(8) Too large of endotracheal tube
b. Signs and symptoms (Table 31-5)
c. Management
(1) Begins with prevention
(a) Avoid endotracheal intubation when possible.
(b) Ensure smooth intubation.

■ TABLE 31-5
■ ■ **Signs and Symptoms of Postextubation Laryngeal Edema**

Symptoms	Early	Late
Airway sound	Inspiratory stridor	Biphasic stridor
Appearance	Anxious, alert	Lethargic, obtunded
Breath sounds	Decreased bilaterally	
Cough	Barking, brassy	
Dysphagia	Difficulty swallowing, sore throat	
Heart rate	Sinus tachycardia	Bradycardia
Oxyhemoglobin saturation	Decreases with exhaustion	
Phonation	Dysphonia	Aphonia
Respiratory rate	Tachypnea	Bradypnea
Retractions	Suprasternal	Suprasternal, intercostals, subcostal
Voice changes	Hoarseness	

      (c) Avoid endotracheal intubation in children with upper respiratory tract infection when possible.

      (d) Ensure audible leak around cuffless endotracheal tube at 25 to 35 cm H_2O peak airway pressure.

      (e) Avoid endotracheal tube movement.

      (f) Prevent coughing or bucking on endotracheal tube.

  (2) Calm, reassuring support to alleviate fear and anxiety

  (3) Allow child to assume position of comfort (e.g., high Fowler or in caregiver's lap).

  (4) Supplemental oxygen as indicated to prevent hypoxemia according to patient acceptance

  (5) Cool humidity in conjunction with supplemental oxygen therapy or room humidifier to soothe the inflamed laryngeal mucosa and thus minimize coughing

  (6) Aerosolized racemic epinephrine (topical vasoconstrictor)

      (a) For moderate symptoms, 0.5 mL of 2.25% solution in 3 mL of normal saline

      (b) May repeat in 30 minutes (up to three times) and every 2 to 4 hours, as needed

  (7) Dexamethasone 0.5 mg/kg intravenously every 6 hours as needed for moderate symptoms

  (8) Helium 80% and oxygen 20% (Heliox) via nonrebreathing mask to reduce airway resistance for severe symptoms

  (9) If severe symptoms persist

      (a) Positive pressure ventilation with bag-valve-mask and supplemental oxygen synchronized to patient's inspiratory effort

      (b) Consider reintubation with smaller endotracheal tube.

6. Pulmonary aspiration of gastric contents

  a. Incidence of recognized clinical aspiration (bilious secretions or particulate matter in the tracheobronchial tree or presence of new infiltrate on postoperative chest radiograph) is approximately 1.5 to 5 per 10,000 general anesthetics.

  b. Aspiration of sufficiently low gastric fluid pH (<2.5) places patients at risk for aspiration pneumonitis.

  c. Risk factors

    (1) Age extremes (<1 year or >70 years)

    (2) Comorbid diseases (e.g., diabetic gastroparesis)

    (3) Central nervous system deficits

    (4) Chronic alcoholism

    (5) Collagen vascular disease (e.g., scleroderma)

    (6) Hepatobiliary and gastrointestinal diseases

    (7) Renal dysfunction

    (8) Pregnancy

    (9) Recent oral intake

   (10) Opioid administration

   (11) Pain; anxiety and depression

   (12) Gastrointestinal obstruction or dysfunction

   (13) Obesity

   (14) Depressed level of consciousness

   (15) Previous esophageal dysfunction

   (16) Head injury or neurological dysfunction

   (17) Lack of coordination of swallowing and respiration

   (18) Ascites

   (19) Procedures that increase intra-abdominal pressure

  d. Signs and symptoms: depends on severity of pulmonary aspiration

    (1) Coughing

    (2) Wheezing

    (3) Rhonchi

    (4) Hypoxemia

(5) Bilious secretions or particulate matter upon tracheal aspiration

(6) Presence of new infiltrate on postoperative chest radiograph

  e. Management

(1) When regurgitation occurs, gastric contents should be removed from the pharynx by:

(a) Rapidly lowering the head

(b) Turning head to the side

(c) Suctioning the pharynx with a tonsil-tip suction catheter

(2) Support ventilation and oxygenation as required.

(3) Suction trachea and bronchi (but do not instill saline). If particulate matter found or suspected, bronchoscopy is indicated to remove any large aspirated pieces.

(4) Prophylactic antibiotics and steroids are not warranted.

(5) Steroids may increase the risk of pulmonary infection by suppressing the immune response.

(6) Culture tracheal secretions; administer antibiotics if positive culture.

(7) Continue supportive respiratory therapy.

7. Residual neuromuscular blockade

  a. Incidence is up to 9% with intermediate-acting neuromuscular blocking agents (up to 50% with long-acting agents).

  b. Extubation of a partially paralyzed patient results in increased postoperative morbidity.

  c. Consequences of residual weakness include:

(1) Airway obstruction

(2) Hypoventilation

(3) Impaired ventilatory response to hypoxia

(4) Disturbed esophageal motility

(5) Inability to handle vomitus

  d. Risk factors

(1) Use of long-acting neuromuscular blocking agents

(2) Not administering anticholinesterase reversal agents when indicated

(3) Plasma cholinesterase deficiency

(4) Atypical plasma cholinesterase

  e. Signs and symptoms

(1) Air hunger

(2) Writhing

(3) Uncoordinated movements of the extremities

(4) Dysphagia (implies weakness of pharyngeal muscles)

(5) Spasmodic, paradoxical abdominal motion

(6) Impaired cough (occurs when vital capacity is 66% of normal)

(7) Hypertension

(8) Tachycardia

(9) Pupillary dilation

  f. Management

(1) Is additional anticholinesterase indicated?

(a) Has the patient received the optimal dose of reversal agent?

(2) Support the airway and provide adequate ventilation as indicated.

(a) Consider whether the patient is at high risk for pulmonary aspiration of gastric contents.

(b) If yes, take precautions to prevent aspiration.

(3) Neuromuscular blocking agents do not alter the patient's level of consciousness.

(a) If the patient requires mechanical ventilation, provide sedation, analgesia, or amnesia as indicated.

(4) Assessment for continued ventilatory support and control of airway will be required on an ongoing basis until the patient has sufficiently recovered from the neuromuscular blocking agent.

8. Opioid-induced ventilatory depression
   a. Opioid therapy is the primary vehicle for pain management in the surgical patient.
   b. Providing adequate and satisfactory pain relief with the least amount of risk is an important adjunct to patient recovery.
   c. Patient comfort and safety are essential and can be attained through proper monitoring and administration of opioids.
   d. Respiratory depression secondary to opioid administration occurs despite optimal patient care and must be diagnosed and managed appropriately.
   e. Risk factors
      (1) Opioid naïve: a person who does not take opioids regularly may be expected to require less opioid than those who are exposed to potent analgesics.
      (2) Chronic respiratory disease
      (3) Opioid elimination may be delayed in patients with severe liver or renal disease.
      (4) Renarcotization: naloxone has a duration of action approximating 30 to 45 minutes, which might be shorter than the duration of action of the administered opioid, therefore exhibiting recurrence of opioid ventilatory depression in this circumstance.
      (5) Extremes in age
         (a) Neonates, especially premature infants, due to:
            (i) Immature respiratory mechanisms
               [a] Chest wall instability
               [b] Increased tendency for alveolar collapse
               [c] Respiratory pauses
               [d] Periodic ventilation
         (b) Older patients at risk secondary to prolonged drug elimination
   f. Signs and symptoms
      (1) Mental obtundation
      (2) Bradypnea
      (3) Hypoxemia: may be a late sign especially in the patient receiving supplemental oxygen therapy
      (4) Bradycardia
      (5) Chest wall rigidity
   g. Management
      (1) Prevention: use of alternative pain relief methods may lead to a reduced need for opioid therapy.
         (a) Nonopioid analgesics
         (b) Transcutaneous electrical nerve stimulation (TENS)
         (c) Massage therapy
         (d) Distraction therapy
      (2) Stir-up regimen: tactile and verbal stimulation of the patient may be sufficient to maintain adequate spontaneous ventilation.
      (3) Opioid antagonism (e.g., naloxone, naltrexone, nalmefene)
         (i) Intravenous reversal of opioid-induced ventilatory depression
         (ii) Observe patient for renarcotization phenomenon.
         (iii) Intramuscular naloxone should be considered when longer-acting opioids have been administered.
      (4) Ventilation: short-term controlled ventilation may be indicated to normalize $Paco_2$ until opioid antagonism therapy can be instituted.
F. Postthoracotomy pain management
   1. Appropriate pain management is integral to patient care after pulmonary surgery.
      a. Degree of therapy is influenced by the:
         (1) Patient
         (2) Surgical procedure
         (3) Preexisting conditions

    b. Goals of postthoracotomy pain management include:
      (1) Promoting patient comfort
      (2) Preserving pulmonary function by promoting deep breathing and coughing
      (3) Reducing sympathetic stimulation secondary to pain which may contribute to myocardial ischemia
      (4) Promoting mobilization thus maintaining pulmonary function
      (5) Reducing deep venous thrombosis and resultant pulmonary embolus
    c. Pain may be subjectively assessed using a scale from 0 to 10, with 0 reflecting no pain and 10 reflecting the worst pain imaginable.
      (1) Reasonable postthoracotomy pain score goals would be less than 3 at rest and less than 5 while coughing.
      (2) Various modalities can be used alone or in combination to facilitate the goals of postthoracotomy pain management.
  2. Thoracic epidural analgesia
    a. A dilute concentration of long-acting local anesthetic in conjunction with opioids may be continuously infused to improve postthoracotomy pain.
    b. Reduces the risk for postoperative respiratory complications after pneumonectomy
  3. Paravertebral analgesia
    a. Before chest closure, surgeon can place a catheter in the paravertebral space and bring the tube out of the chest wall by a separate intercostal puncture.
    b. Administration of a bolus of local anesthetic, followed with a continual infusion of local anesthesia, affords analgesia comparable to epidural analgesia.
  4. Extrapleural analgesia
    a. Via a separate intercostal puncture in the chest wall, the surgeon can place a catheter between the parietal pleura and the endothoracic fascia.
    b. Management is similar to that of the paravertebral approach.
  5. Intercostal nerve blocks
    a. Usually done by the surgeon intraoperatively under direct vision
    b. May be administered as a bolus or continuous infusion with long-acting local anesthetic agents
    c. Preservation of pulmonary function and oxygenation are better after thoracotomy with fewer side effects (e.g., nausea and vomiting, hypotension) when compared with thoracic epidural anesthesia.
  6. Intrathecal opioid
    a. Morphine, when administered before thoracotomy, has been shown to be effective in reducing postoperative pain; provides pain relief for 18 to 24 hours
  7. Intermittent opioid administration
    a. Judicious use of opioids either intermittent intravenous or via patient-controlled analgesia if required.
  8. Cryoanalgesia
    a. Long-lasting (3–4 weeks) intercostal nerve block obtained by intercostal nerve freezing with a cryoprobe
  9. Nonsteroidal anti-inflammatory drugs
    a. Ketorolac, 15 to 30 mg every 6 hours, over the first 24 to 48 hours, with supplemental opioid for breakthrough pain may be all that is required for thoracoscopy pain.
    b. Used with caution in:
      (1) Elderly patients
      (2) Patients with renal insufficiency
      (3) Patients with history of gastric bleeding
G. Management of the respiratory surgical patient
  1. Chest tubes

a. Air leak and pleural space management
   (1) Air leaks are common after lung resection.
   (2) Most resolve within the first 3 postoperative days.
b. Purpose: chest tube made of sterile vinyl or silicone catheter inserted into the pleural space or mediastinum to:
   (1) Facilitate the drainage of air, blood, or fluid using gravity, suction, or both
   (2) Restore negative pressure in the pleural space and promote reexpansion of a collapsed lung
   (3) Instill medication
c. Indications
   (1) Pneumothorax (i.e., open, closed, tension)
   (2) Hemothorax
   (3) Hemopneumothorax
   (4) Cardiac tamponade
   (5) Empyema
   (6) Chylothorax (an accumulation of lymphatic fluid in the pleural space caused by chest trauma, tumors, mediastinal surgery, or trauma)
   (7) Pleural effusion
   (8) Pleurodesis
       (a) Indication: to instill medications (i.e., chemotherapy or sclerosing agents) to decrease recurrent pleural effusions by creating a pleuritis that causes the parietal and visceral pleura to adhere to each other, thus preventing the effusion
d. Chest tube insertion
   (1) For air drainage: anterior chest near the apex of the lung, at the second or third intercostal space, midclavicular line
   (2) For fluid drainage: base of lung, fourth or fifth intercostal space, midaxillary line; mediastinum
e. Chest drainage systems
   (1) Specific system used will depend on anticipated use.
   (2) Standard closed water seal
       (a) Traditional chest drainage unit that can handle large amounts of drainage; can drain both fluid and air
       (b) Suction control
           (i) Wet: amount of achieved suction in pleural cavity regulated by the height of a water column in suction control chamber, not the setting of suction source
           (ii) Dry: dial set to desired suction level (typically −20 cm H_2O) until float appears in indicator window to signify that the desired suction level has been achieved
               [a] Requires no regulation of water in the suction column
               [b] Some dry suction systems use traditional water seal.
               [c] Others use dry-dry drains that eliminate the need for water, except to fill the air-leak indicator.
               [d] Safe if accidentally tipped over
       (c) Components of closed water seal drainage units
           (i) Collection chamber
               [a] This drainage unit connects directly to the chest tube to collect chest drainage.
               [b] Permits collection and documentation of fluid drainage via a calibrated column.
           (ii) Water seal chamber
               [a] Allows air or fluid to exit from the pleural space on exhalation
               [b] Prevents air from reentering the pleural space or mediastinum on inhalation to help re-establish normal negative intrapleural pressure
               [c] Chamber must be filled with sterile water to 2-cm line.

[1] Levels >2 cm increase the work of breathing.

[2] Levels <2 cm may allow air to reenter the pleural space.

[d] To maintain an adequate seal, closed water seal unit must remain upright and the water level monitored for evaporative loss.

[e] Tidaling

[1] Fluctuations on water seal chamber fluid level that corresponds to respirations

[2] With spontaneous respirations:

[i] On inspiration, increased negative intrapleural pressure increases the water level

[ii] On expiration, decreased pleural pressure decreases the water level

[iii] Tidaling fluctuations reversing with positive pressure mechanical ventilation indicates a patent pleural chest tube.

[iv] Tidaling and air leak may be more apparent when suction turned off briefly.

[f] Air leak meter

[1] Bubbling in air leak meter indicates an air leak.

[2] Meter registers between 1 (minimal leak) and 7 (significant leak).

[3] Initially, air egress out of the chest tube is anticipated with pneumothorax or after thoracic surgery (i.e., open lung biopsies, lobectomies); if bubbling in water seal chamber is continuous, suspect a system leak.

[4] Determine location of air leak by briefly clamping off tubing with a padded clamp.

[5] If air leak stops, leak is inside patient.

[6] If it doesn't stop, leak is somewhere in drainage system.

(iii) Suction control chamber: provides negative pressure to facilitate removal of air or fluid.

[a] Gravity drainage: suction may be turned off with water seal intact for ambulation, transfer, or weaning.

[b] If suction is discontinued, the suction port or tube must remain uncapped/unclamped to allow air to exit, thus minimizing the risk of tension pneumothorax.

(3) Heimlich valve

(a) One-way flutter valve that prevents air reflux into the pleural cavity

(b) Less expensive and easier to use than traditional chest drainage units.

(c) On exhalation:

(i) Air exits the chest, creating positive pressure.

(ii) Positive pressure opens the valve so air can escape.

(iii) Collapses on itself to prevent air from reentering pleural space.

(iv) Distal end may be connected to drainage bag for collection of fluids.

(4) Indwelling pleural catheter

(a) Used to drain chronic pleural effusions

(b) May be used by patient at home

(c) May improve patient's quality of life for malignant conditions

(5) Portable chest drainage unit

(a) Incorporates mechanical one-way valve instead of water seal chamber

(b) Indication: for ambulatory patient requiring chest tube for drainage but not suction to re-expand the lung

(6) Glass bottle water seal method
    (a) Older method
    (b) Increased risk of contamination and breakage

f. Care of patient with a chest tube
    (1) Assessment and documentation
        (a) Vital signs: blood pressure; heart rate and rhythm; respiratory rate, pattern, and depth; oxyhemoglobin saturation; temperature, pain level and location; skin appearance
        (b) Air leak: observe for fluctuations/air leak. Determine the location and degree of air leak. Notify physician of any new or increased air leak.
        (c) Tidaling: assess for presence or absence of tidaling with respirations in the water seal chamber. Absence may indicate complete reexpansion of the lung or obstruction of chest tube (i.e., clots or kinks).
        (d) Suction level
            (i) Confirm suction setting at ordered level and functioning correctly.
            (ii) Check water level in water seal and suction chambers for evaporation and fill according to manufacturer's directions.
            (iii) Suction should never be applied to a pneumonectomy drain, as this will cause the mediastinum to be pulled to the operative side and result in cardiovascular collapse.
            (iv) A move away from using suction is being seen with the belief that there is a shorter requirement for chest drainage and even a shorter hospital stay.
        (e) Chest tube dressing: check dressing for occlusiveness and drainage from insertion site.
        (f) Drainage: monitor volume, color, and consistency of chest tube drainage. Over time, volume of drainage should decrease and color of fluid should lighten.
        (g) Connections: ensure connections of chest tube unit are tight and secure.
        (h) Drainage system positioning
            (i) Maintain chest drainage system so that it is positioned upright and below the level of the heart at all times.
            (ii) Avoid kinking or occlusion of tubing.
            (iii) Avoid any dependent loops because fluid accumulates, causing resistance to flow out of the chest.
            (iv) Properly lay tubing horizontally across bed before dropping vertically into chest drainage system.
        (i) Palpation
            (i) Palpate around chest tube site, chest, face, and neck for crepitus (indicative of subcutaneous emphysema).
            (ii) If new subcutaneous emphysema, notify the physician.
            (iii) Mark the crepitus edges and reassess for any increase.
            (iv) Crepitus may occur if chest tube is improperly placed or dressing is not occlusive and air is getting pulled into tissues around the insertion site.
            (v) Subcutaneous emphysema involving face and neck may cause airway compromise.
        (j) Patient positioning
            (i) Semi-Fowlers, as tolerated, to facilitate gravity drainage of fluid from pleural or mediastinal space, and air to rise and be expelled from the pleural space
            (ii) Semi-Fowlers also facilitates diaphragmatic excursion, thus optimizing ventilation.
            (ii) Reposition patient every 2 hours or per facility policy.
        (k) Chest radiograph: after chest tube insertion or removal

(l) Monitor patient for:
  (i) Respiratory distress or change in baseline
  (ii) Tension pneumothorax: hypotension, pulsus paradoxus, contralateral tracheal deviation
  (iii) Cardiac tamponade or injury with mediastinal tubes
  (iv) Bleeding: establish acceptable chest tube output.
  (v) Lung injury
  (vi) Bronchopleural fistula (rare)
(2) Interventions/troubleshooting
  (a) Never clamp chest tube, except briefly (i.e., <1 minute) for:
    (i) Changing the collection chamber
    (ii) Assessing for air leak location
    (iii) Determining patient's tolerance for removal of chest tube (only with physician order)
    (iv) Chest tube becomes disconnected: if there has been no air leak, the tube may be clamped with two padded hemostats for a short time.
      [a] If an air leak was present, do not clamp chest tube because a tension pneumothorax can rapidly develop.
      [b] Instead, submerge chest tube in sterile water or saline until new unit can be obtained.
  (b) Chest tube becomes occluded.
    (i) If sudden cessation of drainage, air leak, or tidaling, check for chest tube occlusion.
    (ii) If suspected, check for chest tube kinks, dependent loops, and fluid build-up within the tubing.
      [a] Have patient take a deep breath and cough.
      [b] Change patient position.
      [c] Gently milk tubing (squeezing tube between fingers and relaxing every 5 cm while advancing the length of chest tube).
      [d] Do not strip (squeeze) the chest tube in its entirety without releasing because this may cause dangerous increase in negative intrathoracic pressure.
  (c) Chest tube becomes dislodged.
    (i) Immediately cover chest site with sterile dressing (petroleum jelly gauze, sterile 4 × 4 dressings).
    (ii) Call physician.
    (iii) If air leak present:
      [a] Tape the chest dressing only on two or three sides to allow air to escape the chest wall opening and prevent tension pneumothorax.

2. Intravenous fluid therapy
  a. Patients are kept relatively dry (e.g., 1 mL/kg/h of balanced crystalloid solution) until the patient resumes oral intake.
  b. Patients have a tendency to retain fluid during the first few days postthoracotomy.
  c. Relative oliguria, in a normothermic and stable patient, should not be treated aggressively with fluid therapy.
3. Hypothermia
  a. Patients with a temperature less than 35.5° C are at risk for myocardial ischemia and should be warmed to 36.5° C with a forced air warmer.
4. Bleeding
  a. Blood loss into the pleural space is anticipated but should not exceed 500 to 600 mL in 24 hours.
  b. Etiology
    (1) Inadequate perioperative hemostasis

(2) Postoperative coagulopathy

(3) Pulmonary artery rupture or slipped tie or clip

c. Signs and symptoms

(1) Chest tube drainage >100 mL/hr, or if new bleeding occurs, notify the physician. Chest tube output >1000 mL in 1 hour requires an immediate return to the operating room with concomitant correction of any coagulopathy.

(2) Hypotension

(3) Decreased filling pressures

(4) Tachycardia

(5) Restlessness

(6) Decreased cardiac output

d. Interventions

(1) Monitor chest tube output upon admission and at frequent intervals.

(2) Inspect dressing for excessive drainage.

(3) Frequently assess vital signs.

(4) Notify physician of:

(a) Chest tube drainage as noted previously

(b) Sudden increase in wound or chest tube drainage

(c) Abrupt decrease in chest tube drainage

(d) Falling hematocrit

5. Cardiovascular complications (see Chapter 32)

a. Dysrhythmias

(1) Pathophysiology

(a) Greater than 25% of patients undergoing cardiothoracic surgery will have postoperative dysrhythmias.

(b) Atrial fibrillation/flutter: occurrence >12%; the most common dysrhythmia

(2) Risk factors

(a) Certain thoracic operations at high risk for atrial fibrillation

(i) Mediastinal tumor resection (e.g., thymectomy)

(ii) Lobectomy

(iii) Bilobectomy

(iv) Pneumonectomy

(b) Male sex

(c) Advanced age

(d) COPD

(e) Heart rate >72 beats/min

(3) Prevention: evaluate potential for side effects to determine appropriate management in individual patients.

(a) Calcium channel blockers

(b) Beta-adrenergic blockers

(c) Magnesium sulfate

(4) Interventions

(a) Assess hemodynamic stability.

(b) Assess for precipitating factors.

(i) Acid-base disturbances

(ii) Alteration in oxygenation and ventilation

(iii) Electrolyte imbalance

(iv) Adverse effect of bronchodilators

(c) Treatment

(i) Correct electrolyte imbalance.

(ii) Ensure adequate oxygenation and ventilation.

(iii) ECG evaluation

(iv) Pharmacological therapy for stable rhythms

(v) Cardioversion, pacing for unstable rhythms

b. Myocardial ischemia/infarction
c. Thromboembolism
  (1) Pathophysiology: one fourth of patients undergoing thoracotomy have thromboembolic events during their hospitalization.
  (2) Risk factors
    (a) Malignancy
    (b) Major surgery
  (3) Prevention
    (a) Compression stockings
    (b) Low-molecular-weight heparin started evening before surgery such that it does not interfere with insertion of epidural catheter
  (4) Treatment
    (a) Unfractionated heparin for massive embolism unless contraindicated
    (b) Unfractionated heparin or low-molecular-weight heparin for submassive embolism
    (c) Warfarin typically started along with heparin to achieve an INR of 2 to 3.
      (i) Heparin discontinued, usually after about 5 days, once warfarin takes effect
    (d) Acute surgical embolectomy may be considered for proximal pulmonary branch emboli in which:
      (i) There is a massive pulmonary embolism.
      (ii) Patient is unstable despite heparin and other resuscitative measures.
      (iii) There is contraindication to or failure of thrombolytic therapy.
    (e) Inferior vena cava filters indicated for patients in whom anticoagulation contraindicated or who have recurrent pulmonary emboli
d. Cardiac herniation
  (1) Pathophysiology
    (a) Displacement of heart through pericardial defect
    (b) Twisting of great vessels obstructs inflow and outflow tracts of heart.
    (c) May be precipitated by:
      (i) Change in position
      (ii) Coughing
      (iii) Positive-pressure ventilation
    (d) Signs and symptoms
      (i) Cardiovascular collapse
      (ii) Jugular venous distention, upper body cyanosis
      (iii) Tachycardia, myocardial ischemia
      (iv) Displaced point of maximum intensity
      (v) Cyanosis
  (2) Treatment
    (a) Check for positioning restrictions, especially with pneumonectomy patient or any time pericardium has been opened.
    (b) Alert physician of precipitating factors of cardiovascular collapse.
    (c) Reposition patient if turning causes symptoms. May be positioned in lateral decubitus position with operative side up.
    (d) Confirm that suction has not been applied to pneumonectomy drains.
    (e) Prepare patient for emergent surgical reduction.

BIBLIOGRAPHY

1. Cole D, Schlunt R: *Adult perioperative anesthesia: The requisites in anesthesiology*, Philadelphia, 2004, Mosby.
2. Demmy TL, ed: *Thoracic surgery clinics*, Philadelphia, 2006, Saunders.
3. Gardenhire DS: *Rau's respiratory care pharmacology*, Philadelphia, 2008, Mosby.
4. Grippi MA, Litzky LA, Manaker S, eds: *Pulmonary science and medicine: A review of fundamental principles*, Baltimore, 2001, Lippincott Williams & Wilkins.
5. Hagberg CA: *Benumof's airway management*, ed 2, Philadelphia, 2007, Mosby.
6. Hung O, Murphy MF: *Management of the difficult and failed airway*, New York, 2008, McGraw-Hill.
7. Kaplan JA, Slinger PD: *Thoracic anesthesia*, Philadelphia, 2003, Churchill Livingstone.
8. Mason RJ, Broaddus VC, Murray JF, et al, eds: *Murray and Nadel's textbook of respiratory medicine*, ed 4, Philadelphia, 2005, Saunders.
9. Papadokos PJ, Lachmann B: *Mechanical ventilation: Clinical applications and pathophysiology*, Philadelphia, 2008, Saunders.
10. Sidebotham D, McKee A, Gillham M, et al: *Cardiothoracic critical care*, Philadelphia, 2007, Butterworth Heinemann.
11. Slinger P, ed: *Anesthesiology clinics*, Philadelphia, 2008, Saunders.
12. Stoelting RK, Dierdoff SF: *Handbook for anesthesia and co-existing disease*, ed 2, New York, 2002, Churchill Livingstone.
13. Zaglaniczny K, Aker J, eds: *Clinical guide to pediatric anesthesia*, Philadelphia, 1999, WB Saunders.

32 Cardiovascular Care

GARY GUSICK

OBJECTIVES

At the conclusion of this chapter, the reader will be able to:

1. Describe components of a detailed cardiovascular assessment, including normal and abnormal findings.
2. Identify possible cardiopulmonary complications occurring in the perioperative period.
3. Describe pharmacotherapy of drugs used in emergency situations.
4. Identify indications, precautions, and techniques for defibrillation and cardioversion.
5. Compare indications and perioperative considerations for various modes of temporary and permanent cardiac pacing.
6. Explain the interrelationship of preload, afterload, contractility, and heart rate in the determination of cardiac output.
7. Describe effects of congenital heart defects on the hemodynamics of the cardiovascular system.
8. Identify complications and risk factors associated with coronary artery disease.
9. Describe diagnostic studies used to examine the cardiovascular system.
10. Describe preoperative assessment of the cardiovascular surgical patient.
11. Implement nursing process for a postoperative cardiovascular patient in the post anesthesia care unit (PACU).
12. Identify use of an intra-aortic balloon pump (IABP) and management of a patient with an IABP.
13. Identify use of a ventricular assist device (VAD) and management of a patient with a VAD.

I. CARE OF THE POSTOPERATIVE CARDIOVASCULAR PATIENT
   A. Depends on thorough understanding of the concepts of oxygenation
      1. Maximize oxygen delivery to body tissues
      2. Minimize oxygen consumption (i.e., workload) of the heart.
   B. Depends on sound understanding of normal aspects of postoperative nursing care
      1. Cardiac physiology
      2. Pathophysiology
      3. Pharmacology
      4. Psychosocial
   C. Depends on knowledge base and assessment skills of the nurse, which are the primary determinants of positive outcomes after surgery
II. CARDIAC ANATOMY AND PHYSIOLOGY
   A. Structure and function (Figure 32-1)
   B. Conduction system (Figure 32-2)
      1. Sinoatrial (SA) node: pacemaker of the heart
      2. Internodal tracts and Bachmann's bundle
         a. Electrical pathways in atria
         b. Conducts impulse through atria and to atrioventricular (AV) node
      3. AV node: impulse briefly delayed to allow for mechanical event of atrial contraction
      4. Ventricular conduction
         a. Bundle of His

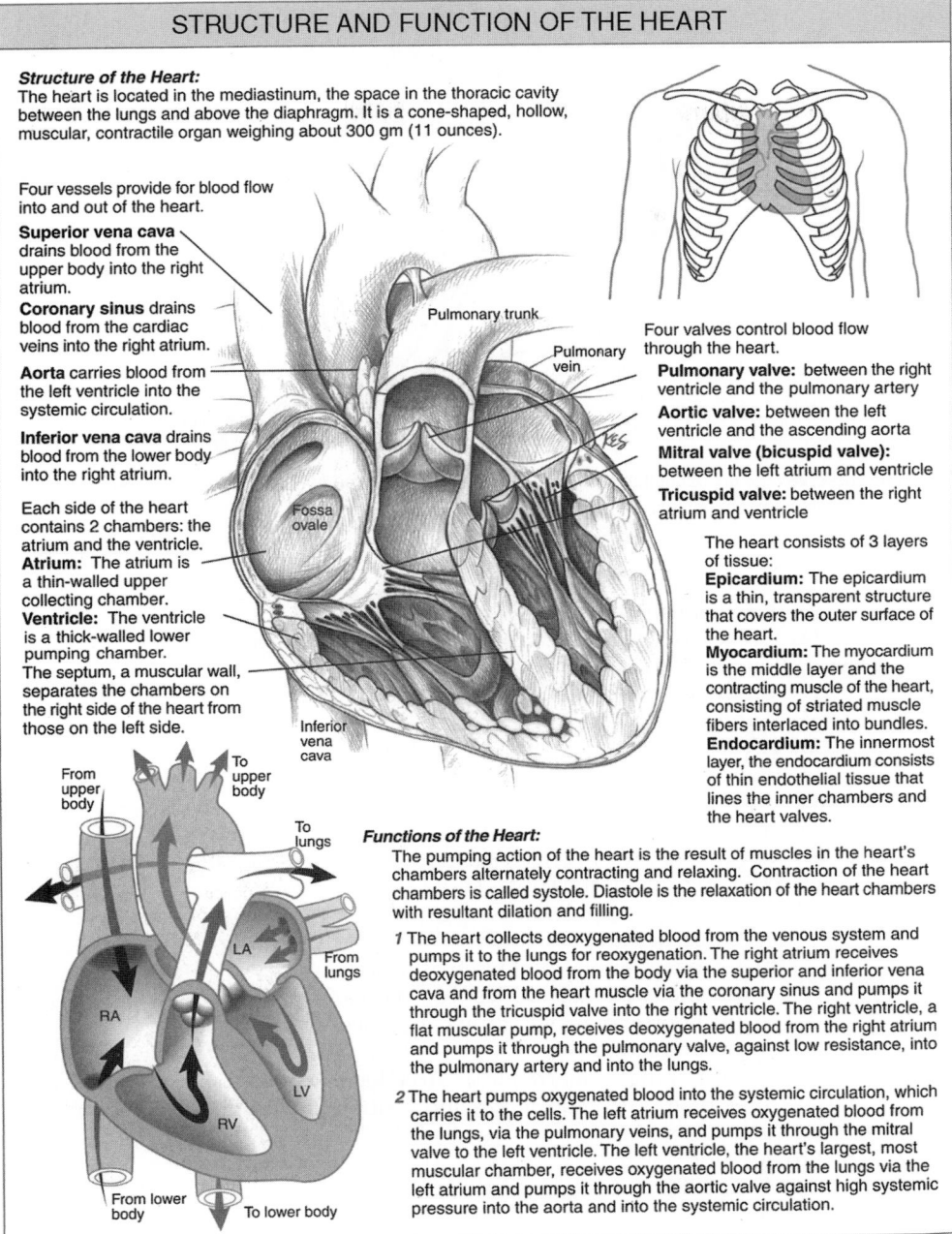

STRUCTURE AND FUNCTION OF THE HEART

Structure of the Heart:
The heart is located in the mediastinum, the space in the thoracic cavity between the lungs and above the diaphragm. It is a cone-shaped, hollow, muscular, contractile organ weighing about 300 gm (11 ounces).

Four vessels provide for blood flow into and out of the heart.
Superior vena cava drains blood from the upper body into the right atrium.
Coronary sinus drains blood from the cardiac veins into the right atrium.
Aorta carries blood from the left ventricle into the systemic circulation.
Inferior vena cava drains blood from the lower body into the right atrium.

Each side of the heart contains 2 chambers: the atrium and the ventricle.
Atrium: The atrium is a thin-walled upper collecting chamber.
Ventricle: The ventricle is a thick-walled lower pumping chamber.
The septum, a muscular wall, separates the chambers on the right side of the heart from those on the left side.

Pulmonary trunk

Pulmonary vein

Fossa ovale

Inferior vena cava

Four valves control blood flow through the heart.
Pulmonary valve: between the right ventricle and the pulmonary artery
Aortic valve: between the left ventricle and the ascending aorta
Mitral valve (bicuspid valve): between the left atrium and ventricle
Tricuspid valve: between the right atrium and ventricle

The heart consists of 3 layers of tissue:
Epicardium: The epicardium is a thin, transparent structure that covers the outer surface of the heart.
Myocardium: The myocardium is the middle layer and the contracting muscle of the heart, consisting of striated muscle fibers interlaced into bundles.
Endocardium: The innermost layer, the endocardium consists of thin endothelial tissue that lines the inner chambers and the heart valves.

From upper body
To upper body
To lungs
From lungs
LA
RA
LV
RV
From lower body
To lower body

Functions of the Heart:
The pumping action of the heart is the result of muscles in the heart's chambers alternately contracting and relaxing. Contraction of the heart chambers is called systole. Diastole is the relaxation of the heart chambers with resultant dilation and filling.

1 The heart collects deoxygenated blood from the venous system and pumps it to the lungs for reoxygenation. The right atrium receives deoxygenated blood from the body via the superior and inferior vena cava and from the heart muscle via the coronary sinus and pumps it through the tricuspid valve into the right ventricle. The right ventricle, a flat muscular pump, receives deoxygenated blood from the right atrium and pumps it through the pulmonary valve, against low resistance, into the pulmonary artery and into the lungs.

2 The heart pumps oxygenated blood into the systemic circulation, which carries it to the cells. The left atrium receives oxygenated blood from the lungs, via the pulmonary veins, and pumps it through the mitral valve to the left ventricle. The left ventricle, the heart's largest, most muscular chamber, receives oxygenated blood from the lungs via the left atrium and pumps it through the aortic valve against high systemic pressure into the aorta and into the systemic circulation.

FIGURE 32-1 ■ The structure and function of the heart. (From Luckman J, ed: *Saunders manual of nursing care,* Philadelphia, 1997, WB Saunders.)

   b. Left and right bundle branches
      (1) Deliver impulse to the Purkinje fibers
      (2) Fibers carry impulse to the ventricular muscle
 C. Cardiac cycle
   1. Systole
      a. Isovolumetric contraction
         (1) Ventricular pressure is generated but has not exceeded vascular pressure.
         (2) Pulmonic and aortic valves closed

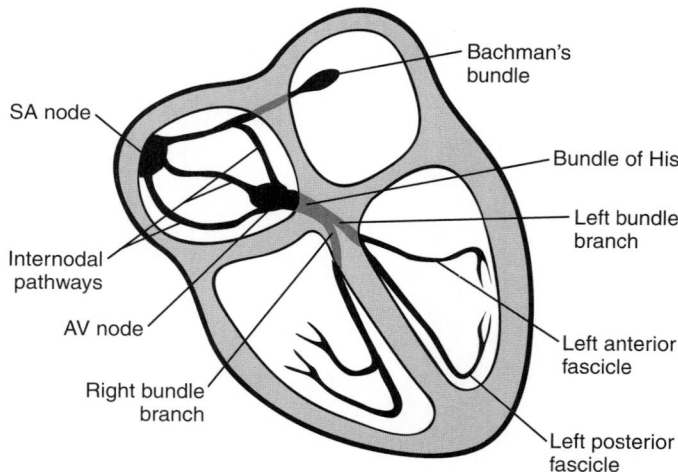

FIGURE 32-2 ■ The conduction system. (From Van Riper S, Luciano A: Basic cardiac arrhythmias: A review for postanesthesia care unit nurses. *J Perianesth Nurs* 9[1]:3, 1994.)

   (3) Tricuspid and mitral valves closed
   (4) Highest oxygen consumption phase of the ventricle ~66%
   b. Systolic ejection
      (1) Ventricular pressure exceeds vascular pressure.
      (2) Pulmonic and aortic valves opened
      (3) Tricuspid and mitral valves closed
      (4) Blood ejected into the vasculature
   2. Diastole
      a. Ventricular relaxation
         (1) Ventricular pressure decreases to less than vascular pressure.
         (2) Pulmonic and aortic valves shut.
         (3) Mitral and tricuspid valves open.
            (a) Ventricles fill passively.
            (b) Coronary artery blood flow is optimal.
               (i) Elevated diastole, less coronary artery filling
               (ii) Shorter diastole, (tachycardia) less coronary filling
         (4) Atrial contraction
            (a) End filling is referred to as atrial kick.
            (b) Atrial pressure decreases and ventricular volume and pressure increases.
      b. Provides for:
         (1) Myocardial perfusion
         (2) Ventricular filling
D. Functional properties of cardiac muscle
   1. Excitability: ability of a nerve to produce an action potential
   2. Automaticity: spontaneous depolarization and generation of an action potential
   3. Conductivity: ability to conduct electricity
   4. Refractoriness: resistance to stimulation while heart is still contracting from an earlier stimulus
   5. Contractility: ability to shorten when stimulated
   6. Extensibility: ability to stretch when heart fills with blood during diastole
   7. Rhythmicity
      a. Ability to function with a definite rhythm
      b. Stimulation—transmission—contraction—relaxation
   8. Irritability: ability to be stimulated

E. Effects of anesthesia on the heart
   1. Tachydysrhythmias and bradydysrhythmias
   2. Decreased contractility
   3. Decreased cardiac output (CO)
   4. Premature beats
   5. Changes in inotropy and vascular tone

III. VASCULAR STRUCTURE AND FUNCTION
   A. Structure (Figure 32-3)
   B. Function
      1. Arteries
         a. Transport oxygenated blood from the heart to the tissues
         b. Exception: pulmonary artery (PA) transports deoxygenated blood from the right ventricle (RV) to the lungs.
      2. Capillaries: thin-walled structures allow for the exchange of nutrients and wastes between the blood and cells.
      3. Veins
         a. Transport deoxygenated blood from the tissues to the right side of the heart
         b. Exception: pulmonary vein transports oxygenated blood from the lungs to the left atrium.

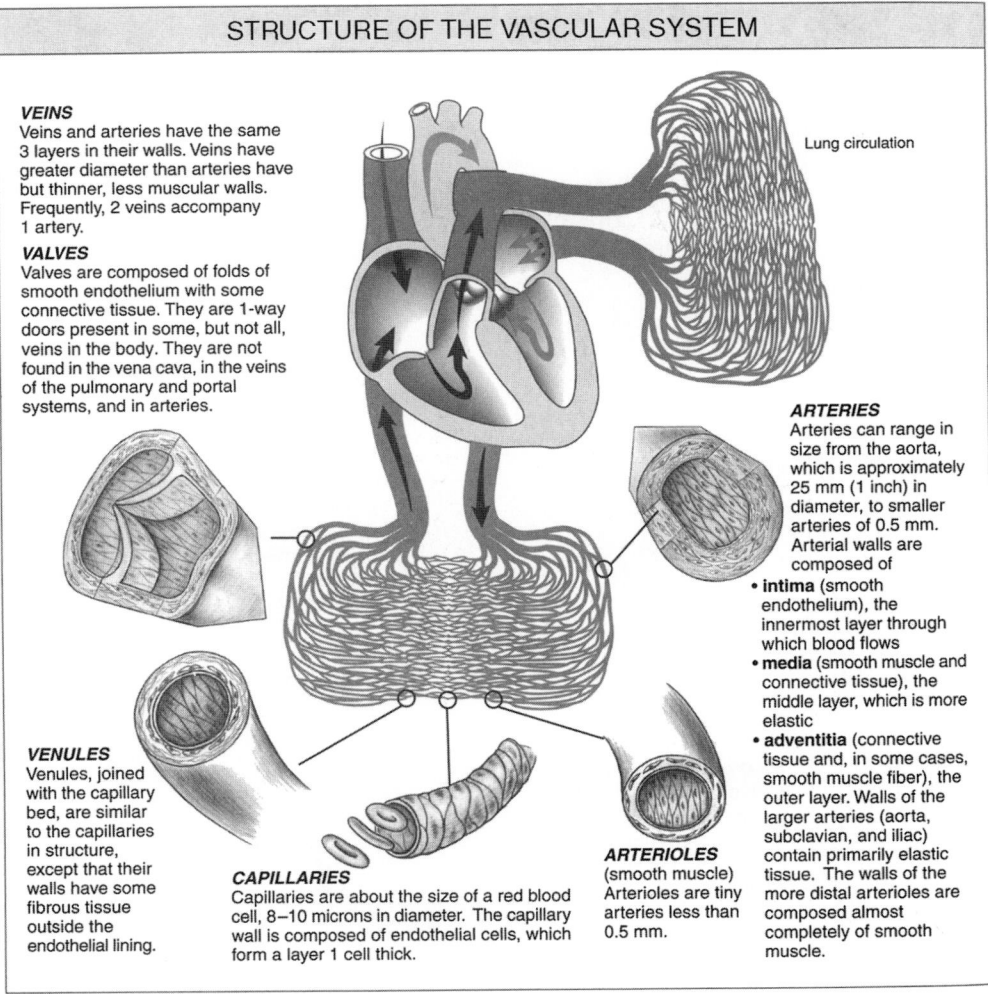

STRUCTURE OF THE VASCULAR SYSTEM

VEINS
Veins and arteries have the same 3 layers in their walls. Veins have greater diameter than arteries have but thinner, less muscular walls. Frequently, 2 veins accompany 1 artery.

VALVES
Valves are composed of folds of smooth endothelium with some connective tissue. They are 1-way doors present in some, but not all, veins in the body. They are not found in the vena cava, in the veins of the pulmonary and portal systems, and in arteries.

Lung circulation

ARTERIES
Arteries can range in size from the aorta, which is approximately 25 mm (1 inch) in diameter, to smaller arteries of 0.5 mm. Arterial walls are composed of
- **intima** (smooth endothelium), the innermost layer through which blood flows
- **media** (smooth muscle and connective tissue), the middle layer, which is more elastic
- **adventitia** (connective tissue and, in some cases, smooth muscle fiber), the outer layer. Walls of the larger arteries (aorta, subclavian, and iliac) contain primarily elastic tissue. The walls of the more distal arterioles are composed almost completely of smooth muscle.

VENULES
Venules, joined with the capillary bed, are similar to the capillaries in structure, except that their walls have some fibrous tissue outside the endothelial lining.

CAPILLARIES
Capillaries are about the size of a red blood cell, 8–10 microns in diameter. The capillary wall is composed of endothelial cells, which form a layer 1 cell thick.

ARTERIOLES
(smooth muscle) Arterioles are tiny arteries less than 0.5 mm.

FIGURE 32-3 ■ Structure of the vascular system. (From Luckman J, ed: *Saunders' manual of nursing care*, Philadelphia, 1997, WB Saunders.)

    c. Approximately 75% of total blood volume found in the venous system at any given time

    d. Venous return controlled by several factors

       (1) Valves (Figure 32-4)

          (a) Prevent backflow of blood, allowing flow to occur only in the direction toward the heart

          (b) Become incompetent when vein walls have been overstretched by excessive venous pressure

          (c) Muscle pump

          (d) Gravity

       (2) Venous elasticity

          (a) Venous walls less elastic than arterial walls, thus allowing distention or pooling to occur

          (b) Known as venous capacitance

       (3) Intrathoracic pressure

          (a) Negative intrathoracic pressure enhances flow into the heart by decreasing resistance.

          (b) Positive intrathoracic pressure reduces flow into the heart by increasing resistance.

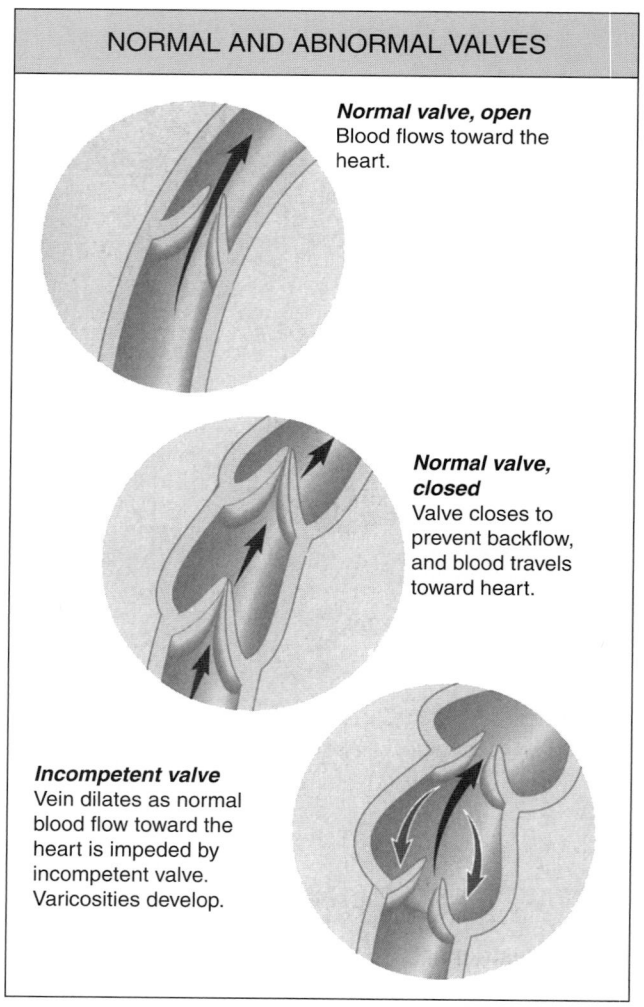

NORMAL AND ABNORMAL VALVES

Normal valve, open
Blood flows toward the heart.

Normal valve, closed
Valve closes to prevent backflow, and blood travels toward heart.

Incompetent valve
Vein dilates as normal blood flow toward the heart is impeded by incompetent valve. Varicosities develop.

FIGURE 32-4 ■ Normal and abnormal valves. (From Luckman J, ed: *Saunders' manual of nursing care,* Philadelphia, 1997, WB Saunders.)

      4. Arteriovenous anastomoses: channels where arterioles and venules connect without capillaries

  C. Control of blood flow

     1. Neural control

       a. Baroreceptors (stretch receptors) and chemoreceptors on the aortic arch, internal carotid sinus, and in the right atrium

         (1) Sense changes in blood pressure (BP) and chemical composition

         (2) Send messages to the vasomotor center in the medulla

         (3) Stimulate the sympathetic nervous system (SNS) cardioaccelerator to respond

           (a) Low pressure: epinephrine and norepinephrine released (SNS)

           (b) Causes:

              (i)   Vasoconstriction

              (ii) Increased heart rate (HR)

              (iii) Increased contractility

         (4) Stimulate the parasympathetic nervous system (PNS) cardio-decelerator to respond

           (a) High pressure: acetylcholine released (PNS)

           (b) Causes vasodilation

     2. Humoral control

       a. Also stimulated by SNS in reaction to changes in blood flow, as well as other substances in the body

         (1) Low-flow states

           (a) Corticotropin released, leading to:

              (i)   Sodium and water reabsorption in renal tubules

              (ii) Increased intravascular volume

           (b) Renin-angiotensin-aldosterone system (RAAS) stimulated

              (i)   Marked constriction of peripheral arteries

              (ii) Sodium and water retention

           (c) Antidiuretic hormone released: increased water reabsorption in the renal tubules, resulting in increased intravascular volume

         (2) High-flow states

           (a) Bradykinin (plasma protein): potent vasodilator

           (b) Histamine: vasodilator released after mast cell injury

         (3) Feedback systems

           (a) Brain natriuretic peptide (BNP), a natural antagonist to RAAS, is released by the myocardial myocyte in response to volume overload.

     3. Local control: autoregulation

       a. Blood vessels' ability to respond to tissue needs by dilating or constricting

       b. Used mainly by arterioles as a result of:

         (1) Decreased oxygen availability

         (2) Increased metabolic demand at the tissue level

IV. FOUNDATIONS OF TISSUE OXYGENATION

  A. Effective postoperative care and positive outcomes depend on a thorough understanding of oxygenation.

  B. Every assessment and intervention focused toward optimizing tissue perfusion

  C. Tissue perfusion optimized by:

     1. Maximizing oxygen delivery (Dao_2)

     2. Minimizing oxygen consumption (Vo_2)

  D. Key ingredients of Dao_2

     1. CO

     2. Hemoglobin (Hb)

     3. Arterial oxygen saturation (Sao_2)

  E. Key ingredients of CO

     1. CO = Stroke volume (SV) × HR

     2. CO is the major contributor (or detractor) of Dao_2.

     3. Control factors for HR

      a. SNS (epinephrine) increases rate.
        (1) HR greater than 130 beats/min decreases:
          (a) Diastolic filling time
          (b) Myocardial perfusion
      b. PNS (acetylcholine) decreases rate.
        (1) HR less than 50 beats/min may decrease CO.
    4. Control factors for SV
      a. Preload
        (1) End-diastolic ventricular volume
        (2) Measured by pressure
        (3) Controls "stretch" of myocardial fibers
        (4) Increase in preload
          (a) Stretches myocardial fibers
          (b) Improves contractility (Frank-Starling's law)
        (5) Excessive preload
          (a) Overstretches fibers
          (b) Results in decreased contractility
        (6) Preload affected by:
          (a) Volume returning to ventricle
          (b) Volume leaving ventricle
      b. Afterload: resistance to ejection of blood from the ventricle
        (1) Increased by:
          (a) Peripheral arterial vasoconstriction
          (b) Obstruction of flow
            (i) Valvular stenosis
            (ii) Pulmonary embolus
          (c) Increased ventricular diameter (i.e., congestive heart failure [CHF])
          (d) Blood viscosity (i.e., increased hematocrit)
        (2) Decreased by:
          (a) Peripheral arterial vasodilation
          (b) Incompetent valves
          (c) Hemodilution
      c. Contractility: inherent ability of myocardial muscle fibers to shorten and contract
        (1) Increased by:
          (a) Sympathetic nervous stimulation
        (2) Decreased by:
          (a) Ischemia/hypoxia
          (b) Hypothermia
          (c) Imbalances
            (i) Hypocalcemia
            (ii) Hypomagnesemia
            (iii) Hypokalemia
          (d) Acidosis/hypercapnia
          (e) Cellular changes
            (i) CHF
            (ii) Cardiomyopathy

V. ASSESSMENT AND MANAGEMENT
  A. Preoperative baseline assessment
  B. Cardiac-focused assessment
    1. Chest pain
      a. Stable
      b. Unstable
    2. Dyspnea (most common symptom of organic heart disease)
    3. Paroxysmal nocturnal dyspnea (PND)
    4. Syncope
    5. Unexplained weakness or fatigue
    6. Weight loss or gain

7. Dependent edema
8. Orthopnea
9. Coughing at night (assess for angiotensin converting enzyme [ACE] inhibitor use)
10. Hemoptysis
11. Rapid heartbeat or palpitations
12. Nocturia
13. Intermittent claudication

C. Peripheral vascular–focused assessment
  1. Skin
    a. Turgor
    b. Edema
    c. Compare temperature at different sites.
    d. Inspect for lesions or ulcerations.
    e. Determine history of slow wound healing.
    f. Inspect for varicose veins: visibly engorged, palpable subcutaneous veins.
    g. Differentiate between venous and arterial insufficiency.
      (1) Arterial insufficiency
        (a) Loss of hair
        (b) Pallor
        (c) Translucent, waxy appearance of skin
      (2) Venous insufficiency
        (a) Skin thickened
        (b) Reddish-brown pigmentation
        (c) Ulceration
  2. Vasculature and circulation
    a. Arterial
      (1) Capillary refill
        (a) Brisk: <3 seconds
        (b) Sluggish: >3 seconds
      (2) Bruits: low-pitched blowing sound from turbulent flow
        (a) Indicative of atherosclerosis
        (b) Assess with bell of stethoscope at:
          (i) Carotid arteries
          (ii) Femoral arteries
          (iii) Abdominal aorta
      (3) Determine strength of peripheral pulses.
        (a) Absent: 0
        (b) Weak and thready: 1
        (c) Normal: 2
        (d) Full and bounding: 3
      (4) Neurovascular assessment: five *P*'s, indicative of arterial insufficiency
        (a) Pain
        (b) Pulselessness
        (c) Pallor
        (d) Paresthesia
        (e) Paralysis
        (f) Ankle-brachial index: inexpensive, noninvasive bedside assessment of arterial perfusion (atherosclerosis)
          (i) Obtain brachial BP in both arms (use the higher systolic pressure for the calculation).
          (ii) Obtain ankle BP in the questionable extremity.
          (iii) Divide the systolic ankle pressure by the systolic brachial pressure.
          (iv) Index >0.95: normal perfusion
          (v) Index <0.90
            [a] Early asymptomatic disease

        [b] Difficulty with wound healing
        [c] Increased risk for cardiovascular event (i.e., myocardial infarction [MI] or death)
    (vi) Index <0.60
        [a] Wound probably will not heal.
        [b] More advanced atheroma
        [c] Greater risk for cardiovascular event or death
    (vii) Index >1.3: indicative of calcified arteries (usually associated with diabetes)

b. Venous
  (1) Superficial thrombophlebitis: subcutaneous cords with overlying erythema
  (2) Deep vein thrombosis (DVT)
    (a) Silent at onset
    (b) Shooting pain at moment of embolism, with numbness and weakness followed by signs of ischemia
    (c) Homan's sign
      (i) Positive: pain in popliteal fossa and upper posterior calf on dorsiflexion of foot
      (ii) Helpful but not specific for DVT

D. Preexisting disease states
  1. Atherosclerotic heart disease
  2. Diabetes
  3. Hypertension
  4. Chronic obstructive pulmonary disease
  5. Previous MI
  6. CHF

E. Specific allergies
  1. Shellfish
  2. Iodine
  3. Contrast media

F. Cardiac auscultation
  1. Normal heart sounds
    a. S1 (first heart sound)
      (1) Represents closure of tricuspid and mitral AV valves
      (2) Occurs at the end of atrial contraction and with the onset of ventricular contraction
      (3) Loudest at the apex
      (4) Slightly longer and lower pitch than S2
      (5) Occurs as ventricles contract; almost synchronous with carotid pulse
    b. S2 (second heart sound)
      (1) Caused by closure of aortic and pulmonic valves at end of ventricular contraction
      (2) Signals the beginning of diastole
      (3) Loudest at the base
      (4) Higher pitch than S1, so is louder and transmits better
    c. Split heart sounds
      (1) Split S1: occurs if right and left AV valves do not close at precisely the same time
      (2) Split S2: occurs if semilunar valves do not close simultaneously
      (3) Slight time variance normal caused by inspiration; wide variance in time between right-and left-sided valve closure possibly related to conduction defects or obstruction to flow
  2. Extra heart sounds
    a. S3 (ventricular gallop, Figure 32-5)
      (1) Immediately follows S2; sounds like "lubb-dup-up" or "Ken-tuc-ky"
      (2) Dull and low-pitched
      (3) Normal finding in children and healthy young adults

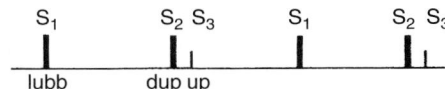

FIGURE 32-5 ■ Auscultated cadence of the third heart sound. (From Darovic GO, ed: *Hemodynamic monitoring: Invasive and noninvasive clinical application,* ed 3, Philadelphia, 2002, WB Saunders.)

(4) Best heard with bell of stethoscope at:
    (a) Apex
    (b) Patient in left lateral position
(5) Occurs when AV valves open and atrial blood rushes into ventricles
(6) Usually indicates decreased compliance of ventricles commonly associated with heart failure
(7) May also indicate mitral or tricuspid AV valve incompetence
(8) Signifies ventricular failure in older adults
  b. S4 (atrial gallop, Figure 32-6)
    (1) Immediately precedes S1; sounds like "la-lubb-dup" or "Ten-nes-see"
    (2) Very low pitch
    (3) Best heard at apex with bell of stethoscope
    (4) Produced by atrial contraction when the ventricle is resistant to filling
    (5) Heard in patients with:
      (a) Decreased compliance of ventricles as seen in:
        (i) Myocardial ischemia
        (ii) Pulmonary hypertension
        (iii) Heart failure
      (b) Increased SV as seen with severe anemia and hyperthyroidism
      (c) Delayed conduction between atria and ventricles
3. Murmurs
  a. Caused by increased turbulence or blood flow through the heart
  b. Causes
    (1) Stenosis: valves will not open properly.
    (2) Regurgitant (incompetent, insufficient): valves will not close properly to prevent backward flow of blood.
    (3) Presence of a congenital defect between chambers
    (4) Dilated heart chamber
    (5) Other
      (a) Increased blood flow: pregnancy, hyperthyroidism
      (b) Decreased blood viscosity
  c. Murmur description should include:
    (1) Primary location related to valve where best auscultated
    (2) Area of radiation or site of maximum intensity
    (3) Timing as related to cardiac cycle
    (4) Pitch
    (5) Configuration or shape as determined by intensity over time
    (6) Quality
      (a) Blowing
      (b) Rumbling
      (c) Musical
      (d) Harsh
      (e) Intensity

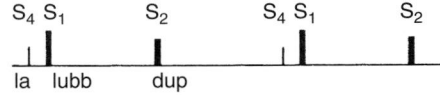

FIGURE 32-6 ■ Auscultated cadence of the fourth heart sound. (From Darovic GO, ed: *Hemodynamic monitoring: Invasive and noninvasive clinical application,* ed 3, Philadelphia, 2002, WB Saunders.)

        (7) Intensity (loudness)
           (a) Grade I: very faint, heard only after a period of intent listening
           (b) Grade II: quiet and faint, but heard immediately upon placing the stethoscope on the chest
           (c) Grade III: moderately intense
           (d) Grade IV: loud, associated with a thrill
           (e) Grade V: very loud, can be heard with the stethoscope partially off the chest wall
           (f) Grade VI: very loud, can be heard with the entire chest piece just removed from the chest wall
    4. Pericardial friction rub
      a. Occurs if the pericardium becomes inflamed
      b. A scratchy "to-and-fro"; should be heard with each heartbeat
      c. Best auscultated with patient sitting upright and leaning forward
  G. Laboratory studies
    1. Arterial blood gases (ABGs) as indicated
    2. Cardiac enzymes and markers (if history significant for myocardial ischemia) (Table 32-1)
      a. Creatine Kinase–MB isoenzyme (CK-MB; cardiac specific)
        (1) Normal within 3 days: compromised ability for late diagnosis of MI
        (2) >10 to 13 U/L or >3% to 5% total CK activity
      b. Biochemical markers cardiac troponin I (cTnI) and cardiac troponin T (cTntT)
        (1) Efficient for diagnosis of MI because it rises within one hour
        (2) Remain elevated for 7 to 10 days: compromise ability to diagnose recurrent infarction if used alone
    3. Electrolytes critical to cardiac function
      a. Potassium
      b. Sodium
      c. Magnesium
      d. Calcium
    4. Coagulation profile
      a. Prothrombin time (PT)
      b. Partial thromboplastin time (PTT)
      c. International normalized ratio
    5. BNP levels >100 mcg/mL: highly significant for heart failure (volume overload)

■ TABLE 32-1
■ ■ **Cardiac Marker Activity After Myocardial Infarction**

Marker	Onset of Elevation (h)	Peak Elevation (h)	Return to Normal (days)
Troponin I (cTnI)* Normal <3.1 ng/mL	Within minutes	1	7–10
CK 12–80 U/L males 10–70 U/L females	3–6	12–24	24–48
CK-MB (cardiac specific) 0%–3% total CK	4–8	18–24	3
LDH 45–90 U/L	24–72	72–96	10–14
LDH$_1$ (cardiac specific) 20%–30% total LDH	12–24	48	10–14
LDH$_1$ to LDH$_2$ ratio <1 (i.e., LDH$_2$ >LDH$_1$)	12–24	48	10–14

*Considered most diagnostic of myocardial injury.
CK, Creatine kinase; *CK-MB,* Creatine Kinase–MB isoenzyme; *LDH,* lactate dehydrogenase.
From Hicks FD: *Core curriculum for postanesthesia nursing practice,* ed 4, Philadelphia, 1999, Saunders.

H. Noninvasive diagnostic studies
  1. Chest x-ray (CXR)
  2. Electrocardiogram (ECG)
    a. Twelve-lead ECG
    b. Determines or detects:
      (1) Disturbances of rate, rhythm, or conduction
      (2) Ischemia or infarction
      (3) Electrolyte abnormalities
      (4) Anatomic orientation of heart
      (5) Chamber enlargement
      (6) Drug toxicity
  3. Echocardiography
    a. Ultrasonic exam
    b. Detects abnormalities of anatomy and/or motion and blood flow
  4. Radionuclide imaging
    a. Uses radioactive tracer injected into bloodstream
      (1) Thallium-201 [TI-201]
      (2) Technetium-99m [Tc-99m]
    b. May be performed at rest or with exercise stress or pharmacologic vasodilation
      (1) Infarction scintigram: detects regional perfusion deficits that represent areas of ischemic or infarcted cardiac muscle
      (2) Left ventricular (LV) angiography—assesses ventricular:
        (a) Size
        (b) Volume
        (c) Ejection fraction
        (d) Wall abnormality
      (3) Positron emission tomography (PET): uses biologically active radiopharmaceuticals to distinguish dysfunctional but viable myocardium from infarcted tissue
  5. Exercise electrocardiography (stress testing)
    a. Most widely used method for assessing the presence and severity of coronary artery disease (CAD)
    b. Observation, measurement and recording of ECG, BP, and HR in response to progressively increasing, graded levels of work
    c. May combine or use pharmacological stressing for individuals unable to perform physically
I. Invasive diagnostic studies
  1. Cardiac catheterization: fluoroscopically guided placement of catheters in the heart to measure:
    a. Intracardiac pressures
    b. Valve function
    c. Saturation
    d. Angiography—injection of radiographic contrast material into:
      (1) Cardiac chambers (ventriculography)
      (2) Coronary arteries
      (3) Valve roots (aortography)
      (4) Great vessels
  2. Electrophysiology studies—fluoroscopically guided intracardiac placement of catheters to assess:
    a. Spontaneous function
    b. Responses to stress
    c. Vulnerability to induced tachydysrhythmias
    d. Diagnostic modality for characterizing:
      (1) Dysrhythmic disorders
      (2) Stratifying risk
      (3) Directing therapy for chronic dysrhythmic disorders

3. Endomyocardial biopsy: acquisition of a small piece of myocardium for microscopic analysis using a specially designed catheter
   a. Diagnostic technique for evaluating cardiac failure of unknown cause and response to cardiac transplantation
   J. Medications
   1. Types
   2. Dosages
   3. Consult with anesthesia or surgeon as to necessity of taking cardiac and antihypertensive medications the morning of surgery.
   4. If unable to obtain consult, have patient bring medications on the morning of surgery.
VI. CARDIOVASCULAR OPERATIVE PROCEDURES
   A. Coronary artery revascularization
   B. Valvular repair or replacement
   C. Permanent pacemaker implantation (for detailed information on evidence-based guidelines for permanent pacemakers, (see ACC/AHA/HRS guidelines for implantation of permanent pacemakers and antidysrhythmia devices)
   1. Indications
      a. Complete heart block
      b. Symptomatic bradycardia associated with sinus node dysfunction or second-degree heart block
      c. Acute MI with persistent, advanced second- or third-degree heart block
      d. Recurrent syncope associated with hypersensitive carotid sinus syndrome
      e. Advanced block with atrial fibrillation or flutter and symptomatic slow ventricular rate
      f. Symptomatic bradycardia secondary to pharmacological therapy
   2. Pacing modes (Table 32-2)
      a. Single chamber
         (1) AAI—demand atrial pacemaker
         (2) VVI—demand ventricular pacemaker
      b. Dual chamber
         (1) DDD—demand atrial and ventricular pacemaker
      c. Resynchronization for patients with heart failure
   3. Implantation
      a. May be same-day procedure; overnight hospital stay more typical
      b. Preoperative considerations
         (1) Education and informed consent
            (a) Postprocedure restrictions
            (b) Anticoagulants discontinued for several days (may have to initiate heparin therapy for patients with prosthetic valves)
         (2) Laboratory tests: chemistries and coagulation studies
         (3) CXR
         (4) Antibiotics (preoperative and postoperative)
      c. Intraoperative considerations
         (1) Catheterization laboratory or operating room (OR)

■ TABLE 32-2
■ ■ **Three-Position Pacemaker Code**

Chamber Paced	**Chamber Sensed**	**Mode of Response***
V = Ventricle	V = Ventricle	I = Inhibited
A = Atrium	A = Atrium	T = Triggered
D = Atrium and ventricle	D = Atrium and ventricle	D = Atrial triggered and ventricle inhibited
0 = None	0 = None	0 = None

*Inhibited = will not pace on sensing spontaneous cardiac activity. Triggered = delivers stimulus just after spontaneous depolarization and resets timing immediately on sensing spontaneous cardiac activity.

   (2) Local anesthesia with mild sedation

   (3) Inserted through right or left subclavian or jugular vein

   (4) Pulse generator placement below the clavicle in a pocket between the pectoral muscle fascia and the overlying subcutaneous tissue

    (a) Depends on patient factors such as:

     (i) Previous surgeries (e.g., mastectomy)

     (ii) History of radiation

     (iii) Central line placement

     (iv) Infection

     (v) Dermatitis

     (vi) Vein occlusion

     (vii) Patient's hobbies and dominant hand

 d. Postoperative considerations

  (1) Complications

   (a) Perforation of the subclavian vein or RV

   (b) Pneumothorax

   (c) Pacemaker failure

   (d) Electromagnetic interference (EMI): any signal, biological or nonbiological, that is detected by the pacemaker and results in rate alteration or sensing abnormalities. Possible causes are:

    (i) Welding equipment

    (ii) Store security equipment: maintain safe distance; do not lean on equipment.

    (iii) Electric generators

    (iv) Microwave ovens considered safe for use

   (e) Pacemaker syndrome: hemodynamic compromise with VVI pacing as a result of intermittent loss of AV synchrony

    (i) Reprogram pacemaker.

    (ii) Replace generator.

   (f) Cross-talk: inappropriate sensing of output in dual-chamber pacemakers from one lead by the other with inhibition of pacing

    (i) Reprogram pacemaker.

   (g) Pacemaker-mediated tachycardia: circular reentrant tachycardia induced by an ectopic ventricular impulse that is conducted retrograde to the atria in dual-chamber pacemakers with atrial sensing

    (i) Apply a magnet over the pulse generator to disable atrial sensing.

    (ii) Reprogram pacemaker.

   (h) Infection

   (i) Frequently produce fistula formation and chronic infection until removal of the pulse generator and as much of the leads as possible is accomplished

  (2) Nursing care and follow-up

   (a) Bed rest for 6 to 12 hours

   (b) Limited arm movements on affected side

   (c) Limited activity requiring vigorous arm movement for several weeks (e.g., golf, tennis)

   (d) Written and verbal instruction regarding descriptive information and pacemaker identification (patient given a temporary wallet card)

   (e) Device registered with manufacturer for patient notification in the event of device recall

   (f) Comprehensive pacemaker performance evaluation

D. Implantable cardioverter-defibrillator (ICD), automatic ICD (AICD)

 1. Indications

  a. Cardiac arrest not the result of a reversible cause

      b. Spontaneous, sustained ventricular tachycardia (VT) or ventricular fibrillation (VF)

      c. Syncope of undetermined origin with clinically relevant, hemodynamically significant, sustained VT or VF

      d. Nonsustained VT with CAD, prior MI, LV dysfunction and inducible VF or sustained VT at electrophysiology study not suppressed by a class I antidysrhythmic

  2. ICD therapies

      a. All current ICDs have the ability to:

        (1) Defibrillate

        (2) Cardiovert

        (3) Provide antitachycardia and antibradycardia pacing

      b. Preoperative considerations

        (1) Same as for pacemaker except:

          (a) May be hospitalized preoperatively because of cardiac arrest or sustained VT

          (b) Potential for significant lifestyle changes (e.g., driving) because of the possibilities of injury with syncope or working in an area with EMI

          (c) Education regarding possibility of discomfort with cardioversion

      c. Intraoperative considerations

        (1) Transvenous implantation in catheterization laboratory or OR

        (2) Local anesthesia and sedation and analgesia; occasional need for deep sedation or general anesthesia

        (3) External defibrillation patches placed on chest before draping patient

        (4) Implantation site determination same as for pacemaker; generator occasionally placed in abdomen

        (5) Early complications

          (a) Difficult or unobtainable venous access

          (b) Pneumothorax

          (c) Tamponade

          (d) Excessive defibrillation threshold

          (e) Refractory VF

      d. Postoperative considerations

        (1) Nursing care and follow-up

          (a) Bed rest for 6 to 18 hours in a monitored setting

          (b) Standard transthoracic defibrillation in the event of sustained VT or VF. Do not place paddles directly over generator.

          (c) Limited arm movement on affected side

          (d) CXR

          (e) Discharge day of or day after implantation

          (f) Written and verbal instructions regarding device description (temporary identification card given), activity restrictions, and instructions for what to do if device is discharged

            (i) Driving typically restricted for 6 months

            (ii) Magnetic resonance imaging (MRI) prohibited

          (g) Family support and teaching

            (i) BLS training prior to discharge to alleviate anxiety

        (2) Late complications

          (a) Lead dislodgment

          (b) Pocket hematoma

          (c) Poor wound healing

          (d) Worsening of dysrhythmia

          (e) Anxiety and depression: early psychological intervention suggested for patients identified with significant anxiety and emotional distress

VII. CARDIAC COMPLICATIONS
   A. Hypotension
      1. Definition: systolic BP >20% below baseline
      2. Assessment findings
         a. Low BP
         b. Decreased urine output (oliguria to anuria)
         c. Tachycardia, tachypnea
         d. Pale, cool, clammy extremities
         e. Disorientation to unconsciousness
         f. Nausea
         g. Chest pain
      3. Potential causes
         a. Decreased intravascular volume
         b. LV failure
         c. Decreased vascular tone
         d. Exhaustion of catecholamines (e.g., prolonged pain)
      4. Treatment
         a. Oxygen therapy
         b. Assess and replace intravascular volume.
         c. For ventricular failure
            (1) Coronary vasodilators
            (2) Decrease afterload
            (3) Inotropic support
         d. Maximize vascular tone.
            (1) Discontinue vasodilators.
            (2) Administer vasoconstrictive agents.
         e. Pain management
      5. Prevention through:
            (1) Monitoring of preoperative, intraoperative, and postoperative volume status
            (2) Titration of vasoactive and cardiac medications
   B. Hypertension
      1. Definition: BP >20% to 30% above baseline BP
      2. Assessment findings
         a. Elevated BP
         b. Signs of sympathetic stimulation
         c. Headache
         d. Decreased level of consciousness with disruption of cerebral autoregulation and cerebral hemorrhage
         e. Signs of ventricular failure and pulmonary edema with long-standing elevations (>190/100 mm Hg for 3 hours or more)
      3. Potential causes
         a. Preexisting disease
         b. CNS damage
         c. Cardiovascular impairment
         d. Excess catecholamine production (e.g., pain, emotional stress)
         e. Hypoxemia and hypercarbia
         f. Endocrinopathies
         g. Hypothermia
         h. Excess intravascular volume
         i. Sudden withdrawal or overdose of medications
         j. Visceral distention
         k. Preeclampsia
      4. Treatment
         a. Assess for and alleviate cause.
            (1) Restart antihypertensives.
            (2) Maximize cardiac function.
            (3) Pain and stress management

(4) Maximize respiratory function.

(5) Rewarming

(6) Correct fluid overload (fluid restriction and diuretics).

(7) Decrease visceral distention (Foley catheter, nasogastric tube).

5. Prevention
   a. Assess for potential causes early.
   b. Patients to take antihypertensives on day of surgery

C. Cardiac dysrhythmias

1. Causes
   a. Disturbances in automaticity—speeding and slowing
   b. Disturbances in conduction—too slow or fast
   c. Combinations of altered automaticity and conduction

2. Normal ECG (Figure 32-7)
   a. P wave—represents origination of impulse in sinus node; abnormality indicates impulse origination in some other area of heart; atrial depolarization
   b. PR interval—represents conduction through atria and AV node and into bundle of His
   c. QRS complex—represents conduction through bundle branches; ventricular depolarization
   d. T wave—ventricular repolarization

3. Rhythm assessment
   a. Electrode placement
      (1) Lead I: positive left arm; negative right arm
      (2) Lead II: positive left leg; negative right arm
      (3) Lead III: positive left leg; negative left arm
   b. Evaluate rate.
      (1) Bradycardia (<60 beats/min)
      (2) Tachycardia (>100 beats/min)
   c. Evaluate regularity.
      (1) R-R interval
      (2) P-P interval
   d. Evaluate P waves.
      (1) Presence: does a P wave precede every QRS complex?
      (2) Morphology: do all the P waves look alike?
      (3) Relationship to QRS complex
         (a) PR interval (normal = 0.12-0.20 seconds)
         (b) Length and consistency

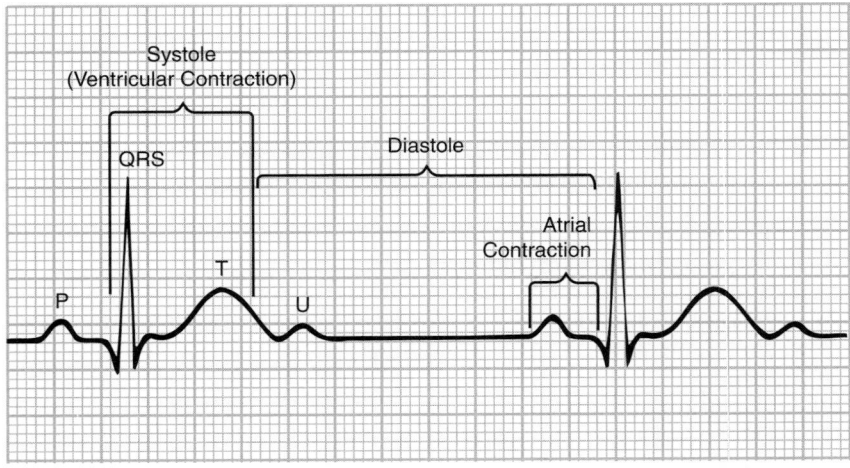

FIGURE 32-7 ■ Normal ECG. (From Grauer K: *A practical guide to ECG interpretation,* ed 2, St Louis, 1998, Mosby.)

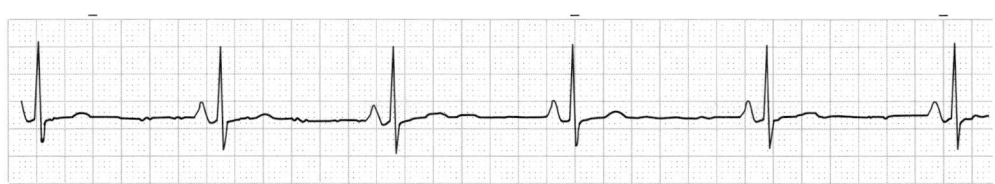

FIGURE 32-8 ■ Sinus bradycardia. (From Paul S, Hera J, eds: *The nurse's guide to cardiac rhythm interpretation,* Philadelphia, 1998, WB Saunders.)

    e. Evaluate QRS complex.
      (1) Width (normal = 0.12 seconds)
  4. Dysrhythmia recognition and treatment
    a. Bradycardias
      (1) Sinus bradycardia (Figure 32-8)
        (a) Description: characterized by decrease in HR caused by slowing of sinus node. May be a result of:
          (i) Sinus node disease
          (ii) Increased parasympathetic tone
          (iii) Drug effects (beta-blockers, digitalis)
        (b) ECG criteria
          (i) Rate: <60 beats/min
          (ii) Rhythm: regular
          (iii) P waves: upright
        (c) Treatment—if symptomatic, consider:
          (i) Atropine, 0.5 to 1 mg IV to a total of 0.03 mg/kg
          (ii) Transcutaneous pacing
          (iii) Dopamine, 5 to 20 mcg/kg/min
          (iv) Epinephrine, 2 to 10 mcg/min
      (2) First-degree block (Figure 32-9)
        (a) Description: delayed conduction through AV node between atria and ventricles
        (b) ECG criteria
          (i) Regular rhythm
          (ii) P wave followed by QRS
          (iii) Prolonged PR interval (>0.20 sec)
          (iv) QRS normal
        (c) Treatment: none, does not result in symptoms
      (3) Second-degree type I: Wenckebach block (Figure 32-10)
        (a) ECG criteria
          (i) Ventricular rate less than atrial rate
          (ii) Rhythm usually irregular
          (iii) P waves normal and followed by QRS except for dropped beat
          (iv) PR interval gets progressively longer until ventricular beat is dropped.
          (v) QRS normal

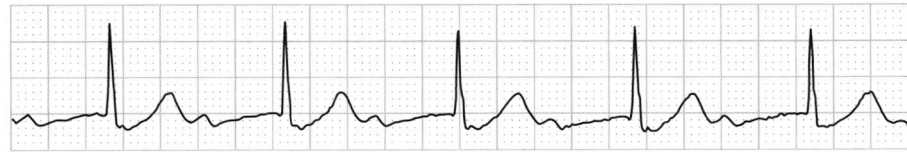

FIGURE 32-9 ■ First-degree AV block. (From Paul S, Hera J, eds: *The nurse's guide to cardiac rhythm interpretation,* Philadelphia, 1998, WB Saunders.)

Lead II

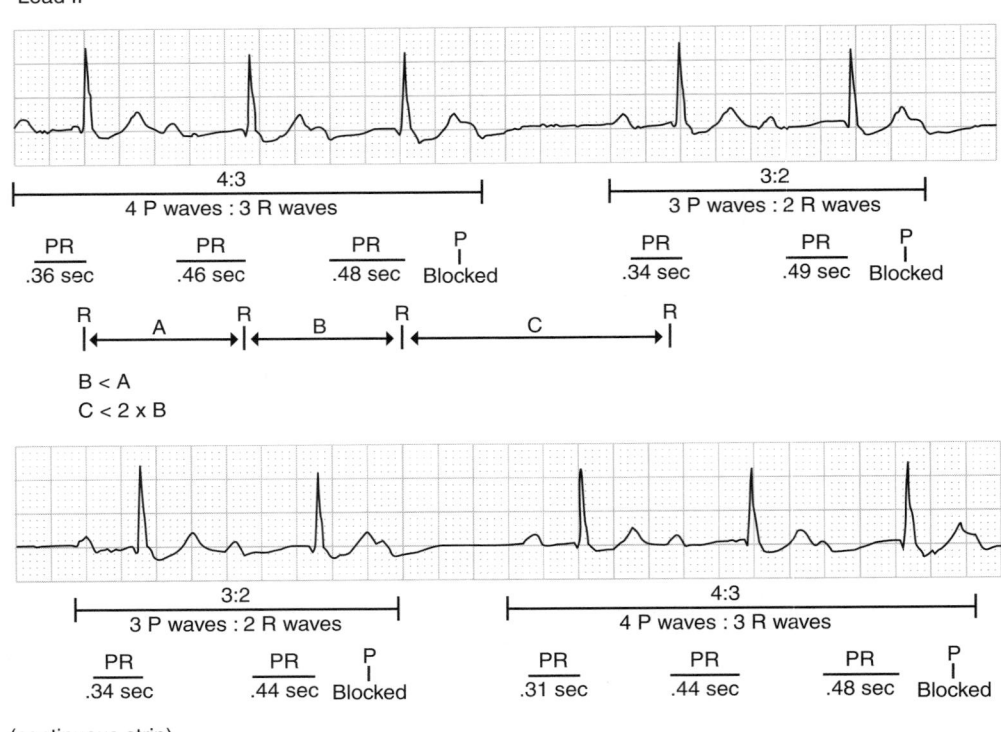

(continuous strip)

FIGURE 32-10 ■ Second-degree type I (Wenckebach) block. (From Paul S, Hera J, eds: *The nurse's guide to cardiac rhythm interpretation,* Philadelphia, 1998, WB Saunders.)

    (b) Treatment
        (i)   None needed because generally not symptomatic
        (ii) Look for underlying cause.
        (iii) Monitor rhythm.
  (4) Second-degree type II Mobitz block (Figure 32-11)
    (a) ECG criteria
        (i)   Ventricular rate less than atrial rate
        (ii) Rhythm regular or irregular (block may be variable)
        (iii) P waves normal and PR interval consistent for conducted beats
        (iv) Intermittent P wave not followed by a QRS
        (v) QRS normal
    (b) Treatment
        (i)   Same as symptomatic sinus bradycardia
        (ii) Avoid atropine.
        (iii) Use transcutaneous pacing.
        (iv) Sympathomimetic drugs (prevent progression to a higher-grade block)

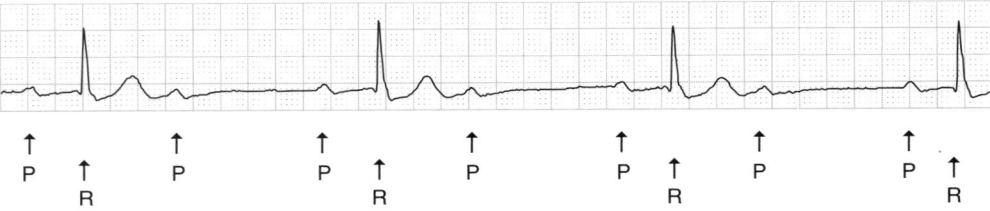

FIGURE 32-11 ■ Second-degree type II block. (From Paul S, Hera J, eds: *The nurse's guide to cardiac rhythm interpretation,* Philadelphia, 1998, WB Saunders.)

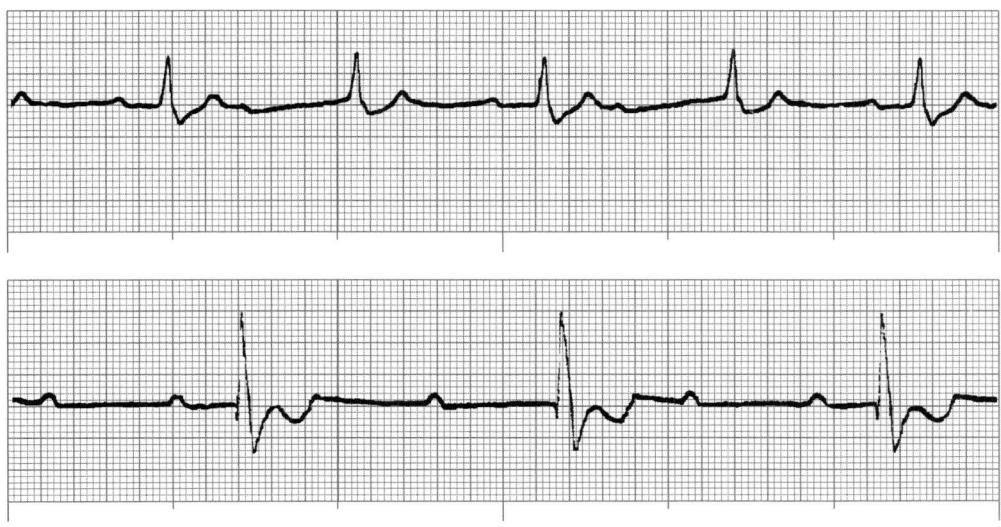

FIGURE 32-12 ■ Third-degree AV block. (From Aehlert B: *ECG's made easy,* St Louis, 1995, Mosby.)

        (5) Third-degree block (Figure 32-12)
           (a) Description: atrial and ventricular asynchrony
               (i)   Total loss of electrical conduction between atria and ventricles
           (b) ECG criteria
               (i)   Ventricular rate: 40 to 60 beats/min
               (ii) Atrial rate: 60 to 100 beats/min
               (iii) P waves normal
               (iv) QRS may be normal or widened.
               (v) P waves and QRS unrelated to each other
           (c) Treatment
               (i)   Same as symptomatic sinus bradycardia
               (ii) Avoid atropine.
               (iii) Use transcutaneous pacing.
               (iv) Sympathomimetic drugs
    b. Narrow complex tachydysrhythmias
        (1) Evaluate patient for serious signs and symptoms caused by tachycardia.
        (2) If unstable: sedation if conscious and synchronized cardioversion
           (a) For monophasic: 100 to 200 joules
               (i) Escalate second and subsequent shocks as needed.
           (b) For biphasic: 100 to 120 joules
               (i) Escalate second and subsequent shocks as needed.
        (3) Have available at bedside:
           (a) Pulse oximetry (Spo_2) monitor
           (b) Suction device
           (c) IV line
           (d) Intubation equipment
        (4) If stable, attempt to slow and diagnose rhythm via:
           (a) Vagal maneuvers
           (b) Adenosine, 6 mg IV push followed by fluid bolus (12-mg dose may be repeated twice after initial 6 mg dose)
        (5) Sinus tachycardia (Figure 32-13)
           (a) Characterized by normal-looking QRS
           (b) Rate >100 beats/min
           (c) Regular rhythm
           (d) Upright P waves in leads I, II, and AVF (augmented voltage left leg)

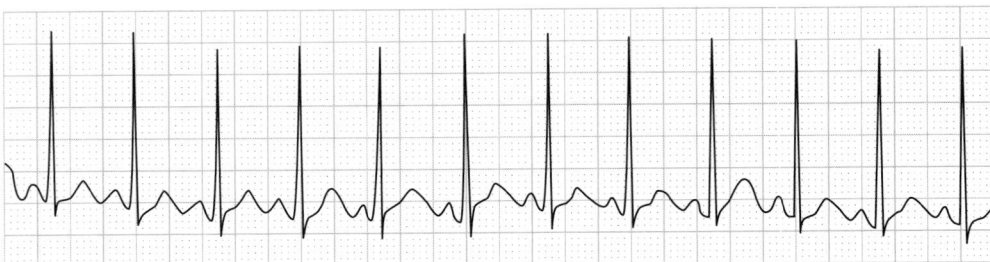

FIGURE 32-13 ■ Sinus tachycardia. (From Paul S, Hera J, eds: *The nurse's guide to cardiac rhythm interpretation,* Philadelphia, 1998, WB Saunders.)

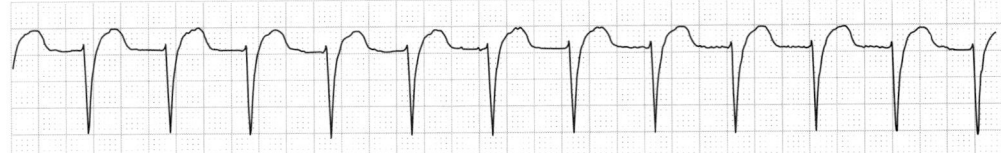

FIGURE 32-14 ■ Junctional tachycardia. (From Paul S, Hera J, eds: *The nurse's guide to cardiac rhythm interpretation,* Philadelphia, 1998, WB Saunders.)

        (e) Evaluation and treatment of causes usually sufficient to resolve (pain, hypoxemia, hypovolemia)
    (6) Junctional tachycardia (Figure 32-14)
        (a) Rate >100 beats/min
            (i) Normal-looking QRS
            (ii) P waves either absent, inverted, or after the QRS complex
        (b) Best treated by pharmacological suppression of AV node
            (i) Avoid cardioversion.
        (c) Assess for drug effects (often related to digoxin toxicity).
    (7) Paroxysmal supraventricular tachycardia (Figure 32-15)
        (a) Rate >100 beats/min with:
            (i) Normal-looking QRS
            (ii) Regular rhythm
            (iii) Sudden onset frequently initiated with a premature beat
        (b) Synchronized cardioversion effective in those with poor ejection fraction
        (c) Often converts with adenosine
        (d) May use medications to slow rate
            (i) Calcium channel blockers
            (ii) Beta-blockers

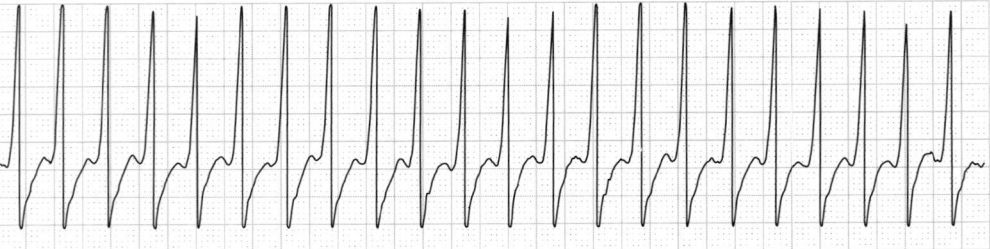

Lead II

FIGURE 32-15 ■ Paroxysmal supraventricular tachycardia. (From Paul S, Hera J, eds: *The nurse's guide to cardiac rhythm interpretation,* Philadelphia, 1998, WB Saunders.)

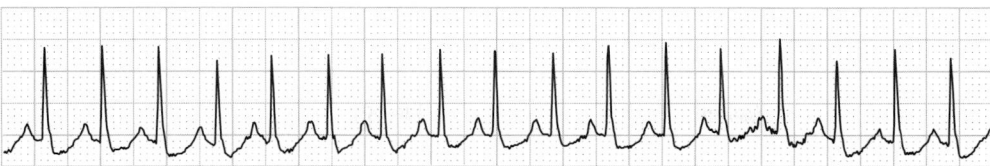

FIGURE 32-16 ■ Multifocal atrial tachycardia. (From Paul S, Hera J, eds: *The nurse's guide to cardiac rhythm interpretation,* Philadelphia, 1998, WB Saunders.)

(8) Multifocal atrial tachycardia (Figure 32-16)
  (a) Characterized by:
    (i)   Rate >100 beats/min
    (ii) At least three different morphologies of the P wave
    (iii) Normal-appearing QRS
  (b) Best treated with medications to slow rate; avoid cardioversion.
  (c) Typically, underlying pulmonary disease present
  (d) Select slowing agents according to origin of tachycardia and pumping ability of myocardium.
    (i)   Amiodarone
      [a] 150 mg/100 mL D$_5$W (5% dextrose in water) over 10 minutes
      [b] Followed by 1-mg/min infusion for 6 hours
      [c] Then 0.5 mg/min for a maximum daily dose of 2 g
    (ii) Beta-blocking agents
    (iii) Calcium channel blocking agents
    (iv) Digoxin
(10) Atrial fibrillation and flutter (Figures 32-17 and 32-18)
  (a) Atrial fibrillation
    (i)   Atrial rate too rapid to be counted
    (ii) No organized atrial activity, therefore no P waves
    (iii) Irregular ventricular rhythm
    (iv) Normal QRS unless aberrant conduction present
  (b) Atrial flutter
    (i)   Atrial rate usually 300 beats/min but may range from 220 to 350 beats/min
    (ii) Atrial rhythm regular
    (iii) Ventricular rhythm usually regular but may be irregular
    (iv) P waves resemble flutter and saw tooth waves.
  (c) Determine if duration >48 hours.

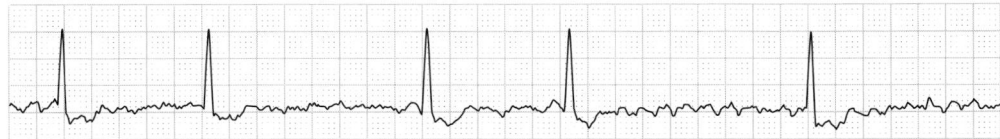

FIGURE 32-17 ■ Atrial fibrillation. (From Paul S, Hera J, eds: *The nurse's guide to cardiac rhythm interpretation,* Philadelphia, 1998, WB Saunders.)

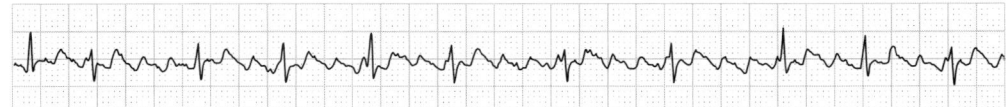

FIGURE 32-18 ■ Atrial flutter. (From Paul S, Hera J, eds: *The nurse's guide to cardiac rhythm interpretation,* Philadelphia, 1998, WB Saunders.)

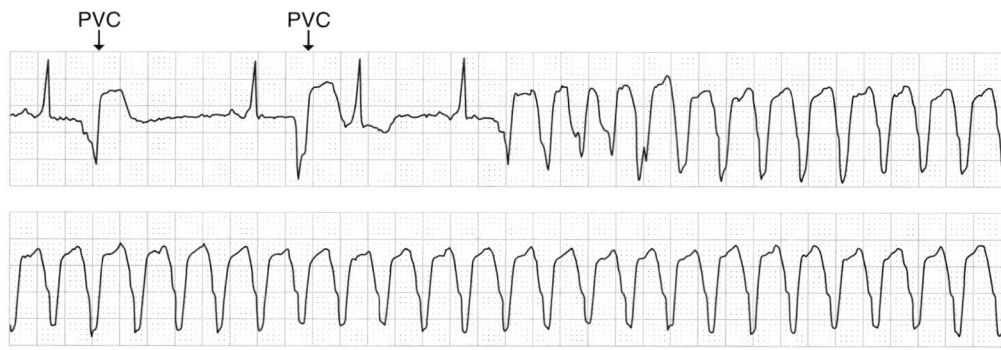

FIGURE 32-19 ■ Ventricular tachycardia. (From Paul S, Hera J, eds: *The nurse's guide to cardiac rhythm interpretation,* Philadelphia, 1998, WB Saunders.)

> (d) Slow rate with appropriate agent depending on myocardial contractility.
> (e) Initiate anticoagulation.
> (f) Synchronized cardioversion only if unstable
>
> **c.** Wide complex
> (1) Ventricular tachycardia (Figure 32-19): three or more beats of ventricular origin in a row with a rate >100 beats/min
> (2) ECG criteria
>   (a) Rate: 100 to 220 beats/min
>   (b) Rhythm: usually regular
>   (c) P waves: difficult to detect
>   (d) QRS complex: wide and bizarre
>   (e) Monomorphic: regular with consistent appearance to complexes, usually ischemic in origin
>   (f) Polymorphic: complexes are inconsistent and may be related to a prolonged QT interval, resulting in a thick and thin spindle pattern.
>   (i) Commonly referred to as torsades de pointes (Figure 32-20)
> **d.** Premature ventricular complex
> (1) Abnormal QRS usually wider than 0.12 seconds
> (2) Full compensatory pause (Figure 32-21)
> (3) Indicative of ventricles firing prematurely
> (4) May occur isolated or in pairs (couplets) (Figure 32-22)
> (5) May also occur from different foci in ventricles (multifocal/multiformed) (Figure 32-23)
> (6) May occur:
>   (a) Every other beat (bigeminy) (Figure 32-24, *A*)
>   (b) Every third beat (trigeminy) (Figure 32-24, *B*)
>   (c) Every fourth beat (quadrigeminy)
>   (d) Too close to T wave resulting in VT or VF (Figure 32-25)

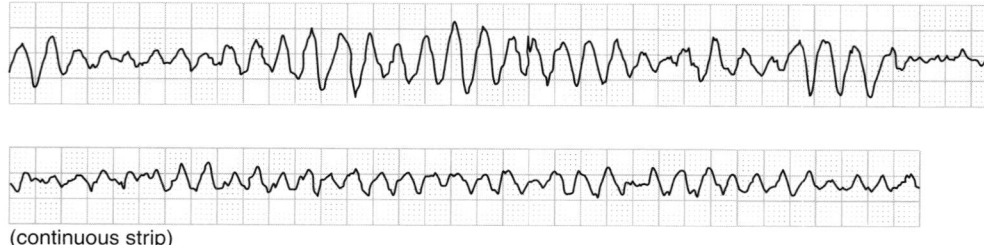

(continuous strip)

FIGURE 32-20 ■ Torsades de pointes degenerating into ventricular fibrillation. (From Paul S, Hera J, eds: *The nurse's guide to cardiac rhythm interpretation,* Philadelphia, 1998, WB Saunders.)

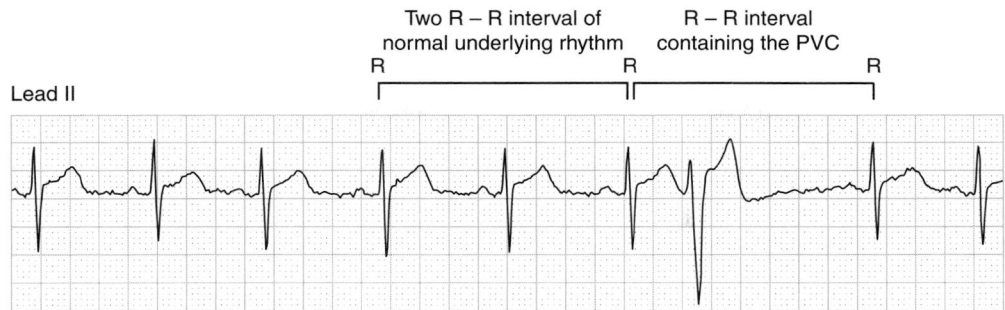

FIGURE 32-21 ■ Premature ventricular complexes with compensatory pause. (From Paul S, Hera J, eds: *The nurse's guide to cardiac rhythm interpretation,* Philadelphia, 1998, WB Saunders.)

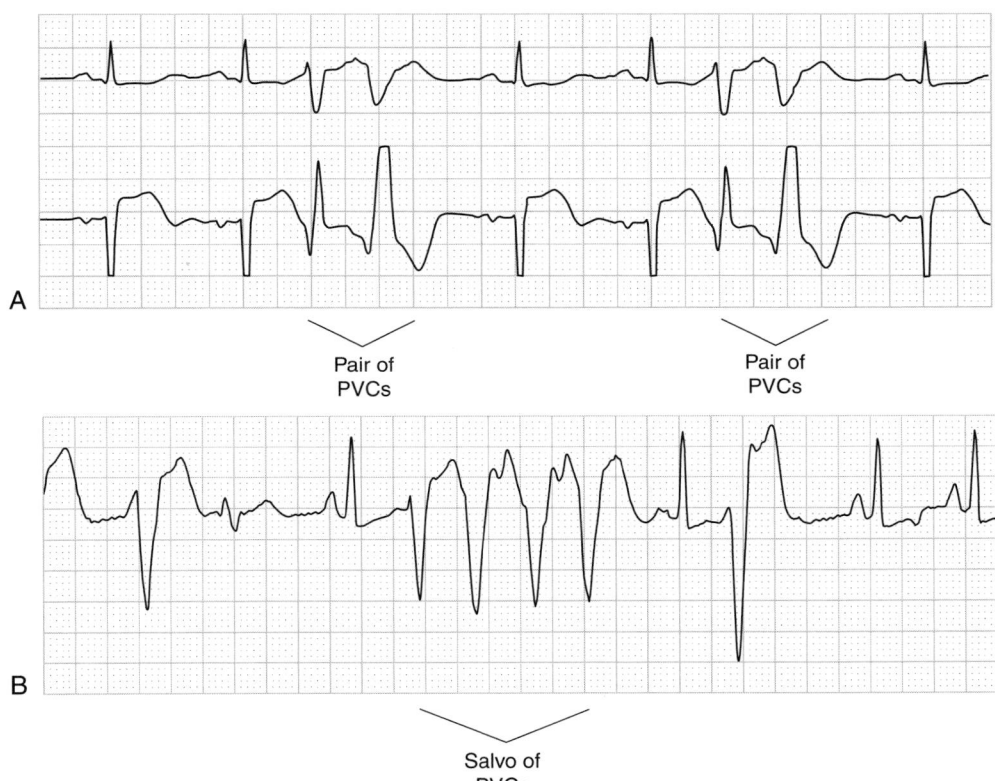

FIGURE 32-22 ■ Ventricular pairs (couplets). (From Paul S, Hera J, eds: *The nurse's guide to cardiac rhythm interpretation,* Philadelphia, 1998, WB Saunders.)

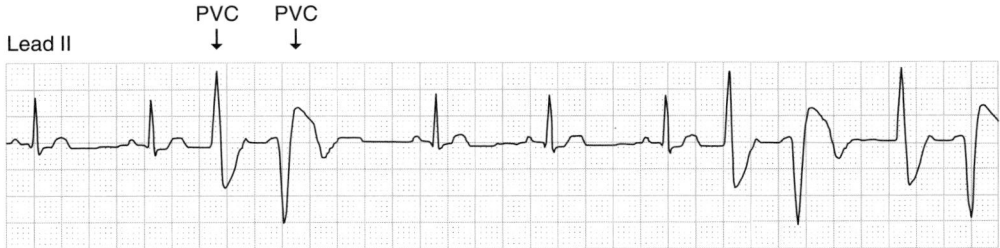

FIGURE 32-23 ■ Multiformed (multifocal) premature ventricular complexes. (From Paul S, Hera J, eds: *The nurse's guide to cardiac rhythm interpretation,* Philadelphia, 1998, WB Saunders.)

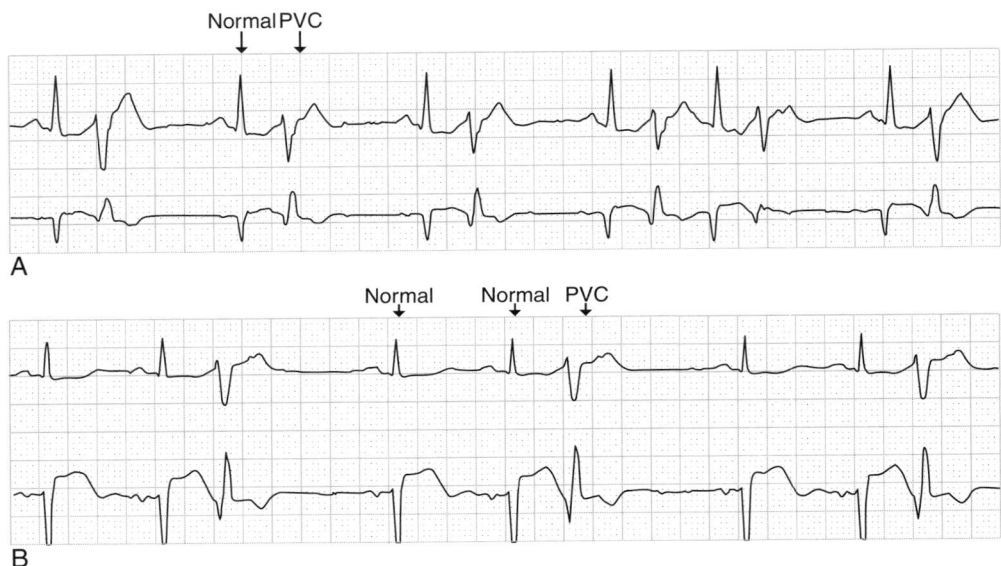

FIGURE 32-24 ■ **A,** Ventricular bigeminy. **B,** Ventricular trigeminy. (From Paul S, Hera J, eds: *The nurse's guide to cardiac rhythm interpretation,* Philadelphia, 1998, WB Saunders.)

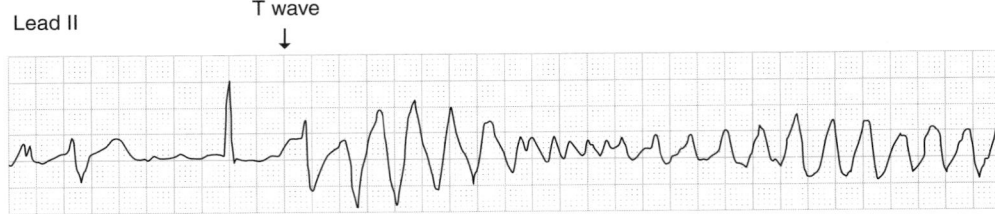

FIGURE 32-25 ■ R on T phenomenon. (From Paul S, Hera J, eds: *The nurse's guide to cardiac rhythm interpretation,* Philadelphia, 1998, WB Saunders.)

    e. Pulseless electrical activity (electromechanical dissociation)
       (1) Description: can be any rhythm on ECG (except VT/VF); however, no pulse and no BP can be detected.
       (2) Treatment
         (a) Initiate primary and secondary assessment.
         (b) Initiate CPR.
         (c) Assess for and treat reversible causes (five *H*'s and five *T*'s).
           (i)   Hypovolemia
           (ii)   Hypoxia
           (iii)   Hydrogen ion–acidosis
           (iv)   Hyperkalemia, hypokalemia
           (v)   Hypothermia
           (vi)   Tablets (drug overdose, accidents)
           (vii) Tamponade, cardiac
           (viii) Tension pneumothorax
           (ix)   Thrombosis, coronary
           (x)   Thrombosis, pulmonary (embolism)
         (d) Epinephrine, 1 mg IV or by endotracheal tube (ETT) (twice the IV dose)
           (i) Repeat every 3 to 5 minutes, or
           (ii) Vasopressin, 40 units IV single dose
    f. Ventricular fibrillation (Figure 32-26)

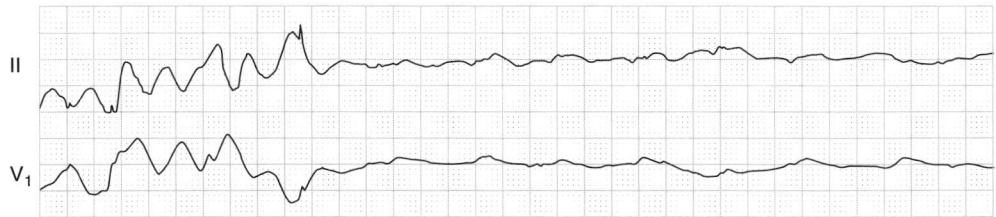

FIGURE 32-26 ■ Coarse ventricular fibrillation degenerating into fine ventricular fibrillation. (From Paul S, Hera J, eds: *The nurse's guide to cardiac rhythm interpretation,* Philadelphia, 1998, WB Saunders.)

   (1) Description
      (a) ECG with no organized rhythm
      (b) No CO
      (c) Coarse or fine refers to amplitude.
   (2) ECG criteria
      (a) Rate: rapid and too disorganized to count
      (b) Rhythm: irregularly irregular
      (c) No P wave, QRS complex, ST segment, or T wave
   (3) Treatment
      (a) Initiate primary and secondary assessment.
      (b) Immediate cardiopulmonary resuscitation (CPR) until defibrillator arrives, then defibrillation: 1 shock 200 joules for biphasic and 360 joules for monophasic
      (c) Epinephrine, 1 mg intravenously (IV) every 3 minutes while arrest persists; or vasopressin, 40 units IV single dose; or epinephrine may be given by endotracheal tube (ETT) at 2 to 2.5 mg diluted in 10 mL normal saline.
      (d) Assess for shockable rhythm every 5 cycles of CPR, and defibrillate if VF persists.
      (e) Consider antidysrhythmics.
         (i) Amiodarone, 300 mg IV
         (ii) Lidocaine, 1 to 1.5 mg/kg IV or by ETT (twice the IV dose)
         (iii) Magnesium, 1 to 2 g IV
      (f) Resume attempts to defibrillate.
      (g) Continue epinephrine, 1 mg IV every 3 min followed by CPR and defibrillation.
 g. Asystole (Figure 32-27)
   (1) Description
      (a) Total absence of ventricular electrical activity
      (b) No pulse or BP
   (2) ECG criteria: complete absence of activity; "flat line"
   (3) Treatment
      (a) Initiate primary and secondary assessment.

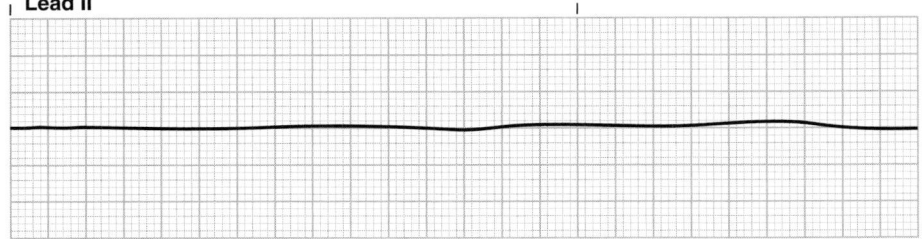

FIGURE 32-27 ■ Asystole. (From Huszar RJ: *Pocket guide to basic dysrhythmias,* ed 3, St Louis, 2002, Mosby.)

       (b) Initiate CPR.

       (c) Epinephrine, 1 mg IV or by ETT (twice the IV dose)

          (i) Repeat every 3 to 5 minutes

          (ii) Vasopressin, 40 units IV single dose

       (d) Consider withholding or ceasing resuscitative efforts.

5. Defibrillation and cardioversion

  a. Defibrillation

    (1) Monophasic defibrillators

      (a) Deliver one polarity of current

      (b) Use the traditional energy settings of 100, 200, 300, 360 joules

    (2) Biphasic defibrillators

      (a) Deliver energy via different waveforms

      (b) Able to terminate VF at lower energy levels

    (3) Because of different energy levels:

      (a) Consult manufacturer's recommendation.

      (b) If information absent, start at 200 joules.

    (4) Indications

      (a) VF—initial intervention

      (b) Pulseless VT—initial intervention

    (5) Technique

      (a) Confirm dysrhythmia.

      (b) Apply electrodes, or if using paddles apply conductive gel, or use saline or gelled pads.

      (c) Turn on defibrillator.

      (d) Select energy level.

        (i) Adults

          [a] 200 joules

          [b] If ineffective, progress to 300, then 360 joules.

        (ii) Pediatric patients

          [a] 2 joules/kg of body weight

          [b] Progress to 4 joules/kg if ineffective.

      (e) Apply paddles to chest.

        (i) One paddle just below right clavicle on chest

        (ii) One paddle to left of nipple in midaxillary line

        (iii) Use 25-lb paddle pressure on both paddles.

      (f) Charge defibrillator.

      (g) Clear personal contact with patient verbally and visually.

      (h) Deliver countershock.

      (i) Evaluate rhythm and pulse.

      (j) Repeat as necessary; select energy level.

    (6) Precautions

      (a) Know how defibrillator works in advance of need.

      (b) Defibrillation most effective when done promptly

      (c) Clear area to avoid delivering shock to others.

      (d) Always confirm rhythm and pulse before and after shock.

  b. Cardioversion

    (1) Indications

      (a) Treatment of choice for hemodynamically unstable tachydysrhythmias

        (i) VT

        (ii) Supraventricular tachycardias

    (2) Technique

      (a) If patient conscious, consider sedation or analgesia; provide explanation.

      (b) Procedure is same as with defibrillation except:

        (i) Unit set on synchronous mode

          [a] Adults: initial setting 50 to 100 joules

            [1] Advance to 200, 300, and 360 joules if ineffective.

           [b] Pediatrics: initial setting 0.5 to 1.0 joules/kg of body weight
               [1] Advance to 2 joules/kg if ineffective.
      (3) Precautions
         (a) Same as defibrillation
         (b) Recognition that VF may occur
            (i)   Turn off synchronous mode.
            (ii) Charge unit to defibrillation energy level.
            (iii) Defibrillate.
            (iv) Prepare to initiate CPR.
         (c) Monitor per institution's sedation and analgesia policy.
  6. Cardiac pacing
    a. Temporary pacing
      (1) Single chamber: use of a pulse generator to provide electrical stimulation of either the atria or the ventricle to produce an action potential resulting in myocardial contraction
         (a) Indications
            (i)   Intermittent AV nodal dysfunction or sinus bradycardia
            (ii) Suppression of ventricular ectopy
      (2) Dual chamber: sequential pacing of the atrium and ventricle
         (a) Indications
            (i)   Hemodynamically compromised patients with AV nodal dysfunction
      (3) Rapid atrial pacing: delivery of pacing discharges at rates of up to 800 beats/min resulting in atrial overdrive
         (a) Indications
            (i)   Paroxysmal atrial tachycardia or atrial flutter
      (4) Transcutaneous: electrical energy delivered using a defibrillator with pacing capabilities via gel pads applied to the chest wall in the anterior and posterior (preferred) or sternal and apex position
         (a) Indications: emergency treatment of symptomatic bradycardic dysrhythmias
      (5) Transvenous: pacing wires inserted through a central venous access (i.e., femoral, subclavian, internal jugular, or brachial)
         (a) Indications: short-term therapy or bridge to permanent pacer implantation
         (b) Removal
            (i)   Turn off generator.
            (ii) Gently apply continuous tension to wires and remove in one continuous motion. Stop if resistance felt.
            (iii) Maintain digital pressure at insertion site until hemostasis achieved. Apply dressing.
            (iv) Observe rhythm, pulse, and BP, insertion site and distal extremity every 15 minutes four times, then every 30 minutes two times.
      (6) Epicardial: application of pacing wires to surface of epicardium via a surgical incision; most commonly done related to cardiac bypass or valvular surgery
         (a) Removal
            (i)   Day before discharge
            (ii) Put patient in supine position and apply gentle traction after severing the skin suture.
            (iii) If unable to remove with gentle traction, swab entry site with antiseptic solution and cut wire off at skin while applying gentle traction on wires.
            (iv) Complications: cardiac tamponade
            (v)   Assess patient at 5-, 15-, and 30-minute intervals after removal.
      (7) Precautions and common problems (Table 32-3)
         (a) Direct stimulation of myocardium resulting in VF
            (i)   Insulate external pacing wire with needle cap, finger cot, or nonconductive tape and secure to chest when not in use.

■ TABLE 32-3
■ ■ **Troubleshooting Temporary Pacemakers**

Problem	Actions
Failure to capture	1. Check lead connections. 2. Check lead placement by x-ray if transvenous. 3. ↑ Milliamperage (mA). 4. Change battery. 5. Reposition patient. 6. Prepare to switch from transvenous to transcutaneous if applicable.
Failure to sense	1. ↑ Sensitivity. 2. Change battery.
Failure to pace	1. ↓ Sensitivity. 2. Switch to asynchronous mode. 3. ↑ Rate.

        (ii) Protect wire from moisture.

    (b) Failure to pace or capture: absent pacer spikes or spikes that are not followed by a QRS complex (Figure 32-28)

        (i) Examine all pacing wire connections.

        (ii) Increase milliamps.

        (iii) Replace battery and/or pacing generator.

        (iv) Assess for metabolic and acid-base abnormalities.

        (v) Inform physician and prepare to support patient with transcutaneous pacing and pharmacological agents (may be caused by pacer wire fracture or detachment from myocardium).

    (c) Failure to sense (Figure 32-29)

        (i) Undersensing of inherent patient complexes (pacer spikes occurring closely adjacent to or on inherent complexes)

        (ii) Oversensing (inhibition of pacer spikes in relation to movement or artifact)

        (iii) Adjust sensitivity setting while observing rhythm.

        (iv) Change battery and/or pulse generator.

        (v) Undersensing: conversion from unipolar to bipolar or vice versa

  b. Permanent (see Permanent Pacemaker Implantation, section VI.C)

    (1) Indications

      (a) Complete heart block

      (b) Symptomatic bradycardia associated with:

        (i) Sinus node dysfunction

        (ii) Second-degree heart block

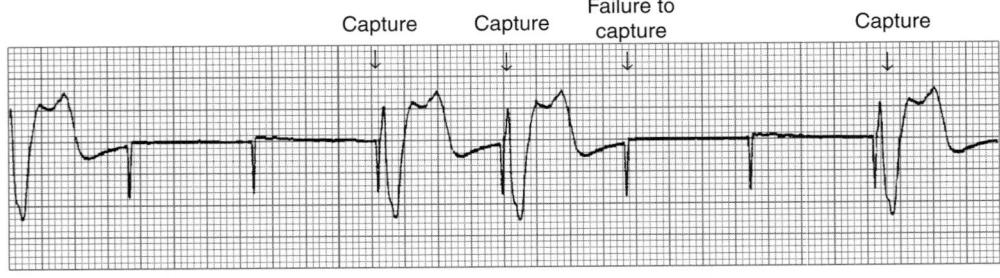

FIGURE 32-28 ■ Failure to capture. (From Aehlert B: *ECG's made easy,* ed 3, St Louis, 2006, Mosby.)

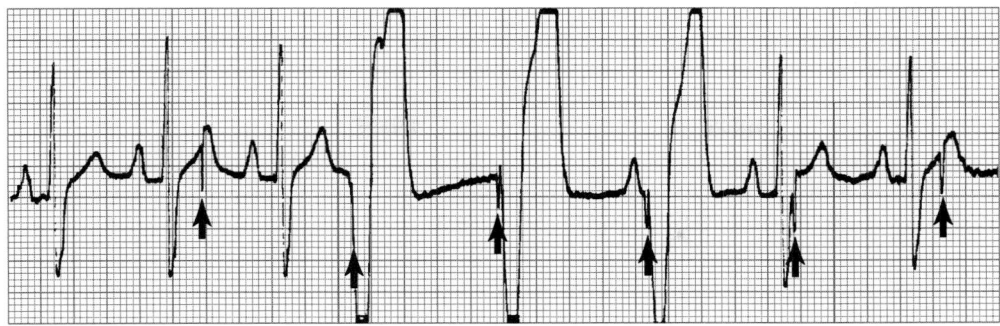

FIGURE 32-29 ■ Failure to sense. (From Aehlert B: *ECG's made easy*, ed 3, St Louis, 2006, Mosby.)

      (c) Acute MI with persistent, advanced second- or third-degree heart block
      (d) Recurrent syncope associated with hypersensitive carotid sinus syndrome
      (e) Advanced block with atrial fibrillation or flutter and symptomatic slow ventricular rate
      (f) Symptomatic bradycardia secondary to pharmacological therapy

D. Hemorrhage
  1. Definition: loss of intravascular volume
  2. Assessment findings
    a. Visible blood on dressings, in drains, emesis
    b. Restlessness
    c. Swelling at surgical site
    d. Hypotension
    e. Signs of hypovolemia (tachycardia)
    f. Ear, nose, and throat
      (1) Frequent swallowing
      (2) Hemoptysis
      (3) Vomiting blood
    g. Abdominal
      (1) Increased girth
      (2) Abdominal pain
      (3) Hardness
  3. Potential causes
    a. Loss of vascular integrity
    b. Coagulation disorders
  4. Treatment
    a. Stop active bleeding.
    b. Support circulation—transfusion usually not indicated unless:
      (1) Hb <7 g/dL
      (2) Hematocrit <21%
      (3) Autologous blood available
      (4) Patient symptomatic (patients with cardiac dysfunction will need transfusion earlier because of the increased need for oxygen-carrying capacity)
    c. Patient comfort measures
      (1) Decrease anxiety
      (2) Keep warm
      (3) Pain management
  5. Prevention
    a. Assess for bleeding disorders preoperatively.
    b. Assess for medications that interfere with coagulation and discontinue before surgery (include over-the-counter and herbal preparations).
    c. Maintain normothermic body temperatures.

  d. Investigate all elevations in HR for cause (i.e., pain, stress response, bleeding).

  e. Monitor closely postoperatively for unexplained or excessive bleeding.

 E. Peripheral circulatory compromise

  1. Definition: decreased or absent blood flow to an extremity

  2. Assessment findings

   a. Color changes of extremity (pale, flushed to blue)

   b. Swelling if obstructed venous return

   c. Diminished or absent pulses

   d. Delayed or absent capillary refill

   e. Pain, paresthesia

   f. Temperature different from other extremity, usually cooler

  3. Potential causes

   a. Bandage, splint, cast too tight

   b. Occurrence of thrombus or embolus

  4. Treatment

   a. Relieve restriction to blood flow by loosening constricting bandages.

   b. Possible return to surgery for thrombectomy or embolectomy

  5. Prevention

   a. Use caution when applying circumferential bandages.

   b. Evaluation of surgical site extremities

 F. MI (see Section XI)

 G. CHF

  1. New York Heart Association classification of heart failure (Table 32-4)

  2. Preoperative considerations

   a. Weight gain may indicate worsening failure.

   b. Prone to electrolyte imbalances

   c. Must have preoperative ECG and CXR

  3. Intraoperative considerations

   a. Prone to dysrhythmias

   b. Preload sensitive

    (1) Myocardial function dependent on volume status usually overloaded

    (2) Prone to pulmonary edema with volume overload

   c. May develop myocardial ischemia with small to moderate loss of Hb

  4. Postoperative considerations

   a. Phase I

    (1) Tachycardia may indicate decreased CO.

    (2) Narrowing pulse pressure may be an indication of decreasing SV.

■ TABLE 32-4
■ ■ **New York Heart Classification of Cardiovascular Disease**

Class Subjective	Assessment	Prognosis
I	Normal cardiac output without systemic or pulmonary congestion: asymptomatic at rest and on heavy exertion	Good
II	Normal cardiac output maintained with a moderate increase in pulmonary-systemic congestion; symptomatic on exertion	Good with therapy
III	Normal cardiac output maintained with a marked increase in pulmonary-systemic congestion; symptomatic on mild exercise	Fair with therapy
IV	Cardiac output reduced at rest with a marked increase in pulmonary-systemic congestion; symptomatic at rest	Guarded despite therapy

From Killip T, Kimball JT: Treatment of myocardial infarction in a coronary care unit. A two year experience with 250 patients. *Am J Cardiol* 20:457, 1967.

(3) Monitor ECG closely for changes consistent with myocardial ischemia (ST changes).
(4) Monitor fluid status closely.
  b. Phase II
(1) Teaching to include signs and symptoms of heart failure
(2) Instruct in daily weight and need to contact physician for weight gain of 3 lb or more.

VIII. DRUG ADMINISTRATION IN EMERGENCY SITUATIONS
Note: Consider patient's do-not-resuscitate (DNR) and do-not-intubate (DNI) status (Box 32-1).
  A. Know the drugs to be given; this is the principle of continuing education and advanced cardiac life support (ACLS) repeat evaluation.
  B. IV drugs require circulation.
    1. Via CPR
    2. Effective, independent rhythm
    3. BP >60 mm Hg systolic
  C. IV drugs require:
    1. IV line
    2. Some require a central line.
    3. Get IV access early in emergency situation in largest vein possible.
  D. In absence of IV line, certain medications may be given by ETT, including:
    1. Lidocaine
    2. Epinephrine
    3. Atropine
    4. Naloxone
    5. Remember these drugs with the acronym LEAN.
      a. Word spelled by the first letters of the drugs
  E. If medications are given by ETT:
    1. Dilute into 10 mL of saline or distilled water.
    2. Give as distally as possible.
    3. Follow with immediate Ambu bagging to force medications into lungs.
    4. Double the IV dose when administering per ETT.
  F. IV infusions of vasoactive medications—recommend arterial line placement to monitor BP changes.
  G. Route, dosage, and time of all medications given should be documented along with patient response and associated rhythm; use of an arrest record can facilitate documentation.
  H. Cardioactive drugs (Table 32-5)

■ BOX 32-1
■ **AMERICAN SOCIETY OF PERIANESTHESIA NURSES POSITION STATEMENT ON THE PERIANESTHESIA PATIENT WITH A DO-NOT-RESUSCITATE ADVANCE DIRECTIVE**

"The American Society of PeriAnesthesia Nurses (ASPAN) recommends that at the time of surgery and prior to receiving any anesthetic medication, a patient with an active do-not-resuscitate advance directive and/or patient representative will be asked to clarify wishes about resuscitation during the perianesthesia period.

To limit potential for ethical dilemmas, the patient's informed consent will include discussion of the advance directive, living will, or physician order that specifies do-not-resuscitate (DNR) or do-not-intubate (DNI) during a candid and well-documented conversation with physicians and appropriate significant other(s).

Each facility establishes and communicates a policy that identifies resources and procedures that detail the management of a patient's DNR/DNI status during the perianesthesia period."

From American Society of PeriAnesthesia Nurses: *Standards of perianesthesia nursing practice 2008-2010*, Thorofare, NJ, 2008, American Society of PeriAnesthesia Nurses.

TABLE 32-5
■ Cardioactive Drugs

Drugs	Mechanism of Action	Indications	Dosage and Route	Precautions
INOTROPIC AGENTS				
Epinephrine	Alpha and beta activity (beta greater than alpha) resulting in increased SVR, BP, automaticity, HR, coronary and cerebral blood flow, myocardial contraction, and myocardial oxygen consumption	Drug of choice in asystole PEA Circulatory shock	***Adult*** 1 mg of 1:10,000 solution IV every 3 to 5 minutes Double dose by ETT Infusion, 4 mg/250 mL D_5W; start at 1 mcg/min and titrate to effect. **Pediatric** IV and IO: 0.01 mg/kg of 1:10,000 solution every 3 to 5 minutes ETT: 0.1 mg/kg	Not compatible with sodium bicarbonate Excessive effects can produce ischemia, hypertension, and ventricular ectopy.
Norepinephrine	Alpha$_1$-agonist, alpha$_2$-agonist, and beta$_1$-agonist (alpha greater than beta) resulting in increased myocardial contractility and vasoconstriction	Hemodynamically significant hypotension that does not respond to epinephrine or dopamine	IV infusion: 1-4 mg/250 mL D_5W. Begin at 2 mcg/min, and titrate to desired effect.	Strict BP monitoring requires use of arterial line. Increases myocardial oxygen needs May precipitate dysrhythmias Ischemic necrosis if extravasation occurs; cannot be infused through a peripheral line
Dobutamine	Potent beta$_1$-agonist, mild beta$_2$-agonist resulting in increased cardiac output, HR, and possible peripheral and coronary vasodilation	Pulmonary congestion and low cardiac output with systolic BP of 70-100 mm Hg and no sign of shock	Infusion, 500 mg in 250 mL D_5W 2-20 mcg/kg per minute; titrate to effect (limit dose so that HR does not exceed >10% of baseline).	May cause tachycardia, dysrhythmias Myocardial ischemia at high doses May exacerbate hypotension

Drug	Action	Indications	Administration	Adverse Effects/Considerations
Milrinone lactate (Primacor)	Phosphodiesterase III inhibitor that results in dose-dependent positive inotrope and vasodilator with minimal chronotropic response, decreases pulmonary capillary wedge pressure and SVR, and increases cardiac output	Severe heart failure or cardiogenic shock (not adequately responsive to standard therapy)	IV infusion: 50 mg/250 mL normal saline Loading dose of 50 mcg/kg over 10 minutes, then infusion of 0.375 to 0.750 mcg/kg per minute for 2-3 days; titrate to effect.	Ventricular dysrhythmias Hypotension
Dopamine	Dose-dependent $beta_2$-agonist, $alpha_1$-agonist, and $alpha_2$-agonist, and dopaminergic agonist. Dose of 2-5 mcg/kg per minute: Dopaminergic stimulation may cause vasodilation of renal, mesenteric, and cerebral arteries. Dose of 5-10 mcg/kg per minute: $Beta_1$ stimulation results in increased cardiac output ($beta_1$ effects), mild to moderate peripheral vasoconstriction (alpha effects). Dose of 10-20 mcg/kg per minute: stimulation results in profound increase in peripheral vasoconstriction ($alpha_1$ effects) and myocardial contractility and HR ($beta_1$ effects)	Hemodynamically significant hypotension; systolic BP of 70-100 mm Hg with signs of shock Symptomatic bradycardia if atropine ineffective and in the absence of a pacer	Infusion, 400 or 800 mg in 250 mL D_5W, NS, or lactated Ringer's solution Begin at lowest appropriate dose for intended receptor stimulation and titrate to BP, urine output, and signs of organ perfusion.	May result in extreme tachycardia leading to severe dysrhythmias, especially if hypovolemic; always optimize volume status first. Increases myocardial oxygen consumption at high doses Tissue necrosis if extravasation occurs Incompatible with sodium bicarbonate

Continued

TABLE 32-5

■ Cardioactive Drugs—cont'd

Drugs	Mechanism of Action	Indications	Dosage and Route	Precautions
INOTROPIC AGENTS—cont'd				
Digitalis	Cardiac glycoside that also increases AV block and enhances vagal tone, which slows impulse conduction and prolongs the effective refractory period	Atrial fibrillation PSVT CHF	Varies with ventricular rate, urgency, patient age, body size, and renal function IV: Loading dose of 10 to 15 mcg/kg lean body weight Nonemergency situation, oral	Toxicity (dysrhythmias—all types; nausea, vomiting, diarrhea; visual disturbances—yellow halos; more common with hypokalemia, hypomagnesemia, and hypocalcemia) Treatment may require temporary pacemaker. Avoid electrical cardioversion unless condition is life-threatening. Use lower currents (10-20 joules).
BETA-BLOCKING AGENTS				
Class	Block effect of catecholamines on beta-receptors Decrease HR, BP, contractility, bronchoconstriction	Suspected MI and unstable angina in the absence of complications Adjunctive agent with fibrinolytic therapy Supraventricular tachydysrhythmias (PSVT), atrial fibrillation or flutter Hypertension		May cause severe hypotension especially if given concurrently with calcium channel blocking agents Avoid use in bronchospastic disease, symptomatic heart failure, and severe abnormalities in cardiac conduction. Monitor cardiac and pulmonary status vigilantly.
Metoprolol (beta₁ selective)			Initial IV dose, 5 mg administered slowly at 5-minute intervals to a total of 15 mg; oral regimen to follow IV dose: 50 mg twice per day for 24 hours, then increase to 100 mg twice per day if tolerated	

Drug	Class/Action	Indications	Dosing	Special Considerations
Atenolol (beta$_1$ selective)			5 mg slow IV (over 5 minutes). Wait 10 minutes, then give second dose of 5 mg slow IV (over 5 minutes). In 10 minutes, if tolerated, may start 50 mg orally; then 50 mg twice a day	
Propranolol (beta$_1$ and beta$_2$ stimulation)			Total dose, 0.1 mg/kg divided into 3 equal doses at 2- to 3-minute intervals. Do not exceed 1 mg/min.	
Esmolol			0.5 mg/kg over 1 minute, followed by a continuous infusion at 0.05 mg/kg per minute; titrate to effect; short half-life: 2-9 minutes (maximum: 0.3 mg/kg per minute)	
Labetalol (alpha and beta$_1$ selective)			10 mg IV push over 1-2 minutes; may repeat or double dose every 10 minutes to a maximum of 150 mg; may be given as an infusion of 2-8 mg/min after initial bolus. Do not repeat boluses if infusion initiated.	

CALCIUM CHANNEL BLOCKING AGENTS

Class		Indications		Special Considerations
Slow conduction and increase refractoriness in the AV node by blocking the movement of calcium into the cells		Termination of reentrant dysrhythmias Control of ventricular response in atrial fibrillation and flutter and multifocal atrial tachycardia		Do not use for wide-QRS tachycardias of unknown origin. Avoid use in patients with Wolff-Parkinson-White syndrome, sick sinus syndrome, or AV block without a pacemaker. May cause severe hypotension especially with concurrent beta-blocking agent use May exacerbate CHF with severe left ventricular failure

Continued

■ TABLE 32-5
■ Cardioactive Drugs—cont'd

Drugs	Mechanism of Action	Indications	Dosage and Route	Precautions
CALCIUM CHANNEL BLOCKING AGENTS—cont'd				
Diltiazem			15-20 mg (0.25 mg/kg) IV over 2 minutes; may repeat in 15 minutes at 20 to 25 mg (0.35 mg/kg) over 2 minutes; may use as an infusion at 5-15 mg/h titrated to HR	
Verapamil			2.5- to 5.0-mg IV bolus over 2 minutes (give doses over 3 minutes for older patients) Second dose in 15-30 minutes (if needed): 5-10 mg; maximum dose: 20 mg Alternate dosing: 5-mg bolus every 15 minutes to total dose of 30 mg	
ANTIDYSRHYTHMIC AGENTS				
Lidocaine	Class IB antiarrhythmic; stabilizes the cell membrane by blocking the movement of sodium into cardiac conducting cells; suppresses ventricular dysrhythmias and elevates fibrillation threshold; also has a local anesthetic property	Ventricular ectopy (VF/VT) and symptomatic premature ventricular contractions	***Adult*** Initial: 1-1.5 mg/kg IV or by ETT every 3-5 minutes; repeat doses: 0.5-0.75 mg/kg every 5-10 minutes to a maximum of 3 mg/kg Infusion: 2 g/500 mL NS at 1-4 mg/min ***Pediatric*** 1 mg/kg IV, IO, ETT	Excessive doses cause myocardial and circulatory depression. Toxicity (drowsiness, disorientation, twitching) Extreme toxicity can result in seizures.
Amiodarone	Class III antidysrhythmic agent with complex effects on sodium, potassium, and calcium channels as	Ventricular rate control of rapid atrial dysrhythmias in patients with compromised cardiac contractility and preexcited atrial arrhythmias VT or VF	***Adult*** VF or pulseless VT: 300 mg IV push; may be followed by 150 mg IV if defibrillation ineffective after first dose	May cause hypotension and bradycardia Infusion must be mixed in D_5W in a glass bottle.

Drug	Action	Uses	Dosage	Nursing Considerations
	well as alpha-blocking and beta-blocking properties; prolongs the action potential duration	Hemodynamically stable VT; Adjunct to electrical cardioversion of PSVT and atrial tachycardia	Stable VT or atrial dysrhythmias: 150 mg in 200 mL D$_5$W over 10-15 minutes followed by an infusion 1 mg/min for 6 hours, then 0.5 mg/min to a maximum daily dose of 2 g. **_Pediatric_** 5 mg/kg bolus IV or IO	Comes in glass ampule; use filter needle to aspirate. Can cause pulmonary fibrosis with extended use
Procainamide	Class IA antidysrhythmic; stabilizes cell membrane and decreases rates of conduction through the conducting system and ventricular tissue	Recurrent VT and VF, and antidysrhythmic of choice for stable monomorphic VT with an ejection fraction >40%	**_Adult_** IV: 20-50 mg/min to a total of 17 mg/kg. Infusion: 2 g in 500 mL NS at 1-4 mg/min. **_Pediatric_** 15 mg/kg over 30-60 minutes	Stop drug if: Dysrhythmia is suppressed (IV bolus). QRS complex widens by 50% of original width. Hypotension develops.
Magnesium sulfate	Reduces sinoatrial node impulse formation, prolongs myocardial conduction time	Hypomagnesemia; Ventricular dysrhythmias: VF and VT (drug of choice for torsades de pointes)	**_Adult_** Cardiac arrest: 1-2 g of a 50% solution. Torsades de pointes: 1-2 g diluted in 100 mL D$_5$W over 5-60 minutes; follow with infusion of 0.5-1 g/h for up to 24 hours. **_Pediatric_** 20-50 mg/kg IV or IO, maximum of 2 g over 10-20 minutes	Hypotension; Caution with renal failure
Adenosine	Depresses AV and sinus node activity (supraventricular); terminates reentry dysrhythmias (tachydysrhythmias)	First-line treatment for narrow-complex SVT	In the most central vein possible. **_Adult_** Rapid bolus of 6 mg over 1-3 seconds followed by 20-mL saline flush. Repeat a 12-mg dose in 1-2 minutes; may repeat in 1-2 minutes. **_Pediatric_** 0.1 mg/kg IV or IO (maximum first dose: 6 mg). May double and repeat dose once (maximum second dose: 12 mg)	Short half-life (<5 seconds) may result in recurrent SVT. Less effective in patients taking theophylline. Side effects: chest pain, flushing, dyspnea are transient

Continued

■ TABLE 32-5
■ ■ Cardioactive Drugs—cont'd

Drugs	Mechanism of Action	Indications	Dosage and Route	Precautions
ANTIDYSRHYTHMIC AGENTS—cont'd				
Ibutilide	Class III antidysrhythmic; prolongs the action potential duration and increases the refractory period of cardiac tissue	Acute pharmacological conversion of atrial fibrillation or flutter, or as an adjunct to electrical cardioversion	Adults ≥60 kg: 1 mg IV over 10 minutes; dose may be repeated in 10 minutes. Adults ≤60 kg: 0.01 mg/kg over 10 minutes	High incidence of polymorphic VT Continuous monitoring for minimum of 4-6 hours Optimize potassium and magnesium levels before initiating. Patients with impaired left ventricle function at higher risk for dysrhythmias
VAGOLYTIC AGENTS				
Atropine	Parasympatholytic resulting in increased automaticity, AV conduction, and vagolysis	Initial treatment for symptomatic bradycardia May be beneficial in asystole after epinephrine May be beneficial in symptomatic bradycardia and bradycardic PEA	*Adult* Dose of 0.5-1 mg IV every 3-5 minutes to a total of 0.03-0.04 mg or 2-3 mg by ETT *Pediatric* Dose of 0.02 mg/kg (minimum single dose: 0.1 mg); may repeat once	Tachycardia that may result in ischemia or infarction Excessive dosing, VF, or VT
VASODILATORS				
Nitroglycerin	Relaxes vascular smooth muscle resulting in dilation of coronary arteries and decreased SVR (especially in venous smooth muscle)	Drug of choice with angina pectoris or acute MI Drug of choice with CHF	Sublingual with angina: 0.3-0.4 mg; may repeat in 5 minutes to three-dose total IV infusion: 50 mg in 250 mL D_5W; start at 10-20 mcg/min and titrate in 5- to 10-mcg/min increments to effect every 5-10 minutes	Hypotension Bradycardia Recommend arterial line monitoring for infusion therapy. Must be given by infusion pump
Sodium nitroprusside	Potent, rapid-acting arteriolar and venous vasodilator resulting in a decrease	Hypertensive crisis Emergency treatment of heart failure Pulmonary edema	IV infusion: 50 mg/250 mL D_5W Begin at 0.15 mcg/kg per minute; titrate to effect (higher doses may be needed).	Requires arterial line monitoring Can cause profound hypotension resulting in ischemia or infarction Elderly patients more sensitive to effects

Medication	Action	Indication	Dose	Special Considerations
	in right and left ventricular filling (preload) and peripheral arterial resistance (afterload)		Average dose is 3 mcg/kg per minute.	Metabolized to thiocyanate (cyanide toxicity) Keep infusion protected from light (foil wrap). Must be given by infusion pump
VASOPRESSORS Epinephrine (see above) Dopamine (see above) Norepinephrine (see above)			10-20 mcg/kg per minute	
Vasopressin	Naturally occurring antidiuretic hormone; acts as a nonadrenergic peripheral vasoconstrictor at unnaturally high doses by directly stimulating smooth muscle.	VF, pulseless VT Vasodilatory shock	40 units IV push times one dose or an infusion titrated for effect	Extreme vasoconstriction may provoke myocardial ischemia and angina. Not recommended for responsive patients with coronary artery disease
Sodium bicarbonate	Reacts with hydrogen ions to form water and CO_2 to buffer metabolic acidosis	Known, preexisting hyperkalemia Known, preexisting bicarbonate-responsive acidosis (i.e., diabetic ketoacidosis, cyclic antidepressants or cocaine overdose) Prolonged resuscitation after defibrillation, effective cardiopulmonary resuscitation, intubation, hyperventilation with 100% oxygen, epinephrine, and antidysrhythmics	Initial dose of 1 mEq/kg, then 0.5 mEq/kg every 10 minutes	Sodium bicarbonate produces CO_2 and will worsen respiratory acidosis; CO_2 is also a negative inotrope; sodium bicarbonate causes oxyhemoglobin saturation curve to shift to left, decreasing oxygen release into plasma. Use blood gas analysis for monitoring if available.

AV, Atrioventricular; *BP,* blood pressure; *CHF,* congestive heart failure; *CO₂,* carbon dioxide; *D₅W,* 5% dextrose in water; *ETT,* endotracheal tube; *HR,* heart rate; *IO,* intraosseous; *IV,* intravenous; *MI,* myocardial infarction; *NS,* normal saline; *PEA,* pulseless electrical activity; *PSVT,* paroxysmal supraventricular tachycardia; *SVR,* systemic vascular resistance; *SVT,* supraventricular tachycardia; *VF,* ventricular fibrillation; *VT,* ventricular tachycardia.

IX. CONGENITAL HEART DISEASE (CHD)
   A. Malformation of heart or its associated blood vessels during fetal life
     1. Incidence: about 1% of live births
     2. Defects are categorized as:
       a. Acyanotic: increased pulmonary blood flow
       b. Cyanotic: increased or decreased pulmonary blood flow
     3. Three major types
       a. Stenosis: results in obstruction to blood flow
       b. Left-to-right shunt: blood flows directly from the left side of the heart, or aorta, to the right side of the heart, or PA, bypassing the systemic circulation (generally acyanotic).
       c. Right-to-left shunt: blood flows from the right side of the heart, or PA, directly into the left side of the heart, or aorta, bypassing the lungs (generally cyanotic).
     4. Special considerations in CHD
       a. Surgical patients are usually pediatric, but there is an ever-increasing adult population with CHD.
       b. Effective care and positive outcomes mandate a thorough understanding of the unique physiology of each type of defect.
       c. Preoperative concerns
         (1) Preoperative teaching and preparation must be centered on the cognitive and social perception of the child's health.
         (2) Child and family need to meet the staff before surgery.
         (3) Include the child life specialist for assessment and teaching.
         (4) Understand the child's unique words or expressions for:
           (a) Pain
           (b) Thirst
           (c) Fear
           (d) Voiding
           (e) People or objects that comfort the child
         (5) Surgical and anesthetic planning requires knowledge of:
           (a) Weight and body surface area
             (i) Measure and weigh the child on admitting unit's scale the night before surgery if possible.
           (b) Cardiac status
           (c) General health
           (d) Laboratory data
           (e) Chest radiograph findings
           (f) ECG results
         (6) Awareness of other significant congenital defects may influence surgical and postoperative course (e.g., hypoplastic lungs).
       d. Operative and postoperative concerns
         (1) Phases of postoperative recovery
           (a) Support of myocardium to prevent secondary injury to the heart and other organs
           (b) Weaning of external support as the heart and other organs recover from the stress of surgery and cardiopulmonary bypass (CPB)
         (2) Body temperature
           (a) Pediatric patients have a larger body surface area, and care must be taken to control heat loss.
             (i) Hypothermia blanket
             (ii) IV solution warmers
         (3) Patients with severe CHF and little cardiac reserve require narcotic anesthetics.
         (4) Patients with severe outflow obstruction may benefit from ketamine.
           (a) May use a prostaglandin E infusion to decrease pulmonary vascular vasoconstriction
         (5) Heart must be carefully purged of air to prevent embolism.

(6) Complications include those associated with thoracotomy.
  (a) Bleeding
  (b) Atelectasis
  (c) Hemothorax
  (d) Pneumothorax
(7) For optimal postoperative care, personnel must have training in nursing care of the critically ill child.

B. Left-to-right shunts
  1. Patent ductus arteriosus (PDA)—acyanotic (Figure 32-30)
    a. Definition: failure of ductus arteriosus to close during early months of life
    b. In United States, accounts for about 5% to 10% of all types of CHD
      (1) 1 in 1000 to 1 in 2000 full-term live births
    c. Signs and symptoms result from:
      (1) Increased cardiac workload on the left side
      (2) Increased pulmonary blood flow
      (3) Decreased systemic blood flow if PDA large
      (4) May be asymptomatic or experience:
        (a) Tachypnea
        (b) Poor feeding and weight gain
        (c) Frequent respiratory tract infections
        (d) Fatigue
        (e) Diaphoresis
    d. Assessment and diagnostics
      (1) Diastolic murmur present (machinery murmur)
        (a) Best heard over pulmonic area (left second intercostal space close to sternum)
      (2) ABG analysis
      (3) Mixed venous oxygen saturation (Svo_2)
      (4) Echocardiography
      (5) Pulmonary catheterization
    e. Effects on hemodynamics
      (1) Flow of blood from aorta (high pressure) to PA (low pressure) through open ductus arteriosus

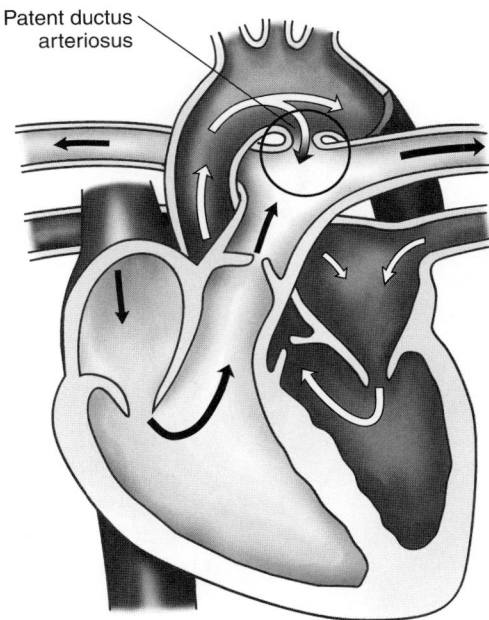

Patent ductus arteriosus

FIGURE 32-30 ■ Patent ductus arteriosus: Acyanotic. (From Kenner C, Lott JW: *Comprehensive neonatal nursing: A physiologic perspective,* ed 3, Philadelphia, 2003, WB Saunders.)

(2) High pulmonary pressures caused by pulmonary congestion lead to increased RV afterload, resulting in RV hypertrophy.

(3) LV hypertrophy results from increased pumping requirements of left ventricle (two or more times CO).

    f. Corrective surgical procedures: ligation or ligation and division of ductus arteriosus

2. Ventricular septal defect (VSD)—acyanotic (Figure 32-31)

    a. Accounts for about 25% of CHD

        (1) Most common congenital cardiac lesion

        (2) Often accompanied by other cardiac defects

    b. Definition: hole in the ventricular septum (may vary in size)

    c. Type based on location

        (1) Conoventricular

        (2) AV canal type

        (3) Muscular

    d. Signs and symptoms (same as PDA—infants; asymptotic until 4-12 weeks when the pulmonary vascular resistance [PVR] begins to fall)

    e. Assessment

        (1) Physical

            (a) RV hypertrophy

            (b) Systolic murmur of VSD shunt

            (c) Presternal thrill

        (2) Chest film

            (a) RV hypertrophy

            (b) PA enlargement

            (c) Left atrial and LV enlargement

        (3) Diagnostic assessment

            (a) Echocardiography (color Doppler)

            (b) Cardiac catheterization

            (c) ABG and Svo_2 analysis

    f. Effects on hemodynamics (depends on size of defect)

        (1) Blood flow from LV to RV

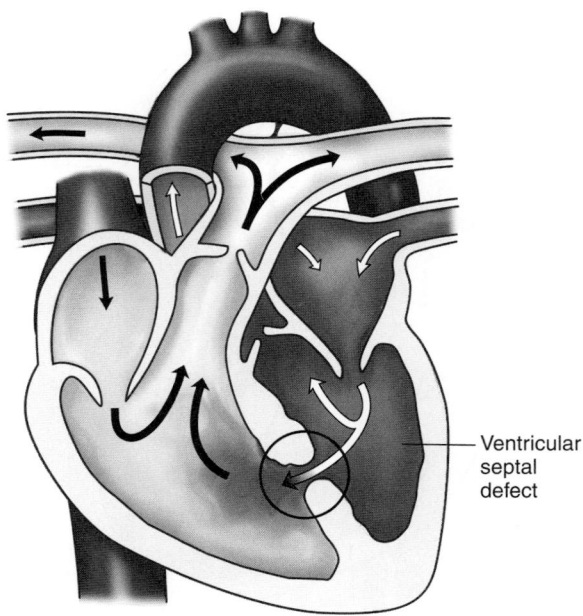

FIGURE 32-31 ■ Ventricular septal defect: Acyanotic. (From Kenner C, Lott JW: *Comprehensive neonatal nursing: A physiologic perspective,* ed 3, Philadelphia, 2003, WB Saunders.)

           (2) Increase in RV volume (increased preload) and pressure results in hypertrophy.

           (3) May develop aortic insufficiency (2%–7%)

    g. Corrective surgical procedure

           (1) Timing is based on:

               (a) Location

               (b) Symptoms

               (c) Incidence of spontaneous closing (generally in first year of life)

           (2) Antibiotic prophylaxis indicated for all VSDs

           (3) Patch closure of defect—requires:

               (a) Median sternotomy

               (b) CPB

               (c) Hypothermia

           (4) PA banding: palliative

  3. Atrial septal defect (ASD) (Figure 32-32)

    a. Accounts for 3% to 4% of congenital heart defects

    b. Definition: communicating hole between left and right atria, which results in blood flow from left to right atrium

    c. Defects classified by location

           (1) Partial or incomplete (ostium primum ASD): two AV valves with a cleft in the mitral

           (2) Intermediate or transitional (ostium secundum ASD): AV valve configuration is between two AV valves and a common AV valve; ASD and no significant VSD (most common)

           (3) Complete (sinus venosus ASD): marked by a single common AV valve orifice as well as an ASD and VSD (least common)

    d. Signs and symptoms

           (1) Usually asymptomatic

           (2) Surgery done to prevent development of pulmonary hypertension that could lead to RV failure

    e. Assessment and diagnostics

           (1) Cardiac catheterization: demonstrates increased oxygen content in right atrium

           (2) Chest film: RV enlargement and prominent main PA

    f. Effects on hemodynamics: increased RV volume (preload)

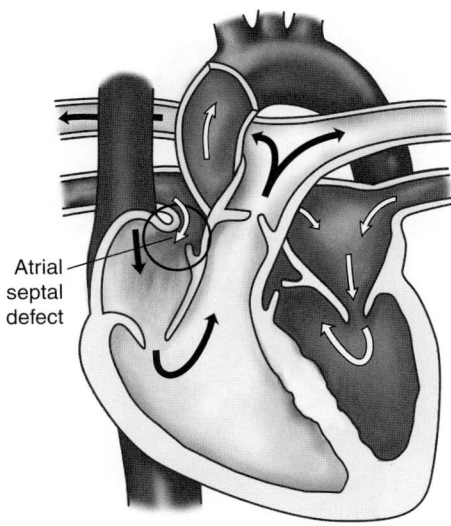

Atrial
septal
defect

FIGURE 32-32 ■ Atrial septal defect: Acyanotic. (From Kenner C, Lott JW: *Comprehensive neonatal nursing: A physiologic perspective,* ed 3, Philadelphia, 2003, WB Saunders.)

        g. Corrective surgical procedure: suture or patch closure of defect
- (1) Asymptomatic: older than 3 months to early childhood but before pulmonary vascular disease develops
- (2) Symptomatic: 3 to 4 months of age
- (3) Requires median sternotomy and usually CPB
- (4) Complications: dysrhythmias—heart block and sick sinus syndrome (usually transient)—and CHF (2%)

C. Right-to-left shunts

  1. Tetralogy of Fallot—cyanotic with decreased pulmonary blood flow (Figure 32-33)

    a. Accounts for 8% to 10% of CHD

    b. Definition: composed of four anatomic defects
- (1) VSD
- (2) Aorta overriding VSD
- (3) RV outflow obstruction: pulmonary stenosis
- (4) RV hypertrophy (develops secondary to pulmonary stenosis)

    c. Presence of cyanosis depends on degree of RV obstruction and shunting caused by obstruction.

    d. If cyanosis present, systemic and venous blood mixing with pulmonary venous blood
- (1) Imperative to eliminate any air in IV tubing because it may proceed to the cerebral circulation and result in stroke

    e. Corrective surgical procedure
- (1) Asymptomatic: scheduled at 2 to 4 months of age and sooner for symptomatic
- (2) Requires CPB
- (3) Aortopulmonary shunt for palliation
- (4) Patch closure of VSD
- (5) RV outflow reconstruction
- (6) Complications
  - (a) Narrow complex tachycardia
  - (b) Varying degrees of heart block
  - (c) Residual VSD
  - (d) Low CO
  - (e) Residual ventricular outflow obstruction
  - (f) Branch PA stenosis
- (7) Mortality for uncomplicated repair: 2% to 5%

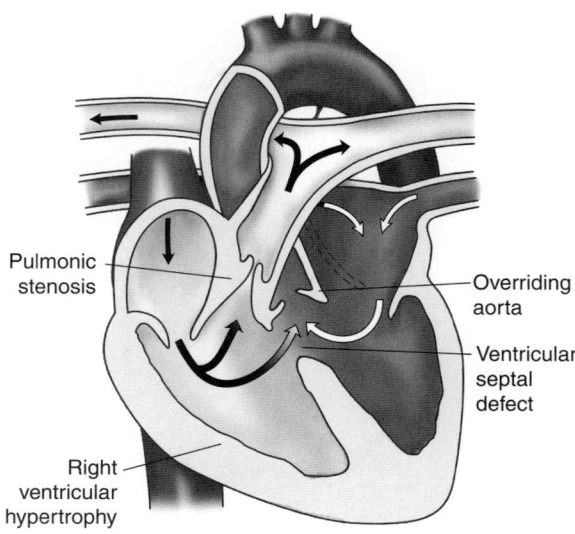

FIGURE 32-33 ■ Tetralogy of Fallot. (From Kenner C, Lott JW: *Comprehensive neonatal nursing: A physiologic perspective,* ed 3, Philadelphia, 2003, WB Saunders.)

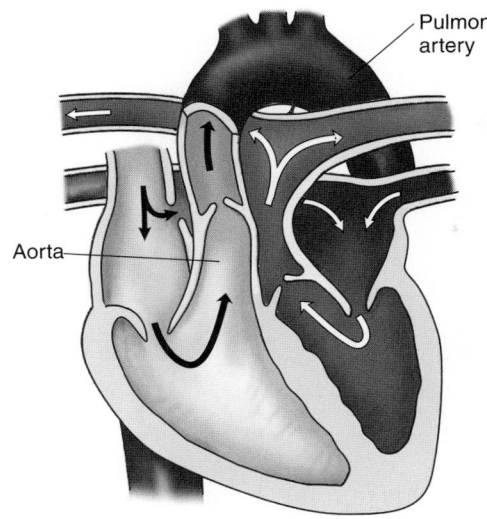

FIGURE 32-34 ■ Transposition of the great vessels: Cyanotic. (From Kenner C, Lott JW: *Comprehensive neonatal nursing: A physiologic perspective,* ed 3, Philadelphia, 2003, WB Saunders.)

2. Complete transposition of great vessels—cyanotic mixing lesion (Figure 32-34)
    a. Accounts for 5% to 7% of CHD
    b. Definition: aorta arises from RV, and PA arises from LV.
    c. Coexisting VSD present in 45% of cases
       (1) Without mixing of oxygenated and venous blood, the patient will die.
    d. Produces chronic arterial desaturation, compensatory polycythemia, and cyanosis
    e. Diagnosis frequently made by ruling out other cyanotic defects
    f. Corrective surgical procedure
       (1) Balloon atrial septectomy for palliation
       (2) Arterial switch procedure: places PA and aorta in their proper anatomic positions over right and left ventricles
          (a) Requires CPB
          (b) Reimplantation of coronary arteries is a critical component.
       (3) Mortality for arterial switch with uncomplicated lesions: 5% to 10%
       (4) Complications
          (a) Low CO related to poor LV function
          (b) Dysrhythmias related to decreased coronary artery perfusion and myocardial ischemia
3. Total anomalous pulmonary venous return—cyanotic (Figure 32-35)
    a. Definition (1% of CHD)
       (1) No pulmonary veins enter the left atrium (pulmonary veins join systemic venous circulation and mixed venous blood returns to heart).
       (2) Anomalous common pulmonary venous channel formed
       (3) ASD (one half have a PDA or patent foramen ovale)
    b. Signs and symptoms
       (1) One half are cyanotic in the first month.
       (2) Two thirds exhibit CHF by 3 months.
       (3) Ninety percent have CHF and cyanosis by first year.
    c. Corrective surgical procedure
       (1) Anastomosis of collecting vein and enlargement of left atrium—requires:
          (a) Median sternotomy
          (b) CPB
          (c) Profound hypothermia (20° C [68° F])
       (2) Requires vigorous management of CHF and endocarditis (perioperative mortality is 90%)

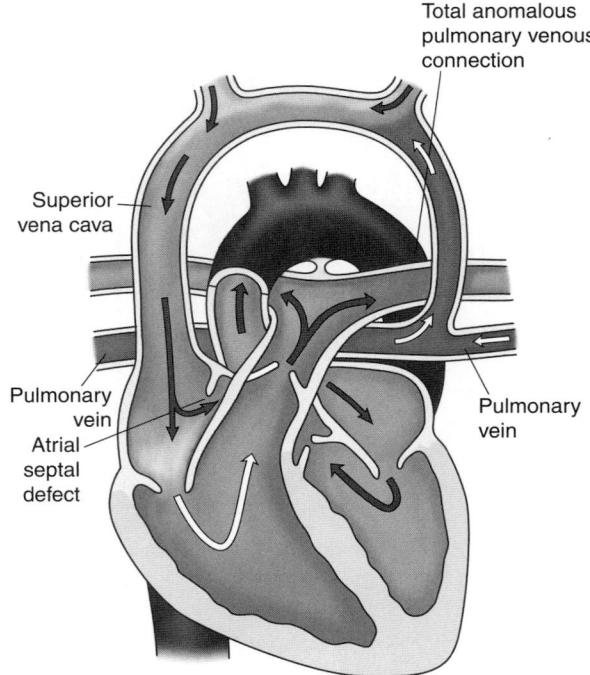

Total anomalous
pulmonary venous
connection

Superior
vena cava

Pulmonary
vein

Atrial
septal
defect

Pulmonary
vein

FIGURE 32-35 ■ Anomalous pulmonary venous return: Cyanotic. (From Kenner C, Lott JW: *Comprehensive neonatal nursing: A physiologic perspective,* ed 3, Philadelphia, 2003, WB Saunders.)

D. Obstruction to blood flow—cyanotic
    1. Valvular pulmonic stenosis (Figure 32-36)
        a. Accounts for 10% of CHD
        b. Definition: thickening of valve with fusion of leaflets at their commissure, resulting in narrowing pulmonary outflow tract and poststenotic dilatation of the PA
        c. VSD or ASD may also be present.
        d. Assessment: cardiac catheterization defines the level of obstruction and identifies other lesions.

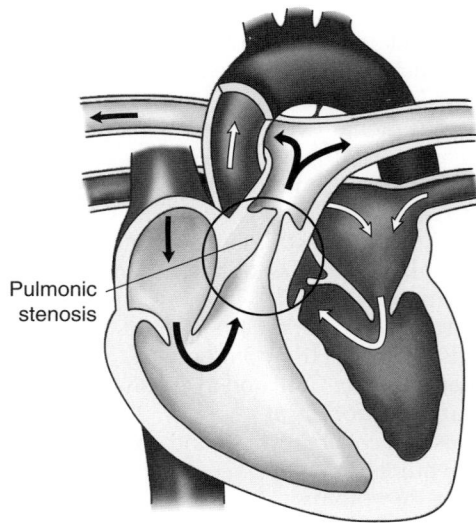

Pulmonic
stenosis

FIGURE 32-36 ■ Pulmonic stenosis: Cyanotic. (From Kenner C, Lott JW: *Comprehensive neonatal nursing: A physiologic perspective,* ed 3, Philadelphia, 2003, WB Saunders.)

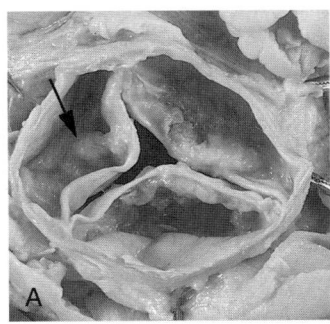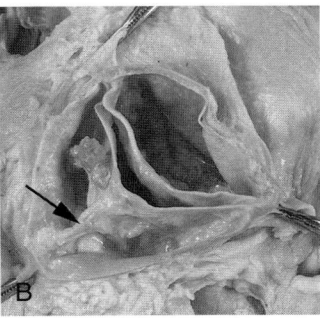

FIGURE 32-37 ■ **A,** Aortic stenosis of a previously normal valve having three cusps. **B,** Calcific aortic stenosis occurring on a congenitally bicuspid valve. (From Kumar V, Abbas AK, Fausto N: *Robbins and Cotran pathologic basis of disease,* ed 7, Philadelphia, 2005, WB Saunders.)

  e. Effects on hemodynamics: increased RV afterload and RV hypertrophy
   (1) Increased pressure gradient between RV and PA
    (a) Mild: 25 to 49 mm Hg
    (b) Moderate: 50 to 70 mm Hg
    (c) Severe: ≥80 mm Hg
  f. Corrective surgical procedure: pulmonary valvotomy—requires CPB
 2. Valvular aortic stenosis (Figure 32-37)
  a. Accounts for 5% to 10% of CHD
  b. Definition: thickened aortic valve, which is generally bicuspid instead of tricuspid, resulting in narrowing of aortic outflow
  c. May be present with PDA, coarctation of aorta, or both
  d. Physical assessment
   (1) Different BP between two arms
   (2) Systolic thrill
   (3) Systolic ejection murmur
   (4) Tachypnea
   (5) Tachycardia
   (6) Cyanosis with severe stenosis
 3. Coarctation of aorta (Figure 32-38)
  a. Accounts for 5% to 10% of CHD, with male-to-female ratio of 2:1

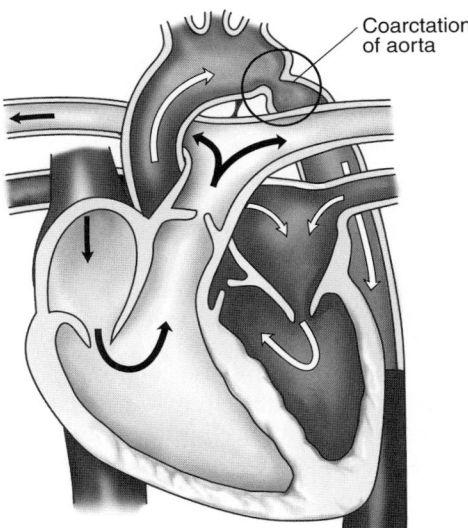

FIGURE 32-38 ■ Coarctation of the aorta: Cyanotic. (From Kenner C, Lott JW: *Comprehensive neonatal nursing: A physiologic perspective,* ed 3, Philadelphia, 2003, WB Saunders.)

       b. Definition: localized narrowing of aortic lumen (usually at ligamentum arteriosum); two types are:

         (1) Preductal (infantile): upper body supplied by LV and lower body supplied by RV through ductus arteriosus

         (2) Postductal (adult): LV supplies upper body, and collaterals develop in utero through intercostal and internal mammary arteries to supply lower body.

       c. May present with:

         (1) PDA

         (2) Valvular aortic stenosis

         (3) VSD

         (4) Other left-sided lesions

       d. Physical assessment

         (1) Classic finding

            (a) Disparity in pulses and BPs between upper and lower extremities

         (2) Right upper extremity is the preferred location for BP checks for accuracy.

         (3) Preductal coarctation

            (a) CHF (may occur early in infancy)

            (b) Cyanosis

            (c) Diminished pulses in lower body

         (4) Postductal coarctation

            (a) Acyanotic

            (b) Upper extremity hypertension

            (c) Diminished pulses in lower body

            (d) Midsystolic ejection murmur

            (e) Leg pain with exercise

            (f) Fatigability

            (g) Headaches

       e. Effects on hemodynamics

         (1) Increased LV afterload from obstruction to flow and increased arteriolar resistance

       f. Corrective surgical procedure

         (1) Patch angioplasty or resection with end-to-end anastomosis

E. Generalized signs and symptoms of CHD

   1. Cyanosis—results from:

      a. Shunting of unoxygenated blood into left side of heart: right-to-left shunt (i.e., Tetralogy of Fallot)

      b. Poor oxygen uptake: CHF, pulmonary edema

   2. Tachypnea

      a. Physiological chemical compensation to low oxygen content in blood

      b. Precipitated by mild exercise

   3. Effort intolerance

      a. Inability of infant to tolerate feedings; respiratory distress

      b. Fatigue with activity, inability to keep up with other children

   4. Failure to thrive

      a. Usually indicates left-to-right shunt or CHF

      b. Growth retardation, inability to gain weight

   5. Miscellaneous findings

      a. Frequent upper respiratory infections with ASD or PDA

      b. Headaches and leg pains with activity—coarctation of aorta

      c. Chest pain on exertion, fainting—aortic stenosis

      d. Clubbing of fingers, hypoxic episodes—Tetralogy of Fallot

X. Coronary artery disease (CAD)

    A. Definition: progressive narrowing or total occlusion of the arterial lumen characterized by accumulation of lipids, fibrous tissue, and calcium deposits in the arterial wall

    B. Angina pectoris

        1. Sensory response (chest pain) to a transient lack of oxygen in the myocardium

        2. Symptom of CAD, not a disease

        3. Exhibited late in disease process

        4. Results from an imbalance between oxygen supply and oxygen demand to myocardium

            a. Factors increasing demand

                (1) Increased afterload (i.e., hypertension)

                (2) Increased preload (i.e., sodium and water retention)

                (3) Dysrhythmias (i.e., tachydysrhythmias)

                (4) Increased contractility

                (5) Increased metabolism (i.e., fever, pain)

            b. Factors decreasing oxygen supply

                (1) Hypotension

                (2) Decreased afterload (i.e., peripheral vasodilation)

                (3) Increased LV preload (i.e., CHF) (increases resistance to coronary artery filling)

        5. Stress of surgery and postoperative pain are two of many precipitants of angina.

        6. Characteristics

            a. Typically lasts 1 to 5 minutes and subsides when precipitating factor is removed

            b. May be described as heaviness in chest, squeezing, burning, aching, or tightness

            c. Location is usually precordial, middle or lower sternum; may radiate to jaw, neck, shoulder, arm or hand, usually on left side.

            d. May be accompanied by dyspnea, diaphoresis, nausea, vomiting, and general fatigue

            e. Usually subsides with rest or is relieved with nitroglycerin within 30 to 90 seconds

        7. Classification

            a. Stable

                (1) Predictable in onset, duration, location, radiation, and quality of pain

                (2) Typically subsides with rest

            b. Unstable (preinfarction)

                (1) Unpredictable with increased frequency

                (2) May require nitrates for relief

                (3) May signify impending infarction

            c. Vasospastic (Prinzmetal's)

                (1) Results from coronary artery spasm

                (2) Anginal pain at rest that is cyclic and unrelated to exertion

                (3) Pain may persist for longer duration and is difficult to relieve.

        8. Diagnostic assessment

            a. ECG may not show ischemia or injury.

            b. Echocardiography (dobutamine stress) may show transient abnormal wall movement or valve function.

            c. Nuclear imaging (scintigraphy) with exercise or pharmacological stress

            d. Coronary catheterization

        9. Noninvasive management

            a. Identify and reduce modifiable risk factors (e.g., diet, smoking, obesity).

            b. Decrease myocardial oxygen demand.

                (1) Beta-blocker therapy

                (2) ACE inhibitors or angiotensin receptor blockers

                (3) Calcium channel blocker therapy

      c. Improve coronary blood flow.
        (1) Acetylsalicylic acid (ASA; aspirin) therapy
        (2) Clopidogrel
        (3) Nitrates
      d. Cholesterol/lipid management: statin therapy
    10. Invasive management
      a. Interventional cardiology
        (1) Percutaneous transluminal coronary angioplasty (PTCA)
        (2) Laser angioplasty
        (3) Stent placement
        (4) Atherectomy
      b. Surgical management
        (1) Coronary artery bypass grafting (CABG)

XI. MYOCARDIAL INFARCTION (MI)
  A. Definition: sustained myocardial ischemia resulting in death of myocardial tissue from sustained oxygen deprivation
  B. Causes
    1. Atherosclerosis of coronary arteries (most common cause)
      a. Atherosclerotic lesions occlude the vessel lumen and restrict flow under resting conditions while making the vessel stiff and unable to dilate.
    2. Coronary artery thrombosis
      a. Thought to be present in almost all acute occlusions
    3. Plaque fissure or hemorrhage
      a. Considered a predisposing factor that initiates response to injury
        (1) Platelet aggregation
        (2) Clotting cascade
        (3) Inflammatory process
    4. Coronary artery spasm
    5. Imbalance of myocardial oxygen demand versus supply (i.e., cocaine abuse, anemia, thyrotoxicosis)
      a. Regardless of cause, the result is decreased driving pressure beyond the site of the lesion and less oxygenated blood available to myocardial cells perfused by that vessel.
  C. Description
    1. Location is described by the affected wall of the heart (i.e., inferior).
    2. Necrosis may:
      a. Extend through the full myocardial wall (ST-segment elevation MI [STEMI])
      b. Affect only the heart's inner lining (Non-STEMI)
    3. Signs and symptoms
      a. Chest pain is generally described as:
        (1) More severe (crushing) in quality than anginal pain
        (2) Unrelieved after 20 to 30 minutes from either nitrates or rest
      b. Pain may be accompanied by symptoms of:
        (1) N/V
        (2) Diaphoresis
        (3) Intense anxiety
        (4) Apprehension
        (5) A feeling of doom
      c. Some patients do not experience chest pain.
        (1) Diabetics, female, and elderly may exhibit associated symptoms such as:
          (a) Fatigue
          (b) Syncope
  D. Assessment
    1. Physical
      a. Inspection may include any of the previously mentioned symptoms (e.g., dyspnea, diaphoresis).

  b. Palpation may reveal:
   (1) Thrill over valvular areas
   (2) Chest wall heaves
   (3) Shift of the point of maximal impulse (PMI)
  c. Auscultation may reveal:
   (1) Crackles
   (2) Gallop rhythms
   (3) Murmurs
   (4) Precordial friction rubs
 2. ECG should be obtained within 10 minutes from onset of symptoms.
  a. ST-segment depression and T-wave inversion indicate:
   (1) Possible ischemia
   (2) Unstable angina
  b. ST-segment elevation indicates pattern of injury.
  c. Q-wave appearance (>0.03-second width) indicates:
   (1) Pattern of necrosis
   (2) Definitive diagnosis of infarction
 3. Laboratory findings
  a. Elevations in cardiac markers
   (1) Creatine Kinase—MB isoenzyme (CK-MB) cardiac specific
   (2) Troponin-I
 4. Effects on hemodynamics
  a. Hemodynamic effects are a direct result of decreased pumping ability of the ventricle, which results in:
   (1) Backup of pressure and volume from the affected ventricle
   (2) Decreased forward flow of blood
  b. Severe LV dysfunction results in cardiogenic shock and pulmonary edema.
  c. Severe RV dysfunction results in:
   (1) LV dysfunction (from decreased volume to the LV)
   (2) Systemic congestion
  d. Dysrhythmia is the number one complication and cause of death.
   (1) Other complications requiring surgical intervention
    (a) Papillary muscle rupture
    (b) Septal defect
    (c) Ventricular aneurysm
 E. Treatment
 1. Goal of treatment is to support the patient while attempting to prevent complications by:
  a. Revascularizing the ischemic myocardium
  b. Limiting the size of the MI
 2. Treatment is categorized between ST elevation and new or presumed new left bundle branch block and ST depression or T-wave inversion.
  a. Revascularization
   (1) Fibrinolytics
   (2) Antithrombin agents
   (3) Antiplatelet agents
    (a) Aspirin
    (b) Glycoprotein IIb/IIIa inhibitors
    (c) Clopidogrel
   (4) Percutaneous coronary interventions
    (a) PTCA
    (b) Coronary stents
   (5) CABG
  b. Inotropic support (see Table 32-5)
   (1) Drugs
    (a) Dobutamine
    (b) Dopamine
    (c) Digoxin
    (d) Norepinephrine

        (2) Mechanical
           (a) IABP
           (b) VAD
    c. Pain control
        (1) Nitrates
        (2) Morphine sulfate
    d. Prevention and treatment of symptoms depend on the manifestations but may include:
        (1) Diuretics
        (2) Antidysrhythmic agents
        (3) Magnesium sulfate
        (4) Beta-blockers
        (5) Calcium channel blockers
        (6) ACE inhibitors

XII. VALVULAR HEART DISEASE
  A. Rheumatic heart disease
    1. Characterized by scarring and deformity of heart valves resulting from rheumatic fever
    2. Rheumatic fever is a diffuse inflammatory disease affecting
      a. Joints
      b. Heart
      c. Skin
      d. Nervous system
      e. Result of an autoimmune process induced by streptococcal antigens
    3. Valves commonly involved
      a. Mitral and aortic (most common)
      b. Tricuspid
      c. Pulmonary (rare)
    4. Extent of cardiac disease depends on several factors.
      a. Duration and severity of inflammation
      b. Location of the valvular insufficiency and/or stenosis and the severity of hemodynamic effect
      c. Frequent recurrences of carditis
      d. Degree of valvular and myocardial scarring after resolution of the inflammation
      e. Presence of valvular disease unrelated to underlying rheumatic inflammation
    5. Signs and symptoms
      a. Will depend on the degree of disease and the valve affected
    6. Diagnostic evaluation
      a. Echocardiography
      b. Cardiac catheterization
    7. Effects on hemodynamics
      a. Dependent on amount of regurgitation or stenosis and which valves are affected
    8. Treatment
      a. Antibiotic therapy: for active streptococccal infections (penicillin)
      b. Anti-inflammatory agents
        (1) Salicylates
        (2) Corticosteroids
      c. Valve surgery indicated if significant hemodynamic effects
  B. Special considerations for valve replacement
    1. Categories
      a. Mechanical (i.e., central flow disk [St. Jude], ball-and-cage [Starr-Edwards], tilting disk [Bjork-Shiley, Lillehei-Kaster, Medtronic Hall])
        (1) Suitable for larger orifices (i.e., aortic and mitral)
        (2) Durable, but thrombogenic, and require long-term anticoagulation
        (3) Suitable for patients with a life expectancy >10 years
        (4) Unsuitable for patients with a questionable ability for compliance with:
          (a) Anticoagulation

(b) Liver dysfunction

(c) Stated desire to bear children

   b. Bioprosthetic

     (1) Porcine, bovine, or homografts

     (2) Low risk of thromboembolic complications without coagulation

     (3) Low durability—8 to 10 years

     (4) Human allografts (homografts)

       (a) Removed and prepared from cadavers

       (b) Stored in a cryopreservation process

       (c) Technically difficult to implant

       (d) Contraindicated with history of an adverse immunological response to human allogenic tissue

       (e) Does not require anticoagulation

C. Nonrheumatic causes of valvular disease

   1. Atherosclerotic heart disease

   2. Congenital abnormalities

   3. Cardiothoracic trauma

   4. Calcification caused by aging

   5. Systemic infections

   6. Tumors

   7. Syphilis

   8. Marfan's syndrome

D. Pathophysiology of valvular disease

   1. Stenosis: narrowing of valve orifice; obstructs blood flow

   2. Insufficiency: incompetent valve that results in regurgitation through the valve orifice

   3. Mixed lesion: stenosis and insufficiency

E. Specific valvular abnormalities

   1. Mitral stenosis (MS; Figure 32-39)

     a. Principal cause is rheumatic fever.

     b. Most common valvular defect, especially in women in their third decades

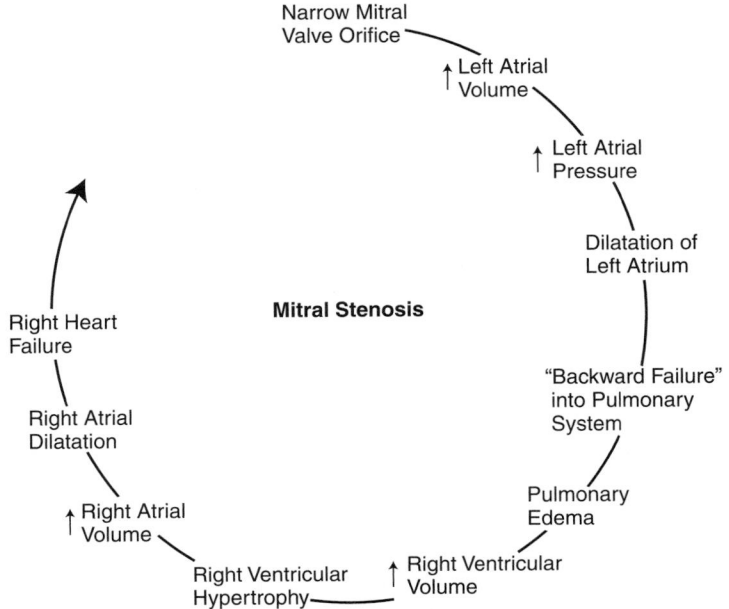

FIGURE 32-39 ■ Mitral stenosis. (From Abranczk EL, Brown MM: *Comprehensive cardiac care,* ed 7, St Louis, 1991, Mosby.)

   c. Pathological findings
     (1) Progressive narrowing of mitral valve from 4 to 6 cm to 1.5 cm
     (2) Fusion of commissures
     (3) Scarring of anterior and posterior leaflets' free margins
     (4) Shortening, fusion, and nodularity of chordae tendineae
   d. Signs and symptoms
     (1) Most common
       (a) Dyspnea
       (b) Fatigue
       (c) Palpitations
       (d) Cough
       (e) Hemoptysis
     (2) Less common
       (a) Dysphagia
       (b) Hoarseness
       (c) Chest pain
       (d) Embolic events
       (e) Seizure
       (f) Cerebrovascular accident
     (3) Atrial fibrillation
       (a) Occurs in 40% to 50% of patients with MS
       (b) May decrease CO by as much as 15% to 20%
       (c) Increases likelihood of clot formation caused by incomplete emptying of atria
     (4) Thromboembolism: 80% of patients who develop systemic emboli are in atrial fibrillation.
     (5) Murmur is early diastolic to middiastolic, low-pitched, rumbling sound heard best at the apex.
   e. Diagnostic studies
     (1) ECG (wide, notched P waves)
     (2) Echocardiogram
       (a) Most useful
       (b) Valve appears thick and shows diminished motion and posterior leaflet movement.
     (3) Cardiac catheterization (obtains valvular gradient data)
   f. Effects on hemodynamics
     (1) Increased left atrial (LA) pressures and volumes resulting in atrial strain and dysrhythmias
     (2) Progresses to low CO states
       (a) Increased PA pressures (PAPs)
       (b) Increased PA occlusion (wedge) pressures (PAOPs, PCWPs)
   g. Treatment
     (1) Noninvasive
       (a) Sodium restriction
       (b) Diuretics
       (c) Antidysrhythmics
       (d) Anticoagulation
       (e) Balloon valvulotomy
         (i) Performed on an outpatient basis
         (ii) Risk of damage to mitral valve
         (iii) Would require mitral valve replacement
     (2) Surgical intervention
       (a) Indicated when the patient develops symptoms of:
         (i) Atrial fibrillation
         (ii) Pulmonary edema
         (iii) Pulmonary hypertension
         (iv) Orthopnea
         (v) Fatigue

      (b) Commissurotomy—performed if:
         (i)   Valve is only stenotic with fusion of uncalcified commissures.
         (ii) Chordae tendineae not severely deformed
         (iii) Leaflets mobile
         (iv) No associated insufficiency
      (c) Mitral valve replacement
         (i)   Performed if preoperative catheterization, angiography, and echocardiography indicate valvular or subvalvular calcification and thickening.

   h. Preoperative considerations
     (1) Important to have a thorough evaluation of cardiac disease, including:
       (a) Exertional tolerance
       (b) History of CHF
       (c) Response to drug therapy
     (2) Review of all diagnostic testing, including:
       (a) Cardiac catheterization
       (b) Laboratory tests
       (c) ECG
       (d) X-rays
       (e) Cardiac catheterization data become immensely useful in patient management postoperatively.
     (3) Baseline system evaluation with emphasis on:
       (a) Neurological
       (b) Pulmonary
       (c) Renal
     (4) Patient teaching should include the criteria for selection of valve type (mechanical vs bioprosthesis) and long-term considerations.
       (a) Intraoperative and postoperative considerations
     (5) Pulmonary hypertension common
     (6) Generally have insertion of PA catheter, possibly fiberoptic
     (7) Preload management is important to maintain adequate CO and avoid pulmonary edema.
       (a) Generally, use crystalloid or synthetic colloid fluid for volume replacement.
       (b) Very useful to know the preoperative PAP
     (8) Control of dysrhythmia is essential for CO (prone to atrial dysrhythmias).

 2. Mitral insufficiency (Figure 32-40)
   a. Second most common valvular defect
   b. Causes
     (1) Heart failure (annular dilation from dilated LV)
     (2) Bacterial endocarditis
     (3) Ruptured chordae tendineae
     (4) Rupture or dysfunction of a papillary muscle
     (5) Rheumatic heart disease
     (6) Prolapse (prolapse and CAD most common causes)
     (7) Trauma
     (8) Calcification (common in elderly women)
   c. Pathological findings
     (1) Backward leakage of blood from the LV into the LA during systole
     (2) Scarring and calcification
     (3) Bacterial destruction of uninvolved tissue
     (4) Dilation of the annulus
   d. Signs and symptoms
     (1) Blowing, high-pitched, pansystolic murmur heard best at PMI, with radiation to the left axilla or infrascapular areas
     (2) Atrial pulsation at the third left intercostal space
     (3) Weakness and fatigue

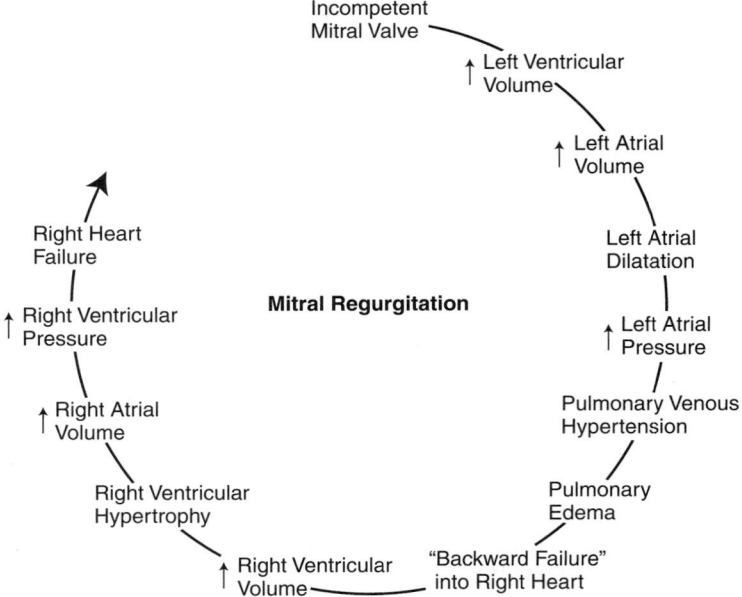

FIGURE 32-40 ■ Mitral regurgitation. (From Abranczk EL, Brown MM: *Comprehensive cardiac care,* ed 7, St Louis, 1991, Mosby.)

      (4) Atrial fibrillation
      (5) Pulmonary edema
      (6) CHF
      (7) Chest pain (usually atypical)
   e. Diagnostic studies (same as MS)
      (1) ECG (altered P waves and QRS amplitude and nonspecific ST changes)
      (2) CXR (LV and LA enlargement)
      (3) Echocardiogram and echo Doppler (decreased ventricular wall motion and estimates severity of regurgitation)
      (4) Cardiac catheterization (LV end-diastolic pressure [LVEDP] and wall motion)
   f. Effects on hemodynamics
      (1) Backward flow of blood from LV to LA during ventricular systole:
         (a) Increases LA and LV volumes (preload) and pressures
            (i) Causes a backup of pressure and volume into the pulmonary vasculature (increased LVEDP [PAOP, PCWP] and PAP)
      (2) Increased pulmonary pressures result in pulmonary edema.
      (3) Over time, pulmonary edema and hypertension can result in failure of the right side of the heart (increased right arterial pressure).
   g. Treatment
      (1) Noninvasive (same as for MS)
      (2) Surgical interventions
         (a) Surgery should be timed to occur before irreversible LV dysfunction has developed.
         (b) Mitral valve replacement with removal of the mitral valve apparatus
         (c) Mitral valve replacement with preservation of at least part of the mitral valve apparatus
         (d) Mitral valve repair (valvuloplasty)
            (i) Preservation of the mitral valve apparatus helps to maintain LV performance and avoids the risks of a prosthesis.
           (ii) Results of valvuloplasty are better in nonrheumatic valves.

   h. Preoperative considerations (same as MS)
   i. Intraoperative and postoperative considerations
      (1) Both LA and LV usually volume overloaded and dilated
      (2) Goals of anesthesia
         (a) Maintain HR at normal levels.
         (b) Control afterload with vasodilators.
      (3) Generally have a PA catheter inserted after the initiation of anesthesia
      (4) Requires heart-lung bypass and myocardial preservation techniques
      (5) Usually performed via a medial sternotomy: insertion of mediastinal chest drainage tubes and sometimes a left pleural drainage tube
      (6) Patients are preload sensitive and require higher filling pressures (vigilant hemodynamic monitoring and fluid maintenance).
      (7) Postoperative goal is rapid extubation and ambulation (pulmonary problems common).
3. Aortic stenosis (AS; Figure 32-41)
   a. A narrowing of aortic valve orifice, which obstructs the ejection of blood from the LV
   b. Three times more common in men than women
   c. Causes
      (1) Congenital abnormalities (generally in patients younger than 30 years)
      (2) Rheumatic fever (30–70 years of age)
      (3) Idiopathic calcification
         (a) Aging (older than 70 years)
         (b) Hypertrophic obstructive cardiomyopathy
   d. Pathological findings
      (1) Narrowing of normal valve orifice (2.6–3.5 cm²)
         (a) A valve orifice of 0.5 cm² may still prove functional if it develops over several years with LV compensation.
         (b) A valve orifice of 0.4 cm² with peak systolic pressure gradients above 50 mm Hg results in a critical obstruction.
      (2) Congenital malformations may include:
         (a) Unicuspid

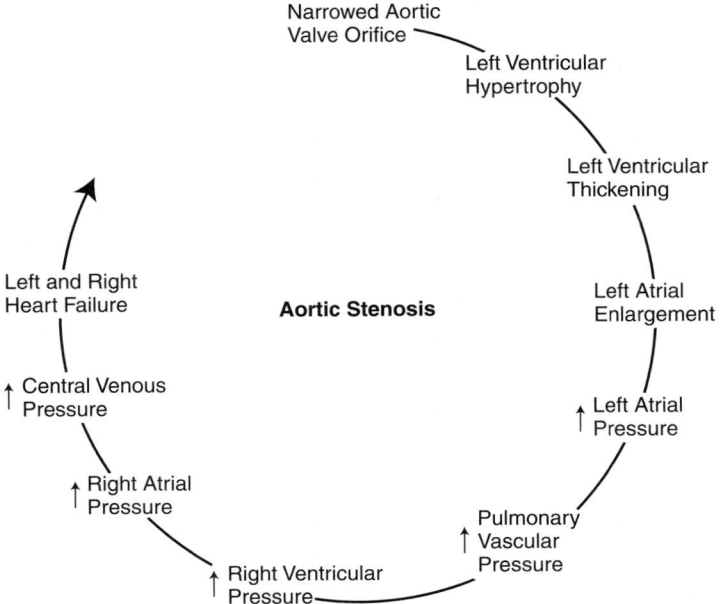

FIGURE 32-41 ■ Aortic stenosis. (From Abranczk EL, Brown MM: *Comprehensive cardiac care*, ed 7, St Louis, 1991, Mosby.)

      (b) Bicuspid
         (i) One percent of Americans born with a bicuspid aortic valve
      (c) Multicuspid
      (d) Unequal aortic valve leaflets

  e. Signs and symptoms
    (1) Most patients with AS initially asymptomatic
      (a) Risk of death rapidly increases with the development of symptoms.
    (2) Classic manifestations
      (a) Fatigue
      (b) Chest pain (approximately 50% experience exertional angina)
      (c) Syncope (15%-30% as consequences of dysrhythmia or an abrupt fall in systemic vascular resistance [SVR])
    (3) Harsh, high-pitched systolic crescendo-decrescendo murmur
      (a) Best heard at right sternal border at second intercostal space
      (b) May radiate to neck or apex
      (c) Intensity of murmur usually decreases as:
         (i) Disease progresses
         (ii) CO falls
    (4) Systolic thrill over apex
    (5) Narrowed pulse pressure

  f. Diagnostic studies
    (1) ECG
      (a) LV hypertrophy
      (b) First-degree AV block
      (c) Left bundle branch block
    (2) CXR
      (a) LV enlargement
      (b) Poststenotic dilatation of the aorta
      (c) Calcification of valve cusps
      (d) Pulmonary congestion
    (3) Echocardiogram
      (a) LV thickening
      (b) Reduced mobility and calcification of cusps
    (4) Nuclear scans
      (a) Ventricular function
      (b) Ejection fraction
    (5) Cardiac catheterization
      (a) Determines the gradient
      (b) Evaluates LV function
      (c) Identifies the presence of other valvular lesions and CAD

  g. Effects on hemodynamics
    (1) Increase in afterload leads to LV hypertrophy and elevated LVEDP, resulting in:
      (a) Elevated pulmonary vascular pressures
      (b) Left-sided heart failure
      (c) Eventual right-sided heart failure

  h. Treatment
    (1) Symptomatic AS is lethal if not treated.
    (2) Noninvasive
      (a) Patients must be asymptomatic or clearly nonsurgical candidates.
      (b) Prophylactic antibiotics recommended for high-risk patients before dental and invasive medical procedures.
      (c) Nitrates for chest pain should always be administered cautiously because the vasodilation may result in:
         (i) Hypotension
         (ii) Syncope
         (iii) Decreased CO

(3) Surgical intervention
  (a) Even patients with advanced heart failure and severe LV dysfunction may still benefit from aortic valve replacement, especially if the gradient exceeds 30 mm Hg.
  (b) Aortic valve replacement (most common procedure)
  (c) Indicated for patients who develop:
    (i) Gradient >50 mm Hg with CHF, angina, or exertional syncope
    (ii) Calculated aortic valve area index <0.8 cm^2/m^2
  (d) Requires use of extracorporeal circulation and the selection of a valvular prosthesis
  (e) Criteria for selection of mechanical or bioprosthesis is the same as for MS.
  (f) Approximately 20% of patients with a bioprosthetic aortic valve require a second valve replacement within 8 years.
(4) Valvuloplasty
  (a) Indicated in patients who are severely symptomatic but are not candidates for aortic replacement to decrease the gradient and relieve symptoms
  (b) Does not decrease mortality
i. Preoperative considerations (same as MS)
j. Intraoperative and postoperative considerations
  (1) Most difficult to manage of all valvular diseases
  (2) Extremely preload sensitive
    (a) Replacement of valve greatly decreases the afterload the ventricle must pump against to eject blood.
    (b) The decreased resistance allows the ventricle to easily eject, therefore decreasing:
      (i) Volume (preload)
      (ii) Stretch of the myocardium
    (c) This can significantly impact ventricular filling and CO by decreasing contractility.
  (3) PA catheter inserted; pay special attention to following parameters:
    (a) Preload (right atrial [RA])
    (b) PAOP (PCWP)
    (c) Afterload SVR
    (d) PVR
  (4) Prone to atrial fibrillation and tachycardia
4. Aortic insufficiency (AI; Figure 32-42)
  a. Backward flow of blood from the aorta into the LV during ventricular diastole
  b. Causes
    (1) Result from pathophysiology of the aortic root or the valve leaflet
    (2) Most common valvular causes
      (a) Endocarditis—most common cause
      (b) Rheumatic heart disease
    (3) Most common aortic root causes
      (a) Idiopathic dilation (annuloaortic ectasia) associated with hypertension and aging
      (b) Marfan's syndrome
      (c) Aortic dissection
      (d) Syphilis
      (e) Collagen vascular disease
      (f) Trauma
  c. Signs and symptoms
    (1) Patients with normal LV function may be remarkably asymptomatic, even during strenuous exertion.
    (2) Symptoms usually those of left-sided failure
    (3) May develop angina because of the relative diastolic hypotension resulting in decreased coronary filling pressure
      (a) Angina usually associated with vasodilation and flushing

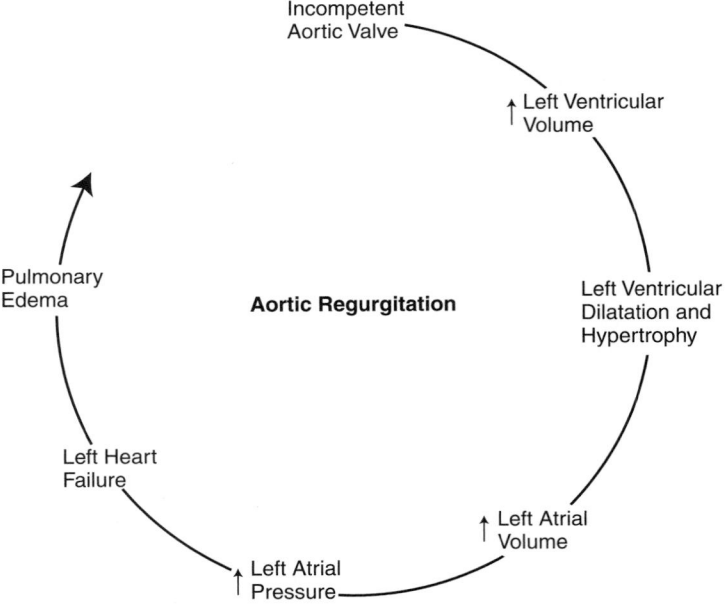

FIGURE 32-42 ■ Aortic regurgitation. (From Abranczk EL, Brown MM: *Comprehensive cardiac care*, ed 7, St Louis, 1991, Mosby.)

      (4) Presenting signs and symptoms of acute AI
         (a) Tachycardia
         (b) Dyspnea
         (c) Pulmonary edema
         (d) Peripheral vasoconstriction
         (e) Cyanosis
         (f) Midpitched, short, diastolic murmur
         (g) Audible third heart sound
      (5) Presenting signs and symptoms of chronic AI
         (a) Exertional dyspnea
         (b) Orthopnea
         (c) High-pitched, blowing crescendo diastolic sound heard best at second right intercostal space while patient sitting
         (d) Third or fourth heart sound may be audible depending on degree of regurgitation.
      (6) Patient may also have a rapid upstroke and downstroke of the carotid pulse (Corrigan's pulse).
   d. Diagnostic studies
      (1) ECG
         (a) Chronic—LV hypertrophy (increased amplitude of the QRS and ST-T wave strain pattern)
            (i) AV conduction prolonged
         (b) Acute—ST-T wave changes consistent with myocardial ischemia
      (2) CXR
         (a) Chronic—dilatation of LV with elongation of apex inferiorly and posteriorly
            (i) May see a prominent ascending aorta with Marfan's syndrome
         (b) Acute—normal-sized heart, but may show pulmonary edema
      (3) Echocardiogram
         (a) May visualize vegetation formation on valve leaflets from endocarditis
         (b) Quantifies amount of regurgitation
         (c) Promptness of exam mandatory in acute AI

    (4) Cardiac catheterization
        (a) Estimates the severity of regurgitation and evaluates extent of LV failure
        (b) Generally not indicated in young patients where acute AI results from endocarditis
  e. Effects on hemodynamics
    (1) Produces LV volume overload
    (2) With chronic AI, the increase in LVEDV results in a more forceful LV contraction.
        (a) Force of contraction maintained by LV hypertrophy and dilation
    (3) Eventually, increased LVEDP is reflected backward to:
        (a) LA
        (b) Pulmonary vasculature
        (c) Right side of the heart
        (d) Results in:
           (i)   Pulmonary edema
           (ii) Right-sided heart failure
    (4) With acute AI, the LV does not have time to hypertrophy and increase the force of contraction.
        (a) Increased LVEDP may:
           (i)   Exceed LA pressure
           (ii) Cause the mitral valve to close prematurely
        (b) This results in pulmonary venous hypertension and pulmonary edema.
  f. Treatment
    (1) Noninvasive
        (a) Antibiotic prophylaxis
        (b) Treat CHF with:
           (i)   Diuretics
           (ii) Digoxin
           (iii) Vasodilators
           (iv) Preload and afterload reducers
        (c) Important to remember AI is a fluid volume overload problem, whereas AS is a pressure overload disturbance.
    (2) Surgical valve replacement
    (3) Must be performed before the development of irreversible LV dysfunction
    (4) Indications
        (a) Symptomatic chronic AI
        (b) Asymptomatic—"55 rule"
           (i)   Good outcome can be expected if LV end-systolic diameter <55 mm and LV ejection fraction 55% or greater.
        (c) Acute
           (i)   Mortality rate if treated medically: 75%
           (ii) Mortality rate if treated surgically: 25%
    (5) Prosthesis selection (same as mitral)
        (a) Incidence of prosthetic infective endocarditis is 1% to 2% regardless of the prosthesis selected.
  g. Preoperative considerations (same as MS)
    (1) Important to know degree of LV failure preoperatively to guide postoperative care
  h. Intraoperative and postoperative considerations
    (1) Severe volume overload
    (2) Prevent bradycardias because they prolong filling time and result in volume overload.
    (3) Use afterload reduction.
        (a) Nitroglycerin
        (b) Nitroprusside

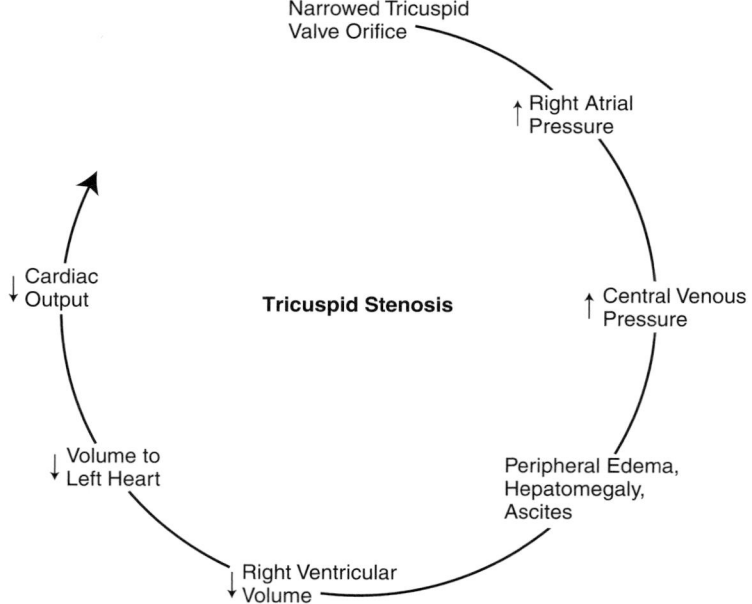

FIGURE 32-43 ■ Tricuspid stenosis. (From Abranczk EL, Brown MM: *Comprehensive cardiac care,* ed 7, St Louis, 1991, Mosby.)

      (4) Mechanical valves carry a 2% to 5% incidence of thromboembolic and bleeding complications.
   5. Tricuspid stenosis (TS; Figure 32-43)
     a. Causes
       (1) Rheumatic heart disease
       (2) Frequently associated with MS
       (3) RA tumors
       (4) Congenital abnormalities
     b. Pathological findings
       (1) Reduction of the normal tricuspid valve orifice of 7 cm^2 to 1.5 cm^2 or less
     c. Signs and symptoms
       (1) Major symptoms: dyspnea and fatigue
       (2) Peripheral edema and neck pulsation (especially when RA pressure ≥10 mm Hg)
       (3) Murmur is a low-pitched diastolic rumble best heard at fourth intercostal space to the left of the sternal border
         (a) Increases in intensity with inspiration
     d. Diagnostic studies
       (1) ECG: large P waves
       (2) CXR: prominent RA
       (3) Echocardiogram: fibrosis, calcifications, and obstruction
       (4) Echo Doppler: estimates the diastolic gradient
       (5) Cardiac catheterization: confirms a gradient of greater than 1 mm Hg between RA and RV
     e. Effects on hemodynamics
       (1) Increased RA volume (preload) and pressure
       (2) Decreased CO because less blood fills RV and therefore less blood reaches left side of the heart
     f. Treatment
       (1) Noninvasive
         (a) Antibiotic prophylaxis
         (b) Peripheral edema may not respond to diuretics because the edema is a result of pressure overload and not volume overload.

(2) Surgical intervention
    (a) Valve replacement
    (b) Long-term anticoagulation warranted because of the high thrombogenic rate and therefore negates the benefit of a bioprosthesis.
g. Preoperative considerations (same as MS)
h. Intraoperative and postoperative considerations
  (1) Potential for valve infection is a persistent problem.
  (2) Will require extensive education regarding:
    (a) Anticoagulation
    (b) Signs and symptoms of endocarditis
  (3) May have considerations of other valvular diseases if have concomitant disease (e.g., mitral stenosis)
6. Tricuspid insufficiency (Figure 32-44)
  a. Causes
    (1) Infective endocarditis
      (a) Occurs in 10% of the general endocarditis population, but increases to 50% among illicit IV drug users who develop endocarditis
      (b) RV dilatation and failure secondary to LV failure and pulmonary hypertension
      (c) Congenital abnormality
  b. Signs and symptoms
    (1) Generally well tolerated by the RV
    (2) Presence worsens the symptoms of RV failure (i.e., fatigue, edema, and ascites)
    (3) Atrial fibrillation common
    (4) Murmur
      (a) High-pitched
      (b) Blowing
      (c) Holosystolic
      (d) Heard best at fourth intercostal space at the left sternal border or xiphoid area
      (e) Intensifies with inspiration

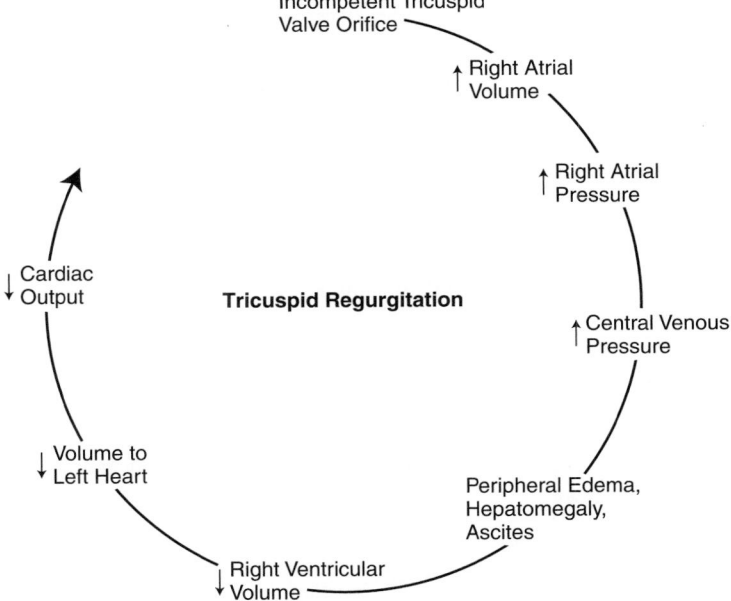

FIGURE 32-44 ■ Tricuspid regurgitation. (From Abranczk EL, Brown MM: *Comprehensive cardiac care,* ed 7, St Louis, 1991, Mosby.)

    c. Diagnostic studies
       (1) ECG: atrial fibrillation or right bundle branch block
       (2) CXR: RA and RV enlargement
       (3) Echocardiogram: recognition of vegetative lesions, ruptured chordae and papillary muscles, and the back-and-forth motion of the valve
       (4) Doppler: estimates severity of regurgitation
       (5) Cardiac catheterization: prominent V wave in the RA
    d. Effects on hemodynamics
       (1) Backward flow of blood into RA increases RA volume (preload) and pressure.
       (2) Decreased CO resulting from a diminished amount of blood reaching the left side of the heart
    e. Treatment
       (1) Noninvasive
         (a) Alleviation of RV failure
         (b) Improvement of diseases responsible (e.g., endocarditis)
       (2) Surgical intervention (same as TS)
         (a) May have to replace a concurrent stenotic mitral valve
    f. Preoperative considerations (same as MS)
    g. Intraoperative and postoperative considerations will have:
       (1) Right-sided volume overload
       (2) Long-term anticoagulation considerations
  7. Pulmonic valvular disease
    a. Stenosis: most common cause is congenital abnormality (Figure 32-45)
    b. Insufficiency: most common cause is dilatation of the valve ring resulting from pulmonary hypertension (Figure 32-46)
    c. May be tolerated for years without difficulty unless it is complicated by pulmonary hypertension
    d. Signs and symptoms
       (1) Stenosis
         (a) Dyspnea, fatigue, and syncope proportional to severity of disease

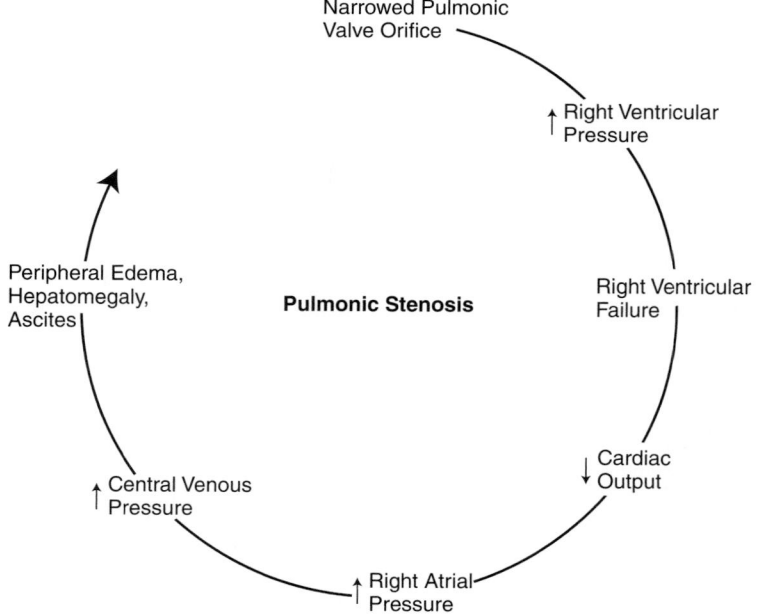

FIGURE 32-45 ■ Pulmonic stenosis. (From Abranczk EL, Brown MM: *Comprehensive cardiac care*, ed 7, St Louis, 1991, Mosby.)

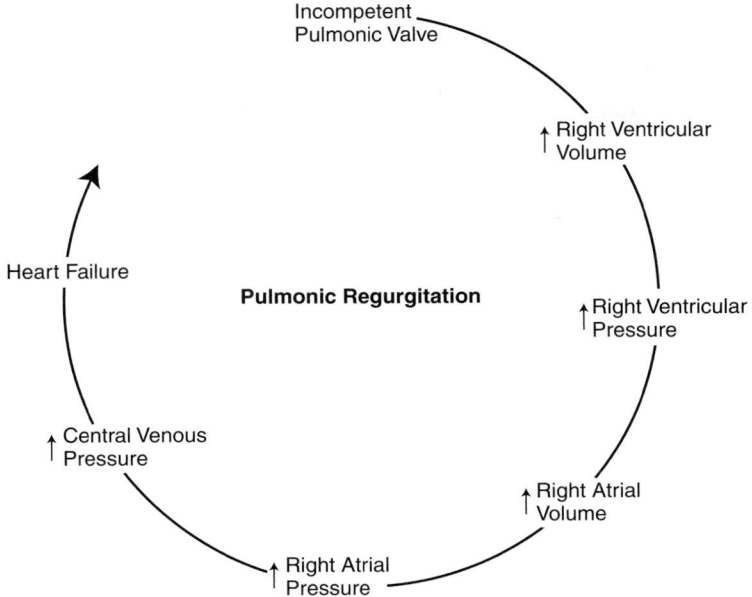

FIGURE 32-46 ■ Pulmonic regurgitation. (From Abranczk EL, Brown MM: *Comprehensive cardiac care,* ed 7, St Louis, 1991, Mosby.)

        (b) Murmur is a sharp, systolic crescendo-decrescendo best heard at left sternal border at second or third intercostal space.
           (i) Second heart sound may be widely split or absent.
    (2) Insufficiency
        (a) No symptoms except those of pulmonary hypertension
        (b) Murmur is high-pitched with pulmonary hypertension and moderately pitched without pulmonary hypertension.
           (i) Blowing sound most optimally auscultated at fourth or fifth intercostal space to the left of the sternal border
           (ii) Hard to distinguish from AI
  e. Diagnostic studies
    (1) Thorough history
    (2) Echocardiography is the most valuable noninvasive tool.
  f. Effects on hemodynamics
    (1) Stenosis is a right-sided pressure overload, while insufficiency is a right-sided volume overload.
        (a) Both are evidenced by elevated RA pressures and eventual heart failure.
        (b) Stenosis will show evidence of diminished CO earlier than insufficiency.
  g. Treatment
    (1) Noninvasive intervention is aimed at:
        (a) Alleviation of symptoms with insufficiency
        (b) Prevention of recurrent endocarditis and emboli with stenosis
    (2) Surgical replacement of a stenotic valve is rare.
    (3) Replacement prosthesis will be a bioprosthesis because of the high incidence of emboli associated with mechanical valves.
    (4) Valvotomy is the preferred invasive treatment for stenosis.
  h. Preoperative considerations (same as MS)
  i. Intraoperative and postoperative considerations
    (1) Hemodynamic monitoring and intervention will be focused on:
        (a) Presence of pulmonary hypertension
        (b) Decreased CO
        (c) RV overload and failure
    (2) Same considerations as any mechanical valve replacement

        8. Multivalvular disease

           a. Common with rheumatic heart disease

           b. Should undergo right- and left-sided heart catheterizations for full assessment before surgery

           c. Common types

               (1) Mitral stenosis and aortic insufficiency

               (2) Mitral stenosis and aortic stenosis

               (3) Aortic stenosis and mitral insufficiency

               (4) Aortic and mitral insufficiency

           d. Management

               (1) Double valve replacement

                   (a) Operative mortality: 5.4%

                   (b) Fifteen-year survival: 57%

               (2) Triple valve replacement

                   (a) Complicated with severe heart failure

                   (b) Surgical correction generally the only option

                   (c) Operative mortality: 18% to 40%

               (3) Preoperative considerations

                   (a) Patients and families have extensive needs.

                       (i) Educational

                       (ii) Psychosocial

                       (iii) Physiological

                   (b) Generally present with complex medical history and treatment regimens

               (4) Intraoperative and postoperative considerations

                   (a) Effective postoperative care and outcome require a thorough understanding of all the valvular pathologies and complications.

                   (b) Hemodynamic measurements may be confounded by multivalvular disease.

XIII. MISCELLANEOUS ACQUIRED LESIONS

    A. Unrelated to rheumatic or atherosclerotic disease

    B. Primary myocardial diseases

        1. Cardiomyopathy

           a. Heart muscle diseases that primarily affect the structural and/or functional capacity of the myocardium

           b. Primary (no known cause—idiopathic)

           c. Secondary: common causes

               (1) Ischemia

               (2) Viral infections

               (3) Alcohol

               (4) Pregnancy

           d. Functional classifications (Box 32-2)

               (1) Dilated

                   (a) Characterized by systolic dysfunction

                   (b) Cardiomegaly with ventricular dilatation

                   (c) Impairment of systolic function

■ BOX 32-2

■ **FUNCTIONAL CLASSIFICATIONS OF CARDIOMYOPATHY**

Dilated	**Hypertrophic**	**Restrictive**
▪ Systolic dysfunction	▪ Diastolic dysfunction	▪ Diastolic dysfunction
▪ Cardiomegaly	▪ Ventricular hypertrophy	▪ Cardiac muscle stiffness
▪ Atrial enlargement	▪ Rapid LV contraction	▪ ↓ Cardiac output
▪ LV stasis	▪ Impaired relaxation	
	▪ Intracavity systolic pressure gradients	

LV, Left ventricular.

           (d) Atrial enlargement
           (e) Stasis of blood in LV
       (2) Hypertrophic
           (a) Characterized by diastolic dysfunction
           (b) Ventricular hypertrophy (with normal or small ventricles and
               dilated atria)
           (c) Rapid contraction of LV, impaired relaxation
           (d) Intracavity systolic pressure gradients
       (3) Restrictive (least common)
           (a) Diastolic dysfunction
           (b) Principal characteristic is cardiac muscle stiffness caused by
               infiltrative changes in heart muscle.
           (c) Diminished CO
   e. Signs and symptoms
       (1) Dilated
           (a) CHF
           (b) Fatigue
           (c) Weakness
           (d) Pulmonary and systemic emboli
       (2) Hypertrophic
           (a) Dyspnea (most common)
           (b) Angina
           (c) Fatigue
           (d) Syncope
       (3) Restrictive: similar to dilated
           (a) Exercise intolerance the most common
   f. Diagnostic studies: echocardiogram the most useful tool for diagnosis
   g. Effects on hemodynamics (Table 32-6)
   h. Treatment
       (1) Noninvasive
           (a) Goals
               (i) Reduce workload of the heart.
               (ii) Improve symptoms of CHF.
           (b) May use beta-blocking agents and calcium-blocking agents for
               hypertrophic presentation
           (c) Restrictive presentations may require pacemaker insertion for
               treatment of AV blocks.
       (2) Surgical intervention
           (a) Dilated: cardiac transplantation or implantable LV assist devices
               (LVADs; i.e., Novacor and Heartmate)
           (b) Hypertrophic: septal myotomy-myectomy (excision of a part of the
               hypertrophied septum)
           (c) Restrictive
               (i) Excision of the thickened endomyocardial plaque
               (ii) Mitral or tricuspid valve replacement

■ TABLE 32-6
■ ■ **Cardiomyopathy Effects on Hemodynamics**

	Contractility	LV Filling Pressure
Dilated	↓↓↓	↑↑
Hypertrophic	↑↑→↓	Normal
Restrictive	Normal →↓	↑

LV, Left ventricular.
From Kinney MR, Packa DR, Andreoli KG, et al, eds: *Comprehensive cardiac care,* ed 7, St Louis, 1991, Mosby.

      i. Preoperative considerations
        (1) Cardiac transplantation
        (2) All patients present with advanced signs and symptoms of failure.
        (3) Will have to deal with implications of end-stage cardiac disease
        (4) Imperative that patients and families understand risks, alternative and benefits, and the level of ongoing care required postoperatively (must assess willingness to comply with treatment regimen postoperatively)
      j. Intraoperative and postoperative considerations
        (1) Dependent on procedure performed, but will have all the implications of any cardiac surgery performed on an extremely debilitated patient in end-stage cardiac failure
        (2) Likely to require complex and comprehensive hemodynamic monitoring and titration of vasoactive medications
        (3) Likely to require mechanical support postoperatively if not transplanted (i.e., IABP or LVAD)
2. Pericardial disease (pericarditis)
    a. Clinical syndrome caused by inflammation of pericardial membrane
    b. Principal cause is viral infection; can also be caused by:
      (1) Postpericardiectomy syndrome
      (2) Trauma
      (3) Tumor
    c. Signs and symptoms
      (1) Pleuritic, substernal chest pain
      (2) Dyspnea
      (3) Pericardial friction rub
    d. Diagnostic studies
      (1) Transthoracic echocardiography is the most sensitive and accurate tool for detection and quantification of pericardial fluid.
      (2) ECG: acute pericarditis—ST elevation is concave upward and usually present in all leads except V1 and aVR (diagnostic).
    e. Effects on hemodynamics
      (1) Build-up of pericardial fluid or blood leads to constriction around the heart and results in tamponade.
        (a) Hypotension
        (b) Plateauing of all heart pressures
        (c) Decreased CO
    f. Treatment
      (1) Noninvasive: anti-inflammatory agents
      (2) Invasive intervention
        (a) Pericardiocentesis: subxiphoid needle aspiration of pericardial fluid (may leave a catheter with stopcock in place)
        (b) Subxiphoid limited pericardiotomy
        (c) Pericardiectomy or pericardial window: surgical resection of all or part of the pericardium
    g. Preoperative considerations
      (1) Dependent on cause
    h. Intraoperative and postoperative considerations
      (1) Pericardiectomy will require median sternotomy or thoracotomy.
        (a) Will have mediastinal tubes and/or pleural drainage tubes
      (2) Pericardial window will require a small subxiphoid incision with mediastinal drain to vacuum initially, then gravity.
      (3) Pericardiotomy may have catheter left in for aspiration of fluid and infusion of antibiotics.
      (4) Tamponade remains the most worrisome complication.
3. Traumatic heart disease
    a. Types
      (1) Blunt
      (2) Penetrating

b. Potential injuries
    (1) Lacerations to the heart muscle
    (2) Myocardial contusions
    (3) Aortic dissection
c. Potential complications
    (1) Dysrhythmias
    (2) Hemorrhagic shock
    (3) Cardiogenic shock
    (4) Tamponade
d. Presentation and effects on hemodynamics depend on extent of injuries acquired.
e. Diagnostic studies: same as other pathologies but also includes:
    (1) Computed tomography
    (2) MRI
    (3) Emergent presentations may be self-obvious and be taken immediately to the OR.
f. Surgical intervention: repair of injury, depends of type of injury
g. Intraoperative and postoperative considerations
    (1) Dependent on type of surgical repair
    (2) Some injuries (ruptured aortic dissection) may require massive blood products and fluid resuscitation.
    (3) May require CPB
    (4) Likely to have multiple injuries (initial surgical intervention will only address life-threatening injuries)

4. Cardiac tumors
  a. Primary or metastatic
  b. Complications
    (1) Pericardial effusion
    (2) Restrictive disease
    (3) Obstruction to blood flow
    (4) Impaired contractility
  c. Surgical intervention
    (1) Depends on location of tumor and hemodynamic effects
  d. Preoperative considerations
    (1) Whether treatment is palliative or curative
    (2) May be dealing with psychosocial implications of cancer
  e. Intraoperative and postoperative considerations
    (1) Depends on surgical intervention
    (2) May have experienced radiation and/or chemotherapy preoperatively (may be immunocompromised and have depressed cardiac function related to cardiotoxic effects of chemotherapy agents)

5. Aneurysms
  a. Defined as lumen enlargement, which results in weakening of the aortic wall
  b. Sometimes confused with dissection
    (1) Creation of a channel between inner and outer portions of the wall of the aorta by the surging column of blood
    (2) Dissection can occur in a previously aneurysmal segment.
    (3) Dissection can lead to aneurysm formation if the false lumen continues to expand.
  c. Location
    (1) Thoracic (ascending, arch, or descending)
      (a) Ascending may involve the aortic valve.
    (2) Abdominal (suprarenal or infrarenal)
    (3) Thoracoabdominal (aneurysm that extends above and below the diaphragm)
  d. Causes—most common are:
    (1) Atherosclerosis

(2) Trauma

(3) Common with Marfan's syndrome

e. Signs and symptoms

(1) Asymptomatic unless dissecting

(2) Tearing abdominal pain

(3) Profound hypotension

f. Diagnostic studies

(1) CXR

(2) Transesophageal echocardiography

(3) MRI

g. Treatment

(1) Noninvasive: aimed at aggressive BP control with beta-blocking agents

(2) Aortic endoscopic grafting

(3) Surgical intervention (aneurysmectomy with graft replacement)

    (a) Indications (Table 32-7)

    (b) Risk of rupture

        (i) 10%: <4.0 cm

        (ii) 45%: 7.0 to 10.0 cm

        (iii) 60%: >10.0 cm

h. Preoperative considerations

(1) Need a comprehensive assessment

    (a) Cardiac

    (b) Pulmonary

    (c) Renal

i. Intraoperative and postoperative considerations

(1) Generally have insertion of arterial and/or central line; may have PA line

(2) Will require vigorous BP control

    (a) Hypertension can cause graft dehiscence.

    (b) Hypotension may cause organ failure (renal).

(3) Typically, require large amounts of fluid resuscitation postoperatively to maintain preload

(4) Aortic cross-clamp

    (a) Aortic cross-clamp time may result in:

        (i) Renal failure

        (ii) Paralysis

        (iii) Neurological injury

    (b) May insert an intrathecal catheter with thoracic aneurysm repair and use to monitor and maintain intrathecal pressures ≤15 mm Hg by drainage of cerebrospinal fluid

---

■ TABLE 32-7

■ ■ **Aortic Aneurysms: Criteria for Surgical Intervention**

Ascending Thoracic	Descending Thoracic	Thoraco-Abdominal	Abdominal
Pain	Pain	As for descending thoracic or abdominal aorta	Pain, tenderness
Severe aortic regurgitation	Compression of adjacent structures		Athero-emboli
Size ≥6 cm	Size ≥6 cm		Size ≥5 cm
Marfan's ≥5 cm	Growth ≥1 cm/yr		Growth ≥1 cm/yr
Growth ≥1 cm/yr			

From Braunwald E, ed: *Atlas of heart diseases,* Philadelphia, 1996, Current Medicine.

(c) May use spinal cord cooling

(d) May use left-sided heart bypass

(e) May use organ perfusion strategies (cold lactate to renals)

XIV. CLASSIFICATIONS OF CARDIOVASCULAR DISEASE
  A. New York Heart Association guidelines (see Table 32-4)
  B. American Society of Anesthesiologists' Physical Status Classification
    1. Descriptive analysis of patient status
    2. Often used to classify patient's status relative to risks of operative intervention (P1 → P6)
    3. Classes
       a. Class P1
          (1) Patient has no organic, physiological, biochemical, or psychiatric disturbances.
          (2) Pathological process for which operation is to be performed is localized and does not entail systemic disturbance.
       b. Class P2
          (1) Mild to moderate systemic disturbance
          (2) Caused by either condition to be treated surgically or other pathophysiological process
       c. Class P3
          (1) Severe systemic disturbance or disease from whatever cause
          (2) May not be possible to define degree of disability with finality
       d. Class P4
          (1) Severe systemic disorders that are already life-threatening
          (2) Not always correctable by operation
       e. Class P5
          (1) Moribund patient who has little chance of survival
          (2) Has submitted to operation in desperation
       f. Class P6
          (1) Declared brain death patient whose organs are being removed for donor purposes
       g. Emergency operation (E)
          (1) Any patient in one of the classes listed previously
          (2) Operated on as an emergency
          (3) Considered to be in less-than-optimal physical condition
          (4) The *E* placed after the numeric classification

XV. PACU ADMISSION (PHASE I)
  A. Major goals of patient care
    1. Maintain adequate cardiac function by minimizing oxygen demand of the myocardium and maximizing oxygen delivery to all body tissues.
  B. What you want to know from OR
    1. Type of surgical procedure
    2. Type of anesthesia and combinations of agents and reversal agents used
    3. Hemodynamic data and problems
    4. CPB (or cross-clamp) time
    5. Recent laboratory data
       a. Hb
       b. Hematocrit
       c. Potassium
       d. Activated clotting time (ACT)
    6. EBL and fluids and blood products given
       a. Empty or mark all drainage devices, and ensure patency of tubes.
    7. Reversal of anticoagulation
    8. Pertinent medical history, especially pulmonary and cardiovascular
  C. Respiratory support
    1. Mechanical ventilator settings or high-flow humidified O_2 as ordered
    2. Monitor continuous Spo_2 and regular ABGs: acidosis increases myocardial oxygen demand and reduces contractility.

D. Cardiac support
  1. Assess for and select best lead to detect dysrhythmias.
    a. V_1 for VT/supraventricular tachycardia
    b. Multilead ST analysis for ischemia
  2. Monitor measured and derived hemodynamic parameters: ensure accuracy by leveling and zeroing transducer and record baseline data.
  3. Assess for abnormal heart sounds.
  4. Obtain baseline rhythm strips of all waveforms.
  5. Be prepared to support HR with pacing.
    a. Type: transcutaneous, transvenous epicardial
    b. Mode: ventricular, atrial, AV sequential
    c. Sensitivity
      (1) Demand: senses intrinsic cardiac rhythm
      (2) Asynchronous: does not sense intrinsic cardiac rhythm
XVI. IMMEDIATE PATIENT MANAGEMENT
  A. Dysrhythmias
    1. Identify and treat cause if possible.
      a. Be alert for electrolyte imbalance related to:
        (1) Diuresis
        (2) CPB
        (3) Acidosis
        (4) Irritable myocardium
      b. Treat per ACLS protocol.
      c. Be prepared to use pacing.
  B. Bleeding
    1. Be concerned for:
      a. 100 to 200 mL/hr for the first 3 to 4 hours
      b. 1500 mL/4 hrs
    2. Causes of postoperative bleeding
      a. Clotting abnormalities: preexisting or after CPB
      b. Hypothermia
      c. Excessive hypertension
      d. Disrupted suture lines
      e. Protamine rebound
      f. Preoperative antiplatelet therapy (ASA, clopidogrel)
    3. Nursing interventions
      a. Stat laboratory tests as indicated (i.e., Hb and hematocrit, PTT, PT or ACT, and platelet count)
        (1) Be concerned for:
          (a) PTT >40 seconds, ACT >120 seconds
          (b) Platelets <50,000/μL
          (c) Hb <8 g/dL
          (d) Hematocrit may be hemodiluted.
            (i) Ideally, hematocrit should be 28% to 30%.
        (2) Replace blood products as ordered.
      b. Rewarm to 96.8° F (36° C).
        (1) Convection
        (2) Warmed blankets
        (3) Atmosphere
      c. Treat hypotension.
        (1) Mean arterial pressure (MAP) <70 mm Hg
        (2) Rewarming will also cause vasodilation, which decreases MAP.
      d. Consider adding positive end-expiratory pressure (PEEP) up to 10 cm H_2O if hemodynamically stable.
      e. If fibrinolysis suspected, administer:
        (1) Protamine (heparin reversal agent)
        (2) Aminocaproic acid (Amicar)

   4. Tamponade
      a. Fluid accumulation within the pericardial space, which causes:
         (1) Elevation and equilibration of intracardiac filling pressures
         (2) Progressive limitation of ventricular diastolic filling
         (3) Reduction of SV and CO
      b. Monitor for:
         (1) Beck's triad (classic findings)
            (a) Increased central venous pressure
            (b) Muffled heart tones
            (c) Pulsus paradoxus
         (2) Associated signs and symptoms may include:
            (a) Tachycardia
            (b) ↓ Voltage of QRS complex
            (c) Narrow pulse pressure
            (d) Equalizing pressures (RA, PAP, PAOP [PCWP])
            (e) Sudden cessation of drainage from mediastinal tubes
            (f) Decreased Svo_2 and CO
            (g) Jugular venous distention
         (3) Intervention
            (a) Cardiac tamponade in the cardiac surgery patient can be a true surgical emergency.
               (i) Be prepared for possibility of open sternotomy at the bedside and/or emergent return to OR.
            (b) Strip mediastinal tubes.
            (c) Supportive fluid and blood product replacement
C. Low CO states
   1. Be concerned for cardiac index <2.2 L/min/m².
   2. Assess for cause and treat accordingly.
      a. Assess and treat HR and rhythm disturbances.
      b. Assess and treat preload.
         (1) Most common cause and should be assessed for and treated first
         (2) Be concerned for RA pressures <6 mm Hg and PAOP (PCWP) <10 mm Hg.
         (3) Lactated Ringer's or normal saline usually the crystalloids of choice
         (4) Hespan (hetastarch) is a frequent synthetic colloid used.
         (5) Blood products as indicated
         (6) Be sure to assess for tamponade.
      c. Afterload
         (1) Make sure patient normothermic
         (2) Strive to keep SVR at 900 to 1200 dynes/sec/cm⁵.
            (a) Keep low normal for dysfunctional myocardium.
         (3) Nitroprusside is a common agent used.
      d. Contractility
         (1) LV stroke work index is an indirect indicator of contractility.
            (a) Normal value: 40 to 75 g/m²/beat
         (2) Medical interventions
            (a) Assess and treat electrolyte imbalance.
               (i)   Hypokalemia
               (ii) Hypomagnesemia
               (iii) Hypocalcemia
            (b) Assess and treat acidosis: respiratory and metabolic.
            (c) Assess and treat hypoxia.
            (d) May use:
               (i)   Dobutamine
               (ii) Milrinone
               (iii) Possibly sympathomimetic agents such as:
                  [a] Dopamine
                  [b] Epinephrine
                  [c] Norepinephrine

    3. IABP
      a. Temporary mechanical VAD
        (1) Augments systemic and coronary circulation
        (2) "Unloads" the heart through the diastolic inflation and systolic deflation of a catheter-mounted balloon placed in descending thoracic aorta
      b. Inserted through the femoral artery (most common) or surgical transthoracic implantation
      c. Two major functions
        (1) Increase coronary artery perfusion
        (2) Decrease afterload
      d. Most common complications
        (1) Ischemia to the extremity distal to insertion
        (2) Bleeding
        (3) Obstruction of blood flow to kidneys
      e. Patient management should include (Box 32-3):
        (1) Frequent assessment of insertion site and extremity perfusion
        (2) Hourly urine output
        (3) Continuous hemodynamic monitoring
    4. VAD
      a. Extracorporeal ventricular flow assist device that provides temporary circulatory support for single or biventricular failure
      b. May be a right or left VAD (RVAD or LVAD) or both (BIVAD)
      c. Requires surgical cannulation of the atrium or ventricle and either PA or aorta
      d. Blood is removed from the atrium or ventricle and directed to the appropriate artery.
      e. Primary goals
        (1) Myocardial tissue recovery
        (2) Bridge to transplant
        (3) Destination therapy

◼ BOX 32-3
◼ **CARE OF THE PATIENT ON AN INTRA-AORTIC BALLOON PUMP**

Rationale for Use
- ↑Coronary artery perfusion (balloon inflation)
- ↓ Afterload (balloon deflation)

Placement
- Catheter placed via the femoral artery with the tip of the catheter just distal to left subclavian artery

Timing
- Inflate: On or near the dicrotic notch of the arterial waveform
- Deflate: Slightly before systole (specific criteria to assess proper timing)

Triggering
Uses the ECG, arterial waveform, or pacemaker artifact as a reference point to the cardiac cycle

Troubleshooting
Improper timing
Early inflation
Late inflation
Early deflation
Late deflation

Inadequate augmentation
Patient or device related
Catheter malposition
Catheter leak/gas loss

   f. Most common types
      (1) Temporary
         (a) Pulsatile AB5000
         (b) Centrifugal Tandem Heart
         (c) Bio-Medicus Bio-Pump
      (2) Permanent
         (a) Pulsatile Heartmate XVE
         (b) Axial flow Jarvik flowmaker
         (c) Heartmate II
   g. Most common complications
      (1) Bleeding
      (2) Embolus
      (3) Infection
   h. Patient management requires advanced training related to the specific device.
D. Hypertension
   1. Goal: maintenance of an adequate perfusion pressure for cellular oxygenation
      a. MAP: 65 to 100 mm Hg
      b. SVR: 900 to 1200 dynes/sec/cm^5
   2. Excessive arterial pressures (increased afterload) increase the workload on the heart and put excessive pressure on suture lines.
   3. Assessment and treatment
      a. Ideal assessment is continuous arterial pressure line monitoring of MAP.
      b. Preload should always be assessed and treated first.
         (1) Use of vasodilators in a low preload situation will result in patient deterioration.
      c. Vasodilators
         (1) Nitroglycerin (preload)
         (2) Nitroprusside (afterload)
E. Impaired oxygenation and ventilation
   1. Goal: oxygen delivery sufficient to meet cellular oxygen demand needed to maintain aerobic metabolism
   2. Oxygen demand is specific to the individual and requires invasive and noninvasive monitoring.
      a. Respiratory rate
      b. Spo_2
      c. ABG analysis
      d. Urine output
      e. Skin color and temperature
      f. Pulses
   3. Treatment
      a. Airway maintenance
      b. Administration of appropriate fraction of inspired oxygen (Fio_2)
      c. Mechanical support of ventilation
F. Impaired renal functioning
   1. Kidneys are underperfused early in a low perfusion state.
   2. Intrarenal damage usually results from a prolonged MAP <70 mm Hg.
      a. Mild reversible injury: ≤25 minutes of ischemia
      b. Severe damage: 40 to 60 minutes of ischemia
      c. Irreversible damage: 60 to 90 minutes of ischemia
   3. Most sensitive indicator of renal perfusion is urine output.
      a. Be concerned for urine outputs <0.5 mL/kg per hour.
   4. Treatment depends on whether decreased urine output is a result of a prerenal or intrarenal cause.
      a. Prerenal cause: volume replacement and support of CO
      b. Intrarenal cause: loop diuretics
      c. Renal failure may progress to the point of the need for hemofiltration.

G. Impaired neurological functioning
    1. Most common causes
        a. Air embolism
        b. Preexisting cerebrovascular disease
        c. Hypoxemia and hypercapnea
    2. Preoperative neurological assessment is invaluable for postoperative assessment.
    3. Any change is significant and should be reported and investigated.
    4. Cornerstone of treatment is adequate oxygenation.

XVII. SPECIAL CONSIDERATIONS FOR CABG
    A. Indications: failure of medical management to control the pain and related sequelae of coronary heart disease
    B. Goal: relief of symptoms and improved quality of life
    C. Selection criteria
        1. Angina interfering with activity of daily living and/or evidence of severe ischemia
        2. Left main stenosis of at least 50% (least disputed)
        3. Proximal left anterior descending stenosis of at least 70% with other major and significant coronary artery stenosis
        4. Proximal three-vessel disease of at least 50%
        5. Multivessel stenosis of at least 50% with moderate to severe LV dysfunction
        6. Failed PTCA or stent
    D. Conventional CABG
        1. Median sternotomy approach
        2. Uses internal mammary artery, vein grafts (saphenous), or other artery grafts (i.e., radial or gastroepiploic arteries)
        3. CPB
            a. Purpose: to provide a dry, quiet operative field while achieving myocardial preservation
            b. Blood diverted from entering the heart by a single catheter placed in RA or by catheters placed in inferior and superior vena cava
            c. Blood directed back to the patient from the heart-lung machine through an arterial cannula placed in the ascending aorta
            d. Main structures
                (1) Pump
                (2) Oxygenator with reservoir
                (3) Plastic circuitry
            e. Myocardial protection (incidence of intraoperative MI, 2%-4%)
                (1) Hypothermia: core cooling ($28°C$ to $32°C$) induced by the heart-lung machine via a heat exchanger and topical cooling to the myocardium ($10°C$)
                (2) Cardioplegia
                    (a) A cold ($0°C$ to $4°C$) solution composed of a concentration of electrolytes, albumin, blood, and oxygenated crystalloid (some surgeons use warm cardioplegia, especially in patients with active ischemia)
                    (b) Infused into aortic root, coronary arteries, and myocardium, resulting in immediate electromechanical asystole
                (3) Global ischemic arrest with topical cooling
                    (a) Iced saline instilled into pericardial cavity
                    (b) Left side of the pericardium protected to avoid phrenic nerve injury
                (4) Coronary perfusion
                    (a) Antegrade: injection of cardioplegic solution into each new graft as the distal anastomosis is sutured
                    (b) Retrograde: injection of cardioplegic solution into coronary sinus and coronary veins
                (5) Hemodilution—decreases:
                    (a) Blood viscosity
                    (b) SVR

          (c) Hemolysis

          (d) Use of blood products

          (e) Promotes postoperative diuresis

       (6) Anticoagulation

          (a) Reduces sludging of blood in capillaries

          (b) Reduces blood cell trauma

          (c) Reduces incidence of thromboemboli

          (d) Accomplished using heparin, which is reversed by protamine at the termination of CPB

E. Minimally invasive CABG

   1. Defined as either a small incisional field or absence of CPB

      a. Minimally invasive CABG (Mini CAB)

        (1) Vein grafting visualized and performed through laparoscopes inserted through the chest wall or a left thoracotomy approach

        (2) Heart continues to beat but may be slowed with pharmacological agents (i.e., beta-blockers).

        (3) Technically difficult

        (4) Limited to anterior anastomosis

      b. Off-pump CABG (OPCAB) or beating heart bypass

        (1) Uses a median sternotomy but does not rely on CPB or cardiac arrest

        (2) A stabilizing "foot" used directly over the artery being sutured to stabilize the myocardium

        (3) Able to access more areas because of greater visibility

   2. Benefit: avoids complications associated with CPB, which may decrease recovery time and days of hospitalization

   3. Downside

      a. Heart may be irritable postoperatively from manipulation without hypothermia.

      b. Intraoperative preload and contractility may be difficult to maintain.

F. Preoperative consideration

   1. Thorough history and physical exam with emphasis on:

      a. Medications

      b. Respiratory status

      c. Neurological status

      d. GI status

      e. Renal status

      f. Include pulmonary function studies.

   2. Laboratory tests

      a. Complete blood count with differential

      b. Electrolytes

      c. Coagulation studies: PT, PTT, bleeding times

      d. Type and crossmatch

      e. ABGs (room air)

   3. Preoperative teaching is highly individualized and may be difficult as a result of an emergency presentation.

   4. Many cardiac medications may be continued up to the time of surgery.

      a. Warfarin must be discontinued several days before surgery.

      b. Aspirin should be withheld for 1 week.

   5. Patients generally given a bath or shower with a germicidal agent the evening before surgery

   6. Broad-spectrum prophylactic antibiotics

      a. Administered immediately within 1 hour of incision

      b. Continued for 24 hours postoperatively

G. Intraoperative and postoperative considerations

   1. Goal

      a. First hour: stabilization

        (1) Rewarm.

        (2) Stabilize vital signs.

      (3) Stabilize hemodynamics.

      (4) Provide adequate oxygenation.

  2. Anesthesia uses a combination of inhalation and short-acting IV agents in the lowest possible doses to enhance a rapid emergence from anesthesia.

    a. Patients may be extubated in OR (particularly minimally invasive).

    b. Pain must be anticipated and addressed quickly in recovery phase.

  3. Fast-track extubation (may vary with physician and facility)

    a. Goal: extubation within 4 to 6 hours of arrival to recovery area

      (1) Weaning criteria

        (a) Warm (36.8° C)

        (b) Able to lift head upon request

        (c) Spontaneous respirations

        (d) Negative inspiratory force of at least 20 cm H_2O/20 seconds

        (e) ABGs and related parameters adequate

        (f) Hemodynamically stable

      (2) Acceptable extubation parameters

        (a) Alert and follows commands

        (b) Respiratory rate <30 breaths/min

        (c) Tidal volume >50% of predicted (>5 mL/kg)

        (d) PEEP/continuous positive airway pressure (CPAP) <5 cm H_2O

        (e) Sao_2 >91%, Fio_2 <40%

        (f) Hemodynamically stable

      (3) Acceptable extubation gases

        (a) pH 7.33 to 7.46

        (b) Partial pressure of carbon dioxide in arterial blood ($Paco_2$) ≥33 to 49 mm Hg

        (c) Partial pressure of oxygen in arterial blood (Pao_2) ≥65 mm Hg

    b. Extubate to nasal cannula and stay with patient for 15 to 30 minutes to assess tolerance.

  4. Typical placement of IV and monitoring lines in the holding area or OR suite

    a. Two large-bore (14 gauge) peripheral IV accesses

    b. Central line

    c. Optional PA catheter with CO and Svo_2 monitoring

    d. Radial arterial line

    e. Foley urinary catheter (may have temperature probe)

  5. Median sternotomy incisions will have mediastinal tubes and possibly a pleural tube connected to approximately 25 cm H_2O suction.

    a. Assess drainage every 15 minutes until less than 200 mL an hour.

    b. Elevate head of bed 15 degrees to 25 degrees to promote drainage.

  6. Monitor closely for electrolyte imbalances from massive diuresis postoperatively (be concerned with diuresis of 300 mL or greater for 2 consecutive hours).

  7. Address comfort as soon as possible; typical agents and routes are IV fentanyl or morphine sulfate, and oral analgesics after extubation.

  8. If extubation extended, may be on DVT and stress ulcer prophylaxis.

XVIII. SPECIAL CONSIDERATIONS FOR TRANSPLANT

  A. Potential therapy for patients with end-stage disease refractory to medical and surgical therapy

  B. Recipient criteria (Box 32-4)

    1. Fifty percent of potential recipients are disabled from dilated cardiomyopathy, with the remainder from ischemic cardiomyopathy.

    2. United Network for Organ Sharing Status grouping for allocation of donor hearts (Box 32-5)

  C. Preoperative considerations

    1. Goal: provide the patient and family with factual, realistic information.

    a. Procedure, intensive care, recovery, change in diet, exercise, impact of immunosuppressive therapy, and risk of infection and rejection

    b. Emotional support vital

■ BOX 32-4
■ **RECIPIENT CRITERIA FOR HEART TRANSPLANTATION**

Acceptance Criteria
- Absence of reversible or surgically amenable heart disease
- New York Heart Association Class III-IV symptoms despite optimal medical management
- Maximal O_2 consumption <14 mL/kg/min
- Estimated 1 year survival without transplant <50%
- Age <65 years
- Stable family support system
- Ability to adhere to complex medical regimen
- Normal renal and hepatic function

Exclusion Criteria
- Pulmonary hypertension
- Pulmonary artery systolic pressure α >70 mm Hg, despite nitroprusside
- Age >65
- Acute, unresolved malignancy
- Recent pulmonary infarction
- Active infection
- Active peptic ulcer disease
- Type I diabetes mellitus with significant end-organ damage
- Symptoms of cerebrovascular accident
- Irreversible end-organ failure
- Active substance abuse
- Psychological instability
- Morbid obesity

Data from McKellar SH: *Cardiomyopathy/cardiac transplant donor and recipient selection.* Available at: www.ctsnet.org/doc/4499. Accessed July 10, 2009.

2. Operative procedure
   a. Donor heart excised, preserving the SA node, and passed through a series of cooled saline baths (if transported, it is placed in iced saline solution [4° C])
   b. Ischemic time <4 hours
   c. Orthotopic (95%): recipient's heart removed, and donor heart implanted in its place in normal anatomical position in the chest
   d. Uses CPB and a median sternotomy
   e. Transplanted heart rewarmed, and epicardial pacing wires, chest tubes, and invasive lines placed

■ BOX 32-5
■ **UNITED NETWORK FOR ORGAN SHARING (UNOS) STATUS GROUPING FOR ALLOCATION OF DONOR HEARTS**

Status	Severity of Illness
1A	Candidate admitted to listing transplant center hospital with at least one of the following devices or therapies ■ VAD implanted for ≤30 days, TAH, IABC, or ECMO* ■ Mechanical ventilation* Continuous infusion of intravenous inotrope and continuous hemodynamic monitoring of left ventricular filling pressure[†]
1B	Candidate with at least one of the following devices or therapies ■ VAD implanted for >30 days ■ Continuous infusion of intravenous inotropes
2	Candidate does not meet criteria for status 1A or 1B listing.
7	Candidate is considered temporarily unsuitable to receive a thoracic organ transplant.

*Must be recertified every 14 days.
[†]Valid for 7 days.
From UNOS, 2002 Amended UNOS Policy 3.7 (Allocation of Thoracic Organs). Effective November 15, 2002, Richmond, VA.
ECMO, Extracorporeal membrane oxygenator; *IABC,* intra-aortic balloon counterpulsation; *TAH,* total artificial heart; *VAD,* ventricular assist device.

   3. Postoperative considerations
   a. Early function affected by length of ischemic insult
   b. Neural control
      (1) There is no direct neural control of the conduction system.
      (2) Adrenal hormones exert primary stimulation of the heart by exciting adrenergic receptors of donor myocardium with circulating catecholamines.
      (3) Denervated donor heart may be less sensitive to drugs such as atropine and digoxin.
   c. Immediate postoperative care similar to any open-heart surgery
   d. Frequent use of inotropic and vasodilating drugs (i.e., dobutamine and isoproteronol)
      (1) Common use is 3 to 5 days.
      (2) Transplanted heart has a relatively fixed SV; therefore, CO very dependent on rate.
      (3) Calcium channel blockers and beta-blockers should be used with caution because of negative inotropic activity.
   e. Rhythm disturbances: uncommon in initial postoperative period unless there has been significant ischemia
      (1) May have bradycardia 2 to 3 days postoperatively if the recipient received amiodarone preoperatively (accumulates rapidly in transplanted myocardium and peaks during second postoperative week)
      (2) Adenosine for tachydysrhythmias should be used at one-quarter to one-half normal dose because of increased sinus node sensitivity.
   f. Immunosuppression: immune response can occur by either humoral or cell-mediated mechanisms.
      (1) Patient may be isolated.
      (2) Infection is leading cause of death in first 3 months.
   g. Increased risk of tamponade
      (1) Preoperative warfarin for severe LV dysfunction
      (2) Previous cardiac operations
      (3) Diminished coagulation factors from chronic liver congestion
      (4) Donor heart may not fill the enlarged pericardial space.
   h. Intensive care unit 2 to 3 days and discharged in 7 to 10 days
   i. Require vigilant follow-up
   j. Morbidity: three major types
      (1) Rejection (acute and chronic)
      (2) Infection
      (3) Coronary artery vasculopathy
   k. Classic signs of rejection
      (1) Development of S3 and/or S4
      (2) Weakness, fatigue, malaise
      (3) Hypotension
      (4) Elevated atrial pressures
      (5) Decreased urine output
      (6) Weight gain
      (7) Dysrhythmias
   l. Mortality
      (1) Early operative (<30 days): 5% to 10%
      (2) One-year survival rate: 79%
XIX. PSYCHOSOCIAL FACTORS
   A. Goal of nursing care: provision of holistic nursing care
   B. Psychosocial concepts to consider when planning and implementing care for the cardiac surgery patient
   1. Body image and self-concept perception
   2. Self-esteem
   3. Stress

    4. Fear and anxiety

    5. Pain

    6. Sensory deprivation or overload

    7. Cost

    8. Death

  C. Structured preoperative family and patient teaching enhances understanding.

    1. Surgical procedure information specific to the patient

    2. Tour of postoperative unit and visiting hours

    3. Sequence of events of operative day: premedication, time of procedure, surgical waiting area for family

    4. Identification of equipment to be used postoperatively

    5. Procedure for coughing and deep breathing, stressing rationale for importance

    6. Review of expected postoperative course

    7. Adequate time for discussion to allow patient and family to ask questions and verbalize concerns

  D. Postoperative support of psychosocial factors

    1. Allow family to see patient as soon as appropriate in the recovery phase.

    2. Reinforce preoperative teaching.

    3. Use systems that allow for the family to get rest and nutrition: pagers, sleep rooms, for example.

    4. Use ancillary support services (e.g., social services, pastoral care, family liaisons)

    5. Use a child life specialist if a child needs to be allowed into the critical care area to visit a family member.

BIBLIOGRAPHY

1. ACC/AHA/HRS 2008 guidelines for device based therapy of cardiac rhythm abnormalities: Executive summary. *Circulation* 117:2820–2840, 2008.
2. Aehlert B: *ECG's made easy*, St Louis, 2005, Mosby.
3. Ahrens TS, Kleinpell R, Prentice D, eds: *Critical care nursing certification: Preparation, review, and practice exams*, ed 5, New York, 2006, McGraw-Hill.
4. Burden N, ed: *Ambulatory surgical nursing*, ed 2, Philadelphia, 2000, WB Saunders.
5. Chung MK: Cardiac surgery: Postoperative arrhythmias. *Crit Care Med* 28(Suppl 10): N136–N144, 2000.
6. ECC Committee, Subcommittees and Task Forces of the American Heart Association: 2005 American Heart Association guidelines for cardiopulmonary resuscitation and emergency cardiovascular care. *Circulation* 112(24 Suppl):IV1–IV203, 2005.
7. Finberg L, ed: *Saunders manual of pediatric practice*, ed 2, Philadelphia, 2002, Saunders.
8. Finkelmeier BA, ed: *Cardiothoracic surgical nursing*, ed 2, Philadelphia, 2000, Lippincott.
9. Gahart BL, Nozareno AR: *2010 Intravenous medications: A handbook for nurses and health professionals*, ed 26, St Louis, 2010, Mosby.
10. Hudak CM, Gallo BM, Morton PG, eds: *Critical care nursing: A holistic approach*, ed 9, Philadelphia, 2008, Lippincott.
11. Huszar RJ: *Pocket guide to basic dysrhythmias*, ed 3, St Louis, 2007, Mosby.
12. Karnath BM: Preoperative cardiac risk assessment. *Am Fam Physician* 66 (10): 1889–1896, 2002.
13. Lee J, Lee PC: *Cardiology at a glance*, New York, 2002, McGraw-Hill.
14. McCance KL, Huether SE: *Pathophysiology: The biologic basis for disease in adults and children*, ed 6, St Louis, 2010, Mosby.
15. Quinn DM, Schick L, eds: *Ambulatory surgical nursing core curriculum*, Philadelphia, 2004, WB Saunders.
16. Rollant PD, Ennis DA, eds: *Medical-surgical nursing*, St Louis, 2001, Mosby.
17. Seifert PC: *Cardiac surgery: Perioperative patient care*, St Louis, 2002, Mosby.
18. Thompson JM, McFarland GK, Hirsh JE, et al, eds: *Mosby's clinical nursing*, ed 5, St Louis, 2002, Mosby.

OBJECTIVES

At the conclusion of this chapter, the reader will be able to:

1. Describe the anatomy and physiology of the central nervous system (CNS).

2. Describe the anatomy and physiology of the spinal cord.

3. Identify various neurodiagnostic tools and testing procedures.

4. Discuss the assessment and perianesthesia nursing care for the neurological patient.

5. Explain the medical and nursing management of the patient with increased intracranial pressure (ICP).

6. Describe the pathophysiology, diagnosis, and treatment of the most common neurological disorders.

7. Describe appropriate neurological assessment and patient monitoring for potential complications.

I. ANATOMY AND PHYSIOLOGY OF THE CNS
  A. Cellular structure (Figure 33-1)
  1. Neuron: basic structural unit
    a. Nerve cell: receives and conducts impulses
    b. Functions
      (1) Afferent, or sensory, neurons conduct impulses from receptors to CNS.
      (2) Efferent, or motor, neurons conduct impulses from CNS to effector organs.
    c. Structure
      (1) Cell body contains:
        (a) Nucleus
        (b) Cytoplasm
        (c) Cell membrane
      (2) Nerve cell processes
        (a) Dendrites: short processes with multiple projections
          (i) Conduct impulses toward the cell body
          (ii) Receive information
        (b) Axon: longest process of cell body
          (i) Conducts impulses away from the cell body
          (ii) Sends information
          (iii) Myelinated (insulated)
          (iv) Unmyelinated
    d. Functions (Figure 33-2)
      (1) Sensory (afferent—sensory pathway toward the CNS from the peripheral receptor organs)
        (a) Special senses
          (i) Smell
          (ii) Taste
          (iii) Vision
          (iv) Auditory
        (b) Pain and temperature
        (c) Proprioception (position sense and vibration)

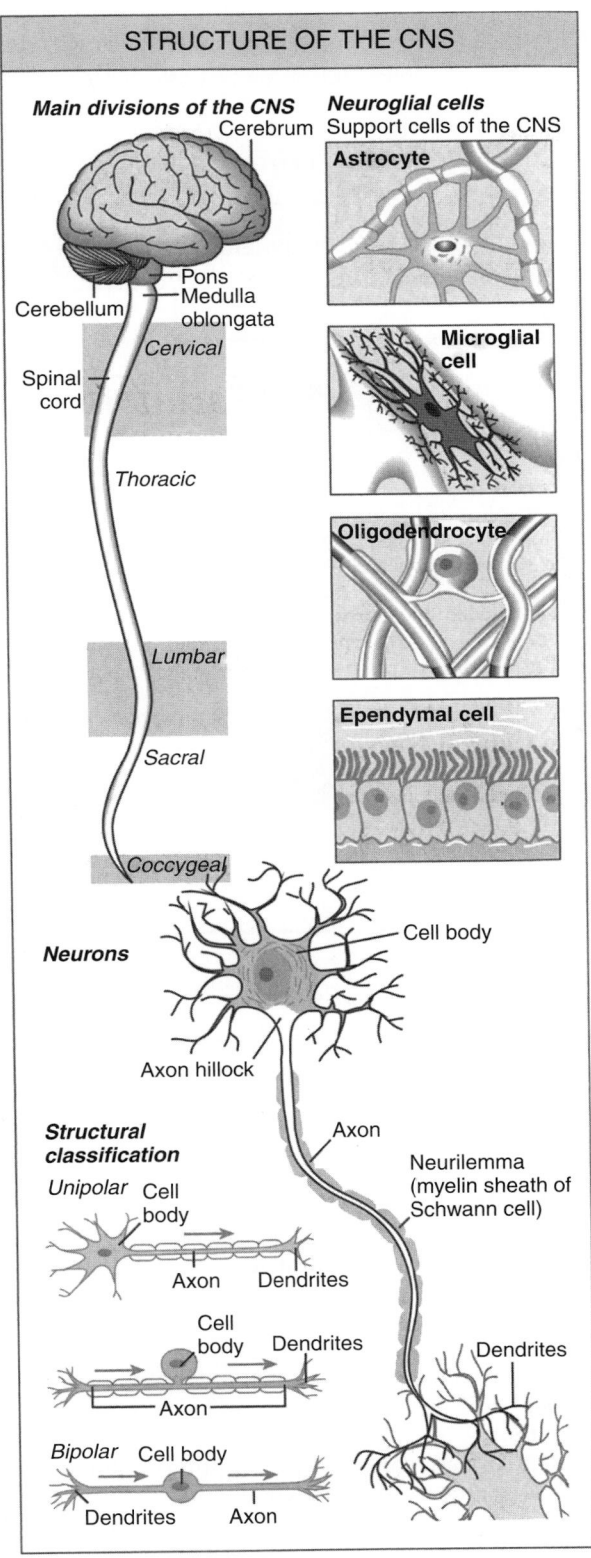

FIGURE 33-1 ■ Structure of the CNS. (From Luckmann J: *Saunders manual of nursing care*, Philadelphia, 1997, WB Saunders.)

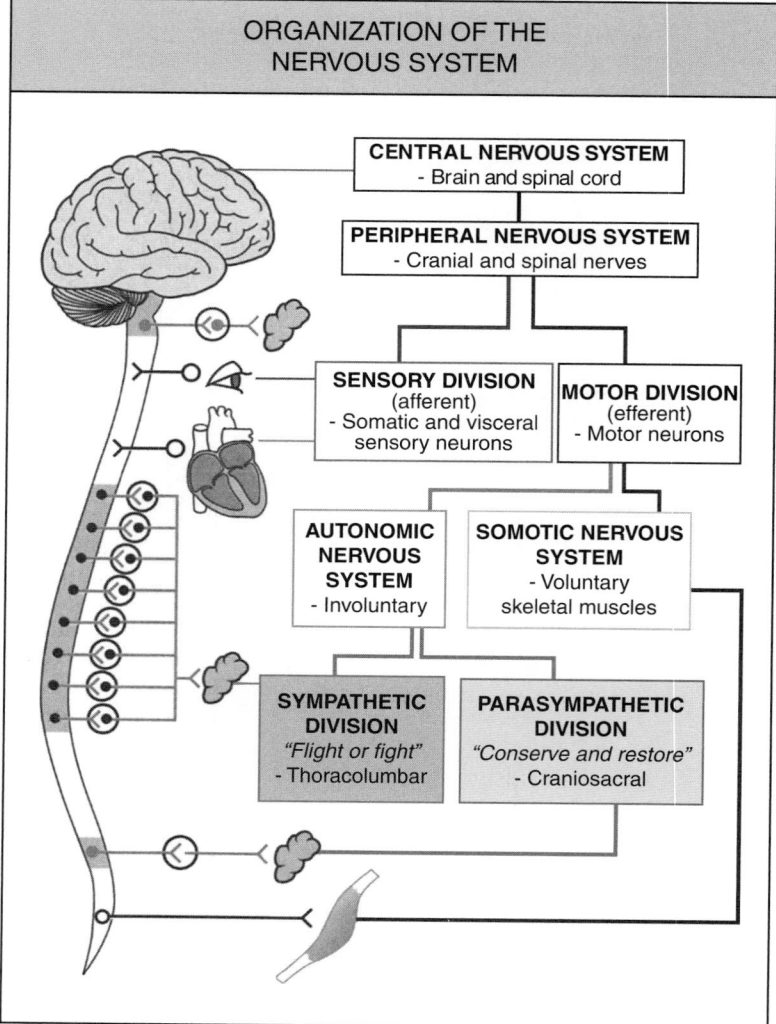

FIGURE 33-2 ■ Organization of the nervous system. (From Luckmann J: *Saunders manual of nursing care,* Philadelphia, 1997, WB Saunders.)

(d) Vibration
(e) Touch (light and deep)
(2) Motor (efferent—motor pathway from the CNS toward the peripheral end organs
(3) Special (interneurons)
e. Transmission
(1) Electrical impulse
(a) Depolarization: potassium ion (K^+) influx, sodium ion (Na^+) outflow
(b) Repolarization: K^+ pump, Na^+ pump restore membrane potential
(c) Axonal versus saltatory conduction
(i) Axonal: entire axon must be depolarized, such as in unmyelinated fibers, making conduction slow.
(ii) Saltatory: sections of a myelinated axon are depolarized, impulse jumping from the node of Ranvier, leading to more rapid impulse conduction.

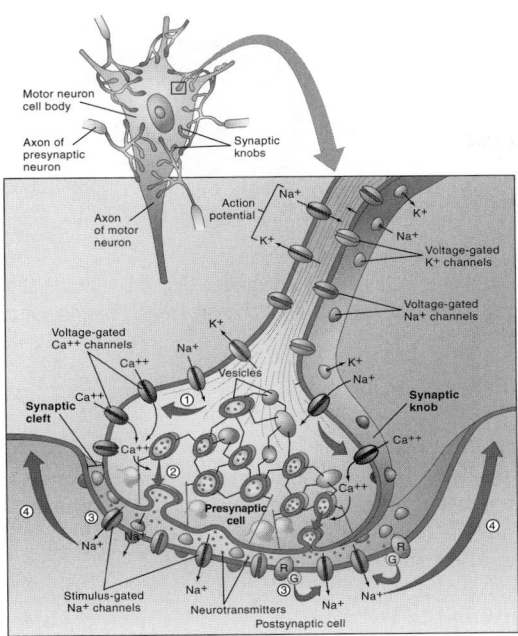

FIGURE 33-3 ■ Structure of a synapse. (From Thibodeau GA, Patton KT: *Anatomy & Physiology*, ed 5, St Louis, 2003, Mosby.)

      (2) Chemical transmission (Figure 33-3)
          (a) Synapse: vesicles release neurotransmitter from the presynaptic membrane into the synaptic cleft, which attaches to receptor sites on the postsynaptic membrane of the target organ (i.e., another neuron, muscle, other organs), resulting in the appropriate response (i.e., muscle contraction or relaxation) or communication points between two neurons.
          (b) Neurotransmitters: protein substances that stimulate, facilitate, or inhibit impulse transmission across synapses
              (i)   Adrenergic
                    [a] Dopamine
                    [b] Norepinephrine
                    [c] Epinephrine
              (ii)   Cholinergic: acetylcholine
              (iii) Serotonin
              (iv) Gamma-aminobutyric acid (GABA)
              (v)   Alpha-endorphins
              (vi) Beta-endorphins
              (vii) Histamine
              (viii) Substance P
  2. Gray matter: cortex of brain; contains cell bodies and dendrites of CNS (Figure 33-4)
  3. White matter: contains myelinated axons and neuroglia; supporting tissue (see Figure 33-4)
  4. Neuroglia: support cells of CNS
      a. Nonexcitable
      b. More numerous than neurons
          (1) Astrocytes
              (a) Small cell bodies with numerous projections
              (b) Projections end on blood vessels, ependyma, and pia mater.
              (c) Form the blood-brain barrier and provide structure

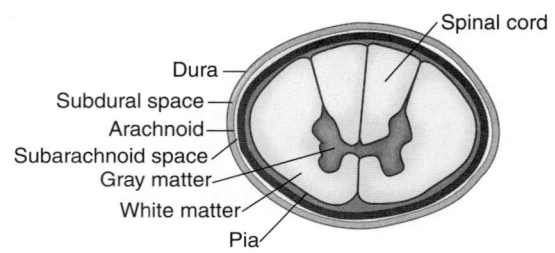

FIGURE 33-4 ■ Illustrations of the gray and white matter. Circulation of the cerebrospinal fluid (CSF) in the brain and spinal cord. (From Drain CB, Odom-Forren J: *Perianesthesia nursing: A critical care approach,* ed 5, St Louis, 2009, WB Saunders.)

       (2) Oligodendrocytes
          (a) Smaller and more delicate than astrocytes
          (b) Responsible for formation of myelin covering of axons
       (3) Microglia
          (a) Smallest neurological cells
          (b) Scavenger cells
       (4) Ependymal cells
          (a) Line cerebrospinal fluid (CSF) pathways (brain and spinal cord)
          (b) Single layer of cuboid cells with villi
          (c) Facilitate movement of CSF
   B. Composition of the CNS
     1. Brain (Figure 33-5)
       a. Primary center for control
       b. Primary regulator for nervous system functions
       c. Three major structures
          (1) Forebrain (prosencephalon) contains:
            (a) Telencephalon (cerebrum) with its hemispheres
            (b) Diencephalon
          (2) Midbrain (mesencephalon) contains:
            (a) Cerebral peduncles
            (b) Corpora quadrigemina
            (c) Cerebral aqueduct (aqueduct of Sylvius)
          (3) Hindbrain (rhombencephalon) contains:
            (a) Medulla oblongata
            (b) Pons
            (c) Cerebellum
            (d) Fourth ventricle
     2. Spinal cord
   C. Extracerebral structures
     1. Scalp: protects integrity of skull
     2. Skull (Figure 33-6)
       a. Protects brain from external forces
       b. Composition
          (1) Frontal bone (1)
          (2) Parietal bones (2)
          (3) Temporal bones (2)
          (4) Occipital bone (1)
          (5) Ethmoid bone (1)
          (6) Sphenoid bone (1)
       c. Compartments: fossas (Figure 33-7)
          (1) Anterior fossa—contains:
            (a) Frontal lobes
            (b) Olfactory nerves

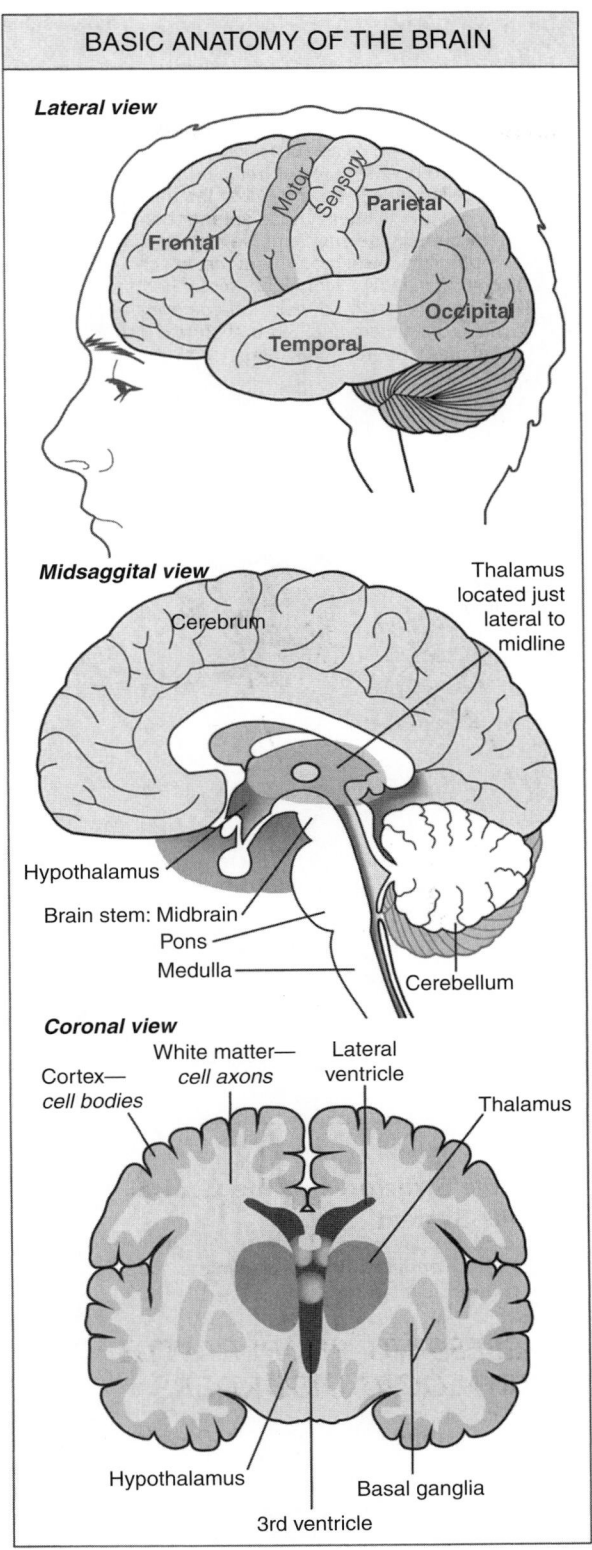

BASIC ANATOMY OF THE BRAIN

Lateral view

Motor
Sensory
Parietal
Frontal
Occipital
Temporal

Midsaggital view

Thalamus located just lateral to midline

Cerebrum

Hypothalamus

Brain stem: Midbrain
Pons
Medulla

Cerebellum

Coronal view

White matter—
cell axons

Cortex—
cell bodies

Lateral ventricle

Thalamus

Hypothalamus

Basal ganglia

3rd ventricle

FIGURE 33-5 ■ Basic anatomy of the brain. (From Luckmann J: *Saunders manual of nursing care*, Philadelphia, 1997, WB Saunders.)

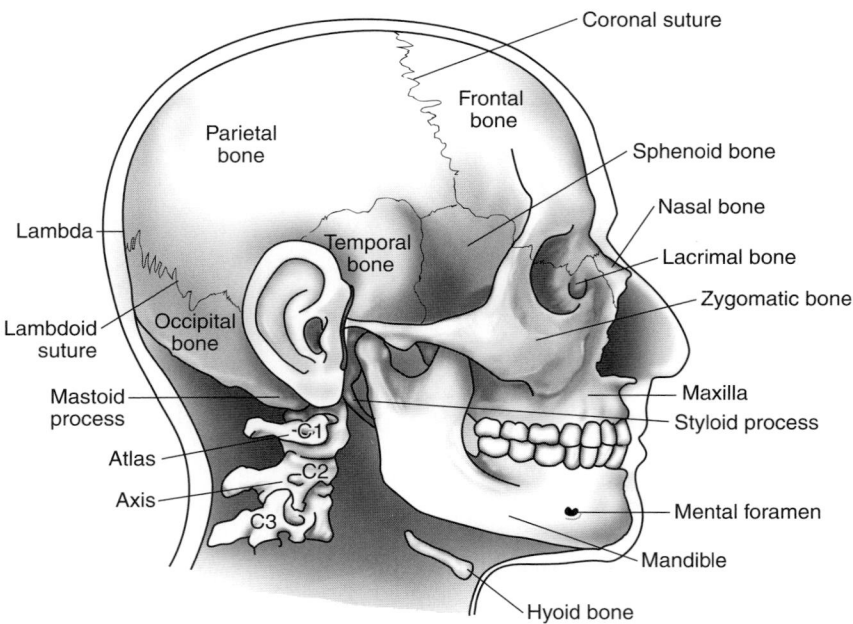

FIGURE 33-6 ■ Lateral view of the skull. (From Drain CB, Odom-Forren J: *Perianesthesia nursing: A critical care approach,* ed 5, St Louis, 2009, WB Saunders.)

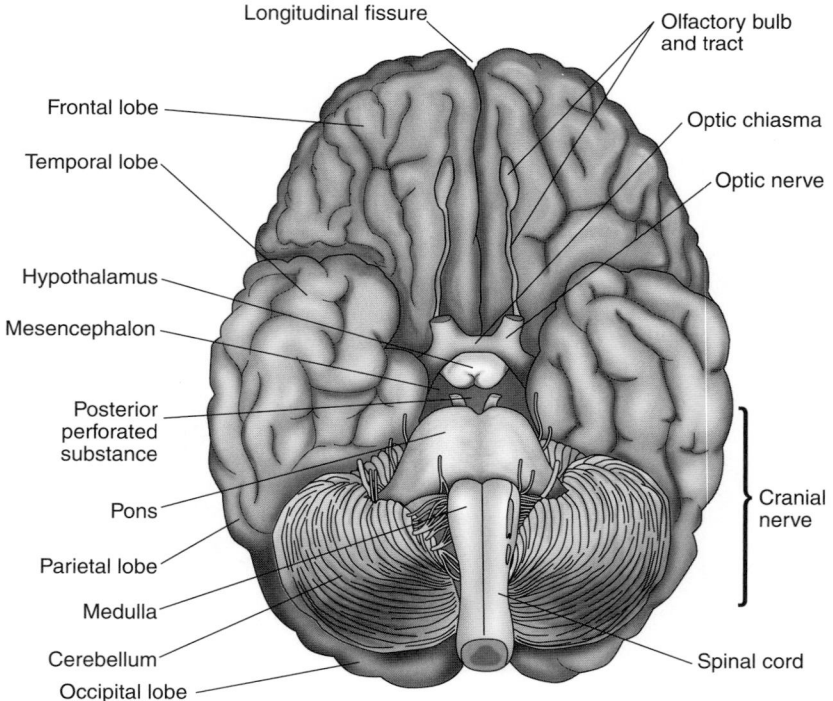

FIGURE 33-7 ■ Basal view of the brain. (From Drain CB, Odom-Forren J: *Perianesthesia nursing: A critical care approach,* ed 5, St Louis, 2009, WB Saunders.)

(2) Middle fossa: contains lobes
    (a) Temporal
    (b) Parietal
    (c) Occipital
(3) Posterior fossa—contains:
    (a) Cerebellum
    (b) Brainstem—composed of:
        (i) Midbrain
        (ii) Pons
        (iii) Medulla

3. Meninges
  a. Function
    (1) Protection for brain and spinal cord
    (2) Support underlying structures
  b. Layers from outermost layer inward
    (1) Dura mater ("tough mother")
      (a) Skinny, dense, fibrous, inelastic membrane
      (b) Double-layered, tough, fibrous covering of the brain
        (i) Outer layer (periosteal): periosteum of skull
        (ii) Inner layer (meningeal): creates intracranial compartments
      (c) Dural folds: divide cranial vault into compartments
        (i) Falx cerebri: separates right and left cerebral hemispheres
        (ii) Tentorium cerebelli: supports and separates the occipital and temporal lobes of cerebrum from cerebellum
        (iii) Falx cerebelli: separates right and left cerebellar hemispheres
    (2) Arachnoid membrane (weblike)
      (a) Fine, thin, delicate, elastic, fibrous
      (b) Closely adheres to dura mater and pia mater
      (c) Separated from dura mater by subdural space
      (d) Contains blood vessels of varying sizes
      (e) Connects to pia mater by trabeculae
      (f) Arachnoid granulations and villi enable CSF to move from subarachnoid space to venous system.
      (g) CSF circulates through the "web."
    (3) Pia mater ("soft mother") (Figure 33-8)
      (a) Innermost layer, one-cell-layer thick, not visible
      (b) Rich in blood, choroid plexuses, and mesothelial cells
      (c) Meshlike, vascular membrane
      (d) Follows sulci, gyri, and fissures
      (e) Inseparable from brain's surface, in direct contact with brain and spinal cord
  c. Spaces
    (1) Epidural
      (a) Potential space
      (b) Must be created by force (e.g., trauma, surgical dissection)
    (2) Subdural
      (a) Potential space
      (b) Below dura, above arachnoid
      (c) Subarachnoid—contains:
        (i) CSF
        (ii) Arteries
        (iii) Veins
      (d) Cisterns: pockets of arachnoid filled with CSF

D. Cerebral vasculature
  1. Arterial system: two paired systems of blood vessels (anterior and posterior) that combine to form circle of Willis (Figures 33-9 and 33-10)
    a. Anterior arterial circulation

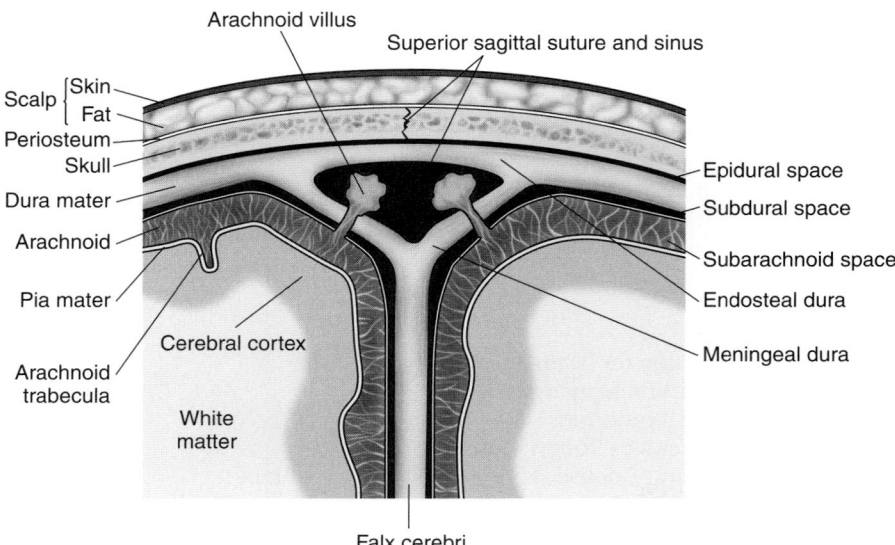

FIGURE 33-8 ■ Coronal section of the skull, brain, meninges, and superior sagittal sinus. (From Drain CB, Odom-Forren J: *Perianesthesia nursing: A critical care approach,* ed 5, St Louis, 2009, WB Saunders.)

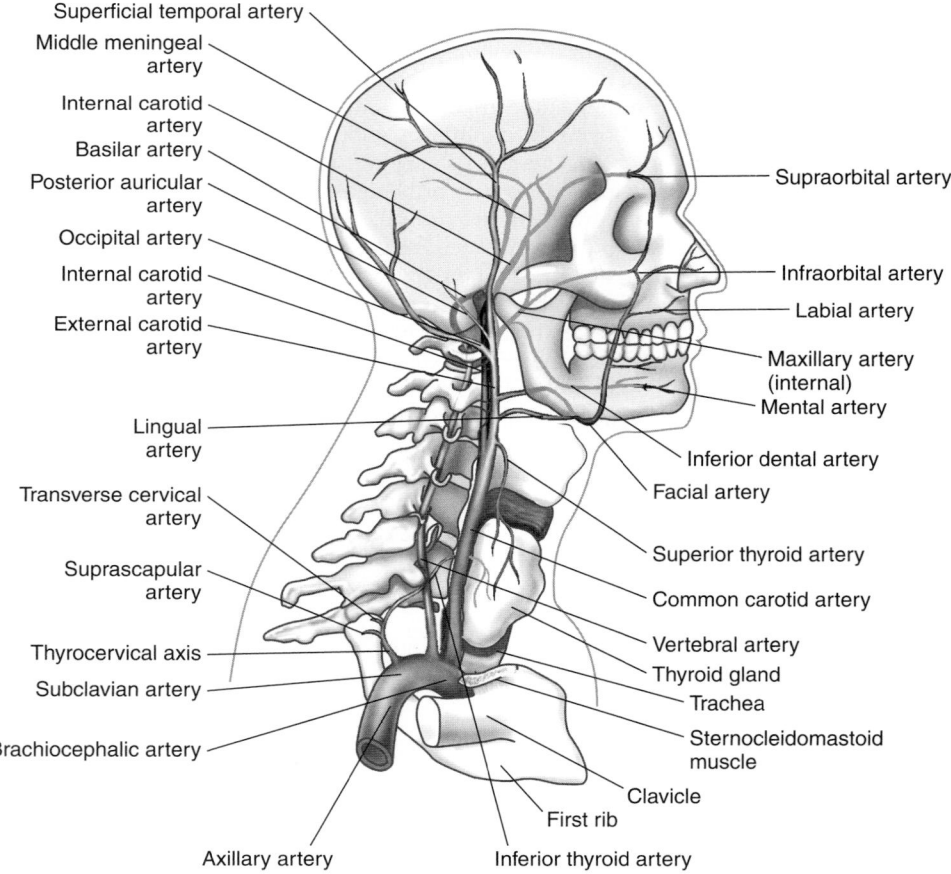

FIGURE 33-9 ■ Arterial supply to the neck and head. (From Drain CB, Odom-Forren J: *Perianesthesia nursing: A critical care approach,* ed 5, St Louis, 2009, WB Saunders.)

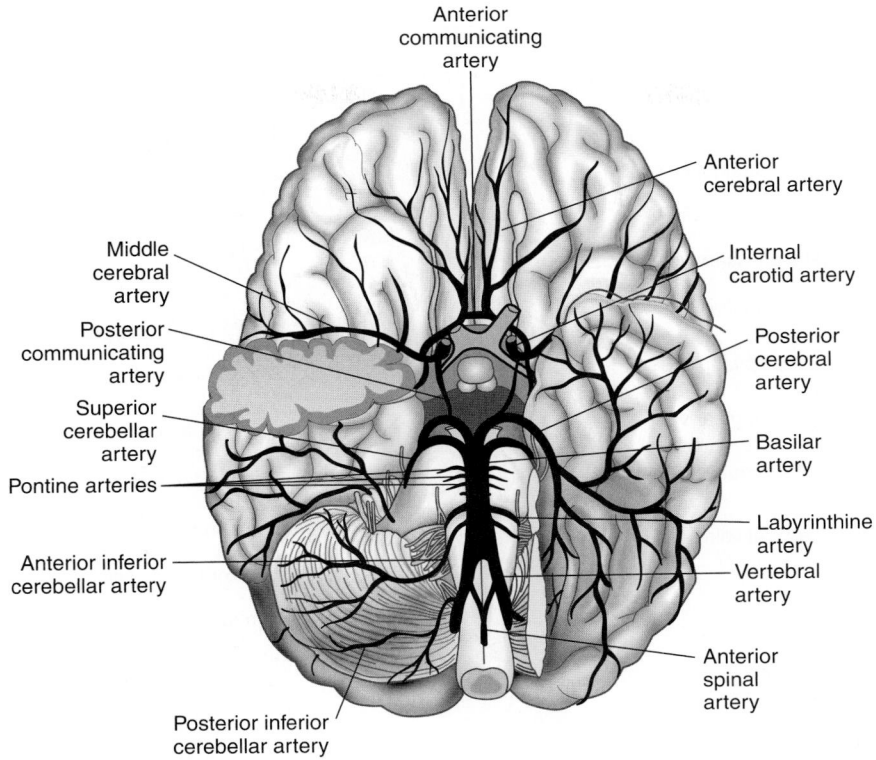

FIGURE 33-10 ■ Major arteries as seen on the base of the brain. (From Drain CB, Odom-Forren J: *Perianesthesia nursing: A critical care approach,* ed 5, St Louis, 2009, WB Saunders.)

 (1) Common carotid: branches into external and internal carotid arteries
 (2) Internal carotid artery: enters cranial cavity at petrous portion of temporal bone; supplies most of hemispheres (except occipital lobe, basal ganglia) and upper two thirds of diencephalons
 (3) External carotid artery: supplies skin and muscles of face, scalp
 (4) Anterior cerebral artery: supplies medial surfaces of frontal and parietal lobes
 (5) Anterior communicating artery: connects anterior cerebral arteries
 (6) Middle cerebral artery
  (a) Largest branch of internal carotid artery
  (b) Supplies two thirds of cerebral hemispheres (lateral surface)
b. Posterior arterial circulation
 (1) Vertebral arteries
  (a) Paired arteries arising from subclavian artery
  (b) Enter cranial vault through foramen magnum
  (c) Branches supply:
   (i) Spinal cord
   (ii) Underside of cerebellum
   (iii) Medulla
   (iv) Choroid plexus of fourth ventricle
  (d) Two arteries merge to form basilar artery.
 (2) Basilar artery
  (a) Branches into posterior cerebral arteries and smaller vessels supplying posterior fossa
 (3) Posterior cerebral artery—supplies:
  (a) Brainstem
  (b) Occipital lobe
  (c) Inferior and medial surfaces of temporal lobe

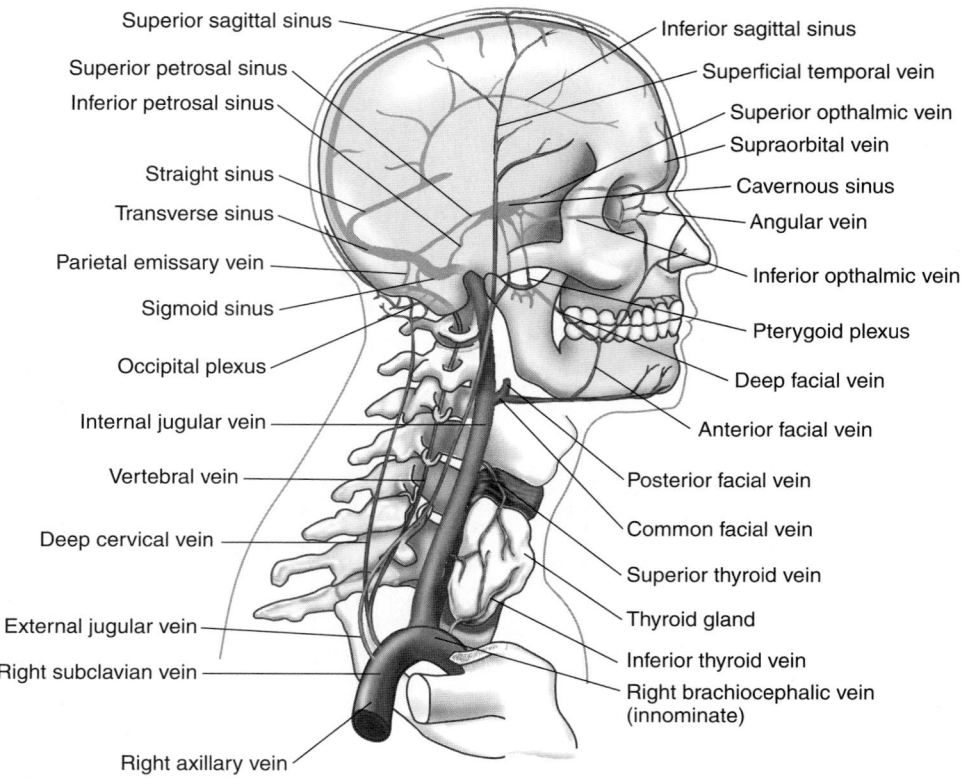

FIGURE 33-11 ■ Venous drainage of the brain, head, and neck. (From Drain CB, Odom-Forren J: *Perianesthesia nursing: A critical care approach*, ed 5, St Louis, 2009, WB Saunders.)

   2. Venous drainage: valveless, thin-walled system of superficial and deep veins and venous sinuses (Figure 33-11)
      a. Superficial veins: drain external surfaces of brain into superior sagittal, cavernous, sphenoparietal, and petrosal sinuses
         (1) Superior cerebral veins
         (2) Middle cerebral veins
         (3) Inferior cerebral veins
      b. Deep veins: drain internal areas of brain
         (1) Basal veins: connect superficial and deep cerebral veins
         (2) Vein of Rosenthal
         (3) Great cerebral vein (great vein of Galen)
      c. Venous sinuses: located between two layers of dura mater
         (1) Posterior (superior) group
            (a) Superior sagittal
            (b) Inferior sagittal
            (c) Straight
            (d) Transverse
            (e) Sigmoid
            (f) Occipital
         (2) Anterior (interior) group
            (a) Cavernous
            (b) Superior petrosal (2)
            (c) Inferior petrosal (2)
            (d) Basilar plexus
   E. Ventricular system (Figure 33-12)
      1. Formation of CSF
         a. Approximately 500 mL/day produced (0.37 mL/min)
         b. Volume of 150 mL in system at one time

VENTRICLES OF THE BRAIN AND CEREBROSPINAL FLUID CIRCULATION

The ventricles are 4 fluid-filled cavities within the brain. They connect with one another and with the spinal canal, which descends down the center of the spinal cord.

These chambers and the spinal canal are filled with cerebrospinal fluid (CSF), a total volume of 135 mL.

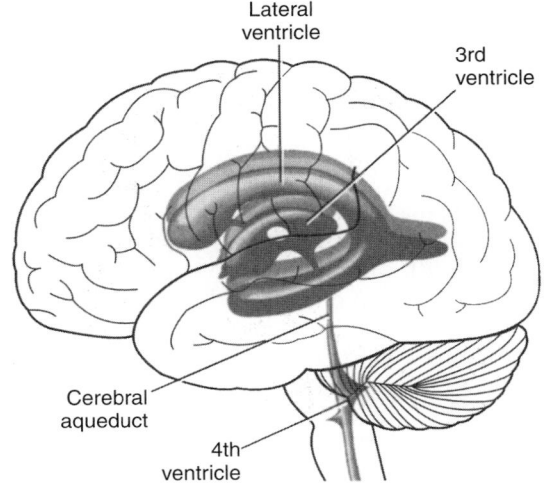

CSF circulates from the lateral ventricles, where most of it is formed, to the 3rd and 4th ventricles, down the spinal canal and throughout the subarachnoid space that surrounds the brain and spinal cord.

CSF provides cushioning for the central nervous system, allows fluid to shift from the cranial cavity to the spinal cavity, and carries nutrients to the brain. It returns to the general circulation primarily through the arachnoid villi, tiny projections of the subarachnoid space, which extend into the intradural venous sinuses. The venous sinuses collect venous blood as well as CSF and pass this mixture into the jugular veins.

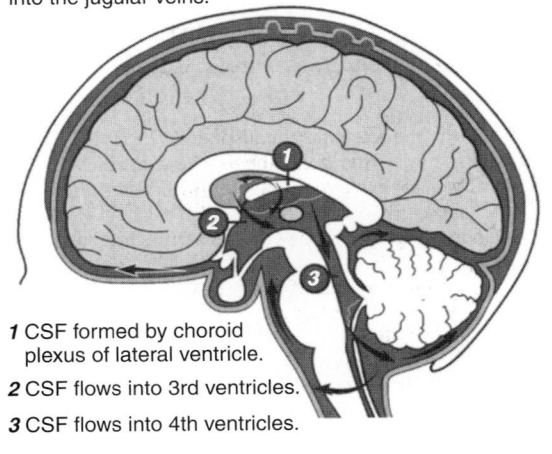

1 CSF formed by choroid plexus of lateral ventricle.

2 CSF flows into 3rd ventricles.

3 CSF flows into 4th ventricles.

FIGURE 33-12 ■ Ventricles of the brain and cerebrospinal fluid (CSF) circulation. (From Luckmann J: *Saunders manual of nursing care,* Philadelphia, 1997, WB Saunders.)

    c. Secreted by choroid plexus
    d. Choroid plexus located in:
        (1) Temporal horns of lateral ventricles
        (2) Posterior portion of third ventricle
        (3) Roof of fourth ventricle
  2. Function
    a. Supports and cushions CNS
    b. Medium for exchange of nutrients and excretion pathways for cerebral metabolic waste products
    c. Maintains stable chemical environment
    d. Facilitates intracerebral transport
  3. CSF properties
    a. Appearance
        (1) Clear
        (2) Colorless
        (3) Odorless
    b. Protein: 15 to 45 mg/dL
    c. Glucose
        (1) 50 to 75 mg/dL
        (2) Two thirds of serum glucose
    d. Chloride 120 to 130 mcg/L
    e. White blood cells: 0 to $5/mm^3$
    f. Red blood cells: none
    g. pH: 7.35 to 7.40
    h. Specific gravity: 1.005 to 1.009
    i. Pressure: 0 to 15 mm Hg or 50 to 150 mm H_2O (depending on the type of monitoring system used)
  4. Blood-brain barrier
    a. Composed of network of endothelial cells (cells of capillaries) and projections from astrocytes close to neurons
        (1) Located throughout brain, except in:
            (a) Hypothalamus
            (b) Pineal gland area
            (c) Floor of fourth ventricle in upper medulla
        (2) More permeable in newborn than adult
    b. Tight junctions between endothelial cells and astrocytes
    c. Functions
        (1) Preserves homeostasis of CNS
        (2) Selectively permeable to facilitate entry of needed metabolites and remove toxic or unnecessary metabolites
        (3) Permeable to:
            (a) Water
            (b) Oxygen
            (c) Carbon dioxide
            (d) Other gases
            (e) Glucose
            (f) Lipid-soluble substances
        (4) Breakdown of blood-brain barrier by inflammation, tumors, and toxins allows large molecules to pass directly into CNS.
  5. Cerebral hemispheres
    a. Cerebral cortex: outermost layer, composed of gray matter
        (1) Gyri or convolution: raised projections
        (2) Sulci: grooves between gyri
            (a) Shallow: sulcus
            (b) Deeper: fissure
        (3) Left cortex: deals with symbols and symbolic material, including:
            (a) Language
            (b) Mathematics

(c) Abstractions

(d) Reasoning

(e) Analytical aspect

(4) Right cortex: deals with visual-spatial tasks, processing of whole sensory experiences such as:

(a) Dancing

(b) Art appreciation

(c) Creative aspect

b. Lobes

(1) Frontal lobes (2)

(a) Motor cortex: controls voluntary and fine motor movement

(b) Sensory cortex: sensory association areas integrate and interpret sensory input.

(c) Memory, attention span

(d) Personality and emotional behavior

(e) Complex intellectual functioning, goal-directed behavior

(f) Broca's area

(i) Left hemisphere

(ii) Expressive speech (producing language)

(2) Parietal lobes (2): posterior to central sulcus of Rolando

(a) Sensory discrimination

(b) Tactile receptive area (i.e., soft, hard texture, smooth, etc.)

(c) Body image, association area (allows body/self awareness/orientation in space)

(3) Temporal lobes (2): located under fissure of Sylvius

(a) Hearing

(b) Olfaction

(c) Sensory speech (Wernicke's area), left hemisphere

(d) Short-term memory

(e) Sound interpretation, right hemisphere

(4) Occipital lobe (1): integrates visual cortex reception

c. Corpus callosum

(1) Bundle of nerve fibers

(2) Connects cerebral hemispheres

(3) Allows transfer of information from one hemisphere to the other

d. Basal ganglia (cerebral nuclei) (Figure 33-13)

(1) Group of deep subcortical gray matter

(2) Buried deep in hemispheres near thalamus and lateral ventricle

(3) Group of neuron cell bodies lying within the CNS

(4) Link cerebral cortex to certain thalamic nuclei

(5) Connect with hindbrain areas for coordination of muscle movements

(6) Modulate voluntary body movements, especially in hands and legs (as seen in Parkinson's syndrome)

e. Internal capsule

(1) White matter pathways

(2) Carries ascending and descending motor and sensory fibers

6. Limbic system (limbic lobe/rhinencephalon)

a. Two rings of limbic cortex and other tissue surrounding ventricles

b. "Visceral" or "emotional" brain and other behavioral response (anger, aggression)

c. Interconnections with other cerebral structures and hemispheres

d. Damage affects:

(1) Emotional responses

(2) Sexual behavior and drive

(3) Motivation

(4) Biological rhythms

7. Diencephalon: second major division of the forebrain, located within cerebrum and continuous with midbrain

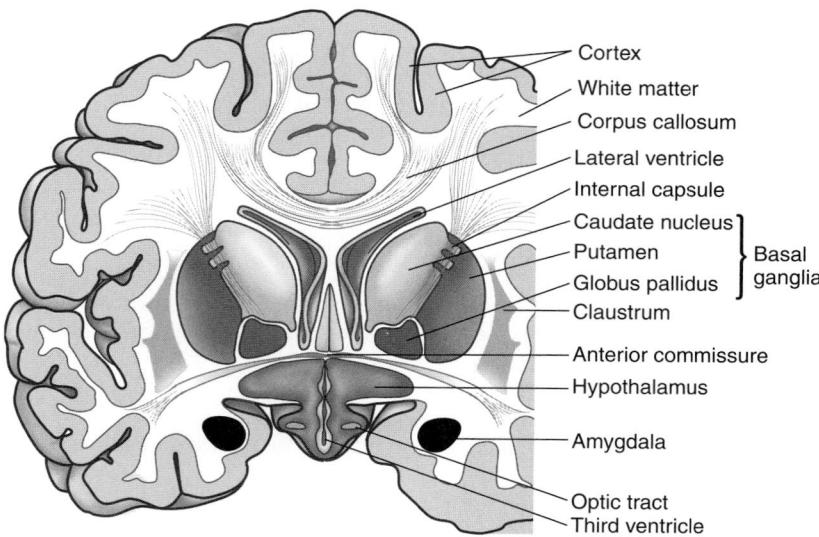

FIGURE 33-13 ■ Section of the cerebrum showing the basal ganglia. (From Drain CB, Odom-Forren J: *Perianesthesia nursing: A critical care approach,* ed 5, St Louis, 2009, WB Saunders.)

    a. Epithalamus
      (1) Narrow band forming roof of diencephalons
      (2) Contains pineal body that secretes melatonin
      (3) Associated with reproductive activity, inhibition or delay of gonadal development
    b. Thalamus (sensory relay station)
      (1) Located on both sides of third ventricle
      (2) Consist of right and left egg-shaped masses of gray matter
      (3) Greatest bulk of diencephalon
      (4) Acts as relay center for all incoming sensory (except for taste and smell) and motor tracts
      (5) Perception of primary sensations of pain, touch, pressure, temperature
      (6) Contributes to emotional activities, attentive processes, and behavioral expression
      (7) Coordinates and regulates functional activity of cerebral cortex
    c. Subthalamus
      (1) Located below the thalamus and above the midbrain
      (2) Correlation center for the optic and vestibular impulses
    d. Hypothalamus
      (1) Connected to pituitary gland by hypophyseal stalk (infundibulum)
      (2) Forms base of diencephalons and part of the third ventricle
      (3) Maintains internal body homeostasis and temperature control
        (a) Regulates:
          (i) Body temperature
          (ii) Endocrine activities
          (iii) Water balance
          (iv) Carbohydrate and fat metabolism
        (b) Has role in maintaining awake state
        (c) Hormonal feedback system (growth and sexual maturity)
        (d) Secretes:
          (i) Neurohormones (hypothalamic releasing and inhibiting factors)
          (ii) Oxytocin
          (iii) Vasopressin (antidiuretic hormone)
        (e) Sympathetic control (pulse rate, blood pressure)

(4) Influences behavior patterns
    (a) Helps control primitive responses such as fear, instinct, self-preservation
    (b) Physical expression of emotions and emotional behavior
    (c) Enhances CNS activity
(5) Cardiovascular regulation
(6) Anterior and posterior pituitary hormone release (e.g., pitocin, growth hormone)

8. Brainstem (Figures 33-14 and 33-15)
  a. Motor and sensory pathways
  b. Relays messages between cerebral structures and spinal cord
  c. Gives rise to cranial nerves (CNs) third through twelfth (III to XII)
  d. Holds respiratory control centers
  e. Composition
    (1) Midbrain (mesencephalon)
      (a) Short, narrow segment that connects the forebrain with the hindbrain
      (b) Conduction pathway and reflex control center
      (c) Connects to cerebrum through diencephalons
      (d) Control of various visual, auditory, postural, and righting reflexes
        (i) Third CN (oculomotor) dorsal or posterior portion
          [a] Moves eyes up, down, and medially
          [b] Opens lid
          [c] Parasympathetic outflow constricts pupil.
          [d] Sympathetic outflow dilates pupil.
        (ii) Fourth CN (trochlear)
          [a] Moves eye down and in

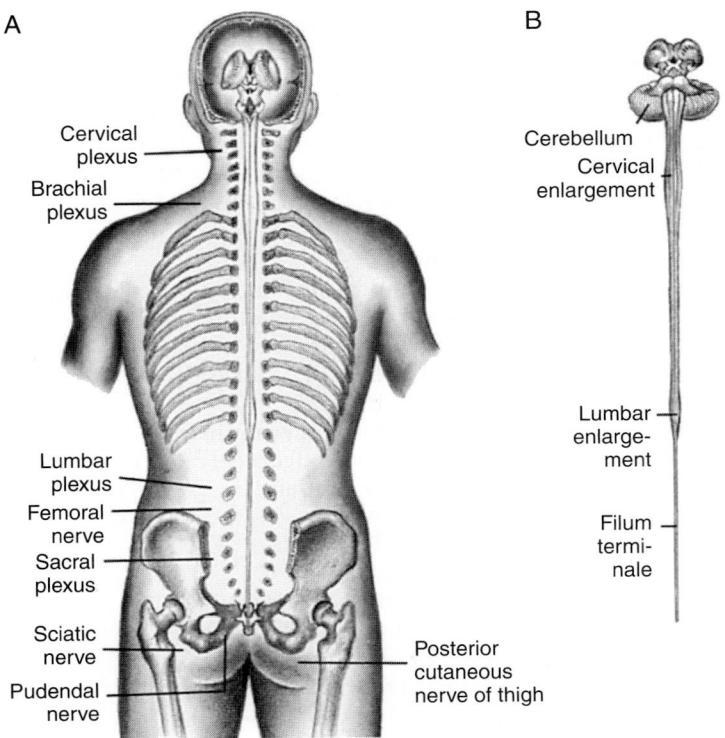

FIGURE 33-14 ■ **A,** Posterior view of brainstem. **B,** Anterior view of brainstem and spinal cord. (From Thompson J: *Mosby's clinical nursing,* ed 5, St Louis, 2002, Mosby.)

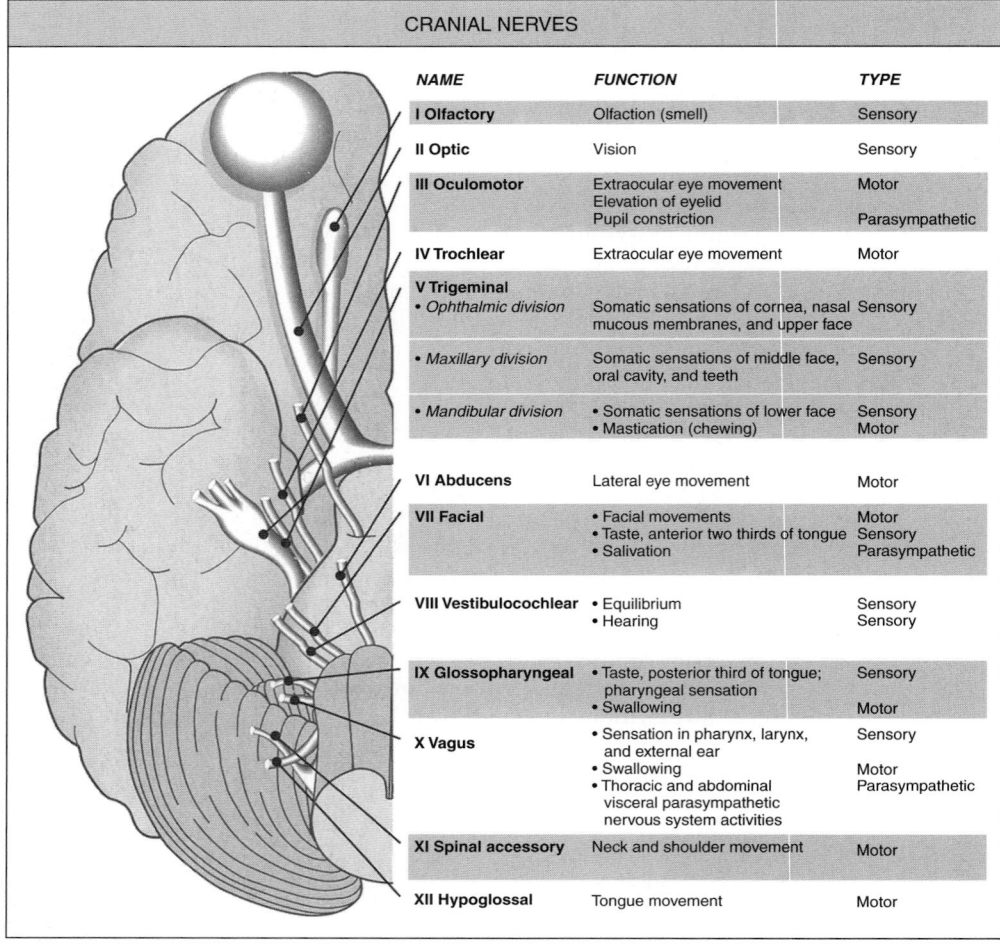

CRANIAL NERVES		
NAME	**FUNCTION**	**TYPE**
I Olfactory	Olfaction (smell)	Sensory
II Optic	Vision	Sensory
III Oculomotor	Extraocular eye movement Elevation of eyelid Pupil constriction	Motor Parasympathetic
IV Trochlear	Extraocular eye movement	Motor
V Trigeminal • *Ophthalmic division*	Somatic sensations of cornea, nasal mucous membranes, and upper face	Sensory
• *Maxillary division*	Somatic sensations of middle face, oral cavity, and teeth	Sensory
• *Mandibular division*	• Somatic sensations of lower face • Mastication (chewing)	Sensory Motor
VI Abducens	Lateral eye movement	Motor
VII Facial	• Facial movements • Taste, anterior two thirds of tongue • Salivation	Motor Sensory Parasympathetic
VIII Vestibulocochlear	• Equilibrium • Hearing	Sensory Sensory
IX Glossopharyngeal	• Taste, posterior third of tongue; pharyngeal sensation • Swallowing	Sensory Motor
X Vagus	• Sensation in pharynx, larynx, and external ear • Swallowing • Thoracic and abdominal visceral parasympathetic nervous system activities	Sensory Motor Parasympathetic
XI Spinal accessory	Neck and shoulder movement	Motor
XII Hypoglossal	Tongue movement	Motor

FIGURE 33-15 ■ Cranial nerves. (From Luckmann J: *Saunders manual of nursing care,* Philadelphia, 1997, WB Saunders. Tabular material from Black JM, Matassarin-Jacobs E, eds: *Luckmann and Sorensen's medical-surgical nursing: A psychophysiologic approach,* ed 4, Philadelphia, 1993, WB Saunders.)

    (2) Pons (metencephalon)
        (a) Bridge between the midbrain and the medulla oblongata
        (b) Roof contains portion of reticular formation.
        (c) Lower pons regulates respiration.
        (d) Contains nuclei of CNs V, VI, VII, and VIII
           (i) Fifth CN (trigeminal)
              [a] Sensation of face (three branches)
              [b] Sensation to cornea (corneal reflex)
              [c] Muscles of mastication
           (ii) Sixth CN (abducens)
              [a] Moves eye laterally
           (iii) Seventh CN (facial)
              [a] Movement of facial expression
           (iv) Eighth CN (auditory or acoustic)
              [a] Auditory branch (hearing)
              [b] Vestibular branch (balance)
    (3) Medulla oblongata (myelencephalon)
        (a) Lower portion of brainstem
        (b) Located between the foramen magnum and pons

(c) Connects to cervical spinal cord
(d) Regulatory centers for:
  (i) Cardiac
  (ii) Respiratory
  (iii) Vasomotor
  (iv) Rhythmicity functions
(e) Contains nuclei of CNs IX, X, XI, and XII
(f) Center for protective reflexes: coughing, gagging, sneezing, swallowing, vomiting (respiratory and vomiting center)
  (i) Ninth CN (glossopharyngeal)
    [a] Taste—anterior two thirds of tongue
    [b] Sensory to tongue and soft palate
  (ii) Tenth CN (vagus)
    [a] Parasympathetic outflow
    [b] Sensory to posterior pharynx
  (iii) Eleventh CN (spinal accessory)
    [a] Shoulder shrug
  (iv) Twelfth CN (hypoglossal)
    [a] Extends tongue

9. Cerebellum
   a. Overlaps the pons and the medulla oblongata
   b. Located at base of brain, below occipital lobes
   c. No sensory function and does not initiate movement
   d. Right and left hemispheres connected at midline
   e. Connected to brainstem by three sets of cerebellar peduncles
     (1) Superior
     (2) Middle
     (3) Inferior
   f. Receives input from brainstem and spinal cord nuclei
   g. Functions
     (1) Coordinates muscle tone
     (2) Coordinates voluntary movements
     (3) Controls equilibrium posture and balance
     (4) Motor gracefulness
   h. Damage to a part of the cerebellum can result in nystagmus and a reeling gait.
   i. Arnold-Chiari malformation: cerebellar tonsillar pillars protrude through foramen magnum.

10. The fourth ventricle
    a. Diamond-shaped space
    b. Located between cerebellum, pons, medulla oblongata
    c. Contains CSF

11. CNs (Figure 33-15, Table 33-1)
    a. Help in remembering names of CNs (Table 33-2)
    b. Help in remembering whether CNs are sensory, motor, or both (S, M, B) (Table 33-3)

12. Autonomic nervous system (Table 33-4, Figure 33-16)
    a. Part of peripheral nervous system
    b. Implications for patient undergoing intracranial surgery should be considered.
    c. Overall purpose: regulation of involuntary functions of internal organs
    d. Sympathetic nervous system
      (1) Originates in thoracic area of spine and upper lumbar segments of spinal cord
      (2) Impulses travel from CNS to ganglia (relay stations outside spinal column), along postganglionic (adrenergic) fibers to effector organs where catecholamines are released (norepinephrine).

■ TABLE 33-1
■■ **Rapid Neurological Evaluation of Cranial Nerve Function**

Nerve	Origin	Function	Method of Testing	Site of Involvement	Abnormal Findings	Frequency
I Olfactory	Olfactory bulb	Sensory—sense of smell	Identify odors, one nostril at a time	Fracture of cribriform plate or in ethmoid area	Anosmia	Uncommon
II Optic	Lateral geniculate body	Sensory—vision and circuit for light reflex	Acuity—Snellen chart or newspaper; test each eye separately Visual fields—confrontation method, each eye separately; move finger from eight cardinal points and indicate when it was seen	Direct trauma to orbit or globe, or fracture involving optic foramen	Loss of both direct and consensual pupillary constriction when light flashed in affected eye; unaffected eye has normal direct and consensual response	Common
III Oculomotor	Midbrain	Motor—pupillary constriction, elevation of upper eyelid, extraocular movements conjointly with III, IV, and VI	Light flashed in affected eye Light flashed in unaffected eye	Pressure on geniculate body; laceration or intracerebral clot in temporal, parietal, occipital lobes Pressure of herniating uncus on nerve just before it enters cavernous sinus, or fracture involving cavernous sinus	Absence of blink when hand brought suddenly from ide; indicates visual field defect (always homonymous) Dilated pupil, ptosis; eye turns down and out Direct pupil reflex absent; consensual reflux present Direct pupil reflex absent; consensual reflux absent	Common Very frequent
IV Trochlear	Midbrain	Motor—extraocular movements of eye downward and inward (oblique muscles)	Follow fingers, using eight cardinal points	Course of nerve around brainstem	Eye fails to move down and out	Infrequent

Cranial Nerve	Origin	Function	Method of Testing	Cause of Damage	Clinical Manifestation	Frequency
V Trigeminal	Pons	*Sensory* Ophthalmic: cornea of eye and above Maxillary: cheek and upper lips Mandibular: lower lip and chin *Motor* Masseter and temporal muscles: biting down and chewing, lateral movement of jaw	Touch cotton to both sides along divisions, corneal reflex	Direct injury to terminal branches, particularly second division in roof of maxillary sinus	Loss of sensation of pain and touch Paresthesias	Uncommon (exception: trigeminal neuralgia)
VI Abducens	Pons	Motor—extraocular movements of eye laterally	Follow fingers using eight cardinal points; test III, IV, VI together	As with III, IV	Eyes fail to move laterally	Infrequent
VII Facial	Pons	Motor—facial muscles around eyes, mouth, and forehead	"Wrinkle your forehead"	Supranuclear: intracerebral clot	Forehead wrinkles because of bilateral innervation of frontalis; otherwise paralysis of facial muscles as below	Frequent
				Peripheral: laceration or contusion in parotid area	Paralysis of facial muscles; eye remains open; angle of mouth droops; forehead fails to wrinkle	Frequent
		Sensory—taste on anterior two thirds of tongue	Identify flavors—does food taste the same?	Peripheral: fracture of temporal bone	As above, plus associated involvement of acoustic nerve (see below), dry cornea, and loss of taste on anterior two thirds of tongue	Frequent

Continued

■ TABLE 33-1
■ ■ **Rapid Neurological Evaluation of Cranial Nerve Function—cont'd**

Nerve	Origin	Function	Method of Testing	Site of Involvement	Abnormal Findings	Frequency
VIII Acoustic	Pons	*Sensory* Cochlear division: hearing Vestibular division: maintenance of equilibrium and posturing of head	In children and unresponsive patients, clap hands close to ears Weber's test: bone conduction with tuning fork Rinne's test: air conduction using mastoid process Caloric test	Fracture of petrous portion of temporal bone; CN VII often involved Caloric test negative	Startle reflex Sound not heard by involved ear	Common
IX Glossopharyngeal	Medulla	Motor—constrictor muscle of the pharynx used in swallowing Sensory—taste receptors on posterior one third of tongue	Touch walls of pharynx with tongue blade Identify tastes	Brainstem or deep laceration of neck	Loss of taste to posterior one third of tongue Loss of sensation on affected side soft palate	Rare Rare
X Vagus	Medulla	Sensory—pharynx and larynx Motor—pharynx and larynx, movement of soft palate and uvula; conjointly with IX, ability to speak clearly	Touch with tongue blade to emit gag reflex Watch movement of uvula when patient says "ahhh"	Brainstem or deep laceration of neck Compression by herniation	Sagging of soft palate; deviation of uvula to normal side Hoarseness from paralysis of vocal cords	Rare
XI Spinal accessory	Medulla	Motor—sternocleidomastoid, trapezius, and rhomboid muscles	Shrug shoulders against resistance, turn head against resistance, flex chin	Laceration of neck	Inability to shrug shoulders or turn head	Rare
XII Hypoglossal	Medulla	Motor—tongue	"Stick out tongue, wiggle tongue"	Neck laceration, usually associated with major vessel damage	Tongue protrudes toward affected side; dysarthria	Rare

■ TABLE 33-2
■ ■ **Help in Remembering Names of Cranial Nerves**

Mnemonic	CN Number Name
O (n)	I Olfactory
O (ld)	II Optic
O (lympus)	III Oculomotor
T (owering)	IV Trochlear
T (ops)	V Trigeminal
A	VI Abducens
F (inn)	VII Facial
A (nd)	VIII Auditory
G (erman)	IX Glossopharyngeal
V (iewed)	X Vagus
S (ome)	XI Spinal accessory
H (ops)	XII Hypoglossal

CN, Cranial nerve.

■ TABLE 33-3
■ ■ **Help in Remembering Whether Cranial Nerves Are Sensory, Motor, or Both**

Mnemonic	CN Number Name
S (ome)	I Olfactory
S (ay)	II Optic
M (arry)	III Oculomotor
M (oney)	IV Trochlear
B (ut)	V Trigeminal
M (y)	VI Abducens
B (rother)	VII Facial
S (ays)	VIII Auditory
B (ad)	IX Glossopharyngeal
B (usiness)	X Vagus
M (arry)	XI Spinal accessory
M (en)	XII Hypoglossal

B, Both; *CN*, cranial nerve; *M*, motor; *S*, sensory.

  (a) Regulates body's energy expenditures
  (b) Prepares body for stress (fight or flight)
 e. Parasympathetic nervous system
  (1) Cell bodies located in extreme ends of spinal cord (brainstem, sacrum)
  (2) Transmits impulses from CNS along preganglionic fibers to ganglia located in or near effector organs
   (a) Nerves are cholinergic.
   (b) Acetylcholine is released.
  (3) Helps in conservation of body's energy
  (4) Affects localized, discrete areas rather than whole body
 II. ANATOMY AND PHYSIOLOGY OF THE SPINE AND SPINAL CORD
  A. Vertebral column (Figure 33-16)
   1. Purpose
    a. Supports head and trunk
    b. Protects spinal cord
    c. Flexibility for movement

■ TABLE 33-4
■ ■ **Effects of Autonomic Nervous System**

Effector Organ	Sympathetic (Adrenergic Effect)	Parasympathetic (Cholinergic Effect)
Pupil	Dilates	Constricts
Salivary glands	Decreases secretion	Increases secretion
Bronchi	Dilates	Constricts
Respiratory rate	Increases	Decreases
Heart		
Pulse	Increases	Decreases
Contraction	Strengthens	Weakens
Blood pressure	Increases	Decreases
Stomach	Decreases contractions	Increases contractions
Adrenal glands	Stimulates secretion of epinephrine, norepinephrine	Decreases secretions
Digestive tract	Decreases motility	Increases motility
	Contracts sphincters	Relaxes sphincters
	Inhibits secretions	Stimulates secretions
Bladder	Relaxes	Contracts
	Relaxes sphincter	
Sweat glands	Increases activity	Decreases activity
Hair	Piloerection	Relaxes
Blood vessels		
Coronary	Dilates	No significant effect
Skeletal muscle	Dilates	Constricts
Skin	Constricts	No significant effect

2. Unique aspects
   a. Atlas (C1): sits on odontoid process
   b. Axis (C2)
3. Divisions (Figure 33-17)
   a. Composed of 33 vertebrae
     (1) Cervical (7 vertebrae)
       (a) Smallest vertebrae
       (b) Supports head and neck
     (2) Thoracic or dorsal (12 vertebrae)
       (a) Supports the chest muscle
       (b) Articulates with the ribs
       (c) Intermediate in size
       (d) Becomes larger as descends
   b. Lumbar (5 vertebrae)
     (1) Supports the lower back muscle
     (2) Largest segment
     (3) Strongest vertebrae
   c. Sacral (5 vertebrae)
     (1) Fused vertebrae into one
     (2) Form a large triangular bone
   d. Coccygeal (4 vertebrae): fused as one
4. Essential parts of vertebrae
   a. Body: anterior, flat, round, solid segment separated by disks
   b. Arch: posterior segment; consists of:
     (1) Pedicles (2): short, thick pieces of bone
     (2) Laminae (2): broad plates of bone
     (3) Articular processes (4 facets): two on either side, provide spine stability

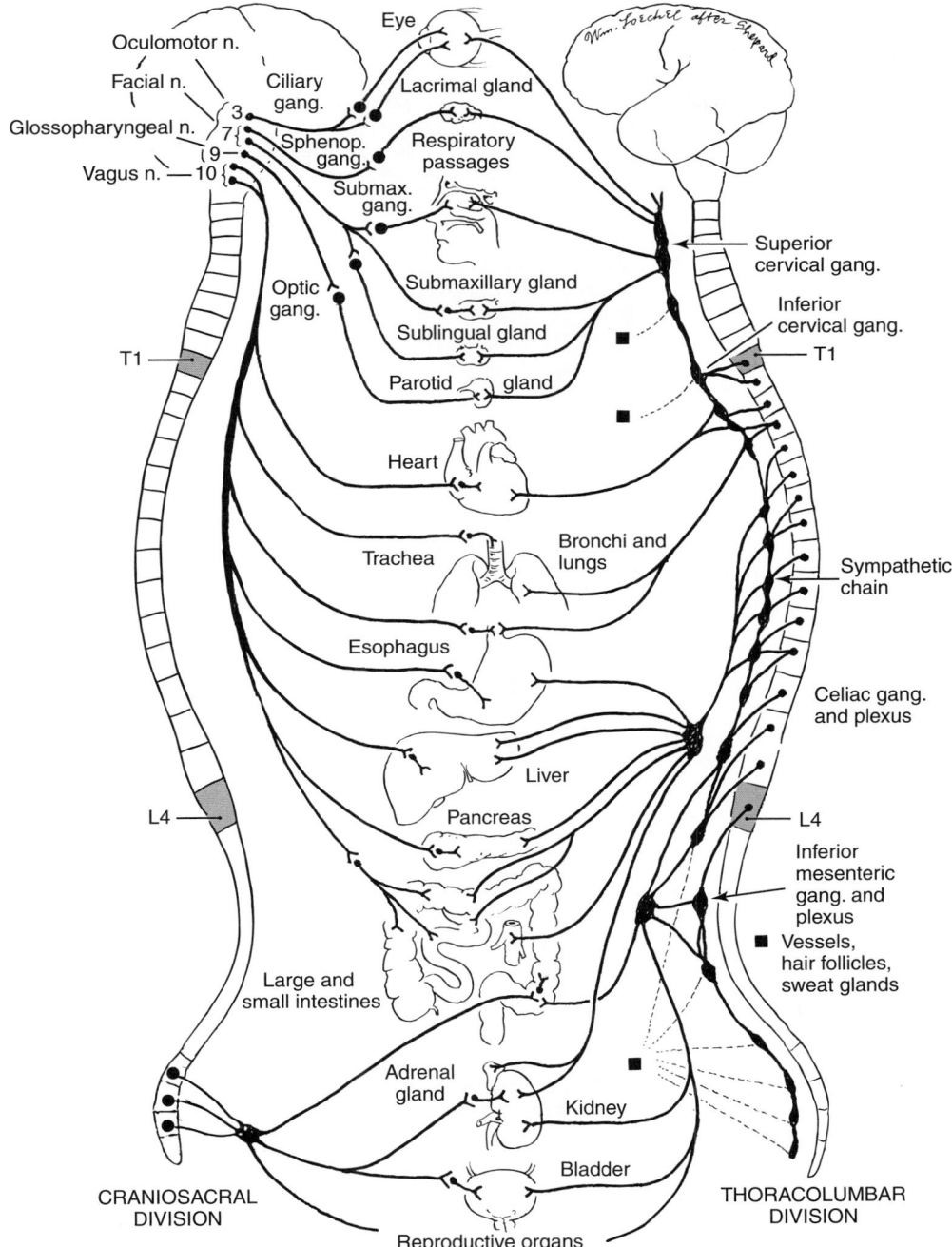

FIGURE 33-16 ■ Diagram of the autonomic nervous system. *gang.*, Ganglion; *n.*, nerve. (From Nagelhout JJ, Plaus KL: *Nurse anesthesia,* ed 4, Philadelphia, 2010, Saunders.)

       (4) Transverse processes (2 facets): points of attachment for muscles and ligaments

       (5) Spinous process (1): midline projection from rear of arch, serves as attachment for muscles and ligaments

  c. Foramen

       (1) Opening where vertebral arch meets vertebral body

       (2) Allows for passage of spinal cord

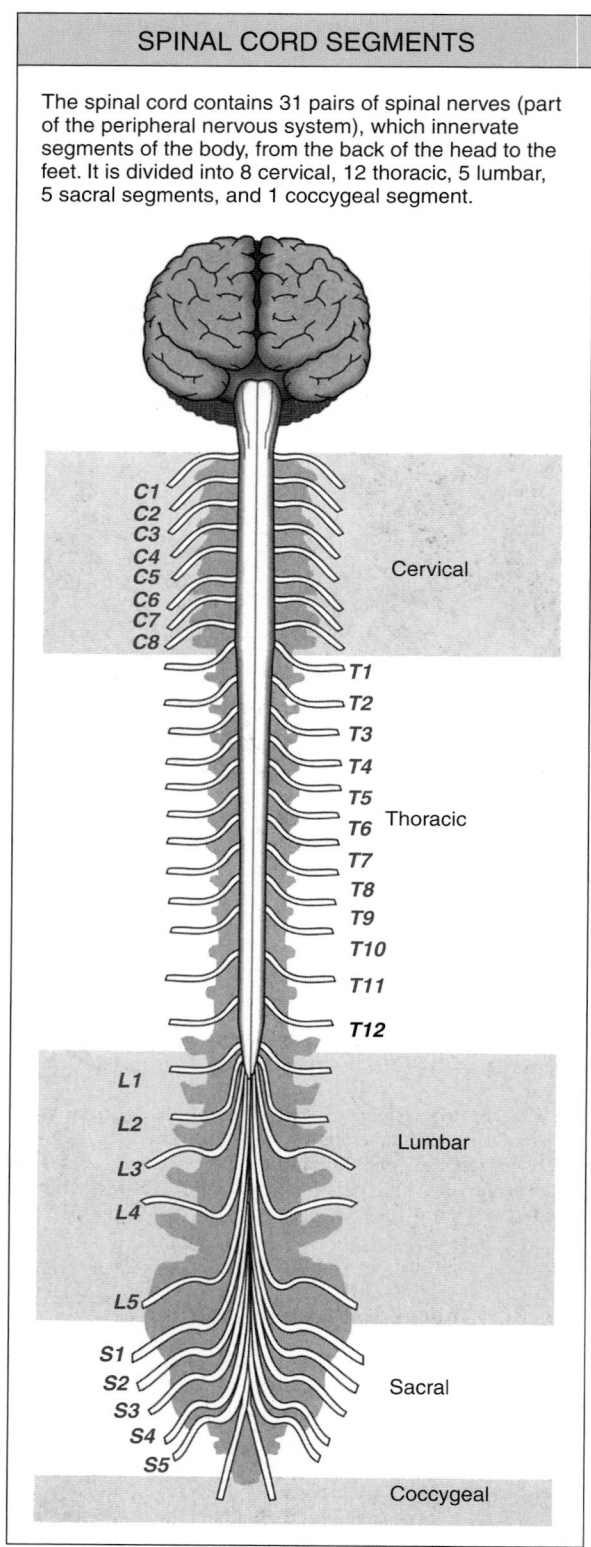

SPINAL CORD SEGMENTS

The spinal cord contains 31 pairs of spinal nerves (part of the peripheral nervous system), which innervate segments of the body, from the back of the head to the feet. It is divided into 8 cervical, 12 thoracic, 5 lumbar, 5 sacral segments, and 1 coccygeal segment.

Cervical

Thoracic

Lumbar

Sacral

Coccygeal

FIGURE 33-17 ■ Spinal cord segments. (From Luckmann J: *Saunders manual of nursing care,* Philadelphia, 1997, WB Saunders.)

5. Spinal ligaments
   a. Anterior longitudinal ligament
      (1) Fibers attach to anterior surface of vertebral body and intervertebral disks.
      (2) Broad, strong
      (3) Extends from occipital bone and anterior tubercle of atlas to sacrum
   b. Posterior longitudinal ligament
      (1) Attaches to posterior surface of vertebral bodies within spinal canal
      (2) Thick, strong
      (3) Extends from occipital bone to coccyx
   c. Ligamenta flava
      (1) Yellow elastic fibers connecting lamina of adjacent vertebrae
      (2) Extend from axis to first segment of sacrum
      (3) Help hold body erect
      (4) Thin, broad, and long in cervical area
      (5) Thicker in thoracic area
      (6) Thickest in lumbar region
   d. Supraspinous ligament
      (1) Joins the spinous process tips from C7 to sacrum
   e. Interspinous ligament
      (1) Connects adjacent spinous process from tips to roots
6. Intervertebral disks (Figure 33-18)
   a. Located between vertebral bodies from second cervical vertebra to sacrum
   b. Fibrocartilaginous, disk-shaped structures
   c. Vary in size, thickness, and shape at different spinal levels
   d. Serve as cushions between bony surfaces of vertebral bodies
   e. Parts

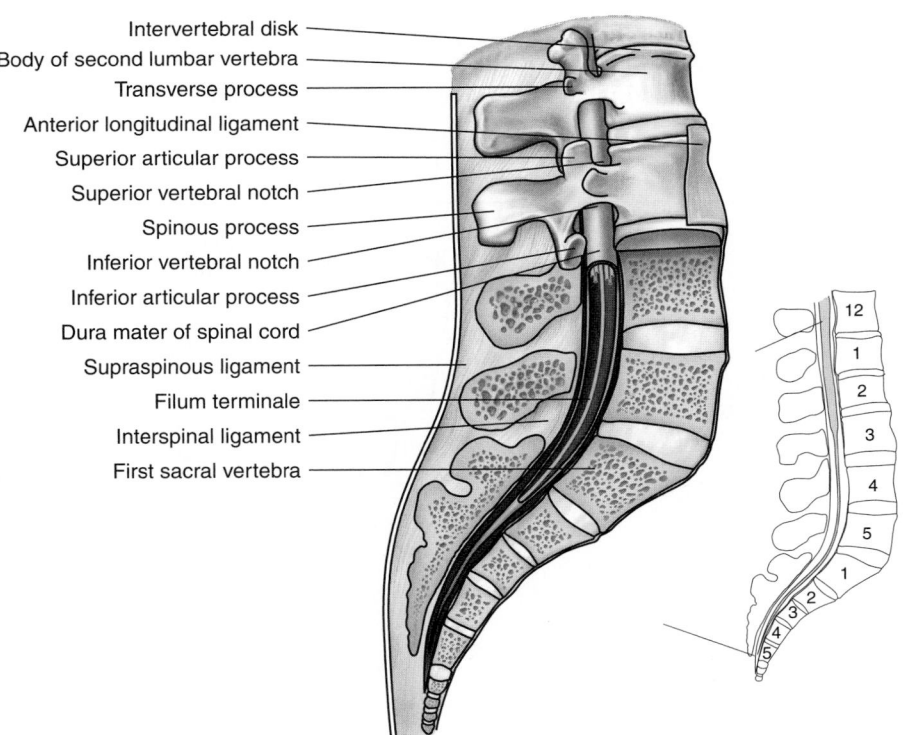

FIGURE 33-18 ■ Vertebral column showing structure. (From Drain CB, Odom-Forren J: *Perianesthesia nursing: A critical care approach*, ed 5, St Louis, 2009, WB Saunders.)

          (1) Nucleus pulposus
             (a) Central, spongy core
             (b) Loses resiliency with age
          (2) Annulus fibrosus
             (a) Fibrous capsule that surrounds nucleus pulposus
             (b) Degenerative changes can occur in middle and later life.

B. Spinal cord

  1. Characteristics

    a. Size: 1 cm in diameter; average length of 42 to 45 cm

    b. Originates at foramen magnum and ends at L2

    c. Elongated mass of nerve tissue that occupies upper two thirds of vertebral canal; continuous with medulla oblongata

    d. 31 segments, each with a pair of spinal nerves

    e. Surrounded by meninges for protection

    f. Central canal contains CSF.

  2. Purposes

    a. Conducts sensory and motor impulses to and from brain

    b. Controls many reflexes

  3. Arterial blood supply

    a. From vertebral arteries

    b. Anterior spinal artery: runs full length of cord, midventrally

    c. Posterior spinal arteries: run full length of spinal cord along each row of dorsal roots

  4. Venous drainage

    a. Intradural vein: follows arterial pattern

    b. Extradural intravertebral veins: form plexus from cranium to pelvis with communication to veins of neck, thorax, abdomen

  5. Transverse section (Figure 33-19)

    a. White matter

      (1) Longitudinal myelinated fibers

      (2) Comprises bulk of spinal cord

      (3) Encases gray matter

      (4) Each half divided into three longitudinal columns (funiculi)

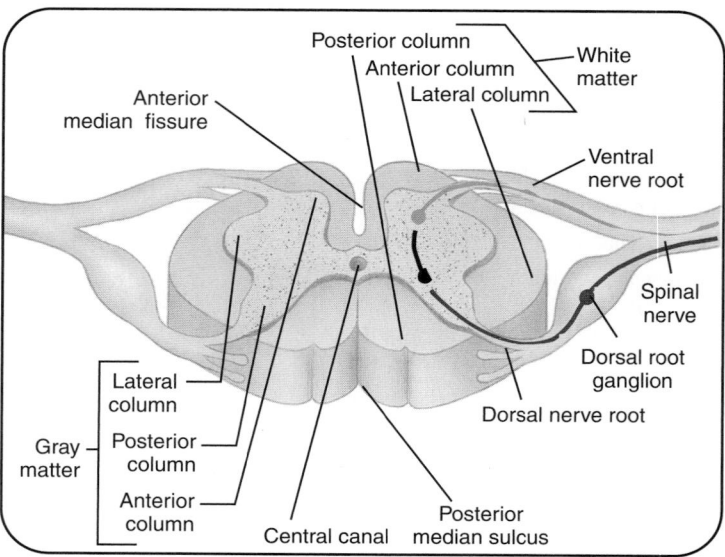

FIGURE 33-19 ■ Transverse section of the spinal cord. (From Lewis SM, Heitkemper MM, Dirksen SR: *Medical surgical nursing: Assessment and management of clinical problems,* ed 5, St Louis, 2000, Mosby.)

(a) Ascending (sensory): pathways to the brain for impulse

(b) Lateral

(c) Descending (motor) tracts: transmit impulses from brain to the motor neurons of the spinal cord

b. Gray matter

(1) Unmyelinated fibers

(2) H-shaped appearance of inner core

(3) H divided into columns (horns) containing ascending (sensory) and descending (motor) tracts

(a) Anterior (ventral) column

(i)   Motor

(ii) Efferent fibers

(b) Posterior (dorsal) column

(i)   Sensory

(ii) Afferent fibers

(iii) Axons from peripheral sensory neurons

(c) Lateral horns

(i)   Thoracic and upper lumbar segments only

(ii) Sympathetic nervous system cell bodies

6. Ascending tracts (Figure 33-20, Table 33-5)

a. Spinothalamic

(1) Carry sensations of:

(a) Pain

(b) Temperature

(c) Light touch

(d) Pressure

(2) Originate in posterior gray column on opposite side and terminate in thalamus

b. Spinocerebellar

(1) Carry impulses of proprioception (knowledge of position and body parts) or kinesthesia from lower body

(2) Originate in posterior gray horns and terminate in cerebellum

c. Fasciculus gracilis and fasciculus cuneatus

(1) Carry impulses of proprioception from:

(a) Muscles

(b) Joints

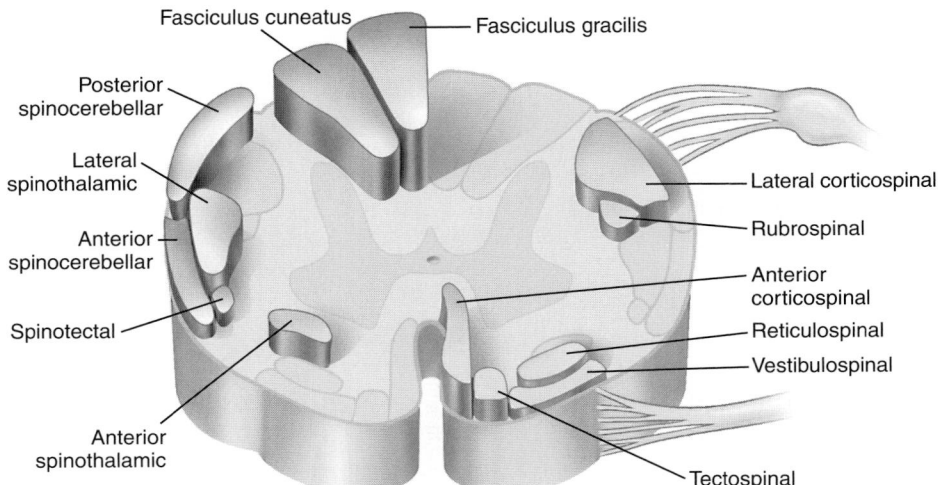

FIGURE 33-20 ■ Major ascending (sensory) and descending (motor) tracts of the spinal cord. (From Thibodeau GA, Patton K: *Anatomy and physiology,* ed 6, St Louis, 2007, Mosby.)

■ TABLE 33–5
■ **Major Spinal Cord Tracts**

Name	Origin	Termination	Cross	Function
ASCENDING TRACTS				
Posterior dorsal columns: fasciculus gracilis and fasciculus cuneatus	Fasciculus gracilis: spinal cord at the lumbar and sacral levels Fasciculus cuneatus: Spinal cord at the cervical and thoracic levels	Medulla → thalamus → sensory strip of the cerebral cortex	Ascend in the posterior funiculus and cross over in the lower medulla	Conveys position and vibratory sense, joint and two-point discrimination, tactile localization, pressure, and discriminating touch Fasciculus gracilis: Carries impulses from the lower body Fasciculus cuneatus: Carries impulses from the upper body
Lateral spinothalamic tract	Posterior horn	Thalamus → cerebral cortex	Crosses over in the spinal cord to the contralateral anterolateral funiculus before ascending	Conveys pain and temperature sensation
Anterior spinothalamic tract	Posterior horn	Thalamus → cerebral cortex	Crosses over the spinal cord to the contralateral anterolateral funiculus before ascending	Conveys light touch and pressure sensation
Posterior spinothalamic tract	Posterior horn	Cerebellum	Ascends uncrossed in the lateral funiculus	Conveys proprioceptive data that influence muscle tone and synergy necessary for coordinated muscle movements
Anterior spinocerebellar tract	Posterior horn	Cerebellum	Mostly crosses in the spinal cord before ascending in the lateral funiculus	Conveys proprioceptive data that influence muscle tone and synergy necessary for coordinated muscle movements
Spinotectal tract	Posterior horn	Tectum (roof) of the midbrain	Ascends crossed in the lateral funiculus	Conveys general sensory information that influences pupil reaction and head and eye movement in response to stimuli

DESCENDING TRACTS

Rubrospinal tract	Red nucleus of the midbrain	Anterior horn	Crosses in the midbrain and descends in the lateral funiculus	Conveys impulses to control muscle tone and synergy and to maintain posture
Lateral corticospinal tract	Cerebral cortical motor areas	Anterior horn	Up to 90% crosses in the medulla and descends in the lateral funiculus	Carries impulses for voluntary movement
Anterior corticospinal tract	Cerebral cortical motor areas	Anterior horn	Descends in the anterior funiculus and crosses in the cord at the level at which it terminates	Carries impulses for voluntary movement
Tectospinal tract	Superior collicus of the midbrain	Anterior horn in the cervical spinal cord	Crosses in the midbrain and descends in the anterior funiculus	Mediates optic and auditory reflexes (e.g., reflexive head turning in response to visual or auditory stimuli)

From American Association of Critical Care Nurses: *Core curriculum for critical care nursing*, ed 6, Philadelphia, 2006, Saunders.

            (c) Light touch from skin
            (d) Discrete localization
            (e) Two-point discrimination
            (f) Vibratory sense
            (g) Stereognosis
        (2) Originate in posterior white columns and terminate in medulla where they cross and continue to thalamus

    7. Descending tracts
      a. Lateral corticospinal (pyramidal)
        (1) Voluntary motor movement, especially contraction of small muscle groups such as hands, fingers, feet, toes
        (2) Originate in motor areas of cerebral cortex on opposite side and terminate in anterior gray columns

    8. Upper motor neurons (UMNs)
      a. Located entirely in CNS
      b. Neurons and their fibers
      c. Extend from cerebral centers to cells in spinal cord
      d. Facilitating and inhibitory descending pathways that modify lower motor neurons
      e. UMN lesions cause:
        (1) Spastic paralysis
        (2) Clonus
        (3) Increased muscle tone and spasticity
        (4) Little to no atrophy of muscles involved
        (5) Hyperactive deep tendon reflexes
        (6) Babinski's sign

    9. Lower motor neurons (LMNs)
      a. Located in anterior horn cells and spinal and peripheral nerves
      b. Receive impulses from different levels of CNS and channels to muscles
      c. LMN lesions cause:
        (1) Flaccid paralysis
        (2) Total loss of voluntary muscle control with complete transection
        (3) Decreased muscle tone and flaccidity
        (4) Diminished or absent reflexes
        (5) Absence of pathological reflexes
        (6) Local twitching of muscle groups
        (7) Progressive atrophy of atonic muscles

  10. Spinal roots
      a. Dorsal (posterior) roots: convey afferent (sensory) impulses from skin segments (dermatomal areas) to dorsal root ganglia
      b. Ventral (anterior) roots: convey efferent (motor) impulses from spinal cord to body
      c. Dorsal and ventral roots meet and join to form spinal nerve.

III. ANATOMY AND PHYSIOLOGY OF THE PERIPHERAL NERVOUS SYSTEM
  A. Spinal nerves (Figure 33-21)
    1. Thirty-one symmetric nerve pairs exit from spinal cord.
      a. Cervical (8): exit above corresponding vertebrae
      b. Thoracic (12): exit below corresponding vertebrae
      c. Lumbar (5): exit below corresponding vertebrae
      d. Sacrum (5): exit below corresponding vertebrae
      e. Coccyx (1): exits below corresponding vertebrae
    2. Formed by union of anterior and posterior roots attached to spinal cord
    3. Spinal segment made up of corresponding spinal cord segment plus spinal nerves
  B. Dermatomes (Figure 33-22): skin areas supplied by the dorsal root of a spinal nerve
  C. Plexuses (Table 33-6)

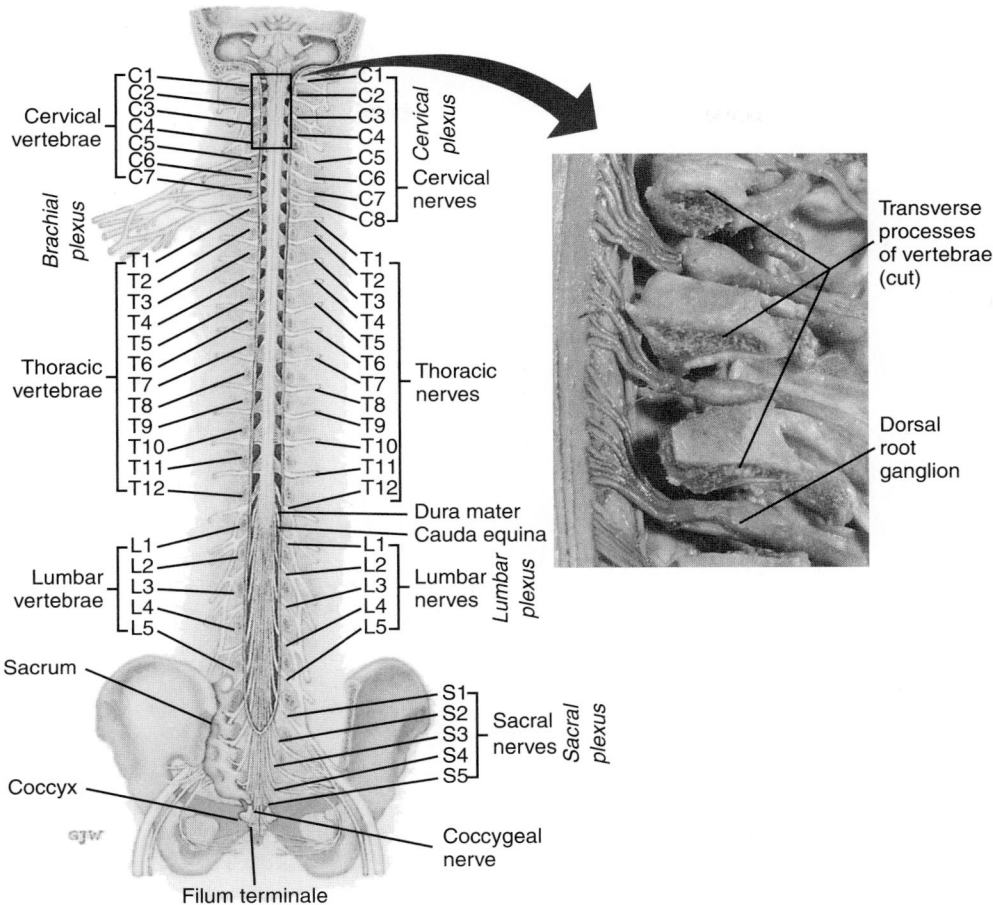

FIGURE 33-21 ■ Spinal nerves. Each of the 31 pairs of spinal nerves exits the spinal cavity from the intervertebral foramina. The names of the vertebrae are given on the left and the names of the corresponding spinal nerves on the right. Note that after leaving the spinal cavity, many of the spinal nerves interconnect to form plexuses. (From Thibodeau GA, Patton K: *Anatomy and physiology,* ed 6, St Louis, 2007, Mosby.)

     1. Network of interlacing spinal nerve roots formed by primary branch of nerves or by terminal funiculi
     2. Cervical (C1-C4)
       a. Innervates muscles of neck and shoulders
       b. Gives rise to phrenic nerve, which supplies diaphragm
     3. Brachial: radial and ulnar nerves merge (C5-C8 and T1).
     4. Lumbar: gives rise to femoral nerve (L1-L4)
     5. Sacral: gives rise to sciatic nerve (L4-5 & S1-S4)
IV. ASSESSMENT
   A. Spinal cord function
     1. Motor function
       a. Muscle size: inspect for atrophy, hypertrophy.
       b. Muscle strength: as described in neurological assessment
       c. Muscle tone
       d. Coordination
         (1) Rapid alternating movements
         (2) Heel to shin
         (3) Finger to nose

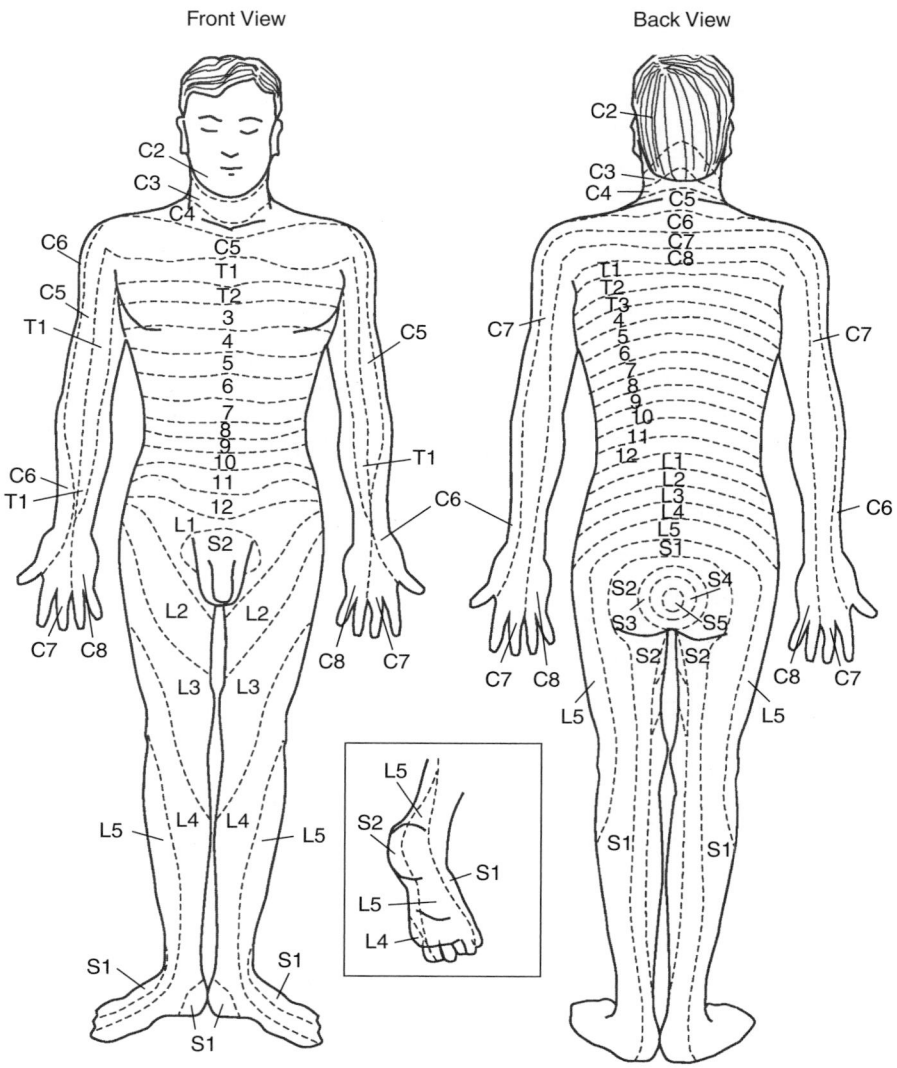

FIGURE 33-22 ■ Dermatomes. (From McQuillan KA, Von Rueden KT, Hartsock RL, et al [eds]: *Trauma nursing from resuscitation through rehabilitation,* ed 3, Philadelphia, 2002, Saunders.)

2. Sensory function
   a. Superficial sensation
      (1) Light touch (cotton wisp)
      (2) Pain (pinprick)
   b. Deep sensation
   c. Technique
      (1) Have patient close eyes.
      (2) Begin at feet and work upward systematically.
      (3) Compare findings on both sides.
      (4) Ask patient to tell you when sensation is felt.
      (5) Note dermatome level.
3. Reflexes
   a. Superficial
      (1) Abdominal
      (2) Cremasteric

■ TABLE 33-6
■ ■ **Plexuses and Their Locations and Areas of Innervation**

Name	Spinal Nerve Anterior Branches That Comprise Plexus	Location of Plexus	Important Nerves That Emerge	Areas of Innervation
Cervical	C1-C4	Deep within the neck	Portion of the phrenic nerve	Muscles and skin of a portion of the head, neck, and upper shoulders; diaphragm
Brachial	C5-C8 and T1	Deep within the shoulder	Phrenic, circumflex, musculocutaneous, ulnar, median, and radial nerves	Shoulder, arm, and hand; diaphragm
Lumbar	L1-L4	Lumbar region of the back	Femoral cutaneous, femoral and genitofemoral branches	Anterior abdominal wall and genitalia; thigh and leg
Sacral	L4 and L5, and S1-S4	Inner surface of the posterior pelvic wall	Tibial, common peroneal, sciatic, and pudendal nerves	Skin of the leg; muscles of the posterior thigh, leg, and foot

From American Association of Critical Care Nurses: *Core curriculum for critical care nursing,* ed 6, Philadelphia, 2006, Saunders.

       (3) Bulbocavernosus
       (4) Perianal reflex (anal wink)
       (5) Plantar
   b. Deep tendon reflexes
       (1) Biceps
       (2) Triceps
       (3) Brachioradial
       (4) Patellar
   c. Pathological
       (1) Corticospinal tract involvement
          (a) Babinski's reflex positive
B. Neurological
   1. Nursing history of patient's current health status
      a. Medical history
         (1) Family history
         (2) Social history
         (3) Allergies (medications, food, etc.)
      b. Medication history
         (1) Over-the-counter drugs
         (2) Prescription drugs
         (3) Herbal supplements
         (4) Nutritional supplements
         (5) Note use of:
            (a) Analgesics
            (b) Anticonvulsants
            (c) Sedatives
            (d) Anticoagulants
            (e) Stimulants
            (f) Antihypertensive drugs
            (g) Cardiac drugs
            (h) Tranquilizers
            (i) Other medications

    c. Surgical history

      (1) Any past surgery performed

      (2) Any procedures performed

  2. Baseline status: necessary to determine improvement or deterioration in patient's condition

    a. Levels of consciousness (LOC): defining elements

      (1) Full consciousness

        (a) Awake, alert, and oriented to time, place, and person

        (b) Able to express ideas verbally or in writing

        (c) Comprehends spoken words

      (2) Confusion

        (a) Disoriented to time, place, or person

        (b) Shortened attention span

        (c) Difficulty with memory

        (d) Difficulty in following commands

        (e) Bewildered easily

        (f) Alterations in perception of stimuli

        (g) Hallucinations; agitated, restless, and irritable

        (h) Increased confusion at night

      (3) Lethargy

        (a) Oriented to time, place, and person

        (b) Very slow and sluggish in speech, mental processes, and motor activities

        (c) Responds to painful stimuli

      (4) Obtunded

        (a) Arousable with stimuli, drowsy

        (b) Responds verbally with a word or two

        (c) Follows simple commands when stimulated

      (5) Stupor

        (a) Lies quietly, with minimal spontaneous movement

        (b) Unresponsive except to vigorous and repeated stimuli

        (c) Responds appropriately to painful stimuli

      (6) Coma

        (a) Sleeplike state with eyes closed

        (b) Unresponsive to stimuli

        (c) Does not make any verbal sounds

    b. Assessment technique

      (1) Arouse patient to maximum level of wakefulness.

      (2) Begin by calling patient by familiar name.

      (3) Assess motor and sensory function.

      (4) If no response, shake patient.

      (5) If no response, apply noxious stimuli, being careful not to injure patient.

        (a) Nail bed pressure

        (b) Supraorbital pressure

        (c) Pinching trapezius muscle

        (d) Pressure to Achilles tendon

        (e) Sternal pressure

      (6) Assess orientation to environment.

        (a) Ask alert, verbal patient to tell you where he or she is.

        (b) Use yes-or-no questions to assess intubated patients.

        (c) For patients who may be confused, give choices similar to yes-or-no questions for intubated patients (i.e., "Is this place a hospital? Is this place your home?").

        (d) Loss of orientation begins with loss of time, then place, then person.

        (e) Avoid using "squeeze my hand" to assess strength or ability to follow commands.

      (i) Patients with diffuse cerebral injury, particularly frontal lobe problems, retain strong hand grasp reflex similar to infant.

      (ii) Give patient a single step command (e.g., "show me two fingers").

      (iii) If you do ask patient to squeeze your hand, also ask patient to let go of your hand.

    (f) Assess for behavioral changes such as restlessness, irritability, combativeness.

  c. Pupillary reactivity (Figure 33-23)

    (1) Oculomotor nerve (CN III) and brainstem control pupil size and reaction.

    (2) Sluggish pupils indicate pressure on CN III, which runs parallel to brainstem.

    (3) Assessment technique

      (a) Observe size, shape, equality, and reaction to light.

      (b) Assess and compare pupils bilaterally.

      (c) Record pupil size as small, medium, or large unless reference is available to measure exact size (Figure 33-24).

    (4) Be aware of effect of anesthetic agents and preoperative medications on pupil size and reactivity.

      (a) Constricting agents (miotic)

        (i) Opiates and narcotics

        (ii) Cholinergic agents

          [a] Optical miotics (pilocarpine)

          [b] Neostigmine bromide (Prostigmin)

          [c] Barbiturates

          [d] Edrophonium chloride (Tensilon)

          [e] Pyridostigmine bromide (Mestinon)

      (b) Dilating agents (mydriatic)

        (i) Anticholinergic agents

          [a] Atropine sulfate

          [b] Naloxone hydrochloride

          [c] Scopolamine

          [d] Glycopyrrolate

      (c) Topical mydriatics

      (d) Adrenergic agents (sympathomimetic or dilate pupils for exam)

        (i) Catecholamines

          [a] Dobutamine (Dobutrex)

          [b] Dopamine (Intropin)

          [c] Epinephrine (Adrenalin)

          [d] Isoproterenol (Isuprel)

          [e] Norepinephrine (Levophed)

        (ii) Noncatecholamine agents

          [a] Ephedrine

          [b] Metaraminol (Aramine)

          [c] Phenylephrine (Neo-Synephrine)

    (5) Pupil size can be altered by direct eye trauma or congenital malformations.

    (6) Any new change in pupil size or reactivity should be reported to physician at once (Figure 33-25).

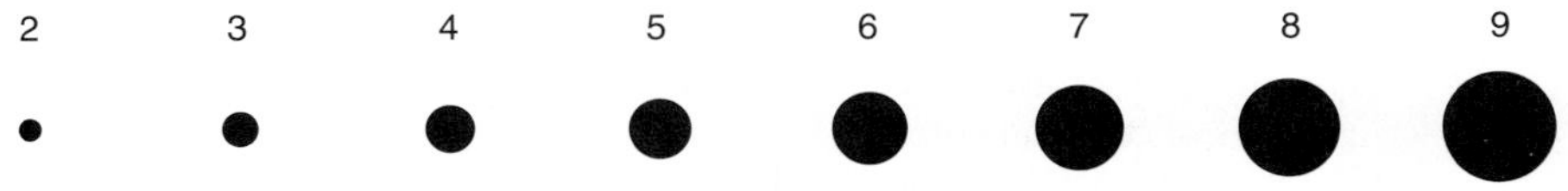

2	3	4	5	6	7	8	9

FIGURE 33-23 ■ Pupil gauge (millimeters).

In assessing pupillary size using either descriptive terms or a gauge, each pupil is assessed individually and then the findings for each pupil are compared. This is very important because pupils are normally equal.

Descriptive Term	Definition	Findings
Pinpoint 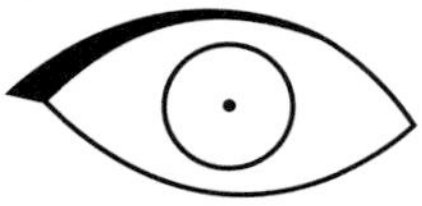	The pupil is so small that it is barely visible or appears as small as a pinpoint.	Seen with opiate overdose, pontine hemorrhage, ischemia.
Small 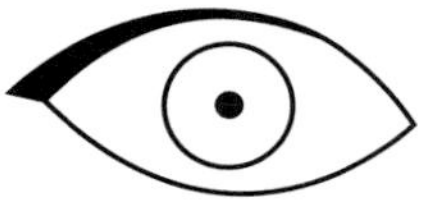	The pupil appears smaller than average, but larger than pinpoint.	Seen normally if the person is in a brightly lit place; also seen with miotic ophthalmic drops, opiates, pontine hemorrhage, Horner's syndrome, bilateral diencephalic lesions, and metabolic coma.
Midposition 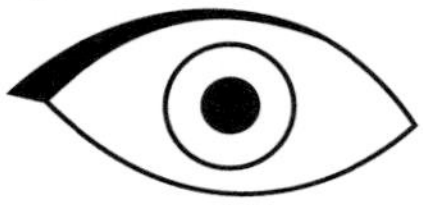	When the pupil and iris are observed, about half of their diameter is iris and half is pupil.	Seen normally; if pupils are midposition and nonreactive, midbrain damage is the cause.
Large 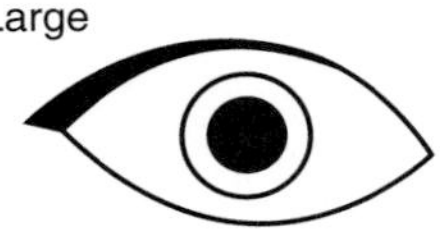	The pupils are larger than average, but there is still an appreciable amount of iris visible.	Seen normally if room is dark; may be seen with some drugs, such as amphetamines; glutethimide (Doriden) overdose; mydriatics; cycloplegic agents; and some orbital injuries.
Dilated 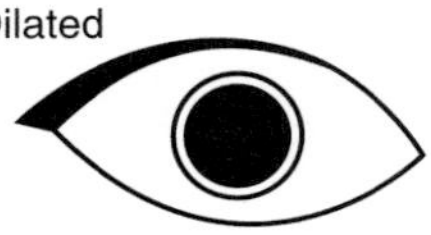	When the pupil and iris are observed, one is struck by the largeness of the pupil with only the slightest ring of iris, which is barely visible.	Abnormal finding; bilateral, fixed, and dilated pupils are seen in the terminal stage of severe anoxia-ischemia or at death.

FIGURE 33-24 ■ Assessing pupillary size. (From Hickey JV: *The clinical practice of neurological and neurosurgical nursing,* ed 5, Philadelphia, 2003, Lippincott.)

  d. Motor function
    (1) Voluntary motor movement controlled by fibers originating in frontal lobes of cerebral cortex
    (2) Fibers descend through brainstem; mostly at level of medulla and continue to spinal cord
    (3) Assessment technique for alert patient

(a) Test strength of all muscle groups against resistance and gravity (Box 33-1, Table 33-7).

(b) Upper extremities: palmar (pronator) drift method
    (i) Ask patient to close eyes and extend arms in front, with palms up.
    (ii) Paretic arm will slowly drift downward and palm will turn upward.

(c) Muscle strength assessed by testing active, passive, and active resistive movement
    (i) Upper extremities
        [a] Grasp: have patient squeeze your first and second fingers; compare right with left.

(Note: Compare findings with previous assessment data, document, and report new findings to the physician.)

OCULOMOTOR NERVE COMPRESSION

Observation

One pupil (R) is larger than the other (L), which is of normal size. The dilated pupil (R) does not react to light, although the other pupil (L) reacts normally. Ptosis may be seen in the dilated pupil.

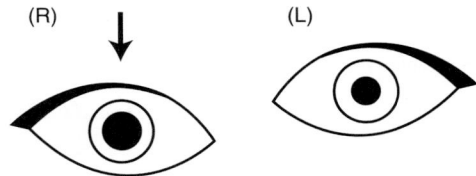

(R)   (L)

Interpretation

A dilated, nonreactive (fixed) pupil indicates that the control for papillary constriction is not functioning. The parasympathetic fibers of the oculomotor nerve control papillary constriction. The most common cause of interruption of this function is compression of the oculomotor nerve, usually against the tentorium or posterior cerebral artery.

Action

Compare with data from previous assessments. If the dilated pupil is a new finding, it should immediately be reported to the physican, because the process of rostral-caudal downward pressure must be treated without delay. In this situation, changes in LOC, motor function, sensory function, and possible vital signs would be expected.

BILATERAL DIENCEPHALIC DAMAGE

Observation

On examination, the pupils appear small but equal in size, and both react to direct light, contracting when light is introduced and dilating when light is withdrawn.

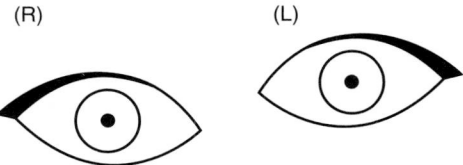

(R)   (L)

Interpretation

The sympathetic pathway that begins in the hypothalamus is affected. Because both pupils are equal in size and respond equally to light, the damage is bilateral. Therefore, it can be assumed that there is bilateral injury in the diencephalons (thalamus and hypothalamus). Because metabolic coma can also result in bilaterally small pupils that react to light, this diagnostic possibility must be ruled out.

Action

Compare findings with previous assessments to determine change. Consider metabolic coma by reviewing blood chemistry findings and other data. For example, diabetic acidosis may result in a metabolic coma because of a high blood glucose level.

FIGURE 33-25 ■ Common abnormal pupillary responses. (From Hickey JV: *The clinical practice of neurological and neurosurgical nursing,* ed 5, Philadelphia, 2003, Lippincott.)

HORNER'S SYNDROME

Observation

(R)   (L)

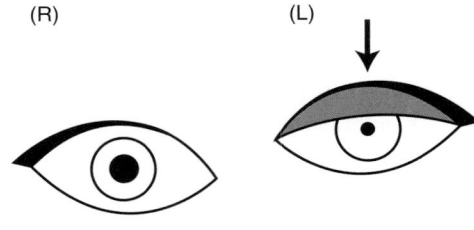

One pupil (L) is smaller than the other (R), although both pupils react to light. The eyelid on the same side as the smaller pupil (L) droops (ptosis). Inability to sweat (anhidrosis) on the same side of the face as the ptosis is common. The symptoms of a small reactive pupil, ptosis, and anhidrosis combine to form Horner's syndrome.

Interpretation

There is an interruption of the ipsilateral sympathetic innervation to the pupil that can be caused by hypothalamic damage, a lesion of the lateral medulla, or the ventrolateral cervical spinal cord, and, sometimes, by occlusion of the internal carotid artery.

Action

If this is a new finding, it should be reported.

MIDBRAIN DAMAGE

Observation

(R)   (L)

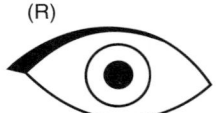 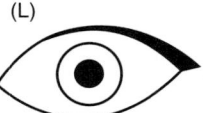

Both pupils are at midposition and nonreactive to light.

Interpretation

With midposition, nonreactive pupils, neither sympathetic nor parasympathetic innervation is functional. This finding is often associated with midbrain infarction or transtentorial herniation.

Action

Compare findings with previous asessment data. Consider also changes in other components of the assessment. The pupils should be evaluated in conjunction with other neurological assessments. Report new findings to the physician.

PONTINE DAMAGE

Observation

(R)   (L)

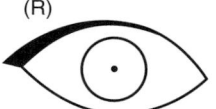 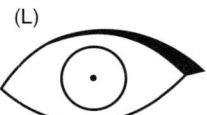

Very small (pinpoint), nonreactive pupils are seen.

Interpretation

This finding indicates focal damage of the pons, often due to hemorrhage or ischemia. *Bilateral* pinpoint pupils may occur from opiate drug overdose, so this possibility should be ruled out.

Action

Compare findings with previous assessment data. Report findings to the physician immediately. Other changes in neurological status, such as decreased LOC and respiratory abnormalities, would be expected.

FIGURE 33-25—cont'd.

          [b] Extension: patient extends arms in front with palms up, eyes closed; observe for arm drift, indicating mild weakness.
     (ii) Lower extremities
          [a] Leg lift: lying in bed, able to lift one leg at a time to clear bed and hold without wavering; compare left with right.

■ BOX 33-1
■ **STRENGTH SCALE**

5 points: full strength, no deficit or weakness
4 points: able to lift extremity against gravity and maintain position without wavering
3 points: able to lift extremity against gravity, but wavers and cannot sustain
2 points: able to slide along support surfaces such as bed or chair
1 point: flicker or trace movement
0 points: no movement

■ TABLE 33-7
■ ■ **Muscle Groups, Associated Level of Spinal Cord Innervation, and Method of Testing**

Muscle(s) Tested	Primary Level(s) of Spinal Nerve Innervation	Method of Testing
Deltoids	C5	Raising of arms
Biceps	C5	Flexion of elbow
Wrist extensors	C6	Extension of wrist
Triceps	C7	Extension of elbow
Hand intrinsics	C8-T1	Hand squeezing, finger flexion, finger abduction
Iliopsoas	L1, L2	Hip flexion
Hip adductors	L2-L4	Adduction of hips (squeezing legs together)
Hip abductors	L4, L5, S1	Abduction of hips (separating hips)
Quadriceps	L3, L4	Knee extension
Hamstrings	L5, S1, S2	Knee flexion
Tibialis anterior	L4, L5	Dorsiflexion of foot
Extensor hallucis longus	L5	Extension of great toe
Gastrocnemius	S1	Plantar flexion of foot

In American Association of Critical Care Nurses: *Core curriculum for critical care nursing,* ed 6, Philadelphia, 2006, Saunders.
Adapted from Bader MK, Littlejohns LR, eds: *AANN core curriculum for neuroscience nursing,* ed 4, St Louis, 2004, Saunders.

      (iii) Trunk
        [a] Able to sit on side of bed independently
      (iv) Sensory (always compare right and left sides and test with patient's eyes closed)
        [a] Touch: eyes closed, identifies where touched; test opposite side to see whether each side "feels the same."
      (v) Pain and temperature: eyes closed, identifies if pinprick is sharp and back of pin is dull, or identifies ice chip as cold
    (4) Assessment technique for unconscious patient: apply noxious stimuli and observe response.
      (a) Purposeful movement, such as pushing away stimulus, indicates intact neuraxis.
      (b) Localization of gross location of stimulus indicates cortical dysfunction.
      (c) Check for Babinski's sign, an indicator for disease along the voluntary motor pathways.
      (d) Nonpurposeful responses indicate dysfunction deeper in cerebral hemispheres and midbrain area.
        (i) Incomplete removal of stimulus
        (ii) Slight movement without moving away from stimulus

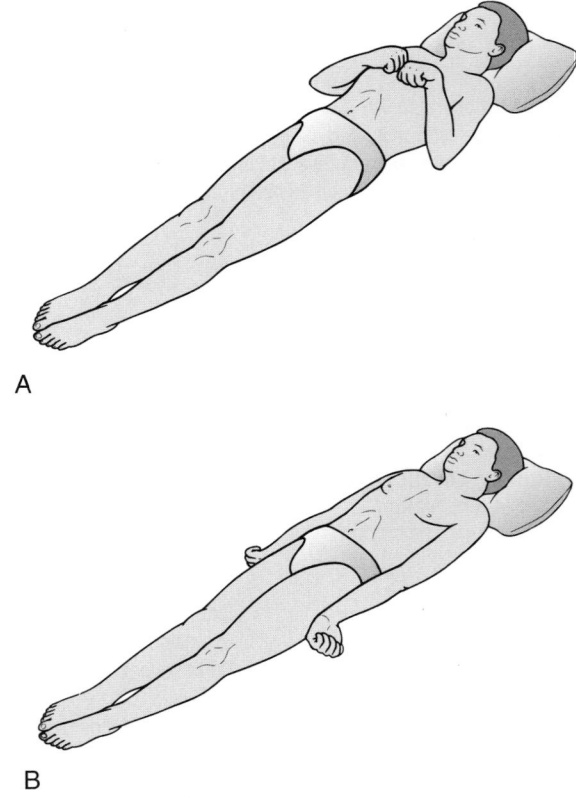

A

B

FIGURE 33-26 ■ **A,** Decorticate posturing. **B,** Decerebrate posturing. (From Lewis SM, Heitkemper MM, Dirksen SR: *Medical-surgical nursing: Assessment and management of clinical problems,* ed 5, St Louis, 1999, Mosby.)

       (iii) Withdrawal of only the part stimulated
       (iv) Lower extremities flex at knees
    (e) Decorticate posturing (flexion response; Figure 33-26, *A*)
       (i)   Occurs with disruption of corticospinal pathways
       (ii) Loss of cerebral cortex influence over movement
    (f) Decerebrate posturing (extension response; Figure 33-26, *B*)
       (i)   Indicates damage in deeper cerebral hemispheres and upper brainstem
       (ii) Indicative of severe brain dysfunction with poor prognosis
  e. Reflexes that reflect integrity of neuraxis
    (1) Oculocephalic reflex (doll's eyes)
      (a) Can only be elicited in patients with depressed LOC
      (b) Alert patients override reflex.
      (c) Tests integrity of brainstem between CN III and CN VIII
      (d) Technique
       (i)   Hold patient's eyes open.
       (ii) Briskly turn patient's head side to side.
       (iii) Pause to assess eyes on each side.
      (e) Interpretation
       (i)   Normal (doll's eye reflex present)
         [a] Conjugate eye deviation to direction opposite direction head is turned; eyes move in orbits.
         [b] In comatose patient, indicates brainstem is intact between CN III and CN VIII.

(ii) Abnormal (doll's eye reflex absent)
[a] Disconjugate eye movements
[b] Eyes move with head; eyes do not move in orbits.
[c] Eyes appear fixed, like painted eyes of a china doll.
[d] Indicative of severe lesion in brainstem
[e] Contraindicated in actual or suspected cervical injuries
(2) Oculovestibular reflex (cold calorics)
(a) Provides information about integrity of brainstem and connections to cerebral cortex
(b) Contraindicated in patients with ruptured tympanic membrane
(c) Technique
(i) Assess integrity of tympanic membrane.
(ii) Cold water (50 mL) slowly injected into external auditory canal
(iii) Observe eye movement (two phases).
[a] Normal: eyes initially deviate to side of stimulus, followed by rapid component of nystagmus deviating toward opposite side.
[b] Eye deviation is common in brainstem; poor prognosis.
f. Vital signs
(1) Changes usually seen late in clinical course; should not be relied on to signal impending neurological clinical problems
(2) Observe for widening pulse pressure: systolic blood pressure increases while diastolic pressure decreases.
(3) Observe for changes in respiratory rate and rhythm.
(4) Observe for Cushing's triad (reflex), a sign of increased ICP.
(a) Increased systolic blood pressure
(b) Decreased diastolic blood pressure
(c) Decreased pulse rate (bradycardia)
(5) Assessment of CN function may be needed, depending on underlying neurological problem.
g. Documentation
(1) Variety of assessment tools available, but most include parameters of Glasgow Coma Scale
(2) Frequency of neurological assessment may be dictated by unit protocol and patient condition.
(a) Report abnormal findings to physician.
(b) Be alert to subtle changes in any of the above parameters.
(3) Give specific descriptions of stimulus used and resulting response of patient.
V. DYNAMICS OF INCREASED ICP
A. Monro-Kellie hypothesis
1. Skull is closed container with fixed volume of blood, CSF, and brain tissue contained within nondistensible skull.
2. If the volume of one intracranial constituent increases, a reciprocal decrease in the volume of the other constituents must occur or the ICP will increase.
3. Contents of skull
a. Blood: 10%
b. CSF: 10%
c. Brain tissue: 80%
4. Volume-pressure relationship (elastance)
a. Small increases in volume more readily compensated for in uninjured or noncompromised brain
b. Increases in volume over extended period more readily compensated for than comparable volume over shorter period
c. Little room in skull for slack
d. In traumatized or injured brain, even small increases in volume can produce drastic elevations in ICP.

5. Compensatory mechanisms: increase in one intracranial volume must be compensated for by a decrease in one of the remaining volumes.
   a. Displacement and reduction of CSF volume
   b. Reduction in blood volume
   c. Displacement of brain tissue
6. Normal intracranial pressure
   a. 0 to 15 mm Hg—with invasive monitoring
   b. 50 to 150 mm H_2O with external manometer
7. Causes of increased ICP
   a. Abnormal production, circulation, or absorption of CSF
      (1) Hydrocephalus
         (a) Communicating
         (b) Noncommunicating
      (2) Congenital abnormalities: hydrocephalus, Arnold-Chiari malformation
      (3) Obstructive masses: tumors, abscesses
   b. Amount of volume increase
   c. Total volume within the intracranial cavity
   d. Rate of volume change (the faster volume added, the greater the rise in ICP)
   e. Intracranial compliance or the capacity for compensation
   f. Increase in intracranial blood volume
      (1) Hemorrhage
      (2) Hyperthermia: increases metabolic demands and thus blood volume
      (3) Venous drainage impairment
      (4) Hypercapnia: increases in partial pressure of carbon dioxide in arterial blood ($Paco_2$) or hydrogen ion (H^+) levels
      (5) Vascular abnormalities
         (a) Aneurysms
         (b) Arteriovenous malformations (AVMs)
      (6) Vasodilating drugs
         (a) Anesthetic gases
            (i) Halothane
            (ii) Enflurane
            (iii) Isoflurane
            (iv) Nitrous oxide
            (v) Sevoflurane
            (vi) Desflurane
         (b) Some antihypertensives
         (c) Some histamines
   g. Increase in brain tissue volume
      (1) Tumors
      (2) Infectious processes
      (3) Edema
   h. Other
      (1) Respiratory
         (a) Intubation
         (b) Positive end-expiratory pressure
         (c) Increased airway pressure
      (2) Body positions
         (a) Trendelenburg
         (b) Prone
         (c) Extreme hip flexion
         (d) Neck flexion
      (3) Coughing
      (4) Isometric muscle exercises
      (5) Valsalva maneuver
      (5) Noxious stimuli
      (6) Emotional upset
      (7) Pain

(8) Seizure activity
(9) Rapid eye movement sleep or arousal from sleep
(10) Shivering
(11) Vomiting
(12) Straining/coughing on endotracheal tube
(13) Clustering care activities

8. Autoregulation: ability of cerebral circulation to maintain relatively constant cerebral blood flow and pressure needed to provide oxygen and nutrients to brain tissue
   a. Cerebral perfusion pressure (CPP): primarily dependent on mean arterial pressure (MAP)
      (1) Determines cerebral blood flow
      (2) CPP = MAP − ICP (or central venous pressure [CVP], whichever is greater)
      (3) As ICP increases and approaches the MAP, CPP decreases.
      (4) Respiratory gas tension (i.e., the relationship between $Paco_2$ and cerebral blood flow)
      (5) Temperature changes: cerebral blood flow changes 5% to 7% per 1° C change in temperature.
      (6) Interpretation of CPP values (Box 33-2)
   b. Invasive ICP monitoring needed to calculate CPP; can estimate CPP by using CVP also.
   c. CPP calculation should be part of neurological assessment.

9. Clinical presentation of signs of increased ICP
   a. Depends on location, cause, and degree of compensation
   b. Damage to brain tissue
      (1) Tissue ischemia as a result of decreased cerebral blood flow
      (2) Brain structures compressed by increasing pressure
   c. Symptoms
      (1) Deterioration in LOC
      (2) Pupillary dysfunction
      (3) Changes in motor status
      (4) Changes in vital signs
         (a) Cushing's triad:
            (i) Hypertension
            (ii) Bradycardia
            (iii) Respiratory disturbances
         (b) Reflex: periodic increase in arterial blood pressure with reflex slowing of the heart (often observed and correlated with abrupt increase in ICP lasting 1–15 minutes)
      (5) Seizures
      (6) Headaches
      (7) Vomiting
      (8) Papilledema
      (9) CN palsies
      (10) Sensory changes

■ BOX 33-2
■ **INTERPRETATION OF CPP VALUES**

70 to 100 mm Hg: normal
60 mm Hg: provides minimally adequate blood supply
<50 mm Hg: autoregulation begins to fail
<40 mm Hg: cerebral blood flow decreases by 25%
<30 mm Hg: incompatible with life: neuronal hypoxia and cell death

CPP, Cerebral perfusion pressure.

  (11) Posturing

  (12) Altered breathing patterns

  (13) Bulging fontanelles in infants

  (14) Impaired brainstem reflexes

 10. Herniation syndromes: increasing pressure causes displacement of brain tissue (Figure 33-27).

  a. Transcalvarial herniation

   (1) Occurs at surgical incision site or through site of gunshot or stab wound or fracture site

   (2) Risk of infection

  b. Cingulate herniation

   (1) One of cerebral hemispheres displaced laterally across midline, with blood vessels and tissue compressed

   (2) Not life-threatening but a sign of brain decompensation

  c. Central transtentorial herniation

   (1) Downward displacement of cerebral hemispheres through tentorial notch located at level of tentorium cerebelli, which separates cerebellum from cerebral hemispheres

   (2) Life-threatening

  d. Uncal (lateral) herniation

   (1) Displacement of medial tip of temporal lobe (uncus) through tentorium, compressing midbrain

   (2) Most common herniation syndrome

   (3) Life-threatening when hemorrhage or brainstem compression occurs.

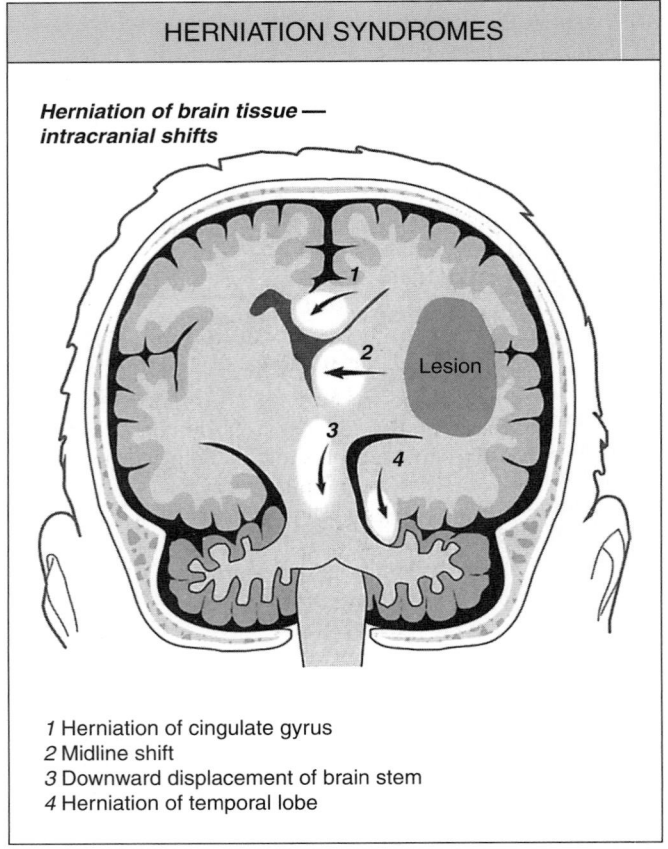

FIGURE 33-27 ■ Herniation syndrome. (From Luckmann J: *Saunders manual of nursing care*, Philadelphia, 1997, WB Saunders.)

      e. Infratentorial herniation
         (1) Compression of brainstem, cerebellum
         (2) Medullary collapse
         (3) May be life-threatening
 B. Medical-surgical interventions
   1. Direct: remove cause by surgical intervention.
   2. Indirect
      a. Maintain patent airway.
      b. Provide oxygen.
      c. Maintain normal fluid and electrolyte balance.
         (1) Adequate fluid management with saline, to avoid dehydration and hypotension
         (2) Serum osmolarity kept between 290 and 320 mOsm/kg
         (3) Monitor serum glucose, electrolytes.
      d. Avoid administration of narcotics; may lead to hypercapnia.
      e. Give diuretics.
         (1) Osmotic diuretics: mannitol
            (a) Draws water from extracellular space of edematous brain into plasma
            (b) Does not cross blood-brain barrier
            (c) Can cause fluid and electrolyte imbalances
         (2) Furosemide (Lasix)
            (a) Thought to decrease CSF production
            (b) Decreases systemic fluid volume
            (c) Manage rebound effect of mannitol
            (d) Monitor electrolytes (K^+)
         (3) Acetazolamide (Diamox): carbonic anhydrase inhibitor
            (a) Decreases CSF production
            (b) Vasoconstrictor
            (c) Monitor electrolytes (K^+).
      f. Administer corticosteroids.
         (1) Controversial with head trauma or cerebral infarction with edema, but useful with brain tumors
         (2) Dosage tapered before discontinued
      g. Initiate therapeutic hyperventilation.
         (1) Maintain Pco_2 between 27 and 33 mm Hg.
         (2) Should be done with mechanical ventilation
         (3) Short-term use recommended (<72 hours); not for prophylaxis
         (4) Manual hyperventilation with Ambu recommended only emergently for patients with "pressure signs" until ventilator available
      h. Reduce cerebral stimulation and metabolic demand.
         (1) Control pain.
         (2) Maintain normothermia: if using hypothermia blankets, prevent shivering, which will increase metabolic demands and ICP.
         (3) Control seizures with phenytoin sodium.
         (4) Control hyperactivity with sedation.
         (5) Neuromuscular blockade for severe agitation in intubated patients
   3. Ventriculostomy to drain CSF
   4. Operative decompression: surgical removal of mass, lesion, blood, or tumor causing the increased ICP
 C. Nursing interventions
   1. Goals
      a. Protect patient at risk from sudden increases in ICP.
      b. Prevent permanent brain damage.
         (1) Maintenance of patent airway
         (2) Ongoing neurological assessment
   2. Positioning
      a. Elevate head of bed 30° to 45°.
      b. Maintain head in neutral position with sandbags or Philadelphia collar.

      c. Avoid prone position.

      d. Patients with infratentorial craniotomies may be positioned flat or slightly elevated.

   3. Prevent Valsalva maneuver by having patient exhale.

   4. Prevent isometric muscle contraction by assisting patient in turning.

   5. Avoid clustering of nursing activities—space nursing care to give patient frequent rest periods, which decreases stimulation.

D. ICP monitoring

   1. Purpose

      a. Monitor trends in ICP (normal ICP, 0–15 mm Hg).

      b. Measure CPP.

      c. Test intracranial compliance.

   2. ICP monitoring techniques (Figure 33-28)

      a. Intraventricular catheter: inserted through anterior horn of lateral ventricle on nondominant side

         (1) Most accurate measurement of ICP

         (2) Allows for sampling of CSF

         (3) Intrathecal administration of medications

         (4) Use as ventriculostomy to decrease increased ICP.

         (5) Increased risk of infection and hemorrhage

         (6) Catheter placement difficult with small ventricles

      b. Subarachnoid bolt (Richmond or Becker bolt): inserted into subarachnoid space through cranial burr hole

         (1) Less risk of infection

         (2) Placement is easier and can be used in patients with small ventricles.

         (3) Inability to sample CSF and test compliance

         (4) Does not allow for intrathecal administration of medications

         (5) Questionable reflection of actual ICP

      c. Epidural or subdural sensors or catheters: inserted into epidural or subdural space

         (1) Easily inserted

         (2) Decreased risk of infection

         (3) Brain or subarachnoid space not penetrated

         (4) Questionable reflection of actual ICP because of pressure from adjacent dura

         (5) Inability to sample CSF

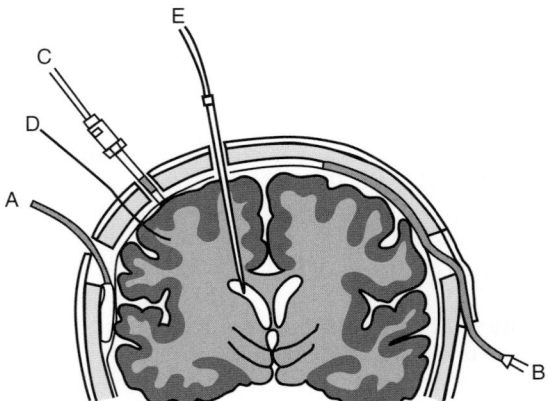

FIGURE 33-28 ■ Coronal section of the brain showing potential sites for placement of intracranial pressure monitoring devices. **A,** Epidural. **B,** Subdural. **C,** Subarachnoid. **D,** Intraparenchymal. **E,** Intraventricular. (From Clochesy JM, Breu C, Cardin S, et al [eds]: *Critical care nursing,* ed 2, Philadelphia, 1996, Saunders.)

   d. Fiberoptic transducer–tipped catheter
      (1) Easily inserted and requires small hole
      (2) Versatile—can be inserted into:
         (a) Ventricles
         (b) Subarachnoid space
         (c) Brain parenchyma
         (d) Subdural space
      (3) Zero balancing required only at time of insertion
      (4) Decreased risk of infection
      (5) Does not allow for CSF sampling or drainage
      (6) Periodic replacement of probe may be necessary.
      (7) Expensive
3. ICP waveforms (Figure 33-29)
   a. Mechanism is transmission of pressure to transducer that converts pressure waves into waveform visible on oscilloscope.
   b. Produced by vascular or arterial pulsations
   c. Normal ICP waveform has three characteristic peaks of decreasing amplitude:
      (1) P_1 (percussion wave): has a fairly consistent amplitude
      (2) P_2 (tidal wave): has variable amplitude
         (a) Most clinically significant
         (b) Rounded appearance from when ICP rises
         (c) When amplitude of P2 greater than P1, indicative of a decrease in compliance
      (3) P_3 (dicrotic wave): tapers to baseline
4. Nursing considerations
   a. Strict aseptic technique
   b. Observe for leaks and breaks in system.
   c. Close observation of waveforms
   d. Troubleshooting of dampened waveforms
   e. Recalibration of system according to unit protocol
   f. Never irrigate system.
   g. Goals of care
      (1) ICP remains below 20 mm Hg.
      (2) CPP remains above 60 mm Hg or as ordered.
      (3) Cerebral blood flow or cerebral oxygenation remains within the desired range (approximately 50–60 mL/100 g/min) if monitored.
   h. Calculation of intracranial compliance is physician's responsibility.
   i. Removal of system is by physician only.
VI. NEUROLOGICAL COMPLICATIONS
   A. Headache
      1. Migraine (may be triggered by many factors involved with surgical procedures)
         a. Careful history should reveal method of treatment.
         b. Analgesics, narcotics, serotonin

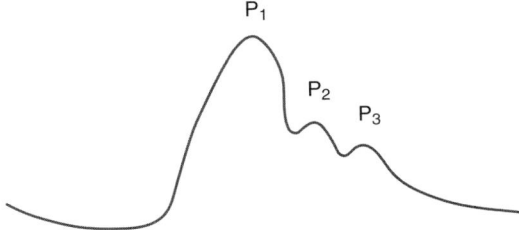

FIGURE 33-29 ■ Components of an intracranial pressure wave. (From McQuillan KA, Von Rueden KT, Hartsock RL, et al [eds]: *Trauma nursing from resuscitation through rehabilitation,* ed 3, Philadelphia, 2002, Saunders.)

     c. Ice or cool cloth to head or back of neck

     d. Treat mild hypoglycemia.

     e. Maintain fluid intake (nausea and vomiting may occur).

  2. Muscle tension (may be related to surgical position)

     a. Neutral head position

     b. Massage and topical creams

     c. Encourage range of motion of neck and shoulders.

     d. Relaxation techniques (deep breathing, etc.)

B. Seizures

  1. Generalized

     a. Generalized tonic-clonic

       (1) Description

         (a) Tonic phase

           (i) Lasts 1 to 2 minutes

           (ii) Patient is rigid, with increased muscle tone.

         (b) Clonic phase

           (i) Usually lasts 1 to 2 minutes

           (ii) Patient has jerking movements that gradually slow, then stop.

           (iii) Breathing stops for 30 seconds to 1 minute.

         (c) Postictal phase

           (i) Does not remember seizure

           (ii) Confused, usually wants to sleep

           (iii) May be combative when stimulated

       (2) Medical emergency: notify physician immediately.

         (a) Lasts more than 5 minutes

         (b) One seizure occurs after another (status epilepticus).

       (3) Treatment

         (a) Do not restrain.

         (b) Do not force anything into the mouth.

         (c) Turn to side.

         (d) Protect from self-harm and the environment.

           (i) Put pillow under head.

           (ii) Remove harmful objects.

         (e) Padded "bite" may be placed between molars if patient opens mouth.

         (f) May use oxygen if available

         (g) Suction as needed; do not force into mouth.

       (4) Assessment

         (a) What was patient doing when seizure started?

         (b) What was the first indication that a seizure had begun (confusion, jerking in any part of the body, etc.)?

         (c) Length of seizure

         (d) Physical appearance (body position, limb movement)

         (e) Bowel or bladder incontinence

         (f) Obtain stat glucose and electrolytes.

     b. Petit mal

       (1) Sometimes called "absence"

       (2) More common in children

       (3) Description

         (a) Short (5–20 seconds) seizure of blinking spells

         (b) May occur 30 or more times per day

       (4) Medical concern if number of seizures reduces quality of life

  2. Complex partial (temporal lobe)

     a. Description

       (1) Appears awake, but confused

       (2) May turn to examiner when name called

       (3) Automatisms

         (a) Repetitive activity

        (b) Not goal-oriented
           (i)   Rubbing
           (ii) Rocking
           (iii) Pulling
           (iv) Pulling at clothes or bed linens
     (4) Activity is not goal-oriented.

b. Medical emergency: notify physician immediately.
     (1) If no history of epilepsy
     (2) If lasts more than 5 minutes
     (3) If one occurs after another
     (4) Obtain stat glucose and electrolytes.
     (5) Observe closely for secondary generalization.

c. Treatment
     (1) Do not restrain; patient may become hostile and perceive intervention as a threat.
     (2) Redirect activity or ambulation by placing barriers (i.e., close doors, place chairs in patient's path).

d. Assessment
     (1) What was patient doing just before seizure?
     (2) Length of time seizure lasts
     (3) Automatisms
     (4) Was patient able to speak?

C. Stroke (cerebrovascular accident)
  1. Definition: a neurological syndrome with gradual or rapid, nonconvulsive onset of neurological deficits that last for more than 24 hours. This occurs when the oxygen supply to a localized area is interrupted, leading to neural tissue destruction, then brain damage.
  2. Description
    a. Third leading cause of death
    b. Risk increases with age (two thirds occur after age 65).
    c. Affects more than 40% of the population older than 80
  3. Classification
    a. Ischemic (cerebral infarction)—85%
      (1) Thrombotic (most common)
        (a) May progressively worsen over time
      (2) Embolic
        (a) Sudden onset
    b. Hemorrhagic—15%
      (1) Subarachnoid
      (2) Intracerebral
  4. Transient ischemic attacks (TIAs)
    a. Temporary focal or retinal deficits
    b. Caused by vascular disease that can clear completely in less than 24 hours
    c. Shorter and reverses completely within 1 hour
    d. Most important warning signs of stroke
  5. Late warning signs (compared with TIAs—early)
    a. Loss of strength and/or sensation, usually on one side of the body
    b. Decreased vision, dimness of vision, loss of vision in one eye, double vision
    c. Difficulty talking or understanding speech
    d. Difficulty swallowing
    e. Severe headache
    f. Sudden dizziness, nausea, and/or vomiting
  6. Treatment
    a. Notify physician/surgeon immediately.
    b. Notify stroke alert team if unable to locate physician.
    c. Start oxygen or maintain patent airway.
    d. Monitor vital signs, especially blood pressure control.

     e. Start acetylsalicylic acid (aspirin) and/or thrombolytics.

     f. Prepare for neurointerventional radiology testing.

     g. Stat brain computed tomography (CT) scan without contrast and/or MRI

     h. Maintain normotension for cerebral perfusion (do not overtreat elevated blood pressure).

     i. Neuroassessment every 5 to 15 minutes

     j. Apply oxygen.

     k. Control blood pressure.

     l. Elevate head of bed to 30° to maintain venous outflow.

     m. Position to facilitate oral secretion drainage; avoid hip flexion and prone position.

     n. Maintain normothermia.

     o. Monitor level of sensation.

     p. Patch one eye at a time to control diplopia.

     q. Provide tactile stimuli to affected hands and limbs with decreased sensation.

     r. Avoid activities that increase ICP.

VII. DIAGNOSTIC TOOLS

  A. Neuroimaging techniques

    1. Skull series

      a. Indications

        (1) Fractures

        (2) Skull erosions

        (3) Deviated pineal gland

      b. Few contraindications (check with physician)

    2. Cerebral angiography (conventional and magnetic resonance angiography [MRA])

      a. Purpose

        (1) To detect abnormalities of cerebral circulation

        (2) To locate lesions distorting cerebral vessels

      b. Indications

        (1) Cerebral vascular abnormalities

        (2) Aneurysms

        (3) AVMs

        (4) Visualization of cerebral arteries and veins

      c. Contraindications

        (1) Allergy to contrast dye

    3. Radionuclide scan

      a. Uses gamma scintillation counter and injection of radioisotope

      b. Radioisotope uptake increased in pathological tissue

      c. Indications

        (1) Brain tumors or masses

        (2) Cerebral infarction

        (3) Headaches

        (4) Seizure disorders

        (5) Other major neurological disorders

      d. Contraindications

        (1) Uncooperative patient

        (2) Pregnancy

        (3) Breast-feeding patients

    4. CT scan

      a. Noninvasive test, but contrast media may be injected to facilitate visualization of vasculature

      b. Provides clear, cross-sectional brain images

      c. Uses computer reconstruction

      d. Contrast media, gadolinium, may be used for enhancement.

      e. Axial CT without contrast shows indications of mass effect and probable increased ICP.

      f. Contraindications
        (1) Uncooperative patient
        (2) Allergy to contrast dye or shellfish
  5. MRI
      a. Tomography technique using magnetic properties of protons in body tissues
      b. High-resolution images are very clear.
      c. Indications: any neurological condition
      d. Contraindications
        (1) Pregnancy
        (2) Uncooperative patient
        (3) Any metallic implants (e.g., pacemakers, orthopedic devices, clips)
      e. Sedation may be required because of claustrophobic nature of scanner.
  6. Myelogram
      a. Visualization of the spinal column and subarachnoid space for suspected lesion
      b. Injection of contrast dye via lumbar or cisternal puncture into the subarachnoid space
      c. Keep head slightly elevated for 4 to 6 hours to prevent water-soluble metrizamide (Amipaque) dye from migrating into the cerebrum.
      d. Keep flat for 4 to 8 hours if oil-based iophendylate (Pantopaque) used
  7. Positron emission tomography (PET) scan
      a. Uses principles of CT scan and radionuclide scanning
      b. Evaluation of biochemical brain substances
      c. Maps metabolic brain activity
      d. Expensive
      e. Indications—limited diagnostic purposes
        (1) Psychiatric disorders
        (2) Epilepsy
        (3) Alzheimer's disease
        (4) Cerebrovascular disease
        (5) Cerebral injuries
      f. Contraindications
        (1) Pregnant patients
        (2) Breast-feeding patients
B. Evoked potentials
  1. Measure changes in brain's electrical activity in response to variety of sensory stimulation.
      a. Visual
      b. Auditory
      c. Somatosensory
  2. Indications
      a. Neuromuscular disorders
      b. Cerebrovascular disease
      c. Head and spinal cord injury
      d. Tumors
      e. Peripheral nerve disease
C. Other diagnostic tools
  1. Lumbar puncture
  2. Electrocardiogram
  3. Electroencephalogram: assists in diagnosis of seizure activity, brain death
  4. Echoencephalogram: detects shifts of midline structures
  5. Radiographs of other body systems as indicated
  6. Cerebral blood flow studies
  7. Electromyogram
  8. Laboratory testing
      a. Blood
      b. Urine
      c. Cultures (as needed)
      d. CSF studies

VIII. DISORDERS POTENTIALLY REQUIRING SURGICAL INTERVENTION
- **A.** Brain tumors
  - **1.** Pathological condition: damage to brain tissue through expansion, infiltration, or destruction
  - **2.** Classification: no universally accepted system
    - **a.** Benign versus malignant
    - **b.** Malignancy depends on:
      - (1) Rate of growth
      - (2) Infiltration
      - (3) Location
      - (4) Grade I and II shows well to moderate differentiated cells.
      - (5) Grading III to IV
        - (a) Very poorly differentiated
        - (b) Has lost characteristics of cell of origin
        - (c) Poor prognosis
  - **3.** Clinical findings: dependent on location of tumor and degree of increased ICP
    - **a.** Headache
      - (1) Characteristically worse in morning
      - (2) Intensified by activity
    - **b.** Seizures: adults with first-time seizure are considered to have brain tumor until proven otherwise.
    - **c.** Papilledema
    - **d.** Vomiting
    - **e.** Sensory and motor dysfunctions
    - **f.** Speech impairments
    - **g.** Changes in personality or mental function
  - **4.** Diagnostic tools
    - **a.** History and physical assessment
    - **b.** Skull films
    - **c.** CT scan
    - **d.** MRI
    - **e.** Angiography
  - **5.** Treatment modalities
    - **a.** Radiation therapy: initially to shrink tumor
    - **b.** Chemotherapy
    - **c.** Craniotomy
    - **d.** Radiosurgery: gamma knife
- **B.** Brain abscess
  - **1.** Pathological condition: pocket(s) of exudates formed from infections of adjacent tissue or hematogenous spread
  - **2.** Clinical findings
    - **a.** Headache
    - **b.** Focal signs
    - **c.** Signs of increased ICP
  - **3.** Diagnostic tools
    - **a.** History and physical assessment
    - **b.** Skull films
    - **c.** CT scan
    - **d.** MRI
    - **e.** Culture of abscess exudates through stereotactic approach
    - **f.** Routine laboratory studies
  - **4.** Treatment modalities
    - **a.** Aspiration or excision of abscess
    - **b.** Intravenous (IV) antibiotic therapy
    - **c.** Treatment of increased ICP
- **C.** Trigeminal neuralgia (tic douloureux)
  - **1.** Pathological condition
    - **a.** Cause unknown

      b. Most common in middle and later life

      c. A symptom and not a disease

  2. Clinical findings

      a. Explosive, severe pain in distribution of CN V

      b. Pain may spontaneously remit and recur.

      c. Pain may cause patient to avoid activities that intensify it, such as eating, hygiene.

  3. Treatment modalities

      a. Pharmacological

         (1) Carbamazepine (Tegretol)

         (2) Phenytoin (Dilantin)

         (3) Baclofen (Lioresal)

      b. Alcohol block of one or more branches

      c. Surgical retrogasserian rhizotomy

      d. Sensory root decompression (Taarnhoj procedure)

      e. Microsurgical decompression of trigeminal root (Jannetta procedure)

      f. Radiofrequency percutaneous electrocoagulation

      g. Vascular decompression of CN V through posterior fossa craniotomy

D. Craniocerebral trauma

  1. Mechanism of injury

      a. Deceleration: head hits stationary object.

      b. Acceleration: head struck by moving object

      c. Acceleration-deceleration (coup-contrecoup): head hits object; brain rebounds inside cranium against opposite cranial bones.

      d. Shear strain: twisting, sliding motions of brainstem

  2. Types of injuries

      a. Primary (impact) injury: damage produced by blow

         (1) Concussion: transient loss of consciousness lasting several minutes

         (2) Contusion: actual bruising of brain tissue resulting in structural damage

         (3) Laceration: actual tearing of brain tissue

         (4) Fractures

            (a) Linear

            (b) Comminuted

            (c) Depressed

            (d) Basilar

      b. Intracranial secondary injury: damage that follows impact injury

         (1) Hematomas

            (a) Epidural: bleeding, usually from middle meningeal artery; accumulates between skull and dura

            (b) Subdural: venous bleeding beneath dura mater; may be acute, subacute, or chronic

         (2) ICP increased

         (3) Brain swelling

         (4) Cerebral edema

      c. Extracranial secondary injury

         (1) Hypoxia

         (2) Systemic hypotension

  3. Clinical findings (variable depending on type of injury) (Figure 33-30)

      a. Epidural hematoma

         (1) Momentary loss of consciousness

         (2) "Lucid interval"

         (3) Rapid deterioration

         (4) Signs of increased ICP

      b. Subdural hematoma

         (1) Drowsiness

         (2) Agitation

         (3) Slow cerebration and confusion

         (4) Signs of increased ICP

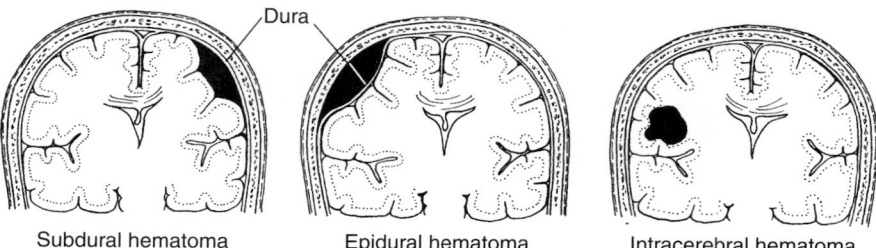

FIGURE 33-30 ■ Types of hematomas. (From Luckmann J, Sorensen KC: *Medical-surgical nursing: A psychophysiologic approach,* ed 3, Philadelphia, 1987, WB Saunders.)

    c. Intracerebral hematoma
       (1) Immediate neurological deficits
       (2) Signs of increased ICP
       (3) Loss of consciousness usually occurs from onset of injury.
    d. Skull fractures (signs and symptoms depend on anterior or middle fossa)
       (1) Basilar fracture most common
       (2) Involves bones of floor of cranial vault
       (3) Otorrhea, rhinorrhea
       (4) Battle's sign: ecchymosis over mastoid process
       (5) Raccoon's eyes: periorbital ecchymosis
       (6) Otorrhagia
       (7) Test ear or nasal drainage for glucose, and observe for concentric circles (halo or ring sign) on dressing or linens.
    e. Open head injuries
       (1) Gunshot and stab wounds
       (2) High potential for infection
  4. Diagnostic tools
    a. History and physical assessment
    b. Skull films
    c. CT scan
    d. MRI (not for initial diagnosis; may be used for follow-up)
    e. Routine laboratory studies
       (1) Alcohol and drug screen
       (2) Arterial blood gases (ABGs)
    f. Cervical spine films
  5. Treatment modalities
    a. Surgical evacuation of hematoma usually needed, depending on size and presence of signs of increased ICP
    b. Debridement
       (1) Removal of bone fragments, foreign objects, infarcted tissue
       (2) Permits inspection of skull fractures and penetrating wound
E. Intracranial hemorrhage
  1. Pathological condition
    a. Arterial aneurysm rupture: dilation of weakened arterial wall, causing blood-filled sac
    b. AVM rupture
       (1) Congenital communication of arteries and veins without intervening capillaries
       (2) Forms tangled, interwoven mass
       (3) Occurs more often in younger patients
       (4) Vessels rupture more easily than normal vessels.
    c. Hypertensive hemorrhage

2. Clinical findings
    a. Subarachnoid hemorrhage
        (1) Sudden, violent headache: "worst headache of my life"
        (2) Altered LOC
        (3) Signs of increased ICP
        (4) Nausea and vomiting
        (5) Meningeal irritation
            (a) Kernig's sign: resistance and pain when patient's leg is flexed at hip and knee
            (b) Brudzinski's sign: flexion of hips and knees in response to passive flexion of neck
        (6) Focal signs depending on location of bleeding
        (7) Bloody CSF
        (8) Hunt and Hess classification of aneurysms (Table 33-8)
    b. Intracerebral hemorrhage
        (1) Abrupt changes in LOC
        (2) Signs of increased ICP
        (3) Headache
        (4) Nausea and vomiting
        (5) Focal signs dependent on site of bleeding
3. Diagnostic tools
    a. History and physical assessment
    b. Lumbar puncture and CSF analysis
    c. Arteriogram, MRA
    d. CT scan
    e. Routine laboratory studies
4. Treatment modalities
    a. Medical
        (1) Minimize increases in ICP.
        (2) Promote cerebrovascular perfusion.
        (3) Prevent complications.
    b. Surgical
        (1) Craniotomy for evacuation of hematomas, clipping of aneurysm
        (2) Carotid endarterectomy
        (3) Extracranial-intracranial bypass
        (4) Embolization of AVM, aneurysm
        (5) Gamma knife radiosurgery
        (6) Interventional neuroradiology
            (a) Insertion of balloons and coils
            (b) Angioplasty and stenting

■ TABLE 33-8
■ ■ **Hunt and Hess Classification of Aneurysms**

Grade 0	Unruptured aneurysm
Grade I	Asymptomatic or minimal headache, slight nuchal rigidity
Grade I-A	Fixed neurological deficit but not acute meningeal signs
Grade II	Moderate to severe headache; nuchal rigidity present; CN III palsy, but no other neurological deficits
Grade III	Drowsy, confused, mild focal deficits
Grade IV	Stupor, moderate to severe hemiparesis, early decerebrate rigidity, vegetative disturbances
Grade V	Deep coma, decerebrate rigidity, moribund

    F. Hydrocephalus
        1. Pathological condition
            a. Noncommunicating hydrocephalus
                (1) Obstruction of CSF flow within ventricular system, resulting in lack of communication within subarachnoid space
                (2) Etiology
                    (a) Congenital malformation of ventricular system
                    (b) Adhesions caused by inflammatory processes (e.g., meningitis)
                    (c) Obstructive, space-occupying lesions
            b. Communicating hydrocephalus
                (1) Obstruction of CSF flow in subarachnoid space or basilar cisterns
                (2) Too few or nonfunctioning arachnoid villi cannot reabsorb CSF sufficiently.
                (3) Etiology
                    (a) Congenital malformations
                    (b) Adhesions caused by inflammatory disorders
                    (c) Overproduction of CSF
                    (d) Occlusion of arachnoid villi by particulate matter (blood, pus)
        2. Clinical findings: dependent on patient's age and type of hydrocephalus
            a. Infants
                (1) Enlarged head
                (2) Thin, fragile, shiny-looking scalp
                (3) Weak, underdeveloped neck muscles
                (4) Poor sucking reflex
                (5) "Sunset" eyes
                (6) Signs of increased ICP
            b. Older children and adults
                (1) Impaired mental function
                (2) Gait disturbances
                (3) Signs of increased ICP
                (4) Papilledema
                (5) Incontinence
                (6) Nausea and vomiting
        3. Diagnostic tools
            a. History and physical assessment
            b. Skull series
            c. CT scan
            d. MRI
            e. Isotope cisternogram (flow study)
            f. Lumbar puncture
            g. Transillumination of infant's skull
        4. Treatment modalities
            a. Removal of obstruction
            b. Ventriculostomy with external ventricular drainage for temporary relief
            c. Insertion of shunt
IX. SELECTED OPERATIVE PROCEDURES
    A. Burr hole (trephination)
        1. Procedure: removal of isolated or multiple small, circular portions of cranium for purposes of clot removal or in preparation for a craniotomy where a series of burr holes are made and connected
        2. Purpose
            a. Evacuation of extracerebral clot
            b. Removal of subdural fluid
            c. Drainage of CSF
            d. Aspiration of CSF
            e. Instillation of medications
            f. Instillation of air for ventriculography
    B. Craniotomy

1. Procedure
    a. Series of burr holes made into skull
    b. Burr holes connected with saw
    c. Bone flap created
    d. Opening kept as small as possible without restricting surgical approach
    e. Bone flap may or may not be replaced.
2. Purpose
    a. Removal of tumor, mass, or clot
    b. Clipping of an aneurysm
        (1) Ruptured aneurysm
        (2) Unruptured aneurysm
        (3) AVMs
    c. Repair of a cerebral injury
    d. Protection of cranial contents
    e. Improvement of cosmetic appearance
    f. Usually done only in supratentorial area because neck muscles protect infratentorial areas
    g. Triple H postoperative therapy
        (1) Hypovolemia
        (2) Hemodilution
        (3) Hypotension
C. Cranioplasty
    1. Procedure
        a. Repair of skull defects to reestablish the contour and integrity of the skull
    2. Purpose
        a. Protection of cranial contents
        b. Improvement of cosmetic appearance
        c. Usually done only in supratentorial area because neck muscles protect infratentorial areas
D. Craniectomy
    1. Procedure
        a. Excision of a portion of the skull without replacement
    2. Purpose
        a. Surgical access
        b. Decompression after cerebral debulking
        c. Removal of bone fragments from skull fracture
        d. Removal of skull growths (e.g., dermoid cysts)
E. Microsurgery
    1. Procedure
        a. Surgery performed with the assistance of an operating microscope
    2. Purpose
        a. Provides magnification of various intensities
F. Transsphenoidal hypophysectomy
    1. Procedure
        a. Access to the pituitary gland by an incision inside the superior upper lip, in front of the hard palate
        b. Removal of pituitary gland through transnasal or sublabial approach
        c. Often requires collaboration of neurosurgeon and ear, nose, and throat specialist
    2. Purpose
        a. Removal of pituitary tumors, adenomas, or craniopharyngiomas
        b. Preservation of pituitary gland, infundibular stalk, and normal vital structures
        c. Palliation for breast cancer
        d. Identification of tumor tissue
        e. Decompression
        f. Control of bone pain in metastatic cancer
G. Shunts
    1. Procedure
        a. Placement of primary catheter, one-way valve reservoir

        b. Connection of reservoir to tubing emptying into distal site

   2. Purpose

        a. Used to treat hydrocephalus

        b. Provide drainage of excessive CSF from the brain

        c. Improvement or preservation of neurological status by providing alternative CSF pathway

        d. Emergency reduction of increased ICP

        e. Instillation of antibiotics, analgesics, omega reservoir

        f. Sampling of CSF

   3. Types

        a. Ventriculoperitoneal

        b. Ventriculoatrial

        c. Lumbar-peritoneal

        d. External lumbar drain

        e. Multiple shunt sites (ureter, pleura, etc.)

   4. Components of shunting system

        a. Primary catheter: into lateral ventricle through burr hole

        b. Reservoir: rests on mastoid bone to collect CSF

        c. One-way valve: at reservoir to prevent CSF reflux

        d. Terminal catheter: tunneled under skin to termination point and secured in position

H. Stereotactic procedures ("stereo" means three-dimensional; "tactic" means touch)

   1. Procedure

        a. Fiducials placed preoperatively in MRI/CT

        b. Precise localization of lesion through use of three-dimensional coordinates, stereotactic frame, and instrumentation

        c. Involves intraoperative use of CT scans, radiographs

   2. Purpose

        a. Precise localization and treatment of deep brain lesions (thalamic lesions) for biopsy and/or removal of lesions

        b. Evacuation of intracerebral hemorrhage

        c. Catheter placement for drainage of deep lesions, colloid cyst, or abscess

        d. Ventricular catheter shunt placement

        e. Placement of electrodes for epilepsy

        f. Implantation of radioactive seeds into brain tumor

        g. Ablative procedures for extrapyramidal diseases (Parkinson's disease)

        h. Especially useful with intractable, chronic pain with deep brain stimulator

I. Carotid endarterectomy

   1. Procedure

        a. Incision made in neck area

        b. Heparinization and clamping of artery above and below obstruction

        c. Small incision made into artery

        d. Obstruction removed

        e. End-to-end anastomosis, suturing of artery, or patching of artery with autologous vein or Gortex graft

   2. Purpose

        a. Removal of stenotic vessel area

        b. Removal of plaques in vessels

        c. Primarily involves carotid bifurcation and junction of carotid and vertebral vessels with aorta or subclavian and innominate arteries

        d. Bypass of occlusion by use of grafts

        e. Primary purpose is to restore flow to cerebral circulation and prevent stroke if vessel is more than 70% occluded.

J. Microradiosurgery

   1. Procedure

        a. Gamma knife

           (1) Precise destruction of deep and inaccessible lesions during single session using 201 radially distributed, sealed, radioactive, sharply focused sources of cobalt 60 radiation; surrounding healthy tissue not harmed

(2) Minute measurement and precise patient positioning
(3) Purpose
    (a) Excessive risk for conventional surgical procedure
    (b) Surgical inaccessibility of lesion (acoustic neuromas)
    (c) Prior surgical failure
    (d) Patient refusal to undergo conventional craniotomy
(4) Used for:
    (a) AVMs
    (b) Tumors
    (c) Other intracranial lesions for which conventional surgery is inappropriate
(5) Time between treatment and results long
(6) Time required for treatment limits centers to one or two patients per day.
(7) Procedure can be done with local anesthesia, but patient needs to be cooperative.

  b. Cyberknife
    (1) Used in conjunction with a frameless computerized guidance system
  c. Lasers
    (1) Types
      (a) Carbon dioxide
      (b) Argon
      (c) Neodymium-doped yttrium aluminum garnet (Nd:YAG)
    (2) Precise dissection without traumatizing surrounding tissues
    (3) Formerly inaccessible anatomical areas can be reached.
    (4) Dissect tissue by:
      (a) Vaporizing
      (b) Coagulating blood vessels
      (c) Shrinking tumors

  2. Patient selection an important aspect

K. Seizure surgery
  1. Procedure
    a. Phase 1: noninvasive scalp monitoring
    b. Phase 2: placement of depth electrodes
    c. Phase 3: placement of grids and resection of epileptogenic focus
    d. Deep brain stimulators
  2. Purpose
    a. Localization of seizure focus
    b. Removal of epileptogenic focus without causing neurological deficits
  3. Selection criteria
    a. Refractory to medical management
    b. Unilateral focus
    c. Significant alteration in quality of life

X. DISORDERS POTENTIALLY REQUIRING SPINAL SURGERY
  A. Herniated intervertebral disk (Figure 33-31)
    1. Major cause of severe and chronic back pain
      a. Disruption of annulus with leakage of nucleus pulposus
      b. May extrude into epidural space and compress nerve roots
    2. Often referred to as HNP (herniated nucleus pulposus)
    3. Cervical and lumbar regions most susceptible to injury and stress (especially lumbar disk disease)
    4. Patients often admitted with diagnosis of radiculopathy, disease of spinal nerve roots, complaining of arm and leg pain
    5. Occurs more in men
    6. Occurs most often in 30 to 50 year-old age group
    7. Etiology
      a. Trauma (50%)
        (1) Lifting

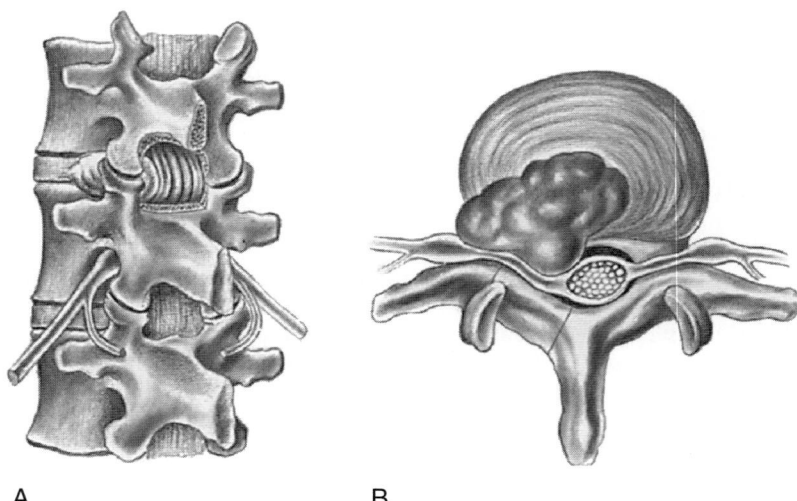

FIGURE 33-31 ■ Herniated nucleus pulposus **(A)** and laminectomy **(B)**. (From Thompson J: *Mosby's clinical nursing,* ed 5, St Louis, 2002, Mosby.)

      (2) Slipping
      (3) Falling on buttocks or back
      (4) Suppressing a sneeze
   b. Degenerative processes such as:
      (1) Aging
      (2) Osteoarthritis
      (3) Ankylosing spondylitis
   c. Congenital anomalies (scoliosis) can predispose to disk injury.
   d. Obesity
8. Signs and symptoms
   a. Lumbar (90%-95% at L4 to S1 level)
      (1) Pain aggravated by:
         (a) Sneezing
         (b) Coughing
         (c) Stooping
         (d) Straining
         (e) Standing
         (f) Jarring movements while walking or riding
      (2) Postural deformity
         (a) Lumbar lordosis absent (60%)
         (b) Restriction in lateral flexion
         (c) Limited lumbar spine movement
         (d) Painful when climbing stairs
      (3) Motor changes
         (a) Hypotonia
         (b) Atrophy of affected muscles
         (c) Paresis
         (d) Footdrop
         (e) Difficult micturition and sexual activity
      (4) Sensory deficits
         (a) Paresthesias
         (b) Numbness of leg and foot with or without pain
         (c) Tenderness over L5 and S1
      (5) Alteration in reflexes (diminished knee or ankle reflexes)
      (6) Other diagnostic signs
         (a) Straight leg raising test (Lasegue's sign)

        (b) Neri's sign (patient bends forward after knee flexion on affected side)

        (c) Naffziger's test (pain when both jugular veins simultaneously compressed while standing)

        (d) Kernig's sign (unable to extend knee to normal range while in dorsal recumbent position)

  b. Cervical (most commonly C6 to C7, then C5 to C6)

    (1) Pain

    (2) Paresthesias

    (3) Reflex loss

    (4) Motor weakness in hand, forearm

    (5) Restricted neck movement

    (6) Atrophy of affected muscles

    (7) Tenderness when pressure exerted over cervical area of spine

9. Diagnostic tools

  a. History and physical assessment

  b. Spinal films

  c. Contrast myelography

  d. MRI

  e. CT scan

B. Spinal cord injury (Figure 33-32)

  1. Mechanisms of injury

    a. Hyperflexion (e.g., head-on collision and diving incident)

    b. Hyperextension (e.g., rear-end collision, elderly who fell and struck chin)

    c. Axial loading (e.g., falling from height and land on feet or buttocks)

    d. Rotational (e.g., extreme flexion or twisting of head and neck)

    e. Penetrating (e.g., bullets penetrate spinal column or soft tissue)

  2. Classifications of injury

    a. Concussion—jarring resulting in temporary loss of function

    b. Compression—distortion of normal curvatures

    c. Contusion—bruising, edema, and necrosis from compression

    d. Laceration—actual tear resulting in permanent injury

    e. Transection—severing of cord (complete or incomplete)

    f. Hemorrhage—blood in or around spinal cord

    g. Damage to blood vessel—results in ischemia and possible necrosis

  3. Spinal cord injury syndromes

    a. Quadriplegia

      (1) Lesion involves one or more cervical segments.

      (2) Loss of motor and sensory function below level of lesion, usually upper and lower extremities

      (3) Bowel, bladder, and sexual dysfunction

      (4) Respiratory dysfunction

    b. Paraplegia

      (1) Lesion involves one or more of thoracic, lumbar, or sacral regions.

      (2) Loss of motor and sensory function below level of lesion, usually lower extremities

      (3) Bowel, bladder, and sexual dysfunction

    c. Complete lesion: implies total loss of motor and sensory function below the injury

    d. Incomplete lesion

      (1) Preservation of motor or sensory function, or both, below level of lesion

      (2) Classified according to area of damage

        (a) Central cord syndrome

          (i)   More motor deficits in upper extremities than lower extremities

          (ii) Sensory loss varies.

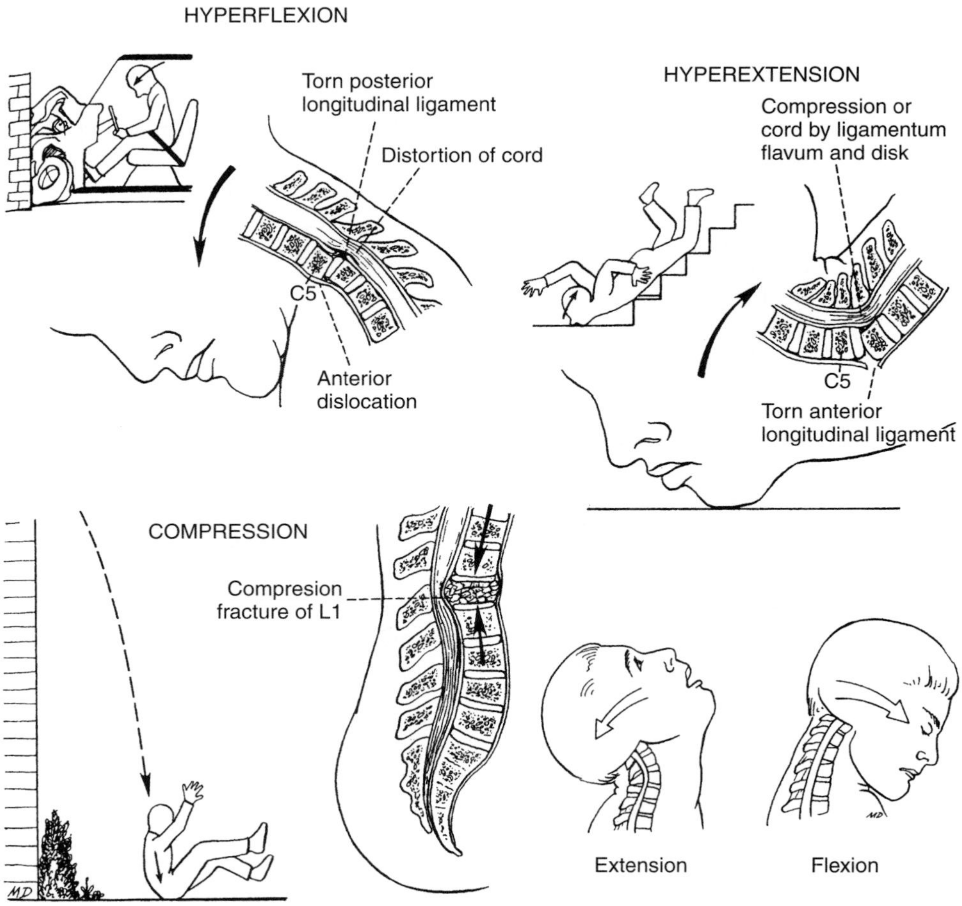

FIGURE 33-32 ■ Closed spinal injury mechanism. (From Clochesy J, Breu C, Cardin S, et al: *Critical care nursing,* ed 2, Philadelphia, 1996, WB Saunders.)

        (iii) Bowel, bladder dysfunction variable, or function may be completely preserved.

        (iv) Injury to central area of spinal cord, usually cervical area

    (b) Anterior cord syndrome

        (i) Loss of perception of pain, temperature, and motor function below level of lesion

        (ii) Light touch, position, vibration intact

        (iii) Injury to anterior spinal artery through trauma, hyperflexion

        (iv) Injury in anterior part of spinal cord including spinothalamic tracts (pain), corticospinal tracts (temperature), anterior gray horn motor neurons

    (c) Brown-Séquard syndrome (lateral cord syndrome)

        (i) Ipsilateral paralysis or paresis

        (ii) Ipsilateral loss of touch, pressure, and vibration

        (iii) Contralateral loss of pain and temperature

        (iv) Transverse hemisection of cord, usually as a result of knife or missile injury or acute ruptured disk

    (d) Posterior cord syndrome

        (i) Rare syndrome

        (ii) Position and vibration senses of posterior columns involved

        (e) Root syndrome (peripheral syndrome)
- (i) Tingling, pain, motor weakness of selected muscles; absent or decreased reflexes in involved area
- (ii) Sacral roots: bowel and bladder dysfunction
- (iii) Cervical roots: tingling and weakness in arm; pain radiating down arm and into shoulder
- (iv) Compression or vertebral subluxation with compression of nerve roots

        (f) Horner's syndrome
- (i) Seen with partial transection at T1 level or above
- (ii) Associated with miosis, ptosis, loss of sweating on ipsilateral side (anhydrosis)
- (iii) Lesions of preganglionic sympathetic trunk or cervical postganglionic sympathetic neurons

4. Treatment
- **a.** Medical: dependent on patient's symptoms and severity of injury
  - (1) High-dose steroid for acute cord injury
  - (2) Immobilization
  - (3) Bed rest
- **b.** Surgery
  - (1) May be delayed
    - (a) Allow for decrease in cord edema.
    - (b) Allow for immobilization and realignment of vertebral column.
    - (c) Allow for reduction of fracture dislocation.
  - (2) May occur within 12 to 72 hours if any of following are present:
    - (a) Compression of spinal cord
    - (b) Progressive neurological deficits
    - (c) Bony fragments with compound fractures (because they could penetrate cord)
    - (d) Penetrating wounds
    - (e) Bone fragments in spinal cord
  - (3) Purpose
    - (a) Decompress spinal cord or spinal nerves to prevent the following:
      - (i) Pain
      - (ii) Loss of neurological function
      - (iii) Ischemia or necrosis of neural tissue
    - (b) Stabilization
  - (4) Procedures
    - (a) Decompression laminectomies with fusion
    - (b) Posterior laminectomy using acrylic wire mesh and fusion
    - (c) Insertion of Harrington rods or instrumentation for stabilization

5. Complications: affect all body systems
- **a.** Neurological
  - (1) Spinal shock
  - (2) Autonomic dysreflexia
  - (3) Spinal instability
  - (4) Pain
  - (5) Spasticity
- **b.** Respiratory
  - (1) Hypoxia
  - (2) Aspiration
  - (3) Pulmonary embolus
  - (4) Pneumonia
  - (5) Atelectasis
- **c.** Cardiovascular
  - (1) Bradydysrhythmias
  - (2) Orthostatic hypotension
  - (3) Deep vein thrombosis

      d. Orthopedic, musculoskeletal, integumentary
         (1) Contractures
         (2) Osteoporosis
         (3) Pressure ulcers
      e. Gastrointestinal
         (1) Bleeding
         (2) Fecal impaction or incontinence
         (3) Paralytic ileus
      f. Genitourinary
         (1) Urinary tract infections
         (2) Urinary calculi
         (3) Urinary retention or incontinence
         (4) Sexual dysfunction
  6. Spinal shock
      a. Condition occurring immediately after injury; may last hours to months, depending on severity of injury
      b. Commonly lasts 1 to 6 weeks after injury
      c. Characteristics
         (1) Loss of motor, sensory, reflex, and autonomic activity below level of injury
         (2) Flaccid paralysis of all skeletal muscle
         (3) Loss of pain perception, light touch, temperature, and pressure below level of injury
         (4) Loss of ability to perspire
         (5) Absence of somatic and visceral sensation
         (6) Bowel and bladder dysfunction
         (7) Hypotension, bradycardia
      d. Resolution of spinal shock
         (1) Gradual process (4–6 weeks)
         (2) Varies with patient and level of injury
  7. Autonomic dysreflexia
      a. Usually occurs after resolution of spinal shock and return of reflex activity
      b. Occurs most often with lesions at T6 or above
      c. Results from uninhibited sympathetic discharge
      d. Causes
         (1) Bladder distention
         (2) Fecal impaction
         (3) Noxious stimuli (vary with individual patient)
      e. Symptoms
         (1) Pounding headache
         (2) Hypertension (can be dangerously high)
            (a) Changes in mental status
            (b) Seizures
            (c) Intracerebral hemorrhage
         (3) Profuse sweating above level of lesion
         (4) Nasal congestion
         (5) Flushed skin above level of lesion
         (6) Pallor below level of lesion
         (7) Piloerection (goose pimples) below level of lesion
         (8) Anxiety
         (9) Visual disturbances
      f. Treatment
         (1) Assess patient.
         (2) Remove stimulus.
         (3) Elevate head of bed.
         (4) Notify physician immediately.
         (5) Fast-acting antihypertensive medications may be ordered.

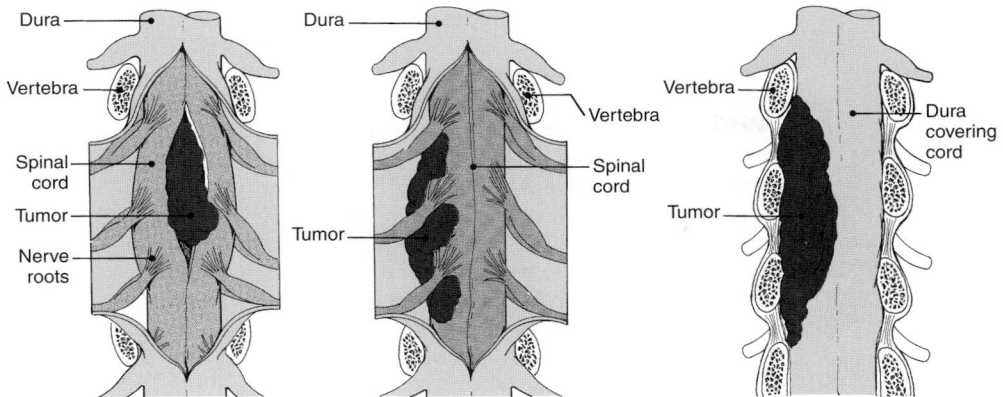

FIGURE 33-33 ■ Spinal cord tumors. (From Thompson J: *Mosby's clinical nursing*, ed 5, St Louis, 2002, Mosby.)

C. Spinal cord tumors (Figure 33-33)
   1. Less common than brain tumors
   2. Usually occur in young and middle-aged adults, with men and women equally affected
   3. Sites
      a. Cervical: 30%
      b. Thoracic: 50%
      c. Lumbosacral: 20%
   4. Classification
      a. Intramedullary
         (1) Within spinal cord tissue
         (2) May compress cord and nerve roots and destroy cord tissue
         (3) Usually malignant
         (4) Types
            (a) Astrocytoma
            (b) Ependymoma
            (c) Oligodendroglioma
            (d) Hemangioblastoma
         (5) Characteristics
            (a) Slow growing
            (b) May extend over more than one spinal segment
            (c) Loss of pain and temperature
            (d) Caudal area tumors may precipitate sexual, bladder, and bowel dysfunction.
         (6) Compression is usually on central portion of spinal cord, rather than on nerve roots.
      b. Extramedullary
         (1) Can occur inside or outside dura, but do not occur within spinal cord parenchyma
            (a) Extradural: occur outside the spinal dura, within the epidural space
               (i)   Symptoms occur rapidly.
               (ii) Mostly malignant
               (iii) Pain is a common symptom and may occur before signs of spinal cord compression.
               (iv) Metastatic tumors (from lungs, breast, prostate, kidneys, gastrointestinal tract)
               (v)   Multiple myeloma
               (vi) Lymphoma, chordomas, and sarcomas

        (b) Intradural: occur within the spinal dura but not within the spinal cord
- (i) Most common spinal cord tumor
- (ii) Most frequently seen in thoracic area
- (iii) Gradual onset of symptoms of cord compression
- (iv) Pain may not always be present.
- (v) Meningioma
- (vi) Neurofibroma
- (vii) Congenital: dermoid, epidermoid

5. Symptoms
- **a.** Etiology
  - (1) Destruction of spinal cord parenchyma
  - (2) Compression of spinal cord or spinal nerves
  - (3) Compression or occlusion of spinal blood vessels
  - (4) Obstruction of CSF flow
- **b.** Dependent on the following:
  - (1) Level of lesion
  - (2) Tumor type

6. Diagnostic tools
- **a.** History and physical assessment
- **b.** Spinal films
  - (1) Assess destruction of bony structures.
  - (2) Assess presence of vertebral column lesions.
- **c.** Contrast myelography
  - (1) Identifies obstruction of spinal CSF pathway (subarachnoid space)
  - (2) Identifies location, size, boundaries of lesion
  - (3) Considered hallmark of diagnostic armamentarium
  - (4) May be scheduled immediately before surgery, so patient may proceed directly from myelogram to operating room
- **d.** CT scan: identifies location, size, boundaries of lesion
- **e.** MRI
  - (1) Identifies location, size, boundaries of lesion
  - (2) Identifies destruction of bony structures
- **f.** CSF analysis
  - (1) Routine analysis as discussed with cranial space-occupying lesions
  - (2) CSF collected from below level of lesion may show increases in protein, absence of large amounts of cells, rapid coagulation.
- **g.** Spinal angiogram: assists in differentiating vascular lesions
- **h.** Electromyogram: used for differential diagnosis
- **i.** Other laboratory test or x-ray films as indicated by patient's symptoms and condition

XI. COMMON SPINAL OPERATIVE PROCEDURES
- **A.** Laminectomy
  - **1.** Most frequent surgical procedure
  - **2.** Procedure
    - **a.** Removal of:
      - (1) Laminae
      - (2) Part of posterior arch of vertebrae
      - (3) Attached ligamentum flavum
    - **b.** Hemilaminectomy: excision of part of laminae
  - **3.** Purpose
    - **a.** Decompression of spinal cord or spinal nerves
    - **b.** Allow for diskectomy
  - **4.** Spinal fusion may be performed at the same time for stability of spinal column.
  - **5.** Approaches
    - **a.** Posterior (traditional): with cervical surgery, incision made through back
    - **b.** Anterior: with cervical surgery, incision made anteriorly through throat and neck area

  B. Hemilaminectomy
    1. Removal of part of the lamina and posterior arch
  C. Diskectomy
    1. Procedure
      a. Lumbar
        (1) Posterior approach always used
        (2) Entire disk and cartilaginous plate removed
      b. Cervical
        (1) Posterior approach: only extruded disk fragments removed
        (2) Anterior approach: total disk removed
    2. Purpose: removal of nuclear disk material with or without laminectomy
  D. Microdiskectomy
    1. Procedure and purpose: microscopic surgical technique
      a. Allows for easier identification of anatomic structures
      b. Improves precision in removing small fragments
      c. Decreases tissue trauma and pain: smaller incision
    2. Patient able to ambulate sooner
    3. Advantages
      a. Decreases risk of CSF leak through dural laceration
      b. Improved hemostasis: decreases vascular trauma and hematoma formation
      c. Decreases muscle spasms by decreasing traction on spinal nerve roots
      d. Less risk of stripping muscle from fascia
      e. Decreases risk of infection
  E. Percutaneous diskectomy
    1. Procedure and purpose: endoscopic lumbar surgical technique
      a. Posterolateral approach
      b. High-power suction shaver and cutter system
      c. Local anesthesia
    2. Alternative to microdiskectomy
    3. Indicated in disk-related root compression with minor deficits
  F. Microendoscopic diskectomy (lumbar disk removal)
    1. Disorder
      a. Characteristics
        (1) Ruptured intravertebral disk with resulting pressure on a nerve
        (2) Associated health factors: no clear indication of a particular risk factor except age; disk rupture in most cases thought to be caused by the weight loading of an erect posture
          (a) Misuse of back
          (b) Static positions at work
            (i)   Sitting at a desk or work station
            (ii) Standing at a work station
            (iii) Sedentary lifestyle
          (c) Weight-loading phenomenon
            (i)   Load that is too heavy
            (ii) Load that is too bulky
        (3) Age-related phenomenon
          (a) Greatest risk between 30 and 50 years of age
          (b) Peak occurrence in the 40s
      b. Symptoms
        (1) Pain
          (a) Sharp, stabbing, burning
          (b) Radiates into a dermatome and can be fairly accurately traced by the patient
          (c) Pain increases with any straining, Valsalva's maneuver, sneezing, coughing.
        (2) Paresthesia may exist anywhere along the affected dermatome.
        (3) Weakness and atrophy may become evident in the muscles innervated by the specific nerve root.

(4) Decreased or loss of reflexes specific to the innervation of the involved nerve root

(5) Specific nerve root involvement (disk rupture at one level may involve more than one root, and with individual anatomic variations symptoms may vary)

    (a) Pressure on L4, L5, or S1 nerve root (sciatica)

        (i) Pain radiating down one buttock, possibly into the ipsilateral posterior thigh, knee, calf, and may extend all the way into the foot

        (ii) Usually more comfortable with leg flexed

        (iii) Sitting may be particularly painful.

        (iv) Weakness

           [a] L5—unable to walk on heels because of weakness of dorsiflexion

           [b] S1—unable to walk on toes because of weakness of plantar flexion

        (v) L4 and L5—most common areas of disk herniation in the lumbar spine

    (b) Pressure on L2 or L3 nerve root (more rare)

        (i) Pain radiating into the groin, anterior thigh, and medial calf of affected leg

        (ii) Will usually assume a position of knee and hip flexion with lateral rotation of the hip

c. Conservative treatment

(1) Activity restrictions

    (a) Bed rest

    (b) Avoid sitting for more than 30 minutes at a time.

(2) Steroid or anti-inflammatory treatment

    (a) Topical

    (b) Oral medication

(3) Traction

(4) Exercise

(5) Heat and massage

(6) Ice massage or ice application

(7) Sleeping position and mattress adjustments

(8) Ergonomic evaluation of work environment

2. Procedure

a. A small 15-mm incision is made over the site (left or right of the midline).

b. The endoscope is positioned and verified with x-ray.

c. Part of the lamina is removed to allow access to the nerve root.

d. The nerve root is identified and protected as the loose pieces of disk are removed.

e. The nerve root is verified as being "free" without pressure.

f. A foraminotomy may be performed (bone along the neural foramen can be drilled away, leaving a slightly larger area for the nerve to pass through).

g. Benefits

(1) Can be done under local or epidural anesthesia

(2) Minimal tissue damage to skin, muscle, and other tissue at entry site

(3) Minimal scarring, therefore less morbidity

3. Postprocedure

a. Assessment

(1) Description of pain, paresthesia, numbness; compare with preoperative

(2) Pain scale score; compare with preoperative

(3) Weakness

    (a) Walk on heels

    (b) Walk on toes

    (c) Difficulty ambulating

(4) Band-Aid intact without bleeding
(5) Able to void
b. Care
(1) Remove Foley catheter.
(2) Teach to get out of bed "statue style."
(a) Turn to unaffected side.
(b) Lower legs off bed, while pushing upper body up with upper extremities, keeping back straight.
(3) Ambulate increasing distances and to bathroom, to ensure ambulation ability at home.
G. Spinal fusion—with or without instrumentation
1. Procedure: insertion of bone chips between vertebrae; variety of surgical hardware (rods, screws, bolts) may also be used.
2. Purpose
a. Immobilization of vertebral column
b. Stabilization of weakened vertebral column
3. Types
a. Lumbar
(1) Motion increased above level of lesion
(2) Patient often unaware of permanent area of stiffness
b. Cervical
(1) Increased limitation of movement
(2) Anterior approach: used when cervical area of spine is unstable
(3) Often performed with anterior laminectomy and diskectomy
H. Foraminotomy
1. Procedure: surgical enlargement of intervertebral foramen to accommodate exit of spinal nerves
2. Purpose
a. Decrease pressure on spinal nerve
b. Release entrapped spinal nerve
3. Most often done in cervical area where foramen is smaller in diameter
I. Chemonucleolysis
1. Procedure
a. Injection of chymopapain, enzyme found in papaya plant, into nucleus pulposus
b. Fluoroscopy and local anesthesia used
2. Purpose
a. Decreases size of disk by hydrolysis
b. Decreases pain
3. Fallen out of favor
a. Increased incidence of pain recurrence
b. Adverse reactions to chymopapain
J. Rhizotomy
1. Procedure: destruction of sensory nerve roots at entrance to spinal cord
2. Purpose: interruption of transmission of pain
3. Types
a. Closed
(1) Percutaneous insertion of catheter to destroy nerve root through coagulation
(2) Injection of neurolytic chemicals
(3) Cryodestruction
b. Open
(1) Requires laminectomy
(2) Nerve roots isolated and destroyed
K. Chordotomy
1. Procedure: pain pathways transected at midline portion of spinal cord before impulse ascends through spinothalamic tract
2. Purpose: interruption of transmission of pain

XII. OTHER OUTPATIENT PROCEDURES
    A. Carpal tunnel release (example of peripheral median nerve entrapment)
        1. Disorder
            a. Characteristics
                (1) Results from pressure on the median nerve
                (2) Associated health factors
                    (a) Diabetes mellitus
                    (b) Pregnancy
                    (c) Premenstrual fluid retention
                    (d) Obesity
                    (e) Arthritis
                (3) Most common in women ages 40 to 60
            b. Symptoms
                (1) Pain, paresthesia ("pins and needles"), numbness in the hand that may radiate up the arm
                (2) Exacerbation of pain upon wrist flexion, often interrupting sleep from normal wrist flexion during sleep
                (3) Weakness in the thumb, first, second, and third fingers
        2. Procedure
            a. Anesthesia may be with:
                (1) Local infiltration
                (2) Bier block
                (3) Axillary block
                (4) General
            b. Carpal ligament sectioned vertically over the median nerve
            c. Incision
                (1) Along the ulnar or medial side of the thenar groove (most common)
                (2) Along the median groove
                (3) Endoscopic procedure (½-inch incision)
        3. Postprocedure
            a. Assessment: check all fingers, but most particularly the thumb, index, and middle fingers every 15 minutes for 1 hour, then every 30 minutes for 1 hour, then every hour until discharged.
                (1) Sensation to touch
                (2) Sensation to pin prick or temperature; this is intact if patient is describing pain.
                (3) Blanching of fingertips—compare with uninvolved fingertips
                (4) Assess dressing for drainage and increasing tightness.
            b. Care
                (1) Keep hand elevated at level of, or higher than, the heart.
                (2) If dressing becomes constrictive, request or have standing order to clip dressing ½ to 1½ inches on back of hand.
                (3) Do not take blood pressure in affected arm.
                (4) Use sling for elevation and protection only when ambulating.
                (5) Keep elbow free of pressure.
                (6) Exercise the fingers throughout the day.
                (7) Check fingers for movement, sensation, and color (compare with uninvolved hand) several times a day (upon arising, at each meal, and at bedtime).
                (8) Avoid soiling dressing or hand; use unaffected hand or ask for assistance.
    B. Epidural blood patch
        1. Disorder
            a. Characteristics
                (1) Follows a lumbar puncture (LP)
                    (a) Postmyelogram
                    (b) Post-LP for diagnostic tests
                    (c) Post–intrathecal catheter removal

    (d) Post–intrathecal injection of medication

   (2) Most often related to large-bore LP needle >20 gauge

  b. Symptoms

   (1) Severe headache (postural)

    (a) Worsens when up but subsides when supine

    (b) May extend into neck

    (c) Prevents activities

   (2) Nausea and vomiting

  c. Conservative treatment

   (1) Bed rest

   (2) Fluid challenge

   (3) Analgesics and antiemetics

   (4) Abdominal binder

   (5) Caffeine

 2. Procedure

  a. Have patient lie down in quiet, dark room with limited visitors.

  b. Patient may be too ill to listen to detailed instructions; limit information.

  c. Detailed explanations may be given to significant other.

  d. Establish at least one IV route (two sites may be needed if severely dehydrated).

  e. Prepare to obtain 15 to 20 mL of blood under careful aseptic technique for patch (physician may prefer to obtain blood).

   (1) Intermittent IV access for blood retrieval

   (2) Prepare site for phlebotomy.

    (a) Povidone preparation

  f. Place patient prone (pillow under abdomen).

   (1) May be done under fluoroscopy

  g. Epidural puncture is performed.

   (1) Anesthesia

    (a) Local infiltration

    (b) IV sedation and analgesia

  h. Assist with LP preparation.

  i. Obtain or assist with blood for patch.

  j. Blood is injected into epidural space.

  k. Band-Aid applied

 3. Postprocedure

  a. Assessment

   (1) Severity of headache (pain scale)

   (2) Description of headache (observe for changes)

   (3) Observe for nerve root irritation.

    (a) Symptoms worsen.

    (b) Pain in legs or groin area

    (c) Inability to void

  b. Care

   (1) Force fluid, caffeinated (IV fluid bolus if nausea persists).

   (2) Caffeine

    (a) Beverages

    (b) Tablets

    (c) IV (caffeine, sodium benzoate)

   (3) Bed rest with head of bed flat

   (4) Establish ability to void.

   (5) At any point, if symptoms return, bed rest must be resumed (patch procedure may be repeated).

C. Excision of neuroma

 1. Disorder

  a. Characteristics

   (1) Results from trauma to the nerve, particularly the axon

    (a) Surgical or traumatic incision

          (b) Amputation sites

          (c) Repeated trauma

              (i)   Oral from dentures

              (ii) Wrist or hand from repetitive work injuries

              (iii) Morton's neuroma from trauma to the digital nerve

              (iv) Any traumatized nerve

      (2) Associated health factors

          (a) Traumatic injuries

          (b) Familial tendency

          (c) Poorly fitted shoes

      (3) Morton's neuroma more common in adult women

   b. Symptoms

      (1) Pain at neuroma site

      (2) Numbness and tingling around neuroma and distally

   c. Conservative treatment

      (1) Injection with various medications and saline

      (2) At operative and amputation sites, many methods have been and are currently being tried to prevent neuroma formation.

      (3) Morton's neuroma

          (a) Padding in shoes

          (b) Limiting walking and standing

          (c) Proper fitting footwear, avoiding heels >1 inch

  2. Procedure

   a. Anesthesia may be:

      (1) Local infiltration

      (2) Nerve block

      (3) Epidural

      (4) Spinal

      (5) General

   b. Neuroma is excised, and the nerve ending may be buried into bone or muscle, or other attempts made to prevent reoccurrence.

   c. Morton's neuroma

      (1) Incision

          (a) Vertical plantar

          (b) Dorsal

  3. Postprocedure

   a. Assessment: check extremity distal to surgical site every 15 minutes for 1 hour, every 30 minutes for 1 hour, and every hour until discharge.

      (1) Sensation to touch distal to surgical site (consider type of anesthesia, document resolution)

      (2) Sensation to pain and temperature distal to surgical site: compare preoperative pain score and description with postoperative pain score and description (consider type of anesthesia, document resolution).

      (3) Capillary refill and warmth of digits compared with unaffected extremity (capillary refill <3 seconds)

      (4) Assess dressing for drainage and increasing tightness.

   b. Care

      (1) Keep extremity elevated at level or above heart.

      (2) If dressing becomes constricting, obtain order or have standing order to clip ½ to 1½ inches on opposite surface of incision.

      (3) If upper extremity, avoid taking blood pressure in affected arm.

XIII. POSTANESTHESIA CARE FOR SPINAL SURGERY

  A. Postoperative assessment

   1. Ongoing, frequent, and careful observation

   2. Specific spinal cord assessment form may assist in consistent documentation of improvement or deterioration.

   3. Assess for signs of meningeal irritation.

     a. Headache

        b. Photophobia

        c. Nuchal rigidity

        d. Kernig's sign: resistance and pain when patient's leg is flexed at hip and knee

        e. Brudzinski's sign: flexion of hips and knees in response to passive flexion of neck

    4. Hemodynamic monitoring: especially useful for patient with spinal cord injury who may be in spinal shock

        a. Thermodilution catheter

        b. Arterial lines

        c. Central venous pressure line

    5. Respiratory status

        a. Especially important with cervical lesions

        b. Assess rate, use of accessory muscles, nasal flaring.

        c. Breath sounds

        d. Ability to handle secretions

        e. For patients with anterior cervical approach (may have damage to laryngeal nerves, vocal cords, hematoma formation)

            (1) Hoarseness

            (2) Tracheal deviation (edema)

            (3) Stridor

        f. Pulse oximetry

        g. ABGs

    6. Neurovascular checks

    7. Urinary elimination

        a. Voiding pattern

        b. Intake and output

        c. Palpate abdomen for distention.

    8. Auscultate bowel sounds, presence of distention.

B. Postoperative complications

    1. Increase in existing deficits

    2. Motor loss: paralysis of upper or lower extremities

    3. Sensory loss

    4. Urinary retention

    5. Paralytic ileus

    6. Leakage of CSF fistula

    7. Nerve root injury

    8. Postural deformity

    9. Hematoma at operative site (will increase neurological deficits)

    10. Arachnoiditis: inflammation of arachnoid layer of meninges

    11. Infection

    12. Respiratory distress

    13. Spinal cord–injured patients may experience any of the complications indicated in discussion of spinal cord injury.

C. Signs of deterioration in status

    1. Increase in existing deficits

    2. Appearance of new deficits

    3. Spinal shock

    4. Autonomic dysreflexia

    5. Respiratory distress

D. Nursing interventions after spinal injury

    1. Maintain patent airway.

        a. Coughing and deep breathing

        b. Use of incentive spirometry

        c. Supplemental oxygen

        d. Assistance with mechanical ventilation may be needed with cervical lesions.

    2. Frequent assessment of neurological status: note deviations from patient's baseline

    3. Positioning

      a. Factors

         (1) Type of surgery

         (2) Type of lesion

         (3) Site of lesion

         (4) Presence of complications

      b. Reduce pressure on operative site.

      c. Reposition every 2 hours once specified by surgeon.

      d. Log rolling

         (1) Maintains alignment

         (2) Decreases pain

         (3) Decreases muscle spasms

         (4) Use of turning sheet decreases stress on caregiver and helps ensure alignment.

      e. Avoid twisting.

      f. Proper body alignment

      g. Stryker frame

         (1) May be used for a variety of spinal surgeries depending on patient condition and severity of injury

         (2) May be used in conjunction with halo apparatus or Gardner-Wells tongs

            (a) Maintain traction.

            (b) Observe pin sites.

            (c) Assess stability of halo apparatus and security bolts.

         (3) Physician must be present first time patient is turned down.

         (4) Psychosocial and emotional support needed, because patients frequently are afraid and anxious on frame.

      h. Cervical collar or Philadelphia collar

   4. Maintain skin and mucous membrane integrity.

      a. Monitor incision site.

         (1) Hematoma development

         (2) Edema at surgical site

         (3) CSF leakage

            (a) Test for glucose.

            (b) Look for halo or ring sign.

      b. Pad bony prominences.

      c. Frequent repositioning for paralyzed patients

   5. Pain control

      a. Assess pain.

         (1) Level, location, duration

         (2) Use of pain scale

      b. Patient-controlled analgesia (PCA) often used with spinal surgery

      c. Frequent repositioning

      d. Maintenance of stabilizing devices

      e. Administration of pain medications if PCA not used

      f. Alternative methods of pain relief

         (1) Relaxation

         (2) Imagery

   6. Antiembolic stockings or sequential compression devices

   7. Psychosocial and emotional support

      a. Reassure patient frequently.

      b. Inform patient when assessing, performing procedures.

      c. Keep family informed of patient's condition.

      d. Answer patient's and family's questions as honestly as possible.

BIBLIOGRAPHY

1. American Association of Critical Care Nurses: *Core curriculum for critical care nursing*, ed 6, Philadelphia, 2006, Saunders.

2. American Association of Neuroscience Nurses: *Clinical guidelines series: Intracranial pressure monitoring*, Chicago, 2007, American Association of Neuroscience Nurses.

3. American Heart Association: *Heart attack, stroke and cardiac arrest warning signs.* Available at: www.americanheart.org. Accessed February 11, 2008.

4. Bader MK, Littlejohns L: *AANN core curriculum for neuroscience nursing*, ed 4, St Louis, 2004, Saunders.

5. Barker E: *Neuroscience of nursing: A spectrum of care*, ed 2, St Louis, 2007, Mosby.

6. Chipps E, Clanin N, Campbell V: *Neurologic disorders*, St Louis, 1992, Mosby.

7. DeMyer W: *Neuroanatomy*, ed 2, Baltimore, 1998, Williams & Wilkins.

8. Dennison RD: *Pass CCRN!*, ed 3, St Louis, 2007, Mosby.

9. Drain C, Odom-Forren J: *Perianesthesia nursing: A critical care approach*, ed 5, Philadelphia, 2009, Saunders.

10. Hickey JV: *The clinical practice of neurological and neurosurgical nursing*, ed 5, Philadelphia, 2003, Lippincott Williams and Wilkins.

11. Lazar M: Neurological consultants, Inc. Available at: http://neurosurgerydallas.com/1_3_4.html. Accessed July 15, 2008.

12. Luckmann J, Sweeney K: *Saunders manual of nursing care*, Philadelphia, 1997, Saunders.

13. Marshall BA, Miller RH: *Essentials of neurosurgery: A guide to clinical practice*, New York, 1995, McGraw-Hill.

14. McNair ND: Intracranial pressure monitoring. In Clochesy JM, Breu C, Cardin S, et al, eds: *Critical care nursing*, ed 2, Philadelphia, 1996, Saunders.

15. McQuillan KA, Von Rueden KT, Hartsock RL, et al: *Trauma nursing from resuscitation through rehabilitation*, ed 3, St Louis, 2002, Saunders.

16. Morton P, Fontaine O, Hudak C, Gallo B: *Critical care nursing: A critical care approach*, ed 8, Philadelphia, 2005, Lippincott Williams & Wilkins.

17. Nagelhout JL, Plaus KL: *Nurse anesthesia*, ed 4, St Louis, 2010, Saunders.

18. National Institute of Neurologic Disorders and Stroke: *NINDS brain and spinal tumors information page.* Available at: www.ninds.nih.gov/disorders/brainandspinaltumors/brainandspinaltumors.htm. Accessed February 11, 2008.

19. Neck Reference: Available at: www.neckreference.com. Accessed on February 11, 2008.

20. Ozuna JM: Nursing assessment neurologic system. In Lewis SM, Heitkemper MM, Dirksen SR, eds: *Medical surgical nursing assessment and management of clinical problems*, ed 5, St Louis, 2000, Mosby.

21. Patton KT, Thibodeau GA: *Anatomy and physiology*, ed 7, St Louis, 2010, Mosby.

22. Roisen M, Fleisher L: *Essence of anesthesia practice*, ed 2, Philadelphia, 2002, Saunders.

23. Spinal Cord Injury Information Network: Available at: www.spinalcord.uab.edu. Accessed February 11, 2008.

OBJECTIVES

At the conclusion of this chapter, the reader will be able to:

1. Describe the basic function of the endocrine system including the hormones produced by the thyroid, parathyroid, pituitary, and adrenal glands.

2. Identify the signs, symptoms, and diagnostic testing used to assess endocrine gland function.

3. Identify the surgical procedure and perioperative considerations for the patient with hyperthyroidism, hypothyroidism, pheochromocytoma, hypersecretion and hyposecretion of the pituitary and adrenal glands.

4. Identify the postanesthesia plan of care for the patient having subtotal thyroidectomy, bilateral adrenalectomy, hypophysectomy, and parathyroidectomy.

5. Discuss the postanesthesia considerations of the patient with endocrine dysfunctions: thyrotoxicosis, hypercalcemia, Cushing's syndrome, Addison's disease, diabetes insipidus, syndrome of inappropriate antidiuretic hormone.

6. Discuss the postanesthesia care of the diabetic patient and diabetic emergencies: hypoglycemia, diabetic ketoacidosis, and hyperglycemic hyperosmolar syndrome.

I. THYROID GLAND
  A. Anatomy and physiology (Figure 34-1)
    1. Location
      a. Sits in anterior portion of the neck
      b. Right lobe below the larynx
      c. Left lobe beside the trachea
      d. Middle portion called the isthmus lies at the base of the neck between second and fourth tracheal rings.
    2. Blood supply from external carotid arteries
    3. Nerve supply from cervical sympathetic trunk
    4. Functions of thyroid gland
      a. Regulates energy, metabolism and growth, and development
        (1) Hormone production from the hypothalamic-pituitary-thyroid axis
          (a) Hypothalamus secretes thyrotropin-releasing hormone (TRH)→stimulates the anterior pituitary to secrete thyroid-stimulating hormone (TSH)→increases the production of the thyroid hormones (THs) thyroxine (T_4) and triiodothyronine (T_3) and the uptake of iodide
        (2) Negative feedback loop (Figure 34-2)
          (a) Hypothalamus secretes TRH to regulate the synthesis and release of TSH.
          (b) When TH levels decrease, TSH and TRH levels increase.
          (c) Conversely, if TH levels increase, TSH and TRH levels decrease.
      b. T_3 has a short half-life, and T_4 has a half-life of 5 to 7 days.
      c. Peripheral tissue converts T_4 to T_3.
      d. T_3 considered the true tissue TH
      e. T_4 considered a plasma prohormone

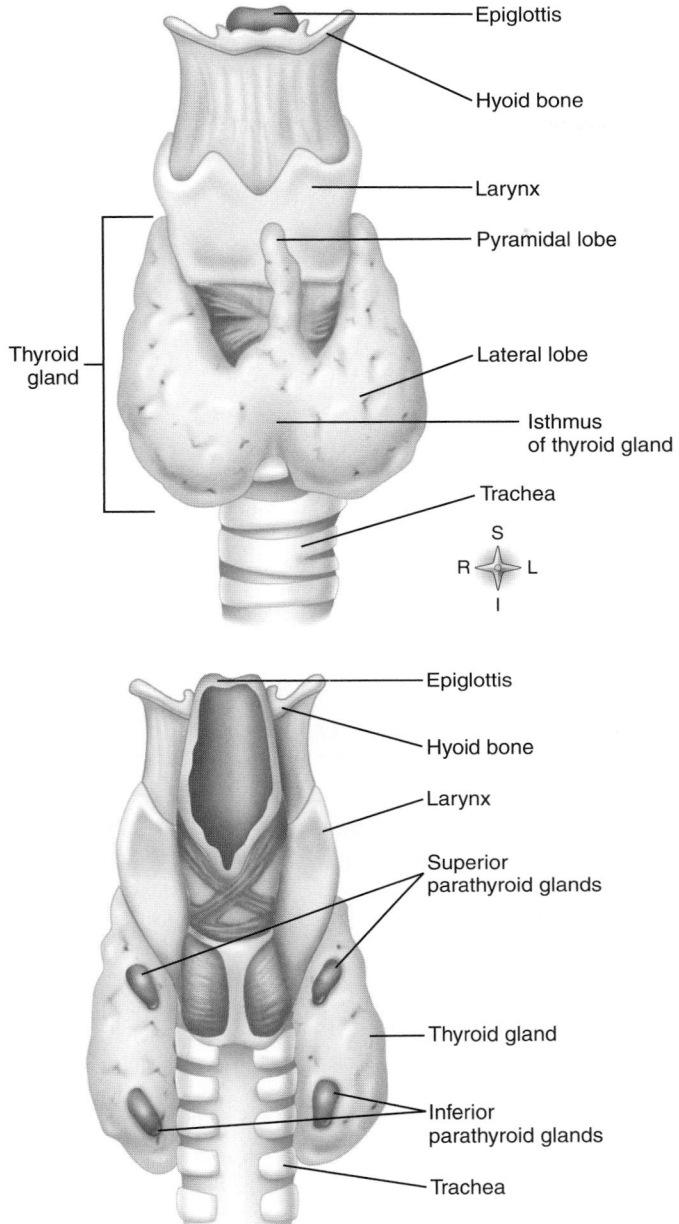

FIGURE 34-1 ■ Anatomy of thyroid and parathyroid gland. (From Thibodeau GA, Patton KT: *Anatomy & physiology,* ed 6, St Louis, 2007, Mosby.)

    B. Comparison of hyperthyroid and hypothyroid conditions (Table 34-1)

    C. Medical therapy: goal is to promote a euthyroid state.

        1. Hyperthyroid conditions

            a. Inhibition of TH synthesis

                (1) Propylthiouracil: 600- to 1000-mg loading dose followed by 200 to 250 mg every 4 hours

                    (a) Blocks conversion of T_4 and T_3

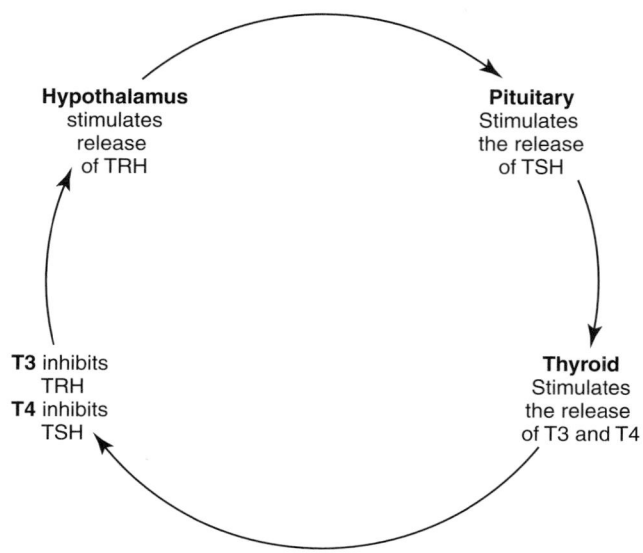

FIGURE 34-2 ■ Hypothalamus-pituitary-thyroid axis.

■ TABLE 34-1
■ ■ **Comparison of Hyperthyroid and Hypothyroid Conditions**

	Hyperthyroid	**Hypothyroid**
Description	Excessive secretion of thyroid hormones	Insufficient secretion of thyroid hormones
Causes	Multinodular, toxic, diffuse enlargement (goiter)—Graves' disease Malignancy Thyroiditis Viral, autoimmune Excessive iodine intake Amiodarone toxicity secondary to high concentrations of iodine; inhibits the conversion of T_4 to T_3	Chronic thyroiditis—progressively destroys thyroid function (Hashimoto's thyroiditis) Autoimmune diseases Iodine deficiency Surgical removal of thyroid Secondary dysfunction related to pituitary problems Tertiary dysfunction related to hypothalamus problems
Signs and symptoms	***Cardiopulmonary*** Hypertension Tachycardia or new atrial fibrillation Low blood pressure—fluid loss Potential heart failure Tachypnea ***Eyes/Ears/Nose/Throat*** Exophthalmos Enlarged thyroid /goiter Hoarseness/difficulty swallowing ***Gastrointestinal*** Weight loss Increased peristalsis Diarrhea and abdominal pain ***Musculoskeletal*** Body thinness Muscle atrophy and weakness	***Cardiopulmonary*** Bradycardia Decreased cardiac output High blood pressure—fluid retention Peripheral vasoconstriction Increased cholesterol levels ***Eyes/Ears/Nose/Throat*** Puffy eyes, enlarged tongue Goiter Hoarseness/difficulty swallowing ***Gastrointestinal*** Weight gain Constipation ***Musculoskeletal*** Muscle weakness Joint pain

■ TABLE 34-1
■ ■ **Comparison of Hyperthyroid and Hypothyroid Conditions—cont'd**

	Hyperthyroid	Hypothyroid
Signs and symptoms—cont'd	**Skin** Diaphoresis Fine, silky, thin hair Hyperpigmentation **Nervous System** Hyperactive emotional state Heat intolerance Insomnia **Genitourinary** Menstrual cycle changes Infertility	**Skin** Dry Alopecia Myxedema (late) **Nervous System** Fatigue, inability to concentrate Miscellaneous Cold intolerance **Genitourinary** Heavy menstrual bleeding Infertility
Diagnostic tests	TSH decreased T_3 increased Free T_4 increased Thyroid scan: radioactive iodine uptake Ultrasonography: identification of tumor type Fine-needle aspiration	TSH increased T_3 decreased Free T_4 decreased
Operative procedures to correct condition	**Purpose:** remove tracheal/esophageal obstructions or malignancy Subtotal thyroid lobectomy (partial lobe) Thyroid lobectomy (total lobe) Total thyroidectomy (removal of entire gland)	No specific surgery Comorbid condition
Preoperative objectives	**Promote a euthyroid state by:** Regulating antithyroid drugs Controlling hyperdynamic cardiac status Educate patient and family related to type of surgery/procedure, incision site, drains, and pain. Thyroid surgery–specific head and neck support when turning	**Promote a euthyroid state by:** Regulating thyroid replacement Educate patient and family related to type of surgery/procedure, incision site, drains, and pain.
Anesthesia concerns	Corneal drying or abrasions Considerations of agents based on euthyroid state Stability of cardiac status Airway status Oxygen requirements increased with hypermetabolic state and increased temperature Vocal cord visualization for injury to recurrent laryngeal nerves	Predisposition to hypothermia, cardiac failure, and delayed gastric emptying Metabolism of medications may be delayed. Adrenal insufficiency: may consider glucocorticoids to correct insufficiency Neuromuscular weakness may affect weaning. Potential difficult intubation secondary to predisposition for an enlarged tongue

T_3, Triiodothyronine; T_4, thyroxine; *TSH,* thyroid-stimulating hormone.

      (b) Administered at least 6 to 12 weeks preoperatively to achieve euthyroid state
      (c) Avoid acetylsalicylic acid because it displaces T_3 from protein binding.
    (2) Methimazole: 60 to 120 mg/day in divided doses
      (a) Blocks uptake of iodine
      (b) Administered 6 to 12 weeks preoperatively to achieve euthyroid state

        b. Inhibition of TH release
           (1) Saturated solution of potassium iodide
              (a) 50 mg iodine per drop: 1 to 2 drops three times per day
              (b) Iodide blocks T_4 release from the thyroid gland.
              (c) Acute management
           (2) Lugol's solution (5% iodine, 10% potassium solution)
              (a) 8 mg iodine per drop
              (b) Acute management: 4 to 8 drops Lugol's solution or saturated solution of sodium iodide every 6 to 8 hours; administer at least 2 to 3 hours after initial dosing of inhibitors of TH synthesis.
           (3) Lithium carbonate: 300 mg every 6 hours
        c. Inhibition of sympathetic nervous system innervation
           (1) Beta-blockers first choice
              (a) Propanolol: 0.5 to 1 mg intravenously (IV) every 15 minutes as needed, as loading dose until onset of action of oral propranolol (60-80 mg every 4 hours)
              (b) Esmolol: loading dose of 250 to 500 mcg/kg followed by infusion of 50 to 100 mcg/kg per minute
           (2) Calcium channel blockers if unable to tolerate beta-blockers
        d. Prevent peripheral conversion of T_4 to T_3 during acute thyrotoxic storm.
           (1) Hydrocortisone: 300 mg initially, followed by 100 mg every 8 hours IV
           (2) Dexamethasone: 2 mg IV every 6 hours
           (3) Prednisone: 40 mg/day—amiodarone-induced thyrotoxicosis
     2. Hypothyroid conditions
        a. Replace hormone
           (1) Chronic—levothyroxine: 1 to 1.5 mcg/kg per day orally initially; adjust as needed every 6 weeks until TSH in normal range; average dosage 1.6 to 1.8 mcg/kg per day (1.3 mcg/kg per day in the elderly)
           (2) Acute—myxedema coma: initial dosage 200 to 500 mcg IV daily; reduce dosage to 50 to 100 mcg IV daily until patient is able to take medication orally.
  D. Postanesthesia nursing plan of care (Boxes 34-1 and 34-2)
II. PARATHYROID GLANDS (see Figure 34-1)
  A. Anatomy and physiology
     1. Consists of four small ovoid masses of tissue lying behind the thyroid gland
     2. Parathyroid hormone (PTH) secreted from parathyroid glands
        a. PTH and vitamin D responsible for the regulation of calcium and phosphorous
        b. Serum calcium maintained by:
           (1) Regulating bone turnover
           (2) Absorption of calcium from the gut (with vitamin D)
           (3) Release of calcium in the urine

■ BOX 34-1

■ **DIFFERENCES BETWEEN THYROTOXIC CRISIS AND MALIGNANT HYPERTHERMIA**

	Thyrotoxic Crisis	**Malignant Hyperthermia**
Trigger	Increase in circulating thyroid hormones due to physiological stress	Exposure to anesthetic agents such as succinylcholine and/or volatile inhalation agents
Acute signs and symptoms	Hyperthermia Tachycardia Hypercarbia No muscle rigidity	Hyperthermia Tachycardia Hypercarbia Muscle rigidity
Treatment	Beta Blockers Steroids	Dantrolene sodium

■ BOX 34-2
■ **POSTANESTHESIA NURSING PLAN OF CARE: THYROID SURGERY/CONDITIONS**

Managing Hyperthyroid Conditions After Thyroid Surgery
Nursing Diagnosis
- Ineffective airway clearance related to edema of surgical area
- Impaired gas exchange related to increased metabolic demands
- Alteration in tissue perfusion related to hyperdynamic metabolic state
- Ineffective thermoregulation related to hyperdynamic metabolic state

Interventions
Airway Management
- Assess for signs of distress resulting from edema of the glottis or hematoma formation: dyspnea, cyanosis, stridor, retraction of neck muscles, tracheal deviation.
- Manage secretions to decrease strain on incision line caused by coughing.
- Manage oxygenation secondary to increased metabolic demands with supplemental humidified oxygen.
- Manage ventilation by monitoring rate, depth, and acid-base balance (arterial blood gases).

Cardiac Status
- Assess cardiac status secondary to hypermetabolic state, activation of the sympathetic nervous systems from the stress of surgery.

Wound Management
- Assess incision line for wound hemorrhaging (early complication) and report immediately.
- Monitor drainage devices if used.
- Assess laryngeal nerve damage by quality of vocalization and ability to swallow.

Positioning
- Maintain proper positioning after surgery.
  30° or higher head positioning
  Proper neck support by avoiding extreme head flexion or extension

General
- Monitor for tetany and hypocalcemia if combined with removal of parathyroid glands.
  Laryngeal spasm, tingling in toes, fingers, mouth
  Positive Chvostek's sign: twitching of facial muscles if cheek is tapped over facial nerve
  Positive Trousseau's sign: carpopedal spasm if circulation in arm is impeded with blood pressure cuff
- Monitor for thyrotoxic crisis (storm) versus malignant hyperthermia (see Box 34-1).

Managing Hypothyroid Conditions After Surgery
Nursing Diagnosis
- Impaired gas exchange related to decreased metabolism of medications
- Ineffective airway clearance related to neurological weakness
- Ineffective thermoregulation related to decreased metabolic state
- Alteration in tissue perfusion related to decreased metabolic state

Interventions
Airway Management
- Assess for signs of distress related to neurological weakness, sensitivity to medications, and predisposition for an enlarged tongue.
- Manage oxygenation secondary to decreased metabolism of medications.
- Manage ventilation by monitoring rate, depth, and acid-base balance (arterial blood gases).

Cardiac Status
- Assess for signs and symptoms of low cardiac output/heart failure.
- Assess for bradycardia.

Thermoregulation
- Monitor temperature secondary to predisposition to hypothermia.

        c. PTH release inhibited by rising serum calcium level

        d. PTH release dependent on normal serum magnesium levels

    B. Hyperparathyroid disease (Table 34-2)

    C. Postanesthesia nursing plan of care (Box 34-3)

III. PITUITARY GLAND

    A. Anatomy and physiology

        1. Location: pituitary gland located at the base of the skull in the sphenoid bone

            a. Lies within the sella turcica, near the hypothalamus and the optic chiasm

            b. Connected to the hypothalamus by the pituitary stalk, which links the endocrine and nervous systems

            c. Composed of anterior (80% of gland) and posterior lobes (20% of gland)

■ TABLE 34-2
■ ■ **Hyperparathyroid Disease**

	Primary Hyperparathyroidism	Secondary Hyperparathyroidism
Description	Excessive secretion of PTH, resulting in hypercalcemia	Hyperplasia of the parathyroid secondary to the dysfunction of another organ or secondary to another condition
Causes	Adenomas (single or multiple gland) most common Hyperplasia of one or more glands Malignancies (rare) Previous head or neck radiation	Vitamin D conditions (deficiency, malabsorption, metabolism, osteomalacia [i.e., rickets]) Calcium disorders Phosphate disorders Chronic renal failure
Signs and symptoms	Result from hypercalcemia: ***Cardiopulmonary*** Hypertension Dysrhythmias ***Nervous System*** Irritability Somnolence Lethargy ***Genitourinary*** Renal calculi Polyuria ***Musculoskeletal*** Osteopenia and osteoporosis Muscle weakness Joint or back pain ***Gastrointestinal*** Abdominal pain Constipation Nausea Risk for gastric ulcers and pancreatitis	

LABORATORY TESTS*

PTH	Normal: 10–65 mg/mL Hyperparathyroid conditions: Elevated
Ionized calcium	Normal: 4.5–5.6 mg/dL Hyperparathyroid conditions: Elevated

*Normal values vary with laboratories.

■ TABLE 34-2
■ ■ **Hyperparathyroid Disease—cont'd**

	Primary Hyperparathyroidism	Secondary Hyperparathyroidism
LABORATORY TESTS—cont'd		
Calcium	Normal: 9.0–10.5 mg/dL	
	Hyperparathyroid conditions: Elevated	
Phosphorus	Normal: 2.5–4.5 mg/dL	
	Hyperparathyroid conditions: Decreased	
Operative procedures to correct condition	Surgical removal of parathyroid Total parathyroidectomy: removal of all glands Partial parathyroidectomy: removal of up to 3.5 of 4 glands Minimally invasive parathyroidectomy	
Preoperative objectives	Treat hypercalcemia and correct associated conditions. Saline hydration and furosemide administration for rapid correction Calcitonin Mithramycin for thrombocytopenia and renal problems Prednisone Dysrhythmia management Educate patient and family related to type of surgery/procedure, incision site, drains, and pain. Parathyroid surgery–specific head and neck support when turning	
Anesthesia concerns	Intravascular volume changes Postoperative airway obstruction related to recurrent laryngeal nerve injury or bleeding Renal, cardiac, and nervous system abnormalities Consider prophylaxis with H_2 receptor blockers.	

H_2, Histamine type 2; *PTH,* parathyroid hormone.

    B. Pathophysiology
      1. Causes of glandular dysfunction
        a. Adenomas
        b. Malignancies
        c. Congenital abnormalities
        d. Hypothalamic dysfunction
      2. Hormones of the anterior and posterior pituitary gland (Table 34-3)
    C. Clinical considerations of the anterior and posterior pituitary gland (Tables 34-4 and 34-5)
    D. Postanesthesia plan of care: pituitary surgery/conditions (Box 34-4)
  IV. ADRENAL GLANDS
    A. Anatomy and physiology
      1. Location
        a. Lie retroperitoneal beneath the diaphragm capping the medial aspect of the superior pole of each kidney
        b. Right adrenal is triangular and adjacent to the inferior vena cava.
        c. Left adrenal is round or crescent shaped and sits posterior to the stomach and the pancreas.
      2. Adrenal medulla
        a. Ten percent of the gland secretes catecholamines.
      3. Adrenal cortex
        a. Ninety percent of the gland secretes steroids and hormones.

■ BOX 34-3
■ **POSTANESTHESIA NURSING PLAN OF CARE: PARATHYROID SURGERY**

Nursing Diagnosis
- Ineffective airway clearance related to edema of surgical area
- Impaired gas exchange related to postoperative bleeding or swelling or inability to move secretions
- Alteration in fluid and electrolyte balance secondary to total or partial removal of parathyroid gland(s)
- Alteration in tissue perfusion related to cardiac dysrhythmias
- Altered sensory perception related to postoperative hypocalcemia

Interventions
Airway Management
- Assess for signs of distress resulting from edema of the glottis or hematoma formation: dyspnea, cyanosis, stridor, retraction of neck muscles, tracheal deviation.
- Manage secretions to decrease strain on incision line caused by coughing.
- Manage oxygenation secondary to increased metabolic demands with supplemental humidified oxygen.
- Manage ventilation by monitoring rate, depth, and acid-base balance (arterial blood gases).

Cardiac Status
- Assess cardiac status secondary to hypocalcemia.

Wound Management
- Assess incision line for wound hemorrhaging or hematoma and report immediately.
- Assess laryngeal nerve damage by quality of vocalization and ability to swallow.
- Maintain proper positioning after surgery.
  30° or higher head positioning
  Proper neck support by avoiding extreme head flexion or extension

General
- Monitor for tetany and hypocalcemia with removal of parathyroid glands (immediate to 72 hours postoperatively).
  Laryngeal spasm, tingling in toes, fingers, mouth
  Positive Chvostek's sign: twitching of facial muscles if cheek is tapped over facial nerve
  Positive Trousseau's sign: carpopedal spasm if circulation in arm is impeded with blood pressure cuff
- Consider treatments for hypocalcemia.
  Calcium chloride IV administration
  Vitamin D to replace PTH to increase serum calcium level

IV, Intravenous; *PTH,* parathyroid hormone.

B. Pathophysiology
   1. Normal regulation of adrenal hormones
      a. Regulated by the release of corticotropin from the hypothalamus
      b. Functions of glucocorticoids (cortisol)
         (1) Carbohydrate metabolism
         (2) Protein metabolism
         (3) Promotes lipolysis
         (4) Increases tissue responsiveness to other hormones
         (5) Anti-inflammatory effects
      c. Functions of mineralocorticoids (aldosterone)
         (1) Control blood pressure by regulating sodium and water reabsorption
         (2) Increases potassium secretion
   2. Medullary hormones
      a. Catecholamines (epinephrine, norepinephrine, dopamine)
         (1) Control blood pressure and heart rate by regulation of sympathetic nervous system
         (2) Regulation of gluconeogenesis and lipolysis

■ TABLE 34-3
■ **Hormones of the Anterior and Posterior Pituitary Gland**

Hormone	Normal Physiology	Hypersecretion Conditions	Hyposecretion Conditions
ANTERIOR PITUITARY			
Growth hormone	Stimulates protein synthesis and lipolysis and promotes growth by working with other hormones	Acromegaly	Dwarfism
Adrenocorticotropic hormone (ACTH; corticotropin)	Stimulates adrenal glands to produce and release corticosteroids: cortisol (glucocorticoid) and aldosterone (mineralocorticoid)	Cushing's syndrome	Addison's disease
Thyroid-stimulating hormone (TSH)	Stimulates thyroid gland to produce thyroid hormones	Hyperthyroid conditions Graves' disease	Hypothyroid conditions Myxedema
Luteinizing hormone (LH) Follicle-stimulating hormone (FSH) (gonadotropins)	Stimulates ovaries and testes to produce estrogen and testosterone Responsible for ovulation and spermatogenesis	Polycystic ovary conditions	Infertility Amenorrhea Decreased sperm production
Prolactin (PRL)	Stimulates mammary glands to produce milk	Galactorrhea: an increase in milk production in men and non–breast-feeding women Suppresses production of LH and FSH	Reduction in milk production
POSTERIOR PITUITARY			
Antidiuretic hormone (ADH) Vasopressin	Regulation of water by increasing water permeability in renal collecting duct, controlling extracellular fluid osmolality Regulation of blood pressure by constricting arterioles	Syndrome of inappropriate antidiuretic hormone (SIADH)	Diabetes insipidus

■ TABLE 34-4
■ ■ **Clinical Considerations with Anterior Pituitary Disorders**

	Hypersecretion	Hyposecretion
Clinical signs and symptoms	Acromegaly Bone overgrowth or malformations usually of the mandible causing the jaw to protrude Larynx cartilage may thicken, causing a deep voice Tongue enlargement Barrel chest Joint pain Coarse body hair Enlarged sweat glands causing excessive perspiration Enlarged heart Headaches Nerve disturbances Menstrual changes	Dwarfism Hypothyroidism Obesity Headaches Decreased secondary sexual characteristics Lethargy
Diagnostic evaluation	CT/MRI scan of pituitary gland Increase in hormonal levels of human growth hormone/ACTH levels	CT/MRI scan of pituitary gland Decrease in ACTH or human growth hormone levels
Treatments	Hypophysectomy—removal of pituitary gland Craniotomy Transsphenoidal through the nasal floor	Management of target organ disease state Surgical resection of adenoma
Anesthesia /operative concerns	Airway management secondary to soft tissue/bone overgrowth Management of blood pressure secondary to increases in ACTH and TSH Management of hyperglycemia secondary to increases in ACTH (glucocorticoid release) Management of dysrhythmias secondary to increases in ACTH and TSH Management of fluids and electrolytes related to stimulation of ACTH (aldosterone release) Risk for infection secondary to surgical procedure	Airway management secondary to obesity Management of bradydysrhythmias secondary to decreases in ACTH and TSH Management of hypoglycemia secondary to decreases in ACTH Management of core temperature secondary to hypometabolism Metabolism of medications may be delayed. Neuromuscular weakness may effect weaning.

ACTH, Adrenocorticotropic hormone (corticotropin); *CT*, computed tomography; *MRI*, magnetic resonance imaging; *TSH*, thyroid-stimulating hormone.

    C. Adrenal gland conditions (Table 34-6)
    D. Postanesthesia nursing plan of care: adrenal gland surgery/conditions (Box 34-5)
  V. DIABETES MELLITUS IN THE SURGICAL PATIENT
    A. Pathophysiology
      1. Etiology
        a. Deficits in insulin secretion, action, or both
        b. Chronic hyperglycemia can lead to dysfunction and failure of various organs, especially the eyes, kidneys, nerves, heart, and blood vessels.
        c. Diabetic patient at higher risk for surgery and anesthetic complications than nondiabetic patient
      2. Types of diabetes mellitus
        a. Type 1 (ketosis prone)

■ TABLE 34-5
Clinical Considerations with Posterior Pituitary Disorders

	Hypersecretion	Hyposecretion
Clinical signs and symptoms	SIADH Water intoxication/fluid overload Headache Decreased LOC Decreased urine output Seizures secondary to hyponatremia Elevated BP, HR, CVP Heart failure Nausea, vomiting, and diarrhea	DI Neurogenic: insufficient synthesis of ADH Nephrogenic: inability to respond to ADH Dehydration Headache, lethargy Visual disturbances Increased HR Decreased BP, CVP, and cardiac output Polydipsia Polyuria
Diagnostic evaluation	CT/MRI scan of pituitary gland for tumors Increase in plasma levels of ADH Increased urine osmolality greater than serum osmolality Decreased urine aldosterone Dilutional serum hyponatremia	CT/MRI scan of pituitary gland Decrease in ACTH or human growth hormone levels Hemoconcentrated hypernatremia Decreased serum ADH with neurogenic DI Increased serum ADH with nephrogenic DI Decreased urine osmolality
Treatments	Hypophysectomy—removal of pituitary gland Surgical resection of tumors Restrict fluids. Sodium level >125 mEq/L: fluid restriction of 800–1000 mL/day. Demeclocycline (Declomycin) can be administered: allows excretion of water because it inhibits the effect of ADH on renal tubules. Sodium level <105 mEq/L: administer hypertonic (3% saline) infusion over 2–3 hours Furosemide to increase urinary water excretion	Management of target organ disease state Surgical resection of adenoma Treat with exogenous ADH (vasopressin/Pitressin). 5–10 units Pitressin subcutaneously or IM Thiazide diuretics Replace volume lost by titrating hypotonic or dextrose fluids to urine output.
Anesthesia /operative concerns	Management of volume secondary to systemic fluid retention Manage or prevent seizure activity secondary to hyponatremia. Limit the use of drugs that may increase ADH release (morphine, barbiturates, beta-adrenergics).	Management of volume secondary to signs of intravascular dehydration Management of BP secondary to dehydration Management of cardiac status secondary to vasopressin administration (potent vasoconstrictor)

ADH, Antidiuretic hormone; *BP*, blood pressure; *CT*, computed tomography; *CVP*, central venous pressure; *DI*, diabetes insipidus; *HR*, heart rate; *IM*, intramuscular; *LOC*, level of consciousness; *MRI*, magnetic resonance imaging; *SIADH*, syndrome of inappropriate antidiuretic hormone (secretion).

■ BOX 34-4
■ **POSTANESTHESIA PLAN OF CARE: PITUITARY SURGERY/CONDITIONS**

Nursing Diagnosis
- Potential impaired gas exchange secondary to difficult intubation
- Ineffective thermoregulation related to changes in metabolic demands
- Potential for infection related to impaired glucocorticoid levels and surgery
- Impaired fluid and electrolyte balance related to fluid volume excess or deficit
- Potential alteration in neurological status

Interventions

Airway
- Assess for signs of distress: dyspnea, cyanosis, stridor, retraction of neck muscles, tracheal deviation.
- Manage secretions.
- Manage oxygenation secondary to increased metabolic demands with supplemental humidified oxygen.
- Manage ventilation by monitoring rate, depth, and acid-base balance (arterial blood gases).

Thermoregulation
- Monitor for hyperthermia (hypothalamic influences)
- Monitor for hypothermia (from decreased thyroid-stimulating hormone levels).

Infection
- Monitor blood glucose levels to range between 80 and 120 mg/dL.
- Monitor incisions for signs and symptoms of infection.

Fluid and Electrolytes
- Fluid restriction as indicated
- Monitor intake, output, and weight.
- Monitor electrolytes.
- Manage dysrhythmias.
- Mouth care to protect mucous membranes
- Monitor for signs and symptoms of fluid overload or deficit.
- Monitor mental status as a result of fluid status and electrolyte (sodium) imbalance.
- Monitor urine specific gravity.

Neurological Status
- Monitor for signs of changes in level of consciousness.
- Monitor for signs of seizure activity.
- Monitor for cerebrospinal fluid leakage at incision site/transsphenoidal approach.

(1) Characteristics
    (a) Insulin deficient
    (b) Ketotic
    (c) Children and young adults
    (d) Rarely obese
    (e) Prone to other autoimmune disorders
    (f) Accounts for 5% to 10% of the population with diabetes
(2) Causes
    (a) Genetic
    (b) Autoimmune destruction of pancreatic beta cells (insulin-producing cells)
    (c) Environmental
  b. Type 2
    (1) Characteristics
        (a) Insulin resistance and insulin deficiency
        (b) Nonketotic

TABLE 34-6

Adrenal Gland Conditions

	Hyperaldosteronism	Addison's Disease	Cushing's Syndrome	Pheochromocytoma
Definition	**Primary** Overproduction of aldosterone **Secondary** High renin activity from other pathological conditions and hypertension	Hyposecretion of cortisol and aldosterone	Hypersecretion of corticosteroids	Overproduction of catecholamines
Physiology	Adrenal cortex	Adrenal cortex	Adrenal cortex	Adrenal medulla
Etiology	**Primary** Adenomas Adrenocortical malignancies Adrenocortical hyperplasia **Secondary** Ascites Hypertension Heart failure Obstructed renal artery disease	**Primary** Autoimmune reaction Infection Secondary effect from other glandular conditions Secondary from steroid therapy for other conditions Congenital disorders	Adenomas Carcinomas Overstimulation of adrenal cortex by ACTH release from pituitary gland (negative feedback loop) Prolonged use of glucocorticoids Congenital disorders	Benign tumor of adrenal medulla Tumors that secrete high levels of catecholamines (epinephrine and norepinephrine)
Effects of conditions	**Primary** Hypernatremia Hypervolemia Hypertension Hypokalemia Weakness Paresthesias Tetany Hyperglycemia **Secondary** Hypovolemia Hyponatremia Hypokalemia	**From Aldosterone Deficiency** Hypernatremia Hypokalemia Weakness Dizziness Polyuria **From Corticosteroid Deficiency** Hypoglycemia Hyperpigmentation from excessive corticotropin stimulation as a result of pituitary stimulation (negative feedback loop) Addisonian crisis Prolonged hypotension and cardiac dysrhythmias Shock Lack of response to vasopressors	**From Corticosteroid Hypersecretion** Altered distribution of body fat primarily to the back of the neck ("buffalo hump") and the trunk of the body (centripetal) "Moon face" Ecchymosis Osteoporosis Poor wound healing	Severe hypertension Hyperglycemia Hypermetabolism Increased levels of norepinephrine and epinephrine Tachycardia Palpitations Nausea Weight loss Abdominal pain Irritability Diaphoresis Headaches Visual disturbances

Continued

■ TABLE 34-6
■ ■ Adrenal Gland Conditions—cont'd

	Hyperaldosteronism	Addison's Disease	Cushing's Syndrome	Pheochromocytoma
Diagnostic evaluation	Elevated sodium Decreased potassium Increased urinary excretion of aldosterone Hyperglycemia and glycosuria ECG changes secondary to electrolyte imbalance CT/MRI scan of adrenal gland Hyperglycemia clinical signs	Elevated potassium Decreased sodium CT/MRI scan of adrenal gland ACTH stimulation test: failure to stimulate ACTH helps with confirming diagnosis of Addison's disease Hypoglycemia	Elevated cortisol levels Decreased potassium levels Increase plasma ACTH levels (if pituitary cause) Decrease in eosinophils CT/MRI scan of adrenal gland Dexamethasone suppression test: failure to suppress cortisol helps to confirm a diagnosis of Cushing's syndrome	Increase in serum catecholamines (epinephrine and norepinephrine) Increase in urine catecholamines CT/MRI scan of adrenal gland Clonidine administration: decreases plasma norepinephrine
Treatments	Adrenalectomy (unilateral or bilateral)	Corticosteroid administration	Adrenalectomy (unilateral or bilateral)	Adrenalectomy
Anesthesia/ operative/ post-anesthesia concerns	Management of blood pressure Assess lung expansion postoperatively Hypertension Antihypertensive agents Vasodilators Angiotensin-converting enzyme inhibitors Hypotension Volume expanders (blood, albumin) Vasopressors Dysrhythmia management secondary to potassium changes and catecholamine releases	Management of corticosteroid administration Preoperative usage from preexisting conditions such as arthritis, colitis, asthma Inadequate corticosteroid replacement during and after surgical procedures	Airway management Compromised lung expansion secondary to truncal obesity or moon face Positioning for exposure and preventing stress fractures or skin trauma Managing blood pressure Managing hyperglycemia	Avoidance of medications causing histamine release of sympathetic stimulation Management of blood pressure before and after excision of tumor Before: hypertensive management with vasodilators After: rebound hypotension with vasopressors, blood expanders, cortisol replacement

ACTH, Adrenocorticotropic hormone (corticotropin); *CT*, computed tomography; *ECG*, electrocardiogram; *MRI*, magnetic resonance imaging.

■ BOX 34-5
■ **POSTANESTHESIA NURSING PLAN OF CARE: ADRENAL GLAND SURGERY/CONDITIONS**

Nursing Diagnosis
- Potential for alterations in neurological status secondary to hypertension, increased circulating catecholamines, or rapid removal/change in circulating catecholamines after removal of a pheochromocytoma
- Potential for impaired gas exchange related to postoperative atelectasis/pneumothorax secondary to 12th rib resection during adrenalectomy
- Altered cardiac output secondary to activation or inactivation of the sympathetic nervous system
- Alteration in tissue perfusion secondary to cardiac dysrhythmias related to electrolyte disturbances
- Alteration in fluid and electrolyte balance secondary to adrenalectomy/excision of pheochromocytoma
- Potential for infection secondary to hyperglycemia

Interventions
Neurological Status
- Monitor for signs/sudden changes in level of consciousness.
- Assess pupils for reactivity/light accommodation.

Airway Management
- Assess for signs of distress secondary to risk of atelectasis/pneumothorax: dyspnea, cyanosis, stridor, retraction of neck muscles, tracheal deviation.
- Manage secretions to minimize risk of hypoxemia.
- Evaluate lung expansion by chest x-ray verification.
- Manage oxygenation with supplemental humidified oxygen.
- Manage ventilation by monitoring rate, depth, and acid-base balance (arterial blood gases).

Cardiac Management
- Assess and treat hyper/hypotension
  - Administer vasoactives as needed to maintain hemodynamics secondary to decreased circulating catecholamines.
  - Administer vasodilators as needed secondary to hypertension caused by pheochromocytoma.
- Monitor for bleeding.
- Monitor for rebound epinephrine shock secondary to insensitive receptors and impaired vascular reflexes.
- Maintain hemodynamics as indicated.
- Monitor laboratory values: changes in serum sodium, potassium, and glucose.
- Administer IV fluids (hypertonic saline for low serum sodium levels), blood products, albumin as indicated.

Wound Management
- Assess incision line for wound hemorrhaging or hematoma and report immediately.
- Monitor for signs and symptoms of infection: redness, swelling, increased tenderness.
- Monitor for trends in WBC counts

IV, Intravenous; *WBC*, white blood cell.

(c) Overweight/obese
(d) Accounts for 90% to 95% of the population with diabetes
(2) Causes
   (a) Resistance to insulin action
   (b) Inadequate compensatory insulin secretory response
   (c) Risk factors:
      (i)   Age
      (ii) Obesity
      (iii) Inactivity
      (iv) Hypertension
      (v) Dyslipidemia

    3. Other types of diabetes mellitus
        a. Gestational
        b. Drug or chemical induced
        c. Genetic defects in beta-cell function
        d. Genetic defects in insulin action
        e. Diseases of the exocrine pancreas
        f. Infections
        g. Endocrinopathies
  B. Perioperative considerations
    1. Preoperative evaluation
        a. Assess for macrovascular complications secondary to diabetes.
            (1) Coronary artery disease (CAD) (see Chapter 32)
                (a) Common cause of mortality in diabetic patients
                (b) Assess for pain/electrocardiogram changes, serum troponin values secondary to incidence of painless angina.
                (c) Lipid profile
            (2) Peripheral vascular system
                (a) Shiny taut skin
                (b) Diminished or absent pulses
                (c) Loss of hair on lower extremity
                (d) Cool extremities
                (e) Leg pain at rest/night
                (f) Intermittent claudication
                (g) Color changes in legs with positioning (red with legs dependent; white with legs elevated)
            (3) Cerebral circulation
                (a) History of transient ischemic attacks/stroke
                (b) Confusion/disorientation
                (c) Chronic hypertension
        b. Assess for microvascular complications.
            (1) Diabetic nephropathy
                (a) Serum creatinine
                (b) Blood urea nitrogen
                (c) Albumin levels in urine
                (d) Urinary output
            (2) Diabetic retinopathy
                (a) Presence of cataracts
            (3) Diabetic neuropathy
                (a) Postural hypotension
                (b) Sensory motor impairment
                (c) Genitourinary impairment
                (d) Delayed gastric emptying
        c. Assess laboratory values.
            (1) Glucose levels before surgery
            (2) Glycosylated hemoglobin (hemoglobin A1C) to determine long-term (3 months) control of diabetes
            (3) Electrolytes
                (a) Potassium
                (b) Sodium
                (c) Chloride
                (d) Bicarbonate
            (4) Creatine Kinase
            (5) Troponin
        d. Assess for medications associated with altering glucose levels.
            (1) Medications associated with contributing to hyperglycemia
                (a) Thiazides and loop diuretics
                (b) Glucocorticoids
                (c) Dilantin

        (d) Calcium channel blockers

        (e) H$_2$ receptor blockers

        (f) Beta-adrenergic receptor agonists

        (g) Morphine sulfate

     (2) Medications associated with contributing to hypoglycemia

        (a) Insulin

        (b) Sulfonylureas

        (c) Beta-adrenergic receptor antagonists

        (d) Angiotensin-converting enzyme inhibitors

        (e) Alcohol

2. Intraoperative and anesthesia considerations

    a. Glycemic control to target range during surgery

     (1) Stress of surgery contributes to insulin resistance in all patients.

     (2) Prevent diabetic emergencies such as diabetic ketoacidosis and hyperglycemic hyperosmolar syndrome.

        (a) Frequent blood glucose monitoring intraoperatively

        (b) Maintain patient in well-hydrated anabolic state.

    b. Anesthetic agents

     (1) No specific anesthetic for diabetic patients

     (2) Inhalation agents may cause less pronounced changes in blood glucose.

     (3) Regional blocks may be considered because they cause fewer metabolic disturbances.

    c. Avoidance of hypoglycemia and serious cerebral dysfunction

     (1) Maintain blood glucose levels for diabetic patients undergoing surgery to target ranges (American Diabetes Association recommends 80–110 mg/dL; Box 34-6).

     (2) Monitor for signs of hypoglycemia during surgery.

        (a) Elevated heart rate

        (b) Decrease in urinary output

        (c) Seizure activity

    d. Avoidance of hyperglycemia

     (1) Assess for increase in urine output.

     (2) Assess for risk of intravascular dehydration secondary to osmotic diuresis.

     (3) Assess for hyperglycemia with administration of vasoactive agents such as epinephrine.

    e. Avoidance of cardiopulmonary complications

     (1) Prevent myocardial infarction.

        (a) Consider perioperative beta-blockers.

        (b) Monitor electrolytes: potassium, magnesium.

        (c) Maintain hemodynamics.

        (d) Monitor and treat dysrhythmias.

     (2) Prevent hypotension caused by increased urinary output by administering IV fluid.

     (3) Prevent hypoxemia.

        (a) Assess glycosylated hemoglobin: increased levels influence tissue oxygenation.

        (b) Assess oxygen saturations: oxygen consumption increased secondary to increased shunting as a result of general anesthesia.

    f. Avoidance of injury

     (1) Maintain proper positioning during surgery secondary to peripheral neuropathy.

     (2) Monitor for risk of aspiration secondary to impaired gastric emptying (gastroparesis).

        (a) Consider rapid sequence induction.

        (b) Elevate the head to decrease the risk when possible.

3. Diabetic emergencies (Table 34-7)

4. Postanesthesia nursing plan of care: diabetes mellitus (Box 34-7)

■ BOX 34-6
■ **EVIDENCED-BASED PRACTICE CONSIDERATIONS FOR PATIENTS WITH DIABETES MELLITUS**

According to the American Diabetic Association (2008) position statement titled *Standards of Medical Care in Diabetes Mellitus*, targeting glucose control in the hospital can potentially improve mortality, morbidity, and health economic outcomes. The patient can manifest hyperglycemia from the stress of the hospitalization or the procedure, the withholding of antihyperglycemic medications or the administration of hyperglycemia-provoking agents such as glucocorticoids or vasopressors, or the decompensation of type 1, type 2 diabetes. Many studies have looked at varying populations of hospitalized patients and the effects of targeted glucose on morbidity and mortality. It is recommended that the target glucose for critically ill patients should be 80-110 mg/dL. The incidence of hypoglycemia was found to be higher in medical critically patients compared with surgical critically ill patients.

Specific to perianesthesia care, most of the studies on glycemic control have been done on the cardiac surgical population. These patients experienced the lowest mortality rates and risks of sternal wound infections with a target blood glucose <150 mg/dL. This can translate to perioperative hyperglycemia as a predictor of infection in patients with diabetes.

From this review, many variations of insulin protocols and regimens have been created.

Each patient's clinical situation should be evaluated and goals for glycemic control targeted and achieved. It is recommended that hospital facilities develop standards for glycemic control and provide support to achieve the goals. In addition, quality improvement initiatives should be developed to evaluate progress and facilitate improvement.

VI. PANCREAS TRANSPLANTATION
   A. Overview
      1. Select criteria/considerations for patient selection for pancreas transplantation
         a. Frequent episodes of hypoglycemia, marked hyperglycemia, ketoacidosis requiring medical attention
         b. Clinical and emotional problems with exogenous insulin therapy or administration
         c. Consistent failure of insulin-based management to prevent acute complications
         d. Diabetes for at least 20 years
         e. Risks of secondary complications of diabetes mellitus are greater than those of the surgical procedure and the posttransplant immunosuppression.
      2. Goals of pancreas transplantation
         a. Improve the quality of life of people with diabetes, by eliminating the acute complications commonly experienced by patients with type 1 diabetes (hypoglycemia, marked hyperglycemia, and ketoacidosis).
         b. Eliminate the need for exogenous insulin, frequent daily blood glucose measurements, and many of the dietary restrictions.
         c. Reverse or stabilize the long-term renal and neural complications of diabetes.
         d. Frequently combined with kidney transplant
   B. Preoperative assessment
      1. Health history
         a. Absence of infection
            (1) Screened for remote infection (i.e., urinary tract infection, respiratory, dental)
            (2) Preoperative antibiotics
         b. Central nervous system
            (1) Evaluate mental/emotional illness secondary to postoperative compliance.
            (2) Evaluate for autonomic neuropathy.
               (a) Gastroparesis
               (b) Cystopathy
               (c) Orthostatic hypotension

TABLE 34-7

■ Diabetic Emergencies

	Hypoglycemia	DIABETIC KETOACIDOSIS	HYPERGLYCEMIC HYPEROSMOLAR SYNDROME
Characteristics/ clinical signs	Shakiness/tremors Diaphoresis Tachycardia Irritability Decreased level of consciousness Confusion Slurred speech Seizures Coma	Type 1 diabetics Polydipsia Polyuria Polyphagia Decreased level of consciousness Warm and dry Decreased blood pressure Elevated heart rate ECG changes: tall, peaked T waves Abdominal pain Nausea and vomiting Kussmaul's respirations Fruity acetone breath	Type 2 diabetics Polydipsia Polyuria Polyphagia Decreased level of consciousness Warm and dry or cool and moist Normal or decreased blood pressure Normal heart rate Abdominal pain Nausea and vomiting
Possible causes	Interactions with other drugs Alcohol Insulin overdose or incorrect dosages Inadequate food intake Hormonal deficiencies Renal diseases Neoplasms	Infection Poorly controlled type 1 diabetes Insulin omission Surgical stress Medications that interfere with insulin	Precipitated by an acute illness Poorly controlled type 2 diabetes Infection: pneumonia and urinary tract infections most common Surgical stress Medications that interfere with insulin
Laboratory values	Glucose <60 mg/dL	Glucose 250–800 mg/dL pH <7.3 HCO_3 <15 mEq/L Serum and urine ketones >2+ Elevated potassium	Glucose >800 mg/dL pH >7.3 HCO_3 >15 mEq/L Serum and urine ketones <2+

Continued

TABLE 34-7
■ Diabetic Emergencies—cont'd

	Hypoglycemia	DIABETIC KETOACIDOSIS	HYPERGLYCEMIC HYPEROSMOLAR SYNDROME
Treatments	***Mild Reactions*** Administer 10–15 g carbohydrate (i.e., 4 oz of orange juice) or inject 1 mg glucagon or via feeding tube, administer a liquid source of glucose (soda). ***Moderate and Severe Reactions*** Administer 50% dextrose equivalent to 25 g glucose and follow with continuous IV infusion. Monitor glucose levels frequently for several hours.	Treatment goals are similar for both DKA and HHS. ***Administer fluids.*** 0.9% normal saline at rapid rates (adjusted for other comorbidities and corrected sodium levels) Titrate with consideration to urine output, blood pressure, and central venous pressures. Administer 5% dextrose in 0.45% normal saline once the blood glucose level reaches 250 mg/dL. ***Treat hyperglycemia (protocols may vary).*** Initiate IV bolus of regular insulin recommended at 0.15 units/kg as IV bolus. Continuous IV insulin infusion recommended at a rate of 0.1 units/kg per hour. Titrate to target ranges as indicated. Decrease insulin infusion at a glucose level of 250 mg/dL to decrease the risk of hypoglycemia and to protect against cerebral edema. ***Replace electrolytes IV as needed.*** Potassium Magnesium Calcium ***Replace lost bicarbonate as needed.***	

DKA, Diabetic ketoacidosis; *ECG,* electrocardiogram; *HCO₃,* bicarbonate; *HHS,* hyperglycemic hyperosmolar syndrome; *IV,* intravenous.

■ BOX 34-7
■ **POSTANESTHESIA NURSING PLAN OF CARE: DIABETES MELLITUS**

Nursing Diagnosis (Actual or Potential)
- Alteration in cerebral circulation secondary to hypoglycemia or hyperglycemia
- Impaired gas exchange secondary to hypoxemia
- Decreased cardiac output secondary to cardiovascular complications from diabetes
- Fluid volume deficit secondary to hyperglycemia
- Infection secondary to diabetes

Interventions
- Monitor and manage serum glucose to target range.
- Assess for and treat diabetic emergencies as indicated.

Neurological Management
- Assess level of consciousness.
- Assess for changes in cerebral function.
  Slurred speech
  Seizure activity
  Irritability

Airway Management
- Assess for signs of distress secondary to hypoxemia: dyspnea, cyanosis, stridor, retraction of neck muscles, tracheal deviation.
- Manage secretions to increase oxygenation.
- Manage oxygenation secondary to hypoxemia with supplemental humidified oxygen.
- Manage ventilation by monitoring rate, depth, and acid-base balance (arterial blood gases).

Cardiovascular Management
- Assess for dysrhythmias secondary to electrolyte imbalance.
- Assess extremities for color, sensation, and motor function.
- Maintain hemodynamics.

Fluid Volume Management
- Monitor intake and output.
- Continue hydration as indicated.
- Monitor electrolytes.

Infection
- Monitor for signs and symptoms of infection.
- Assess incision site and/or invasive line site for erythema, pain, purulent drainage.
- Assess WBC counts for trends.

WBC, White blood cell.

  c. Coronary artery disease
  d. Renal disease
  e. Peripheral vascular disease
  f. Sensory neuropathies
 2. Preoperative preparation
  a. Patient/family education to long-term management
  b. Invasive lines
C. Anesthesia/operative concerns
 1. Rapid induction may be considered secondary to gastroparesis.
 2. Control serum glucose levels during surgery to range of 80 to 110 mg/dL.
 3. Manage electrolyte levels, with primary emphasis on maintaining potassium at levels of 3.5 to 5.3 mEq/L.

    4. Administration of immunosuppressive agents before graft reperfusion
      a. High-dose immunosuppressants administered
        (1) Antilymphocyte antibody induction therapeutic agents intraoperatively and early postoperatively
        (2) Steroid agents/immunosuppressants for maintenance
    5. Positioning secondary to long surgical time
    6. Operative techniques
      a. Provide adequate arterial blood flow to the pancreas and duodenal segment during transplantation.
      b. Provide adequate venous outflow of the pancreas via the portal vein.
      c. Pancreas graft arterial revascularization using the recipient right common or external iliac artery
      d. The Y-graft portal vein anastomosed to iliac vein
  D. Postanesthesia concerns
    1. Control of glucose level to 80 to 110 mg/dL
      a. Insulin infusion indicated versus bolusing to maintain a steady euglycemic state
      b. Decrease in insulin infusion after surgery common secondary to euglycemic condition after transplantation
    2. Manage volume as indicated by patient condition.
      a. Blood products may be indicated.
      b. IV hydration as appropriate to clinical condition
      c. Monitor urine output.
    3. Wound management
    4. Pain management
    5. Skin and sensory perception management secondary to prolonged positioning
    6. Postoperative complications
      a. Thrombosis secondary to low-flow states of the graft: first 24 to 48 hours after surgery
      b. Pancreatitis: frequent and temporary; seen 48 to 96 hours postoperatively; evidenced by elevated serum amylase level

BIBLIOGRAPHY

1. American Diabetes Association: Diagnosis and classification of diabetes mellitus. *Diabetes Care* 31(Suppl 1):S55–S60, 2008.
2. American Diabetes Association: *Position statement standards of medical care in diabetes mellitus.* Available at: http://care.diabetesjournals.org/cgi/content/full/31/Supplement_1/S12#SEC8. Accessed January 31, 2008.
3. Brunton L: *Goodman & Gilman's the pharmacological basis of therapeutics*, ed 11, New York, 2006, McGraw-Hill.
4. Chulay M, Burns S: *AACN essentials of critical care nursing: Endocrine system*, New York, 2006, McGraw Hill.
5. Flomenbaum N, Goldfrank L, Hoffman R, et al, eds: *Goldfrank's toxicological emergencies*, ed 8, New York, 2006, McGraw-Hill.
6. Kaufman DB: *Pancreas transplantation.* Available at: www.emedicine.com/med/topic2605. Accessed January 12, 2008.
7. Klein I, Danzi S: Thyroid disease and the heart. *Circulation* 116(15):1725–1735, 2007.
8. Noble K: Thyroid storm. *J Perianesth Nurs* 21 (2):119–122, 2006.
9. Porter R, Kaplan J, Homeier B, et al, editors: *Merck manual online: Endocrine and metabolic disorders*, Whitehouse Station, NJ, 2006, Merck.
10. Rothrock J: *Alexander's care of the patient in surgery*, ed 13, St. Louis, 2007, Mosby.
11. Townsend C, Beauchamp RD, Evers BM, et al: *Sabiston's textbook of surgery*, ed 18, Philadelphia, 2007, Saunders.

35 Gastrointestinal Care

DENISE O'BRIEN

Acknowledgement: I thank Lisa Colletti, MD, for her assistance in preparing this chapter.

OBJECTIVES

At the conclusion of this chapter, the reader will be able to:

1. List name and locate the major anatomical components of the gastrointestinal tract and the accessory organs of digestion.

2. Identify the major functions of each of the divisions of the gastrointestinal system and the accessory organs of digestion.

3. Describe the fluid and electrolyte problems most frequently encountered in the patient with a gastrointestinal disorder.

4. Incorporate the care of the other body systems into the postoperative management of the gastrointestinal surgery patient.

5. Describe two specific system complications of the gastrointestinal surgery patient.

6. State the rationale for placement of tubes and drains in the gastrointestinal surgery patient.

7. State the rationale for observations necessary in postanesthesia care of the patient undergoing gastrointestinal surgery.

I. ANATOMY AND PHYSIOLOGY
  A. Major anatomic components (Figure 35-1)
    1. Mouth
      a. Begins mechanical breakdown of food
      b. Secretion of saliva
      c. Tongue
      d. Teeth
    2. Pharynx
    3. Esophagus
      a. Carries food to stomach through peristalsis
      b. Lower esophageal sphincter
    4. Stomach
      a. Main site of digestion
      b. Produces digestive enzymes
      c. Cardiac sphincter
        (1) Prevents backflow of food and digestive enzymes
      d. Fundus
        (1) Begins digestion of proteins
      e. Pylorus
        (1) Contracts to empty stomach contents into small intestine
      f. Pyloric sphincter
        (1) Prevents food and digestive enzymes from entering the small intestine before digestion is completed

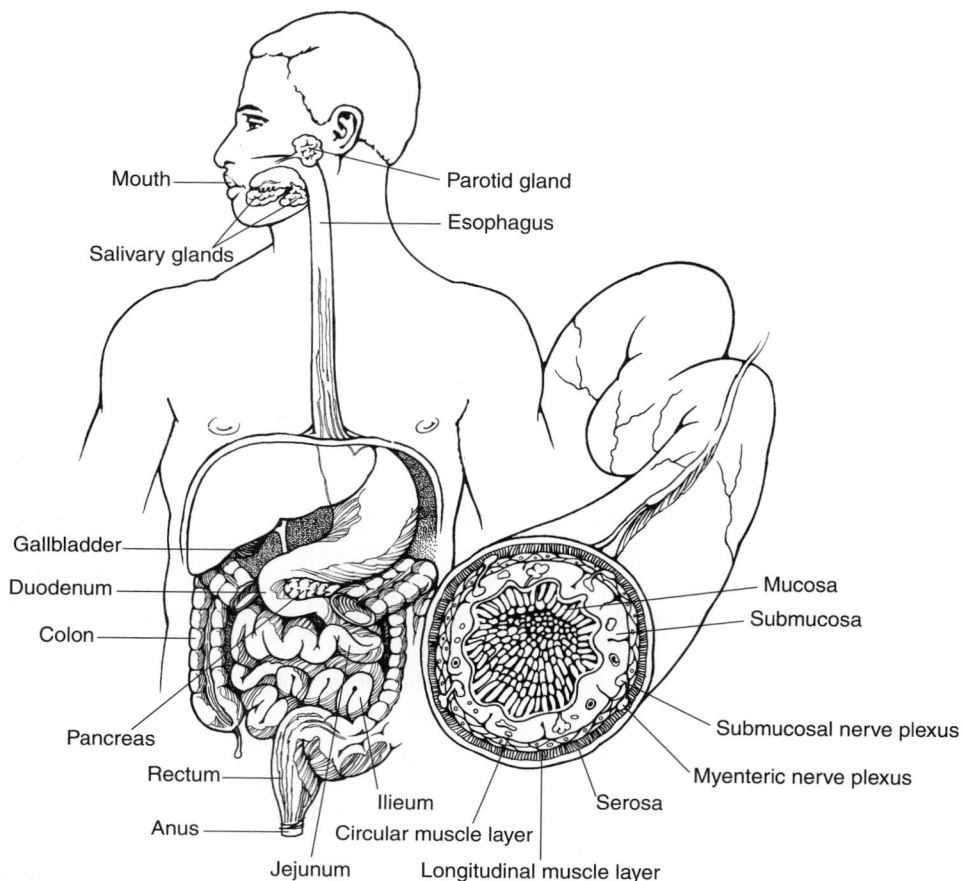

FIGURE 35-1 ■ The gastrointestinal system. (From Ignatavicius DD, Bayne MV: *Medical-surgical nursing,* ed 4, Philadelphia, 2002, WB Saunders.)

    g. Rugae
      (1) Provide the stomach with increased surface area
      (2) Expands with food
  5. Small intestine
    a. Duodenum
      (1) Chemical digestion occurs
        (a) Neutralizes stomach acids
        (b) Breaks down carbohydrates and fats
    b. Jejunum
      (1) Absorbs most nutrients
    c. Ileum
      (1) Absorbs water and vitamins
    d. Villi
  6. Large intestine
    a. Absorbs remaining water and vitamins
    b. Appendix
    c. Colon
    d. Rectum
    e. Anus
 B. Accessory organs of digestion
  1. Salivary glands
    a. Produce amylase
    b. Begins chemical breakdown of starch

        c. Provides lubrication

    2. Liver

        a. Detoxifies

        b. Neutralizes stomach acid

        c. Produces bile

    3. Gallbladder

        a. Stores bile

    4. Pancreas

        a. Produces insulin

        b. Produces digestive enzymes that are released into the duodenum

II. PATHOPHYSIOLOGY

  A. Neoplasms and growths

    1. Malignancies

        a. Primary

        b. Metastatic

    2. Polyps: a benign proliferation of cells lining the gastrointestinal tract

        a. Some with potential for malignant transformation

    3. See Strictures (II.C.1) and Adhesions below (II.C.2).

  B. Calculi

    1. Calculi or stones (e.g., cholelithiasis), primarily resulting from supersaturation of bile with cholesterol

  C. Strictures or obstructions

    1. Stricture: abnormal narrowing of gastrointestinal passage

        a. Neoplasms commonly cause strictures; for example:

            (1) Colon

            (2) Biliary tree

        b. Strictures can:

            (1) Progress to obstruction (blockage of gastrointestinal passage)

            (2) Be caused by adhesions

    2. Adhesions: union of two normally separate surfaces or a fibrous band that connects them

        a. Occasionally, produce obstruction or malfunction of an organ

        b. Result of the formation of scar tissue

        c. Abdominal surgery results in the formation of:

            (1) Adhesions

            (2) Scar tissue

            (3) Magnitude of these adhesions or scar tissue varies.

        d. Approximately 5% of cases associated with adhesions occur in persons who have had no previous abdominal surgery.

            (1) Virtually always the result of some other previous or ongoing pathological process, such as:

                (a) Pelvic inflammatory disease

                (b) Appendicitis

                (c) Diverticulitis

  D. Ulceration

    1. Ulcer disease

        a. Peptic ulcer disease

            (1) *Helicobacter pylori (H. pylori)*

            (2) Medications

                (a) Aspirin

                (b) Steroids

                (c) Nonsteroidal anti-inflammatory agents

        b. Stress ulceration, resulting from the following:

            (1) Surgical stress

            (2) Burns

            (3) Cranial trauma

            (4) Sepsis associated with multisystem failure

    E. Perforations
       1. Caused by ulceration
       2. Resulting from trauma
       3. Can also result from vascular compromise or obstruction
    F. Inflammation
       1. Regional enteritis (Crohn's disease)
       2. Cholecystitis
       3. Pancreatitis
       4. Appendicitis
       5. Diverticulitis
       6. Esophagitis
       7. Gastritis
       8. Ulcerative colitis
    G. Altered innervation
       1. Achalasia
    H. Congenital defects
       1. Hirschsprung's disease
       2. Tracheoesophageal fistula
       3. Imperforate anus
       4. Pyloric stenosis
       5. Arteriovenous malformation
    I. Ischemia: arterial or venous infarction
       1. Complication after abdominal aortic aneurysmectomy
       2. After repair of coarctation of aorta
       3. After coronary artery bypass
       4. Embolic
       5. Related to atherosclerosis of the abdominal vasculature; can result in mesenteric ischemia
       6. Low flow states: either related to cardiac disease, especially congestive heart failure, or sepsis
    J. Gastroesophageal reflux disease (GERD)
       1. Results from the reflux of stomach contents into the esophagus
       2. Symptoms may include:
         a. Heartburn
         b. Gastric regurgitation
         c. Dysphagia
         d. Pulmonary manifestations
           (1) Asthma
           (2) Coughing
           (3) Wheezing
           (4) Laryngeal inflammation
III. DIAGNOSTIC TESTS OR PROCEDURES
    A. Tests ordered depend on gastrointestinal area thought to be involved.
    B. Laboratory tests
       1. Basic hematology and electrolyte studies
       2. Serum enzyme levels
         a. Amylase
         b. Lipase
         c. Liver function tests or hepatic function panel
           (1) Albumin
           (2) Bilirubin (total and direct)
           (3) Aspartate aminotransferase (AST)
           (4) Alanine aminotransferase (ALT)
           (5) Alkaline phosphatase
           (6) Total protein
       3. Serum markers
         a. CA 19-9 for pancreatic cancer
         b. Alpha-fetoprotein (AFP) for hepatocellular cancer

       c. Carcinoembryonic antigen (CEA) for different types of cancer
- (1) Pancreas
- (2) Large intestine (colon and rectum)
- (3) Breast
- (4) Lung

  4. Coagulation studies
- **a.** If liver involvement suspected
- **b.** With malabsorption syndromes
  - (1) Cause malabsorption of vitamins that can compromise metabolism of coagulation factors produced by liver

C. Endoscopic procedures
- **1.** Motility studies (e.g., esophageal manometry)
- **2.** Esophagogastroduodenoscopy (EGD)
- **3.** Endoscopic retrograde cholangiopancreatography (ERCP)
  - **a.** With or without stents
  - **b.** With or without sphincterotomy
  - **c.** Purpose
    - (1) To remove retained common duct stones before or after biliary tract surgery
    - (2) As an emergency measure in patients with common bile duct obstruction (single or multiple stones) resulting in cholangitis
    - (3) May be done preoperatively to explore common bile duct in patients needing:
      - (a) Laparoscopic cholecystectomy
      - (b) Temporary or permanent treatment for biliary obstruction and jaundice
        - (i) Pancreatic malignancies
        - (ii) Biliary malignancies
  - **d.** Description—by use of side-viewing fiberoptic endoscope:
    - (1) Pancreatic and biliary ducts cannulated through ampulla of Vater
    - (2) Ducts visualized fluoroscopically after retrograde injection of radiopaque contrast medium
- **4.** Colonoscopy
- **5.** Sigmoidoscopy
- **6.** Twenty-four-hour pH monitoring with probe for reflux

D. Radiological examinations
- **1.** Barium swallow
- **2.** Upper gastrointestinal series—may also include a small bowel follow-through to evaluate:
  - **a.** Small intestine
  - **b.** Stomach
  - **c.** Duodenum
- **3.** Cholangiogram—typically done as part of:
  - **a.** ERCP
  - **b.** Percutaneous transhepatic cholangiography (PTC)
  - **c.** Operatively
- **4.** PTC
- **5.** Barium enema
- **6.** Flat plate of abdomen
- **7.** Visceral angiography
  - **a.** Angiography
  - **b.** Carbon dioxide (CO_2) digital subtraction angiography
- **8.** Computed tomography (CT) scan

E. Other modalities
- **1.** Endoscopic ultrasonography
  - **a.** Endoscopic ultrasonography of:
    - (1) Esophagus
    - (2) Stomach

    (3) Pancreas

    (4) Biliary tree

   b. Transanal ultrasonography

  2. Radionuclide

   a. Gastrointestinal studies

   b. Liver and spleen studies

   c. Hepatobiliary iminodiacetic acid (HIDA) scan for acute cholecystitis or to detect biliary leak

   d. Labeled red blood cells to check site of bleeding

  3. Magnetic resonance imaging

  4. Magnetic resonance angiography: used to evaluate vasculature

  5. Magnetic resonance cholangiopancreatography

 F. Tissue biopsies as indicated with cytological or histological studies; typically done with ultrasound or CT guidance

IV. INTRAOPERATIVE CONCERNS

 A. Proper positioning

  1. Maintain neurovascular integrity.

   a. Padding and support of all body parts with particular attention given to vulnerable areas (e.g., elbows, sacrum, heels, occiput)

   b. For comfort

   c. Proper alignment in presence of arthritis, lumbar disorders, and contractures

   d. Preserve integrity of popliteal nerve and/or ulnar and brachial nerve plexus when lithotomy or exaggerated arm abduction is used.

  2. Prevent complications.

   a. Proper application of electrosurgical grounding pads to prevent cautery burns; avoid contact with metal or hard surfaces.

   b. Careful positioning changes of anesthetized patient (to and from Trendelenburg or lithotomy position) to prevent adverse alterations in tidal volume and cardiac output; position of padding and support rechecked after each change

   c. Protect skin from shearing while positioning and moving.

 B. Cardiovascular stability

  1. Factors influencing altered fluid volume, electrolyte, and nutritional status

   a. Chronic bleeding

   b. Diarrhea

   c. Vomiting

   d. Increased secretions

   e. Fluid loss

    (1) Nasogastric suctioning

    (2) Fistula drainage

    (3) Bowel preparation

    (4) Length of operative procedure

  2. Problems with preceding factors if not corrected preoperatively

   a. Hypotension: caused by deficits in circulating volume

    (1) Poorly tolerated in pediatric, elderly, and debilitated patients vulnerable to adverse effects of hypotension because of decreased body reserve necessary to handle crises

    (2) Potential rapid fluid (blood) loss because of rich intestinal blood supply and its proximity to aorta and vena cava

    (3) Rapid fluid resuscitation with crystalloid or colloid solution can result in overhydration, leading to pulmonary edema and congestive heart failure in compromised patient.

   b. Altered electrolyte balance: cardiac dysrhythmias can occur with abnormal potassium or calcium levels.

   c. Clotting abnormalities caused by poor nutritional status or hemodilution or in presence of liver disease

           (1) Decreased vitamin K, leading to decreased levels of factors V, VII, IX, and X

           (2) Prolonged prothrombin times

  C. Thermal regulation (see Chapter 24)

    1. Hyperthermia

      a. Elevated temperature on arrival in the operating room, possibly as a result of:

        (1) Infection

        (2) Peritonitis

        (3) Other inflammatory process

      b. Anesthesia care provider must observe for signs and symptoms of possible adverse reaction to anesthetic agents and muscle relaxants, which may lead to malignant hyperthermia, either in operating room or in post anesthesia care unit (PACU).

    2. Hypothermia

      a. Prolonged exposure of abdominal viscera causes loss of body heat.

        (1) Procedures of 3 or more hours

        (2) Extensive gastrointestinal resection

      b. Large-volume fluid or blood/blood product resuscitation without adequately warming fluids

      c. Temperature control methods

        (1) Room temperature control

        (2) Use of warming mattresses, convective warming devices, and protective coverings

        (3) Warming of intravenous (IV) and irrigating fluids

  D. Drug interactions and other concerns

    1. Nondepolarizing muscle relaxants (see Chapter 22)

      a. Antagonized by hypothermia

      b. Patients may reparalyze with postoperative warming.

      c. May have slowed return of neuromuscular function because of:

        (1) Hypothermia

        (2) Decreased elimination of some relaxants (those eliminated by Hofmann elimination)

      d. Potentiated by broad-spectrum antibiotics (mycins, aminoglycosides)

    2. Metabolism and excretion of medications impaired in presence of:

      a. Liver dysfunction

      b. Renal failure

      c. Obesity

    3. Avoid use of histamine-releasing agents such as morphine sulfate.

      a. Histamine release can cause hypotension in hypovolemic patient.

    4. All opioids increase biliary tract pressure, which may cause spasm of sphincter of Oddi, producing severe right upper quadrant or substernal pain in the patient with biliary obstruction or disease.

      a. Severity of symptoms (pain, nausea, diaphoresis, hypotension) requires that myocardial infarction be ruled out.

      b. Symptoms usually abate with administration of naloxone (Narcan) or glucagon.

    5. Rapid sequence induction ("crash" induction): possible indications

      a. History of gastroesophageal reflux

      b. Stricture of gastroesophageal sphincter

      c. History of recent eating before emergency surgery

      d. Bowel obstruction

      e. History of gastroparesis

    6. Spillage of feces or bile into peritoneal cavity is potential cause of chemical or bacterial peritonitis and should be documented.

V. GASTROINTESTINAL OPERATIVE PROCEDURES

  A. Esophageal procedures

    1. Cervical esophagostomy

     a. Purpose—often done as part of first-stage repair in infants for:

        (1) Tracheoesophageal fistula

        (2) Esophageal atresia

     b. Description: surgical formation of opening into esophagus at cervical level

     c. Preoperative phase I assessment and concerns

        (1) At risk for aspiration; gastrostomy tube placed as soon as atresia or fistula identified

        (2) May have multiple anomalies of cardiovascular, gastrointestinal systems

     d. Postanesthesia phase I priorities

        (1) Maintain normothermia.

        (2) Tracheal leak may be present.

        (3) Pain management

     e. Complications

        (1) Pulmonary aspiration

        (2) Vocal cord paralysis

2. Esophagectomy with colon or gastric interposition

     a. Purpose: used in presence of esophageal atresia or for esophageal damage anywhere, except very proximal cervical esophagus

        (1) Commonly performed for:

            (a) Esophageal malignancies

            (b) End-stage achalasia

     b. Description: usually a piece of colon or stomach (more common) is used to establish continuity between esophagus and stomach.

     c. Preoperative assessment and concerns

        (1) May have recurrent aspiration pneumonia from gastric reflux

        (2) Malnutrition related to dysphagia or anorexia

        (3) Evaluation of cardiovascular and respiratory status (may be compromised in patients with esophageal malignancies because these patients often are smokers and drink excess alcoholic beverages)

     d. Intraoperative concerns

        (1) Hypothermia

        (2) Positioning to avoid neural injuries or soft tissue damage

     e. Postanesthesia phase I priorities

        (1) At risk for aspiration and atelectasis; head of bed elevated

        (2) Pain management: consider thoracic epidural continuous analgesia.

        (3) Assess for hypoventilation, pneumothorax, anastomotic leak.

        (4) Patient may be hoarse.

     f. Complications

        (1) Aspiration

        (2) Atelectasis, hypoventilation

        (3) Hemorrhage

        (4) Pneumothorax

        (5) Esophageal anastomotic leak

        (6) Recurrent laryngeal nerve injury

3. Esophageal dilation

     a. Purpose: to allow free passage of food and fluids into stomach; used to correct:

        (1) Achalasia

        (2) Esophageal spasms

        (3) Strictures

     b. Description: dilating instruments (bougies or balloons) passed in increasingly larger sizes or inflated to enlarge lumen of esophagus

     c. Preoperative assessment and concerns

        (1) Nothing by mouth (NPO) before procedure

     d. Intraoperative concerns

        (1) Procedure may be done with sedation and analgesia or with general anesthesia.

     e. Postanesthesia priorities

        (1) Phase I

(a) Minimal postprocedure pain expected

(b) Observe for:

(i) Subcutaneous emphysema

(ii) Pain

(iii) Aspiration

(c) Monitor temperature.

(2) Phase II

(a) Assess gag reflex before giving fluids.

(b) Review appropriate instructions with patient, family, and responsible accompanying adult.

f. Psychosocial concerns

(1) May require frequent dilations

(2) May prefer particular type of sedation or anesthesia for procedure based on past experience

g. Complications

(1) Esophageal perforation

(2) Pain

(3) Hemorrhage

(4) Bacteremia or sepsis

4. Esophagomyotomy (Heller procedure)

a. Purpose: to allow food to pass from esophagus to stomach when a segment of esophagus is narrowed, causing functional obstruction

b. Description: surgical division or anatomical dissection of muscles at distal esophagogastric junction, leaving mucosa intact

5. Herniations (see Chapter 36)

a. Part of stomach protruding through an opening, or hiatus, in diaphragm

b. Surgical repair of hiatal or diaphragmatic hernias accomplished through either an abdominal or a thoracic approach

c. Hiatal hernia is not a true hernia, while diaphragmatic hernia is.

(1) Hiatal hernia occurs when the gastroesophageal junction slides up and down between the chest and abdomen.

(2) Tends to be associated with GERD

(3) No indication to fix hiatal hernia unless patient also has GERD

d. Diaphragmatic hernia is a true hernia and should always be repaired because of risk of incarceration or strangulation of the stomach.

e. Purposes

(1) To restore herniated part below diaphragm for diaphragmatic hernias

(2) For patients with GERD and hiatal hernias

(a) To narrow esophageal hiatus

(b) To recreate esophagogastric angle to enhance lower esophageal sphincter function

(c) To stop reflux of gastric contents

f. Description (these procedures are done for GERD and not specifically for a hiatal hernia)

(1) Collis-Belsey and Collis-Nissen repairs: esophageal lengthening with antireflux wrap of distal esophagus

(2) Hill repair: abdominal approach that narrows esophageal orifice and fixes esophagogastric junction in intra-abdominal position; includes 180° wrap of stomach around esophagus

(3) Belsey Mark IV repair: performed through incision in left side of chest

(a) Consists of 240° wrap of distal portion of esophagus with fundus of stomach

(b) This partial fundoplication is technically difficult.

(c) Risk of leakage or diverticulum developing in esophagus is higher because sutures are required in esophageal wall.

(d) Newer procedure: modified thoracoscopic Belsey repair

    (4) Nissen fundoplication: transabdominal or laparoscopic (similar to open approach and most common procedure for this condition) treatment for sliding esophageal hiatal hernia

        (a) Portion of fundus of stomach is mobilized and completely wrapped around (360°) distal portion of esophagus.

        (b) Prevents stomach displacement into posterior portion of mediastinum through diaphragmatic defect

    (5) Toupet partial fundoplication: alternative antireflux procedure; fundal wrap reduced to 180° to 270°

  g. Preoperative assessment and concerns

    (1) Possible recurrent aspiration pneumonia

    (2) Antacid and antireflux prophylaxis recommended

  h. Intraoperative concerns

    (1) Aspiration risk during induction and emergence

    (2) Hemorrhage

    (3) Visceral injury

    (4) Hypothermia

  i. Postanesthesia priorities

    (1) Phase I

        (a) Nausea and vomiting

        (b) Shoulder pain (if laparoscopic approach)

        (c) Pain management

        (d) Hypoventilation

    (2) Length of stay usually 2 to 3 days for Nissen fundoplications

  j. Complications

    (1) Gastric perforation

    (2) Bleeding, hemorrhage

    (3) Pneumothorax

    (4) Aspiration

    (5) Hypoventilation

    (6) Wrap too tight, with resultant dysphagia and difficulty eating/swallowing

6. Esophageal band ligation

  a. Purpose: to obliterate esophageal varices to reduce risk of bleeding or hemorrhage

  b. Description: endoscopic procedure involves placing a band around (ligation) varices in esophagus.

  c. Preoperative assessment and concerns

    (1) NPO before procedure

  d. Intraoperative concerns

    (1) Procedure may be done with sedation and analgesia or with general anesthesia.

  e. Postanesthesia priorities

    (1) Phase I

        (a) Minimal postprocedure pain expected

        (b) Observe for:

            (i)   Subcutaneous emphysema

            (ii) Severe pain

            (iii) Aspiration

        (c) Monitor temperature.

        (d) Watch for bleeding.

    (2) Phase II

        (a) Assess gag reflex before giving fluids.

        (b) Review appropriate instructions for postsedation or postanesthesia care with patient, family, and responsible accompanying adult.

        (c) Verify that patient and caregiver are aware of potential for bleeding and when to notify surgeon.

    f. Psychosocial concerns
       (1) Patient may require repeat procedures.
       (2) Patient may prefer particular type of sedation or anesthesia for procedure based on past experience.
    g. Complications
       (1) Esophageal perforation
       (2) Aspiration pneumonitis
       (3) Hemorrhage
       (4) Bacteremia and sepsis

B. Gastric procedures
    1. Gastrectomy
      a. Purpose: to remove all or a portion of diseased organ; most commonly performed for cancer
      b. Description: surgical removal of whole or a part of stomach
       (1) Antrectomy
        (a) Involves almost a 50% distal gastrectomy
        (b) Antral mucosa (site of gastrin formation) removed, usually in conjunction with truncal vagotomy
        (c) Remaining portion of stomach anastomosed to duodenum or jejunum
       (2) Billroth I (gastroduodenostomy): type of reconstruction used with an antrectomy
        (a) First portion of duodenum sewn to remaining portion of stomach (Figure 35-2)
       (3) Billroth II (gastrojejunostomy): reconstruction used with an antrectomy
        (a) First portion of duodenum is unable to reach remaining portion of stomach.
        (b) First portion of the duodenum is sewn shut.
        (c) Loop of jejunum just distal to ligament of Treitz is brought up and sewn to remaining stomach remnant (Figure 35-2).
       (4) Total gastrectomy: done for cancer of stomach or abdominal esophagus; reconstruction after total gastrectomy usually by esophagojejunostomy
       (5) Near total gastrectomy: may be done for treatment of gastroparesis
       (6) Roux-en-Y gastrojejunostomy: reconstruction procedure for the stomach
        (a) May be used for reconstruction after antrectomy or after total gastrectomy
        (b) Used as a bypass procedure for unresectable pancreatic cancer
        (c) More commonly a loop gastrojejunostomy used in this situation (a loop of jejunum is sewn to stomach to bypass an obstructed distal stomach or duodenum)
      c. Preoperative assessment and concerns
       (1) Rehydration
       (2) Possible transfusion because of bleeding
       (3) Possible hyperalimentation for nutritional deficits
       (4) Electrolyte abnormalities
      d. Intraoperative concerns
       (1) Volume status
       (2) Anticipate significant third space losses.
       (3) Acute hemorrhage
      e. Postanesthesia phase I priorities
       (1) Low thoracic epidural for pain management; patient-controlled analgesia also an option
       (2) Maintain nasogastric tube patency and position.
    2. Gastric bypass (see Chapter 48)
    3. Laparoscopic adjustable gastric banding (see Chapter 48)
    4. Gastroenterostomy (Figure 35-2)

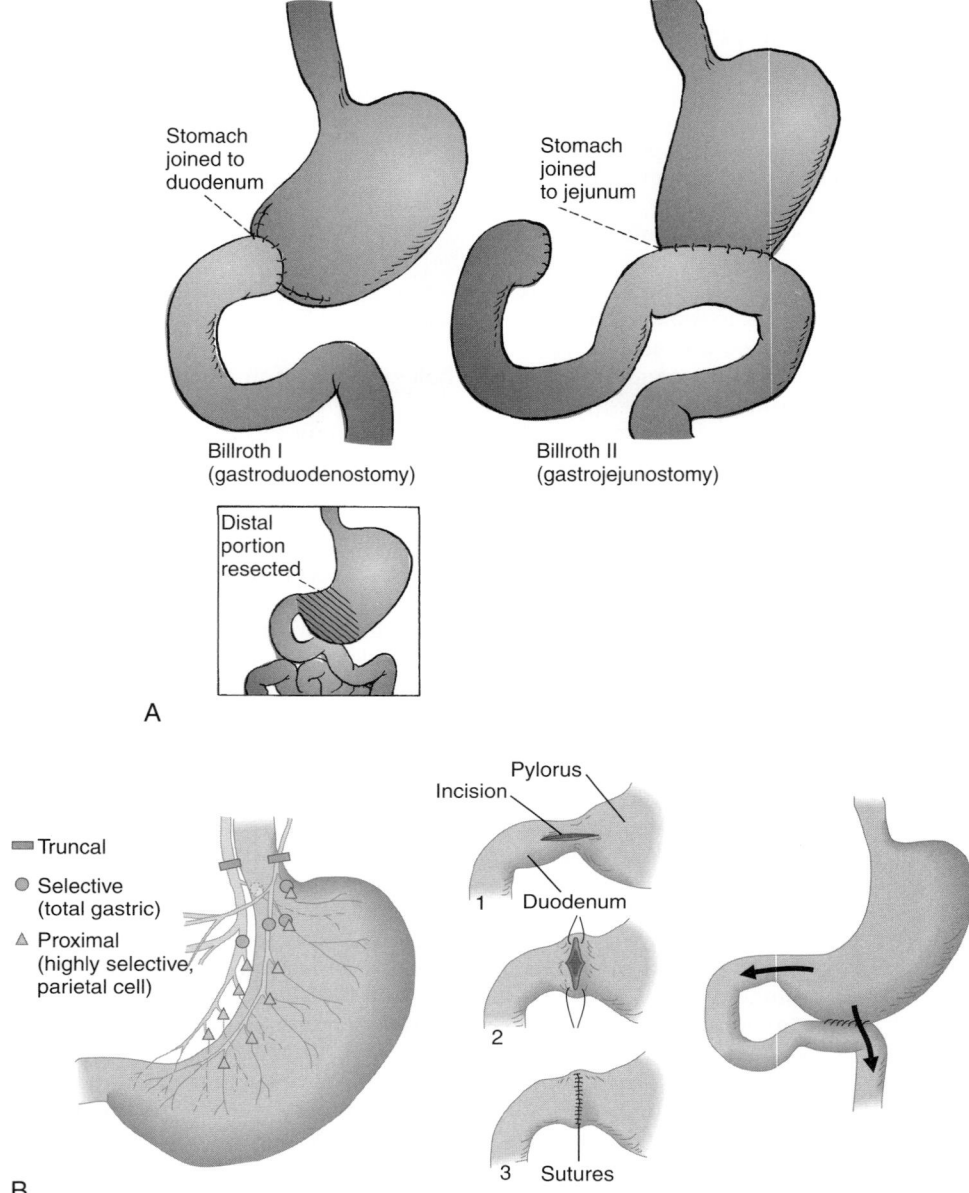

FIGURE 35-2 ■ Gastric surgical procedures. **A,** Billroth I, Billroth II. **B,** Vagotomy *(left)*; pyloroplasty *(middle)*; gastroenterostomy *(right)*. (From Black JM, Hawks JH: *Medical-surgical nursing: Clinical management for positive outcomes,* ed 7, Philadelphia, 2005, Saunders.)

    a. Purpose: to create an artificial passage between stomach and small intestine

    b. Description: surgical anastomosis between stomach and small intestine, usually jejunum, for unresectable pancreatic cancer with gastric outlet obstruction

  5. Gastrostomy

    a. Purpose: used for long-term stomach decompression or to introduce food into gastrointestinal system

    b. Description: creation of gastric fistula or opening through abdominal wall, usually with a tube in place

(1) May be done operatively or endoscopically (insertion of gastrostomy tube through incision made at point where anterior portion of stomach wall is tented with endoscope, making contact with parietal peritoneum)

(2) Traction on tube maintains contact between stomach and abdominal wall.

c. Percutaneous endoscopic gastrostomy (PEG)

(1) Endoscopic procedure performed with local anesthesia

(2) Relative and/or absolute contraindications to PEG

(a) Prior gastric surgery

(b) Portal hypertension with varices and/or ascites

(c) Ascites from other causes

(d) Prior abdominal surgery

6. Pyloromyotomy

a. Purpose: to widen pyloric opening

b. Description: muscle fibers of outlet of stomach are cut without severing mucosa.

7. Pyloroplasty (see Figure 35-2)

a. Purpose: to increase size of pyloric opening in presence of pyloric stenosis or scarring caused by ulcer disease; usually performed in conjunction with vagotomy when done for latter

b. Description: repair of pylorus used to establish opening in presence of pyloric or prepyloric obstruction

8. Vagotomy (see Figure 35-2): since recognition of *H. pylori*, almost never done anymore

a. Purpose: to reduce amount of gastric acid secreted and lessen chance of recurrence of peptic ulcer

b. Description: sectioning of vagus nerve or its branches; choices of vagotomy include:

(1) Truncal

(2) Selective

(3) Proximal (highly selective, parietal cell)

(4) May be accomplished by laparoscopic approach

c. Needs to be performed in conjunction with an "emptying procedure," either pyloroplasty or partial gastrectomy (antrectomy)

C. Biliary, hepatic, and pancreatic procedures

1. Surgical correction of biliary atresia (condition in which extrahepatic bile ducts are nonpatent, seen primarily in infants) or any type of biliary obstruction in adults

a. Stones

b. Strictures

c. Surgical injury (lap chole injury)

d. Distal biliary obstruction due to chronic pancreatitis

e. Sclerosing cholangitis

f. Biliary carcinoma

2. Roux-en-Y procedure

a. Purpose—used when:

(1) Proximal extrahepatic bile ducts patent

(2) Distal ducts occluded

(3) For bypass in cancer of bile duct and pancreatitis

b. Description: distal end of divided jejunum anastomosed to patent remnant of proximal bile duct

3. Hepatic portoenterostomy (Kasai procedure): typically done in infants/children for biliary atresia

a. Purpose: used when proximal extrahepatic ducts are totally occluded

b. Description: removal of entire extrahepatic biliary tree; bile drainage established by anastomosis of intestinal conduit to transected ducts at liver hilus

      c. Preoperative assessment and concerns

         (1) May have impaired elimination of drugs because of hepatic dysfunction

         (2) Coagulation values need to be evaluated.

      d. Intraoperative concerns

         (1) Potential for large third-space losses

      e. Postanesthesia/phase I priorities

         (1) Monitor volume status.

      f. Complications: cholangitis

  4. Cholecystectomy (see Chapter 36)

      a. Purpose: to treat cholelithiasis and cholecystitis

      b. Description: removal of gallbladder and its cystic duct

         (1) May be through traditional "open" approach or by laparoscopy

         (2) Laparoscopic approach may use the following to remove the gallbladder from liver bed and ligate vessels and ducts:

            (a) Laser

            (b) Electrosurgical cautery

            (c) Harmonic scalpel

      c. Intraoperative concerns

         (1) High incidence of postoperative nausea and vomiting; prophylactic antiemetics recommended before end of case

         (2) Pneumoperitoneum if laparoscopic; risk of gas embolism

      d. Postanesthesia priorities

         (1) Phase I

            (a) Postoperative nausea and vomiting management

            (b) Shoulder pain (both open and laparoscopic approaches)

         (2) Phase II

            (a) Minimal nausea and vomiting for discharge home

            (b) Oral analgesics initiated as needed for pain management before discharge

            (c) Instruct patient and companion regarding:

               (i) Diet

               (ii) Incision sites

               (iii) Care of incisions

  5. Cholecystostomy

      a. Purpose: to decompress gallbladder of debilitated patient with acute cholecystitis or cholelithiasis unable to tolerate cholecystectomy at that time

      b. Description: formation of opening into gallbladder through abdominal wall

         (1) If stones present, approach may be by angiography with lithotripsy to break up stones.

         (2) Usually done with local anesthesia and sedation

      c. Preoperative assessment and concerns

         (1) Dehydration from the following may require fluid resuscitation before operative procedure:

            (a) Fever

            (b) Vomiting

            (c) Decreased oral intake

         (2) Peritonitis

         (3) Sepsis

  6. Choledochotomy

      a. Purpose: usually for removal of stones

      b. Description: incision of common bile duct

      c. Preoperative assessment and concerns

         (1) As in preceding section (V.C.5.c)

  7. Common bile duct exploration

      a. Purpose

         (1) To check for stones and/or strictures

         (2) Frequently performed at time of cholecystectomy

    b. Description: exploration of common bile duct

       (1) T-tube drain left in place for a period of time postoperatively to ensure patency of common bile duct

       (2) Can use laparoscopic approach

  8. Hepaticojejunostomy

    a. Purpose

       (1) To repair stricture of common bile duct after laparoscopic or open cholecystectomy

       (2) May also be done for patients with bile duct cancer

    b. Description: creation of anastomosis between hepatic duct and jejunum

  9. Portal systemic shunt: rarely done now; transjugular intrahepatic portosystemic shunt (TIPS) procedure more commonly done in radiology

    a. Purpose—primarily used for treatment of:

       (1) Portal hypertension

       (2) Decompression of esophagogastric varices

    b. Increasing use of TIPS procedures reduces the number of older shunt procedures.

    c. Since liver transplantation more commonly performed, these patients also treated with hepatic transplantation, rather than shunting

       (1) TIPS commonly used as a bridge to transplantation

    d. Description: shunts divert, either partially or totally, portal venous blood flow to liver

       (1) Types of shunts include:

          (a) End-to-side

          (b) Side-to-side

          (c) Interposition

          (d) Sarfeh portacaval

          (e) Interposition (adult) or direct (pediatric) mesocaval

          (f) Distal splenorenal

          (g) Mesoatrial (Budd-Chiari syndrome management)

       (2) Sugiura procedures (combines esophageal transection, extensive esophagogastric devascularization, and splenectomy, while paraesophageal collateral vessels are preserved)

         (a) Done for varices in patients who are not candidates for shunt procedures

         (b) Procedure not a shunt procedure

  10. TIPS

    a. Purpose: definitive treatment for patients who bleed from portal hypertension

       (1) Major limitation is that up to 50% have shunt stenosis or shunt thrombosis within the first year.

       (2) May be ideal therapy for patients needing short-term portal decompression (those awaiting liver transplantation who fail sclerotherapy)

    b. Description

       (1) Nonoperative

          (a) Functions similarly to a side-to-side portosystemic shunt (effective in treating ascites)

          (b) Adverse side effects include:

             (i) Total portal diversion

             (ii) Encephalopathy

    c. Procedure

       (1) Needle advanced from a hepatic vein to a major portal branch

       (2) Guide wire placed

       (3) Hepatic parenchymal tract created by balloon dilation

       (4) Expandable metal stent placed, creating shunt

    d. Preoperative assessment and concerns

       (1) Hypoxemia secondary to ascites

  (2) Portal hypertension
  (3) Risk for bleeding from esophageal and gastric varices
  (4) Risk of bleeding from coagulopathy due to liver dysfunction
  (5) Renal failure
  (6) Anemia
  (7) Altered drug elimination
  (8) Electrolyte disturbances
  e. Intraoperative concerns
  (1) Anticipate large blood loss for open procedures.
  (2) Pulmonary artery catheter for monitoring
  f. Postanesthesia/phase I priorities
  (1) Intensive care monitoring usual following these procedures
  g. Complications
  (1) Coagulopathy
  (2) Encephalopathy
  (3) Renal failure
11. Hepatectomy: excision of all or part of liver
  a. Increasing use of segmentectomies and wedge resections for patients with liver metastases
  b. Cryotherapy or radiofrequency ablation also used to treat:
  (1) Primary liver cancer
  (2) Hepatic metastases
12. Hepatic lobectomy: surgical removal of one of the two (right, left) lobes of liver; each lobe is then divided into several segments (eight total)—if a segment is removed, segmentectomy; may be accomplished with total vascular occlusion intraoperatively
  a. Intraoperative concerns (for hepatectomy and hepatic lobectomy)
  (1) Potential for large blood loss
  b. Postanesthesia phase I priorities
  (1) Epidural analgesia for pain management
  (2) May remain intubated and ventilated
  (3) Anticipate intensive care monitoring
  c. Complications
  (1) Massive hemorrhage
  (2) Disseminated intravascular coagulopathy
  (3) Hypoglycemia
  (4) Electrolyte imbalance
  (5) Pulmonary insufficiency
  (6) Encephalopathy
  (7) Liver failure
  (8) Renal failure
13. Peritoneovenous shunts (e.g., LeVeen or Denver); not commonly used
  a. Purpose
  (1) Used in an attempt to control ascites by reinfusing peritoneal fluid into venous system
  (2) Patients with limited hepatic reserve who may not tolerate blood being shunted away from liver are candidates.
  (3) Used to palliate patients with malignant ascites
  b. Description
  (1) Unidirectional silicone elastomer valve and catheter inserted into peritoneum
  (2) Other end tunneled subcutaneously up to neck and inserted into internal jugular vein
  (3) Catheter then threaded into superior vena cava or right atrium
  c. These shunts have significant problems with occlusion.
  (1) Particularly in patients with malignant ascites
  (2) Due to high cell and protein levels
  (3) Shunts need to be frequently pumped to maintain patency.

14. Liver transplant
  a. Purpose
      (1) Replacement of diseased liver with donor liver
      (2) May use cadaveric or living-related (split-liver) organs
  b. Description
      (1) Native liver removed and replaced with whole liver (cadaveric)
          or liver segment (split liver or liver segment from a living
          donor)
      (2) Effective approach for treatment of liver failure of various causes
          because of:
          (a) Development of improved surgical techniques
          (b) Venous bypass method
          (c) Newer antirejection agents
  c. Preoperative assessment and concerns
      (1) Fifteen percent of all liver transplant recipients in the United States are
          children.
      (2) Premedications used with care
      (3) Avoid intramuscular injections.
  d. Intraoperative concerns
      (1) Monitoring includes:
          (a) Arterial line
          (b) Central venous pressure
          (c) Pulmonary artery catheter
          (d) Transesophageal echocardiogram
      (2) Warming essential
      (3) Massive blood loss and subsequent transfusion
      (4) Volume management
  e. Postanesthesia phase I priorities
      (1) May remain intubated and mechanically ventilated; extubation
          may occur in operating room or immediately postoperatively in
          hemodynamically stable patients.
      (2) Monitored in intensive care setting or specialized transplant unit
      (3) Pain can be severe.
  f. Psychosocial concerns
      (1) Psychological preparation essential
      (2) Provide family support.
  g. Complications
      (1) Bleeding
      (2) Neurological deficits
      (3) Hepatic artery and/or portal vein thrombosis
      (4) Bile leaks
      (5) Rejection: primary or delayed
      (6) Renal failure
      (7) Electrolyte abnormalities
      (8) Pulmonary complications
      (9) Liver failure
15. Pancreatectomy
  a. Purpose—to treat:
      (1) Cancer
      (2) Necrosis
      (3) Abscess
      (4) Pseudocysts
      (5) Intractable pain from injury or pancreatitis
      (6) Most commonly used to treat pancreatic cancer
  b. Description
      (1) Partial resection or total removal of pancreas
      (2) Total removal results in diabetes and other metabolic difficulties.
      (3) May use jejunal loop to drain

16. Pancreaticoduodenectomy (Whipple's procedure)
    a. Purpose
       (1) Treat cancer of head of pancreas.
       (2) For resectable localized cancers of:
          (a) Ampulla
          (b) Distal common bile duct
          (c) Duodenum
          (d) Also used to treat chronic pancreatitis
    b. Description—removal of:
       (1) Proximal portion of pancreas adjoining duodenum
       (2) Lower portion of stomach, gallbladder, and common bile duct
17. Distal pancreatectomy
    a. Used to treat:
       (1) Malignancies
       (2) Benign (but symptomatic) neoplastic cysts
       (3) Pancreatic pseudocysts
       (4) Distal pancreatitis
       (5) Combined with splenectomy, especially if done for malignancy, in order to resect lymph nodes and spleen for staging purposes
18. Cystogastrostomy, cystoduodenostomy, cystojejunostomy
    a. Purpose: to treat pancreatic pseudocysts that do not disappear spontaneously
    b. Description: decompressive procedures for internally draining pseudocysts that are fixed to retrogastric area or duodenum or not in proximity to either stomach or duodenum
    c. Preoperative assessment and concerns (for pancreatectomy, pancreaticoduodenectomy, and cystogastrostomy)
       (1) Jaundice and abdominal pain may be present.
       (2) Electrolyte abnormalities
       (3) Blood glucose monitoring
    d. Intraoperative concerns
       (1) Anticipate large fluid loss.
       (2) Invasive monitoring usually required
    e. Postanesthesia phase I priorities
       (1) Epidural analgesia for pain management
       (2) Glucose monitoring; prone to hyperglycemia
       (3) For patients with chronic pancreatitis, pain management can often be difficult because of long-term use of opioids for chronic pain associated with chronic pancreatitis.
    f. Complications
       (1) Hypovolemia
       (2) Hyperglycemia
       (3) Hypocalcemia
19. Pancreas transplant
    a. Purpose: to treat diabetes mellitus; establishes an insulin-independent euglycemic state
    b. Description
       (1) Donor pancreatic tissue transplanted into recipient
       (2) Achieved through various techniques
          (a) Whole organ
          (b) Segmental graft
          (c) Duct management occluded or drained into a hollow viscus; usually combined with a renal transplant procedure
    c. Preoperative assessment and concerns
       (1) Absence of infection, dental evaluation completed
       (2) Blood glucose assessment and monitoring
       (3) If on dialysis, may need dialysis before procedure

    d. Intraoperative concerns
       (1) Increased risk for aspiration
       (2) Blood glucose monitoring
    e. Postanesthesia phase I priorities
       (1) Pain management: use caution with opioids if renal failure or nonfunctioning renal transplant.
       (2) Blood glucose monitoring: early return to euglycemic state possible after surgery
    f. Complications
       (1) Rejection
       (2) Graft thrombosis
  20. Splenectomy or splenorrhaphy
    a. Purpose: treat
       (1) Traumatic injuries to spleen
       (2) Thrombocytopenic purpura refractory to other treatment
       (3) Anemias
       (4) Myeloproliferative disorders (e.g., leukemia)
       (5) Splenorrhaphy only used for traumatic injuries; all other listed disorders (including trauma) treated with total splenectomy
    b. Description
       (1) Excision or repair of spleen, either by open or laparoscopic approach
       (2) Laparoscopic approach generally not used for trauma
D. Small intestine
  1. Duodenojejunostomy
    a. Purpose: relieve duodenal obstruction
    b. Description: creation of opening or passage from obstructed or stenosed duodenum into jejunum
  2. Feeding jejunostomy
    a. Purpose: allow access for alimentation in presence of functioning gastrointestinal tract.
    b. Description: permanent opening or fistula into jejunum through abdominal wall, usually with placement of a tube
  3. Ileostomy
    a. Purpose—created after total proctocolectomy for:
       (1) Crohn's disease
       (2) Ulcerative colitis
       (3) Less frequently for:
         (a) Multiple colorectal carcinomas
         (b) Familial polyposis coli
         (c) Ischemia
         (d) Trauma
         (e) Congenital anomalies in which colon remains intact
    b. Description: creation of passage through abdominal wall into ileum
    c. Psychosocial concerns
       (1) Acceptance of stoma and stoma care
       (2) Concerns related to social and physical activities
  4. Continent ileostomy (Kock pouch or Barnett continent intestinal reservoir)
    a. Purpose: create a reservoir for feces after total proctocolectomy
    b. Description: construction of an intestinal reservoir created by joining a loop of terminal ileum and forming a nipple valve; after healing is complete, patient controls expulsion of feces and gas by emptying reservoir or pouch with catheter.
    c. Postanesthesia phase I priorities
       (1) Maintain patency of decompression tube after creation of continent ileostomy; gently irrigate pouch with normal saline solution (30 mL every 3 hours is commonly ordered).
       (2) Surgically created pouch is fragile until healed and matured because of many anastomoses.

   5. Small bowel resection
    a. Purpose: treat
      (1) Trauma
      (2) Mesenteric thrombosis
      (3) Regional enteritis
      (4) Radiation enteropathy
      (5) Strangulated small bowel obstruction
      (6) Neoplasm
      (7) Congenital atresia
      (8) Enterocutaneous fistulas
    b. Description: excision of varying lengths of small intestine; profound consequences with resection of more than 75% of small intestine (e.g., "short-gut" syndrome)
      (1) In general, patients need 150 cm of small intestine without their ileocecal valve or 100 cm of small intestine with their ileocecal valve.
      (2) Less small intestine than this generally results in "short-gut" syndrome and the need for supplemental total parenteral nutrition.

E. Colon or large intestine
  1. Abdominoperineal resection
    a. Purpose
      (1) Generally performed for cancer of rectum
      (2) Occasionally for severe Crohn's, especially in the presence of severe perianal disease
    b. Description: surgical procedure in which anus, rectum, and sigmoid colon are removed en bloc through incision extending from pubis to above umbilicus
      (1) Segment of lower bowel mobilized and divided
      (2) Proximal end exteriorized through separate stab wound as a single-barreled colostomy or ileostomy
      (3) Distal end pushed into hollow of sacrum, and rectum removed through perineal route via a perineal incision
    c. Preoperative assessment and concerns
      (1) Patients may experience significant dehydration subsequent to extensive bowel preparation.
    d. Complications
      (1) Ureter or bladder injury
      (2) Wound dehiscence or infection
  2. Cecostomy
    a. Purpose: temporary measure to relieve obstruction distal to cecum
    b. Description: construction of opening into cecum, generally by placing a tube
  3. Colectomy
    a. Purpose: treat
      (1) Tumors
      (2) Bleeding
      (3) Inflammation
      (4) Trauma of large intestine
    b. Description: surgical removal of all or part of colon
  4. Restorative proctocolectomy (total proctocolectomy with ileal reservoir and anal anastomosis)
    a. Purpose
      (1) Maintain the anal sphincter muscles and allow the patient to avoid a permanent ileostomy.
      (2) Patient with a good to excellent result has 4 to 12 bowel movements per day.
      (3) Used for selected patients with ulcerative colitis or familial polyposis coli
    b. Description: pouch made from terminal ileum is created and then anastomosed to rectum at or just above dentate line; J-shaped ileoanal or larger W-shaped reservoir is most common; also S shaped

5. Colostomy
   a. Purpose: incision of colon to create fistula between bowel and abdominal wall
   b. Description
      (1) Either temporary or permanent
      (2) Placement of ostomy site is individualized.
      (3) Location depends on:
         (a) Pathological condition involved
            (i) Transverse colostomy
            (ii) Sigmoid colostomy
         (b) Patient's anatomy and lifestyle
      (4) Mucous fistula may also be created for decompression of cancer-caused obstruction of lower colon.
6. Low anterior resection
   a. Purpose: treat malignancies of rectosigmoid area or diverticulitis.
   b. Description
      (1) Rectum-containing tumor excised
      (2) Rectal stump and proximal bowel anastomosed either with suture or with staples
7. Omphalocele (excision): rare defect of periumbilical abdominal wall seen primarily in premature infants; omphalocele sac may contain small and/or large bowel, liver, or spleen.
   a. Primary closure
      (1) Purpose: used for omphaloceles with small abdominal defects
      (2) Description: omphalocele sac excised, and abdominal wall muscles and skin edges reapproximated.
   b. Staged repair
      (1) Purpose: used for large omphaloceles
      (2) Description: omphalocele is encased in silicone elastomer mesh sack that is sutured in place around defect; viscera are gradually moved into abdominal cavity in stages.
   c. Preoperative assessment and concerns
      (1) Often associated with other anomalies
      (2) Decompression of stomach to prevent regurgitation or aspiration
   d. Intraoperative concerns
      (1) Closure may be primary or staged depending on size of defect, abdominal tension.
   e. Postanesthesia phase I priorities
      (1) Patients with large defects may remain intubated and mechanically ventilated.
      (2) Fluid management
   f. Psychosocial concerns
      (1) Parental support
   g. Complications
      (1) Circulatory and renal dysfunction
      (2) Infection
8. Polypectomy
   a. Purpose: to remove isolated gastrointestinal polyps
   b. Description: using snare and electrocautery, polyps removed endoscopically; large polyps may require open colectomy.
F. Rectal and anal procedures
   1. Transanal excision of polyps or masses
      a. Purpose: to remove polyps or masses from the anal or rectal areas
      b. Description: excision of polyps or masses using a transanal approach
   2. Lateral internal sphincterotomy
      a. Purpose: to treat chronic anal fissures
      b. Description: cutting of anal sphincter; anoplasty normally required to reestablish anal tissue and mucosal integrity

    c. Botulinum toxin injection is an alternative procedure that is done without anesthesia.

  3. Anal fistulotomy or fistulectomy

    a. Purpose: treat, by either incision or excision, fistulous tracts in anal canal.

    b. Description: infection of anal duct gland creates fistula in ano.

      (1) May be incised and drained or excised and packed to heal by granulation

      (2) Usually has presenting condition of a perianal abscess, which is incised and drained

      (3) Chronic draining tract may develop, which communicates with the anal canal.

      (4) Treated with fistulotomy (opening the fistula) if not deep and crossing the sphincters

      (5) If deep and cross multiple sphincters, more complicated anorectal procedures required to repair the defect

  4. Duhamel and Soave operations

    a. Purpose: treat congenital megacolon (Hirschsprung's disease) in children.

    b. Description: in both Duhamel and Soave procedures:

      (1) Aganglionic bowel resected

      (2) Proximal, healthy colon pulled through and anastomosed to rectum

    c. Preoperative assessment and concerns

      (1) Present with prior colostomy

      (2) Mildly malnourished with associated malabsorption state

      (3) Diarrhea may be present.

    d. Intraoperative concerns

      (1) Potential for large third-space losses

    e. Postanesthesia phase I priorities

      (1) Continuous epidural analgesia for pain management

VI. GENERAL POSTANESTHESIA CARE CONCERNS

  A. Routine immediate postanesthesia assessment following American Society of PeriAnesthesia Nurses *Standards of Perianesthesia Nursing Practice* and American Society of Anesthesiologists *Standards for Postanesthesia Care*

  B. General postanesthesia observation and care for gastrointestinal procedures

    1. Cardiovascular system

    a. Monitor vital signs per unit routine; check perfusion to extremities.

      (1) Risk for radical shifts in body fluids as result of:

        (a) Inadequate fluid replacement

        (b) Excessive replacement

        (c) Preoperative status

        (d) Presence of fistula

        (e) Vomiting

        (f) Diarrhea

        (g) Intestinal obstruction

        (h) Third spacing

        (i) Nasogastric drains and tubes

      (2) Sequestered fluid in gastrointestinal tract resulting from:

        (a) Tumor

        (b) Stricture

        (c) Adhesions

        (d) Paralytic ileus

        (e) Surgical manipulation

      (3) Sequestered fluid is lost to circulating volume of body.

        (a) It is in a potential or "third" space.

        (b) Third-space fluid generally does not begin to mobilize until second or third postoperative day.

      (4) Stress responses resulting in hormonal alterations can lead to retention of fluids and potential for fluid overload postoperatively.

    b. Observe for hemostasis; observe for and document coagulation deficiencies.
      (1) Oozing
      (2) Bruising
      (3) Petechiae
      (4) In patients with a history of coagulation problems or those who have received massive transfusions, coagulation difficulties can occur.
      (5) Clotting also affected by:
        (a) Malabsorption
        (b) Impaired digestion
        (c) Altered liver function
    c. Deep vein thrombosis (DVT)
      (1) Formation is potential complication of immobility.
      (2) Laparoscopic procedures increase risk of emboli as result of:
        (a) Air insufflation
        (b) Resultant increase in intra-abdominal pressure
        (c) Decreasing venous return, particularly from the lower extremities
      (3) Prevention
        (a) Leg exercises
        (b) Range of motion (ROM) at least every hour as part of "stir-up" regimen
        (c) Antiembolism stockings
        (d) Intermittent pneumatic or sequential compression devices
        (e) Low-dose anticoagulation as ordered
      (4) Active ROM exercises stimulate venous return from extremities.

2. Genitourinary system
    a. Monitor intake and output every hour and specific gravity every 4 hours.
      (1) Potential for decreased urine output as result of fluid shifts
    b. Assess bladder distention if no indwelling catheter in place.
      (1) Bladder distention is common postoperative problem.
      (2) Palpation of bladder or bladder ultrasound may be used.
    c. Note color of urine.
      (1) Retraction or pressure placed on bladder or kidney during surgery can traumatize bladder or kidney.

3. Endocrine system
    a. Document blood glucose levels, urine glucose, and ketones as appropriate.
      (1) Surgical intervention and operative stress on body systems alter pancreatic enzymes and insulin production.
        (a) Patients with diabetes are observed for same reasons.
      (2) Blood glucose can be monitored with point-of-care blood glucose checks

4. Respiratory system
    a. Document routine postanesthesia nursing interventions ("stir-up" or "wake-up" regimens) and their results concerning:
      (1) Lung auscultation
      (2) Deep breathing
      (3) Incentive spirometry
      (4) Coughing to mobilize and expectorate secretions
      (5) Turning
      (6) ROM exercises
      (7) Prevention of decreased lung expansion leading to:
        (a) Atelectasis
        (b) Congestion
        (c) Hypostatic pneumonia
      (8) Reasons for decreased lung expansion
        (a) Oversedation
        (b) Lack of sedation
        (c) Hypoxia

      (d) Fluid overload

      (e) Decreased ventilatory excursion

  b. If central line (central venous or pulmonary artery catheter) is placed intraoperatively or in PACU, obtain chest film.

    (1) Demonstration of correct catheter placement

    (2) Confirmation of presence or absence of pneumothorax

  c. Document chest drainage and chest tube function.

    (1) Follow PACU routine for care of chest tubes for patients undergoing pulmonary approach for upper gastrointestinal surgery.

      (a) Esophageal resection

      (b) Hiatal herniorrhaphy

5. Gastrointestinal system

  a. NPO

    (1) Nausea and vomiting may be present because of effects of:

      (a) Anesthesia

      (b) Decreased intestinal motility

      (c) Malfunctioning nasogastric tube

      (d) Disease process

  b. Nasogastric tube assessment

    (1) Check for proper tube placement by auscultating with stethoscope over gastric area while inserting 20 to 50 mL air into tube.

      (a) If nasogastric tube was placed intraoperatively under direct visualization:

        (i)   Check with surgeon before irrigating or repositioning.

        (ii) If tube is properly placed, rush of air should be heard.

    (2) Secure tube to nares with correct taping technique.

      (a) Taping or securing tube properly decreases:

        (i)   Risk of necrosis or damage of nares

        (ii) Inadvertent dislodgment of tube

        (iii) Alar necrosis is disfiguring and difficult to repair if it occurs.

  c. Maintain patency of nasogastric or gastrostomy tube.

    (1) To decrease tension on gastric suture line

    (2) Notify surgeon of excessive drainage from tubes or drains so that IV fluid and rates can be adjusted.

    (3) Initial 24-hour drainage may be bloody, changing to dark serosanguineous to bile colored over the next 24 to 72 hours.

    (4) Color and consistency vary with location of surgery.

      (a) If esophageal or gastric surgery, expect bloody drainage.

      (b) If hepatic, biliary, or intestinal surgery, drainage should not be bloody.

  d. Irrigation or manipulation of nasogastric tubes

    (1) Do not irrigate or manipulate nasogastric tube unless specifically ordered.

      (a) Nasogastric tube lies close to anastomosis (gastric resection, some pancreatic procedures involving stomach).

    (2) Check, if nasogastric tube to dependent drainage, for proper securing of tube to eliminate manipulation.

      (a) Nasogastric tube may be used as stent anastomosis in esophageal procedures.

    (3) Notify surgeon if nasogastric tube is accidentally removed or becomes displaced.

      (a) Attempts to replace tube can result in esophageal perforation.

  e. Assess abdominal girth (abdominal distention), and auscultate bowel sounds.

    (1) Abdominal distention, nausea, and vomiting may be caused by:

      (a) Anastomotic leak

      (b) Hemorrhage

      (c) Malfunctioning nasogastric tube

      (d) Ileus

      (e) Mechanical obstructions

    f. Observe and document status of:
       (1) Stoma color
          (a) Notify surgeon of any sudden or progressive change in stoma color.
          (b) Altered color may indicate increasing edema, leading to:
             (i) Decreased circulation
             (ii) Generalized poor circulation to bowel
       (2) Drainage from stoma
       (3) Position of stoma to skin
6. Dressings and drains
    a. Document dressing status every hour or as needed.
       (1) Keeping dressing dry promotes wound healing by minimizing potential breeding ground for bacterial contamination.
    b. Reinforce or change dressing per preferred routine or as ordered.
       (1) Dry dressings more comfortable for patient
    c. Monitor amount of drainage on dressings and from drains.
       (1) Establish expected drainage amounts with surgeon when patient arrives in PACU.
       (2) Notify surgeon of excessive or questionable quantities of drainage.
       (3) Significant blood or fluid losses can occur from incisions or drain sites that may require replacement or exploration of site.
    d. Document both abdominal and perineal dressings after abdominoperineal resection.
       (1) Sump or Penrose (cigarette or tube) drains may be present in perineal incision, a likely area for copious serosanguineous drainage.
7. Positioning
    a. Lateral recumbent position
       (1) Side-lying position is usually more comfortable for patients who have had rectal or perineal procedures.
    b. Elevate head of the bed (reverse Trendelenburg, not head up and hips flexed).
       (1) Elevating head decreases weight against diaphragm to:
          (a) Promote improved respiratory excursion.
          (b) Facilitate gas exchange.
8. Temperature
    a. Monitor temperature on admission to PACU.
    b. Warm or cool patient as indicated with:
       (1) Warming lights
       (2) Hypothermia or hyperthermia blankets
       (3) Convective warming devices
    c. Vital signs should include temperature monitoring on PACU admission and every 1 to 2 hours until discharge.
    d. Avoid rectal temperatures with:
       (1) Permanent colostomies
       (2) Ileostomies
       (3) Rectal or anal incisions
       (4) After pull-through or stapled low anterior resections
       (5) Perforation of suture or staple lines is possible if rectal or anal incision exists or if rectum has been totally removed.
9. Pain control (see Chapter 26)
    a. Assessment
       (1) Location
       (2) Pattern
       (3) Intensity
       (4) Duration of pain
       (5) If possible, use pain assessment tool.
          (a) Requires patient to identify quality of pain or discomfort
       (6) Initiate pain relief measures.

(7) Medicate patients according to PACU routine and approved pain guidelines.
  b. Pain management practices will vary from institution to institution.
    (1) Pain is subjective; patient complaining of pain should be believed and comfort measures initiated.
  c. Observe for incisional splinting.
    (1) Splinting can lead to increased partial pressure of carbon dioxide (Pco_2) level because of inadequate gas exchange.
  d. IV route preferred for opioid and analgesic administration
    (1) Absorption time and onset of action less predictable when intramuscular injections administered in cold patient
  e. In selected patients, pain relief can be significant from:
    (1) Patient-controlled analgesia
    (2) Epidural analgesia
    (3) Incisional or field blocks
  f. Adequate pain control may improve:
    (1) Ventilation
    (2) Promote deep breathing and coughing.
    (3) Allow patient to move more easily, especially after procedures with large or upper abdominal incisions.
  g. Pain generally related to incision type
    (1) Midline incisions less painful than transverse or chevron incisions
    (2) Upper midline incisions more painful than lower midline incisions
C. Phase II priorities
  1. Pain management
    a. Initiate oral analgesics to prepare for discharge.
    b. Instruct patients to call if:
      (1) Pain unrelieved by oral medications
      (2) Has severe pain
      (3) Questions related to pain (amount, location, duration)
  2. Diet
    a. Encourage fluids if desired; do not force fluids.
    b. Instruct patients to begin with light foods and progress to full diet as tolerated.
    c. If nauseated or vomiting for more than 6 hours after discharge, instruct patients to call and report nausea and vomiting.
  3. Wound care
    a. Review basic wound care with patients, companions, and families.
    b. Provide written and verbal instructions, especially for specialized incisional and/or drain care.
    c. Instruct patients to call if incision shows signs of infection or a fever is present.
  4. Activity
    a. Generally, activities limited first day postoperatively
    b. Dependent on operative procedure, lifting and activity restrictions may be ordered.
  5. Complications
    a. Provide patient, family, and responsible accompanying adult with information on expected outcomes and complications.
    b. Instruct in appropriate follow-up if needed for complications.
D. Postoperative complications
  1. General complications (not in order of occurrence or severity)
    a. Paralytic (adynamic) ileus: although commonly listed as a complication, it is an expected part of any abdominal or intestinal procedure; all patients who have these procedures will experience ileus.
    b. Atelectasis and respiratory problems
    c. Bladder distention
    d. Hemorrhage or shock

    e. Wound infection
    f. Dehiscence or evisceration
    g. Peritonitis
    h. Hiccups (singultus)
    i. Anastomotic leak
    j. Anastomotic or stomal obstruction
    k. Intestinal fistulas
    l. Electrolyte and fluid imbalances
    m. Stress ulceration
    n. DVT and possible pulmonary embolus
    o. Pancreatitis
    p. Toxic shock syndrome
2. Specific system complications
    a. Pulmonary
        (1) Hypoventilation: most frequent and dangerous pulmonary complication after surgery; various causes
            (a) Preoperative medication
            (b) Anesthetic agents
            (c) Opioid, sedative administration
                (i)   Preoperative
                (ii) Intraoperative
                (iii) Postoperative
            (d) Pain
            (e) Patient position
        (2) Atelectasis: constitutes 90% of all pulmonary complications
            (a) Acute gastric dilation or ascites in advanced cancer can cause elevation of diaphragm, leading to decreased size of chest cavity and atelectasis (can also lead to shock).
            (b) Postoperative splinting resulting from incisional pain is the most common cause of atelectasis.
    b. Cardiovascular
        (1) Venous thrombosis
        (2) Hypotension
        (3) Shock
            (a) Hypovolemic
            (b) Septic
        (4) Myocardial infarction
        (5) Cerebrovascular accident

BIBLIOGRAPHY

1. American Society for Gastrointestinal Endoscopy: Complications of upper GI endoscopy. *Gastrointest Endosc* 55 (7):784–793, 2002.
2. Ball KA: *Endoscopic surgery: Mosby's perioperative nursing series*, St Louis, 1997, Mosby.
3. Black JM, Hawks JH: *Medical-surgical nursing: Clinical management for positive outcomes*, ed 7, St Louis, 2005, Saunders.
4. Guyton AC: *Human physiology and mechanisms of disease*, ed 5, Philadelphia, 1996, WB Saunders.
5. Hulka JF, Reich H: *Textbook of laparoscopy*, ed 3, Philadelphia, 1998, WB Saunders.
6. Jaffe RA, Samuels SI, eds: *Anesthesiologist's manual of surgical procedures*, ed 3, Philadelphia, 2004, Lippincott, Williams & Wilkins.
7. Moody FG, Carey LC, Jones RS, et al, eds: *Surgical treatment of digestive disease*, ed 2, Chicago, 1990, Mosby.
8. O'Brien D: Care of the gastrointestinal, abdominal, and anorectal surgical patient. In Drain CB, Odom-Forren J, eds: *Perianesthesia nursing: A critical care approach*, ed 5, Philadelphia, 2009, WB Saunders.
9. O'Brien D, Walters VA, Burden N: Special procedures in the ambulatory setting. In Burden N, Quinn DMD, O'Brien D, et al, eds: *Ambulatory surgical nursing*, ed 2, Philadelphia, 2000, WB Saunders.
10. O'Hanlon-Nichols T: Book assessment series: Gastrointestinal system. *Am J Nurs* 98 (4):48–52, 1998.

11. Patton KT, Thibodeau GA: *Anatomy & physiology*, ed 7, St Louis, 2010, Mosby.

12. Rakel RE, Bope ET: *Conn's current therapy*, ed 60, Philadelphia, 2008, Saunders.

13. Ray S: Result of 310 consecutive patients undergoing laparoscopic Nissen fundoplication as hospital outpatients or at a free-standing surgery center. *Surg Endosc* 17:378–380, 2003.

14. Roizen MF, Fleisher LA: *Essence of anesthesia practice*, ed 2, Philadelphia, 2002, WB Saunders.

15. Sommers MS, Johnson SA, Beery TA: *Diseases and disorders: A nursing therapeutics manual*, ed 3, Philadelphia, 2007, FA Davis.

16. Standring S: *Gray's anatomy: The anatomical basis of clinical practice*, Philadelphia, 2009, Churchill Livingston.

17. Suter M, Giusti V, Heraief E, et al: Laparoscopic roux-en-Y gastric bypass. *Surg Endosc* 17:603–609, 2003.

18. Thompson J, McFarland G, Hirsch J, et al: *Mosby's clinical nursing*, ed 5, St Louis, 2002, Mosby.

19. Tilkian SM, Conover MH, Tilkian AG: *Clinical nursing implications of laboratory tests*, ed 5, St Louis, 1996, Mosby.

20. Townsend CM, Beauchamp RD, Evers BM, et al: *Sabiston textbook of surgery*, ed 18, Philadelphia, 2007, Saunders.

21. Widmaier E, Raff H, Strang K: *Vander's human physiology*, ed 9, New York, 2003, McGraw-Hill.

22. Wiegand DJLM, Carlson KK: *AACN procedure manual for critical care*, ed 5, St Louis, 2005, Saunders.

36 General Care

MYRNA E. MAMARIL

OBJECTIVES

At the conclusion of this chapter, the reader will be able to:

1. Describe anatomy and physiology relative to selected general surgical procedures.

2. Describe selected laparoscopic and open general surgical procedures.

3. Review assessment considerations before selected surgical procedures.

4. Compare post anesthesia care unit (PACU) phase I and II care and key educational elements specific to selected general surgical procedures.

5. Relate the advantages of minimally invasive procedures.

6. Identify perioperative and perianesthesia issues concerned with minimally invasive procedures.

7. Summarize potential perioperative complications associated with selected general surgical procedures.

I. OVERVIEW
   A. General surgery refers to treatment of:
      1. Disease
      2. Injury
      3. Deformity
   B. Purpose: to prevent or alleviate suffering when a cure is not likely through:
      1. Medical modalities
      2. Medications
   C. General surgery procedures can be done:
      1. Open
      2. Using minimally invasive laparoscopic technique
   D. Reference postanesthesia priorities (see Chapter 50)
II. BREAST
   A. Anatomy and physiology (Figure 36-1)
      1. Bilateral mammary glands
         a. Lie on pectoralis major fascia of anterior chest wall
         b. Surrounded by layers of fat enclosed in envelope of skin
      2. Muscle
         a. Fixed to overlying skin and underlying pectoral fascia with fibrous bands
      3. Lobes
         a. Twelve to 20 lobes subdivided into lobules, composed of acini
         b. Arranged in spiral fashion around nipple
         c. Each lobe drained by duct (12-20) opening on nipple
      4. Nipple
         a. In adult women, is in center of fully developed breast with pigmented areola
         b. Located in fourth intercostal space
         c. Bundles of smooth muscle fibers have erectile properties.

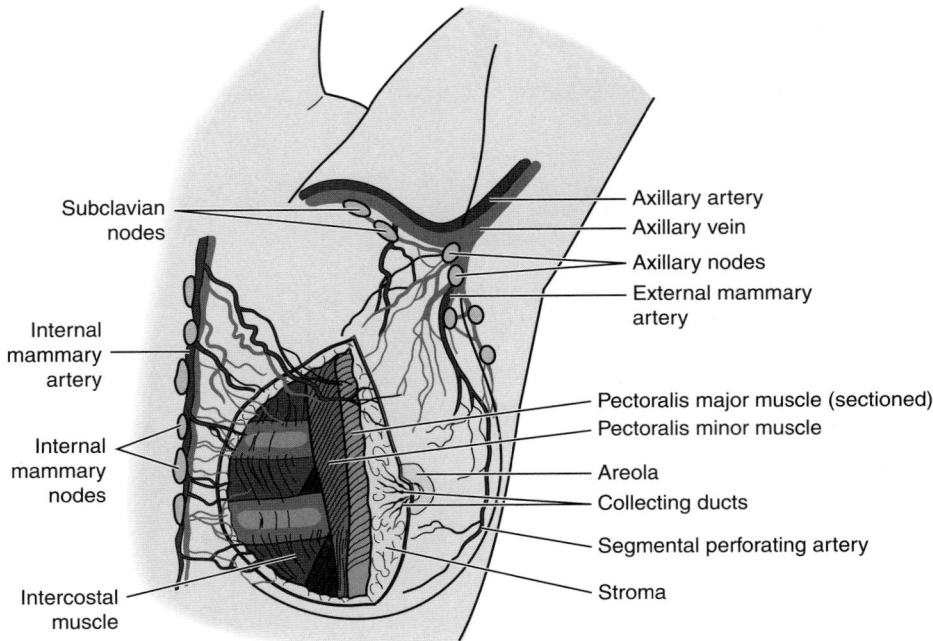

Subclavian nodes

Axillary artery

Axillary vein

Axillary nodes

External mammary artery

Internal mammary artery

Internal mammary nodes

Pectoralis major muscle (sectioned)

Pectoralis minor muscle

Areola

Collecting ducts

Segmental perforating artery

Stroma

Intercostal muscle

FIGURE 36-1 ■ Female breast. (From Phillips NF: *Berry & Kohn's operating room technique,* ed 11, St Louis, 2007, Mosby.)

    d. Fifteen to 20 lactiferous ducts arranged radially under areola
    e. Areolar epithelium contains small hairs and glands.
        (1) Sebaceous glands (Montgomery's glands)
        (2) Sweat glands
        (3) Accessory mammary glands
  5. Blood supply
    a. Arteries
        (1) Internal mammary
        (2) Lateral branches of anterior aortic intercostal arteries
    b. Veins
        (1) Main veins follow arterial pattern.
        (2) Superficial veins frequently dilated during pregnancy or over areas of disease
  6. Lymph system
    a. Generally follows course of blood vessels
    b. Drains into axillary nodes (approximately 53) and into internal mammary nodes (few in number)
  7. Nerve supply
    a. Anterior cutaneous branches of upper intercostal nerves
    b. Third and fourth branches of cervical plexus
    c. Lateral cutaneous branches of intercostal nerves
B. Pathophysiology
  1. Affected by three types of physiological changes related to:
    a. Growth and development
    b. Menstrual cycle
    c. Pregnancy and lactation
  2. Benign breast tumors
    a. Fibrocystic disease
        (1) Accounts for 45% of all biopsied female breast lesions

   b. Adenofibrosis
     (1) Disease of youth: mean age 21 years
   c. Papilloma (intraductal papillomas)
     (1) Grows in terminal portion of duct or throughout duct
   d. Duct ectasia (comedomastitis)
     (1) Disease of large ducts of the breast (in contrast to chronic cystic mastitis, which is a disease of the acini and ductules)
     (2) May result in an indurated area of the breast that is fixed in the skin and is associated with a retracted nipple
     (3) Disease of ducts in subareolar zone
     (4) Disease of aging breast, most commonly in or near menopause
     (5) No demonstrated association with carcinoma
 3. Malignant breast tumors
   a. Early
     (1) Solitary
     (2) Unilateral
     (3) Hard
     (4) Painless
     (5) Solid
     (6) Irregular
     (7) Poorly outlined
     (8) Nonmobile lump located in quadrant
       (a) Upper
       (b) Outer
     (9) Opaque to transillumination
   b. Moderately advanced locally
     (1) Axillary nodes
     (2) Nipple retraction or elevation
     (3) Skin dimpling
     (4) Nipple discharge
   c. Far advanced locally
     (1) Supraclavicular nodes
     (2) Fixation of axillary nodes
     (3) Fixation of tumor to chest wall
     (4) Edema (peau d'orange or redness over more than one third of breast)
     (5) Edema of arm
     (6) Ulceration of skin
     (7) Satellite nodules
   d. Distant metastasis
     (1) Inoperable
     (2) Partial
     (3) Osseous
     (4) Visceral
C. Assessment
 1. Clinical manifestations
   a. Benign breast tumor may include:
     (1) Breast pain and tenderness
     (2) Change in mass size with menstrual cycle
     (3) Palpable masses: firm, round, freely movable
   b. Conditions affecting nipple include:
     (1) Bloody nipple discharge (intraductal papilloma)
     (2) Eczematous or ulcerated nipple (Paget's disease)
     (3) Usually minimal pain
   c. Malignant breast tumor may include:
     (1) Nontender lump, usually in upper, outer quadrant
     (2) Axillary lymphadenopathy (late)
     (3) Fixed, nodular breast mass (late)

    2. Diagnostic studies

      a. Monthly breast self-examination

      b. Annual breast examination by physician

      c. Annual mammography for women 40 years and older

      d. Annual or periodic mammography for younger women if:

        (1) Familial history of breast cancer

        (2) Early menarche

        (3) Multiparous or birth of first child after 34 years of age

        (4) High-fat diet

        (5) Oral contraceptive use

        (6) Radiation exposure

        (7) Presence of other cancer

    3. Laboratory studies

      a. Estrogen receptor protein

      b. Carcinoembryonic antigen

      c. Gross cystic disease protein

      d. Liver function studies

    4. Scans

      a. Bone scan

      b. Brain or computed tomography (CT) scan

      c. Chest x-ray

      d. Ultrasonography

      e. Thermography

D. Operative procedures

    1. Preoperative concerns

      a. Possible malignancy

      b. Losing a body part

      c. Facing negative reaction from spouse and family

      d. Change in self-image

      e. Life expectancy and ability to raise family

    2. Intraoperative concerns

      a. Mammogram films available

      b. Correct side verified

      c. Specimen properly prepared and labeled for pathology

    3. Procedures

      a. Needle biopsy

        (1) Purpose: remove tissue sample for biopsy via needle aspiration.

        (2) Vim-Silverman or disposable cutting-type needle introduced and advanced into breast mass to entrap a core of tissue

        (3) Needle withdrawn and tissue specimen sent for diagnostic examination

        (4) Definitive surgical treatment should only follow formal biopsy.

      b. Incisional biopsy

        (1) Purpose: remove a sample of involved tissue for biopsy.

        (2) Portion of mass surgically excised using a curved incisional line

        (3) Tissue sent for diagnostic examination

      c. Excisional biopsy

        (1) Purpose: remove entire tumor mass for biopsy.

        (2) Needle localization may be done preoperatively to locate mass.

        (3) Specimen sent for diagnostic examination

        (4) Usually done under local anesthesia or intravenous (IV) sedation

        (5) Short delay between biopsy and further treatment does not adversely affect survival.

      d. Sentinel node or primary lymph node biopsy

        (1) Purpose: identify first lymph nodes along lymphatic channel from primary tumor site to determine need for additional or more extensive surgeries and treatments.

        (2) Small amount of radioisotope injected and sentinel node identified during a nuclear medicine scan

(3) Node excised in addition to the malignant breast mass
(4) Less extensive than axillary lymph node dissection
   e. Incision and drainage of abscess
     (1) Purpose: incise inflamed and suppurative area of breast to drain abscess.
     (2) Abscesses occur most frequently in infected lactating breast; chronic abscesses rare.
     (3) Free drainage required with abscesses around nipple or in breast tissue
   f. Partial mastectomy (lumpectomy, segmental resection, quadrant resection, wedge resection) or modified radical (breast tissue, lymph tissue and selective muscle tissue)
     (1) Purpose: remove tumor mass with at least 1 inch of surrounding tissue.
     (2) Appears to provide results equal to more radical procedure when combined with axillary node or sentinel node dissection and irradiation in stages I and II
   g. Subcutaneous mastectomy
     (1) Procedure: removal of all breast tissue with overlying skin and nipple left intact
     (2) Purpose: remove benign subcutaneous involved tissue.
     (3) Recommended for patients who have:
       (a) Central tumors of noninvasive origin
       (b) Chronic cystic mastitis
       (c) Hyperplastic duct changes
       (d) Multiple fibroadenomas
       (e) Undergone several previous biopsies
   h. Simple mastectomy
     (1) Procedure: removal of entire breast without lymph node dissection
     (2) Purpose—performed:
       (a) To remove extensive benign disease
       (b) If malignancy is believed to be confined only to breast tissue
       (c) As a palliative measure to remove an ulcerated advanced malignancy
   i. Procedure: reduction of male breast
     (1) Purpose: performed to relieve gynecomastia
       (a) Occurs primarily after 40 years or during puberty
       (b) Usually related to alterations in normal hormonal balance
       (c) All subareolar fibroglandular tissue removed with reconstruction of resultant defect
       (d) Liposuction may be used to debulk male breast.
E. Postanesthesia care phase I
  1. Monitor and document
   a. Drainage output
   b. Competency of drainage system
   c. Dressing for hemorrhage or oozing
  2. Assess comfort level.
   a. Pain may increase.
     (1) Anxiety
     (2) Feeling of powerlessness
   b. If severe, may limit chest expansion
   c. Assess effectiveness of any analgesics given.
  3. Position for comfort
   a. Usually supine or semi-Fowler's
   b. Affected arm may be elevated on pillow to:
     (1) Decrease swelling
     (2) Enhance circulation
  4. Psychological support
   a. Respond appropriately to patient's verbalized questions and responses.

         b. Avoid making unfounded promises or encouraging false or unreasonable hopes.

         c. Respect patient's privacy.

   F. Postanesthesia care phase II

      1. Assess

         a. Dressing and bra firmness

         b. Security of drain

         c. Emotional feelings

      2. Key educational components

         a. Depends on extent of procedure and diagnosis

         b. Reinforce need for firm-fitting bra without underwire to provide support.

         c. Provide information on range-of-motion exercises as directed by the physician.

         d. Provide information about resources and support systems as appropriate.

      3. Provide written and verbal instructions; assess and ensure patient and family understanding.

      4. Psychosocial concerns

         a. Possible malignancy

         b. Depression

            (1) Loss of a body part

            (2) Change in self-image

            (3) Possible negative reaction from spouse and family

            (4) Possible distancing of friends who "don't know what to say"

            (5) Life expectancy and ability to raise family

      5. Complications

         a. Detached or occluded drain

         b. Hematoma

         c. Hemorrhage or shock

         d. Wound infection

III. GALLBLADDER

   A. Anatomy and physiology (Figure 36-2)

      1. Location

         a. Lies in sulcus on undersurface of right lobe of liver

         b. Terminates in cystic duct

      2. Bile

         a. Becomes concentrated in gallbladder during storage period

         b. Consists of:

            (1) Water

            (2) Salts of bile acids

            (3) Pigments

            (4) Inorganic salts

            (5) Cholesterol

            (6) Phospholipids

         c. Presence of certain foodstuffs, especially fat in duodenum:

            (1) Causes release of cholecystokinin-pancreozymin

            (2) Results in gallbladder contraction

         d. As sphincter of Oddi in ampulla of Vater relaxes, bile pours forth into duodenum to aid digestion.

      3. Blood supply

         a. From cystic artery, a branch of the hepatic artery

   B. Pathophysiology

      1. Cholelithiasis

         a. Precipitating factors for stone formation

            (1) Disturbances in metabolism

            (2) Biliary stasis

            (3) Obstruction

            (4) Infection

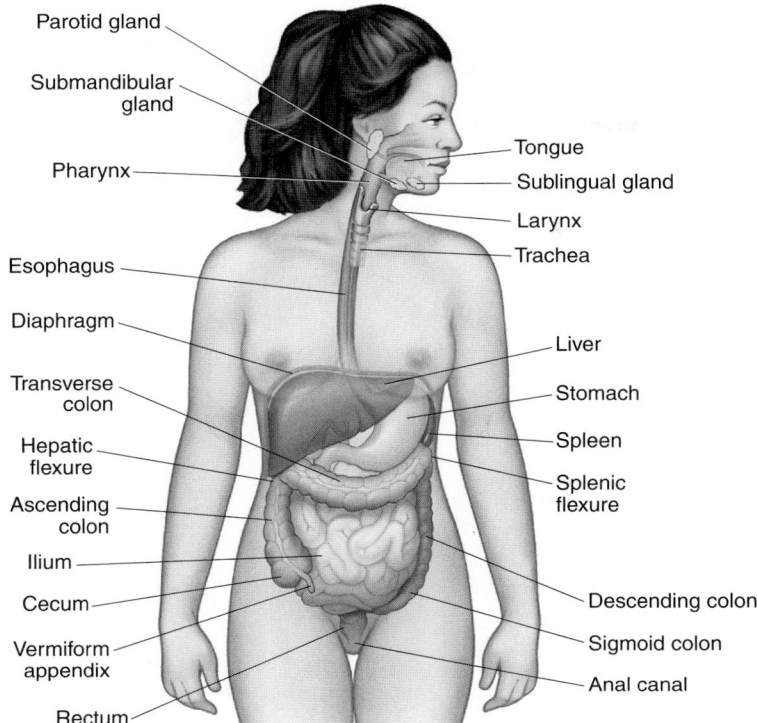

FIGURE 36-2 ■ Alimentary canal. (From Thibodeau GA, Patton KT: *Anatomy & physiology,* ed 6, St Louis, 2007, Mosby.)

     b. Especially prevalent in women who are:
       (1) Multiparous
       (2) Taking estrogen therapy
       (3) Using oral contraceptives
     c. Other risk factors
       (1) Obesity
       (2) Dietary intake of fats
       (3) Sedentary lifestyle
       (4) Familial tendencies
     d. Frequently seen in disease states such as:
       (1) Diabetes mellitus
       (2) Regional enteritis
       (3) Certain blood dyscrasias
     e. Classification
       (1) Cholesterol
         (a) More common in United States
       (2) Pigment stones
         (a) Black-pigment stones associated with cirrhosis and chronic hemolysis
         (b) Brown-pigment stones predominant in native Asians and associated with bacterial infection of the bile
  2. Cholecystitis
     a. Frequently associated with:
       (1) Cystic duct obstruction caused by impacted gallstones
       (2) Stasis
       (3) Bacterial infection
       (4) Ischemia of gallbladder due to trauma, massive burns, or surgery

    C. Assessment

       1. Clinical manifestations

         a. Episodic, cramping pain in right upper abdominal quadrant or epigastrium, possibly radiating to back near right scapular tip (biliary colic)

         b. Nausea and/or vomiting

         c. Fat intolerance

         d. Fever and leukocytosis

         e. Signs and symptoms of jaundice

         f. Heartburn

         g. Flatulence

       2. Laboratory studies

         a. Serum liver enzyme levels

         b. Bilirubin studies, liver function tests, alkaline phosphate

       3. Radiological studies

         a. Flat plate of abdomen

         b. Ultrasonography

         c. Oral cholecystogram

         d. IV cholangiogram

         e. Upper gastrointestinal series

       4. Other studies

         a. Endoscopic retrograde cholangiopancreatography (ERCP)

         b. CT scan

  D. Operative procedures

       1. Cholecystectomy: removal of gallbladder

       2. Purpose: treatment of cholelithiasis or cholecystitis

       3. Preoperative concerns

         a. Anxiety related to impending surgical procedure and knowledge deficit

         b. Self-consciousness about body image if obese

         c. Concern about ability to resume normal activity and work

       4. Intraoperative concerns

         a. Fluid volume deficit related to hemorrhage

         b. Altered body temperature

         c. Infection related to invasive gastrointestinal (GI) procedure

         d. Perforation of bladder, bowel, vascular organs

         e. Injury related to positioning

         f. Long instruments for obese or tall patient

       5. Procedures

         a. Laparoscopic cholecystectomy

           (1) Accomplished through three or four incisions made in abdominal wall

           (2) Rigid fiberoptic laparoscope inserted into peritoneal cavity

           (3) Specialized, long-handled instruments used to resect gallbladder with electrocautery or laser cautery

           (4) Advantages

              (a) Less postoperative pain

              (b) Fewer complications

              (c) More rapid postoperative recovery

           (5) Disadvantages

              (a) Longer surgery time

              (b) Longer exposure to anesthesia

              (c) More costly than open abdominal cholecystectomy

         b. Open abdominal cholecystectomy

           (1) Performed through right subcostal incision that may be extended over the midline

           (2) Performed if laparoscopic cholecystectomy is unsuccessful or contraindicated

           (3) Common duct exploration done if stones suspected

         c. Cholelithotripsy: high-energy shock waves used to fragment gallstones

           (1) Performed under IV sedation or general anesthesia

           (2) Pulverized stone fragments pass through bile duct.

    E. Postanesthesia care phase I
        1. Laparoscopic or open cholecystectomy
           a. Monitor intake and output.
               (1) Assess nasogastric (NG) tube for proper placement; if ordered, discontinue.
               (2) Note patency of urinary catheter, color and amount of urine; if ordered, discontinue.
           b. Assess comfort level.
               (1) Note location of discomfort and position for comfort.
           c. Administer prescribed medications and evaluate relief.
    F. Postanesthesia care phase II
        1. Laparoscopic cholecystectomy
           a. Assess dressings.
           b. Assess abdominal girth and firmness.
           c. Key educational components
               (1) Instruct patient and family about routine care after abdominal surgery.
                   (a) Ambulate regularly.
                   (b) Rest frequently.
                   (c) Gradually increase activity as tolerated.
                   (d) Keep incisions dry.
                   (e) Report redness, increasing pain, or incision drainage.
                   (f) Avoid heavy lifting as ordered.
                   (g) Deep breathing
                   (h) Splint abdomen when coughing.
               (2) Stress importance of follow-up care with surgeon.
               (3) Instruct regarding pneumoperitoneum (retained carbon dioxide [CO_2] under diaphragm).
                   (a) Not to be alarmed if experience shoulder pain or pressure in lower abdomen
                       (i) May help to lie flat
                       (ii) Symptoms may last for several days.
               (4) Stress adequate nutrition; low- to moderate-fat diet.
           d. Provide instructions.
               (1) Written
               (2) Verbal
               (3) Assess and ensure patient and family understanding.
           e. Psychosocial concerns
               (1) Fear of not being able to eat a normal diet without pain
               (2) Body image related to possible obesity
               (3) Resume normal activity and work.
           f. Complications
               (1) Atelectasis and respiratory problems
               (2) Bladder distention
               (3) Hemorrhage or shock
               (4) Wound infection
               (5) Hiccups, especially in laparoscopic procedure
               (6) Pneumoperitoneum in laparoscopic procedure
               (7) Electrolyte and fluid imbalance
        2. Cholelithotripsy
           a. Assess for comfort.
               (1) Position
               (2) Medicate
           b. Key educational components
               (1) Instruct patient and family about routine care after abdominal procedure.
                   (a) Ambulate regularly.
                   (b) Rest frequently.
                   (c) Gradually increase activity as tolerated.

    (d) Avoid heavy lifting as ordered.
    (e) Splint abdomen when coughing.
   (2) Stress importance of follow-up care with physician.
   (3) Take deoxycholic acid daily as ordered to dissolve stone fragments.
  c. Provide instructions.
   (1) Written
   (2) Verbal
   (3) Assess and ensure patient and family understanding.
  d. Psychosocial concerns
   (1) All stones may not be eliminated or may recur.
   (2) Surgery may be necessary.
   (3) Resume normal activity and work.
  e. Complications
   (1) Retained fragments

IV. SPLEEN
 A. Anatomy and physiology (Figure 36-3)
  1. Location
   a. Lies in upper left abdominal cavity beneath dome of diaphragm
   b. Covered with peritoneum and held in place by numerous suspensory ligaments
  2. Blood supply
   a. Splenic artery furnishes arterial blood supply.
   b. Splenic vein drains into portal system.
  3. Function
   a. Largest lymphatic organ of body, having intimate role in immunological defenses of body
   b. Involved in formation of blood elements
   c. Acts as a blood reservoir
   d. Site of red blood cell destruction
 B. Pathophysiology
  1. Hypersplenism
   a. Causes a reduction in circulating quantity of:
    (1) Red blood cells (RBCs)
    (2) White blood cells (WBCs)
    (3) Platelets
    (4) Combination of RBCs, WBCs, and platelets
  2. Splenomegaly
   a. Congestive
   b. Hemolytic

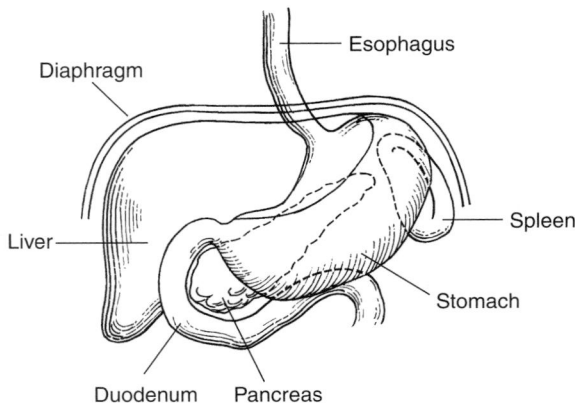

FIGURE 36-3 ■ Organs in upper abdominal cavity. (From Phillips NF: *Berry & Kohn's operating room technique,* ed 11, St Louis, 2007, Mosby.)

3. Hematological disorders
   a. Hemolytical anemia
   b. Thrombocytopenia
4. Tumors or cysts
5. Accessory spleen
6. Trauma
C. Assessment
   1. History of:
      a. Fatigue
      b. Lassitude
      c. Easy bruising
      d. Frequent nosebleed
      e. Hematuria
      f. Blood in stools
      g. Excessive bleeding after minor injuries or dental extractions
   2. Physical examination
      a. Petechiae or bruising
      b. Pallor or cyanosis of skin and mucous membranes
      c. Hepatomegaly
      d. Splenomegaly
      e. Evidence of rupture
         (1) Increased abdominal girth
         (2) Abdominal pain
         (3) Signs and symptoms of shock
   3. Laboratory studies as indicated
      a. Lactate dehydrogenase
      b. Bilirubin
      c. Sickle cell test
      d. Bone marrow aspiration
   4. Radionuclide scanning
   5. Other radiographical studies
D. Operative procedures
   1. Splenectomy: removal of spleen
   2. Purpose
      a. Provide symptomatic relief depending on cause of anemia or hemorrhage
      b. Performed prophylactically to reduce potential for rupture and massive blood loss
   3. Preoperative concerns
      a. Anxiety related to impending surgical procedure and knowledge deficit
      b. Concern about ability to resume normal activity and work
      c. Scheduled splenectomy patients may require preoperative:
         (1) Whole blood immediately before procedure
         (2) Corticosteroids to stabilize cell membranes and decrease inflammatory response
   4. Intraoperative concerns
      a. Fluid volume deficit related to hemorrhage
      b. Altered body temperature
      c. Infection related to invasive GI procedure
      d. Perforation of bladder, bowel, vascular organs
      e. Injury related to positioning
      f. Inflammatory response
   5. Procedures
      a. Laparoscopic splenectomy
         (1) Accomplished through three or four incisions made in abdominal wall
         (2) Rigid fiberoptic laparoscope inserted into peritoneal cavity
         (3) Performed in patients with benign disease

          (4) Advantages
            (a) Less postoperative pain
            (b) Fewer complications
            (c) More rapid postoperative recovery
          (5) Disadvantages
            (a) Longer surgery time
            (b) Longer exposure to anesthesia
            (c) More costly than open abdominal splenectomy
      b. Open abdominal splenectomy
          (1) Left rectus paramedian, midline, or subcostal incision
          (2) Splenic artery and vein often friable

  E. Postanesthesia care phase I
    1. Monitor intake and output.
      a. Assess NG tube for proper placement; if ordered, discontinue.
      b. Note patency of catheter, color and amount of urine; if ordered, discontinue.
    2. Assess comfort level.
      a. Note location of discomfort and position for comfort.
      b. Administer prescribed medications and evaluate relief.
    3. Maintain preoperative corticosteroid treatment if ordered.
    4. Monitor for internal bleeding.
      a. Abdominal girth and distention
      b. Abdominal firmness
      c. Signs and symptoms of shock

  F. Postanesthesia care phase II
    1. Usually stay for extended observation
    2. Key educational components
      a. Instruct patient and family about routine care after abdominal surgery.
         (1) Ambulate regularly.
         (2) Rest frequently.
         (3) Gradually increase activity as tolerated.
         (4) Keep incisions dry.
         (5) Report redness, increasing pain, or incision drainage.
         (6) Avoid heavy lifting as ordered.
         (7) Splint abdomen when coughing and deep breathing.
      b. Stress importance of follow-up care with surgeon.
      c. Stress adequate nutrition.
      d. Stress awareness of susceptibility to infection.
         (1) Prevention
         (2) Need for medical care at earliest possible signs and symptoms of infection
      e. Follow-up as ordered
    3. Provide instructions.
      a. Written
      b. Verbal
      c. Assess and ensure patient, family, and accompanying responsible adult understanding.
    4. Psychosocial concerns
      a. Susceptibility to infection
      b. Fear of germs, obsessive concern about cleanliness
      c. Social isolation and avoidance of social gatherings
      d. Concern about ability to return to normal activity
      e. Concern about ability to return to same line of work or need to change jobs
    5. Complications
      a. Atelectasis and respiratory problems
      b. Hemorrhage or shock
      c. Wound infection
      d. Generalized infection
      e. Inflammatory response
      f. Electrolyte and fluid imbalance

V. ESOPHAGUS-STOMACH
  A. Anatomy and physiology (see Figure 36-2)
    1. Location
      a. Esophagus
        (1) Musculocutaneous canal between pharynx in the throat and the stomach in the abdomen
        (2) Passes through thoracic cavity and enters abdominal cavity through esophageal hiatus of diaphragm
        (3) Lies between liver and aorta and between right and left branches of vagus nerve
      b. Stomach
        (1) Hollow muscular organ situated in upper left abdomen between esophagus and duodenum
        (2) Divided into fundus, body, and pyloric antrum
        (3) Omentum
          (a) Attached to lesser and greater curvatures
          (b) Covers stomach and small intestine
    2. Nerve supply
      a. Autonomic nervous supply from vagus nerve
        (1) Controls reflex activities of movement and secretions of alimentary canal
        (2) Significant in rhythmic relaxation of pyloric sphincter
  B. Pathophysiology
    1. Hiatal or diaphragmatic hernia
      a. Esophagitis
      b. Gastritis
      c. Aspiration of reflux contents
      d. Ulceration
      e. Bleeding
      f. Stenosis
      g. Chest and back symptoms
    2. Barrett's esophagus due to gastric reflux
      a. Ulcerations at distal esophagus
      b. May be precancerous
    3. Obesity
      a. Most common nutritional disorder in United States
      b. Causes
        (1) Social
        (2) Metabolical
        (3) Physiological
        (4) Psychological
  C. Assessment
    1. Clinical manifestations of esophageal reflux
      a. Reflux esophagitis
        (1) After eating
        (2) While sleeping or reclining
        (3) With stress
        (4) With increased intra-abdominal pressure
      b. Heartburn
      c. Belching
      d. Regurgitation
      e. Vomiting
      f. Retrosternal or substernal chest pain (dull, full, heavy)
      g. Hiccups
      h. Mild or occult bleeding and mild anemia
      i. Dysphagia
      j. Pneumonitis caused by aspiration
      k. Peptic stricture

     2. Physical assessment
       a. Not diagnostic
       b. Not usually helpful in making a diagnosis
     3. Diagnostic tests
       a. Barium swallow
       b. Chest x-ray
       c. Upper endoscopy and biopsy
       d. Esophageal motility studies
       e. Gastric analysis
       f. Stool occult blood test
       g. Electrocardiogram
     4. Clinical manifestations of morbid obesity
       a. Weight more than 100 lb (45.4 kg) more than ideal weight
       b. Body mass index (BMI): a measure of body fat based on height and weight using recognized standard metric measurements
         (1) Underweight: BMI <18.5
         (2) Normal weight: BMI = 18.5 to 24.9
         (3) Overweight: BMI = 25 to 29.9
         (4) Obesity: BMI ≥30
       c. Failure to lose weight despite years of medical treatment
       d. Comorbid conditions possibly also present
         (1) Hypertension
         (2) Peripheral vascular disease
         (3) Cardiac disease
         (4) Degenerative arthritis or joint disorders
         (5) Gallbladder disease
         (6) Hiatal hernia
         (7) Diabetes mellitus
         (8) Obstructive sleep apnea
     5. Diagnostic tests
       a. Diagnostic tests for comorbid conditions
         (1) Blood pressure (BP) checks
         (2) Doppler studies for circulatory status
         (3) Cardiac dysfunction studies
         (4) Motion analysis
         (5) GI studies
         (6) Nutritional studies
         (7) Electrolyte studies
         (8) Glucose studies
         (9) Pulmonary function studies
         (10) Psychological studies
  D. Operative procedures
     1. Preoperative concerns
       a. Anxiety related to impending surgical procedure and knowledge deficit
       b. Self-consciousness about body image if obese
       c. Concern about ability to resume normal activity and work
     2. Intraoperative concerns
       a. Adequately sized cart, table, procedural instruments, and equipment
       b. Adequate moving help and mechanical aids
       c. Difficult IV access
       d. Difficult intubation
       e. Respiratory problems, especially during intubation or laryngospasm
       f. Aspiration
       g. Thromboembolism
       h. Fluid volume deficit related to loss of blood and electrolyte-rich gastric and intestinal juices
       i. Altered body temperature
       j. Infection related to invasive GI procedure

      k. Perforation of bladder, bowel, vascular organs

      l. Injury related to positioning

   3. Procedures

      a. Esophageal hiatal herniorrhaphy: repair hiatal hernia.

         (1) Purpose: prevent reflux of gastric contents into esophagus.

         (2) Laparoscopic Nissen fundoplication (one of several common procedures) or new technology that provides a more precise robot-guided laparoscopic repair

            (a) Performed on selected patients

            (b) Performed through five stab wounds in abdomen

            (c) Portion of upper stomach is:

               (i)   Wrapped around distal esophagus

               (ii) Sutured to itself to prevent reflux

            (d) Advantages

               (i)   Less postoperative pain

               (ii) Fewer complications

               (iii) More rapid postoperative recovery

            (e) Disadvantages

               (i)   Longer surgery time

               (ii) Longer exposure to anesthesia

               (iii) More costly than open abdominal fundoplication

         (3) Open abdominal approach

            (a) Accomplished through midline or left subcostal incision, possibly extending over lower rib cage

            (b) Hiatus narrowed and fundus of stomach anchored against diaphragm

 E. Postanesthesia care phase I

   1. Laparoscopic or open Nissen fundoplication

      a. Initiate chest physiotherapy.

         (1) Coughing and deep breathing

         (2) Observe for indications of pneumothorax.

            (a) Dyspnea

            (b) Cyanosis

            (c) Sharp chest pain

      b. Initiate care of chest tubes if present for open procedure.

      c. Monitor intake and output.

         (1) Nothing by mouth (NPO) until:

            (a) Absence of nausea and vomiting

            (b) Bowel sounds present

         (2) Assess NG tube for proper placement; if ordered, discontinue.

         (3) Administer IV fluids and electrolytes as ordered.

         (4) Note patency of urinary catheter, color and amount of urine; if ordered, discontinue.

      d. Monitor for internal bleeding.

         (1) Abdominal girth and distention

         (2) Abdominal firmness

         (3) Signs and symptoms of shock

      e. Assess comfort level.

         (1) Note location of discomfort and position for comfort.

         (2) Administer prescribed medications and evaluate relief.

   2. Laparoscopic or open procedures

      a. Protect airway.

         (1) Elevate head.

            (a) Prevent aspiration.

            (b) Improve ventilation.

         (2) Lateral positioning

         (3) Oxygen

         (4) Cough, deep breathing

         (5) Vigilant observation

    b. Monitor intake and output.

      (1) NPO until:

        (a) Absence of nausea and vomiting

        (b) Bowel sounds present

      (2) Administer IV fluids and electrolytes as ordered.

        (a) Avoid overhydration.

      (3) Note patency of catheter, color and amount of urine.

    c. Provide NG tube care if tube present.

      (1) Ensure patency.

      (2) Anchor tube securely.

    d. Wound care

      (1) Observe for excessive drainage.

      (2) Splint incision when coughing.

      (3) Apply binders as ordered.

    e. Prevent thromboemboli.

      (1) Continue antiembolism stockings and sequential pneumatic devices as ordered.

      (2) Encourage leg movement.

      (3) Avoid groin and popliteal pressure.

    f. Assess comfort level.

      (1) Note location of discomfort and position for comfort.

      (2) Administer prescribed medications and evaluate relief.

      (3) Beware of prolonged somnolence caused by drugs stored in adipose tissue.

        (a) Barbiturates

        (b) Fentanyl

        (c) Sufentanil

        (d) Meperidine

        (e) Diazepam

    g. Provide psychological support.

      (1) Provide privacy.

      (2) Respect dignity.

F. Postanesthesia care phase II

  1. Laparoscopic Nissen fundoplication

    a. Stay for extended observation

    b. Key educational components

      (1) Instruct patient and family about routine care after abdominal surgery.

        (a) Ambulate regularly.

        (b) Rest frequently.

        (c) Gradually increase activity as tolerated.

        (d) Keep incisions dry.

        (e) Report redness, increasing pain, or incision drainage.

        (f) Avoid heavy lifting as ordered.

      (2) Splint abdomen when coughing.

      (3) Instruct in indicators of reflux recurrence.

        (a) Dysphagia

        (b) Hematemesis

        (c) Increased pain

      (4) Instruct in occasional, temporary side effects.

        (a) Inability to vomit may not be temporary

        (b) Gas bloat

        (c) Early satiety

    c. Provide instructions.

      (1) Written

      (2) Verbal

      (3) Assess and ensure patient and family understanding.

    d. Psychosocial concerns

      (1) Persistent GI disorders (bloating, nausea, diarrhea)

      (2) Recurrence of reflux

(3) Inability to enjoy eating

(4) Concern about ability to resume normal activity and work

  e. Complications

    (1) Pneumothorax

    (2) Perforation

    (3) Hemorrhage

    (4) Pneumonia

    (5) Dysphagia

    (6) Reflux, although less severe than before surgery

    (7) Gas bloat

    (8) Inability to vomit

    (9) Early satiety

    (10) Diarrhea common

    (11) Nausea

VI. APPENDIX

A. Anatomy and physiology (see Figure 36-2)

  1. Location

    a. Blind, narrow tube that extends from inferior portion of cecum

    b. Some appendices are retrocecal.

  2. Has no known useful function

B. Pathophysiology

  1. Appendicitis

    a. Most common in adolescents and young adults, especially males

    b. Can imitate other conditions

      (1) Ruptured ovarian cyst

      (2) Ureteral calculus

    c. Usually caused by obstruction of appendiceal lumen

    d. Inflammation and infection result from normal bacteria invading devitalized wall.

  2. Peritonitis

    a. Result of severely inflamed and ruptured appendix

    b. Local or generalized

C. Assessment

  1. Early stage

    a. Epigastric or umbilical pain

    b. Vague and diffuse pain or mild cramping

    c. Fever

    d. Nausea and vomiting

  2. Acute stage

    a. Rebound tenderness in right lower quadrant at McBurney's point

    b. Pain aggravated by walking, coughing, movement

    c. Sensation of constipation

    d. Anorexia

    e. Malaise

    f. Diarrhea

    g. Diminished peristalsis

  3. Acute appendicitis with perforation

    a. Increasing, generalized pain

    b. Recurrent vomiting

  4. Physical examination

    a. Temperature increases

    b. Generalized abdominal rigidity

    c. Rigid position with flexed knees

    d. Tender, palpable mass in the presence of abscess

    e. Possible abdominal distention

  5. Diagnostic tests

    a. Complete blood cell count (CBC) with differential (elevated WBC count)

    b. Urinalysis

        c. Abdominal x-ray

        d. Intravenous pyelogram

        e. Abdominal ultrasound

        f. Abdominal CT scan

D. Operative procedures

  1. Appendectomy: removal of appendix

  2. Purpose

    a. Prevent progression to gangrene.

    b. Prevent perforation of friable tissue with subsequent peritonitis.

  3. Preoperative concerns

    a. Anxiety related to impending surgical procedure and knowledge deficit

    b. Concern about ability to resume normal activity and work

  4. Intraoperative concerns

    a. Potential or actual rupture

    b. Potential peritonitis

    c. Potential bladder or bowel perforation

  5. Procedures

    a. Laparoscopic appendectomy

      (1) Performed through periumbilical incision with additional stab wounds at:

        (a) Suprapubic area

        (b) Left lower quadrant

      (2) May be done incidental to gynecological procedures or for acute or chronic appendicitis

      (3) Advantages

        (a) Earlier ambulation and hospital discharge

        (b) Decreased risk of wound infection

        (c) More aesthetically appealing appearance

        (d) Less pain

      (4) Disadvantages

        (a) Longer surgical time

        (b) Increased general anesthesia exposure time

        (c) Increased cost

    b. Open appendectomy

      (1) Involves a muscle-splitting incision over McBurney's point in right lower quadrant

      (2) After amputation of appendix, stump may be cauterized with phenol and alcohol or wiped with Betadine to reduce contamination.

      (3) Drainage indicated in presence of:

        (a) Abscess

        (b) Appendix rupture

        (c) Gross contamination of wound

E. Postanesthesia care phase I

  1. Monitor intake and output.

    a. NPO until:

      (1) Absence of nausea and vomiting

      (2) Bowel sounds present

    b. Administer IV fluids and electrolytes as ordered.

    c. Note patency of catheter if present, color and amount of urine.

    d. Provide NG tube care if tube present.

      (1) Ensure patency.

      (2) Anchor tube securely.

  2. Administer antibiotics as ordered.

  3. Assess comfort level.

    a. Note location of discomfort and position for comfort.

    b. Administer prescribed medications and evaluate relief.

F. Perianesthesia care phase II

  1. Stay for extended observation

  2. Key educational components

          a. Instruct patient and family about routine care after abdominal surgery.
            (1) Ambulate regularly.
            (2) Rest frequently.
            (3) Gradually increase activity as tolerated.
            (4) Wound care, dressing changes, bathing restrictions if appropriate
            (5) Report redness, increasing pain, or incision drainage.
            (6) Avoid heavy lifting as ordered.
            (7) Splint abdomen when coughing.
          b. Bowel management: if needed for constipation
            (1) Laxatives or stool softeners may be used only as prescribed.
            (2) Avoid enema unless or until approved by physician.
          c. Stress importance of follow-up care with surgeon.
       3. Provide instructions.
          a. Written
          b. Verbal
          c. Assess and ensure patient and family understanding.
       4. Psychosocial concerns
          a. Concern about how soon patient will be able to resume eating
          b. Concern about cosmetic appearance of scar (especially in young females)
          c. Concern about ability to resume normal activity and work
       5. Complications
          a. Wound infection
          b. Peritonitis

VII. INTESTINE
    A. Anatomy and physiology (see Figure 36-2)
       1. Location
          a. Continuous muscular tube of bowel extending from lower end of stomach to rectum
          b. Intestines divided into:
            (1) Small intestine extends from pylorus to ileocecal valve.
               (a) Duodenum (proximal portion)
               (b) Jejunum (middle section)
               (c) Ileum (distal portion joining large intestine)
            (2) Large intestine (colon) extends from ileum to rectum.
               (a) Ascending
               (b) Transverse
               (c) Descending
               (d) Sigmoid
          c. Mesentery
            (1) A peritoneal fold attaching small and large intestines to posterior abdominal wall
            (2) Contains arteries, veins, lymph nodes that supply intestines
       2. Purpose—food and digestive products pass through alimentary canal during:
          a. Digestion
          b. Absorption
          c. Elimination of waste products
    B. Pathophysiology
       1. Inflammation
          a. Diverticulitis
          b. Ulcerative colitis (Crohn's disease)
       2. Intestinal obstruction
          a. Neoplasms
          b. Strangulation from adhesions
          c. Volvulus
    C. Assessment
       1. Signs and symptoms
          a. Severe, cramping abdominal pain
          b. Back pain

      c. Restlessness

      d. Hiccups

      e. Belching

      f. Inability to pass stool or flatus with feeling of fullness

  2. Physical assessment

      a. Abdominal distention

      b. Abdominal tenderness

      c. High pitched and intermittent bowel sounds above point of obstruction

      d. Absent bowel sounds with paralytic ileus

      e. Signs of intravascular volume depletion

          (1) Decreased urinary output

          (2) Poor skin turgor

          (3) Dry skin and mucous membranes

      f. Bleeding on rectal examination

  3. History of:

      a. Abdominal hernia

      b. Recent or past abdominal surgery

      c. GI inflammation or perforation secondary to various disease processes

  4. Diagnostic tests

      a. CBC

      b. Abdominal x-ray

      c. Contrast studies

      d. CT scan of abdomen

      e. Endoscopy

          (1) Sigmoidoscopy

          (2) Colonoscopy

D. Operative procedures

  1. Bowel resection: remove a portion of intestine

  2. Purpose: relieve an obstruction or remove a portion of diseased intestine or adhesions

  3. Preoperative concerns

      a. Anxiety related to impending surgical procedure and knowledge deficit

      b. Concern about ability to resume normal activity and work

  4. Intraoperative concerns

      a. Fluid volume deficit related to hemorrhage

      b. Altered body temperature

      c. Infection related to invasive GI procedure

      d. Perforation of bladder, vascular organs

      e. Injury related to positioning

      f. Long instruments for obese or tall patient

  5. Procedures

      a. Laparoscopic intestinal resection

          (1) Performed through minimal access incision made in abdominal wall

          (2) Large or small bowel mobilized and resected through scope

          (3) Stomas can also be created with this technique.

          (4) Advantages

              (a) Less postoperative pain

              (b) Fewer complications

              (c) More rapid postoperative recovery

          (5) Disadvantages

              (a) Longer surgery time

              (b) Longer exposure to anesthesia

              (c) More costly than open intestinal resection procedure

          (6) Performed through midline abdominal incision

          (7) Peritoneal cavity walled off with intestine incised and clamped

          (8) Continuity reestablished by anastomosis

E. Postanesthesia care phase I
　1. Monitor intake and output.
　　a. NPO until:
　　　(1) Absence of nausea and vomiting
　　　(2) Bowel sounds present
　　b. Assess NG tube for proper placement.
　　c. Administer IV fluids and electrolytes as ordered.
　　d. Note patency of urinary catheter, color and amount of urine.
　2. Monitor for internal bleeding.
　　a. Abdominal girth and distention
　　b. Abdominal firmness
　　c. Signs and symptoms of shock
　3. Assess comfort level.
　　a. Note location of discomfort and position for comfort.
　　b. Administer prescribed medications and evaluate relief.
F. Postanesthesia care phase II
　1. Stay for extended observation
　2. Key educational components
　　a. Instruct patient and family about routine care after abdominal surgery.
　　　(1) Ambulate regularly.
　　　(2) Rest frequently.
　　　(3) Gradually increase activity as tolerated.
　　　(4) Wound care, dressing changes, bathing restrictions if appropriate
　　　(5) Report redness, increasing pain, or incision drainage.
　　　(6) Avoid heavy lifting as ordered.
　　　(7) Splint abdomen when deep breathing and coughing.
　　b. Bowel management: if needed for constipation
　　　(1) Laxatives
　　　(2) Stool softeners
　　　(3) Avoid enema unless or until approved by physician.
　　c. Stress importance of follow-up care with surgeon.
　3. Provide instructions.
　　　(1) Written
　　　(2) Verbal
　　　(3) Assess and ensure patient, family, and responsible accompanying adult understanding.
　4. Psychosocial concerns
　　a. Bowel movements
　　　(1) Possibility of pain
　　　(2) Possibility of constipation
　　b. Eating normal diet
　　c. Bloating or flatus
　　d. Ability to resume normal activity and work
　　e. Resuming sexual activity
　5. Complications
　　a. Wound contamination
　　b. Peritonitis
VIII. ANAL-RECTAL DISORDERS
　A. Anatomy and physiology
　　1. Hemorrhoids
　　　a. Location
　　　　(1) Masses of vascular tissue found in anal canal
　　　　(2) Internal hemorrhoid
　　　　　(a) Found above internal sphincter
　　　　　(b) Covered with columnar mucosa
　　　　(3) External hemorrhoids
　　　　　(a) Found outside external sphincter
　　　　　(b) Covered by anoderm and perianal skin
　　　　(4) May have combination of internal and external hemorrhoids

  b. Classification
    (1) First degree: project slightly into anal canal
    (2) Second degree: prolapse with defecation and reduce spontaneously
    (3) Third degree: prolapse with defecation and reduce manually
    (4) Fourth degree: irreducible
 2. Anal fissure
  a. Small tear in lining of anus resembling slitlike crack
  b. May extend from anal verge to pectinate line
 3. Anorectal fissure
  a. Location
    (1) Hollow, fibrous tunnel or tract with two openings
    (2) Primary, or internal, opening usually at a crypt near pectinate line
  b. May have single or multiple fistulas.
 4. Pilonidal cyst
  a. Midline of upper portion of gluteal fold
  b. Rarely symptomatic until adulthood
B. Pathophysiology
 1. Hemorrhoids
  a. Bleeding: if severe can cause iron deficiency anemia
  b. Strangulation: prolapsed hemorrhoid in which blood supply is cut off by anal sphincter
  c. Thrombosis: clotting of blood within hemorrhoid
 2. Anal fissure
  a. Loss of elasticity of anal canal may predispose
  b. Caused by:
    (1) Laxative abuse
    (2) Scarring from anal surgery
    (3) Chronic diarrhea disease
    (4) Frequent anal intercourse
 3. Anorectal fissure
  a. Infection in crypt progresses to form abscess that drains:
    (1) Spontaneously
    (2) Surgically
  b. Tract preserved as abscess heals
  c. Associated with:
    (1) Traumatic injury
    (2) Crohn's disease
    (3) Cancer
    (4) Radiation therapy
 4. Pilonidal cyst
  a. Sinus channel develops; lined with epithelium and hair
  b. Occurs during embryonic development when small amount of endothelial tissue is included beneath skin
C. Assessment
 1. Hemorrhoids
  a. Clinical manifestations
    (1) External hemorrhoids
      (a) Pruritus
      (b) Pain
    (2) Internal hemorrhoids
      (a) Bleeding
      (b) Thrombosis
      (c) Edema
  b. Diagnostic tests
    (1) Anoscopy
      (a) Visualization of hemorrhoids as instrument is removed
    (2) Sigmoidoscopy
    (3) Barium enema

2. Anal fissure
    a. Clinical manifestations
        (1) Inflammation
        (2) Bleeding
        (3) Burning
        (4) Pain on defecation
    b. Diagnostic tests
        (1) Digital rectal exam
            (a) Induration
            (b) Sphincter spasm
        (2) Anoscopy (proctoscopy)
            (a) Visualization of anorectal fissure
            (b) Superficial tear
                (i) Bleeds easily
                (ii) Has a reddish base
    c. Differential diagnosis
        (1) If fissure not found in midline, rule out:
            (a) Inflammatory disease
            (b) Bowel disease
            (c) Carcinoma
            (d) Tuberculosis
            (e) Syphilis
            (f) Herpes or other venereal disease
3. Anorectal fissure
    a. Diagnostic tests
        (1) Digital rectal examination
        (2) Palpate tract direction internally.
        (3) Anoscopy (proctoscopy)
            (a) May reveal primary opening in a cyst
        (4) Sigmoidoscopy
            (a) Used to rule out other sources of fistula formation
        (5) Fistulography
            (a) Used if tract is of questionable origin
            (b) Rule out colonic, small bowel, or urethral fistulas.
4. Pilonidal cyst
    a. Physical examination
        (1) Hairy dimple in gluteal fold
        (2) Open, draining lesion in sacral region with hair protruding from sinus opening
D. Operative procedures
    1. Hemorrhoidectomy: remove varicosities of veins or prolapsed mucosa of the anus and rectum.
        a. Purpose: relieve discomfort and control bleeding.
        b. Usual procedure
            (1) Sphincter dilated
            (2) Hemorrhoidal pedicle ligated with suture ligatures
            (3) Mass excised with:
                (a) Dissection
                (b) Laser
                (c) Cautery
                (d) Cryosurgical unit
            (4) Petrolatum gauze packed into anal canal
        c. Alternative procedure
            (1) Rubber band ligation placed around base of each hemorrhoid
            (2) Sloughing of avascularized hemorrhoid occurs in 7 to 10 days.
            (3) Can be done as an office procedure under local anesthesia
            (4) Advantages
                (a) Less postprocedure pain

    (b) Fewer complications

    (c) More rapid postprocedure recovery

   (5) Disadvantage

    (a) Local pain

    (b) Potential for hemorrhage

 2. Anal fissurectomy: dilation of anal sphincter and removal of lesion

  a. Purpose: relieve discomfort.

  b. Procedure

   (1) Anal sphincter dilation may be only surgical treatment necessary.

   (2) Scarred tissue removed for chronic conditions

 3. Anorectal fissure

  a. Anal fistulotomy: incision and drainage of a fistulous tract

  b. Anal fistulectomy: excision of fistula

  c. Purpose: prevent spread of infection.

  d. Procedure

   (1) Fistulotomy—tract is:

    (a) Opened

    (b) Packed

    (c) Allowed to drain

    (d) Allowed to heal by granulation

   (2) Fistulectomy—tract is:

    (a) Excised

    (b) Sometimes partially closed with suture

 4. Pilonidal cystectomy: remove cyst with sinus tract.

  a. Purpose: prevent recurrence of infection and abscess formation in pilonidal sinus.

  b. Procedure

   (1) Cyst with sinus tracts removed from intergluteal fold on posterior surface of lower sacrum to prevent:

    (a) Recurrence of infection

    (b) Abscess formation in pilonidal sinus

   (2) Wound may be:

    (a) Packed open

    (b) Closed

    (c) Closed with tissue flaps

 5. Preoperative concerns for above procedures

  a. Embarrassment because of private nature of site

  b. Excessive pain

  c. Fecal incontinence

  d. Painful suture removal

  e. Ability to resume normal activity and work

 6. Intraoperative concerns

  a. Maintaining privacy

  b. Contamination of vagina with bloody anal fluid

  c. If used, laser safety

E. Postanesthesia care phase I

 1. Monitor for urinary retention.

 2. Monitor for bleeding.

 3. Assess comfort level.

  a. Note location of discomfort and position for comfort.

  b. Administer prescribed medications and evaluate relief.

 4. Monitor for hypotension secondary to vasodilation of pelvic blood vessels.

F. Postanesthesia care phase II

 1. Assess dressings.

 2. Key educational components

  a. Pain control

   (1) Analgesics

   (2) Position for comfort.

            (a) Side-lying
            (b) Recumbent
        b. Observe for adequate output.
        c. Wound care
            (1) Packing removal
            (2) Sitz baths as ordered
            (3) Perianal cleansing after each stool
            (4) Dressing changes
        d. Bowel management to avoid constipation
            (1) Adequate hydration
            (2) Exercise
            (3) Fiber intake
            (4) Stool softener
            (5) Mild laxative if ordered
    3. Provide instructions.
        a. Written
        b. Verbal
        c. Assess and ensure patient and family understanding.
    4. Psychosocial concerns
        a. Bowel movements
            (1) Pain and discomfort
            (2) Not eating to postpone the first bowel movement
            (3) Fecal incontinence
        b. Ability to resume normal activity and work
        c. Resuming sexual activity
    5. Complications
        a. Hemorrhage or shock
        b. Urinary retention
        c. Constipation
        d. Diarrhea
        e. External fistulas
        f. Nonhealing wound
        g. Fluid and electrolyte imbalance
IX. HERNIAS
    A. Anatomy and physiology (Figure 36-4)
        1. Sac lined by peritoneum that protrudes through defect in layers of abdominal wall
        2. Type
            a. Acquired
            b. Congenital
        3. Weak places or intervals in abdominal aponeurosis
            a. Inguinal canals
            b. Femoral rings
            c. Umbilicus
        4. Contributing factors
            a. Age
            b. Sex
            c. Previous surgery
            d. Obesity
            e. Nutritional status
            f. Pulmonary and cardiac disease
            g. Loss of skin turgor
                (1) Aging
                (2) Chronic debilitating diseases
    B. Pathophysiology
        1. Internal hernias
            a. Congenital
            b. Associated with failure of intestine to rotate in usual sequence in fetus

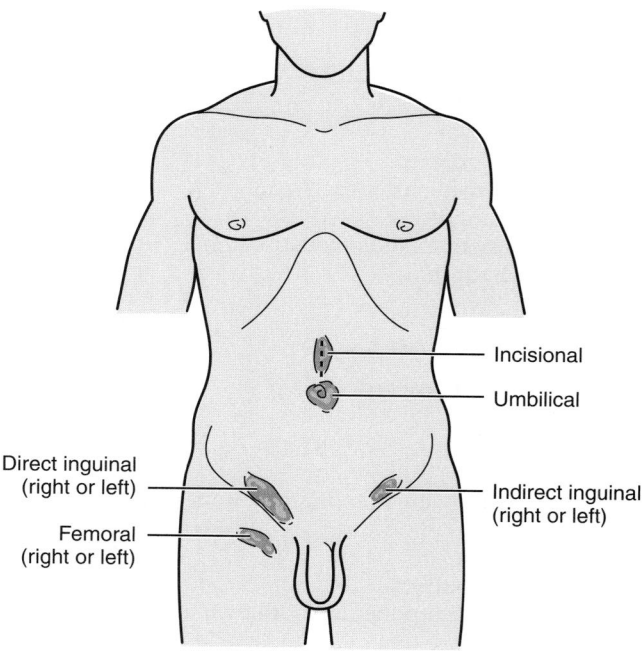

FIGURE 36-4 ■ Common types of herniation. (From Phillips NF: *Berry & Kohn's operating room technique,* ed 11, St Louis, 2007, Mosby.)

2. External hernias
   a. Inguinal hernia
     (1) Most common
     (2) Types
       (a) Indirect: herniation protrudes through inguinal ring and follows round ligament or spermatic cord.
       (b) Direct: herniation goes through posterior inguinal wall.
       (c) Reducible: hernia contents can be returned to the normal cavity by manipulation.
       (d) Irreducible or incarcerated
         (i) Hernia contents cannot be returned to the normal cavity by manipulation.
         (ii) Bowel may lack adequate blood supply.
         (iii) Bowel may become obstructed or strangulated.
   b. Femoral
     (1) More frequent in women
     (2) Protrusion through femoral ring into femoral canal
     (3) Seen as bulge below inguinal ligament
     (4) Can easily strangulate
   c. Ventral
     (1) Associated with muscle weakness from abdominal incisions
     (2) Types
       (a) Epigastric
         (i) Protrusion of fat through defects in abdominal wall
         (ii) Between xiphoid process and umbilicus
       (b) Umbilical
         (i) Child
           [a] Common
           [b] Frequently disappears spontaneously by 2 years of age
         (ii) Adult
           [a] Acquired

[b] Common in females
[c] Increased abdominal pressure
[d] Obesity
[e] Multiparity
(c) Incisional
   (i) Muscle weakness from prior surgeries
   (ii) Poor nutritional state
   (iii) Faulty surgical technique
   (iv) Obesity associated with ascites
   (v) Wound infection
   (vi) Wounds healed by secondary intention

C. Assessment
1. Physical examination of abdomen
   a. Examine supine and sitting.
   b. Often see hernia protrude when:
      (1) Changing position
      (2) Coughing
      (3) Laughing
      (4) Crying
   c. Palpate weakened muscle area.
2. Signs of intestinal obstruction
   a. Abdominal distention
   b. Nausea
   c. Vomiting
3. Signs of strangulation
   a. Pain of increasing severity
   b. Fever
   c. Tachycardia
   d. Abdominal rigidity
D. Operative procedures
1. Herniorrhaphy: repair of weakened abdominal wall
2. Hernioplasty: reinforcement of weakened area with wire, fascia, or mesh
3. Purpose: reduce or repair hernia; may be:
   a. Inguinal
   b. Femoral
   c. Ventral
   d. Umbilical
   e. Incisional
4. Preoperative concerns
   a. Anxiety related to impending surgical procedure and knowledge deficit
   b. Ability to resume normal activity and work
5. Intraoperative concerns
   a. Fluid volume deficit related to hemorrhage
   b. Altered body temperature
   c. Infection related to invasive GI procedure
   d. Perforation of bladder, bowel, vascular organs
   e. Injury related to positioning
   f. Long instruments for obese or tall patient
6. Procedures
   a. Laparoscopic hernia repair
      (1) Transabdominal preperitoneal approach uses intraperitoneal trocars and the creation of a peritoneal flap over posterior inguinal region.
      (2) Totally extraperitoneal approach provides access to the preperitoneal space without entering peritoneal cavity.
      (3) Advantages
         (a) Less oral analgesics required
         (b) Recovery period shorter
         (c) Wound infection rate lower

          (d) Tension-free application of mesh enabled

          (e) Bilateral herniorrhaphy can be performed using same port sites.

          (f) Postoperative adhesions reduced

        (4) Disadvantages

          (a) Surgical time longer

          (b) General anesthesia exposure time increased

          (c) Potential for nerve injury greater

          (d) Cost increased

    b. Open hernia repair

      (1) Incision depends on hernia location and type.

      (2) Principle is same regardless of hernia location and type.

        (a) Free tightly bound hernias.

        (b) Examine contents of hernia for ischemic change.

        (c) Repair hernia defect with or without reinforcement.

E. Postanesthesia care phase I

  1. Laparoscopic or open procedure

    a. Monitor for hematoma formation in laparoscopic procedure or perforation of the following:

      (1) Bowels

      (2) Epigastric vessels

      (3) Ilioinguinal vessels

    b. Monitor for scrotal edema and ecchymosis.

      (1) Ice packs for scrotal edema as ordered

    c. Monitor for sensory and motor alterations.

      (1) Damage of ilioinguinal nerves during manipulation and dissection of various anatomic structures

      (2) Infiltration of incisional area with local anesthesia

    d. Assess for bladder distention.

      (1) Urinary retention

      (2) Perforation of urinary bladder during dissection

    e. Monitor for internal bleeding.

      (1) Abdominal girth and distention

      (2) Abdominal firmness

      (3) Signs and symptoms of shock

    f. Assess comfort level.

      (1) Note location of discomfort and position for comfort.

      (2) Administer prescribed medications and evaluate relief.

F. Postanesthesia care phase II

  1. Key educational components

    a. Instruct patient, family, and responsible accompanying adult about routine care after abdominal surgery.

      (1) Activity

        (a) Ambulate regularly.

        (b) Rest frequently.

        (c) Gradually increase activity as tolerated.

        (d) Avoid coughing, straining, stretching, heavy lifting until approved by physician.

        (e) Splint incision while coughing, sneezing.

        (f) Use proper body mechanics for moving and lifting.

        (g) Avoid sexual activity until approved by physician.

      (2) Wound care

        (a) Dressing changes

        (b) Binder or scrotal support

        (c) Ice to incision or scrotum if ordered

        (d) Bathing restrictions if appropriate

        (e) Signs of infection

          (i)   Redness

          (ii) Fever

     (iii) Tenderness

     (iv) Incisional drainage

    (3) Pain control

    (4) Assess adequate intake and output.

    (5) Bowel management to avoid constipation

     (a) Hydration

     (b) Fiber

     (c) Exercise

     (d) Stool softener

     (e) Mild laxative if ordered

  b. Stress importance of follow-up care with surgeon.

 2. Provide instructions.

  a. Written

  b. Verbal

  c. Assess and ensure patient, family, and accompanying adult understanding.

 3. Psychosocial concerns about

  a. Resuming normal diet

  b. Ability to urinate

  c. Constipation and bowel movements

  d. Ability to resume normal activity and work

  e. Resuming sexual activity

 4. Complications

  a. Pneumoperitoneum in laparoscopic procedure

  b. Atelectasis and respiratory problems

  c. Bladder distention

  d. Paralytic ileus

  e. Hemorrhage or shock

  f. Wound infection

  g. Dehiscence or evisceration

  h. Electrolyte and fluid imbalance

  i. Pulmonary embolus

X. THYROID GLAND

 A. Anatomy and physiology (Figure 36-5)

  1. Location

   a. Butterfly-shaped gland composed of two lobes

    (1) Positioned on either side of trachea

    (2) Joined by isthmus

   b. Isthmus situated near base of neck

   c. Posterior surface of isthmus adherent to anterior surface of tracheal ring

   d. Upper pole of gland beneath upper end of sternothyroid muscle

   e. Lower pole extends to sixth tracheal ring.

   f. Enclosed by pretracheal fascia

  2. Blood supply

   a. Arteries

    (1) External carotid arteries via superior thyroid artery

    (2) Subclavian artery via inferior thyroid arteries

   b. Veins

    (1) Three pairs

    (2) Extend from a plexus formed on surface of gland and on front of trachea

  3. Nerve supply

   a. Superior laryngeal nerve lies bilateral in proximity to superior thyroid artery.

   b. Recurrent laryngeal nerve that supplies vocal cord

    (1) Ascends from mediastinum

    (2) In close association with tracheoesophageal sulcus and interior thyroid artery

   c. Sympathetic and parasympathetic nerves enter gland, probably exerting influence primarily on blood supply.

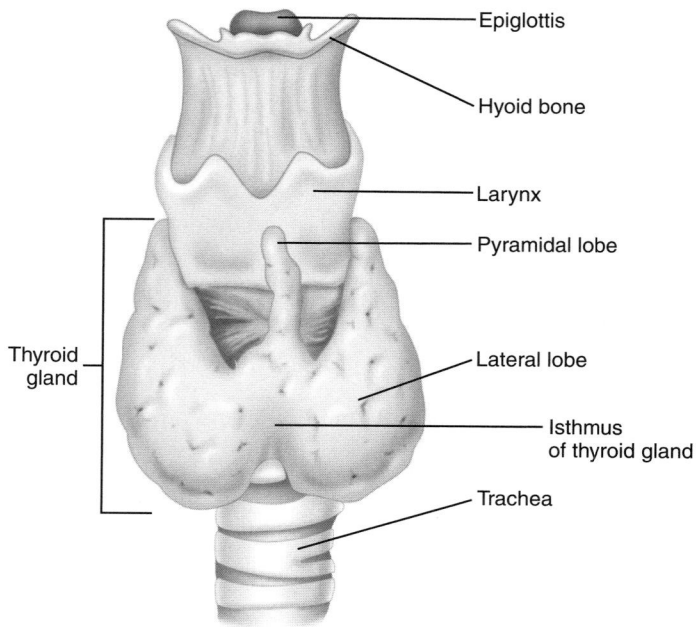

FIGURE 36-5 ■ Thyroid gland. (From Thibodeau GA, Patton KT: *Anatomy & physiology,* ed 6, St Louis, 2007, Mosby.)

4. Physiology
   a. Thyrotropin (also called thyroid-stimulating hormone, or TSH) is released by pituitary gland in response to thyrotropin-releasing hormone (TRH), which is released by the hypothalmus.
   b. In response to TSH, thyroid gland produces thyroxine (T_4) and triiodothyronine (T_3) each day.
      (1) T_3 has short half-life.
      (2) T_4 has half-life of 5 to 7 days.
      (3) Peripheral tissue converts T_4 to T_3.
      (4) T_3 considered as true tissue thyroid hormone, whereas T_4 considered a plasma prohormone.
      (5) Control of hormones exists in hypothalamus and pituitary on negative feedback cycle.
B. Pathophysiology
   1. Multinodular toxic diffuse enlargement (Graves' disease)
   2. Adenomas
   3. Malignancy
   4. Thyroiditis
      a. Viral, autoimmune, or unknown etiology
      b. Immunoglobulins found in serum of hyperthyroid patients mimic TSH.
C. Assessment
   1. Clinical manifestations of hyperthyroidism (also consider thyroid nodules)
      a. Nervousness, irritability, hyperactivity, emotional lability, and decreased attention span
      b. Weakness, easy fatigability, exercise intolerance
      c. Heat intolerance
      d. Weight change (loss or gain), increased appetite
      e. Insomnia, interrupted sleep
      f. Frequent stools, diarrhea
      g. Menstrual irregularities, decreased libido

    h. Warm, sweaty, flushed skin with a velvety-smooth texture; spider telangiectasis

    i. Exophthalmos, retracted eyelids, staring gaze

    j. Tremor, hyperkinesia, hyperreflexia

    k. Hair loss

    l. Goiter

    m. Bruits over thyroid gland

    n. Elevated systolic blood pressure, widened pulse pressure, S_3 heart sound

  2. Diagnostic laboratory tests

    a. TRH stimulation test

    b. Serum T_4 and T_3

    c. Serum free T_4 and T_3

    d. Radioactive T_3 uptake

    e. Radioactive iodine uptake

    f. TSH

    g. Thyroid-stimulating immunoglobulins

D. Operative procedure

  1. Thyroidectomy: removal of all or part of thyroid gland

  2. Purpose: relates to patient's medical diagnosis

    a. Relieve tracheal and esophageal obstruction.

      (1) Graves' disease (hyperthyroidism)

      (2) Hashimoto's thyroiditis (autoimmune disease)

      (3) Nontoxic nodular goiter

      (4) Rule out a malignant nodule of thyroid gland.

    b. Remove malignant tumors.

  3. Preoperative concerns

    a. Anxiety related to disease state and impending surgical procedure with knowledge deficit

    b. Success of surgery

    c. Cosmetic results of surgery

    d. Ability to resume normal activity and work

  4. Intraoperative concerns

    a. Edema resulting in postoperative:

      (1) Impaired swallowing

      (2) Ineffective airway clearance

      (3) Ineffective gas exchange

    b. Ineffective thermoregulation

    c. Laryngeal nerve damage

    d. Positioning to prevent distorted body contour in neck region

  5. Procedures

    a. Unilateral thyroid lobectomy: removal of one thyroid lobe with division at isthmus

    b. Subtotal lobectomy: lobectomy that spares posterior capsule and possibly a portion of adjacent thyroid tissue

    c. Bilateral subtotal thyroidectomy: removal of both lobes of thyroid

    d. Near-total thyroidectomy: total lobectomy with contralateral subtotal thyroidectomy

    e. Total thyroidectomy: removal of both lobes of thyroid and attempted removal of all thyroid tissue present

    f. All procedures performed through a transverse incision parallel to normal skin lines

E. Postanesthesia care phase I

  1. Usually stay for extended observation

  2. Assess and document surgical site.

    a. Neck dressings for signs of hemorrhaging

    b. Presence of drain and drainage

    c. Neck for swelling

        (1) Nerve damage: have patient say "e."
        (2) Obstructed airway
        (3) Vascularity of neck
    d. Encourage patient to remain calm, and prevent neck thrashing.
    e. Importance of remaining silent to rest vocal cords
  3. Key educational components
    a. Instruct patient in signs and symptoms of:
        (1) Hyperthyroidism
            (a) Nervousness, irritability, hyperactivity, emotional lability, decreased attention span
            (b) Weakness, easy fatigability, exercise intolerance
            (c) Heat intolerance
            (d) Weight change (loss or gain), increased appetite
            (e) Insomnia, interrupted sleep
            (f) Menstrual irregularities, decreased libido
            (g) Tremor, hyperkinesia, hyperreflexia
            (h) Exophthalmos, retracted eyelids, staring gaze
            (i) Hair loss
            (j) Palpitations
            (k) Tachycardia
        (2) Hypothyroidism
            (a) Physical and mental sluggishness
            (b) Slow, clumsy movements
            (c) Dry, flaky skin; dry, brittle head and body hair; reduced nail and hair growth
            (d) Weight gain/obesity
            (e) Cool skin and cold tolerance
            (f) Dyspnea
            (g) Fluid retention
            (h) Decreased appetite, constipation
            (i) Muscle aching, stiffness
        (3) Hypocalcemia
            (a) Nervousness
            (b) Muscle cramps
            (c) Paresthesias (especially circumoral, fingers, and toes)
            (d) Tingling and numbness of feet
            (e) Positive Chvostek's sign: abnormal spasm of facial muscles when facial nerve is tapped
            (f) Trousseau's sign (carpal tunnel spasm provoked by ischemia)
            (g) Carpopedal spasms
            (h) Laryngeal stridor
            (i) Convulsions
    b. Wound care
        (1) Report incisional pain.
        (2) Report redness, swelling, drainage, fever.
    c. Teach patient to support head and neck.
        (1) When turning or lifting head
        (2) When rising from a lying position
    d. Establish alternate means of communication (writing, sign language).
    e. Stress importance of follow-up care with physician.
  4. Provide instructions.
    a. Written
    b. Verbal
    c. Assess and ensure patient and family understand.
  5. Psychosocial concerns
    a. Quality of voice
    b. Cosmetic appearance of surgical scar
    c. Ability to resume normal activity and work

6. Complications
   a. Incisional bleeding
   b. Recurrent laryngeal nerve damage with resultant vocal cord impairment or paralysis
   c. Pneumothorax
   d. Tracheal compression from bleeding or edema
   e. Hypothyroidism
   f. Thyroid storm
      (1) Cause
         (a) Severe hyperthyroidism
         (b) Excessive stress
      (2) Symptoms
         (a) Hyperthermia
         (b) Tachycardia, especially atrial tachydysrhythmias
         (c) High-output heart failure
         (d) Agitation or delirium
         (e) Fluid volume depletion
            (i) Nausea and vomiting
            (ii) Diarrhea

XI. PARATHYROID GLANDS
   A. Anatomy and physiology (Figure 36-6)
      1. Consist of four small masses of tissue lying behind or within thyroid gland, inside pretracheal fascia
         a. Upper pair lies behind superior pole of thyroid.
         b. Lower pair lies near pole of thyroid.
      2. Aberrant nodules of parathyroid tissue may be found outside pretracheal fascia as low as superior mediastinum, especially within thymus.
      3. Normally measure 3 to 4 mm in diameter
      4. Blood supply
         a. Superior thyroid arteries
         b. Inferior thyroid arteries

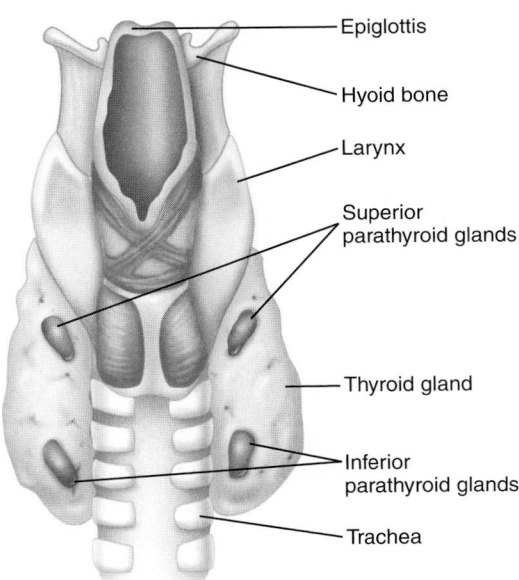

FIGURE 36-6 ■ Parathyroid glands. (From Thibodeau GA, Patton KT: *Anatomy & physiology,* ed 6, St Louis, 2007, Mosby.)

     5. Physiology
        a. Parathyroid hormone (PTH) regulates and maintains:
           (1) Metabolism
           (2) Hemostasis of blood calcium concentration
        b. Regulation of PTH secretion
  B. Pathophysiology
     1. Primary hyperparathyroidism
        a. Characterized by hypercalcemia and hypophosphatemia
        b. Results in major kidney and bone lesions
     2. Secondary hyperparathyroidism
        a. Results from parathyroid hyperplasia
        b. Produces decreased serum calcium levels
     3. Results in:
        a. Bone lesions
        b. Overactivity of one or more parathyroid glands
        c. Excessive secretion of PTH
        d. Imbalance in calcium and phosphate metabolism
  C. Assessment
     1. Surgical site assessment and documentation
        a. Neck dressings for signs of hemorrhage
        b. Presence of drain and drainage
        c. Neck for swelling
           (1) Nerve damage: have patient say "e."
           (2) Obstructed airway
           (3) Vascularity of neck
        d. Encourage patient to remain calm, and prevent neck thrashing.
     2. Neurologic sequelae (parathyroidectomy)
        a. Hyperthermia
        b. Increased intracranial pressure
        c. Cerebrospinal fluid leakage
        d. Convulsions
     3. Clinical manifestations
        a. Fatigue, muscular weakness, listlessness
        b. Frequent fractures
        c. Renal calculi
        d. Anorexia, nausea, abdominal discomfort
        e. Memory impairment
        f. Polyuria, polydipsia
        g. Back and joint pain
        h. Hypertension
     4. Diagnostic laboratory tests
        a. Serum calcium levels
        b. Serum phosphorus (PO_4) levels
        c. Urinary calcium levels
        d. Urinary PO_4 levels
        e. Creatine clearance
        f. Hydroxyproline
        g. Urinary cyclic adenosine monophosphate
  D. Operative procedures
     1. Purpose: relates to patient's medical diagnosis
        a. Presence of adenomas (hypersecreting neoplasms)
        b. Hyperplasia
        c. Carcinomas
           (1) Require surgical excision
           (2) Resection of lymphatics is essential.
        d. Inability to locate glands
        e. Underlying medical conditions

(1) Renal failure
(2) Severe cardiac disorders
(3) Hypercalcemia of nonparathyroid etiology
2. Preoperative concerns
   a. Anxiety related to:
      (1) Disease state
      (2) Impending surgical procedure
      (3) Knowledge deficit
   b. Success of surgery
   c. Cosmetic results of surgery
   d. Ability to resume normal activity and work
3. Intraoperative concerns
   a. Edema resulting in postoperative:
      (1) Impaired swallowing
      (2) Ineffective airway clearance
      (3) Ineffective gas exchange
   b. Ineffective thermoregulation
   c. Laryngeal nerve damage
   d. Positioning to prevent distorted body contour in neck region
4. Procedures
   a. Parathyroidectomy: excision of one or more parathyroid glands
   b. Total parathyroidectomy: removal of all glands
   c. Partial parathyroidectomy: removal of 3½ to 4 glands
      (1) Metal clips left in place to identify remaining glandular tissue
   d. Procedures performed through a transverse incision parallel to normal skin lines
E. Postanesthesia care phase I
   1. Usually stay for extended observation
   2. Key educational components
      a. Instruct patient in signs and symptoms of hypocalcemia.
         (1) Nervousness
         (2) Muscle cramps
         (3) Trousseau sign
            (a) Place blood pressure cuff around the arm and inflated to a pressure greater than the systolic blood pressure
            (b) Inflate for 3 minutes.
            (c) Brachial artery is occluded.
            (d) In the absence of blood flow, hypocalcemia and subsequent neuromuscular irritability will induce spasm of the muscles of the hand and forearm.
         (4) Paresthesias (especially circumoral)
         (5) Tingling and numbness of feet
         (6) Positive Chvostek's sign: abnormal spasm of facial muscles when facial nerve is tapped
         (7) Carpopedal spasms
         (8) Laryngeal stridor
         (9) Convulsions
      b. Wound care
         (1) Report incisional pain.
         (2) Report redness, swelling, drainage, fever.
      c. Activity
         (1) Importance of mobility, especially with irreversible skeletal impairment
      d. Nutrition
         (1) Monitor weight.
         (2) Take dietary supplements containing calcium.
         (3) Take calcium replacement medication.

      3. Provide instructions.
        a. Written
        b. Verbal
        c. Assess and ensure patient, family, and responsible accompanying adult.
      4. Psychosocial concerns
        a. Cosmetic appearance of surgical scar
        b. Ability to resume normal activity and work
      5. Complications
        a. Incisional bleeding
        b. Tracheal compression from bleeding or edema
        c. Tetany
        d. Hyperparathyroid crisis
          (1) Polyuria, polydipsia, kidney stones
          (2) Abdominal pain, constipation, nausea, anorexia
          (3) Joint or back pain
          (4) Muscle weakness and atrophy
          (5) Depression, paranoia, mood swings

XII. LYMPH NODES
    A. Anatomy and physiology (Figure 36-7)
      1. Lymphatic system closely related to circulatory system
      2. Lymphatic system consists of:
        a. Lymphatic vessels
        b. Lymph nodes
      3. Lymph nodes are small, oval bodies enclosed within fibrous connective tissue capsules.
        a. Trap foreign matter
        b. May become enlarged, infected, or the focus of metastatic cancer
      4. Lymphatic vessels
        a. Transport lymph fluid from interstitial spaces to venous bloodstream.
        b. Help protect body from disease.
      5. Nodes occur in clusters in specific regions of body.
        a. Popliteal, inguinal nodes of lower extremity
        b. Lumbar nodes of pelvic region
        c. Cubital, axillary nodes of upper extremity
        d. Thoracic nodes of chest
        e. Cervical nodes of neck
        f. Peyer's patches of mesentery
    B. Pathophysiology
      1. Infectious mononucleosis
      2. Lymphadenopathy
      3. Malignant lymphomas
        a. Hodgkin's disease
        b. Non-Hodgkin's lymphoma
      4. Metastasis
    C. Assessment
      1. Clinical manifestations
        a. Enlarged, painless lump or swelling
        b. Fever, sometimes intermittent
        c. Weakness, malaise
        d. Weight loss
        e. Anemia
        f. Local symptoms caused by pressure or obstruction
          (1) Pain, nerve irritation
          (2) Obliteration of pulse
      2. Diagnostic tests
        a. Chest x-ray
        b. Lymphangiography
        c. Biopsy

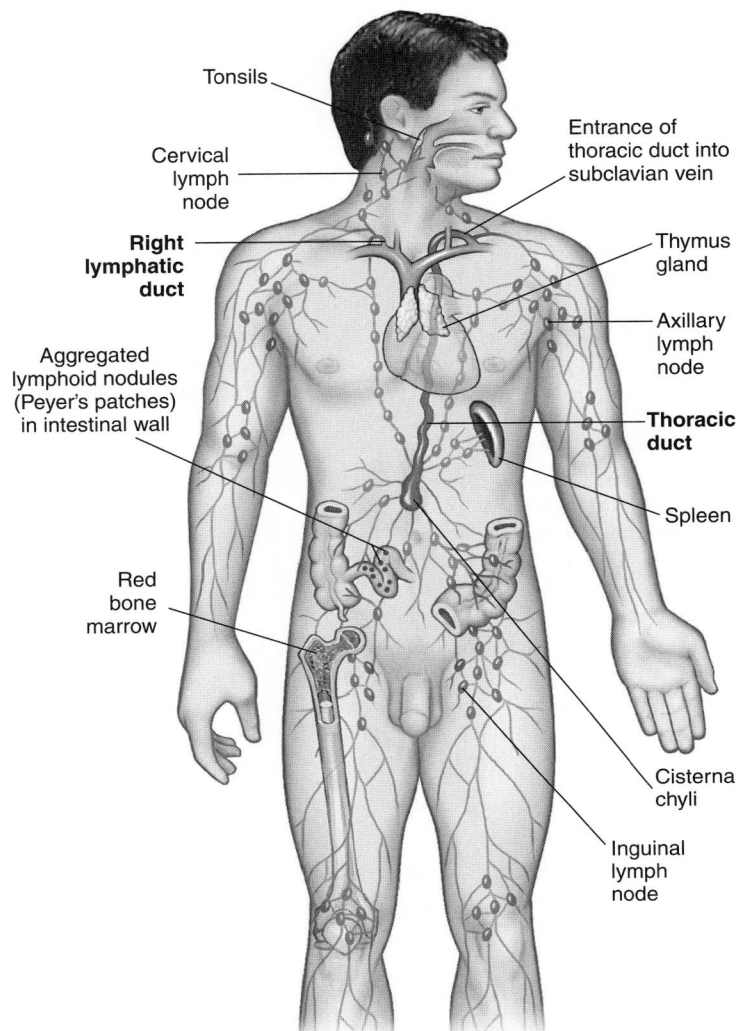

FIGURE 36-7 ■ Schematic representation of lymphatic system. (From Thibodeau GA, Patton KT: *Anatomy & physiology,* ed 6, St Louis, 2007, Mosby.)

D. Operative procedure
  1. Lymph node biopsy—excision of:
    a. One or more lymph nodes
    b. Possibly some surrounding tissue
  2. Purpose: relates to patient's medical diagnosis
  3. Preoperative concerns
    a. Cosmetic appearance of surgical site
    b. Possible malignancy
    c. Life expectancy and ability to raise family
  4. Intraoperative concerns
    a. Lymphangiogram reports available
    b. Correct side verified
    c. Specimen properly prepared and labeled for pathology
  5. Procedure
    a. Depends on site of procedure
    b. Removal of nodes done through small incision

    c. Identification and microscopic examination of nodes determines:

      (1) Diagnosis

      (2) Staging of malignancy

      (3) Need for additional or more extensive surgeries and adjunct treatment

E. Postanesthesia care phase I

  1. Assess surgical site for drainage.

  2. Assess comfort level.

    a. Pain may increase anxiety and feeling of powerlessness.

    b. Assess effectiveness of any analgesics given.

  3. Assess circulation in affected extremity.

  4. Psychological support

    a. Respond appropriately to patient's verbalized questions and responses.

    b. Avoid making unfounded promises or encouraging false or unreasonable hopes.

F. Postanesthesia care phase II

  1. Assess emotional feelings.

  2. Key educational components

    a. Depends on extent of procedure and diagnosis

    b. Provide information on wound care.

    c. Provide information on range-of-motion exercises as directed by the physician.

    d. Provide information about resources and support systems as appropriate.

    e. Stress importance of follow-up with physician.

    f. Educate patient to avoid having BP or venipuncture on operative side of node dissection.

  3. Provide instructions.

    a. Written

    b. Verbal

    c. Assess and ensure patient and family understanding.

  4. Psychosocial concerns

    a. Possible malignancy

    b. Depression

      (1) Change in self-image

      (2) Possible negative reaction from spouse and family

      (3) Possible distancing of friends who "don't know what to say"

      (4) Life expectancy and ability to raise family

    c. Ability to resume normal activity and work

  5. Complications

    a. Hematoma

    b. Wound infection

XIII. SKIN

  A. Anatomy and physiology (Figure 36-8)

    1. Largest organ of body

    2. Composition of integumentary system

      a. Skin

        (1) Epidermis

          (a) Basal layer

          (b) Spiny layer

          (c) Granular layer

          (d) Clear layer

          (e) Hornlike layer

        (2) Dermis

          (a) Papillary layer

          (b) Reticular layer

        (3) Hypodermis (subcutaneous tissue)

          (a) Connects skin to underlying organs

ANATOMIC LAYERS   SKIN GRAFTS   BURNS

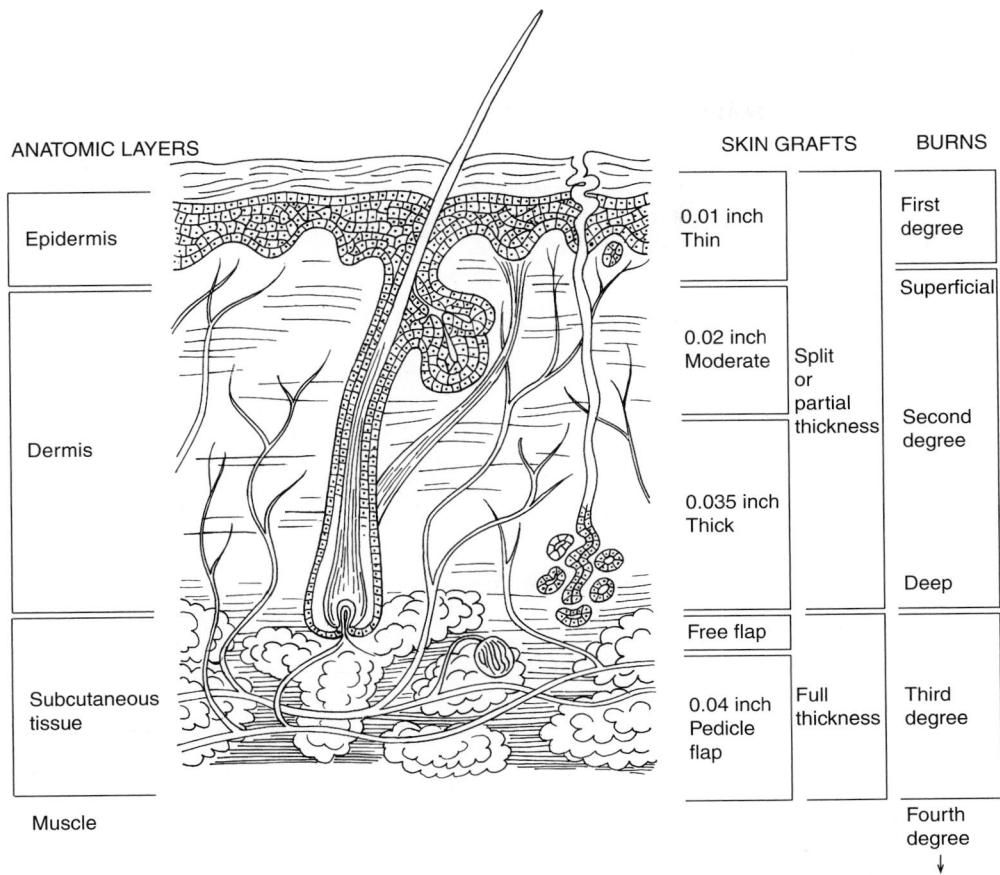

Anatomic Layers	Skin Grafts	Burns
Epidermis	0.01 inch Thin	First degree
		Superficial
Dermis	0.02 inch Moderate — Split or partial thickness	Second degree
	0.035 inch Thick	Deep
	Free flap	
Subcutaneous tissue	0.04 inch Pedicle flap — Full thickness	Third degree
Muscle		Fourth degree ↓

FIGURE 36-8 ■ Cross-section of skin and subcutaneous tissue. (From Phillips NF: *Berry & Kohn's operating room technique,* ed 11, St Louis, 2007, Mosby.)

    b. Epidermal modifications
       (1) Hair
       (2) Glands
       (3) Nails
  3. Physiology
      (1) Functions as protective barrier against physical, chemical, bacterial agents
      (2) Maintains body temperature
      (3) Functions as sensory organ for pressure, touch, temperature, pain
      (4) Prevents loss of body fluid
      (5) Excretes waste from sweat glands
      (6) Contributes to self-concept and body image
B. Pathophysiology
  1. Cuts and punctures
  2. Burns and frostbite
  3. Abrasions
  4. Inflammation and infections
  5. Ulceration
  6. Disease conditions
  7. Neoplasms
    a. Malignant
      (1) Basal cell carcinoma
        (a) Most common skin cancer
        (b) Nodular with ulcerated center or crusted, dermatitis-like

  (2) Squamous cell carcinoma
   (a) Begins as red papule
   (b) Progresses to area that ulcerates, then crusts
   (c) Invades underlying tissue
  (3) Malignant melanoma
   (a) Changes size
   (b) Changes color (brown to black)
   (c) Changes smooth to rough
   (d) Borders become irregular.
   (e) Satellite lesions may be present.
 b. Nonmalignant nevus
  (1) Most common skin lesion
  (2) Round shape
  (3) Brown or black color
  (4) Flat or raised
  (5) With or without hair

C. General assessment
 1. Test requirements individualized according to institutional policy
 2. History and physical
 3. Laboratory tests
  a. Basic hematology and electrolyte studies
  b. Urinalysis
 4. Chest x-ray
 5. Electrocardiogram with follow-up evaluation as dictated by medical history and/or physical findings
 6. Psychological assessment

D. Operative procedure
 1. Skin biopsy and excision of lesion: excision of involved layers of tissue
 2. Purpose: relates to patient's medical diagnosis
 3. Preoperative concerns
  a. Cosmetic appearance of surgical site
  b. Possible malignancy
  c. Life expectancy and ability to raise family
 4. Intraoperative concerns
  a. Correct side verified
  b. Specimen properly prepared and labeled for pathology
 5. Procedure
  a. Excision of involved tissue to:
   (1) Depth of involvement
   (2) Clean margins
  b. Graft may be required depending on:
   (1) Size of lesion
   (2) Depth of lesion

E. Postanesthesia care phase I
 1. Skin physical examination
  a. Color
  b. Texture
  c. Temperature
  d. Moisture or dryness
  e. Turgor
  f. Aging
  g. Sensory reception
  h. Condition of:
   (1) Hair
   (2) Nails
   (3) Glands
 2. Diagnostic tests
  a. Biopsy
  b. Culture and sensitivity

   F. Postanesthesia care phase II
      1. Assess dressings.
         a. Note location and amount of drainage.
         b. Note hematoma formation.
      2. Assess circulation and sensation.
         a. Impaired circulation
         b. Sensation deficit
      3. Assess comfort level.
         a. Note location of discomfort and position for comfort.
         b. Administer prescribed medications and evaluate relief.
      4. Key educational components
         a. Depends on extent of procedure and diagnosis
         b. Wound care
            (1) Dressings
            (2) Signs and symptoms of infection
         c. Impaired circulation or sensation
         d. Medications
            (1) Analgesics
            (2) Antibiotics
         e. Activity limitations or restrictions
      5. Provide instructions.
         a. Written
         b. Verbal
         c. Assess and ensure patient, family, and responsible accompanying adult understanding.
      6. Psychosocial concerns
         a. Cosmetic appearance of surgical site and possible skin graft
         b. Possible malignancy
         c. Depression
            (1) Change in self-image
            (2) Possible negative reaction from spouse and family
            (3) Possible distancing of friends who "don't know what to say"
            (4) Life expectancy and ability to raise family
         d. Ability to resume normal activity and work
      7. Complications
         a. Hematoma
         b. Wound infection
XIV. MINIMALLY INVASIVE SURGERY
    A. Overview
      1. Definitions
         a. Endoscopy—visual examination with an endoscope of interior of a:
            (1) Body cavity
            (2) Hollow organ
            (3) Structure
         b. Endoscope—instrument designed for examination with an optical system in a tubular structure and named for anatomic area it is designed to visualize
         c. Minimally invasive surgery—a variety of surgical modalities, including:
            (1) Endoscopy
            (2) Video technology
            (3) Energies
            (4) Combination of these technologies, used during least disruptive surgical interventions
      2. Types of endoscopic procedures
         a. Through natural orifice
            (1) Mouth
            (2) Anus

        (3) Cervix

        (4) Urethra

    b. Through small skin incision and/or trocar puncture through:

        (1) Joint space

        (2) Abdominal wall

  3. Advantages

    a. Shorter postoperative stay

    b. Decreased postoperative pain

    c. Small incisions enable faster healing.

    d. Decreased infection rate

    e. Shorter rehabilitation time

    f. Quicker return to activities of daily living

  4. Disadvantages

    a. May take longer than open procedures

    b. Longer procedures mean longer exposure to anesthesia.

    c. May be more expensive than open procedures

B. Technology

  1. Endoscopes

    a. Rigid scope

        (1) Hollow tube that permits viewing in a forward direction only

    b. Flexible scope

        (1) Hollow tube that contours the lensed tip into and around anatomic curvatures to permit visualization of all surfaces of the wall of a hollow structure

  2. Laparoscopy equipment (Figure 36-9)

    a. Veress needle or other pneumoperitoneal needles

        (1) Used to penetrate abdomen

        (2) Has outer sharp tip to penetrate abdomen and inner blunt tip to protect underlying tissue

    b. CO_2 insufflator

        (1) Machine that delivers metered flow of CO_2 into peritoneal cavity through disposable tubing connected to needle

        (2) Creates a pneumoperitoneum before laparoscope inserted through abdominal wall

        (3) Pneumoperitoneum expands abdomen and allows for visualization of organs and structures within peritoneal cavity.

    c. Trocar and cannula

        (1) Sharp inner obturator penetrates abdomen.

        (2) Cannula inserted via open laparoscopy technique

        (3) Trocar has valve to maintain pneumoperitoneum.

    d. Laparoscope

        (1) Consists of lenses and channels for fiberoptics and viewing

        (2) Available in various angles for viewing

           (a) Straight ahead

           (b) Around intra-abdominal tissue

        (3) Position maintained by assistant or scope holder

    e. Light source

        (1) Provides illumination through fiberoptic cables to laparoscope

    f. Camera and video

        (1) Permit real-time video imaging

        (2) Videocassette recorder can document procedure.

    g. Instruments

        (1) Disposable or reusable

        (2) Classification

           (a) Grasping

           (b) Retracting

           (c) Cutting

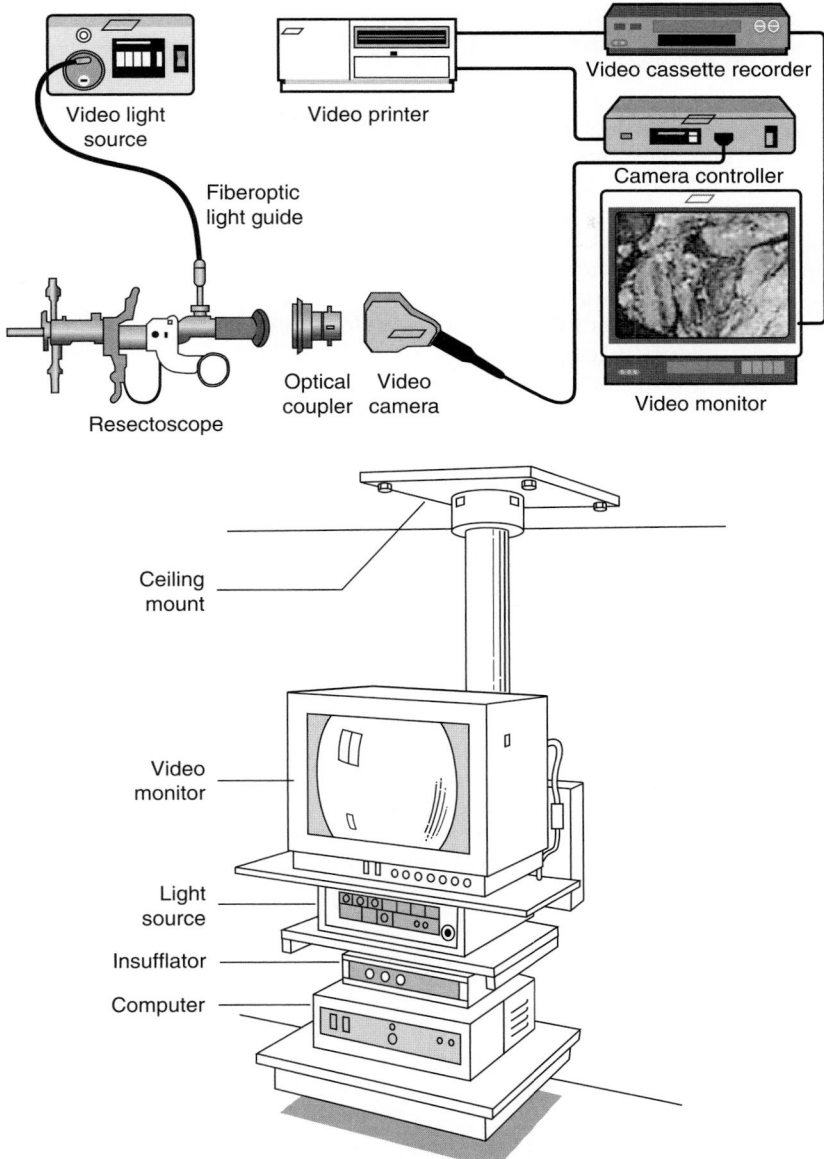

FIGURE 36-9 ■ Endoscopic machinery. Two examples of video system setups. (From Phillips NF: *Berry & Kohn's operating room technique,* ed 11, St Louis, 2007, Mosby.)

       (3) Insulated for use with electrocautery devices
       (4) Nonreflective for use with lasers
  h. Devices being developed for laparoscopy visualization without risk of pneumoperitoneum
       (1) Slings, wires, T-shaped, L-shaped, or fan-shaped devices
       (2) Require additional puncture sites for retractors.
       (3) Enable use of ordinary surgical instruments.
  i. Staples and clips
       (1) Purpose
         (a) Ligate vessels.
         (b) Close abdominal structures with lumens.
         (c) Approximate tissue

      (2) Forms of clips
        (a) Occlusive
        (b) Tacking
      (3) Staples pushed into tissue and closed
      (4) Advantages
        (a) Save time
        (b) Less difficult than laparoscopic knot tying
   j. Resources from Association of periOperative Registered Nurses (AORN) and Society of Gastroenterology Nurses and Associates (SGNA)
      (1) Teaching videos for endoscopic surgery
        (a) Equipment
          (i) Handling
          (ii) Cleaning
          (iii) Care of equipment
      (2) Published information: recommended practices for endoscopic minimally invasive surgery
        (a) Practices that reduce risk of injuries and complications
        (b) Endoscopic instruments and equipment performance and safety criteria

3. Electrosurgical unit (ESU) commonly called Bovie
   a. Adapted for use in laparoscopic procedures
   b. Modes
      (1) Monopolar
        (a) Grounding pad placement
          (i) On same side or close to surgical site
          (ii) Over muscle mass
          (iii) Avoid
            [a] Bony prominences
            [b] Metal implant areas
            [c] Hairy areas
            [d] Pooled prep solution areas
      (2) Bipolar
   c. Action
      (1) Coagulate
      (2) Cut
   d. Risk of "current" leakage

4. Plane expander
   a. Balloon device inserted between tissue layers
   b. Expanded with saline to separate and bluntly open preperitoneal plane of dissection
   c. Balloon then deflated and withdrawn as space then insufflated

5. Laser
   a. Acronym for light amplification by stimulated emission of radiation
   b. Laser-tissue interaction
      (1) Reflection
      (2) Scattering
      (3) Transmission
      (4) Absorption
   c. Laser action
      (1) Cuts
      (2) Vaporizes
      (3) Coagulates
   d. Types
      (1) Argon laser—used on cutaneous lesions in:
        (a) GI procedures
        (b) Ophthalmology
        (c) Otolaryngology

      (d) Gynecology

      (e) Urology

      (f) Neurosurgery

      (g) Dermatology

    (2) CO_2 laser—used primarily in:

      (a) Otolaryngology

      (b) Gynecology

      (c) Plastic surgery

      (d) Dermatology

      (e) Neurosurgery

      (f) Orthopedic surgery

      (g) Cardiovascular surgery

      (h) General surgery

    (3) Excimer laser—used in:

      (a) Ophthalmology

      (b) Peripheral and coronary angioplasty

      (c) Orthopedics

      (d) Neurosurgery

    (4) Diode laser—used in:

      (a) Ophthalmology

      (b) Pain management

    (5) Free electron laser—used to:

      (a) Fragment calculi

      (b) Precisely cut tissue

    (6) Holmium: Yttrium-aluminum-garnet (YAG) laser—used in orthopedics

    (7) Krypton laser—used in ophthalmology

    (8) Neodymium: YAG laser—used in:

      (a) Rhinolaryngology

      (b) Urology

      (c) Gynecology

      (d) Neurosurgery

      (e) Orthopedics

      (f) Ophthalmology

      (g) Thoracic surgery

      (h) General surgery

    (9) Potassium triphosphate laser—used in all surgical specialties for good cutting properties

   (10) Ruby laser—used to eradicate:

      (a) Port wine stain lesions

      (b) Tattoos

   (11) Tunable dye laser—used for photodynamic therapy

e. Laser safety

    (1) Regulatory controls of Department of Health and Human Services

      (a) National Center for Devices and Radiological Health: the regulatory section of the Food and Drug Administration in the Department.

      (b) American National Standards Institute provides for:

        (i) Laser safety officer

        (ii) Education of users

        (iii) Protective measures

        (iv) Management of accidents

      (c) Occupational Safety and Health Administration

      (d) AORN

      (e) State and local agencies

      (f) Facility policy and procedures include but not limited to:

        (i) Credentialing and clinical practice privileges of medical staff

(ii) Initial and ongoing educational laser use and safety programs for perioperative personnel

(iii) Continuous quality improvement

(iv) Documentation

(2) Protective measures

(a) Eye safety measures

(i) Protective eyewear of appropriate optical density for anyone entering area

(ii) Protection (eyewear or moist gauze pads) for patient's eyes

(b) Environmental controls

(i) Mark laser-use area with laser safety symbol.

(ii) Limit traffic.

(iii) Cover glass windows.

(iv) Leave laser key with authorized personnel, not with laser.

(c) Fire safety

(i) Sources of ignition

[a] Surgical drapes

[b] Anesthesia tubing

[c] Surgical sponges

(ii) Contributors to flammability

[a] Oxygen

[b] Anesthetic gases

[c] Vapors from alcohol-based preparation solutions

(iii) Safety measures

[a] Use special drapes and endotracheal tubes.

[b] Keep sponges wet.

[c] Keep oxygen concentrations low.

[d] Prevent preparation solutions from pooling.

[e] Locate laser foot pedal for safe activation by surgeon.

[f] Laser plume

[1] Smoke produced by laser may contain particles of:

[i] Tissue

[ii] Toxins

[iii] Steam

[2] Smoke evacuators remove smoke and particles.

[3] High-filtration masks filter plume not captured by evacuator.

f. Advantages of laser surgery

(1) Precise control for accurate tissue:

(a) Incision

(b) Excision

(c) Ablation

(2) Access to areas inaccessible to other surgical instruments through minimally invasive techniques

(3) Unobstructed view of surgical site

(4) Minimal handling of and trauma to tissues

(5) Dry, bloodless surgical field

(6) Minimal thermal effect on surrounding tissue

(7) Reduced risk of contamination or infection

(8) Prompt healing with minimal postoperative:

(a) Edema

(b) Sloughing of tissue

(c) Pain

(d) Scarring

(9) Reduced operating time

g. Disadvantages of laser surgery

(1) High program start-up expenses

(2) Disposable versus reusable supplies and impact on patient care

(3) Increased medical liability; need for credentialing medical practitioners, and need for continuing education to maintain staff competence
6. Ultrasound
   a. Sound waves are mechanical energy.
   b. Used to remove or reduce tumors in highly vascular, delicate tissue
      (1) Ultrasonic aspirator fragments, irrigates, and aspirates tissue.
      (2) Harmonic scalpel cuts and coagulates.
   c. Used in open or laparoscopic procedures
7. Robotics and telemedicine
   a. Combination of mechanical manipulators and a computer
      (1) Computer controls complex movements of joints and arms of manipulators (da Vinci Robot—surgeon sits at console away from patient).
      (2) Surgeon verbally controls other computer-generated information during surgical procedure.
         (a) Can see diagnostic reports
         (b) Operative report generated by electronic media
      (3) Surgeon sits at console to command verbally multiple robotic arms while many miles away.
   b. Virtual reality training for surgeons
      (1) Surgeon practices procedure without touching real patient.
      (2) Allows for evaluation of surgeon's skill and dexterity
C. Perioperative and perianesthesia issues
   1. Preoperative considerations
      a. Patient selection
         (1) Not all patients appropriate candidates for laparoscopic procedures
         (2) Relative contraindications
            (a) Prior abdominal or pelvic surgery
            (b) Previous peritonitis or pelvic fibrosis
            (c) Obesity
            (d) Umbilical abnormality
            (e) Abdominal or iliac artery aneurysm
            (f) Severe pulmonary disease
            (g) Acute and chronic inflammation
            (h) Uncontrolled coagulopathy
            (i) Pregnancy
         (3) Absolute contraindications
            (a) Hypovolemic shock
            (b) Large pelvic or abdominal mass
            (c) Severe cardiac decompensation
            (d) Congestive heart failure
            (e) Increased intracranial pressure
            (f) Ventricular or peritoneal shunts
      b. Patient education
         (1) Usual preparatory activities
         (2) Method depends on patient's ability and readiness to learn.
         (3) Patients and families tend to trivialize minimally invasive and ambulatory procedures.
         (4) Prepare patients, family, and responsible accompanying adults for:
            (a) Nature of procedure
            (b) Potential complications
            (c) Aftercare required
   2. Intraoperative considerations
      a. Efficient and accessible room layout
      b. Video monitors on either side of patient or at foot of operating room table
      c. Insufflation equipment and ESU or laser easily accessible and observable by surgical team

3. Anesthesia considerations
  a. Types of anesthesia
    (1) Local
      (a) For brief, simple procedures
      (b) Injection of local anesthetic with epinephrine at each trocar site
    (2) Monitored anesthesia care
      (a) In conjunction with local anesthetic
      (b) Advantages
        (i) Avoids general anesthesia risks
        (ii) Less postoperative nausea and vomiting
        (iii) Rapid postoperative recovery
      (c) Disadvantages
        (i) Intraoperative anxiety
        (ii) Respiratory compromise: shoulder and abdominal pain from insufflation
    (3) Epidural
      (a) Used in abdominal procedures
        (i) Viable alternative in selected cases to avoid risks of general anesthesia
      (b) Appropriate for procedures on extremities
    (4) General anesthesia
      (a) Most common technique
      (b) Endotracheal intubation
        (i) Decreases risk of regurgitation and aspiration
        (ii) Allows control of ventilation to compensate for compromised intraoperative pulmonary status
      (c) Gastric considerations
        (i) NPO status confirmed
        (ii) Administration of metoclopramide or histamine receptor antagonists (H_2 blockers) preoperatively
        (iii) Placement of NG tube to decrease risk of injury to stomach
      (d) Placement of catheter (unless patient has voided preoperatively) to reduce risk of injury to bladder
      (e) Goals
        (i) Maintain end-tidal CO_2 <40 mm Hg.
        (ii) Maintain oxygen saturation at least 93%.
  b. Physiological effects of pneumoperitoneum
    (1) Increased pressure in abdominal cavity
      (a) Causes circulatory impairment by decreasing venous return
      (b) Decreases central venous pressure, which is managed with fluids
      (c) Can lead to acute pulmonary edema in patients with cardiac compromise
    (2) CO_2 absorbed from abdomen into circulation
      (a) Leads to hypercarbia and dysrhythmias
      (b) Tidal volume must be increased to compensate.
    (3) Increased tidal volume results in:
      (a) Increased wedge pressures
      (b) Decreased stroke volume
      (c) Decreased cardiac output
    (4) Cardiovascular collapse can occur from:
      (a) CO_2 embolus
      (b) Vagal effects of manipulation of abdominal organs
    (5) Pulmonary effects
      (a) Atelectasis
      (b) Decreased functional residual capacity
      (c) High peak airway pressures

        (6) Renal effects
           (a) Renal cortical perfusion diminished with pressure of 15 mm Hg, resulting in oliguria
           (b) Perfusion rapidly restored when pressure released
           (c) Urinary output may not promptly return because of abdominal compartment syndrome.

4. Complications of endoscopy

    a. Perforation of major organ
        (1) Cause
           (a) Sharp trocars and rigid scopes
           (b) Trendelenburg position shifts intra-abdominal anatomy, causing elevation of major organs of lower abdomen.
        (2) Treatment
           (a) Minor injury controlled with suturing or staples
           (b) Major injury requires suturing, clips, or open repair.
           (c) Thorough irrigation
           (d) Postoperative antibiotics

    b. Bleeding
        (1) Cause
           (a) Perforation of vessel by sharp object
           (b) From biopsy site, pedicle of polyp, or other area where tissue cut
           (c) From dislodged endoscopic sutures or clips
        (2) Signs and symptoms
           (a) Blood apparent at site
           (b) Decrease in BP
           (c) Tachycardia
           (d) Pallor
        (3) Treatment
           (a) Minor vascular injury controlled with pressure
           (b) Major vascular injury requires clips, suturing, or open vascular repair.

    c. Thermal injury
        (1) Cause
           (a) ESU burns
           (b) Laser injury
         (2) Signs and symptoms
           (a) Not always readily apparent until 2 to 3 days postoperatively
              (i)   Abdominal pain
              (ii) Nausea
              (iii) Fever
           (b) Slowed healing process
        (3) Treatment
           (a) Antiemetics
           (b) Antibiotics

    d. Hypothermia
        (1) Cause
           (a) CO_2 gas colder than body temperature
           (b) Exposed skin
           (c) Cold infusion fluids
        (2) Signs and symptoms
           (a) Decreased temperature
           (b) Altered effects of drugs
           (c) Increased incidence of hypothermic coagulopathy
        (3) Treatment
           (a) Forced air warming blankets/gowns
           (b) Warmed IV fluids

    e. Electrical Considerations
        (1) Cause
           (a) Improperly grounded electrical equipment

        (b) Unsuspected current leaks
           (i)   Insulation failure
           (ii) Direct coupling
           (iii) Capacitive coupling
    (2) Signs and symptoms
        (a) Not always readily apparent until 2 to 3 days postoperatively
           (i)   Abdominal pain
           (ii) Nausea
           (iii) Fever
        (b) Slowed healing process
    (3) Treatment
        (a) Antiemetics
        (b) Antibiotics

f. Complications related to pneumoperitoneum
    (1) Pneumothorax and pneumomediastinum
        (a) Cause
           (i)   Air accumulates in pleural space/mediastinal space.
        (b) Signs and symptoms
           (i)   Unilateral breath sounds
           (ii) Confirmed by chest x-ray
        (c) Treatment
           (i)   Decompress pneumoperitoneum.
           (ii) Terminate procedure.
           (iii) Reverse muscle relaxants.
           (iv) Ventilate with oxygen.
           (v) Needle thoracostomy or chest tube insertion
    (2) Subcutaneous emphysema
        (a) Cause
           (i)   Improper positioning of Veress needle
           (ii) In conjunction with pneumothorax, pneumomediastinum, or both
           (iii) Weak areas in diaphragm allow CO_2 to leak through and enter mediastinum.
        (b) Signs and symptoms
           (i)   Increase in end-tidal CO_2
           (ii) Cannot be lowered by:
               [a] Increasing tidal volume
               [b] Increasing rate of ventilation
           (iii) Crepitus upon palpation of head, neck, and chest
           (iv) Facial and conjunctival subcutaneous emphysema
        (c) Treatment
           (i)   Observe for compromised airway.
    (3) Gastric reflux
        (a) Cause
           (i)   Increased risk with history of:
               [a] Obesity
               [b] Hiatal hernia
               [c] Gastric outlet obstruction
           (ii) Increased abdominal pressure associated with pneumoperitoneum
        (b) Signs and symptoms
           (i)   Reflux esophagitis
           (ii)   Heartburn
           (iii)   Belching
           (iv)   Regurgitation
           (v)   Vomiting
           (vi)   Retrosternal or substernal chest pain
           (vii) Hiccups
           (viii) Mild or occult bleeding and mild anemia

             (ix)   Dysphagia
             (x)   Pneumonitis caused by aspiration
         (c) Treatment
             (i)   NG or orogastric tube insertion
             (ii)   Stomach decompression
                 [a] Decreases risk of visceral puncture
                 [b] Improves visualization
                 [c] Decreases risk of aspiration
                 [d] Decreases risk of postoperative nausea and vomiting
             (iii) Pharmacological interventions
                 [a] Metoclopramide, 10 mg IV, preoperatively to promote gastric emptying
                 [b] Metoclopramide, 10 mg IV, at end of procedure to decrease potential for nausea and vomiting
     (4) CO_2 embolus
        (a) Cause
           (i)   Large amount of CO_2 enters central venous circulation through opening in venous channels.
        (b) Signs and symptoms
           (i)   Sudden decrease in BP
           (ii)   Cardiac dysrhythmias
           (iii) Heart murmur
           (iv) Cyanosis
           (v)   Pulmonary edema
           (vi) Increase in end-tidal CO_2
        (c) Treatment
           (i)   Deflate peritoneum immediately.
           (ii)   Place patient in left lateral decubitus position.
           (iii) Position head below level of right atrium.
           (iv) Establish IV access to central circulation to aspirate gas from heart.
     (5) Abdominal wall hematoma
        (a) Cause
           (i)   Injury
        (b) Signs and symptoms
           (i)   Depends on size
           (ii)   Pressure on adjacent organs or vessels
        (c) Treatment
           (i)   Evacuation
     (6) Cardiovascular collapse
        (a) Possible causes
           (i)   Hemorrhage
           (ii)   Pulmonary embolus
           (iii) Myocardial infarction
5. Postoperative considerations
  a. Immediate postoperative assessment (see Chapter 50)
  b. Postoperative care associated with surgical specialties
  c. Postoperative complications
    (1) Observe for any signs and symptoms as noted previously.
    (2) Notify anesthesiologist and surgeon.
    (3) Treat accordingly.
  d. Patient and family teaching
    (1) Regarding signs and symptoms of potential complications
    (2) Specific to procedure
  e. Minimally invasive surgery decreases length of stay. Patients are:
    (1) Ambulatory
    (2) Fast-track
    (3) Extended observation

BIBLIOGRAPHY

1. Association of periOperative Registered Nurses: *Standards, recommended practices and guidelines*, Denver, 2008, Association of periOperative Registered Nurses.
2. Baker CL, Whaley AL: *Clinical sports medicine*, Philadelphia, 2004, Elsevier.
3. Burden N, DeFazio Quinn DM, O'Brien D, et al, eds: *Ambulatory surgical nursing*, ed 2, Philadelphia, 2000, WB Saunders.
4. Carlson MA, Frantzides CT: Complications and results of primary minimally invasive antireflux procedures: A review of 10,735 reported cases. *J Am Coll Surg* 193:428–439, 2001.
5. D'Agostino RB, Vascan RS, Pancina MJ, et al: General cardiovascular risk profile for use in primary care. *Circulation* 117(6): 736–753, 2008.
6. Earnhart SW: What's the best mix of procedures for ASC? *OR Manager* 18:26–27, 2002.
7. Ellis H, Watson CW: *Surgery: Clinical cases uncovered*, St Louis, 2008, Wiley-Blackwell Publishers.
8. Fazio VW, Church, JM, Delaney CP: *Current therapy in colon and rectal surgery*. Philadelphia, 2005, Elsevier Mosby.
9. Fischer CP, Castaneda A, Moore F: Laparoscopic appendectomy: Indications and controversies. *Semin Laparosc Surg* 9:32–39, 2002.
10. Fleisher LA, Yee K, Lillemoe KD, et al: Is outpatient laparoscopic cholecystectomy safe and cost-effective? A model to study transition of care. *Anesthesiology* 90:1746–1755, 1999.
11. Frantzides CT, Carlson MA: *Atlas of minimally invasive surgery*, Philadelphia, 2006, Saunders.
12. Hammond DS: *Atlas of breast surgery*, Philadelphia, 2009, Elsevier.
13. Jones SB, Jones DB: Surgical aspects and future developments of laparoscopy. *Anesthesiol Clin N Am* 19:107–124, 2001.
14. Ignatavicius DD, Workman M, Langue L: *Medical-surgical nursing*, ed 6, Philadelphia, 2008, Saunders.
15. Joshi GP: Complications of laparoscopy. *Anesthesiol Clin N Am* 19:89–105, 2001.
16. Karp SJ, Morris JPG: *Blueprints surgery*, ed 4, Baltimore, 2007, Lippincott Williams & Wilkins.
17. Lawrence PF: *Essentials of general surgery*, ed 4, Philadelphia, 2006, Lippincott Williams & Wilkins.
18. Marcucci C, Cohen NA, Metro DG, et al: *Avoiding common anesthesia errors*, Philadelphia, 2008, Lippincott Williams Wilkins.
19. McCance KL, Huether SE: *Pathophysiology: The biologic basis for disease in adults and children*, ed 6, St Louis, 2010, Mosby.
20. McLaughlin MR, Hail RN, Rodts GE: *Atlas of cervical spine surgery*, Philadelphia, 2008, Elsevier Saunders.
21. Miller MD, Chhabra AB, Hurwitz SR, et al, eds: *Orthopaedic surgical approaches*, Philadelphia, 2008, Saunders Elsevier.
22. Phillips N: *Berry & Kohn's operating room technique*, ed 11, St Louis, 2007, Mosby.
23. Rothrock JC, ed: *Alexander's care of the patient in surgery*, ed 13, St Louis, 2007, Mosby.
24. Smith I: Anesthesia for laparoscopy with emphasis on outpatient laparoscopy. *Anesthesiol Clin N Am* 19:21–41, 2001.
25. Swearingen PL, Ross DG, eds: *Manual of medical-surgical nursing care: Nursing interventions and collaborative management*, ed 6, St Louis, 2006, Mosby.
26. Talamini MA: *Advanced therapy in minimally invasive surgery*, Ontario, Canada, 2006, M C Decker Inc.
27. Wetter PA, Kavic MS, Levinson CJ, et al: *Prevention and management of laparoendoscopic surgical complications*, ed 2, Miami, 2005, Society of Laparoendoscopic Surgeons.

Renal/Genitourinary Care

KIM A. NOBLE

Acknowledgement: I thank Gratia M. Nagle for her original contributions in preparing this chapter.

OBJECTIVES

At the conclusion of this chapter, the reader will be able to:

1. Identify the structure and function of the genitourinary system.
2. Describe the pathophysiological implications of each urological disorder reviewed.
3. Discuss indications for common urological surgical procedures.
4. Describe physical assessment principles as they relate to the nursing process.
5. Identify the specific perianesthesia considerations in patient care by incorporating biological, psychological, social, and cultural assessment of the patient.

I. GENITOURINARY SYSTEM ANATOMY
  A. Genitourinary system
     1. Includes:
        a. Two adrenal glands
        b. Two kidneys
        c. Two ureters
        d. One urinary bladder
        e. A single urethra
        f. Genital organs (Figure 37-1)
     2. Most important structure is the nephron.
        a. Lies within the kidney (Figure 37-2)
        b. Nephron responsible for:
           (1) Removing wastes from the blood
           (2) Regulating fluid and electrolyte content
           (3) Contributing to urine formation and homeostasis (Figure 37-3)
  B. Adrenal gland(s)
     1. Cap each kidney superiorly
        a. Right is triangular, between liver and vena cava.
        b. Left is rounded and crescent shaped, close to aorta, and partially covered by pancreas.
     2. Composed of two layers
        a. Outer adrenal cortex
           (1) Glandular portion of the adrenal gland
           (2) Secretes two hormones via negative feedback control for release
              (a) Glucocorticoid: cortisol
                 (i) Released during times of physical or psychological stress
                 (ii) Stimulates hepatic glucose production, increases fat and protein catabolism, leading to a significant increase in serum glucose
                 (iii) Direct anti-inflammatory action

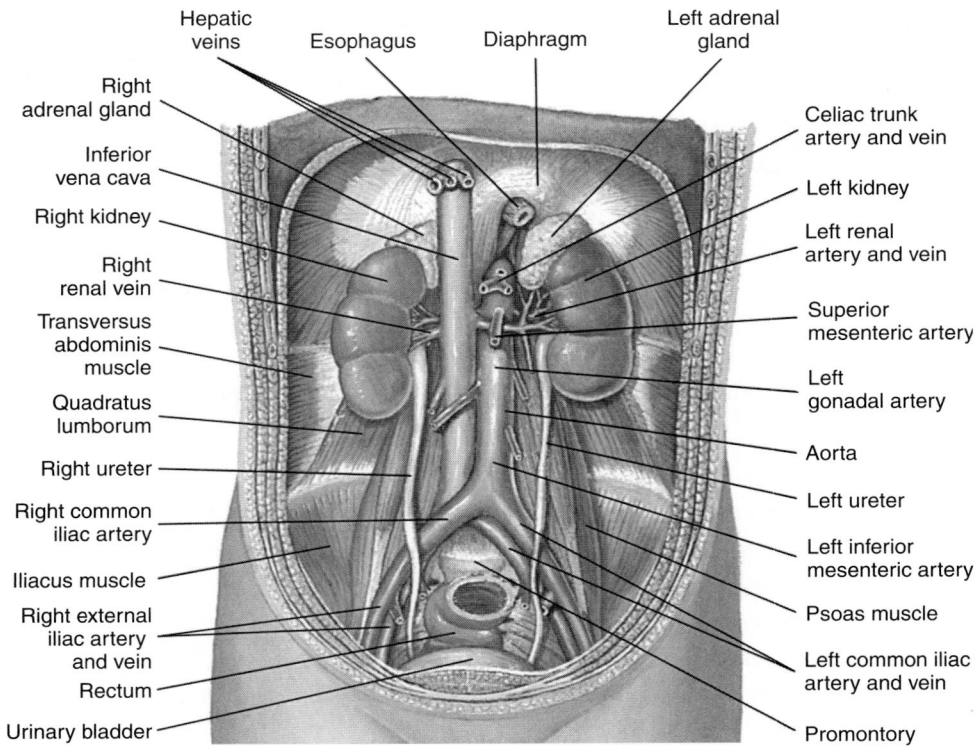

FIGURE 37-1 ■ Location of urinary system organs. (From Rothrock JC: *Alexander's care of the patient in surgery*, ed 12, St Louis, 2003, Mosby.)

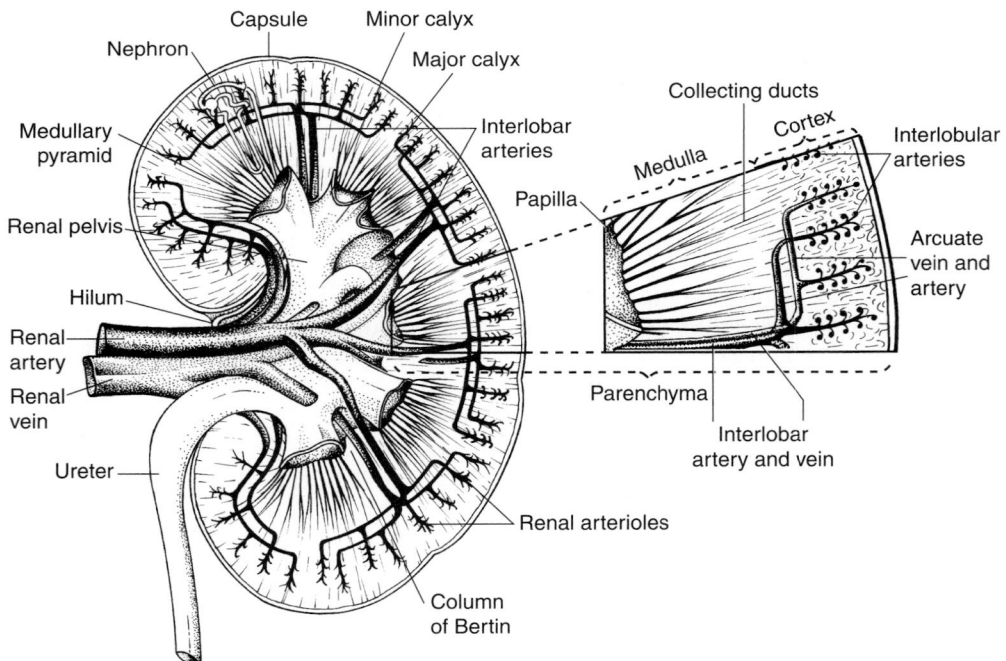

FIGURE 37-2 ■ Bisection of the kidney showing major structures of the kidney. (From Ignatavicius DD, Workman ML, eds: *Medical-surgical nursing: Critical thinking for collaborative care*, ed 4, Philadelphia, 2002, WB Saunders.)

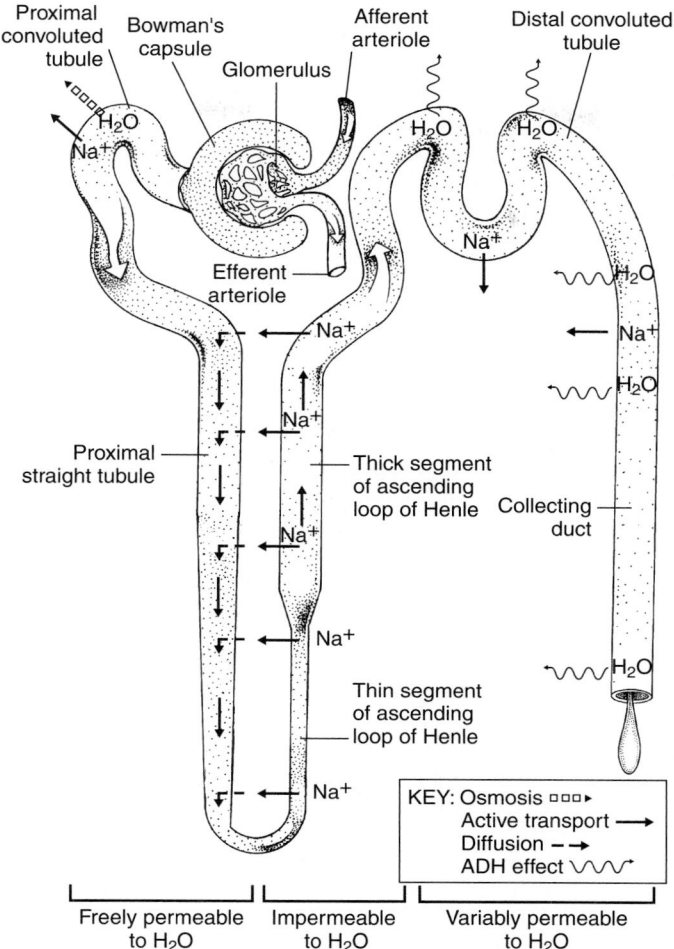

FIGURE 37-3 ■ Sodium and water reabsorption by the tubules of a cortical nephron. (From Ignatavicius DD, Workman ML, eds: *Medical-surgical nursing: Critical thinking for collaborative care,* ed 4, Philadelphia, 2002, WB Saunders.)

       (b) Mineralocorticoid: aldosterone
           (i)   Release stimulated by renin-angiotensin-aldosterone mechanism and ↑ serum potassium (K^+)
           (ii) Promotes sodium (Na^+) reabsorption and excretion of K^+ in the distal renal tubule
           (iii) Aldosterone is the primary mechanism for K^+ excretion.
    b. Inner adrenal medulla
      (1) Portion of adrenal gland that resembles nervous tissue
      (2) Releases two hormones from stimulation by the sympathetic nervous system (SNS)
        (a) Epinephrine and norepinephrine
           (i)   Neurotransmitters used by the SNS
           (ii) Prolongs fight-or-flight response by ↑ heart rate and blood pressure (BP)
3. Arterial blood supply
    a. Enters via the renal hilum, the medial C-shaped indentation on each kidney
    b. Aorta → renal (and suprarenal) artery → inferior phrenic artery

4. Venous blood supply

   a. Right has short vein that empties into inferior vena cava.

   b. Left terminates in left renal vein.

5. Lymphatics

   a. Accompany suprarenal vein

   b. Drain into lumbar lymph nodes

6. Adrenal disease often directly affects renal function.

   a. Adrenal insufficiency

   b. Cushing's disease

   c. Pheochromocytoma

   d. Adenoma

   e. Carcinoma

C. Kidney

   1. Comprises hilum; parenchyma containing medulla, cortex, calices, and nephrons; renal pelvis.

     a. Hilum

       (1) Concave, on medial aspect of kidney

       (2) Pelvis, artery, vein, nerves, and lymphatics enter and exit parenchyma.

     b. Parenchyma is functional tissue of kidney.

       (1) Renal medulla

         (a) Five to 18 cone-shaped pyramids that drain into 4 to 13 minor calices

         (b) Base of pyramids face hilum of kidney, and apices face renal pelvis.

       (2) Renal cortex

         (a) Extends inward between two pyramids

         (b) Forms renal columns that contain nephrons

       (3) Calices

         (a) Minor calices drain into two or three major calices.

         (b) Major calices join in center of medulla, forming and opening directly into renal pelvis.

       (4) Nephron(s)

         (a) Approximately 1.2 million nephrons comprise functional units of each kidney.

         (b) Each nephron contains:

           (i) Glomerulus

             [a] Vascular segment of proximal nephron enclosed in Bowman's capsule

             [b] Tuft of capillaries responsible for blood filtration

             [c] Blood enters via afferent arterioles, to glomerular capillary bed and exits to efferent arterioles to peritubular capillaries.

             [d] Arteriole smooth muscle allows individual nephron to autoregulate blood flow by dilating or constricting arteriole walls.

           (ii) Bowman's capsule (glomerular capsule)

             [a] Tubular portion of nephron begins in Bowman's capsule.

             [b] Interface between tubular epithelium and glomerular endothelium makes up the filtration barrier through which filtrate passes.

             [c] Filtration barrier is permeable to water and solutes (crystalloids) and impermeable to large molecules and plasma proteins.

           (iii) Proximal tubule

             [a] Site of 65% of reabsorption of filtered solutes and water

             [b] Primary site of secretion of nonfiltered substances

           (iv) Loop of Henle

             [a] Reabsorbs 25% of glomerular filtrate

             [b] Mechanisms for Na^+ and water reabsorption are site dependent.

        [c] Divided into three segments
          [1] Descending limb (filtrate descends into renal medulla and water is removed from filtrate)
          [2] Thin ascending limb (filtrate again moves toward renal cortex; Na^+ reabsorbed)
          [3] Thick ascending limb (actively reabsorbs additional Na^+, K^+, and chloride [C])
        [d] Important function for the control of the urine concentration and conservation; such as seen in dehydration and hemorrhage
      (v) Distal tubule
        [a] Contains distal convoluted tubule and collecting ducts
        [b] Site of aldosterone action; primary mechanism for K^+ secretion
        [c] Site for acid-base regulation: hydrogen ion (H^+) secretion and bicarbonate (HCO_3^-) reabsorption
        [d] Site of action of antidiuretic hormone (ADH) leading to water reabsorption
        [e] Collecting ducts empty into minor calyx → major calyx.
    (5) Renal pelvis
      (a) May be intrarenal and extrarenal
      (b) Cone-shaped structure extending from center of medulla, exiting through the hilum, and curving downward to form the ureters
      (c) Left lies at level of first or second lumbar vertebra.
      (d) Right is lower than left because of the presence of the liver.

2. Retroperitoneal location
  a. Parallel to vertebrae and psoas muscle
  b. Covered with a thin fibrous capsule (Gerota's fascia or fascia renalis) and perirenal fat
    (1) Length: 12 to 14 cm
    (2) Width: 5 to 7 cm
    (3) Thickness: 3 cm
    (4) Weight: 150 g
3. One kidney can provide adequate renal function.
4. Autonomic innervation with intraperitoneal organs accounts for gastrointestinal symptoms that accompany genitourinary disease, including nausea, vomiting, and pain.
5. Arterial blood supply
  a. End arteries (absence of collateral connections)
  b. Renal artery
    (1) Arises from abdominal aorta and enters hilum between pelvis and renal vein
    (2) Receives 25% of cardiac output
    (3) Divides into anterior and posterior branches
    (4) Anterior supplies upper and lower poles and anterior surface.
    (5) Posterior supplies posterior surface.
    (6) Divides again into interlobar arteries to glomeruli
6. Venous blood supply
  a. Renal veins paired with renal arteries
  b. Left renal vein three times longer than right
  c. Empties into inferior vena cava
7. Accessory renal vessels
  a. Common, although renal artery and vein usually sole blood supply
  b. May compress ureter to cause hydronephrosis
8. Lymphatics drain into lumbar lymph nodes.
9. Nerve supply
  a. Autonomic nervous innervation: sympathetic and parasympathetic branches
  b. Supplied by splanchnic nerves

D. Ureter(s): paired cylindrical fibromuscular tubes that follow smooth S curve
   1. Lies on psoas muscle, passes medial to sacroiliac joints and lateral near ischial spines
   2. Penetrates base of bladder medially at oblique angle
      a. Posteroinferior to bladder dome
      b. Distance apart: 5 cm
   3. Ureteral narrowing
      a. At ureteropelvic junction
      b. As it crosses over external iliac vessels
      c. As it passes through bladder wall
   4. Averages 26 to 30 cm long and 1 to 6 mm wide in adult
   5. Peristaltic action of small muscle fibers in middle layer of ureter transports urine from renal pelvis to urinary bladder.
   6. Tunneling of the ureter prevents reflux (backflow) of urine from bladder to kidney upon micturition.
E. Bladder
   1. Hollow, muscular, pelvic organ
      a. Inner lining composed of transitional epithelium
      b. Submucosal layer composed of lamina propria (fibroelastic connective tissue) and contains smooth muscle
      c. Muscular layer and detrusor muscle lie outside submucosal layer.
   2. Reservoir for urine
      a. Adult capacity: 350 to 700 mL
      b. Urge to urinate common at 400 to 450 mL
   3. Lies behind symphysis pubis in adult; slightly higher in child
      a. When full, rises above symphysis pubis, especially in children
      b. Easily palpated, especially when full
      c. If overdistended, may cause visible lower abdominal bulge
      d. Postponing urination strains bladder capacity and weakens musculature.
   4. Ureteral orifices are on proximal trigone at extremities of interureteric ridge.
      a. Distance apart: 2.5 cm
      b. Trigone located between ridge and bladder neck
   5. Bladder neck (internal sphincter) formed of interlaced muscle fibers of detrusor on bladder floor
      a. Muscle fibers converge.
      b. Pass distally to form smooth musculature of urethra
   6. Dome and posterior surface covered by peritoneum
   7. Arterial blood supply composed of superior, middle, inferior vesical arteries
      a. From trunk of internal iliac (hypogastric) artery
      b. From obturator and inferior gluteal arteries
      c. In females, also has branches from uterine and vaginal arteries
   8. Venous blood supply rich and empties into internal iliac (hypogastric) veins
   9. Lymphatics drain into:
      a. Vesical
      b. External and internal iliac
      c. Common iliac lymph nodes
   10. Urine storage
      a. Highly coordinated two-phased process of filling and emptying
      b. Controlled by:
         (1) Sympathetic
         (2) Parasympathetic
         (3) Central nervous system
   11. Micturition
      a. Increase in volume of urine in bladder causes slow rise in intravesical pressure.
      b. Stretch receptors in bladder wall convey afferent impulses through pelvic nerve to spinal cord.

        (1) Stimulates sympathetic efferent nerves
        (2) Impulses conveyed back to bladder through hypogastric nerves
        (3) Activates internal sphincter to maintain continence
        (4) Allows for complete bladder filling
    c. When bladder sufficiently distended, nerve impulses transmitted to brain
    d. Brainstem activates micturition.
        (1) Efferent pelvic nerve stimulates bladder to contract.
        (2) Bladder neck and urethra open.
        (3) External urethral sphincter and perineal muscles relax with opening of bladder neck.
    e. Normal micturition dependent on certain factors
        (1) Appropriate bladder sensation during filling stage
        (2) Closed bladder neck at rest
        (3) Absence of involuntary contractions
  F. Urethra
    1. Mucosal tubular structure
      a. Adult male
        (1) Length: 15 to 30 cm with "S"-shaped curve
        (2) Posterior urethra
          (a) Membranous
          (b) Prostatic
        (3) Anterior urethra
          (a) Bulbous
          (b) Penile
          (c) Glandular
        (4) Surrounded by internal and external sphincter
        (5) Curves at strong right angle where bulbous urethra joins prostatic urethra (urogenital diaphragm)
        (6) Empties by contraction of bulbocavernous muscle
      b. Adult female
        (1) Length: 4 cm and slightly curved
          (a) Lies anterior to vagina and beneath symphysis pubis
          (b) Urethral orifice (meatus) lies between clitoris and vaginal introitus (opening).
          (c) Short length common cause of cystitis and urinary tract infection
        (2) Voluntary external sphincter surrounds middle third.
        (3) Composed of submucosa of connective and elastic tissue
          (a) Filled with spongy venous spaces
          (b) Contains many periurethral glands that secrete mucus
        (4) Empties by gravity
    2. Transports urine from bladder to meatus for excretion
II. ADULT MALE ANATOMY
  A. Prostate gland
    1. Encapsulated, glandular, fibromuscular organ lying below and behind bladder; in front of the rectum
      a. Contributes to seminal fluid
      b. Muscular fibers contract during ejaculation.
      c. Transports spermatozoa to ejaculate
      d. Posterosuperior surface adjacent to vas deferens and seminal vesicles
    2. Doughnut configuration surrounds urethra for 2 to 3 cm.
      a. Walnut size
      b. Chestnut shape
    3. Contains 2.5 cm posterior urethra and prostatic urethra
    4. Supported by puboprostatic ligaments, which anchor prostate to pubic bone
    5. Ejaculatory ducts pierce prostate posteriorly and empty through verumontanum.
      a. On floor of prostatic urethra
      b. Proximal to striated external urinary sphincter

    6. Consists of five lobes or zones
      a. Zones can be distinguished both histologically and grossly.
      b. Transition zone enlarges substantially in benign prostatic hypertrophy (BPH).
      c. Peripheral zone is the origination of 90% of prostate cancers.
    7. Prostatic fluid alkaline with high fructose content
      a. Prostatic secretions account for major portion of volume of the normal ejaculate.
      b. Component of semen nourishes sperm cells
      c. Activates sperm cell motility
      d. Protects sperm from acidic vaginal secretion
    8. Blood supply
      a. Arterial blood supply primarily from branches of the hypogastric artery
      b. Venous blood supply drains into periprostatic plexus.
        (1) Connects to deep dorsal vein of penis
        (2) Connects to internal iliac (hypogastric) veins
    9. Nerve supply derived from sympathetic and parasympathetic nerve systems
    10. Lymphatics drain into lymph nodes.
      a. Internal iliac
      b. Sacral
      c. Vesical
      d. External iliac
  B. Cowper's glands (bulbourethral glands)
    1. Pea-sized glands on each side of posterior urethra
    2. Secrete mucus (component of seminal fluid) into ejaculatory ducts and out urethra during ejaculation
  C. Seminal vesicles
    1. Convoluted membranous pouches
    2. Lie under base of bladder and above prostate gland
    3. Each joins corresponding vas deferens to form ejaculatory duct.
    4. Nerve supply mainly from sympathetic system
    5. Lymphatics supply prostate gland.
  D. Spermatic cord
    1. Extends from internal inguinal ring through inguinal canal to testis bilaterally
    2. Contents of each cord
      a. Vas deferens
        (1) Firm cylindrical tubular structure
        (2) Connects epididymis with ejaculatory duct
        (3) Peristaltic contraction of thick muscular walls helps propel sperm through duct.
        (4) Capable of storing sperm cells for as long as 42 days
      b. Internal and external spermatic arteries
      c. Artery of vas (deferential artery)
      d. Venous pampiniform plexus (forms spermatic vein superiorly)
      e. Lymph vessels that empty into external iliac lymph nodes
      f. Autonomic nerves
    3. Enclosed in layers of thin fascia
    4. Serves to suspend testis
    5. Some cremaster nerve fibers penetrate cords in inguinal canal.
  E. Epididymis
    1. Comma-shaped coiled duct that is continuous with vas deferens at its lower pole
    2. Consists of:
      a. Head (upper pole)
      b. Central body
      c. Tail (lower pole)
    3. Connected to posterolateral surface of testis at upper pole
    4. Appendix often found on upper pole

     5. Efferent ductules in head carry spermatozoa from testis to vas deferens.
     6. Storage space for sperm; provides nutrients allowing for sperm maturation
     7. Sperm transported to vas for ejaculation

F. Testis
     1. Essential for male reproductive system
       a. Produces spermatozoa (spermatogenesis)
       b. Secretes testosterone
       c. Housed in scrotal sac to provide lower temperature for sperm viability
     2. Testes are two oval-shaped organs covered by thick fascial layer of tunica albuginea.
       a. Posteriorly forms mediastinum testis
       b. Fibrous septa separate testis into approximately 250 lobules.
       c. Each lobule contains one to three tightly coiled seminiferous tubules.
     3. Covered with and separated from scrotal wall by tunica vaginalis
     4. Appendix testis, similar to epididymis testis, located at upper pole
     5. Seminiferous tubules lie adjacent to interstitial Leydig's cells (essential for testosterone production).
       a. Densely packed within testes
       b. Long, convoluted, threadlike tubules converge into rete testis.
       c. Rete testis leads to epididymis.
       d. Epididymis leads to vas deferens, which converges into ejaculatory ducts.
     6. Shares common embryological origin with kidney and closely associated blood supply
       a. Internal spermatic artery originates in aorta just below renal artery.
       b. Internal spermatic artery joins deferential artery.
       c. Right spermatic vein enters vena cava just below right renal vein.
       d. Left spermatic vein empties into left renal vein.
     7. Lymphatics drain into para-aortic lymph nodes, which are connected to mediastinal nodes.

G. Scrotum
     1. Relaxation and contraction of muscular layer regulate internal temperature.
       a. Temperature generally 1°F to 2°F lower than body temperature
       b. Temperature regulation necessary for fertility
     2. Septum of connective tissue divides internal sac into two pouches.
       a. Dartos (internal septum) consists of superficial fascia and connective tissue.
       b. Median raphe is external central scrotal ridge formed by dartos.
     3. Provides support to testes
     4. Arterial blood supply from femoral, internal pudendal, and inferior epigastric arteries
     5. Veins paired with arteries
     6. Lymphatics drain into subinguinal and superficial inguinal lymph nodes.

H. Penis
     1. Organ of excretion and reproduction
       a. Glans or tip
         (1) Before circumcision, prepuce forms hood over glans (foreskin).
         (2) Prepuce may be smoothed back to expose glans and urethral meatus.
         (3) Contains nerve endings
         (4) Glans formed by distal, expanded end of bulbospongiosus muscle
       b. Shaft or body
         (1) Suspensory ligament from pubic symphysis
         (2) Ligament inserts into fascia of corpus cavernosa.
       c. Two corpus cavernosa and corpus spongiosum underlie
         (1) Corpus cavernosa run along either side of corpus spongiosum along major portion of penile shaft.
         (2) Urethra surrounded by corpus spongiosum
         (3) All contain vascular cavities.
         (4) Corpus cavernosa fills with blood during sexual arousal and produces erection.

    2. Arterial blood supply from internal pudendal arteries
      a. Deep artery of penis supplies corpus cavernosa.
      b. Dorsal artery of penis
      c. Bulbourethral artery supplies:
        (1) Corpus spongiosum
        (2) Glans
        (3) Urethra
    3. Venous blood supply
      a. Superficial dorsal vein
      b. Deep dorsal vein
      c. Drains into internal pudendal vein
    4. Lymphatic system
      a. Lymphatics from penile skin drain into deep and superficial inguinal lymph nodes.
      b. Lymphatics from glans, corpora, and urethra drain into deep inguinal external iliac lymph nodes.
  I. Organs of reproduction
    1. Prostate gland
    2. Seminal vesicles
    3. Testes
    4. Penis
III. ADULT FEMALE ANATOMY
  A. Skene's glands
    1. Open on floor of urethra inside meatus
    2. Stimulate mucus secretion during sexual arousal to lubricate vagina
    3. Inflammation may contribute to urethritis or cystitis.
  B. Bartholin's gland
    1. Small mucus gland opening on each inner aspect of labia minora within vagina (homologue of bulbourethral gland in male)
    2. Supplements lubrication during sexual intercourse
    3. Inflammation may contribute to chronic urethritis or cystitis.
  C. Arterial blood supply
    1. Inferior vesical artery
    2. Vaginal artery
    3. Internal pudendal artery
  D. Venous blood supply empties into internal pudendal veins.
  E. Lymphatic system
    1. Lymphatics from external urethra drain into subinguinal and inguinal lymph nodes.
    2. Lymphatics from deep urethra drain into internal iliac lymph nodes.
  F. External genitalia; also called vulva
    1. Mons pubis
      a. Rounded, skin-covered fat pad
      b. Located anterior to the symphysis pubis
    2. Labia majora
      a. Originate in mons pubis and run posteriorly toward anus
      b. Paired, elongated, hair-covered fatty folds
      c. Analogous with male scrotum
      d. Enclose labia minora
    3. Labia minora
      a. Smaller than labia majora
      b. Medial to labia majora
      c. Composed of skin, fat, and some erectile tissue
    4. Clitoris
      a. Covered by the clitoral hood; formed by the junction of the labia minora
      b. Contains erectile tissue
      c. Contains a rich vascular and nervous supply
      d. Enlarges via blood engorgement during sexual stimulation
      e. Analogous with male penis

G. Internal genitalia
   1. Vagina
   a. Fibromuscular tube that connects the external and internal genitalia
   b. Located behind the urinary bladder and urethra, anterior to the rectum
   c. Does not contain sensory nerve fibers
   d. Uterine cervix projects into the vagina at the superior vaginal end in recesses called the fornices.
   e. Functions of vagina
      (1) Discharge of the menses and other secretions
      (2) Organ of sexual fulfillment and reproduction
   2. Uterus
   a. Pear-shaped structure located between the bladder and the rectum
   b. Hollow, thick-walled muscular organ
   c. Functions of uterus
      (1) Container for pregnancy
      (2) Nutritional supply for pregnancy
      (3) Allows for growth of the fetus
      (4) Delivery of products of conception into the vagina
   d. Uterus can be subdivided into three anatomic parts.
      (1) Fundus
         (a) Upper portion of uterus
         (b) Site for insertion of fallopian tubes
      (2) Body of uterus
         (a) Central portion with a tapered appearance
      (3) Cervix
         (a) Inferior, constricted ending of the uterus
   e. Wall of uterus has three layers.
      (1) Perimetrium
         (a) Outer serous coating of uterus
         (b) Derived from abdominal peritoneum covering the broad ligaments
         (c) Anteriorly, perimetrium extends over bladder forming the vesicouterine pouch
         (d) Extends posteriorly to form the rectouterine pouch
         (e) Because of close proximity with bladder, bladder infections frequently associated with uterine symptoms, especially during pregnancy
      (2) Myometrium
         (a) Middle muscular layer
         (b) Forms major portion of uterine wall
         (c) Continuous with muscular layers of fallopian tubes and vagina
         (d) Extends into all the supporting ligaments with exception of the broad ligament
         (e) Muscle fibers run in a variety of directions, leading to a woven appearance.
         (f) Contraction of myometrium expels menstrual flow and products of conception during miscarriage or childbirth.
      (3) Endometrium
         (a) Innermost layer of uterus
         (b) Continuous with lining of fallopian tubes and vagina
         (c) Consists of two distinct layers that respond to hormonal stimulation
            (i) Basal layer is adjacent to the myometrium and is not sloughed during menstruation.
            (ii) Functional layer arises from basal layer and undergoes proliferative changes and is sloughed during menstruation.
         (d) Endometrial cycle can be divided into three phases:
            (i) Proliferative phase: preovulatory and characterized by growth of functional layer due to estrogen

          (ii) Secretory phase: follows ovulation, with increased vascularization and edema of the endometrium due to progesterone release

          (iii) Menstrual phase: results in sloughing of superficial layer of the endometrium

3. Fallopian tubes
   a. Bilateral, slender, cylindrical projections extending laterally from uterus toward ovary
   b. Supported by upper folds of the broad ligament
   c. Ovarian end of fallopian tube widens with fingerlike projections called fimbriae.
   d. Tube functions to pick up ovum from peritoneal cavity after ovulation.
   e. Ciliated cells and peristalsis propel ovum toward uterus.
   f. Primary site of ovum fertilization
   g. Provides drainage of tubal secretions into uterus

4. Ovaries
   a. Bilateral, flat, almond-shaped structures measuring $4 \times 2.5 \times 1.5\,cm^2$
   b. Located laterally to uterus at termination of fallopian tubes
   c. Suspended by broad ligament and ovarian ligaments bilaterally
   d. Ovarian tissue can be subdivided into four types.
      (1) Stroma is the connective tissue in which the follicles are distributed.
      (2) Interstitial cells
         (a) Estrogen-secreting cells
         (b) Analogous with interstitial cells (Leydig cells) of testes
      (3) Follicles contain female germ cells, termed ova.
      (4) Corpus luteum (yellow-body) develops after ovulation and ejection of ovum from follicle.
   e. Ovarian hormones
      (1) Secreted in a cyclic pattern under negative feedback control with the hypothalamus and anterior pituitary
      (2) There are three ovarian hormones.
         (a) Estrogen
            (i) Secreted throughout menstrual cycle
            (ii) Necessary for normal female physical maturation
            (iii) Provides for reproductive processes of ovulation, implantation of products of conception, pregnancy, parturition, and lactation
            (iv) Maintains normal structure of skin and blood vessels
            (v) Decreases rate of bone resorption
            (vi) Promotes increase in high-density lipoproteins (HDL: "good" cholesterol)
            (vii) Promotes decrease in low-density lipoproteins (LDL: "bad" cholesterol)
            (viii) Causes moderate retention of Na^+ and water
         (b) Progesterone
            (i) Secreted as a normal part of menstrual cycle
            (ii) Responsible for maintenance of pregnancy
            (iii) Initially secreted in large amounts by corpus luteum after eruption of ovum; replaced by secretion by placenta once established
            (iv) Leads to glandular development of breasts and uterine lining
            (v) Responsible for smooth muscle relaxation preventing uterine contractions during pregnancy
            (vi) Increases basal body temperature, leading to temperature spike associated with ovulation
            (vii) Responsible for many of the negative symptoms associated with pregnancy

[a] Edema
[b] Nausea
[c] Constipation
[d] Headaches
(c) Androgens
　(i)　Ovarian: 25%
　(ii)　Adrenal: 25%
　(iii)　Precursor secretion: 50%
　(iv)　Contribute to hair growth during puberty
　(v)　Can be converted to estrogens peripherally, especially in adipose tissue

IV. RENAL PHYSIOLOGY

A. Overview
1. Fluid and electrolyte balance (homeostasis) within kidney maintained through a complex interaction of hormonal systems
2. Renal functions include:
   a. Electrolyte balance
   b. Concentration of body fluid constituents
   c. Autoregulation of renal blood flow
   d. Glomerular filtration
   e. Reabsorption and secretion
   f. Red blood cell (RBC) formation
   g. Calcium formation
   h. Acid-base balance
3. Kidneys filter approximately 180 L of plasma in 25 hours.
   a. One liter becomes urine.
   b. The balance is reabsorbed.
   c. Entire plasma is filtered approximately 60 times per day.
   d. Filtration is affected by blood flowing through the kidney.
      (1) Composition
      (2) Pressure
      (3) Volume
4. Because of importance of adequate blood flow and pressure for renal function, the individual nephron is able to autoregulate blood flow by actions in Bowman's capsule.
5. Renal shutdown may quickly ensue with hypovolemia.
   a. Nephrons become unable to adequately manufacture urine as a result of decreased blood supply to the kidney.
   b. When this occurs, measures must be taken quickly to improve renal blood flow, or acute renal failure may result.

B. Renal endocrine function (hormonal interactions)
1. Renin-angiotensin-aldosterone system (RAA)
   a. Overview
      (1) RAA is major renal hormonal regulator for:
         (a) Systemic BP
         (b) Regional blood flow
         (c) Na^+ and K^+ balance
   b. Renin
      (1) Enzyme secreted by juxtaglomerular apparatus (JGA)
         (a) JGA located at junction of afferent arteriole and distal tubule
         (b) JGA senses filtrate changes indicating ↓ BP, ↓ renal blood flow, or both.
         (c) Renin secreted and released from macula densa cells located in JGA directly into efferent arterial
         (d) Examples of pathophysiological triggers for renin release
            (i)　Hemorrhage (↓ BP, ↓ renal blood flow)
            (ii)　Heart failure (↓ BP)
            (iii)　Dehydration (↓ renal blood flow)
         (e) Renin converts the plasma protein angiotensinogen to angiotensin I.

    c. Angiotensin I

      (1) Inactive mediator; no physiological effect

      (2) Converted to active angiotensin II by angiotensin-converting enzyme (ACE)

      (3) Large concentration of ACE found in pulmonary capillary bed

    d. Angiotensin II

      (1) Powerful arterial vasoconstrictor; directly increases BP

      (2) Stimulates aldosterone release, leading to Na^+ reabsorption in distal tubule

      (3) Dual effect increases renal blood flow and pressure.

        (a) Restoring filtration and renal function

        (b) Negative feedback control would then decrease renin release.

      (4) RAA mechanism has limited compensatory ability to affect alterations in volume.

      (5) Medical management directed toward external efforts

        (a) Appropriate replacement of blood, fluids, electrolytes

        (b) Drug therapy to restore BP and renal perfusion

    e. Aldosterone

      (1) Release from adrenal cortex stimulated by:

        (a) Decreased Na^+ levels

        (b) Increased K^+ levels

      (2) Prompts kidney to:

        (a) Absorb more Na^+

        (b) Excrete more K^+

      (3) Net effect of release

        (a) Conserve Na^+ and water

        (b) Raise blood volume

        (c) Prevent acidosis

      (4) Potential adverse effects

        (a) Systemic vasoconstriction

        (b) Decreased organ perfusion

2. Prostaglandin

  a. Produced, metabolized, and acted on in renal medulla

  b. Maintains renal function by effect on afferent and efferent arterioles of glomerular capillary

  c. Modulates renin release

  d. Affects urine concentration through synergistic activity with arginine vasopressin, an antidiuretic hormone

  e. Nonsteroidal anti-inflammatory agents must be cautiously used.

    (1) Cause Na^+ and water retention

    (2) Acute renal failure can occur in states of dehydration.

3. Erythropoietin

  a. Secreted by kidney in response to decrease in tissue oxygen tension (Pao_2).

  b. Stimulates production of new RBCs

  c. Exerts effect directly on bone marrow

  d. Insufficient levels often found in patients with impaired renal function

  e. Exogenous replacement available

4. ADH (antidiuretic hormone or vasopressin)

  a. Secreted by posterior pituitary gland when significant loss of body water occurs

  b. Acts as messenger in tubules, informing of body's need for water

  c. Exerts effect on distal tubules of nephrons

  d. Results in increased reabsorption of water and decreased urine output

  e. Causes constriction of arterioles, thereby raising BP

5. Vitamin D

  a. Activated in kidney

  b. Deficiency plays major role in chronic renal failure.

    (1) Losses in urine with nephrotic syndrome

(2) Defective enzyme activity in kidney caused by:
  (a) Renal disease
  (b) Diminished parenchymal function
    c. Decreased levels with hypocalcemia
    d. Stimulates intestinal absorption of calcium and phosphate
    e. Increases reabsorption of calcium and phosphorus by kidney
C. Fluid-electrolyte balance (electrolyte interactions)
  1. Na⁺
    a. Kidney regulates total body Na⁺ by varying urinary excretion in relation to intake.
    b. Secretion adjusted in response to alterations in blood volume
    c. Reabsorption accounts for most of energy consumed by kidney.
  2. K⁺
    a. Filtration and excretion independent of one another
      (1) Once filtered, almost totally reabsorbed in proximal tubules and loop of Henle
      (2) Excreted via aldosterone release and secretion in distal nephron
    b. Secretion enhanced by tubular fluid flow rate and increases in Na⁺ reabsorption
  3. Calcium (Ca⁺⁺)
    a. Renal excretion and net intestinal absorption must be equal for proper calcium balance.
    b. Calcium phosphates crystallize in alkaline urine (hereditary distal tubular acidosis).
    c. Ionized in plasma
    d. Two thirds reabsorbed in proximal tubules by bulk flow with Na⁺ and fluids
    e. Direct relation to Na⁺ balance
  4. Phosphates (PO₄)
    a. Ninety percent reabsorbed in proximal tubule through Na⁺-dependent process
    b. Balance reabsorbed in distal tubule
    c. Plasma level constant when renal function is normal
      (1) Excess concentrations of saline decrease proximal reabsorption.
      (2) Phosphate depletion raises reabsorption.
      (3) Excretion depressed with hyperparathyroidism and vitamin D deficiencies
    d. At saturation point, excess load excreted in urine
  5. Glucose in glomerular filtrate completely reabsorbed at normal blood concentrations
D. Glomerular filtration
  1. Nephrons operate in highly sophisticated pressure system.
  2. Pressure gradients affect filtration.
    a. Physical factor(s) assist filtration (movement of fluid from capillary → barrier → tubule).
      (1) Pressure in afferent arteriole is about 90 mm Hg entering glomerular capillary.
      (2) Adequate BP is the primary force promoting filtration.
      (3) Forces promoting filtration must be greater than opposing forces to have filtration take place.
    b. Physical factor(s) opposing filtration (preventing fluid movement into renal tubule)
      (1) Fluid present in tubule already creates hydrostatic pressure at about 15 mm Hg, resisting filtration.
      (2) Presence of protein in plasma (oncotic pressure) opposes filtration.
    c. Osmotic gradient creates difference in hydrostatic pressure of about 30 mm Hg, favoring filtration (movement of fluid from capillary → barrier → tubule).
    d. Net filtration pressure
      (1) Protein-free filtrate forced through filtration barrier into renal tubule

      (2) Filtrate passes into proximal tubule.

      (3) Renal function ceases without filtration.

  E. Urine production

    1. Originates as filtrate in Bowman's capsule

      a. Filtration barrier creates a virtually protein-free filtrate.

      b. Composed basically of water and solutes (ions and dissolved substances)

    2. Filtrate passes into proximal convoluted tubule.

      a. Water and ions and dissolved substances reabsorbed according to body's need.

    3. Loop of Henle concentrates urine.

    4. Distal convoluted tubule can reabsorb or excrete water and solutes.

      a. Reabsorbs only what body requires

      b. Excretes remainder based on ADH and aldosterone secretion

  F. Key points

    1. Kidneys depend on minimum blood flow and pressure for function.

    2. Net filtration pressure can be affected by change in renal artery pressure.

    3. BP has direct effect on urine production by affecting filtration.

    4. Sustained changes in pressure cause compromise normal renal function.

    5. Kidneys are responsible for maintenance of electrolyte balance.

    6. End products of metabolism are excreted in urine.

V. PATHOPHYSIOLOGY

  A. Upper genitourinary system

    1. Adrenal gland

      a. Adrenal insufficiency (Addison's disease)

        (1) Rare disorder caused by autoimmune destruction of adrenal cortex

        (2) Chronic metabolic disorder that requires lifelong hormonal replacement therapy

        (3) Secondary adrenal insufficiency can follow long-term (>2 weeks) exogenous steroid therapy.

        (4) May lead to acute adrenal crisis

          (a) Life-threatening situation

          (b) Follows a stressful episode in a patient with adrenal insufficiency

          (c) Requires rapid treatment with intravenous fluid and steroid replacement

      b. Cushing's disease

        (1) Caused by excessive serum cortisol (hydrocortisone)

          (a) Bilateral adrenocortical hyperplasia from overproduction of adrenocorticotropic hormone (ACTH) in pituitary gland (85%)

          (b) Adrenal adenoma (10%)

          (c) Adenocarcinoma of adrenal gland (5%)

          (d) Also may be seen in exogenous steroid administration

        (2) Signs and symptoms

          (a) Marked muscle weakness, especially in quadriceps

          (b) Obesity with abnormal fat distribution

            (i)   Extremities unaffected

            (ii) Moon face with facial flushing

            (iii) Cervical vertebral hump ("buffalo hump")

            (iv) Central fat leading to obese trunk and pendulous abdomen

            (v) Thin extremities from protein wasting and loss of subcutaneous fat

          (c) Striae

            (i)   Thighs and abdomen

          (d) Poor skin turgor and ulceration

          (e) Hypertension from increased production of aldosterone and Na$^+$ retention

          (f) Calcium loss

            (i)   Osteoporosis

            (ii) Compression fractures of lumbar spine and ribs

            (iii) Renal calculi

        (g) Sleep disturbance
           (i)   Irritability
           (ii) Psychosis
        (h) Diabetic glucose tolerance curve
        (i) Vascular fragility (bruises easily)
        (j) Slow wound healing
    (3) Surgical intervention usually alleviates symptoms with exception of osteoporosis.
        (a) Total bilateral adrenalectomy
        (b) Transsphenoidal hypophysectomy
  c. Pheochromocytoma
    (1) Tumor of the chromaffin cells of adrenal medulla; may be:
        (a) Bilateral
        (b) Extra-adrenal
    (2) Surgically curable hypertensive syndrome
        (a) Severe systolic and diastolic hypertension
        (b) Hypertension may be sustained, or more commonly, paroxysmal.
        (c) Symptoms may be triggered by tyrosine-containing food (i.e., wine, aged cheese).
        (d) Other frequent symptoms
           (i)   Headache (severity directly related to degree of hypertension)
           (ii) Unprovoked diaphoresis with flushing or blanching
           (iii) Tachycardia with palpitations from epinephrine excess
           (iv) Postural hypotension
              [a] Diminished plasma volume
              [b] Ganglionic blockage
              [c] May result in profound weakness
           (v) Weight loss
              [a] Anorexia resulting from elevated blood glucose and fatty acid levels
              [b] Decreased gastrointestinal motility: nausea, vomiting, constipation
    (3) Often occurs in combination with other glandular diseases
    (4) Laboratory analysis
        (a) Elevated hematocrit
        (b) Elevated white blood cells (WBCs)
        (c) Elevated serum protein
        (d) Few lymphocytes
        (e) Elevated fasting glucose level with diabetic glucose tolerance curve
        (f) Urine hormonal analysis reveals elevated epinephrine and sometimes norepinephrine.
    (5) Administration of 1 mg intravenous (IV) glucagon will raise BP and catecholamine in 2 minutes.
2. Kidney
  a. Agenesis
    (1) Absence of one kidney
    (2) Presence of atrophic kidney (not fully developed)
  b. Hypoplasia
    (1) Presence of small kidney with small renal artery
    (2) Contributes to renal hypertension
  c. Polycystic kidneys (hereditary)
    (1) Occurs in renal cortex from defective collecting system
    (2) Bilateral cystic disease leading to progressive functional impairment as cysts enlarge
    (3) Symptoms
        (a) Bilateral flank pain, often with colic
        (b) Hematuria

        (c) Hypertension

        (d) Nodular, palpable kidneys, often tender

     (4) Usually results in need for dialysis and possible transplantation

  d. Congenital ureteropelvic junction obstruction

  e. Glomerulonephritis

     (1) Inflammatory process that attacks glomerulus

     (2) Possible immune reaction

     (3) Contributing causes

        (a) Infectious organisms

           (i)   Streptococci

           (ii) Staphylococci

        (b) Systemic diseases

           (i)   Lupus erythematosus

           (ii) Polyarteritis nodosa—result of:

               [a] Trauma

               [b] Anticoagulants

               [c] Tumor

               [d] Cause of spontaneous subcapsular hematoma

          (iii) Diabetic glomerulosclerosis

          (iv) Amyloidosis

          (v) Alport's syndrome

  f. Nephrotic syndrome (combination of symptoms)

     (1) Massive edema resulting from decreased serum protein and oncotic pressure

     (2) Proteinuria from protein losses in the urine

     (3) Hypoalbuminemia

     (4) Hyperlipidemia

     (5) Lipiduria

  g. Renal artery stenosis

     (1) Plaque formation

     (2) Embolism

     (3) Thrombosis

     (4) Contributes to renal hypertension

  h. Simple (solitary) renal cyst

  i. Pyelonephritis (often a complication of *Escherichia coli* infection elsewhere in body)

  j. Perinephric abscess

  k. High-output renal failure (oliguria)

     (1) Urine output volume insufficient relative to body's excretory need

        (a) Occurs with urine volumes less than 400 mL/day if:

           (i)   Kidney can concentrate to normal specific gravity (1.010-1.025).

        (b) Occurs with urine volumes of 1000 to 1500 mL/day

           (i)   When concentrating ability impaired

           (ii) Causes low specific gravity

     (2) Metabolites retained

     (3) High loss of body water

     (4) Etiology

        (a) Inadequate plasma volume with vasodilation; substantially decreased protein levels

        (b) Normal kidney function compromised by poor perfusion

           (i)   Decreased plasma volume results in decreased perfusion.

           (ii) Poor perfusion accompanies decrease in cardiac contractility.

        (c) Prerenal azotemia (rising serum urea blood levels)

  l. Acute renal failure

     (1) Substantial decrease in glomerular filtration rate results in decrease in clearance of metabolites excreted by kidneys.

        (a) Urea

        (b) K^+

        (c) Phosphate

        (d) Creatinine

    (2) Body retains metabolites in bloodstream.

        (a) Abnormally high creatinine level in bloodstream (best indicator of renal failure)

        (b) Retention produces state known as azotemia (excess of urea in blood).

        (c) Azotemia can be tolerated until treatment interventions are instituted.

        (d) Uremia characterized by progressively higher levels of circulating metabolites

        (e) Uremia (intoxication) seen in advanced nephritis and anuria, incompatible with life

    (3) Causes

        (a) Prerenal

           (i) Dehydration (volume depletion)

              [a] Hemorrhage

              [b] Gastrointestinal losses (vomiting, diarrhea)

              [c] Renal losses (excessive diuretic therapy)

              [d] Burns

              [e] Heat prostration

           (ii) Volume shifts

              [a] "Third space" losses

              [b] Vasodilating drugs

              [c] Gram-negative sepsis

           (iii) Volume expansion

              [a] Congestive heart failure

              [b] Nephrotic syndrome

              [c] Cirrhosis with ascites

           (iv) Vascular anomalies

              [a] Dissecting arterial aneurysms

              [b] Malignant hyperthermia

              [c] Atheroembolism

        (b) Intrarenal (parenchymal) conditions

           (i) Glomerulonephritis

           (ii) Ischemic reaction to vascular compromise

           (iii) Acute tubular necrosis

           (iv) Acute cortical necrosis

           (v) Antibiotic nephrotoxicity

        (c) Postrenal conditions

           (i) Calculus in patients with solitary kidney

           (ii) Bilateral ureteral obstruction: stricture

           (iii) Bladder outlet obstruction: BPH

           (iv) Postrenal trauma

m. Renal insufficiency

    (1) Reduction in functioning nephrons to 25%

    (2) Goal of patient care is the preservation of renal function.

        (a) Prevention of hypotension and reduction in renal BP and blood supply

        (b) Avoidance of nephrotoxic medications.

n. Chronic renal failure

    (1) Irreversible destruction of renal tissue

    (2) Reduced metabolite clearance requiring peritoneal dialysis or hemodialysis

    (3) Chief parameters indicative of renal failure

        (a) Elevated blood urea nitrogen (BUN)

        (b) Elevated serum creatinine

        (c) Decreased creatinine clearance

    (4) Lengthy disease course

        (a) Azotemia

        (b) End-stage renal disease

    (5) Etiology
        (a) Primary causes
            (i)   Glomerulonephritis
            (ii) Pyelonephritis
            (iii) Congenital hypoplasia
            (iv) Polycystic kidney disease
        (b) Secondary causes
            (i)   Diabetes
            (ii) Hypertension
            (iii) Systemic lupus erythematosus
            (iv) Alport's syndrome
            (v) Amyloidosis
                [a] Idiopathic, often malignant condition
                [b] Increased protein levels
                [c] May also involve bladder and prostate
    (6) Treatment modalities
        (a) Maintenance hemodialysis
        (b) Peritoneal dialysis
        (c) Renal transplantation
o. Dialysis
    (1) Therapeutic process
        (a) Replace waste-excretion of renal system
        (b) Removes excess fluid and waste products
        (c) Restores fluid and electrolyte balance
        (d) Eliminate nitrogenous wastes and toxins from the blood
    (2) Indications
        (a) Acute or chronic renal failure
        (b) Severe water intoxication
        (c) Electrolyte imbalance
        (d) Drug intoxication
            (i)   Alcohol
            (ii) Salicylates
            (iii) Lithium
            (iv) Barbiturates
            (v) Poisons
        (e) Hepatic encephalopathy/coma
    (3) Techniques
        (a) Hemodialysis
            (i)   Blood moves through device that exposes to dialysate solution across a semipermeable membrane
            (ii) Uses principles of
                [a] Osmosis
                [b] Diffusion
                [c] Filtration
            (iii) Complications
                [a] Hypotension
                [b] Leg cramps
                [c] Infection
                [d] Cardiac dysrhythmias
                [e] Hemolysis
                [f] Hypoxemia
            (iv) Vascular access (See following section on Arterovenous shunts)
        (b) Peritoneal dialysis
            (i)   Blood component—peritoneal microvasculature; semipermeable membrane—peritoneal lining
            (ii) Uses principles of
                [a] Osmosis
                [b] Diffusion
                [c] Filtration

    (iii) Complications

     [a] Peritonitis

     [b] Hyperglycemia

     [c] Respiratory distress

     [d] Catheter related

      [1] Sluggish fill and emptying times

      [2] Dialysate leakage

      [3] Bowel perforation

    (iv) Peritoneal access

p. Arteriovenous (AV) shunt placement and revision

 (1) Purpose: provide a permanent, internal vascular access for prolonged or long-term dialysis

 (2) Description

  (a) Surgically constructs an AV fistula

  (b) Brings arterial blood flow pressure into the vein that will be used for dialysis

   (i) Significantly increases rate of venous flow to greater than 200 mL/min

   (ii) Allows for completion of dialysis in a reasonable length of time (3-4 hours)

   (iii) Minimum mortality rates

   (iv) Technical failure rate of 10% to 15%

  (c) Preoperative care

   (i) Physical assessment issues

    [a] Respiratory

     [1] Common coexisting disease processes

     [2] Pneumonia

     [3] Pulmonary edema

     [4] Uremic pleuritis

     [5] Assess for:

      [i] Shortness of breath (SOB)

      [ii] Orthopnea

      [iii] Paroxysmal nocturnal dyspnea (PND)

   (ii) Gastrointestinal (GI)

    [a] Common coexisting disease processes

    [b] Delayed gastric emptying

    [c] GI bleeding

    [d] Assess for:

     [1] Regurgitation

     [2] Nausea and vomiting (N/V)

     [3] Early satiety

   (iii) Hematology

    [a] Common coexisting disease processes

    [b] Anemia

    [c] Bleeding disorders

    [d] Assess for:

     [1] SOB

     [2] Bruising

   (iv) Genitourinary and endocrine

    [a] Common coexisting disease processes

    [b] Oliguria or anuria

    [c] Uremia

    [d] Electrolyte and acid-base imbalance

    [e] Diabetes

    [f] Assess for:

     [1] Weight (baseline and highest)

     [2] Hiccoughs

     [3] Anorexia

     [4] N/V

[5] Diarrhea

[6] Loss of skin integrity

[7] Fluid & electrolyte status

    (v) Central nervous system (CNS)

        [a] Common coexisting disease processes

            [1] Encephalopathy

            [2] Seizures

            [3] Neuropathy

            [4] Perform musculoskeletal assessment.

(3) Intraoperative concerns

    (a) Types of internal vascular accesses

        (i) Internal AV fistula

            [a] Creation of an actual fistula

            [b] Not available for immediate use; wound healing must occur and edema subside.

            [c] Usually not accessible for weeks to months after surgery

        (ii) Internal graft AV fistula

            [a] Straight or looped natural or synthetic graft

            [b] Placed in arm or thigh

            [c] Preferred for obese individuals

        (iii) Internal AV graft with external access device

            [a] External access port attached to AV graft

            [b] Alleviates need for repeated needle insertions

    (b) Common graft locations

        (i) Wrist

            [a] "Snuffbox" fistula: antebrachium—cephalic vein to radial artery

        (ii) Forearm: radial, ulnar, or brachial artery to antecubital or brachial vein

        (iii) Upper arm: brachial artery above elbow to basilic or axillary vein

    (c) Anesthesia techniques

        (i) Monitored anesthesia care (MAC)

        (ii) Regional

        (iii) General

    (d) Estimated blood loss (EBL): 25 to 100 mL

    (e) Length of case: 1 to 2 hours

(4) Postanesthesia priorities: phase I PACU

    (a) Avoid venipuncture, BP measurements, and injections in surgical arm.

    (b) Assess for graft AND shunt patency.

        (i) Gently palpate for thrill.

        (ii) Auscultate for bruit.

    (c) Elevate surgical arm to decrease swelling.

    (d) Avoid circumferential dressings, arm bands, on surgical arm.

    (e) Maintain adequate hydration.

        (i) Maintains BP

        (ii) Protects patency of graft

    (f) Assess for bleeding: apply pressure dressing for profuse bleeding.

    (g) Monitor for complications.

        (i) Thrombosis

        (ii) Infection

        (iii) Aneurysm

        (iv) Steal syndrome

            [a] Ischemic pain related to vascular insufficiency as a result of fistula formation

            [b] Assess for:

                [1] Diminished pulses

                [2] Pallor

                [3] Pain distal to graft site

[c] Surgical revision or additional procedures required when this syndrome occurs

(h) Report any suspected or actual complications to physician.

(5) Postanesthesia priorities: phase II
   (a) MAC and regional patients may be admitted directly to phase II.
   (b) Continue phase I level of care.
   (c) Pain management
      (i) Oral analgesia usually effective
      (ii) Average discharge pain score: 1 to 2 (0-10 scale)
   (d) Discharge teaching
      (i) Keep operative arm elevated for several days.
      (ii) Avoid any venipuncture, BP measurements, and injections in operative arm.
      (iii) Avoid wearing constrictive clothing, wristbands on operative site.
      (iv) Instruct patient how to palpate for a thrill.
      (v) Instruct patient in assessment for and management of possible complications.

(6) Postanesthesia priorities: extended observation
   (a) Autogenous fistulas must adequately heal before being used for dialysis.
      (i) Blood flow increases with time.
      (ii) Venous wall must adequately thicken to prevent tears and infiltration during dialysis.
      (iii) Maturation time varies from 3 to 6 weeks.
      (iv) Fistula should not be used for 3 weeks to avoid aneurysm formation.
   (b) Teach importance of rotating injection sites when puncturing for dialysis.
      (i) Prevents aneurysm formation
      (ii) Prevents shredding and eventual breakdown of shunt material
   (c) Instruct patient that arteriovenous hemodialysis accesses have finite lifespan; replacements and revisions common.
   (d) Support patient on waiting list for renal transplantation.
      (i) Optimal therapy for end-stage renal disease
      (ii) Waiting time varies considerably.
   (e) Recommended diagnostic studies
      (i) CXR
      (ii) Platelet count
      (iii) Blood urea nitrogen (BUN) and creatinine
      (iv) Bicarbonate (HCO_3)
      (v) Blood glucose
      (vi) Electrolyte analysis including K^+, Na^+, Cl^-, Mg^{++} & PO_4^+
   (f) Determine nondominant arm.
      (i) Shunt should be easily accessible.
      (ii) Should be placed on nondominant arm when possible
         [a] Allows for easy self-cannulation for home dialysis patients
         [b] Allows for increased patient ease with performance of daily activities

3. Ureter
  a. Congenital abnormalities
    (1) Incomplete ureter
    (2) Duplication of ureter
      (a) Y formation
      (b) Double ureter on one or both sides
    (3) Ureterocele
    (4) Ureteral stricture
    (5) Ureterovesical reflux
    (6) Ureteral stenosis

      b. Acquired condition
        (1) Stenosis
          (a) Surgical trauma
          (b) External trauma
        (2) Metastatic lymph node enlargement
        (3) Endometriosis
        (4) Tumors
        (5) Calculi
B. Lower genitourinary system
  1. Bladder
    a. Exstrophy
      (1) Congenital fusion of bladder wall
      (2) Bladder eversion
    b. Interstitial cystitis
      (1) Multifactorial syndrome of pelvic and/or perineal pain with urinary urgency and frequency
      (2) Loss of normal bladder capacity develops.
      (3) Biopsy of bladder wall may reveal presence of mast cells, thought to be an integral cause of this syndrome.
    c. Stress incontinence
      (1) Leakage of urine with sneezing, coughing, laughing, straining
      (2) Common in older women and after multiple pregnancies
    d. Bladder diverticulum
    e. Bladder tumors
  2. Prostate gland
    a. BPH
      (1) Gland enlarges.
      (2) Evident bladder outlet obstruction necessitates surgical intervention.
    b. Carcinoma
      (1) Nonsurgical treatments
        (a) Androgen therapy
        (b) Radiation
      (2) Surgical modalities
        (a) Orchiectomy
          (i) Testosterone production dramatically reduced
            [a] Adrenal production of testosterone not altered
            [b] Antiandrogen therapy may be required.
          (ii) Alternative to "medical" hormonal therapies
        (b) Prostatectomy
        (c) Cryoablation
        (d) Radioactive seed implantation
  3. Penis and male urethra
    a. Phimosis
      (1) Foreskin unretractable over glans
      (2) Tendency for infection and fibrosis
      (3) Circumcision indicated
    b. Paraphimosis
      (1) Retracted phimotic foreskin
      (2) Painful swelling of glans occurs.
      (3) Dry gangrene can result if severe.
      (4) Circumcision indicated
    c. Balanoposthitis
      (1) Inflamed glans and mucous membrane
      (2) Purulent discharge
      (3) Circumcision indicated
    d. Urethral stricture (stenosis)
      (1) Congenital or acquired condition

(2) Surgical interventions
    (a) Urethral dilation
    (b) Meatotomy
    (c) Urethroplasty
e. Hypospadias
    (1) Congenital anomaly
    (2) Opening of meatus proximal to its normal glandular position at tip of penis
    (3) Requires surgical reconstruction of urethra
f. Epispadias
    (1) Congenital anomaly (often associated with bladder exstrophy)
    (2) Absence of dorsal urethral wall
    (3) Requires surgical correction
g. Carcinoma of penis and/or urethra
h. Trauma (e.g., fractured urethra)
4. Testis, spermatic cord, and scrotum
  a. Cryptorchidism (undescended testis)
    (1) Evident at birth
    (2) Absence of one or both testis in scrotum
    (3) Requires surgical intervention by 1 to 2 years of age
      (a) Sterility ensues when left untreated much beyond this time.
      (b) Maturation will not occur.
      (c) Tendency for cancerous development increases over time if left untreated.
  b. Testicular tumors
    (1) Usually malignant
    (2) Common in 18 to 35 year age group
    (3) Enlargement of testis occurs, usually painless.
    (4) Requires metastatic workup, orchiectomy, and chemotherapy
  c. Spermatocele
    (1) Intrascrotal cystic mass
    (2) Attached to superior head of epididymis
    (3) Caused by obstruction of sperm-carrying tubular system
    (4) Most commonly occurs after vasectomy
  d. Varicocele
    (1) Most often seen on left side
    (2) Veins of spermatic cord become engorged because of venous backflow.
    (3) Often painful
    (4) Uncorrected can affect fertility
  e. Hydrocele
    (1) Collection of fluid within scrotal sac
    (2) May compromise testicular blood supply
  f. Torsion of testis or spermatic cord
    (1) Strangulation of testicular blood supply
    (2) Usually of traumatic origin
    (3) Patient has presenting symptom of extreme pain.
    (4) Requires immediate surgery
5. Female urethra
  a. Urethrovaginal fistula (vesicovaginal fistula)
    (1) Abnormal passageway between urethra and vagina
    (2) Develops after trauma
      (a) Pelvic fracture
      (b) Surgery
      (c) Radiotherapy
    (3) Vaginal urethroplasty performed to correct condition
  b. Urethral diverticulum
    (1) Urethral pouch develops.
    (2) Can be a congenital abnormality

(3) Traumatic causes
- (a) Cystitis
- (b) Urethritis
- (c) Obstetric

(4) Requires excision and plastic repair

c. Urethral carcinoma

d. Urethral caruncle

6. Other female pathophysiology

a. Bartholin's gland cyst and abscess

(1) Occlusion in duct system of gland leads to fluid-filled sac.

(2) Abscess can result if cyst becomes infected and contents become purulent.
- (a) Abscess may become size of orange and reoccur if not treated correctly.
- (b) May be caused by bacterial, chlamydial, or gonococcal infections
- (c) Treatment includes antibiotics, heat application, and surgical incision and drainage.

b. Vulvar intraepithelial neoplasia (VIN)

(1) Age-related differences in appearance of VIN
- (a) Younger women: VIN associated with human papillomavirus (HPV) infection
- (b) Older women: VIN associated with nonneoplastic disorders such as chronic inflammation, lasting on average 6 to 7 years before appearance of neoplasia

c. Vaginitis

(1) Inflammatory disorder causing discharge, burning, redness, swelling, and discomfort

(2) Common causes include:
- (a) Poor hygiene
- (b) Parasites
- (c) Foreign body retention
- (d) Bacterial or fungal infection

d. Cervical polyps

(1) Most common lesion of cervix

(2) Found in all age groups and may protrude through the cervical os (opening)

(3) Most cervical polyps benign, but should be surgically removed

e. Cervical cancer

(1) Readily detected and if treated early, the most easily cured cancer of the female reproductive tract

(2) Worldwide, most common cause of female reproductive cancer death

(3) Decline in incidence in United States from leading cause of cancer death in women 50 years ago to eighth currently due to early diagnosis with Papanicolaou (PAP) smear examination

(4) Cervical cancer considered to be a sexually transmitted disease; frequently caused by HPV infection

(5) HPV immunization available for prevention of multiple strains of HPV infection

C. Voiding dysfunctions

1. Frequency

a. Perception of urge to urinate at more frequent intervals

b. Causes

(1) Residual urine

(2) Inflamed bladder mucosa or submucosa

(3) Inadequate bladder capacity

(4) Bladder instability

(5) Interstitial cystitis

(6) Bladder infection

2. Urgency
   a. Strong sensation of having to void immediately
   b. Causes
      (1) Cystitis
      (2) Bladder instability
3. Nocturia
   a. Need to urinate often during normal sleep time
   b. Often symptom of renal or prostate disease
   c. Causes
      (1) Fluid retention (shift of circulating fluids to kidneys during rest).
      (2) Excess fluid intake before bedtime
      (3) BPH
      (4) Renal calculi
      (5) Cystitis
4. Dysuria
   a. Painful urination
   b. Causes
      (1) Prostatitis
      (2) Cystitis
      (3) Urethritis
      (4) Pyelonephritis
5. Enuresis
   a. Involuntary urination, often during sleep
   b. Normal in first 2 to 3 years of life
   c. Causes
      (1) Delayed neuromuscular maturation
      (2) Organic disease
         (a) Infection
         (b) Urethral stenosis
         (c) Neurogenic bladder
         (d) Pituitary malfunction
      (3) Emotional or behavioral problems
6. Incontinence (includes stress, urge, mixed, and paradoxical or overflow types)
   a. Inability to control urination
   b. Causes
      (1) Exstrophy of bladder
      (2) Epispadias
      (3) Vesicovaginal fistula
      (4) Trauma: childbirth, prostatectomy
      (5) Bladder instability: detrusor, sphincter
7. Hematuria
   a. Presence of gross or microscopic blood in urine
   b. Causes
      (1) Tumors or cysts
      (2) Calculi
      (3) Infection
      (4) Sickle cell disease
      (5) Glomerulonephritis
8. Obstruction and stasis
   a. Backflow of urine may occur, leading to hydronephrosis.
   b. Normal urinary flow blocked or arrested.
      (1) Prostatic obstruction
      (2) Urethral obstruction
      (3) Vesicoureteral reflux
      (4) Pyelonephritis
      (5) Calculi

    c. Contributing causes
       (1) Hypercalciuria
          (a) Increased calcium intake
          (b) Increased vitamin D intake
       (2) Hyperphosphatemia
       (3) Hyperparathyroidism
       (4) Gout
       (5) Cushing's disease
          (a) Increased cortisol production
          (b) Protein loss in urine
 9. Infection
    a. Specific (organisms capable of causing clinical disease)
       (1) Tuberculosis
       (2) Gonorrhea
       (3) Actinomycosis
    b. Nonspecific (similar manifestations among several conditions)
       (1) Gram-negative rods
       (2) Gram-positive cocci
    c. Venereal diseases
       (1) Gonorrhea
       (2) Syphilis
       (3) Lymphogranuloma venereum
       (4) Granuloma inguinale
       (5) Herpes genitalis
       (6) Condylomata acuminata
VI. ASSESSMENT
  A. Inspect (consistent with observation)
    1. Observe for visible signs of pathological conditions.
      a. Abdomen (kidneys, bladder, lungs)
        (1) Costovertebral fullness
        (2) Distention
        (3) Oxygen perfusion
      b. External genitalia
        (1) Edema, crepitus
        (2) Discharge
        (3) Inflammation, rash
        (4) Ulcerations, lesions
        (5) Discoloration
        (6) Alteration in normal shape, size, or position
      c. Operative wounds
        (1) Bleeding
        (2) Drainage
        (3) Assess frequently.
    2. Interview patient for presence of postoperative sequelae.
      a. Collaborate with other perioperative caregivers to promote optimum follow-through.
      b. Compare findings with preoperative psychosocial assessment.
        (1) All patients
          (a) Use comprehensive assessment tools.
          (b) Establish presence of preexisting physical impairments and disease processes.
          (c) Note allergies and need for ancillary drug therapies.
        (2) Pediatric patient
          (a) Age crucial to proper assessment and intervention
          (b) Establish cognitive level of child; note phobias, peculiarities, emotional maturity.
          (c) Allow treasured toy or other "security blanket" to be nearby.
          (d) Evaluate merit of parental comfort.

    c. Expand on preoperative and intraoperative teaching.

        (1) Initiate deep breathing, coughing, mobilization.

        (2) Explain presence of any invasive devices resulting from operative experience.

           (a) Urinary catheters: urge to void, application of traction

           (b) Wound drains

           (c) IV and invasive lines

        (3) Offer medications frequently to control discomfort or agitation.

        (4) Alleviate fears of embarrassment because of altered body image.

           (a) Promote calming environment.

           (b) Provide privacy.

           (c) Provide warmth.

        (5) Communicate as care is being given to patient.

           (a) Wound and drain inspections

           (b) Frequent vital signs

           (c) Oxygen (O_2) therapy

B. Auscultate (first step after inspection of urological patient)

  1. Abdomen

    a. Palpation alters normal peristalsis.

    b. Evaluation of bowel sounds important after abdominal and flank surgeries

    c. Detection of murmurs or bruits associated with aneurysms and renal artery stenosis

  2. Lungs

    a. Evaluate presence and character of breath sounds.

    b. Absence of sounds indicates airway compromise.

    c. Presence of adventitious breath sounds should be investigated and reported.

  3. Heart

    a. Detection of cardiac murmurs or abnormal heart sounds

    b. Note rate and character of apical beats.

C. Palpation

  1. Kidneys

    a. Realistic only in thin adult

    b. Normal kidney is firm and smooth.

        (1) Tenderness should be expected after renal surgery.

        (2) Tenderness or pain may also indicate renal abnormality.

    c. Palpate deeply anteriorly as supine patient inhales deeply.

        (1) Use left hand for left kidney.

        (2) Use right hand for right kidney.

    d. Place palm of hand over costovertebral angle posteriorly, and deliver light blow.

        (1) Necessary for patient to be sitting

        (2) Angle formed by lower thoracic vertebrae and eleventh and twelfth ribs

        (3) Lower poles of kidneys below rib cage bilaterally

           (a) Should be perceived by patient as dull thud

           (b) Sharp tenderness or pain may require further evaluation.

  2. Abdomen

    a. Avoid deep palpation for any perianesthesia patient recovering from abdominal surgery.

    b. Patient should be in supine position.

    c. Note any resistance to light palpation over lower abdomen and suprapubic region.

        (1) May indicate bladder distention

        (2) May indicate bladder infection

        (3) Pelvic mass may elicit similar reaction.

D. Percuss

  1. Kidneys

    a. Rarely achievable

    b. May be possible on child

  2. Bladder
   a. Tympany normal over bladder because of proximity of bowel.
   b. Dullness occurs with distention.
  3. Lungs
   a. Anterior aspects and apices should be resonant.
   b. Posterior aspect resonant to ninth rib
   c. Bases reveal gradual transition from resonance to dullness over borders.
   d. Bases should move downward 5 to 6 cm on inspiration.
 E. Review pertinent preoperative diagnostic data.
  1. Laboratory studies
   a. Urinalysis
    (1) Most fundamental and valuable of all screening methods
    (2) Value dependent on:
     (a) Proper specimen collection
     (b) Prompt delivery of specimens
    (3) Components
     (a) pH (4.6-8.0)
     (b) Appearance (color, clarity)
      (i) Normal clarity is clear.
      (ii) Normal color is straw to amber.
     (c) Odor (aromatic)
     (d) Specific gravity (1.010-1.025)
      (i) Measure of urine concentration
      (ii) Infant (1.001-1.020)
      (iii) Elderly (values decrease with age)
     (e) Protein (albumin, 0-8 mg/dL)
      (i) Normally not present in urine because of filtration barrier
      (ii) Presence of protein indicative of glomerulonephritis
     (f) Glucose (sugar, 0)
      (i) Normally not present in urine because of filtration barrier
      (ii) Present in urine when serum glucose exceeds renal threshold and sugar is spilling into the urine.
      (iii) Glucose in the urine acts as an osmotic diuretic, so urine volume will increase.
     (g) Ketones (0)
      (i) Normally not present in urine
      (ii) Ketones in the urine indicate catabolism of protein as a fuel.
     (h) Blood (RBCs, 0-2; casts, 0)
      (i) Normally not present in urine because of filtration barrier
      (ii) Presence of protein indicative of glomerulonephritis or trauma to urinary drainage system
      (iii) RBCs may also be present in the specimen of a menstruating woman.
     (i) Leukocytes (WBCs, 0)
      (i) Normally not present in urine because of filtration barrier
      (ii) May indicate bacterial infection in urinary system
     (j) Microscopic evaluation
      (i) Casts
      (ii) Crystals
      (iii) Bacteria
      (iv) RBCs
      (v) WBCs
   b. Creatinine clearance
    (1) Urine collected for 24 hours
    (2) First AM voiding discarded, and first voiding of following morning collected
    (3) Requires refrigeration

    c. Urine culture and sensitivities
    d. BUN (10-20 mg/dL)
       (1) Infant or child: 5 to 18 mg/dL
       (2) Above 100 mg/dL: may infer renal function impairment
    e. Urine osmolality
       (1) Monitors electrolyte and water balance
       (2) Evaluate dehydration.
    f. Serum creatinine (0.5-1.2 mg/dL)
       (1) Range for females slightly lower
       (2) Above 1.5 mg/dL: indicates impairment of renal function
    g. Complete blood cell count (CBC) and differential
    h. Serum electrolytes
    i. Cholesterol (120-200 mg/dL)
    j. Coagulation studies
       (1) Prothrombin time
       (2) Partial thromboplastin time
       (3) Platelets
       (4) Bleeding time
2. Diagnostic procedures
    a. Ultrasonography
       (1) Able to focus on particular organ
       (2) Picture of organ displayed on screen
          (a) Measure shape and size.
          (b) High-frequency sound waves
       (3) Affected areas alter image by response to sound waves.
    b. Intravenous pyelogram
       (1) Visualizes entire urinary system through IV administration of contrast dye
       (2) Isolates abnormalities
       (3) Mortality has decreased with use of nonionic dyes.
       (4) Dye may prove nephrotoxic when certain abnormalities are present.
    c. Renal scan (renal isotope studies)
       (1) Evaluates renal flow and function
       (2) Displays space-occupying lesions
    d. Computed tomography
       (1) Retroperitoneal lymph nodes can be evaluated.
       (2) Intra-abdominal and prostate abnormalities revealed
    e. Magnetic resonance imaging (MRI)
       (1) Better contrast between normal and pathological tissue
       (2) Avoids obscuring bone artifacts
       (3) Allows direct imaging of plane
          (a) Transverse
          (b) Sagittal
          (c) Coronal
       (4) Valuable in evaluating renal and prostate abnormalities
       (5) Useful tool in assessing cancer response to radiotherapy and chemotherapy
    f. Cystogram
       (1) Radiopaque dye instilled into bladder through cystoscopy or catheterization.
       (2) Usually performed when reflux suspected
    g. Retrograde pyelogram, ureteroscopy
       (1) Done with cystoscopy using radiopaque dye
       (2) Ureters catheterized
       (3) Direct vision and fluoroscopic views of ureters and kidneys
    h. Angiogram
       (1) Renal arteries catheterized under fluoroscopy
       (2) Demonstrates integrity of renal circulation and great vessels
       (3) Renal artery stenosis and pheochromocytoma may be identified.

       i. Chest x-ray

       j. Flat plate x-ray (kidney, ureter, & bladder (KUB)

       k. Electrocardiogram (ECG)

  F. Establish nursing diagnosis based on data retrieval.

  G. Develop care plan according to findings.

  H. Implement care using criteria of nursing process.

  I. Evaluate patient outcomes.

VII. NURSING DIAGNOSIS

  A. Examples of related categories

    1. Fluid volume imbalance

    2. Altered tissue perfusion

    3. Alteration in urinary elimination

    4. Potential for infection

    5. Electrolyte imbalance

    6. Disturbance of self-esteem

    7. Potential for pain or comfort abnormality

    8. Impaired pulmonary exchange

    9. Potential for anxiety

    10. Potential for positional injury

VIII. RENAL SURGERY

  A. Adrenalectomy

    1. Purpose and procedure

      a. Correct hypersecretion of adrenal hormones.

      b. Remove neoplasms.

      c. Secondary treatment of hormone-dependent carcinomas

        (1) Breast

        (2) Prostate

      d. Surgical approaches

        (1) Transthoracic

        (2) Thoracolumbar

        (3) Upper abdominal

        (4) Flank

        (5) Laparoscopic

    2. Intraoperative concerns

      a. Damage to:

        (1) Liver

        (2) Pancreas

        (3) Spleen

        (4) Pleura

      b. Maintenance of appropriate cortisone levels

      c. Fluid volume imbalance

      d. Inadequate pulmonary perfusion

      e. Hypotension with pheochromocytoma

      f. Potential for deep vein thrombosis/pulmonary embolus

    3. Postanesthesia priorities

      a. Cortisone administration may be indicated if bilateral.

      b. Counteract preoperative antihypertensive agents.

      c. Administer IV fluids to maintain blood volume.

      d. Be alert for signs of hemorrhage and shock.

      e. Maintain adequate pulmonary perfusion.

      f. Closely monitor cardiovascular status.

      g. Monitor hourly urine output.

      h. Monitor electrolyte values as ordered/indicated.

      i. Increased susceptibility to infection requires strict dressing and drain techniques.

      j. Judiciously use narcotics (heightened effect with decreased adrenal function).

    4. Psychosocial concerns

      a. Change in lifestyle

      b. Threat of cancer

     5. Complications

       a. Hypovolemic and hyponatremic shock

       b. Hemorrhage

       c. Dehydration

       d. Infection

B. Renal transplantation

  1. Purpose and procedure

     a. Reverse end-stage renal disease.

     b. Transplantation from cadaver or living donor

     c. Includes anastomosis of renal artery of donor organ to hypogastric or common iliac artery of recipient

     d. Kidney placed in pelvic fossa

     e. Continuity of urinary tract established by implanting donor ureter into recipient bladder

     f. Midline abdominal incision

       (1) Xiphoid to pubis

       (2) Bilateral supraumbilical transverse extensions

  2. Intraoperative concerns

     a. Preoperative elimination of potential sources of infection

       (1) Dialysis cannulas

       (2) Bladder infection

       (3) Dental abscesses

       (4) Upper respiratory infection

       (5) Skin conditions

       (6) Potential for deep vein thrombosis/pulmonary embolus

     b. Minimize shock that adversely affects new kidney's function.

     c. Control hypertension.

     d. Avoid agents metabolized by kidney.

     e. Monitor and control electrolyte balance.

  3. Postanesthesia priorities

     a. Preparation and assembly of patient care supplies

       (1) Blood collection tubes

         (a) CBC

         (b) Clotting factors

         (c) Electrolytes

         (d) BUN

         (e) Creatinine

         (f) Liver enzymes

         (g) Glucose

         (h) Arterial blood gases

       (2) Urine collection containers

       (3) Sterile specimen tubes

       (4) Hemodynamic monitoring equipment

       (5) Intravenous solutions

         (a) D_5 one-half normal saline (5% dextrose in a solution of 0.45% sodium chloride)

         (b) D_5 one-quarter normal saline (5% dextrose in a solution of 0.225% sodium chloride)

         (c) Ringer's lactate

         (d) Plasmanate

         (e) D_5W (5% dextrose in water)

       (6) Medications

         (a) Furosemide (Lasix)

         (b) Sodium bicarbonate

         (c) Methylprednisolone (hydrocortisone)

         (d) Antihypertensive agents

         (e) Immunosuppressive drugs as per hospital protocol (e.g., cyclosporin A)

       (7) Sterile irrigating solutions and syringes

        (8) Protective isolation measures as per hospital protocol (patient immunosuppressed)

  b. Data retrieval

        (1) Establish presence of hepatitis or serum-positive antigens.

        (2) Note times of last steroids and antibiotics.

  c. Monitor all vital signs frequently.

        (1) Patients generally hypertensive

        (2) Temperature may fluctuate.

  d. Monitor central venous pressure lines frequently.

        (1) Assess blood volume.

        (2) Ensure adequate kidney perfusion.

  e. Replace crystalloids and colloids.

        (1) Urinary output may be massive (especially with living donor kidney).

        (2) Measure urinary output scrupulously and at specified intervals.

        (3) Insensible body fluid loss

  f. Maintain patency of catheters.

  g. Initiate pulmonary toilet to combat upper respiratory complications.

  h. Collect ordered laboratory specimens.

        (1) Blood

        (2) Urine

  i. Administer medications as indicated.

        (1) Steroids

        (2) Antibiotics

        (3) Immunosuppressants

        (4) Antihypertensive agents

4. Psychosocial and interfamily concerns

  a. Patient has undergone extreme physical, mental, and psychological strain.

        (1) Hemodialysis

        (2) Transplant seen as last chance for health

        (3) Fear of rejection

        (4) May display excessive concern about renal function

  b. Nurse will need to maintain inner calm and tolerance.

5. Complications

  a. Early onset

        (1) Anuria or oliguria from hypovolemia

            (a) Acute tubular necrosis

            (b) Thrombosis (especially renal artery)

            (c) Operative difficulties

        (2) Hyperacute rejection (immediate nephrectomy mandated)

  b. Delayed onset

        (1) Acute or chronic rejection

        (2) Ureteral obstruction

        (3) Infection

            (a) Constant threat to success of transplant

            (b) Nonpathogenic bacteria and viruses may become opportunistic organisms.

        (4) Steroid reaction

            (a) Gastric bleeding or perforation

            (b) Emotional disturbances or altered body image

            (c) Aseptic bone necrosis

                (i)   Position and turn patient gently.

                (ii) Minimal use of tape due to tissue friability

            (d) Nephrotoxicity to cyclosporin A

C. Nephrectomy (radical nephrectomy, nephroureterectomy)

  1. Purpose and procedure

    a. Reasons for removal of kidney

        (1) Malignancy

        (2) Extensive renal calculi

        (3) Trauma

(4) Renal vascular disease

(5) Infection

(6) Polycystic disease

(a) Medical management and eventual transplant are preferred methods.

(b) Carcinoma may develop from long-term dialysis, requiring organ removal.

b. May include excision of ureter or adrenal gland, or both

c. Surgical approaches

(1) Flank or lumbar incision

(2) Transabdominal

(3) Thoracoabdominal

(4) Laparoscopic (also includes "partial nephrectomy")

(a) Renal cyst decortication

(b) Cryoablation of renal neoplasm

(c) Refer to laparoscopic procedures

2. Intraoperative concerns

a. Flank and lumbar approaches

(1) Position causes compression of dependent side.

(a) Altered pulmonary perfusion

(b) Pressure points on bony prominences

(c) Brachial plexus injuries

(d) Compromise of arterial and venous circulation

(e) Pneumothorax

(2) Potential injury to peritoneum

b. Transabdominal (not commonly used)

(1) Potential injury to:

(a) Liver

(b) Pancreas

(c) Spleen

(2) Proximity to aorta and vena cava

(3) Fluid volume and electrolyte depletion

(a) Increased incidence of third-space losses with this approach

(b) Altered tissue perfusion

c. Thoracoabdominal approach

(1) Same concerns as flank approach

(2) Dependent lung deflated intraoperatively; postoperative chest tube may be indicated.

d. Laparoscopic

(1) Potential injury to liver, spleen, or pleura

(2) Hemorrhage

(3) Concerns related to flank approach

3. Postanesthesia priorities

a. Accurate intake and output records

b. Skin integrity

c. Adequate pulmonary perfusion

d. Fluid volume and electrolyte replacement

e. Maintain comfort level.

(1) Position on affected side to limit stress on suture line.

(2) Pain medication

f. Deep vein thrombosis/pulmonary embolus prophylaxis

4. Psychosocial concerns

a. Threat of disease to remaining kidney

b. Anxiety over potential metastasis

5. Complications

a. Hemorrhage

b. Atelectasis

D. Extracorporeal shock wave lithotripsy

1. Purpose and procedure

a. Noninvasive treatment modality for obstructive renal stone disease

              (1) Patient placed over water-filled cushions

              (2) External shock waves directed at renal and ureteral calculi

              (3) Calculi selectively disintegrated

         b. Remnants pass in urine through forced diuresis.

         c. Ureteral stent placed to maintain patency of ureter (not always required)

      2. Intraoperative concerns

         a. Hemorrhage

         b. Ureteroscopy or percutaneous nephroscopy may be necessary.

         c. Maintenance of pulmonary exchange and heart rate

              (1) Monitored IV sedation, general or spinal anesthesia

              (2) ECG monitored to assess for arrhythmias as result of shock waves

      3. Postanesthesia priorities

         a. Maintain adequate fluid replacement.

         b. Manage postoperative pain.

         c. Strain all urine for stone debris (patient to go home with strainer).

      4. Psychosocial concerns

         a. Altered body image if nephrostomy tube present

         b. Bruising over areas of shock entry

         c. Anxiety over potential postoperative hematuria; may last 2 to 3 days

         d. Anxiety about safety of procedure

      5. Complications

         a. Hemorrhage

         b. Subcapsular hematoma

         c. Steinstrasse ("street of stones," often resulting in obstruction)

         d. Renal colic

         e. Sepsis

         f. Hypertension

         g. Skin bruising

   E. Ureterolithotomy, pyelolithotomy, or nephrolithotomy

      1. Purpose and procedure

         a. Surgical removal of large and adherent renal and ureteral calculi

         b. Flank, supine, prone, or laparoscopic approach

         c. Ureteral stent placed to maintain patency of ureter

      2. Intraoperative concerns

         a. Compression of dependent side (see information on nephrectomy in section VIII.C above)

         b. Hemorrhage

         c. Renal ischemia and parenchymal damage

         d. Hypertension

         e. Potential for deep vein thrombosis/pulmonary embolus

      3. Postanesthesia priorities

         a. Meticulous maintenance of ureteral stents and catheters

         b. Pain management

         c. Adequate pulmonary ventilation

         d. Fluid volume replacement

         e. Intake and output

      4. Psychosocial concerns

         a. Fear of developing more stones necessitating further surgery

         b. Fear of pain postoperatively

      5. Complications

         a. Hemorrhage

         b. Occlusion of ureteral and urethral catheters

         c. Paralytic ileus

   F. Ureteral reimplantation or dismembered pyeloplasty

      1. Purpose and procedure

         a. Repair of ureteral pelvic junction obstructions or reflux

  b. Ureter repositioned at newly created hiatus in bladder or renal pelvis
    (1) Abdominal approach for reimplantation
    (2) Flank or laparoscopic approach for pyeloplasty
  2. Intraoperative concerns
    a. Minimize trauma to involved ureter.
    b. Avoid injury to renal vessels.
    c. Maintain pulmonary and circulatory perfusion in flank position.
    d. Strong fixation of ureter
    e. Integrity of ureteral blood supply
  3. Postanesthesia priorities
    a. Management of catheters, drains, and ureteral stents
      (1) Collection bags labeled
      (2) All drainage devices properly secured
      (3) Report any unexpected color or volume of drainage.
    b. Monitor urinary output.
      (1) Separate record for each catheter
      (2) Assess for blood and sediment.
      (3) All drainage may not equal 30 mL/hr.
      (4) Report any significant drops in output volume.
    c. Administer antibiotics as ordered.
  4. Psychosocial concerns
    a. Patients frequently children
    b. Concern over long-term prognosis of repair
    c. Potential for infection high in early stages of recovery
  5. Complications
    a. Infection
    b. Hemorrhage
    c. Hydronephrosis
    d. Hypertension
    e. Ureteral leak or stricture
    f. Potential for deep vein thrombosis/pulmonary embolus
G. Ureteroscopy and electrohydraulic lithotripsy or laser disintegration of calculi
  1. Purpose and procedure
    a. Diagnose and evaluate patency of ureter.
    b. Remove obstructing calculi.
    c. Involves rigid or flexible instrumentation
    d. Saline irrigation used
  2. Intraoperative concerns
    a. Extravasation of irrigating fluids
    b. Peripheral vascular circulation
    c. Ureteral spasm and perforation
    d. Radiation exposure
  3. Postanesthesia priorities
    a. Monitor electrolyte balance.
    b. Maintenance of stents and catheters
    c. Pain management
  4. Psychosocial concerns
    a. Recurrence of calculi
    b. Threat of long-term treatment for retained stone fragments
  5. Complications
    a. Avulsion or perforation of ureter
    b. Ileus
    c. Urinoma
    d. Ureteral stricture
    e. Alteration in vascular supply to ureter

IX. GENITOURINARY SURGERY
   A. Cystoscopy
      1. Purpose and procedure
         a. Evaluation of:
            (1) Bladder
            (2) Urethra
            (3) Trigone
            (4) Prostate
            (5) Ureteral orifices
         b. Involves flexible or rigid instrumentation
         c. Biopsies may be accomplished.
         d. Method to instill bladder medications
         e. Possible to crush or laser fragment bladder calculi (litholapaxy)
         f. Commonly an outpatient procedure
      2. Intraoperative concerns
         a. Anesthetic may be:
            (1) Local
            (2) General
            (3) Spinal
         b. Bladder perforation, urethral trauma
      3. Postanesthesia priorities
         a. Catheter patency and output
         b. Observe for hemorrhage.
         c. Monitor for dysuria.
         d. Unaltered urinary elimination after procedure or catheter removal
      4. Psychosocial concerns
         a. Fear of cancer
         b. Concern about process of urination
      5. Complications
         a. Incontinence
         b. Hemorrhage
         c. Bladder perforation
         d. Infection
   B. Transurethral resection of bladder tumor or bladder neck
      1. Purpose and procedure
         a. Resection of lesions and contractures
         b. Cystoscopy approach
      2. Intraoperative concerns
         a. Electrocautery safety
         b. Peripheral vascular integrity
         c. Bladder perforation may lead to extravasation of irrigating fluids (very low incidence).
         d. Blood volume and electrolyte balance
         e. If laser used, implementation of appropriate precautions
         f. Hypothermia (irrigation warming units)
         g. Potential for deep vein thrombosis/pulmonary embolus
      3. Postanesthesia priorities
         a. Catheter patency
         b. Continuous irrigation may be indicated.
         c. Monitor urinary output and character.
         d. Infection
         e. Hypothermia
      4. Psychosocial concerns
         a. Fear of cancer
         b. Fear of recurrence
      5. Complications
         a. Urinary retention
         b. Hemorrhage
         c. Electrolyte imbalance

    C. Cystectomy (partial/radical)
       1. Purpose and procedure
          a. Removal of malignancy
          b. Radical required when widespread.
             (1) Involves urinary diversion techniques
             (2) Entire bladder removed with lymphadenectomy
             (3) Lengthy surgery
       2. Intraoperative concerns
          a. Abdominal or laparoscopic approach
          b. Pulmonary and renal function
          c. Fluid and electrolyte balance
          d. Control of body temperature
       3. Postanesthesia priorities
          a. Fluid and electrolyte replacement
          b. Pulmonary perfusion
          c. Catheter maintenance
          d. Nasogastric tube or gastrostomy tube may be present.
          e. Maintenance of wound drains and ureteral stents
       4. Psychosocial concerns
          a. Altered body image
          b. Change in lifestyle
          c. Fear of metastases
       5. Complications
          a. Shock
          b. Hemorrhage
    D. Urinary diversion
       1. Purpose and procedure
          a. Divert ureters before or after radical cystectomy, for neuropathic bladder, or noncompliant interstitial cystitis.
             (1) Diverted to abdominal stoma generally
             (2) Newer techniques create neobladder with internal ureteral diversion and urethral anastomosis.
             (3) Ureteral stents placed to maintain ureteral patency
             (4) Midline abdominal or laparoscopic approach
          b. Segment of ileum generally used
          c. Various types of diversion
             (1) Ileal conduit
             (2) Bladder replacement with section of colon, sigmoid, or ileum
             (3) Continent diversion (Kock pouch, Indiana pouch)
       2. Intraoperative concerns
          a. Fluid and electrolyte balance
          b. Gastric control
          c. Pulmonary and renal function
          d. Patient's body temperature
          e. Peripheral vascular integrity
          f. Potential for deep vein thrombosis/pulmonary embolus
       3. Postanesthesia priorities
          a. Nasogastric or gastrostomy tube
          b. Stomal care
          c. Maintenance of ureteral stents and catheters
          d. Measure intake and output hourly.
          e. Pulmonary perfusion and peripheral circulation
          f. Fluid and electrolyte balance (metabolic acidosis or alkalosis)
          g. Pain management
          h. Central venous pressure and arterial lines
       4. Psychosocial concerns
          a. Depression caused by poor body image
          b. Prognosis may be poor.

      5. Complications
        a. Distention
        b. Mucous plugs
        c. Hemorrhage
        d. Intestinal leaks, ulcers
        e. Infection
        f. Stomal necrosis, obstruction, herniation, or fistula
        g. Vitamins B_{12}, A, and D and iron deficiencies
E. Bladder augmentation
    1. Purpose and procedure
      a. Increase bladder capacity
      b. Neuropathic bladder
      c. Segment of small or large bowel or stomach anastomosed to bladder at dome
    2. Intraoperative concerns
      a. Fecal spills
      b. Fluid and electrolyte balance
      c. Gastric control
      d. Potential for deep vein thrombosis/pulmonary embolus
    3. Postanesthesia priorities
      a. Nasogastric or gastrostomy tube
      b. Hourly urinary output measurements
      c. Pulmonary perfusion
      d. Peripheral vascular circulation
      e. Fluid and electrolyte imbalance
      f. Urinary catheters and irrigations
    4. Psychosocial concerns
      a. Need for intermittent catheterization
      b. Copious mucus discharge
    5. Complications
      a. Metabolic disorders
      b. Hyperchloremic acidosis
      c. Vitamin B_{12} deficiency
      d. Bladder rupture
      e. Urinary retention
F. Bladder neck suspensions
    1. Purpose and procedure
      a. To correct urinary stress incontinence
      b. Various endoscopic techniques require lithotomy position.
        (1) Raz sling
        (2) Stamey or Pereyra endoscopic suspension procedure
        (3) Pubovaginal or tension-free vaginal tape sling
        (4) Laparoscopic modified Burch procedure
        (5) Male sling
      c. Traditional abdominal approach: supine frog-legged or modified lithotomy position
        (1) Marshall-Marchetti-Krantz
        (2) Endoscopy not performed
    2. Intraoperative concerns
      a. Pressure on bony prominences
      b. Peripheral vascular circulation
      c. Bladder perforation
      d. Potential for deep vein thrombosis/pulmonary embolus
    3. Postanesthesia priorities
      a. Maintenance of urinary catheters
      b. Urinary output
    4. Psychosocial concerns
      a. Fear that procedure will be ineffective
      b. Body image

   5. Complications
      a. Urinary retention
      b. Wound infection
      c. Urinary tract infection
      d. Continued incontinence
      e. Retroperitoneal hemorrhage
      f. Organ perforation
G. Artificial urinary sphincter implantation
   1. Purpose and procedure
      a. To correct persistent incontinence and urinary leakage
      b. Most often performed on postprostatectomy patient
      c. Mechanical device placed around bladder neck or bulbous urethra
         (1) Inflation pump in scrotal sac or labia majora
         (2) Reservoir placed behind rectus abdominis muscle
   2. Intraoperative concerns
      a. Maintain body temperature.
      b. Strictly adhere to aseptic technique.
      c. Prevent urethral damage.
   3. Postanesthesia priorities
      a. Catheter care and maintenance
      b. Wound and skin care (skin often raw from persistent leakage of urine)
      c. Fluid and electrolyte balance
      d. Administration of antibiotics as required
   4. Psychosocial concerns
      a. Embarrassment
      b. Low self-esteem
   5. Complications
      a. Infection
      b. Recurrence of persistent stress incontinence
      c. Urinary retention
      d. Cuff erosion
      e. Urethral atrophy
      f. Fluid leaks
      g. Tubing obstruction (kinks)
H. Neuromodulation of voiding dysfunction (InterStim)
   1. Purpose and procedure
      a. Treatment of urinary frequency, urgency, urge incontinence, or
         nonobstructive urinary retention
      b. Pacemaker-type stimulation of sacral nerves ("bladder pacemaker")
      c. Pocket created for pacemaker below waist and adjacent to the pelvic bone
      d. Thin wires tunneled from sacral foramen to pacemaker
      e. MRI contraindicated with implant
   2. Intraoperative concerns
      a. Patient prone
      b. Monitored IV sedation and local injection
      c. Avoid muscle relaxants intraoperatively.
      d. Bipolar cautery preferred
   3. Postanesthesia priorities
      a. Pain management
      b. Edema (ice)
   4. Psychosocial concerns
      a. Fear of injury to device
      b. Fear of dislodging leads
      c. Inability to operate device
   5. Complications
      a. Infection
      b. Persistent pain at pacemaker site
      c. Blunt trauma damage to pacemaker

   I. Pelvic lymph node dissection (lymphadenectomy)

      1. Purpose and procedure

         a. Histological staging of prostatic and bladder carcinomas

         b. Abdominal approach through laparotomy or laparoscopy

         c. Nodes along external iliac, obturator, and hypogastric veins removed

         d. May include removal of nodes along aorta and vena cava (retroperitoneal lymph node dissection) in testicular cancer

         e. Midline abdominal or laparoscopic approach

      2. Intraoperative concerns

         a. Bowel perforation or herniation with laparoscope

         b. Damage to arteries, veins, nerves

         c. Pulmonary perfusion, especially with laparoscopy

         d. Increased intra-abdominal pressure with laparoscopy (pneumoperitoneum)

         e. Hemorrhage

         f. Adequate tissue retrieval

      3. Postanesthesia priorities

         a. Adequate pulmonary perfusion

         b. Intra-abdominal hemorrhage

      4. Psychosocial concerns

         a. Fear of cancer and metastases

         b. Altered body image related to possible future surgery

         c. Anticipation of impotence and sterility

      5. Complications

         a. Lymphocele

         b. Lymph obstruction

         c. Ileus

         d. Wound infection

         e. Pneumonia

         f. Retrograde ejaculation

         g. Infertility and impotence

         h. Scrotal hematoma or pneumoscrotum

   J. Prostatectomies

      1. Purpose and procedure

         a. Transurethral resection of prostate (TURP)

            (1) For BPH

            (2) Done endoscopically with resectoscope

            (3) Laser may be incorporated into procedure for ablation of bleeders.

         b. Retropubic

            (1) Lower abdominal approach to expose and open bladder at urethral juncture with prostate

            (2) Avoids incision into bladder

            (3) Radical procedure for carcinoma of prostate

               (a) Entire gland and seminal vesicles removed, penile vessels ligated

               (b) Nerve-sparing approach become more common

               (c) Significant blood loss may occur.

            (4) Simple retropubic may be done for BPH.

               (a) Seminal vesicles not removed

               (b) Reserved for extremely large glands

         c. Perineal (simple and radical)

            (1) For BPH and carcinoma, respectively

            (2) Patient in lithotomy position

            (3) Incision made behind scrotum between ischial fossae

            (4) Blood loss more easily controlled

         d. Suprapubic (seldom used)

            (1) For BPH when prostate too large to remove endoscopically

            (2) Low abdominal incision to expose and enter bladder

            (3) Enucleation of lateral and medial lobes

    e. Laparoscopic
       (1) For carcinoma of prostate
       (2) Lengthy surgery, 6 to 8 hours
       (3) Requires magnification of laparoscopic image
       (4) Procedure still evolving
2. Intraoperative concerns
    a. TURP
       (1) Fluid and electrolyte balance
          (a) Extravasation, extraperitoneal or intraperitoneal absorption of irrigants (sorbitol, glycine)
             (i)   Transurethral resection syndrome
             (ii)   Newer irrigants have decreased risk.
             (iii) Abdominal pain
             (iv) Restlessness
             (v)   Pallor
             (vi) Diaphoresis
          (b) Blood loss
       (2) Cardiac and pulmonary status
          (a) Hypertension or hypotension
          (b) Bradycardia or tachycardia
          (c) Dyspnea
       (3) Pressure on bony prominences because of lithotomy position
       (4) Peripheral vascular circulation
       (5) Perforation of:
          (a) Bladder neck
          (b) Prostatic capsule
          (c) Bladder wall
    b. Suprapubic
       (1) Suture line integrity
       (2) Bleeding because of vascular nature of gland
    c. Retropubic (radical and simple)
       (1) Bleeding
       (2) Fluid volume depletion
       (3) Hypothermia
       (4) Cardiac status
       (5) Integrity of urethral anastomosis
       (6) Damage to nerves
    d. Perineal (radical and simple)
       (1) Pressure on bony prominences
       (2) Peripheral vascular perfusion
       (3) Integrity of urethral anastomosis
       (4) Pulmonary and cardiac status altered by extreme position
       (5) Bleeding
    e. Laparoscopic
       (1) Perforation of viscera, bowel or bladder
       (2) Pulmonary and cardiac perfusion
       (3) Integrity of vascular ties or clips
       (4) Bleeding
       (5) Security of urethral anastomosis
       (6) Carbon dioxide (CO_2) embolus
3. Postanesthesia priorities (consistent for all; radical and TURP patient at increased risk)
    a. Catheter maintenance and irrigation
       (1) Traction on catheter may be indicated to promote hemostasis of prostatic fossa.
       (2) Observe for occlusion from clots.
       (3) Sudden, excessive bleeding could indicate balloon has slipped into prostatic fossa.

        b. Urinary output
           (1) Be alert for signs of hemorrhage (pink to frank blood).
           (2) Record hourly output volumes.
           (3) Observe for massive diuresis with TURP patient.
        c. Fluid or electrolyte replacement
           (1) Evaluate serum osmolality and other pertinent laboratory data.
              (a) Hemoglobin and hematocrit
              (b) K^+
              (c) Hyponatremia (transurethral resection syndrome)
           (2) Decreased Na^+ values may indicate dilutional syndrome and water intoxication; TURP patient at increased risk.
              (a) Other hyponatremic signs
                  (i)   Shortness of breath, hypoxemia
                  (ii) Mental disorientation (confusion)
                  (iii) Nausea and vomiting
                  (iv) Muscle twitch, apprehension
                  (v) Tachycardia
                  (vi) Hypotension
                (b) Treatment
                  (i)   Administer furosemide to mobilize edema and diurese excess fluid combined with saline drip.
                  (ii) Infuse hypertonic saline (3%-5%) in 100-mL/hr increments for 2 to 4 hours if serum osmolality is low.
                  (iii) Untreated, transurethral resection syndrome has led to seizures and vascular collapse.
        d. Monitor cardiac and pulmonary status.
           (1) Sedate to combat restlessness.
           (2) Evaluate for hypoxemia.
        e. May have nasogastric tube
        f. May have epidural catheter for postoperative pain control
    4. Psychosocial concerns
        a. Impotence
        b. Infertility
        c. Fear of metastases
    5. Complications
        a. Urinary retention
        b. Incontinence
        c. Fistula formation
        d. Urethral calculi formation
        e. Congestive heart failure or pulmonary edema
        f. Dilutional hyponatremia
        g. Delayed wound healing or infection
        h. Hemorrhage
        i. Potential for deep vein thrombosis/pulmonary embolus
        j. Transurethral resection syndrome (often manifested in perianesthesia care unit [PACU])
        k. Erectile dysfunction
        l. Bladder neck contracture
        m. Epididymitis
        n. Osteitis pubis
  K. Minimally invasive surgery for prostate cancer
    1. Cryosurgical ablation of prostate
        a. Purpose and procedure
           (1) Percutaneous transperineal approach
           (2) Uses ultrasound with transrectal transducer
           (3) Multiple small probes placed into prostate gland
           (4) Freezes gland using helium and argon gas (Joule-Thompson effect)
              (a) Argon gas creates freeze.
              (b) Helium causes thaw.

      b. Intraoperative concerns
         (1) Damage to:
            (a) Urethra
            (b) Sigmoid
            (c) Rectum and bladder
         (2) Peripheral vascular injury
         (3) Urethral warming catheter to prevent urethral freeze
      c. Postanesthesia priorities
         (1) Maintain catheter patency.
         (2) Monitor urinary output.
      d. Psychosocial concerns
         (1) Fear of impotence
         (2) Fear of incontinence
         (3) Concern about recurrence
      e. Complications
         (1) Urinary retention secondary to edema
         (2) Sloughing of urethra
   2. Brachytherapy (transperineal implantation of radioactive seeds)
      a. Purpose and procedure
         (1) Percutaneous transperineal approach
         (2) Iodine-125 or palladium-123 seeds
         (3) Uses ultrasound with transrectal transducer and fluoroscopy
      b. Intraoperative concerns
         (1) Risk for seed migration into:
            (a) Urethra
            (b) Bladder
            (c) Perineum
            (d) Neurovascular bundles
            (e) Rectum
         (2) Peripheral vascular compromise (alternating compression stockings)
      c. Postanesthesia priorities
         (1) Pain management
         (2) Maintain catheter patency.
         (3) Monitor urinary output.
         (4) Alpha-blockers may be used to assist voiding.
         (5) Perineal bruising and swelling (ice)
      d. Psychosocial concerns
         (1) Concern over radiation exposure to others
         (2) Fear of recurrence
      e. Complications
         (1) Voiding dysfunction secondary to edema
         (2) Rectal complications
         (3) Urethral stricture
L. Minimally invasive surgery for BPH
   1. Interstitial laser coagulation of the prostate (Indigo)
      a. Purpose and procedure
         (1) Treatment of urinary outflow obstruction secondary to BPH
         (2) May be combined with transurethral incision of the prostate and/or suprapubic cystostomy
         (3) Intended for men older than 50 with prostate glands of 20 to 85 cm^3
            (a) Minimizes risk for impotence and incontinence
            (b) Prostate shrinks over time; no tissue is sloughed.
      b. Intraoperative concerns
         (1) Peripheral vascular injury
         (2) Ultrasound guidance with transrectal transducer
         (3) Monitored IV sedation with local instillation, general or spinal anesthesia
      c. Postanesthesia priorities
         (1) Maintain catheter patency.

    (2) Observe for dysuria.

    (3) Increase intake to minimize bleeding.

   d. Psychosocial concerns

    (1) Fear of cancer

    (2) Fear of recurrence

   e. Complications

    (1) Urinary retention

    (2) Dysuria

  2. Transurethral microwave therapy (Prostatron)

   a. Purpose and procedure

    (1) Microwave therapy applies heat to prostate.

    (2) Able to treat deep transitional zone of gland

   b. Intraoperative concerns

    (1) Cooling catheter in urethra

    (2) Rectal temperature probe

    (3) Monitored IV sedation with local instillation

   c. Postanesthesia priorities

    (1) Maintain catheter patency.

    (2) Observe for signs of discomfort.

    (3) Catheter commonly removed before discharge from hospital

    (4) Patient should demonstrate ability to void.

   d. Psychosocial concerns

    (1) Fear of cancer

    (2) Fear of continued urinary symptoms

   e. Complications

    (1) Urethral burn

    (2) Rectal burn

    (3) Urinary retention secondary to edema

M. Penile implant or penile vein ligation

 1. Purpose and procedure

  a. Correct erectile dysfunction through implant or venous diversion

  b. Techniques for arterial revascularization also being accomplished but less common

 2. Intraoperative concerns

  a. Infection

  b. Hemorrhage

 3. Postanesthesia priorities

  a. Frequent dressing assessment for hemorrhage

  b. Maintenance of urinary catheter

  c. Compression dressings with venous ligations

 4. Psychosocial concerns

  a. Impotence anxiety

  b. Loss of self-esteem

 5. Complications

  a. Wound infection

  b. Erosion of implant

  c. Mechanical failure of implant

  d. Hemorrhage

  e. Persistent pain

N. Circumcision

 1. Purpose and procedure

  a. Correction of constricting foreskin

  b. Surgical excision of redundant foreskin

 2. Intraoperative concerns

  a. Bleeding

  b. Suture line integrity

3. Postanesthesia priorities
    a. Frequent dressing assessment
        (1) Edema
        (2) Hemorrhage
    b. Ice applications as needed
    c. Pain management
4. Psychosocial concerns
    a. Embarrassment
    b. Loss
5. Complications
    a. Excessive scarring
    b. Hemorrhage
O. Hypospadias repair or urethroplasty
    1. Purpose and procedure
        a. Urethral or meatal reconstruction and repositioning
        b. Often a staged procedure
        c. Most frequently found in pediatric populations.
    2. Intraoperative concerns
        a. Urethral damage
        b. Infection
        c. Peripheral circulation or body temperature
    3. Postanesthesia priorities
        a. Catheter care and maintenance
        b. Monitor urinary output.
        c. Fluid and electrolyte balance
        d. Body temperature
        e. Frequent dressing assessment or changes
    4. Psychosocial concerns
        a. Anxiety (most are children)
        b. Parental separation in PACU
    5. Complications
        a. Infection
        b. Urethral stricture
        c. Excessive scarring
        d. Urinary retention
P. Orchiectomy (radical, simple)
    1. Purpose and procedure
        a. Removal of diseased testis
        b. Scrotal or inguinal approach
        c. Adjunct therapy for prostatic carcinoma
        d. Radical may include retroperitoneal lymphadenectomy.
    2. Intraoperative concerns
        a. Cardiac dysrhythmias from traction on spermatic cord
        b. Hypothermia
        c. Hemorrhage
    3. Postanesthesia priorities
        a. Compression dressings
        b. Ice packs
        c. Catheter and drain care
        d. Fluid and electrolyte balance
        e. ECG changes
    4. Psychosocial concerns
        a. Altered body image (loss of manhood)
        b. Concern over fertility
        c. Concern over sexual ability
    5. Complications
        a. Hemorrhage

   b. Shock

   c. Infection

 Q. Penectomy (partial or total)

  1. Purpose and procedure

   a. Carcinoma of the penis

   b. Extent of resection dependent on location and stage of tumor

   c. Prognosis dependent on lymph nodes and metastasis

   d. Inguinal dissection may be necessary.

  2. Intraoperative concerns

   a. Hemostasis

   b. Urinary function

  3. Postanesthesia priorities

   a. Edema (compression and ice)

   b. Pain management

   c. Hemorrhage

   d. Urinary output

  4. Psychosocial concerns

   a. Altered body image (disfigurement)

   b. Fear of metastasis

  5. Complications

   a. Sloughing of tissue

   b. Inability to urinate

   c. Bleeding

   d. Infection

 R. Orchidopexy (orchiopexy)

  1. Purpose and procedure

   a. Placement of undescended testis in normal anatomic position within scrotum

   b. Inguinal approach usually includes hernia repair.

   c. Performed for torsion of the testis to prevent recurrence

  2. Intraoperative concerns

   a. Body temperature (many are small children)

   b. Burns

    (1) Warming blankets

    (2) Preparation solutions

    (3) Electrocautery

   c. Bleeding

  3. Postanesthesia priorities

   a. Traction on testis usually afforded by subdartos pouch.

    (1) Older methods used external fixation with rubber band to inner upper thigh or dental roll to scrotum.

    (2) Older methods increase risk of testicular necrosis.

   b. Titrate small doses of pain remedies as ordered.

   c. Examine frequently for edema and hemorrhage.

   d. Ice packs to scrotum

  4. Psychosocial concerns

   a. Anxiety separation from parents

   b. Fear of surroundings

   c. Promote calm environment to limit activity of child.

  5. Complications

   a. Compromise of testicular blood supply

   b. Torsion of spermatic cord

   c. Hemorrhage

   d. Dislodgment of traction device

 S. Varicocelectomy

  1. Purpose and procedure

   a. Collection of large dilated veins ligated

   b. Commonly in left scrotum

      c. Varicosities affect fertility.

      d. Necessary for pain relief

      e. Scrotal or low inguinal incision

      f. May be performed laparoscopically

   2. Intraoperative concerns

      a. Damage to companion arteries

      b. Bleeding

      c. Injury to vas deferens

   3. Postanesthesia priorities

      a. Edema (ice)

      b. Pain (medication)

      c. Hemorrhage (compressive dressings)

   4. Psychosocial concerns

      a. Infertility

      b. Concern about long-term pain relief

   5. Complications

      a. Scrotal hematoma

      b. Hemorrhage

      c. Continued persistent pain

      d. Injury to vas deferens

T. Spermatocelectomy

   1. Purpose and procedure

      a. Removal of cystic mass at head of epididymis

      b. Not uncommon complication after vasectomy

   2. Intraoperative concerns

      a. Injury to vas deferens

      b. Hemorrhage

      c. Compromise to spermatic vessels

   3. Postanesthesia priorities

      a. Edema (ice)

      b. Hemorrhage (compressive dressings)

      c. Pain (medication, ice)

   4. Psychosocial concerns

      a. Infertility

      b. Pain

   5. Complications

      a. Injury to vas deferens

      b. Scrotal hematoma

U. Hydrocelectomy

   1. Purpose and procedure

      a. Excision of tunica vaginalis

      b. Expression of excessive accumulation of normal fluid between testis and tunica

      c. Generally scrotal incision

   2. Intraoperative concerns

      a. Testicular damage

      b. Drain insertion

   3. Postanesthesia priorities

      a. Pressure dressings

      b. Assess character and amount of drainage.

      c. Scrotal support

      d. Ice to area

         (1) Edema

         (2) Pain

         (3) Hemorrhage

   4. Psychosocial concerns

      a. Embarrassment

      b. Concern about sexual function

      5. Complications
        a. Hematoma
        b. Compromise of testicular blood supply
  V. Detorsion of spermatic cord/testis
      1. Purpose and procedure
        a. Spermatic cord brought into proper position and sutured to scrotal wall
        b. Highest incidence in teenage boys
        c. Bilateral often done to avoid same occurrence in unaffected testis.
      2. Intraoperative concerns
        a. Compromise of blood supply to testis
        b. Testicular hypertrophy
      3. Postanesthesia priorities
        a. Observe for sudden severe pain.
        b. Maintain compressive dressings.
      4. Psychosocial concerns
        a. Anxiety about testicular integrity
        b. Embarrassment
      5. Complications
        a. Hemorrhage (orchiectomy could result if strangulation ensues)
        b. Persistent pain
        c. Sterility
 W. Vasectomy
      1. Purpose and procedure
        a. Elective sterilization
        b. Scrotal approach with patient under any type of anesthesia
      2. Intraoperative concerns
        a. Adequate ligation of bilateral vas deferens
        b. Too high a ligation could result in chronic pain.
      3. Postanesthesia priorities (see information on hydrocelectomy in section IX.U above)
      4. Psychosocial concerns
        a. Ambivalence over decision
        b. Fear of impotence
        c. Association with prostate cancer has been disproved; many patients still express concerns, however.
        d. Concern about continued presence of viable sperm
      5. Complications
        a. Varicocele
        b. Spermatocele
        c. Chronic pain
        d. Migration of vas causing reconnection and resumption of fertility
  X. Vasovasostomy or epididymovasostomy
      1. Purpose and procedure
        a. To reverse previous vasectomy
        b. To correct stenosis of vas deferens or epididymis
        c. Involves microscopic techniques
      2. Intraoperative concerns
        a. Presence of live sperm cells
        b. Stress on anastomosis because of inadequate length
      3. Postanesthesia priorities
        a. Compression dressings
        b. Assess for bleeding.
        c. Ice to control edema
      4. Psychosocial concerns
        a. Desire for fertility
        b. Fear that procedure will not help
      5. Complications
        a. Infection
        b. Fibrosis at anastomosis site

X. LAPAROSCOPY
   A. Recent surgical modality used as alternate operative approach
   B. Purpose or procedures
      1. Large incisions avoided
      2. Postoperative course tends to be shorter.
      3. Procedures currently being performed
         a. Adrenalectomy
         b. Nephrectomy, nephroureterectomy
         c. Ureteropelvic junction repair (pyeloplasty)
         d. Ureteral reimplantation
         e. Ureterolithotomy, pyelolithotomy
         f. Renal cyst decortication
         g. Cryoablation of renal neoplasms
         h. Pelvic lymph node dissection
         i. Retroperitoneal lymph node dissection
         j. Bladder neck suspension
         k. Radical prostatectomy
         l. Radical cystectomy
         m. Ileal conduit, Indiana pouch, and orthotopic neobladder
         n. Varicocelectomy (uncommon presently)
         o. Lymphocele excision
   C. Intraoperative concerns
      1. Improper trocar placement
         a. Subcutaneous emphysema
         b. Preperitoneal insufflation
         c. Vascular injury
         d. Organ perforation
      2. Incorrect positioning can lead to peripheral nerve damage.
         a. Well-padded bony prominences
         b. Pronated hands
         c. Shoulder braces placed over bony aspects, not soft tissue
         d. Extreme hip or sacral positions done cautiously
      3. Cardiac dysrhythmias
         a. Bradycardia
         b. Premature ventricular contractions
         c. Sinus tachycardia
      4. BP fluctuations
         a. Hypotension
         b. Hypertension
      5. Central venous pressure irregularities
      6. Venous gas embolus
      7. Hypoxemia from restricted movement of diaphragm or pulmonary blood pooling
      8. Aspiration from increased abdominal pressure
      9. Pneumothorax if CO_2 enters pleural space
      10. Pneumoscrotum—most common postoperative complaint
      11. Deep vein thrombosis/pulmonary embolus
   D. Postanesthesia priorities
      1. O_2 to assist pulmonary exchange
      2. Pain management to lessen effects of abdominal distention and muscular soreness from position (patient may experience referred shoulder pain from CO_2 mobilization)
      3. Frequent vital signs with attention to BP and respiration
      4. Monitor urinary output.
      5. ECG monitor to assess cardiac status
      6. Compression boot application if not already completed; deep vein thrombosis prophylaxis based on risk

    E. Psychosocial concerns
      1. Fear of cancer
      2. Anxiety over potential internal injury resulting from surgery
    F. Complications
      1. Fever or peritonitis from bowel perforation
      2. Hemorrhage from vessel injury intraoperatively
      3. Incisional hernias
      4. Unrecognized bladder perforation
        a. Ascites
        b. Hyponatremia
        c. Azotemia
      5. Abdominal adhesions caused by excessive manipulation
      6. Pneumoscrotum, pneumothorax, lymphocele, or lymph obstruction

BIBLIOGRAPHY

1. Cancer Treatment Centers of America at Tulsa: *Hormone therapy for prostate cancer.* Available at: www.brachytherapy.com/hormone.html. Accessed August 27, 2001.
2. Donnelly BJ, Saliken JC: Management of radiation failure in prostate cancer: Salvage cryosurgery—how I do it. *Rev Urol* 4(2): 25–29, 2002.
3. Ellsworth P, Heaney JA, Gill O: *100 Questions and answers about prostate cancer,* Sudbury, MA, 2003, Jones & Bartlett.
4. Gillenwater JY, Howards SS, Grayhack JT, et al, eds: *Adult and pediatric urology,* ed 4, St Louis, 2002, Mosby.
5. Graham SD, Glenn JF, eds: *Glenn's urologic surgery,* ed 6, Philadelphia, 2004, Lippincott-Raven.
6. Kirby RS: *An atlas of uro-oncology,* New York, 2002, Parthenon/CRC.
7. Kirby R, Carson C, Goldstein I: *Erectile dysfunction: A clinical guide,* Oxford, UK, 1999, Isis Medical Media.
8. Krane RJ, Siroky MB, Fitzpatrick JM: *Surgical skills: Operative urology,* Philadelphia, 2000, Churchill Livingstone.
9. Kumar U, Gill IS, eds: *Tips and tricks in laparoscopic urology,* London, 2007, Springer-Verlag.
10. Loughlin KR, ed: *Complications of urologic surgery and practice,* New York, 2007, Informa Healthcare.
11. Miller RD, Miller ED, Reves JG, et al: *Anesthesia,* ed 5, Philadelphia, 2000, Churchill-Livingstone-Harcourt.
12. Moore RG, Bishoff JT, Loening S, et al, eds: *Minimally invasive urologic surgery,* New York, 2005, Taylor & Francis.
13. Nagle GM: Genitourinary surgery. In Rothrock JC, ed: *Alexander's care of the patient in surgery,* ed 15, St Louis, 2003, Mosby.
14. Pagana KD, Pagana TJ: *Mosby's diagnostic and laboratory test reference,* ed 9, St Louis, 2008, Mosby.
15. Partin AW, Schell PJ: *eMediguides.com—urology and nephrology: 05/02–04/03,* Princeton, NJ, 2002, Thomson Medical Economics.
16. Perry K, Zisman A, Pantuck AJ, et al: Ablative techniques in the treatment of renal cell carcinoma. *Rev Urol* 4(3):103–111, 2002.
17. Porth CM: *Pathophysiology: Concepts of altered health states,* ed 8, Philadelphia, 2008, Lippincott Williams & Wilkins.
18. Life Extension Foundation: *Prostate cancer (early stage),* 2009. Available at: www.lef.org/protocols/prtcl-093a.shtml. Accessed May 18, 2009.
19. Ragde H, Grado GL, Nadir B, et al: Modern prostate brachytherapy. *CA Cancer J Clin* 50(6):380–393, 2000.
20. Schultz RE, Oliver AW: *Humanizing prostate cancer: A physician-patient perspective,* White Stone, VA, 2000, Brandylane.
21. Tanagho EA, McAninch JW: *Smith's general urology,* ed 15, East Norwalk, CT, 2000, Lange Medical Books/McGraw-Hill.
22. Tanga SS, Smith RB, Ehrlich RM: *Complications of urologic surgery: Prevention and management,* ed 3, Philadelphia, 2001, WB Saunders.
23. Testicular Cancer Resource Center: *Testicular cancer and self-exam,* 2009. Available at: http://tcrc.acor.org/index.html. Accessed May 18, 2009.
24. Walsh P, Retick AB, Darracott VE Jr, et al: *Campbell's urology,* ed 8, Philadelphia, 2002, WB Saunders.
25. Walsh P, Worthington JF: *Dr. Patrick Walsh's guide to surviving prostate cancer,* New York, 2001, Warner.
26. Whitfield HN, Hendry WF, Kirby RS, et al, editors: *Textbook of genitourinary surgery,* ed 2, London, 1998, Blackwell Science.
27. Winkelman C: Assessment of the renal/urinary system. In Ignatavicius DD, Workman ML, eds: *Medical-surgical nursing: Critical thinking for collaborative care,* ed 6, Philadelphia, 2010, WB Saunders.

38 Gynecological and Reproductive Care

LAURA KRIEGER

OBJECTIVES
After completion of this chapter, the reader will be able to:

1. Describe the anatomical and physiological aspects of the female reproductive organs and structures as they pertain to patients undergoing gynecological and reproductive diagnostic or operative procedures.

2. Identify assessment parameters for patients undergoing gynecological and reproductive operative or diagnostic procedures.

3. Define nursing priorities, concerns, and complications in each operative phase.

4. Define nursing care assessments, nursing diagnoses, nursing interventions, and expected patient outcomes.

5. List pertinent patient education and health maintenance tools.

I. OVERVIEW
  A. Patients undergo gynecological operative or diagnostic procedures for:
    1. Acute or chronic reasons
    2. Elective or emergent reasons
  B. Surgical interventions required for a variety of indications ranging from:
    1. Simple diagnostic procedures
    2. Radical excisions for malignancy
  C. Nursing intervention strategies are discussed as they relate to specific diagnostic or operative situations.
II. ANATOMY AND PHYSIOLOGY
  A. External genitalia (Figure 38-1)
    1. Collectively called the vulva
    2. Mons pubis
      a. Mound of adipose tissue overlying symphysis pubis
      b. Covered with pubic hair in the adult
    3. Labia majora
      a. Outer vulval lips
        (1) Two rounded folds of adipose tissue
        (2) Extend from the mons pubis to the perineum
        (3) Covered with hair
        (4) Protect perineum
        (5) Contain large sebaceous glands that maintain lubrication
    4. Labia minora
      a. Inner vulval lips
      b. Anterolateral medial parts
        (1) Join to form prepuce and frenulum
        (2) Folds of skin that cap the clitoris
      c. Posterior union called the fourchette
    5. Clitoris
      a. Small, protuberant organ located beneath the arch of mons pubis

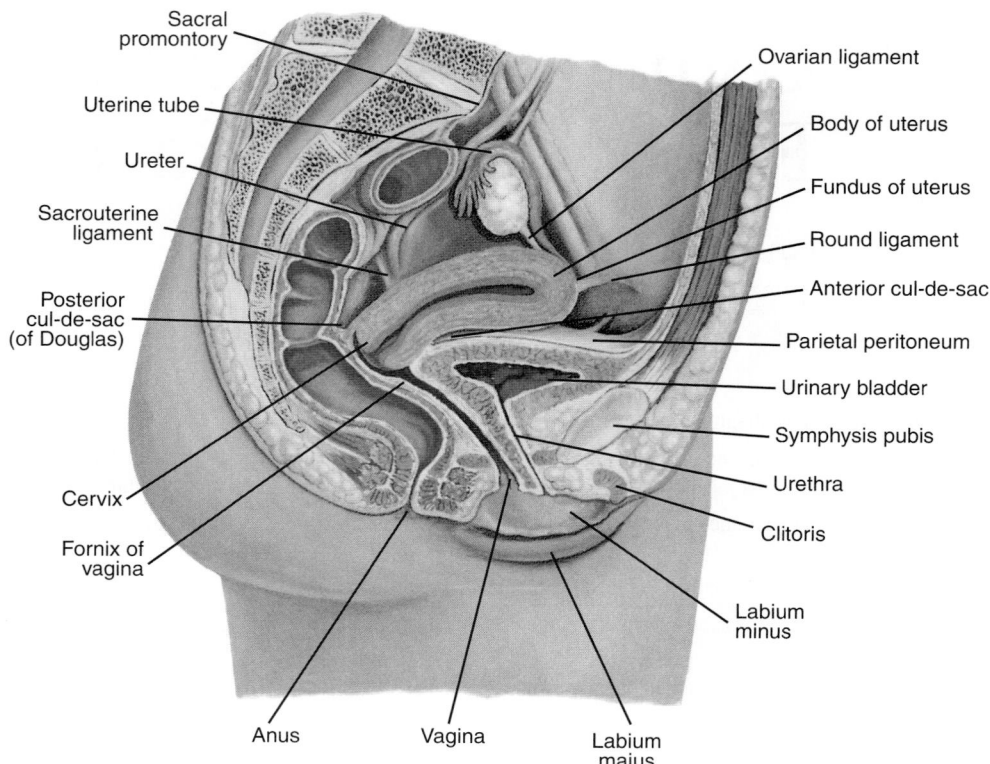

FIGURE 38-1 ■ Midsagittal section of the female pelvis. (From Thibodeau GA, Patton KT: *Anatomy & physiology,* ed 6, St Louis, 2007, Mosby.)

b. Composed of:
   (1) Erectile tissue
   (2) Venous cavernous spaces
   (3) Specialized sensory corpuscles that are stimulated during coitus
c. Urethral opening is a slit below the clitoris.
d. Homologous to the male penis
6. Vestibule
   a. Oval space bordered by:
      (1) Clitoris
      (2) Labia minora
      (3) Fourchette
         (a) Posterior junction of labia majora and labia minora
         (b) Glands lubricate vestibule.
      (4) Skene's glands
         (a) Open on both sides of urethral meatus
         (b) Contain 6 to 31 ducts
         (c) Known as paraurethral glands
         (d) Becomes infected usually from organisms that cause sexually transmitted infections (STIs)
      (5) Bartholin glands
         (a) Open on both sides of vaginal meatus
         (b) Can be palpated when enlarged
         (c) Can become infected usually from organisms that cause STIs
   b. Hymen: thin membrane partially covering vaginal orifice
   c. Perineum
      (1) Anteriorly bordered by top of labial fold
      (2) Posteriorly bordered by anus

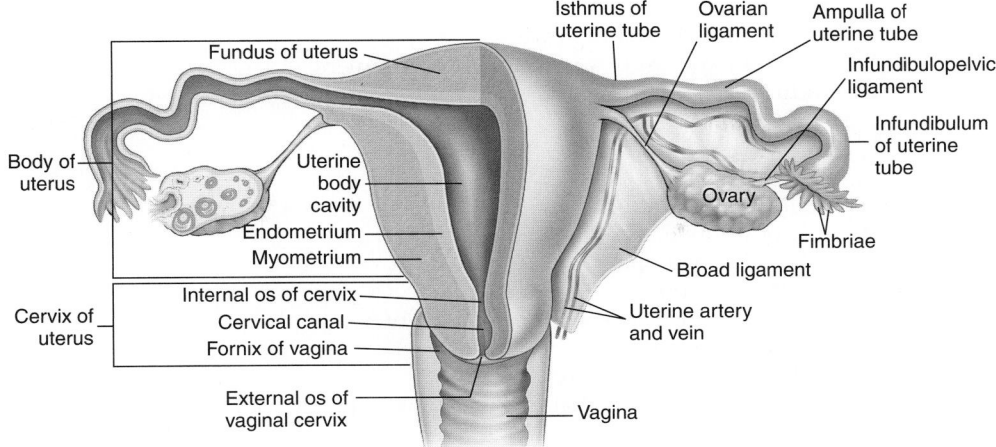

FIGURE 38-2 ■ Uterus and uterine tubes. (From Thibodeau GA, Patton KT: *Anatomy & physiology*, ed 6, St Louis, 2007, Mosby.)

B. Internal structures (Figure 38-2)
1. Vagina
   a. Occupies space between bladder and rectum
   b. Connects uterus with vestibule
   c. Lined with mucous membranes
   d. Conduit for menstrual fluid discharge
   e. Birth canal
2. Cervix
   a. Narrow neck of uterus
   b. Provides passageway between:
      (1) Uterine cavity
      (2) Vagina
3. Uterus
   a. Hollow, pear-shaped muscular organ
   b. Conceptus grows during pregnancy.
   c. Uterine wall consists of:
      (1) Inner mucosal lining (endometrium)
         (a) Undergoes cyclic changes based on hormonal activity
         (b) Facilitates and maintains pregnancy
      (2) Middle muscular lining (myometrium)
         (a) Interlaces uterine and ovarian arteries and veins
         (b) During pregnancy, vasculature expands dramatically.
      (3) Outer serous layer (parietal peritoneum)
         (a) Covers:
            (i)   All of the fundus
            (ii) Part of the corpus
            (iii) Not the cervix
   d. Divided into fundus and cervix, which protrudes into vagina
   e. Lining sheds (menstruation) in monthly cycle in the absence of:
      (1) Fertilization
      (2) Implantation of embryo
4. Fallopian tubes (uterine tubes)
   a. Extend from sides of fundus
   b. Terminate near ovaries
   c. Carry ova to uterus
   d. Facilitate movement of sperm toward ovaries
   e. Move zygote (fertilized ovum) to uterus

5. Ovaries
  a. Two almond-shaped organs
  b. Attached to posterior surface of broad ligament
  c. Produce:
    (1) Ova
    (2) Estrogen
    (3) Progesterone
    (4) Small amounts of androgen
  d. Fully developed after puberty
  e. Shrink after menopause
6. Ligaments of uterus
  a. Wide fold of periosteum that holds the uterus in place
  b. Eight in number
    (1) Two cardinal ligaments
      (a) Fibrous sheets that extend to lateral pelvic wall from:
        (i) Cervix
        (ii) Vagina
      (b) Help prevent prolapse of uterus
    (2) Two lateral or broad ligaments
      (a) Attach uterus to either side of pelvic cavity
      (b) Divide cavity into two portions
        (i) Anterior part—bladder
        (ii) Posterior part—rectum
      (c) Keep uterus in position
    (3) Two uterosacral ligaments
      (a) Lie on either side of rectum
      (b) Connect uterus to sacrum
    (4) Two round ligaments
      (a) Flattened bands between 10 and 12 cm in length
      (b) Situated between layers of the broad ligaments
        (i) In front of uterine tubes
        (ii) Below uterine tubes
7. Peritoneal folds of uterus
  a. One anterior
    (1) Vesicouterine fold of periosteum
    (2) Reflected onto bladder from front of uterus
  b. One posterior
    (1) Rectovaginal fold of periosteum
    (2) Reflected from back of posterior fornix of vagina to front of rectum
8. Vasculature
  a. External genital blood supply
    (1) Vulva
      (a) Blood supply
        (i) External pudendal arteries
        (ii) Internal pudendal arteries
      (b) Venous drainage
        (i) Internal pudendal veins
  b. Internal genital organs
    (1) Vagina
      (a) Blood supply
        (i)   Uterine arteries
        (ii) Vaginal arteries
        (iii) Internal pudendal arteries
      (b) Venous drainage
        (i) Vaginal venous plexus
        (ii) Uterine venous plexus
    (2) Uterus
      (a) Blood supply
        (i) Uterine arteries

        (b) Venous drainage
           (i) Uterine venous plexus into internal iliac vein
     (3) Ovaries and fallopian (uterine) tubes
        (a) Blood supply
           (i) Ovarian arteries from abdominal aorta
           (ii) Uterine arteries from internal iliac artery
        (b) Venous drainage
           (i) Right ovarian vein into inferior vena cava
           (ii) Left ovarian vein into left renal vein
           (iii) Tubal veins drain into:
              [a] Ovarian veins
              [b] Uterine venous plexus

9. Nerves
  a. Superior hypogastric plexus
    (1) Carries sympathetic fibers
    (2) Responsible for innervation of:
      (a) Fundus uteri
      (b) Cervix
      (c) Vagina
  b. Inferior hypogastric plexus
    (1) Three portions representing viscera innervation
      (a) Vesical plexus
        (i) Bladder
        (ii) Urethra
      (b) Hemorrhoidal plexus
        (i) Rectum
      (c) Ureterovaginal plexus
        (i) Uterus
        (ii) Vagina
        (iii) Clitoris
        (iv) Vestibular bulbs
  c. Iliohypogastric
    (1) Innervates skin near iliac crest just above symphysis pubis
  d. Ilioinguinal
    (1) Sensory innervation
      (a) Upper medial thigh
      (b) Mons
      (c) Labia majora
  e. Genitofemoral
    (1) Sensory innervation
      (a) Anterior vulva
      (b) Middle and upper anterior thigh
  f. Posterior femoral cutaneous
    (1) Sensory innervation
      (a) Vulva
      (b) Perineum
  g. Pudendal
    (1) Sensory innervation
      (a) Perianal skin
      (b) Vulva
      (c) Perineum
      (d) Clitoris
      (e) Urethra
      (f) Vaginal vestibule
    (2) Motor innervation
      (a) External anal sphincter
      (b) Perineal muscles
      (c) Urogenital diaphragm

        10. Associated structures
          a. Genitourinary
            (1) Bladder
            (2) Ureters
            (3) Urethra
          b. Sigmoid colon and rectum
          c. Pelvic floor muscles
          d. Lymph nodes

III. PATHOPHYSIOLOGY
    A. Congenital or anatomical abnormalities
      1. Imperforate hymen
        a. Completely closed hymen
      2. Herniations
        a. Abnormal bulging/pouching of organs/tissues
        b. Cystocele
          (1) Herniation of bladder
          (2) Causes anterior vaginal wall to bulge downward
        c. Rectocele
          (1) Formed by protrusion of anterior rectal wall (posterior vaginal wall) into vagina
        d. Enterocele
          (1) Herniation of cud-de-sac of Douglas
          (2) Contains loops of small intestine
        e. Urethrocele
          (1) Pouch-like protrusion of urethral wall
          (2) Thickening of connective tissue around urethra
      3. Uterine displacement
        a. Abnormal position or shape of uterus
        b. Prolapsed uterus
          (1) Collapsed uterus into vaginal opening
      4. Bicornuate uterus
        a. Usually two separate "horns" that form the top of uterus
      5. Septate uterus
        a. Uterine cavity divided by a wall (septum)
        b. Septum may extend only part of the way.
        c. Septum may extend as far as the cervix.
      6. Tubal incompetency: a blockage of one or both fallopian tubes
        a. Complete
        b. Partial
    B. Endocrine (hormonal) dysfunction
      1. Abundant, low, or no secretions of necessary reproductive hormones
      2. Endometriosis (growth of endometrial tissue outside the endometrium)
      3. Dysfunctional uterine bleeding
      4. Stein-Leventhal syndrome (polycystic ovary syndrome)
    C. Growths and neoplasms
      1. Cysts (closed sack or pouch with definite walls that contains fluid, semifluid, or solid material)
        a. Bartholin
        b. Ovarian
      2. Uterine fibroids, myomatas, or leiomyomas—tumors containing muscle tissues
      3. Carcinomas (malignant tumor growth in epithelial tissue)
        a. Vulvar
        b. Cervical
        c. Uterine
        d. Ovarian
      4. Polyps (benign tumors with pediclea). Removed if possibility that it will become malignant
        a. Prone to bleeding (hemorrhage)

    b. Cervical
    c. Uterine
  5. Condylomata (wartlike growths of the skin)
    a. External genitalia
    b. Anal region
  D. Infections and inflammatory processes
    1. Pelvic inflammatory disease (PID)
      a. Affects abdominal organs
      b. May result in infertility
    2. Abscesses (encapsulated infective material)
      a. Perineal region
      b. Abdominal organs
    3. Fistulas (abnormal connection or passageway between two epithelium-lined organs)
      a. Urethrovaginal
      b. Rectovaginal
  E. Pregnancy related (see Chapter 39)
    1. Abortion
      a. Incomplete
        (1) Abortion in which parts of products of conception have been retained in uterus
      b. Missed
        (1) Abortion in which fetus has died before twentieth completed week of gestation
        (2) Products of conception retained in uterus for 8 weeks or longer
      c. Therapeutic
        (1) Abortion performed when mental or physical health of mother is endangered by continuation of pregnancy
    2. Incompetent cervix
    3. Ectopic pregnancy (pregnancy occurring outside uterine cavity)
      a. Commonly occurs in fallopian tube
      b. Life-threatening if ruptured
        (1) Hemorrhage
        (2) Loss of fallopian tube and/or ovary
    4. Hydatidiform mole—degenerative process in chorionic villi that gives rise to:
      a. Multiple cysts
      b. Rapid growth of uterus
      c. Possible hemorrhage
      d. Surgical removal by laparotomy
IV. DIAGNOSTIC/PREOPERATIVE EVALUATION
  A. Physical examination of external genitalia
    1. Pelvic
      a. Inspection of external genitalia and pubic hair to assess sexual maturity
    2. Labia
      a. Gently spread the labia majora and minora and inspect area.
      b. Area should be free from moisture and free from lesions.
      c. May detect a normal discharge that should be:
        (1) Odorless
        (2) Nonirritating to the mucosa
    3. Vestibule
      a. Inspect the area around Bartholin's and Skene's glands.
      b. Check for:
        (1) Swelling
        (2) Redness
        (3) Lesions
        (4) Discharge
        (5) Unusual odor

      c. Inspect the vaginal opening, noting whether hymen:
        (1) Intact
        (2) Perforated
   4. External genitalia
      a. Spread labia with one hand and palpate with the other.
      b. Labia should feel soft.
      c. Note swelling, hardness, or tenderness.
      d. If mass or lesion detected:
        (1) Palpate it to determine its size, shape, and consistency.

B. Physical examination of internal genitalia
   1. Speculum examination of vagina and cervix
   2. Obtain a specimen for a Papanicolaou's test (Pap smear).
      a. Detection and diagnosis of malignant and premalignant conditions
        (1) Vagina
        (2) Cervix
        (3) Endometrium
      b. Obtain wet preparation.
        (1) Yeast infection
        (2) Bacterial infection
        (3) Trichomonas
      c. Cultures for STIs
        (1) Gonorrhea
        (2) Chlamydia
   3. Palpating the internal genitalia
      a. Note tenderness or nodularity in vaginal wall.
      b. Bulging of vaginal walls during "bearing down" may indicate:
        (1) Cystocele
        (2) Rectocele
   4. Bimanual palpation of uterus and ovaries
      a. Performed by advanced practitioners
      b. Allows evaluation of:
        (1) Rectovaginal area
        (2) Posterior part of uterus and pelvic cavity
        (3) Rectum
        (4) Feel the edges of the cervix and lower posterior wall of the uterus.

C. Subjective data
   1. Characteristics (Box 38-1)
      a. Menstrual history
      b. Onset of menses
      c. Length of cycles
      d. Regularity of cycles
      e. Duration, amount, and content of flow
      f. Date of last menstrual cycle
      g. Contraceptive use or absence
   2. Sexual activity, sexual partners
   3. Virilizing features
      a. Hair growth
      b. Irregular or absent periods
   4. Emotional status
      a. Evaluation of adequacies or deficiencies
   5. Psychosocial
      a. Maintain sympathetic and understanding approach.
   6. Special situations
      a. Infertility
        (1) May be associated with:
          (a) Specific psychological problems
          (b) Stress
          (c) Anxiety
          (d) Compulsive-obsessive neurosis

■ BOX 38-1
■ **DEFINITIONS**

Gravidity: pregnancies, full-term deliveries, preterm deliveries
Menarche: beginning of menstrual function
Amenorrhea: absence or abnormal stoppage of menses
Oligomenorrhea: infrequent menstrual flow occurring at intervals of 35 to 180 days
Menorrhagia: hypermenorrhea
Menometrorrhagia: excessive uterine bleeding occurring both during menses and at irregular intervals
Terminations: spontaneous, elective

        b. Loss of desired pregnancy
        c. Surgically induced hormonal changes
        d. Concerns or fears for invasion of privacy
        e. History of sexual abuse and violence
    D. Additional assessment factors
      1. Laboratory data
        a. Hematology values
          (1) Complete blood cell count
          (2) Type and screen
        b. Chemistry values
          (1) Serum electrolytes
          (2) Glucose
          (3) Beta human chorionic gonadotropin (hCG; pregnancy hormone)
        c. Urinalysis
          (1) Bacteria
          (2) Glucose
          (3) Protein
          (4) Ketones
          (5) Red blood cells
          (6) hCG
        d. Cytological studies
          (1) Pap smear
          (2) Previous cryotherapy
          (3) Biopsy reports
      2. Radiological studies
      3. Ultrasonography
      4. Electrocardiography
      5. Physical limitations
        a. May result in alteration of:
          (1) Anesthesia techniques/performance
          (2) Patient positioning
          (3) Immediate- and long-term recovery time and healing
        b. Arthritis
        c. Musculoskeletal disorders
        d. Implanted joints
        e. Autoimmune diseases
        f. Obesity (obese = body mass index [BMI] of 30, morbid obesity = BMI >40)
      6. Allergies to dyes
    E. Risk factor assessment
      1. Deep vein thrombosis or other embolisms
      2. Obesity; level of obesity
      3. Tobacco
      4. Pregnancy
      5. Chronic or acute pain
      6. Pain tolerance alterations
      7. Chronic analgesic use

      8. Developmentally challenged
        a. Potential behavioral problems
        b. Legal authorization appropriately obtained before treatment
        c. Determination of individual learning capability and education needs of patient and caregiver
   F. Pain assessment
   G. Outcome on sexual activity/fertility
   H. Discharge planning
      1. Outpatient versus inpatient
      2. Address:
        a. Clothing
        b. Equipment
        c. Supplies
        d. Medications
        e. Caregiver
        f. Miscellaneous
  V. OPERATIVE PROCEDURES
   A. External
      1. Hymenectomy
        a. Purpose: to enlarge the vaginal orifice
        b. Description: surgical excision of hymen membrane
      2. Hymenotomy
        a. Purpose: to open the vaginal orifice; used to drain hematocolpos
        b. Description: surgical incision of hymen membrane
      3. Excision and drainage of Bartholin cysts
        a. Purpose: surgical drainage of Bartholin gland for relief of pain and/or infection
        b. Description: removal by cutting or systematic withdrawal of fluids or discharges with placement of Word catheter
      4. Bartholinectomy: excision of Bartholin gland
        a. Marsupialization of Bartholin cyst
        b. Purpose: facilitates drainage and healing
        c. Description: creation of open pouch around excised Bartholin gland and cyst
      5. Excision external lesion
        a. Purpose: removal of lesions
          (1) Warts (condylomata)
          (2) Papilloma
          (3) Malignant growths
        b. Description: lesions removed by cutting
          (1) Laser therapy (carbon dioxide [CO_2], neodymium:yttrium-aluminum-garnet [Nd:YAG], argon)
          (2) Electrocautery methods
      6. Vulvectomy
        a. Purpose: treatment for premalignant or malignant lesions of the vulva
        b. Description—excision of:
          (1) Labia majora
          (2) Labia minora
          (3) Surrounding structures
          (4) Requires skin graft
      7. Postanesthesia priorities
        a. Perineal care
        b. Sitz baths may be ordered.
        c. Pain management
   B. Transvaginal
      1. Cervical conization and colposcopy
        a. Purpose: diagnosis or treatment of cervical infection or carcinoma in situ
        b. Description: removal of a cone of cervical tissue (partial excision)

2. Loop electrosurgical excision procedure (LEEP)
   a. Purpose: allows entire specimen to be sectioned for diagnosis
   b. Description: removes intact tissue
      (1) Advantage over CO_2 laser for:
         (a) Diagnostic excision
         (b) Small biopsies
         (c) Ablations of human papillomavirus–related lesions of anogenital tract
      (2) Primarily used for cervical lesions, but may also be used for:
         (a) External warts
         (b) Flat lesions
            (i) Vaginal
            (ii) Vulvar
            (iii) Anal
3. Laser therapy (CO_2, Nd:YAG, argon)
   a. Cervical cancer in situ
4. Dilatation and curettage
   a. Purpose: removal of growths and other materials from uterine cavity
   b. Description
      (1) Stretching the cervix beyond normal dimensions
      (2) Removal of contents from walls of uterine cavity with a curet (spoon-shaped, sharp-edged instrument)
   c. Often performed in conjunction with hysteroscopy
5. Dilatation and evacuation
   a. Purpose: uterine aspiration and emptying
   b. Description: stretching the cervix beyond normal dimensions and removing contents of the uterus by curettage, suction
6. Endometrial ablation and resection
   a. Purpose: treatment of dysfunctional uterine bleeding
   b. Description
      (1) Nd:YAG laser with a hysteroscope
      (2) Roller ball
      (3) Loop electrode with a modified resectoscope
7. Fertility procedures
   a. Cerclage
      (1) Purpose: preservation of uterine contents
      (2) Description: encircling an incompetent cervix uteri with a ring or loop (or a stitch into the cervix)
   b. In vitro fertilization (IVF)
      (1) Purpose: pregnancy
      (2) Description—using transvaginal ultrasound-guided follicle aspiration:
         (a) Healthy, mature oocytes retrieved
         (b) Oocytes and sperm mixed
         (c) Resultant embryo transferred to uterine fundus after 2 days
   c. Transcervical balloon tuboplasty
      (1) Purpose: open obstructed fallopian tubes
      (2) Description: performed under fluoroscopy, sonography, hysteroscopy
         (a) A catheter is passed through the cervix.
         (b) After injection of dye to detect obstruction, the balloon attached to the catheter is inflated inside the fallopian tube.
         (c) Interior of fallopian tube is dilated until recanalization is achieved.
8. Tension-free vaginal tape (TVT)
   a. Purpose: correction of stress incontinence
   b. Description: placement of a synthetic mesh tape under midurethra
      (1) Local anesthesia most commonly used
      (2) General or regional anesthesia used if additional procedures needed
   c. Preanesthesia assessment and concerns
      (1) Patient taught self-catheterization
      (2) May need to self-catheterize postoperatively

    d. Postanesthesia priorities

      (1) Phase II—standard voiding trial before discharge

        (a) May be discharged with indwelling (e.g., Foley) catheter in place

        (b) Patient education: catheter care and removal

    e. Complications

      (1) Bladder perforation

      (2) Hematoma

      (3) Postoperative voiding dysfunction

        (a) Incomplete bladder emptying

        (b) Persistent urgency and urge incontinence

      (4) Urinary tract infection

9. Vaginal hysterectomy

    a. Purpose: removal of uterus

    b. Description: excision of uterus through vagina

    c. Postanesthesia priorities

      (1) May require 23-hour stay (extended recovery) after procedure

10. Anterior colporrhaphy

    a. Purpose: tightens vaginal wall; prevents or corrects bladder herniation into vagina

    b. Description: removal of excess anterior vaginal tissue

11. Posterior colporrhaphy

    a. Purpose: tightens vaginal wall; prevents or corrects rectal herniation into vagina

    b. Description: removal of excess posterior vaginal tissue

12. Culdoscopy: direct visualization of uterus and adnexa through endoscope passed through posterior vaginal wall

13. Culdocentesis

    a. Purpose: used to detect intraperitoneal bleeding or cul-de-sac hematoma

    b. Description: aspiration through vaginal wall of blood or pus from cul-de-sac

    c. Good diagnostic tool to rule out ruptured ectopic pregnancy

C. Endoscopic procedures—laparoscopy

  1. Laparoscopy

    a. Purpose: diagnostic or therapeutic procedures may be performed.

      (1) Biopsies

      (2) Lysis of adhesions

      (3) Sterilization

      (4) Treatment of endometriosis

      (5) Nerve ablative procedures

      (6) Hysterectomy

      (7) Myomectomy

      (8) Cystectomy

      (9) Pelvic reconstructive procedures

    b. Description: examination of interior of abdomen (abdominal and pelvic organs) by means of a lighted endoscope (laparoscope) through small incision(s) in the abdominal wall

      (1) Pneumoperitoneum created using CO_2 to enhance visualization by lifting the abdominal wall

  2. Tubal ligation

    a. Purpose: obliteration of fallopian tubes to cause infertility (sterilization)

    b. Description

      (1) Rings

      (2) Clips

      (3) Ligation (ties)

      (4) Cauterization

  3. Tubal lavage (chromopertubation)

    a. Purpose: ascertains fallopian tube patency

    b. Description: dye injected through fallopian tubes

      (1) Spillage of dye indicates patent tubes.

4. Fertility procedures
    a. Gamete intrafallopian transfer (GIFT)
        (1) Purpose: pregnancy
        (2) Description: follicle stimulation and oocyte retrieval same as for IVF
            (a) Gametes (oocytes and sperm) replaced through the distal fallopian tube
            (b) Via laparoscopically or sonographically guided tubal cannulation
    b. Zygote intrafallopian transfer) (ZIFT—also known as tubal embryo transfer (TET)
        (1) Purpose: pregnancy
        (2) Description: follicle stimulation and oocyte retrieval same as for IVF
            (a) Zygote replaced through the distal fallopian tube
            (b) Via laparoscopically or sonographically guided tubal cannulation
5. Laparoscopic-assisted vaginal hysterectomy (LAVH)
    a. Purpose
        (1) Removal of uterus for myomata
        (2) Abnormal uterine bleeding
        (3) Adenomyosis
        (4) Malignancy
        (5) Pelvic pain
        (6) Endometriosis
    b. Description: hysterectomy begun by laparoscopy and completed vaginally.
6. Myomectomy
    a. Purpose: surgical removal of a myoma (leiomyoma, "fibroids") to preserve uterine integrity and fertility
    b. Description: accomplished by laparoscopic or hysteroscopic technique
7. Oophorectomy: removal of an ovary or ovaries
8. Ovarian cystectomy: excision of ovarian cyst, leaving functioning ovary
9. Salpingectomy: removal of fallopian tube
10. Neosalpingostomy: surgical restoration of patency of fallopian tube
11. Salpingoplasty (tuboplasty)
    a. Purpose: restore patency of fallopian tube
    b. Description: microscopic reconstructive surgery of fallopian tube
        (1) Obstructed portion of fallopian tube may be removed.
        (2) Tube reconstructed to create patency to promote fertilization
        (3) Reversal of tubal ligation
        (4) PID surgery
            (a) Treat tubo-ovarian abscess—drain or remove an abscess
            (b) Treat adhesions—incise scar tissue that cause pain
            (c) Diagnose problem when
                (i) Other tests not done
                (ii) Antibiotic treatment not working
        (5) Adhesions
12. Intraoperative concerns
    a. Considerations unique to laparoscopic procedures
        (1) Pulmonary and cardiovascular changes
            (a) Pneumoperitoneum creates increased intra-abdominal pressures.
            (b) Pulmonary inspiratory pressure increases.
            (c) Compliance decreases.
            (d) Atelectasis develops.
            (e) Functional residual capacity decreases.
        (2) CO_2 absorption from peritoneal cavity into blood can cause:
            (a) Hypercarbia
            (b) Respiratory acidosis
        (3) Trendelenburg positioning can lead to increased:
            (a) Mean arterial pressure
            (b) Pulmonary artery pressure
            (c) Aortic compression

        (d) Systemic vascular resistance

        (e) Parameters accompanied by a drop in cardiac output

    (4) Marked hemodynamic changes may be brought about during the procedure by a significant release of:

        (a) Catecholamines

        (b) Prostaglandins

        (c) Vasopressin

    (5) Stretching of peritoneum and manipulation of viscera can lead to bradycardia, which responds to atropine.

    (6) Pulmonary aspiration is a risk with abdominal insufflation.

13. Postanesthesia priorities—phase I

  a. Pain

    (1) Shoulder pain common after laparoscopy

        (a) Referred pain caused by diaphragmatic irritation from residual CO_2 in abdomen

    (2) Peritoneal surface inflammation after laparoscopy may:

        (a) Be caused by the formation of carbonic acid (reaction between CO_2 and intraperitoneal fluid)

        (b) Persist for 2 to 3 days postoperatively.

    (3) Nonsteroidal anti-inflammatory drugs (NSAIDs) effective in managing postlaparoscopic pain

D. Endoscopic procedures

  1. Hysteroscopy

    a. Purpose

      (1) Examine the endometrium.

      (2) Secure specimens for biopsy.

      (3) Remove foreign bodies (e.g., intrauterine device).

      (4) Remove polyps.

      (5) Remove intrauterine adhesions or submucous fibroids.

      (6) Ablation

      (7) Diagnose uterine abnormalities.

    b. Description: inspection of interior of uterus with an endoscope, using either a liquid or a gaseous distending medium

    c. Intraoperative concerns

      (1) Considerations unique to hysteroscopic procedures

        (a) Fluid (saline, glycine, dextran) used as distending media

        (b) Absorption and resultant circulatory overload

        (c) Dilution can lead to:

          (i) Hyponatremia

          (ii) Hypoproteinemia

          (iii) Transurethral resection syndrome (glycine absorption)

        (d) Disseminated intravascular coagulation (dextran)

        (e) Anaphylaxis (dextran)

      (2) CO_2 used as distending medium

        (a) Abdominal distention from leak via fallopian tubes

        (b) CO_2 absorption leading to acidosis, dysrhythmias

        (c) CO_2 embolism

      (3) Uterine perforation

      (4) Vaginal bleeding

      (5) Careful attention should be paid to:

        (a) Amount of fluid instilled and removed

        (b) Excessive administration can lead to the preceding complications.

    d. Complications

      (1) Fluid overload

        (a) May be result of significant absorption of irrigant through tissue and blood vessels

(b) May lead to:
   (i)   Pulmonary edema
   (ii) Hyponatremia
   (iii) Cerebral edema and subsequent seizures
   (iv) Respiratory arrest
   (v)   Coma
   (vi) Death
(2) Treatment of fluid overload
   (a) Monitor respiratory status.
   (b) Check serum electrolyte levels.
   (c) Diuretics and intravenous (IV) fluid restriction may be needed.

E. Laparotomy (vertical, transverse)
   1. Laparotomy
      a. Purpose: allows for exploration of abdominal cavity
      b. Description—incision of abdominal wall; incision may be:
         (1) Vertical
         (2) Transverse
   2. Abdominal suspension procedures for stress urinary incontinence
      a. Purpose: surgical treatment for relief of stress incontinence
      b. Description
         (1) Marshall-Marchetti-Krantz (MMK)
         (2) Burch procedure
            (a) Preferred
            (b) Paravaginal fascia on each side of urethra, near bladder neck,
                sutured to the ligaments (Cooper's) attached to the pubic bone
            (c) May be performed:
               (i) With a low transverse incision
               (ii) Laparoscopically
   3. Metroplasty
      a. Purpose: repair of septate uterus
      b. Description: reconstructive surgery on the uterus
   4. Hysterectomy
      a. Purpose: excision of uterus
      b. Description: surgical approaches
         (1) Vaginally
         (2) Laparoscopic-assisted vaginal hysterectomy
         (3) Abdominally
   5. Hysterosalpingo-oophorectomy: removal of uterus, fallopian tubes, and ovaries
   6. Radical hysterectomy and lymph node dissection
      a. Purpose: to remove uterus for cervical cancer, preserving the ovaries
      b. Description—laparotomy to remove:
         (1) Uterus
         (2) Tubes
         (3) Upper vagina
         (4) Supporting ligaments
         (5) Pelvic lymph nodes
         (6) Extensive dissection of ureters and bladder
      c. Portions of this procedure may be performed by laparoscopy (e.g., pelvic
         lymph node dissection).
   7. Radical vulvectomy
      a. Purpose: to treat invasive vulvar carcinoma
      b. Description: en bloc dissection of inguinal-femoral region and vulva
         (1) Skin or myocutaneous graft may be needed for closure of wound.
   8. Pelvic exenteration
      a. Purpose: curative; to remove all cancer tissue and reconstruction of
         diversions for urine and possibly colon
      b. Description—pelvic tissues, including:
         (1) Uterus

    (2) Cervix
    (3) Vagina
    (4) Bladder
    (5) Rectum
   c. Preanesthesia assessment and concerns
    (1) Full and thorough mechanical and antibiotic bowel preparation
    (2) Deep vein thrombosis prophylaxis initiated
   d. Postanesthesia priorities—phase I
    (1) Drain and stoma care
    (2) Potential for significant fluid loss and third spacing
    (3) Pain management
    (4) Psychosocial concerns
     (a) Prepare for altered body image.
     (b) Issues associated with cancer diagnosis and prognosis
   e. Complications
    (1) Fluid overload
    (2) Bleeding
    (3) Coagulopathy
    (4) Trauma to kidneys
VI. NURSING PRIORITIES
 A. Anesthesia choice
  1. Depends on operative procedure, patient's needs and physical habitus
  2. Airway used
   a. Endotracheal tube
   b. Laryngeal mask airway
   c. Mask
  3. Use of total IV techniques (propofol and an opioid analgesic)
   a. Can reduce the incidence of postoperative nausea and vomiting (PONV)
  4. Regional; spinal or epidural
  5. Monitored anesthesia care
  6. Sedation and analgesia with local anesthesia
  7. Local anesthesia used alone for minor or office procedures
   a. Paracervical block
   b. Pudendal block
 B. Intraoperative concerns
  1. Lithotomy position
   a. Elevate and lower legs together to avoid strain of back and leg muscles.
   b. Avoid any abnormal movement of the knee or pressure on the knee.
   c. Avoid extreme flexion of hips or popliteal pressure.
   d. Pad lumbar region to prevent pressure.
   e. After positioning, assess neuromuscular status and reposition if compromised.
  2. Arms and hands are safely positioned and shoulders are padded during Trendelenburg position.
  3. Fingers need protection from impingement, especially when positioning and at end of procedure when repositioning for transfer.
  4. Maintain patient's dignity.
  5. Skin integrity (Braden Scale) can be compromised if iodine-based preparation solutions are allowed to pool under the patient; can lead to burns of the skin.
 C. Procedural techniques
  1. Special cautions and care required with each technique
  2. Refer to equipment training and maintenance literature for specific information on precautions, hazards, and safe use of equipment in operating room environment.
  3. Microsurgical
  4. Endoscopic
   a. Laparoscope
    (1) Usually use CO_2 gas as insufflating medium for creation of pneumoperitoneum

        (2) Gasless: uses a mechanical lift method
      b. Hysteroscope
        (1) Rigid scope most commonly used
        (2) Flexible scopes available, not widely used
    5. Laser, cautery, cryotherapy
    6. Transvaginal ultrasonography
    7. Transvaginal fluoroscopy: used infrequently because of risk of radiation exposure to reproductive organs
  D. Intraoperative complications
    1. Gas embolism
    2. Fluid overload, dilutional hyponatremia
    3. Hemorrhage
    4. Perforation of hollow organs or vessels
    5. Thermal injuries
    6. Aspiration
    7. Perioperative neuropathy
VII. POSTANESTHESIA PRIORITIES
  A. Phase I priorities (Box 38-2)
    1. Airway
      a. Spontaneous, unassisted breathing
      b. Adjunct or endotracheal tube in place
      c. Observe for respiratory complications.
        (1) Risk for pulmonary edema after hysteroscopy if excessive irrigant or distending media used
        (2) If intubated, assess location of tube by auscultating chest (dislocation of tube can occur from pneumoperitoneum).
    2. Hemodynamic stability
      a. Vital signs stable, consistent with baseline
      b. Observe for cardiovascular complications.

■ BOX 38-2
■ **PATIENT EDUCATION AND HEALTH OUTCOMES**

Phase I: Patient Will:
- Express feelings of lessened anxiety.
- Describe minimal to tolerable pain.
- Request analgesic to manage pain.

Phase II: Patient Will:
- Tolerate discomfort after administration of oral analgesics.
- Describe wound care after instruction.
- Progress to upright position with minimal orthostatic effects: dizziness, lightheadedness, nausea.

Extended Observation: Patient, Family, and Responsible Adult Accompanying Patient Will:
- Describe follow-up required.
- Identify risks associated with operative procedure: infection, hemorrhage, pain, vomiting.
- Describe wound observation, hand washing, how to change dressing and pads, how to cleanse wounds, and expected drainage.
- Describe at-home activity, restrictions, diet, and pain management.
- Demonstrate knowledge of medications (analgesics, antibiotics, antiemetics, etc.) by describing purpose and administration of each medication prescribed.
- Express understanding of necessity to report uncontrolled bleeding or pain.

3. Bleeding
   a. Vaginal
      (1) Cervical
      (2) Uterine
         (a) Assess uterine firmness after dilatation and evacuation.
            (i) Oxytocin (Pitocin) may be needed in advanced pregnancy termination to control bleeding.
         (b) Methylergonovine (Methergine) for prevention and treatment of postpartum and postabortion hemorrhage
         (c) Rh factor identified for Rh-negative patients to receive Rh immune globulin injection
         (d) Observe for passage of clots.
   b. Incisional
      (1) Oozing or frank bleeding
      (2) Hematoma beneath incision
   c. Internal
      (1) Perforation of organ or vessel
      (2) Operative hemostasis not achieved or oozing
4. Report from anesthesia, surgeon, perioperative nurse
   a. Positioning of patient intraoperatively
   b. Estimated blood loss
   c. Complications
      (1) Perforation
      (2) Burn
      (3) Excessive fluid administration
5. Discomfort
   a. Incisional
   b. Cramping
   c. Significant pain after procedure—suspect:
      (1) Perforation
      (2) Hematoma formation
      (3) Intra-abdominal trauma
   d. Cervical and intrauterine manipulation may result in prostaglandin release.
      (1) Can result in continued postoperative pain
6. Dressing and drains
   a. Abdominal incisions
      (1) Adhesive bandages or no dressing over trocar insertion sites after laparoscopic procedures
      (2) Gauze and tape dressing over longer incisions
   b. Perineal pad in place after cervical, uterine procedures
      (1) Assess on arrival and regularly for type and amount of bleeding.
      (2) Notify surgeon of bleeding—saturating more than a pad an hour.
   c. Vaginal packing: removable, absorbable, hemostatic material
      (1) Observe minimal perineal bleeding.
      (2) Patient may have urge to defecate from pressure of packing.
   d. Drains
      (1) Bartholin cyst incision and drainage or marsupialization
      (2) Vaginal drains include T-tube, Malecot.
      (3) Grenade (Jackson-Pratt)
      (4) Maintain patency of drains.
7. Edema
   a. May observe subcutaneous edema from laparoscopic CO_2 insufflation
   b. External vulvar lesions—swelling may be reduced with application of:
      (1) Ice
      (2) Cold therapy
8. Fluids and nutrition
   a. Do not force fluids, especially when nausea and vomiting present.
   b. Causes of nausea and vomiting (see Chapter 25)

(1) Opioid analgesics
(2) Neuromuscular reversal (neostigmine and pyridostigmine have been associated with increased PONV)
(3) Pain also major cause of nausea after gynecological surgery
(4) Starvation leading to weakness, low blood sugar levels
(5) Controversy exists regarding effect of menstrual cycle and timing of operative procedure on PONV.
  c. Hydrate with IV fluids (replacement and maintenance).
(1) Usual lactated Ringer's (Hartmann's) or dextrose-containing solutions
(2) Long laparoscopic procedures with dry insufflating gases may increase patient's fluid replacement needs.
  d. When nausea or vomiting are present:
(1) Administer antiemetics as ordered; determine whether antiemetic prophylaxis given.
(2) Commonly use:
    (a) Promethazine
    (b) 5-Hydroxytryptamine (serotonin) type 3 (5-HT$_3$) receptor antagonists
      (i) Ondansetron
      (ii) Dolasetron
      (iii) Kytril
  9. Postlithotomy and postlaparoscopy neurovascular checks
    a. Nerve damage secondary to:
(1) Positioning
(2) Retractor injuries
(3) Surgical transection
    b. Pain, numbness, tingling of extremities, and loss of motor function in a given muscle group should be reported.
  10. Urinary distention
    a. Risk after gynecological procedures, which either results in edema surrounding the urethra or injury to urethra and related structures (e.g., vaginal hysterectomy)
    b. Overdistention can cause temporary paralysis of the detrusor muscle, taking several days to resolve.
    c. May require indwelling catheter or intermittent catheterization
  11. Emotional support needed
    a. Adolescents and young adults embarrassed
    b. Pregnancy loss
    c. Negative findings and outcomes
B. Phase II priorities (see Box 38-2)
  1. Determine nursing diagnoses.
  2. Nursing interventions
    a. Operative site
(1) Observe for bleeding, superficial hematoma formation around trocar insertion sites.
(2) Change or reinforce dressing as necessary.
(3) Monitor perineal pad drainage every hour and when patient ambulates first time.
    (a) Note amount and type of drainage.
    (b) Notify surgeon of:
      (i) Significant bleeding
      (ii) Passage of clots
      (iii) Excessive cramping
    b. Discomfort
(1) Gently palpate abdomen.
    (a) Expect soft, slightly tender to touch, slightly distended.

   (b) Notify surgeon of:
    (i) Excessive tenderness
    (ii) Firmness
    (iii) Swelling
    (iv) Suspected hematoma formation
  c. Oral analgesic medications initiated in preparation for discharge home
   (1) May have started in post anesthesia care unit phase I
   (2) Combination of opioid medication and NSAIDs can provide effective analgesia after gynecological procedures.
   (3) Determine effectiveness of medications before patient discharged home on same analgesics.
   (4) Patient with history of chronic pain or analgesia use may require greater support and alteration of usual pain management protocols.
   (5) If ineffective, may need prescription changed or other follow-up
  d. Comfort measures
   (1) Positioning and repositioning to relieve or diminish discomfort
   (2) Back rub or massage may be comforting.
   (3) Continue ice therapy as ordered.
   (4) Promote relaxation techniques.
 3. Urinary retention
  a. Assess bladder status.
  b. Avoid overdistention.
  c. Determine adequate fluid replacement.
  d. May need intermittent catheterization until able to void
 4. Fluids and nutrition
  a. Avoid forced fluid intake if nausea and/or vomiting present.
  b. Dry crackers may help ease nausea.
  c. Maintain IV fluids to ensure adequate hydration.
 5. Education
  a. Includes patient, family, and responsible accompanying adult
  b. Instructions
   (1) Infections—signs and symptoms
   (2) Persistent pain or bleeding
   (3) Be alert for complications.
   (4) Pain relief alternatives
C. Extended observation (see Box 38-2)
 1. Nutrition and diet
  a. Eat lightly after the procedure.
  b. If foods do not sound good, avoid and continue to drink fluids.
  c. Usually can begin regular diet after 24 hours, if not earlier
  d. Encourage fluid intake especially during hot weather.
  e. Avoid constipation through increased dietary fiber, bulking agents.
 2. Nausea and vomiting (see Chapter 25)
  a. Prepare patient, family, and responsible adult for possibility of nausea and vomiting.
  b. Caution patient, family, and responsible accompanying adult to call surgeon or facility if nausea and/or vomiting persists for >6 hours.
 3. Pain
  a. Oral analgesics
   (1) Suggest contacting surgeon if pain:
    (a) Not relieved by prescribed analgesics
    (b) Intolerable
    (c) Increasing
   (2) Unrelieved or increasing pain may indicate:
    (a) Infection
    (b) Peritonitis
    (c) Perforation
    (d) Hematoma

    b. Postoperative deep vein thrombosis can develop after hysterectomy or lengthy lithotomy procedures.
- (1) The following may indicate deep vein thrombosis:
  - (a) Lower extremity pain
  - (b) Edema
  - (c) Erythema
  - (d) Prominent vascular pattern of the superficial veins
- (2) The following are diagnostic of pulmonary embolism:
  - (a) Pleuritic chest pain
  - (b) Hemoptysis
  - (c) Shortness of breath
  - (d) Tachycardia
  - (e) Tachypnea
- (3) Patient should call surgeon immediately and proceed to the nearest medical facility for diagnosis and treatment.

    c. Alternatives
- (1) Intermittent ice for external lesions to help reduce:
  - (a) Swelling
  - (b) Hematoma development
  - (c) Pain
- (2) Sitz baths for easing discomfort of external lesion
- (3) Explore with patient, family, or responsible adult other potential pain management techniques.

4. Medications: instruct on administration and how to apply.
- **a.** Antibiotics
- **b.** Analgesics
- **c.** Vaginal applications
- **d.** Topical sprays and creams

5. Wound care
- **a.** Instruct the patient to wash hands before and after:
  - (1) Changing pads
  - (2) Dressing changes
  - (3) Applying medications
- **b.** Perineal care
  - (1) Change pads every 4 hours or as needed.
  - (2) Note drainage: type, amount, and color.
  - (3) Gently wash the perineum with mild soap and warm water, rinse, and pat dry.
  - (4) Sitz baths or perineal wash as prescribed
- **c.** Incisional care
  - (1) Keep wound clean and dry for minimum of 24 to 48 hours.
  - (2) May be instructed to remove dressing after 24 to 48 hours
  - (3) Observe incision for signs of infection.
    - (a) Redness
    - (b) Swelling
    - (c) Drainage
  - (4) Replace original dressing with fresh gauze or adhesive bandage as needed or as ordered.
  - (5) Report signs and symptoms of infection to surgeon or nurse practitioner.
- **d.** Persistent vaginal bleeding
  - (1) Heavier than a menstrual period must be reported to surgeon.
  - (2) Bleeding may increase 7 to 10 days after cone biopsy and cervical conization.

6. Urinary care
- **a.** Indwelling catheter (e.g., Foley) left in for continued urinary drainage
- **b.** Wash carefully around urinary meatus with gentle soap and warm water, and pat dry.

    c. Keep drainage bag below level of bladder to prevent backflow.

    d. Remove at home if ordered by surgeon.

       (1) Send with 10-mL syringe.

       (2) Instruct how to aspirate balloon and pull catheter.

    e. Arrange return appointment for catheter removal.

7. Activity

    a. Rest

       (1) Limit activity until pain, nausea, and dizziness subside.

       (2) While taking opioid analgesics avoid:

          (a) Operating machinery, automobiles

          (b) Using sharp or potentially injurious articles

          (c) Drinking alcohol

    b. Exercise

       (1) For first 24 hours, exercise is discouraged.

       (2) Defer vigorous activity, heavy lifting.

          (a) Restrict until surgeon allows.

             (i) May be up to 4 weeks after surgery

          (b) Aerobic activity increases heart rate and blood pressure, leading to increased bleeding.

    c. Sexual activity

       (1) Depending on location of incision, operative procedure

       (2) May be advised to avoid douching and coitus for up to 6 weeks

8. Follow-up care

    a. Arrange for return visit with surgeon in specified time interval.

    b. Return to work dependent on:

       (1) Procedure

       (2) Patient's work type

       (3) Usually next day for minor procedures

       (4) After hysterectomy

          (a) Return in 1 to 2 weeks

          (b) When capable

    c. Home visit by a registered nurse may be arranged by the surgeon after certain procedures.

    d. Fever

       (1) Contact surgeon if temperature greater than 100.4° F (38° C).

       (2) As ordered by surgeon

       (3) Check temperature every 4 hours for:

          (a) Two days after procedures such as hysterectomy

          (b) Twice a day after laparoscopic procedures (risk for development of peritonitis)

    e. Particularly with endoscopic procedures, patient should continue to get better every day.

       (1) If not, an injury should be suspected.

    f. Keep surgeon's and surgery facility's telephone number available when questions or concerns arise.

BIBLIOGRAPHY

1. Benrubi G: *Handbook of obstetric emergencies*, ed 3, Philadelphia, 2005, Lippincott Williams & Wilkins.
2. Braveman F: *Obstetric and gynecologic anesthesia: The requisites in anaesthesiology*, Philadelphia, 2006, Mosby.
3. Jenkins G, Kemnitz C, Tortora G: *Anatomy and physiology from science to life*, Hoboken, NJ, 2007, John Wiley & Sons.
4. Moore K, Dalley A: Clinically oriented anatomy, ed 5, Philadelphia, 2006, Lippincott Williams & Wilkins.
5. Nagelhout J, Plaus K: *Nurse anesthesia*, ed 4, St Louis, 2010, Saunders.
6. McCann JS: *Anatomy & physiology made incredibly easy*, ed 3, Philadelphia, 2009, Wolters Kluwer/Lippincott Williams & Wilkins.
7. Rothrock JC: *Alexander's care of the patient in surgery*, ed 13, St Louis, 2007, Mosby.
8. Scanlon V, Sanders T: *Essentials of anatomy and physiology*, ed 4, Philadelphia, 2003, FA Davis.

39 Obstetric Care

JUDITH H. POOLE
JOANNE E. THOMPSON

OBJECTIVES

At the conclusion of this chapter, the reader will be able to:

1. Describe the physiological changes of pregnancy.

2. Describe the pathophysiology, potential problems, assessment parameters, and nursing implications for common complications of pregnancy.

3. Describe commonly used obstetric anesthesia techniques and their impact on pregnancy.

4. Identify various assessment techniques to ascertain fetal well-being.

5. List appropriate nursing interventions in the care of the postanesthesia obstetric patient after low-risk and high-risk vaginal and surgical delivery.

6. Describe the pathophysiology, potential problems, assessment parameters, and nursing implications for various antepartum and postpartum complications.

7. Describe the pharmacology, indications for use, and potential complications of commonly used obstetric medications.

I. PHYSIOLOGICAL CHANGES OF PREGNANCY

A. Cardiovascular system
   1. Anatomical changes
      a. Profound physiological adaptations seen to maximize oxygen (O_2) delivery to maternal and fetal tissues
      b. Heart displaced due to placement of diaphragm and shape of rib cage
         (1) Upward
         (2) To the left
      c. Rotation of heart on its long axis moves the apex slightly laterally, increasing the cardiac silhouette.
      d. Suspected cardiomegaly should be confirmed by echocardiogram when radiographic findings include:
         (1) Straightening of left heart border
         (2) Increased prominence of pulmonary conus
      e. Physiologic myocardial hypertrophy results from:
         (1) Expansion of maternal blood volume early in pregnancy
         (2) Progressive increasing afterload after midpregnancy
         (3) Hypertrophy reverses postpartum.
      f. May be a slight increase in contractility during first and second trimesters
         (1) Contractility (left ventricular function) strongly influenced by changes in:
            (a) Heart rate (HR)
            (b) Preload
            (c) Afterload
         (2) Stroke volume and cardiac output increase in pregnancy, but these changes are not associated with hyperdynamic left ventricular function as measured by:
            (a) Ejection fraction
            (b) Left ventricular stroke work index
            (c) Fractional shortening of the left ventricle

    g. Ventricular wall mass and end-diastolic volume increase without associated increase in end-systolic volume or end-diastolic pressure.

    h. General softening of collagen occurs in entire vascular system.

        (1) Associated with hypertrophy of smooth muscle component

        (2) Results in increased compliance of:

            (a) Capacitive (elastic wall) arteries and veins

            (b) Conductive (muscle wall) arteries and veins

2. Heart sounds

    a. First heart sound becomes louder with exaggerated splitting by end of first trimester.

    b. Second heart sound remains normal.

    c. Third heart sound audible by 20 weeks' gestation (90% of women) due to rapid diastolic filling

    d. Systolic ejection murmur (96% of women)

        (1) Caused by increased blood flow across pulmonic and aortic valves

        (2) Generally midsystolic

    e. Diastolic murmurs uncommon and warrant further evaluation

    f. Continuous murmur in second to fourth intercostal space may be auscultated in second or third trimester due to mammary souffle caused by increased blood flow to breast.

3. Electrocardiography (ECG) changes (see Chapter 32)

    a. Left axis deviation by 15°

    b. Low-voltage QRS may be present.

    c. T wave inversion in lead III

    d. Q waves in leads III and aVF

    e. Premature atrial and ventricular beats may be present.

4. Chest x-ray changes

    a. Straightening of left upper cardiac border

    b. Horizontal position of heart

    c. Increased lung markings

    d. Small pleural effusions early postpartum

5. Echocardiogram changes

    a. Mild increase in left ventricular diastolic dimension with preservation of ejection fraction

    b. Functional tricuspid and mitral valve regurgitation

    c. Small pericardial effusion

    d. Increased left ventricular fiber shortening

6. Hemodynamic changes (see Chapter 27)

    a. Central hemodynamic changes of pregnancy may take up to 12 weeks postpartum to return to prepregnancy values.

    b. Normal central hemodynamic values during pregnancy (Table 39-1)

    c. HR

        (1) Increases noted as early as 5 weeks' gestation and plateaus at about 32 weeks because of increased blood volume and hormonal changes

        (2) Increased rate about 15 to 20 beats/min above nonpregnant rate (approximately 17%)

        (3) HR changes are positional.

            (a) Standing greater than sitting

            (b) Sitting greater than supine

    d. Cardiac output (CO): a measure of functional capacity of heart

        (1) The product of stroke volume (SV) and HR

        (2) Increases progressively by 30% to 50% over nonpregnant values

            (a) Normal CO at term is 6 to 7 L/min at rest.

            (b) Fifty percent of increase occurs by 8 weeks' gestation.

            (c) Small decline in CO seen at term from a decrease in SV

        (3) Increase is the result of:

            (a) Maternal HR increase

■ TABLE 39-1
■ ■ **Normal Hemodynamics During Pregnancy**

Parameter	Normal Value
Central venous pressure (CVP)	1-7 mm Hg
Pulmonary artery pressure (PAP)	Systolic: 18-30 mm Hg
	Diastolic: 6-10 mm Hg
	Mean: 11-15 mm Hg
Pulmonary artery occlusion pressure (PAOP)	6-10 mm Hg
Systemic vascular resistance (SVR)	1210 ± 266 dynes/sec/cm^{-5}
Pulmonary vascular resistance (PVR)	78 ± 22 dynes/sec/cm^{-5}
Cardiac output (CO)	6-7 L/min (at rest)
Cardiac index (CI)	3.2 ± 0.7 L/min
Left ventricular stroke work index (LVSWI)	45 ± 9 gmM/m^2

(i) Primarily responsible for maintaining increase in CO throughout pregnancy
 (b) Increased SV (increases 30%-40% of nonpregnant values)
  (i) Primarily responsible for early increase in CO
 (c) Selective regional distribution
  (i) Uterine blood flow increases 10-fold to between 500 and 800 mL/min; 17% of total CO
  (ii) Renal blood flow increases by 50%.
  (iii) Increased perfusion of breasts and skin
  (iv) No major alteration in blood flow to brain or liver
(4) CO further increased in twin gestations to approximately 20% over that seen with singleton pregnancy
(5) Highest CO seen first 24 to 48 hours postpartum
(6) CO profoundly affected by maternal position
 (a) Highest in lateral or semi-Fowler's with uterine displacement
 (b) Lowest in supine and standing position
  (i) Turning from left lateral recumbent to supine position at term can decrease CO by 25% to 30%
  (ii) Result of vena caval compression by gravid uterus
 (c) Up to 8% of women demonstrate supine hypotensive syndrome.
  (i) Manifested by:
   [a] Sudden drop in blood pressure (BP)
   [b] Bradycardia
   [c] Syncope
  (ii) May result from inadequacy of paravertebral collateral blood supply
  (iii) Symptomatic supine hypotensive syndrome does not appear associated with a decrease in baroreceptor response.
(7) Exacerbation of preexisting cardiac disease with critical period for decompensation occurring:
 (a) Between 24 and 32 weeks' gestation
 (b) In the first 24 to 48 hours of postpartum period
e. Systemic vascular resistance (SVR) and arterial BP
 (1) Basic concepts
  (a) SVR = (Mean Arterial Pressure – Central Venous Pressure) × 80 dyne-sec cm^{-5}/CO
  (b) BP = Force (CO, HR) × Resistance (SVR)
 (2) To accommodate the increased CO, there is a physiological relaxation of smooth muscles causing:
  (a) Vasodilatation
  (b) Reduction in SVR

(3) BP decreases until midpregnancy and then gradually rises until term.

(4) In pregnancies not complicated by gestational hypertension, SV remains 21% lower than prepregnancy values.

(5) Diastolic BP and mean arterial pressure (MAP) decrease more than systolic BP; systolic BP changes minimally.

(6) On average, diastolic BP and MAP decrease 5 to 10 mm Hg.

(7) Like HR, BP changes are affected by maternal position.

    (a) BP is lowest in lateral recumbent position.

    (b) BP should be taken using the left arm in a consistent manner, with the diastolic value determined at fifth Korotkoff sound (silence as the cuff pressure drops below the diastolic BP).

    (c) Automated, noninvasive BP monitors are increasingly inaccurate as BP or pulse rates deviate from normal.

f. Venous pressure

(1) Increases progressively during pregnancy

    (a) Result of:

        (i) Relaxant effect of progesterone or endothelium-relaxant factors on blood vessel smooth muscle

        (ii) Altered elastic properties of venous wall

    (b) Leads to decrease in flow velocity and leads to venous stasis

(2) Upper extremity pressures unchanged

(3) Lower extremity pressures increase progressively until near term secondary to enlarging uterus.

(4) Obstruction of inferior vena cava by enlarged uterus leads to development of:

    (a) Dependent edema

    (b) Varicosities

    (c) Hemorrhoids

    (d) Increased risk for deep venous thrombosis (DVT), including pelvic thrombosis

(5) During pregnancy, women more sensitive to autonomic blockade

    (a) Autonomic blockade results in sudden drop in arterial BP from:

        (i) Further venous pooling

        (ii) Decreased venous return

        (iii) Fall in CO

    (b) Seen in response to:

        (i) Conduction analgesia

        (ii) Anesthesia

        (iii) Ganglionic blockade

g. Central hemodynamic findings during pregnancy

(1) Affected by gestational age and patient positioning

(2) Predisposition to an increased risk for pulmonary edema from:

    (a) Changes in colloid oncotic pressure (COP)

    (b) COP–pulmonary capillary wedge pressure gradient

h. Changes that mimic cardiac disease

(1) Normal physiological adaptations of cardiopulmonary system during pregnancy may mimic cardiac disease.

    (a) Dyspnea

    (b) Decreased exercise tolerance

    (c) Fatigue

    (d) Orthopnea

    (e) Syncope

    (f) Chest discomfort

(2) Clinical findings that warrant further investigation to rule underlying cardiac disease include:

    (a) Hemoptysis

    (b) Syncope or chest pain with exertion

    (c) Progressive orthopnea

    (d) Paroxysmal nocturnal dyspnea

(3) Normal physical findings that may mimic cardiac disease include:
  (a) Peripheral edema
  (b) Mild tachycardia
  (c) Jugular venous distention after midpregnancy
  (d) Lateral displacement of left ventricular apex
  i. Intrapartum and postpartum hemodynamic changes
    (1) Labor significantly alters cardiovascular measurements.
      (a) In first stage of labor, 12% to 13% increase in CO
        (i) Primarily result of 22% increase in SV
      (b) Further increase in CO in second stage of labor (additional 50%)
      (c) Contractions result in transfer of blood from uterine circulation to general circulation (300-500 mL).
      (d) Transient increases seen in BP
        (i) Systolic BP increases by 35 mm Hg.
        (ii) Diastolic BP increases by 25 mm Hg.
    (2) Postpartum changes
      (a) Further increase in CO caused by:
        (i) Release of vena caval obstruction
        (ii) Autotransfusion of uteroplacental blood
        (iii) Rapid mobilization of extravascular fluid
        (iv) Immediate postpartum associated with 80% increase in CO within 10 to 15 minutes of vaginal birth with local anesthesia
        (v) Immediate postpartum cesarean with spinal anesthesia associated with 47% increase in cardiac index and a 39% decrease in systemic vascular index without change in MAP
      (b) Blood loss after birth is:
        (i) Approximately 500 mL with an uncomplicated vaginal birth
        (ii) Approximately 1000 mL with cesarean section
      (c) Left atrial dimensions increase 1 to 3 days postpartum; secondary to mobilization of excessive body fluids and increased venous return
      (d) Atrial natriuretic levels increase.
        (i) Stimulate diuresis
        (ii) Stimulate natriuresis
B. Pulmonary system
  1. Physiological and anatomical changes (see Table 39-1)
    a. Respiratory rate
      (1) Increases 15%
      (2) Rates >24 should be evaluated further.
    b. O_2 consumption increases to accommodate fetus and maternal hyperdynamic function.
      (1) O_2 consumption
        (a) Increases progressively by 10% to 20%
        (b) May increase by 100% during labor
      (2) Women more susceptible to early decompensation
        (a) Asthma
        (b) Pneumonia
        (c) Other respiratory compromise
        (d) Increased O_2 consumption
        (e) Decreased functional residual capacity
    c. Decrease in partial pressure of carbon dioxide (CO_2)
      (1) Hyperventilation facilitates transfer of CO_2 from fetus to mother.
      (2) Partially compensated for by:
        (a) Increased renal secretion of hydrogen ions
        (b) Decrease in bicarbonate (HCO_3)
      (3) Results in shifting of O_2-hemoglobin dissociation curve
        (a) Mild respiratory alkalosis results in left shift of curve.

           (i) Increases affinity of maternal hemoglobin for O_2

           (ii) Reduces O_2 release to fetus

       (b) Compensated for by an alkalosis-stimulated increase in 2,3-diphosphoglycerate (2,3-DPG) in maternal erythrocytes, which:

           (i) Shifts curve to right

           (ii) Facilitates O_2 transfer to fetus

  d. Diaphragm elevated because of compression of enlarging uterus

  e. Anteroposterior and transverse diameters increase.

    (1) Lung volumes

       (a) Tidal volume increases 40%.

       (b) Inspiratory reserve volume (inspiratory capacity − tidal volume)

           (i) No change

           (ii) Slight increase

       (c) Expiratory reserve volume (vital capacity − inspiratory capacity): decreases 20%.

       (d) Residual volume

           (i) Decreases 20%

           (ii) Results in a decrease in total lung capacity

    (2) Lung capacities

       (a) Inspiratory capacity (vital capacity − expiratory reserve volume): increases 5% to 10%

       (b) Vital capacity (total lung capacity − residual volume): no change

       (c) Expiratory capacity: decreases 20%

       (d) Functional residual capacity (residual volume + expiratory reserve volume): decreases 20%

       (e) Total lung capacity (vital capacity + residual volume)

           (i) No change

           (ii) Slight decrease

  f. Weight gain, edema, and mucosal hypervascularity may change anatomy significantly.

    (1) Internal diameter of trachea reduced

    (2) If endotracheal intubation required, a small-caliber endotracheal tube should be used (e.g., a 6.5-mm endotracheal tube).

       (a) Facilitates intubation

       (b) Prevents mucosal trauma

    (3) Should avoid nasotracheal intubation

  g. Nasal and respiratory tract mucosa become:

    (1) Edematous

    (2) Hyperemic

    (3) Nasal congestion and epistaxis common; may obstruct nasal airway

2. Acid-base changes

  a. Pregnancy is a state of compensated respiratory alkalemia.

    (1) Chronic mild hyperventilation results in a lowered partial pressure of CO_2 in arterial blood ($Paco_2$).

    (2) Lowered $Paco_2$ critical to ensure CO_2 transfer at the placental level between fetus and mother

  b. Renal compensation occurs with:

    (1) Increased excretion of HCO_3 (less buffering ability)

    (2) Corresponding decrease in serum HCO_3 levels

  c. Maternal O_2 reserves are decreased because of:

    (1) Increased maternal O_2 consumption

    (2) Decrease in functional residual capacity

  d. Because of lowered O_2 reserves, during intubation or if patient has sleep apnea, pregnant woman less tolerant of periods of:

    (1) Apnea

    (2) Hypoxemia

C. Hematological system
  1. Plasma volume
     a. Pregnancy is a natural hypervolemic state with primary renal sodium and water retention.
     b. Plasma volume progressively increases 40% to 50%; greater with multifetal gestations.
        (1) Responsible for hemodilutional changes seen in:
            (a) Serum hemoglobin
            (b) Hematocrit
            (c) Often referred to as "dilutional anemia"
        (2) Plasma volume expansion is limited with preeclampsia; these women remain hemoconcentrated.
     c. Plasma volume increase:
        (1) Begins by 6 weeks' gestation
        (2) Peaks at 28 to 32 weeks' gestation
        (3) Returns to normal by 6 to 8 weeks postpartum
     d. Pregnancy hypervolemia necessary to provide adequate blood flow to:
        (1) Uterus
        (2) Fetus
        (3) Maternal tissues
        (4) Maintain BP
        (5) Act as protective mechanism against excessive peripartum blood loss
     e. Changes in serum electrolytes and osmolality
        (1) Serum lipids and phospholipids increase 40% to 60%.
        (2) Total plasma protein decreases 10% to 14%.
            (a) Primarily due to hemodilution
            (b) With both absolute and relative decreases in serum albumin
        (3) Decrease in plasma proteins, especially albumin:
            (a) Contributes to a decrease in serum oncotic pressure
            (b) Increases risk for pulmonary edema
        (4) Decrease in serum proteins, including albumin, results in a lower ability to bind with drugs and local anesthetic.
  2. Red blood cell (RBC) mass
     a. Volume increases 20% to 30%.
     b. Greater plasma volume than RBC mass results in physiological hemodilution.
     c. Expansion related to increased hematopoiesis in bone marrow and liver
     d. Iron deficit of approximately 500 mg by midpregnancy created by:
        (1) Physiological hemodilution
        (2) Increased hematopoiesis
        (3) Associated transfer of approximately 300 mg of maternal iron to fetus during third trimester
     e. 2,3-DPG concentration increased during pregnancy, enhancing O_2 transfer to fetus
  3. White blood cells (WBCs)
     a. Volume increases 40% to 50% beginning in first trimester.
     b. Highest increase in WBCs seen in labor and immediate postpartum period; levels return to normal within 2 weeks of birth.
        (1) WBC count of 20,000 to 30,000/mm^3 may be considered normal in labor.
        (2) Increase in WBC count should not be used clinically in determining the presence of infections.
  4. Coagulation system
     a. Pregnancy is a hypercoagulable state related to enhanced potential for coagulation and thrombosis.
        (1) Increases in late pregnancy
        (2) Immediately postpartum

    b. Plasma fibrinolytic activity decreased as result of placental inhibitors but can return to normal within 1 hour after delivery

    c. Tissue thromboplastin released into circulation with placental separation

       (1) Increases chance of thrombosis

       (2) Platelet counts appear to remain in normal range.

D. Renal system

  1. Renal calyces, pelvis, and ureters dilate progressively beginning at twelfth week because of relaxing effects of progesterone, and in late pregnancy because of mechanical compression.

  2. Increased risk of urinary tract infection from urinary stasis

  3. Glomerular filtration rate (GFR) and renal plasma flow (RPF) increase 40% to 50% by 20 weeks' gestation.

    a. Implications for drug metabolism

  4. Blood urea nitrogen (BUN) and serum creatinine levels decrease 40% by midpregnancy because of increased GFR and RPF.

  5. Renal tubular function

    a. Tubular reabsorption of electrolytes and water increases in proportion to GFR.

    b. Glycosuria common in pregnancy related to augmented GFR, which results in filtered load of glucose that exceeds tubular reabsorption capacity

  6. Renin-angiotensin-aldosterone system—all components increase during pregnancy because of their increased regulatory roles in:

    a. Circulatory volume

    b. Sodium balance

E. Gastrointestinal tract (GI)

  1. Anatomical and physiological changes in GI tract predispose pregnant women to silent regurgitation due to effects of progesterone and enlarging uterus.

    a. Lower esophageal muscle tone decreased

    b. Increase in intragastric pressure

    c. Delay in gastric emptying

  2. Increased risk of aspiration, especially during impaired consciousness; all pregnant women considered to have a full stomach

F. Hepatic system

  1. Hepatic blood flow increases, but the percentage of circulating blood volume reaching the liver remains unchanged; metabolism changes in pregnancy lead to liver storage and conversion changes.

  2. See slight increase in:

    a. Serum lactate dehydrogenase (LDH) level

    b. Alkaline phosphatase placental contribution

    c. Leukocyte alkaline phosphatase

  3. Unchanged are serum levels of aspartate aminotransferase (AST) and alanine aminotransferase (ALT).

  4. Serum albumin level decreases.

  5. Serum cholesterol level increases 40% to 50%.

  6. Serum free fatty acid level increases 60%.

G. Central nervous system (CNS)

  1. No major CNS changes during pregnancy

  2. Pain response during intrapartum period

    a. Perception of pain influenced by the following factors:

       (1) Physiological

       (2) Psychological

       (3) Cultural

    b. Specific role of beta-endorphins in pregnancy is unknown.

       (1) Pain during intrapartum period may be modulated by endorphins that alter release of neurotransmitters from afferent nerves and interfere with efferent pathways.

       (2) Endorphins may increase pain threshold.

(3) Lower doses of analgesics and anesthetics during labor may be used because of increased endorphins.

c. Analgesics may cross the placenta to the fetus.

H. Musculoskeletal system

1. Mobility of sacroiliac joints and symphysis pubis increased from relaxin and progesterone effects
2. Distention of abdomen tilts pelvis forward, shifting center of gravity, changing posture and gait.
3. Because of hypermobility of joints, be aware of patient positioning in the surgical suite when using:
   a. Stirrups
   b. Arm boards
   c. Hip wedging

I. Endocrine system

1. Pituitary gland enlarges as result of its function as master of all glandular function.
2. Thyroid gland enlarges in response to need for increased basal metabolic rate.
3. Increased levels of human placental lactogen (HPL)
   a. An insulin antagonist
   b. Lead to diabetogenic state
   c. Insulin requirements increase.

J. Placental physiology

1. Placental perfusion directly related to maternal cardiovascular and hemodynamic status
2. Avoid supine positioning of the pregnant patient because of aorta–vena caval compression syndrome; remember to use a hip wedge.
3. When administering vasoactive drugs, the placenta is part of peripheral circulation.

II. PREGNANCY COMPLICATIONS

A. Nonobstetric surgery during pregnancy

1. Types of procedures
   a. Appendicitis
      (1) Most common nongynecological cause of acute surgical abdomen in pregnancy
      (2) Pain in lower right quadrant
      (3) Rebound tenderness and guarding not always reliable because of laxity of abdominal musculature
      (4) Maternal fever not present in majority of pregnant patients
   b. Cholelithiasis
      (1) Second most common nongynecological surgery
      (2) Clinical presentation same as nonpregnant; Murphy's sign less common
2. Anesthesia (see Obstetric Anesthesia, section III, for further discussion)
3. Nursing assessments and interventions
   a. Call obstetric unit for consultation of care and comanagement.
   b. Maintain lateral position or uterine displacement with hip wedge to increase uterine perfusion.
   c. Assess for adequate oxygenation and need for supplemental O_2 administration.
   d. Maintain intravenous (IV) line for adequate hydration.
   e. Assess risk for DVT and implement DVT prophylaxis as indicated.
   f. Monitor and interpret laboratory values, especially hemoglobin and hematocrit.
   g. Reproductive
      (1) Assess fetal HR (FHR), which has a normal range of 110 to 160 beats/min, through:
         (a) Doppler ultrasonography

            (b) Fetoscope

            (c) Electronic fetal monitoring, if indicated

       (2) Palpate fundus for uterine resting tone and uterine activity; assess for premature contractions.

       (3) Assess for maternal perception of fetal movement if >20 to 22 completed weeks' gestation.

       (4) Administer tocolytic agent if indicated.

    h. Pain management

B. Ectopic pregnancy

  1. Definition

    a. Pregnancy implanted outside uterus

    b. Low human chorionic gonadotropin (HCG) levels compared with intrauterine pregnancy

    c. Ninety percent occur in fallopian tube.

    d. Ultrasonography or laparoscopy for diagnosis

    e. Laparotomy or laparoscopy may be performed after diagnosis.

  2. Potential complications

    a. Ruptured fallopian tube with intrapelvic hemorrhage; sudden and unilateral pain

    b. Shock from rupture, preoperative or intraoperative hemorrhage; referred shoulder pain

    c. Pain management

    d. Rh factor sensitization if Rh negative

    e. Aspiration during intubation and extubation

    f. Emotional crisis

  3. Nursing assessments and interventions

    a. Large-bore IV catheter

    b. Assess for signs and symptoms of shock; hypotension late finding.

    c. Possible Foley catheter, nothing by mouth, intake and output (I&O)

    d. Administer blood or blood products if indicated and as ordered.

    e. Assess and intervene for pain and discomfort.

    f. Assess for postoperative complications related to abdominal surgery or laparoscopy.

    g. Administer Rh immune globulin if woman is Rh negative and a candidate.

    h. Give emotional support for pregnancy loss.

C. Incompetent cervix

  1. Definition

    a. Painless dilation of cervix at or beyond 16 weeks

    b. Cervix mechanically inadequate

    c. Repeated second-trimester spontaneous pregnancy losses in absence of uterine contractions

  2. Surgical intervention

    a. McDonald's suture: Mersilene suture placed at cervicovaginal junction and removed for labor; "purse string"

    b. Shirodkar procedure: Mersilene tape encircles cervix, passed under vaginal mucosa.

       (1) May remove for labor

       (2) If future childbearing desired, will remain intact and birth will be by elective cesarean

       (3) Optimal timing for placement is after first trimester (approximately 14-18 weeks' gestation completed).

       (4) Rescue cerclage higher risk of complications

  3. Potential complications

    a. Uterine contractions

    b. Rupture of membranes

        c. Hemorrhage

        d. Fetal compromise because of anesthesia

        e. Aspiration

    4. Nursing assessments and interventions

        a. Same as for nonobstetric surgery

        b. Slight Trendelenburg position to decrease cervical pressure.

        c. Maintain perineal pad count, monitoring amount, color, and consistency of vaginal discharge.

D. Preterm labor

    1. Definition: cervical change or effacement and uterine contractions that occur between 20 and 36 completed weeks of gestation

    2. Risk factors: more than 50% of women who deliver a preterm infant do not have identifiable risk factors.

        a. Maternal

            (1) Previous preterm birth

            (2) Chronic health problems such as:

                (a) Cardiopulmonary

                (b) Renal disease

                (c) Diabetes

                (d) Hypertensive disease

            (3) Preeclampsia-eclampsia

            (4) Chronic hypertension

            (5) Abdominal surgery during pregnancy

            (6) Abdominal trauma

            (7) Uterine or cervical anomalies

            (8) Maternal infection (systemic, intrauterine)

            (9) Low prepregnancy weight or poor pregnancy weight gain

        b. Fetal

            (1) Multifetal gestation

            (2) Polyhydramnios

            (3) Fetal infection

            (4) Placental abnormalities

    3. Nursing assessments: call obstetric unit for assistance and possible transfer or comanagement.

        a. Maternal

            (1) History especially if previous preterm birth

            (2) Uterine activity

                (a) Uterine contractions

                    (i) By palpation: 4 to 6 per hour

                    (ii) Electronic fetal monitor

                (b) Menstruation-like cramps, including thigh pain

                (c) Pelvic pressure

                (d) Low, dull backache

                (e) Change in vaginal discharge or leaking of fluid

                (f) Abdominal cramping with or without diarrhea

                (g) Thigh pain, cramping

            (3) Cervical status

                (a) Effacement: 80%

                (b) Dilation: 2 cm

                (c) Soft consistency

            (4) Membrane status

            (5) Confirm gestational age of fetus or length of pregnancy.

        b. Laboratory tests

            (1) Complete blood cell count (CBC)

            (2) Electrolytes

            (3) Urinalysis or urine culture or both

        (4) Cervical cultures

        (5) Fetal fibronectin

    c. Fetal

        (1) Ultrasonography for:

           (a) Fetal viability

           (b) Rule out anomalies incompatible with life.

           (c) Cervical length

        (2) Electronic fetal monitor

  4. Management: call obstetric unit for assistance and possible transfer or comanagement.

    a. Initial supportive measures

        (1) Bed rest

        (2) Hydration if evidence of dehydration

        (3) Empty bladder

        (4) Lateral position

    b. Pharmacological interventions (Table 39-2)

        (1) Magnesium sulfate ($MgSO_4$)

        (2) Terbutaline (Brethine)

        (3) Nifedipine

        (4) Nitroglycerin

        (5) Prostaglandin synthetase inhibitors

        (6) Progesterone

■ TABLE 39-2
■ ■ **Commonly Used Obstetric Medications**

Class	Action	Indications	Potential Complications	Special Notes
Oxytocins	Increased uterine contractions	■ Stimulate labor ■ Incomplete abortion	Transient dysrhythmias	Hypertensive crisis possible if Methergine given when patient is hypersensitive
Pitocin *Methylergo-novine maleate* (Methergine)	Stimulate milk ejection	Postpartum bleeding	■ Uterine tetany ■ Water intoxication	Undiluted IV oxytocin produces hypotension; administer as undiluted infusion.
Alprostadil (Prostin)	Increases uterine contractions	■ Second-trimester abortion ■ Postpartum uterine atony unresponsive to oxytocin	■ Fever ■ Chills ■ Nausea and vomiting ■ Diarrhea	Given IM or into myometrium
Magnesium sulfate ($MgSO_4$)	Decreases neuromuscular irritability and CNS irritability	■ Prevents seizures in preeclampsia-eclampsia ■ Inhibits preterm contractions	■ Toxicity ■ Loss of DTRs ■ Respiratory depression ■ Cardiovascular collapse	■ Toxicity reversible with calcium gluconate ■ Careful administration of narcotics, CNS depressants, calcium channel blockers, beta-blockers
Tocolytics Terbutaline	■ Relaxes smooth muscle ■ Beta-agonist	■ Bronchospasm ■ Inhibits preterm labor	■ Tremors ■ Anxiety ■ Dysrhythmais ■ Nausea and vomiting ■ Pulmonary edema	May be given IV, subcutaneously, or orally

■ TABLE 39-2
■ ■ **Commonly Used Obstetric Medications—cont'd**

Class	Action	Indications	Potential Complications	Special Notes
Ritodrine (Yutopar)	■ Decreased uterine contractions ■ Beta-agonist	Preterm labor	■ Tachycardia ■ Hypotension ■ Restlessness and tremors ■ Hyperglycemia or hypoglycemia ■ Pulmonary edema	Contraindicated in abruptio placentae, intrauterine infection, severe preeclampsia, and diabetes
RhoGAM	Decreases immune response	Rh-negative woman after exposure to Rh-positive blood	■ Irritation at site ■ Myalgias ■ Lethargy	Must be given within 72 hours of delivery or abortion
Bromocriptine (Parlodel)	Inhibits prolactin	■ Prevents lactation ■ Parkinson's disease ■ Female infertility	■ Headache ■ Nausea and vomiting ■ Rash ■ Orthostatic hypotension	■ With hypotensive agents, can produce significant hypotension ■ May potentiate hypertension
Anti-hypertensives			■ Reflex tachycardia ■ Headache ■ Nausea and vomiting	
Hydralazine	■ Arteriolar dilator ■ Decreases pulmonary vascular resistance	Essential hypertension, preeclampsia with diastolic BP>110 mmHg	■ Bradycardia ■ Dysrhythmias ■ Nausea and vomiting	Alpha-blocker, beta-blocker
Labetalol	■ Adrenergic antagonist ■ Increases BP	■ Essential hypertension ■ Hypertensive crisis		

    c. Implement management protocol specific to each patient.
       (1) Vital signs
         (a) Monitor for signs of intra-amniotic infection.
         (b) Monitor for signs of pulmonary edema.
       (2) Continuous fetal monitor
       (3) Thorough systems assessment
       (4) Strict measurement of I&O
         (a) Hourly if magnesium sulfate infusing
       (5) Maintain lateral decubitus position or uterine displacement.
       (6) Assess for DVT risk if on bed rest.
    d. Assess for adverse effects of treatment.
    e. Provide psychosocial and emotional support.
    f. Administer corticosteroids to enhance fetal lung maturation if indicated.
  E. Hypertensive disorders
    1. Definitions
      a. Chronic hypertension: hypertension present before pregnancy
        (1) Diagnosed before the 20th week of gestation
        (2) Elevations of BP that persists for more than 12 weeks after delivery
      b. Preeclampsia: pregnancy-specific syndrome of reduced organ perfusion

      c. Eclampsia: seizures or coma in woman with signs and symptoms of preeclampsia; no underlying neurological history

      d. Chronic hypertension with superimposed preeclampsia-eclampsia

      e. Gestational hypertension: development

         (1) New onset of hypertension during pregnancy

         (2) Immediate postpartum period

2. Risk factors

    a. Young primigravida

    b. Older multipara

    c. Maternal age <18 years or >35 years

    d. Weight <100 lb or morbid obesity

    e. Diabetes mellitus

    f. Multifetal gestation, large fetus, fetal hydrops, polyhydramnios

    g. Preeclampsia in previous pregnancy

    h. Familial history of disease

       (1) Renal

       (2) Hypertensive

       (3) Vascular

    i. Presence of:

       (1) Chronic renal disease

       (2) Hypertension

       (3) Vascular disease

       (4) Autoimmune disease

3. Pathophysiology

    a. Early in disease process, increased CO or increased SVR increases BP.

       (1) Increased CO with decreased SVR causes turbulent blood flow through vessels; predisposes to endothelium damage.

       (2) Endothelium damage activates hemostatic system.

       (3) Kidneys respond to hemodynamic changes by inducing vasospasm as protective mechanism initially; later in process, vasospasm causes signs and symptoms seen.

    b. Multiorgan vasospasm

       (1) Autoimmune or immune response occurs.

       (2) Increased vascular tone

       (3) Vasoconstriction caused by:

          (a) Increased thromboxane levels

          (b) Decreased prostacyclin levels

    c. Disease process produces state of decreased uteroplacental perfusion.

       (1) Decreased placental production of prostacyclin

       (2) Activation of intravascular coagulation

       (3) Decreased maternal vascular production of prostacyclin and other vasodilators causes vasoconstriction.

       (4) Increased vascular permeability further decreases COP.

4. Nursing assessments

    a. Signs and symptoms

       (1) Hypertension

          (a) New onset after 20th week of gestation

             (i) Systolic BP = 140 mm Hg

             (ii) Diastolic BP = 90 mm Hg

             (iii) MAP = 105 mm Hg

          (b) Increased maternal and fetal morbidity and mortality

             (i) Systolic BP = 155 to 160 mm Hg

             (ii) Diastolic BP = 105 to 110 mm Hg

             (iii) MAP = 130 mm Hg

             (iv) Indication for antihypertensive therapy

       (2) Edema

          (a) No longer part of diagnostic criteria

   (b) Intracellular and extracellular edema may be present.
   (c) Window into organ integrity and oxygenation status
  (3) Proteinuria
   (a) Late symptom caused by destruction of protein-sparing reticulum in kidney
   (b) Excretion of 1 g/L in random specimen or 0.3 g/L per 24 hours
 b. Clinical features of severe preeclampsia
  (1) On two occasions at least 6 hours apart with patient on bed rest
   (a) Systolic BP = 155 to 160 mm Hg
   (b) Diastolic BP = 105 to 110 mm Hg
  (2) Proteinuria: >5 g/24 hours or 3+ or 4+ on dipstick
  (3) Oliguria: <400 to 500 mL per 24 hours
   (a) <30 mL/hr
   (b) 100 mL per 4 hours
  (4) Cerebral or visual disturbances
  (5) Hepatic, pulmonary, or cardiac involvement
  (6) Thrombocytopenia
  (7) Development of eclamptic seizures
  (8) Development of HELLP (hemolysis, elevated liver enzymes, low platelets) syndrome (see HELLP Syndrome, section II.E.6)
 c. Laboratory studies (abnormalities dependent on severity of disease process and organ systems involved)
  (1) CBC shows hemoconcentration: elevated
   (a) Hemoglobin
   (b) Hematocrit
   (c) Hemolysis
   (d) Thrombocytopenia
  (2) Chemistries
   (a) Elevated
    (i) Serum creatinine (>1 mg/dL)
    (ii) Uric acid
    (iii) BUN
   (b) Reduced
    (i) Creatinine clearance
    (ii) Alkaline phosphatase
  (3) Liver function
   (a) Increased
    (i) LDH
    (ii) ALT
    (iii) AST
   (b) Decreased
    (i) Serum glucose
     [a] Severe hypoglycemia increases risk of maternal mortality.
  (4) Coagulation studies
   (a) Coagulation defects determine whether regional analgesia/anesthesia is contraindicated.
   (b) Decreased
    (i) Fibrinogen (<300 mg/dL)
    (ii) Platelets (<100,000/mL)
   (c) Increased fibrin degradation products, D-dimer, and platelet aggregability
 d. Obtain thorough maternal health history to include medical and obstetric information.
 e. Cardiovascular assessment of risk for pulmonary edema, left ventricular failure
  (1) Vital signs and BP; frequency of assessment dictated by condition of mother and fetus during the antepartum, intrapartum, and postpartum periods
  (2) Daily weight at same time on same scale

(3) Assess skin color, temperature, turgor.

(4) Noninvasive assessments of CO

(5) Capillary refill

(6) ECG and pulse oximetry as indicated by clinical condition

(7) Level of consciousness (LOC), behavior

f. Respiratory assessment of risk for development of pulmonary edema or pulmonary embolism

  (1) Assess respiratory rate, quality, and pattern.

  (2) Auscultate breath sounds at least every shift.

  (3) Assess skin color and mucous membranes for cyanosis.

  (4) Monitor oxygenation status with pulse oximetry as indicated.

  (5) LOC, behavior

g. Renal assessment of risk for renal dysfunction

  (1) Assess urinary output every 1 to 4 hours.

  (2) Evaluate urine for protein.

  (3) Maintain 24-hour urine collection as indicated.

  (4) Strict I&O

h. CNS assessment of risk for cerebral edema, increased intracranial pressure, cerebral hemorrhage

  (1) Assess deep tendon reflexes (DTRs) and clonus hourly (absence of DTRs is earliest sign of magnesium toxicity).

  (2) Assess LOC and changes in behavior.

  (3) Assess for headache or visual disturbances.

  (4) Assess for signs of increasing intracranial pressure and cerebral edema.

i. Reproductive assessment of risk for placental abruption and fetal compromise

  (1) Assess for uterine hypertonicity.

  (2) Assess for postpartum hemorrhage.

  (3) Fetal assessments for well-being or intolerance of intrauterine environment

j. Assess for signs of worsening disease.

  (1) Headache

  (2) Blurred vision

  (3) Nausea and vomiting

  (4) Change in LOC

  (5) Epigastric pain

  (6) Developing coagulopathy

  (7) Multiorgan dysfunction

k. Keep calcium gluconate immediately available (antidote for magnesium sulfate).

5. Management

a. Call obstetric unit for assistance and possible transfer or comanagement.

b. Delivery only cure

c. Magnesium sulfate for seizure prophylaxis (Table 39-2); diazepam no longer used

d. Antihypertensive therapy if systolic BP = 155 to 160 mm Hg, diastolic BP = 105 to 110 mm Hg, or MAP = 130 mm Hg

e. Do not give diuretics.

  (1) Will further deplete an already depleted intravascular volume

  (2) Indicated if cardiogenic pulmonary edema suspected or confirmed

f. Do not give heparin; will increase risk for intracranial hemorrhage.

g. Administration of colloid solutions will increase risk of pulmonary edema.

6. HELLP syndrome

a. Triad consists of hemolysis, elevated liver enzymes, and low platelets.

  (1) Hemolysis

    (a) Vasospasm causes endothelial damage, leading to platelet aggregation and fibrin network formation.

    (b) RBCs forced through fibrin network at increased pressure, causing hemolysis

            (c) Hematocrit decreased; bilirubin and LDH levels increased
            (d) Burr cells and schistocytes may be present on RBC morphology.
        (2) Elevated liver enzymes
            (a) Microemboli form in hepatic vasculature.
            (b) Hepatic blood flow decreases, resulting in ischemia.
            (c) Liver enzymes increase; LDH first to elevate
        (3) Low platelets
            (a) Platelet consumption occurs.
            (b) Thrombocytopenia with platelets <50,000 associated with coagulopathies
            (c) Patients receiving low-dose aspirin therapy will have impaired platelet function irrespective of platelet number.
    b. Signs and symptoms
        (1) Nausea and vomiting
        (2) Epigastric tenderness
        (3) Right upper quadrant pain or tenderness
        (4) Significant hypertension and proteinuria may not be present initially.
        (5) May be present as early as second trimester
    c. Form of severe preeclampsia; management same as outlined above
7. Eclampsia
    a. Complicates ~5% of all pregnancies
    b. Pathological mechanisms implicated in development of eclampsia
        (1) Cerebral vasospasm and ischemia
        (2) Cerebral infarcts and hemorrhage
        (3) Cerebral edema
        (4) Disseminated intravascular coagulation (DIC)
        (5) Hypertensive encephalopathy
        (6) Metabolical encephalopathy
    c. Management
        (1) Call obstetric unit for assistance and possible transfer or comanagement.
        (2) Prevent maternal injury.
        (3) Maintain adequate oxygenation.
            (a) Control airway and ventilation.
            (b) Mechanical ventilation may be required.
        (4) Minimize risk of aspiration.
        (5) Give adequate magnesium sulfate.
            (a) Loading dose: 4 to 6 g IV over 20 minutes; be aware of renal function.
            (b) Then 2 to 4 g/hr IV infusion
            (c) Always administer as secondary infusion.
        (6) Assess for and control elevated increased intracranial pressure.
    d. Goals of therapy
        (1) Control of seizures
            (a) Magnesium sulfate as stated previously
            (b) If seizures persist, give additional 2 g IV bolus of magnesium sulfate slowly at rate not to exceed 1 g/min.
            (c) For seizures refractory to magnesium sulfate, give 250 mg IV sodium amobarbital slowly.
        (2) Correction of hypoxia and acidosis
        (3) Control of severe hypertension (systolic BP >155 to 160 mm Hg, diastolic BP >105 to 110 mm Hg, or MAP >130 mm Hg
            (a) Give antihypertensive agents cautiously because intravascular hypovolemia often accompanies preeclampsia-eclampsia; thus these patients are more sensitive to antihypertensive effects.
            (b) Not necessary to acutely normalize BP; overcorrection may result in uteroplacental hypoperfusion and fetal compromise.
            (c) Maintain diastolic BP of 90 to 100 mm Hg.

(d) Administer calcium channel blockers or beta-blockers with caution in patients receiving magnesium sulfate therapy (can lead to cardiopulmonary collapse).

(4) Delivery if indicated
(a) During acute eclamptic episode, fetal bradycardia common
(b) If fetal bradycardia persists beyond 10 minutes, preparation should be made for cesarean delivery, and abruption should be considered cause for bradycardia.
(c) Often advantageous to fetus to allow intrauterine recovery from maternal seizure, hypoxia, and hypercapnia

e. Nursing responsibilities
(1) Note
(a) Onset of seizures
(b) Progress of seizure
(c) Body involvement
(d) Length of convulsion
(2) Maintain and protect airway.
(3) Administer O_2 by tight face mask at 10 to 12 L/min.
(4) Administer anticonvulsant.
(5) Suction secretions.
(6) Evaluate lungs for aspiration.
(7) Evaluate cardiac status.
(8) Evaluate fetus.
(9) Evaluate uterine activity for possible:
(a) Placental abruption
(b) Precipitous birth
(10) Evaluate for timing and route of birth.
(11) Monitor fluid I&O.

f. Postpartum management: call obstetric unit for assistance and possible transfer or comanagement.
(1) Assessment and intervention continue with same intensity for minimum of 24 hours.
(2) Additional assessments done for:
(a) Recurrent eclampsia
(b) Postpartum hemorrhage
(c) Development of DIC
(d) Development of HELLP syndrome
(e) Development of acute renal failure

F. Hemorrhagic disorders
1. Hemorrhagic disorders in pregnancy are medical emergencies.
a. Hemorrhage remains a leading cause of maternal death.
b. Blood loss may reach 35% before hypovolemic shock occurs.
2. Placenta previa
a. Definition: implantation of placenta in lower uterine segment; either partial or complete
b. Risk factors
(1) Endometrial scarring, including previous uterine surgery
(2) Impeded endometrial vascularization
(3) Increased placental mass
c. Pathophysiology
(1) Normally, blastocyst implants into upper portion of uterus, where blood supply is rich.
(2) With previa, blastocyst implants itself in lower uterine segment, over or near internal os.
d. Signs and symptoms and diagnosis
(1) Painless, continuous or intermittent uterine bleeding, especially during third trimester
(2) Onset while woman at rest or in midst of activity without pain

(3) Normal uterine tone

(4) The earlier in gestation the bleeding, the worse the outcome; fetal effect depends on total blood loss, not number of bleeding episodes.

(5) Preterm labor develops in 30% of pregnancies complicated by placenta previa.

e. Management depends on gestational age, amount of bleeding, and placental location.

(1) Diagnosis by ultrasonography 95% to 99% accurate

(2) Gestational age <37 weeks: manage expectantly if bleeding stops, no labor, and fetal well-being established; home care appropriate for stable patient

(3) Gestational age >37 weeks: deliver

(4) Evidence of maternal or fetal compromise despite gestational age of fetus: deliver

3. Abruptio placentae

a. Definition: premature separation, either partial or total, of normally implanted placenta from decidual lining of uterus after 20 weeks' gestation

b. Bleeding may be concealed or apparent with any classification of abruption.

c. Risk factors

(1) Hypertensive disorders (chronic or preeclampsia-eclampsia)

(2) Multiparity

(3) Previous abruption

(4) Trauma, especially blunt abdominal

(5) Uterine anomaly

(6) Folic acid deficiency

(7) Smoking

(8) Cocaine use

(9) Premature rupture of membranes or sudden decompression of uterus

d. Pathophysiology

(1) Degeneration of spiral arterioles that nourish endometrium and supply blood to placenta

(2) Process leads to rupture of blood vessels, and bleeding quickly occurs.

(3) Separation of placenta takes place in area of hemorrhage.

e. Signs and symptoms and diagnosis

(1) Signs and symptoms related to amount of concealed blood trapped behind placenta and degree of separation

(a) External or concealed dark venous bleeding

(b) Shock greater than apparent blood loss

(c) Pain out of proportion to stage of labor or unrelated to uterine activity

(d) Uterine tenderness and hypertonicity (early finding)

(e) Firm to boardlike uterine fundus (late finding)

(f) Uterus may enlarge and change shape.

(g) Fetal heart tones may or may not be present.

(2) Diagnosis made on basis of presenting symptoms and physical assessment

(a) Severe and moderate abruptions are more easily diagnosed, whereas mild abruptions may be more difficult to diagnose because vaginal bleeding may be only presenting symptom.

(b) Ultrasonographic examination ordered to rule out placenta previa; abruptio placentae may not be diagnosed by ultrasonography.

f. Management depends on degree of abruption suspected, fetal status, and maternal status.

(1) Expectant management: emphasis placed on maintaining cardiovascular status of mother and developing plan for birth of fetus

(2) Emergency management

(a) Restore blood loss quickly.

(b) Maintain vital organ function.

(c) Continuous electronic fetal monitor

(d) Correct coagulation defect or defects if present.

(e) Expedite delivery.

(3) Vaginal delivery if woman hemodynamically stable, fetus stable, or fetal death

(4) Cesarean birth in presence of fetal distress, profuse bleeding, coagulopathy, or increasing uterine resting tone

4. Nursing assessments and interventions for placenta previa and abruptio placentae
   a. Fundamental areas of concern
      (1) Mother's condition as primarily evidenced by degree of obstetric hemorrhage and hemodynamic status; increasing pulse rate indicative of oxygenation/perfusion deficit
      (2) Fetal condition, including gestational age
   b. Nursing assessment plays vital role in this evaluation process.
   c. Intensive observation and monitoring
      (1) Vital signs and noninvasive assessments of cardiovascular status and organ perfusion
      (2) Strict I&O
      (3) Record amount of bleeding.
   d. Fluid resuscitation
      (1) Stable IV site with large-bore catheter (two IV lines possible)
      (2) IV fluid replacement
      (3) Blood replacement therapy
   e. Assessment of renal function
      (1) Strict I&O
      (2) Foley catheter
      (3) Urinary output of at least 30 mL/hr
   f. Fetal evaluation as indicated
   g. Verify maternal Rh status; administer RhoGAM as indicated.

5. Adherent retained placenta (accreta)
   a. Risks
      (1) Associated with increased maternal morbidity and mortality because of hemorrhage leading to hypovolemic shock
      (2) Abnormally adherent placenta may be identified on ultrasound screening.
   b. Types
      (1) Placenta accreta: slight penetration of myometrium by placental trophoblast; most common; may be removed manually
      (2) Placenta increta: deep penetration of myometrium by placental trophoblast; requires surgical intervention
      (3) Placenta percreta: perforation of uterus by placenta; requires surgical intervention
   c. Unusual placental adherence may be partial or complete.

6. Hydatidiform mole
   a. One of three types of gestational trophoblastic neoplasms
      (1) Most often seen in women at both ends of reproductive age spectrum
      (2) Increased risk for development of choriocarcinoma
   b. Signs and symptoms
      (1) Vaginal bleeding may be dark brown (resembling prune juice) or bright red, either scant or profuse.
      (2) Uterine size greater than expected gestational size
      (3) Relatively common findings from uterine distention
         (a) Anemia from blood loss
         (b) Excessive nausea and vomiting (hyperemesis gravidarum)
         (c) Abdominal cramps
      (4) Preeclampsia
         (a) About 15% of cases
         (b) Usually between 9 and 12 weeks' gestation
   c. Management
      (1) May abort spontaneously
      (2) Suction curettage offers safe, rapid, and effective method of evacuation of hydatidiform mole in almost all women.

(3) If woman does not desire preservation of reproductive function, may benefit from primary hysterectomy as method of choice for evacuation of hydatidiform mole and concurrent sterilization

(4) Induction of labor with oxytocic agents or prostaglandins not recommended because of increased risk of hemorrhage

(5) Need to have negative beta-hCG for 6 months

7. Uterine inversion

a. Partial or complete inversion of uterus (turning inside out) after delivery; potentially life-threatening complication

b. Signs and symptoms

(1) Primary presenting sign: hemorrhage

(2) Pelvic mass noted on vaginal examination

(3) No fundus palpable when attempting fundal massage

(4) Patient expresses feeling of fullness in vagina.

(5) Patient symptomatic for hypovolemic shock

c. Management involves all of the following interventions:

(1) Combat shock.

(2) Replace uterus after woman has received tocolysis or deep anesthesia.

(a) Give oxytocic as ordered, only after uterus has been replaced.

(b) Uterus may be packed if inversion seems to recur.

(3) Abdominal or vaginal surgery may be necessary to reposition uterus if successful manual replacement fails.

(4) Give blood replacement therapy as indicated.

(5) Initiate broad-spectrum antibiotic therapy.

(6) Nasogastric tube to minimize paralytic ileus

d. After replacement of uterus, do not massage fundus because inversion may recur.

8. Postpartum hemorrhage

a. Most common and most serious type of excessive obstetric blood loss

(1) Leading cause of maternal morbidity and mortality

(2) Accounts for 10% of nonabortive maternal deaths

(3) Of all deliveries, ~8% complicated by postpartum hemorrhage

b. Definition

(1) Traditionally, loss of >500 mL of blood after delivery

(2) More meaningful definition is:

(a) Loss of 1% or more of body weight

(b) One milliliter of blood weighs 1 g.

c. Pathophysiology

(1) Control of bleeding from placental site accomplished by prolonged contraction and retraction of interlacing strands of myometrium

(2) Most common causes of postpartum hemorrhage, in approximate order of frequency, are:

(a) Mismanagement of third stage of labor

(b) Uterine atony

(c) Lacerations of birth canal

(d) Hematological disorders

(e) Medical complications

(f) Infection

(3) Uterine atony is marked hypotonia of uterus.

(a) Occurs with:

(i) Grand multipara

(ii) Hydramnios

(iii) Fetal macrosomia

(iv) Multifetus gestation

(b) Other causes

(i) Traumatic delivery

(ii) Halogenated anesthesia

(iii) Magnesium sulfate

(iv) Rapid or prolonged labor

            (v)   Chorioamnionitis
            (vi) Use of oxytocin for induction or augmentation of labor
            (vii) Postpartum filling of urinary bladder
        (c) Management goals
            (i)   Eliminate cause.
            (ii)   Administer oxytocic agent.
            (iii) Maintain contraction of uterine muscle.
    (4) Lacerations of birth canal
        (a) Second only to uterine atony as major cause of postpartum hemorrhage
        (b) Continued bleeding despite efficient postpartum uterine contractions demands inspection or reinspection of birth passage (labia, perineum, vagina, cervix).
        (c) Causative factors
            (i)   Operative delivery (forceps or vacuum extraction)
            (ii)   Aseptic or uncontrolled spontaneous delivery
            (iii) Congenital abnormalities of maternal soft tissue
            (iv) Contracted pelvis
            (v)   Fetal size or position
            (vi)   Prior scarring
            (vii) Varices
        (d) Management depends on identification of source of bleeding and repair of laceration.

9. Diagnosis and management of hemorrhage
  a. Call obstetric unit for assistance and possible transfer or comanagement.
  b. Identify source of bleeding early.
  c. ORDER
    (1) **O** = Oxygenation: administer supplemental O_2 as needed to maintain O_2 saturation levels.
    (2) **R** = Replace intravascular volume with crystalloids or blood products.
    (3) **D** = Drug therapy as needed to maintain hemodynamic status
    (4) **E** = Evaluate patient status and effectiveness of treatment.
    (5) **R** = Remedy underlying cause.
  d. REACT
    (1) **R** = Resuscitation: assessments, stabilization, venous access
    (2) **E** = Evaluate: did initial actions improve patient status?
    (3) **A** = Arrest hemorrhage: eliminate cause of hemorrhage, including traditional pharmacological management or surgical intervention.
    (4) **C** = Consultation: care may require collaboration with medicine or anesthesia, transfer to critical care unit.
    (5) **T** = Treat complications: anticipate complications that occur because of hypovolemia, hypotension, and shock.
  e. Treat cause.
    (1) Atony
        (a) Fundal compression
        (b) Oxytocin: 10 to 40 units/L as IV infusion; never given as undiluted IV push bolus
        (c) Methylergonovine (Methergine): 0.2 mg intramuscularly (IM); contraindicated in patient with history of hypertension
        (d) Alprostadil (Prostin/15M): 0.25 to 1.5 mg IM; use with caution in women with:
            (i)   History of reactive airway disease
            (ii)   Asthma
            (iii) Cardiac disease
            (iv) Hepatic disease
            (v)   Systemic lupus erythematosus
        (e) Misoprostil (Cytotec): 800 to 1000 mcg intravaginally or rectally

      (f) Tamponade balloon
         (i) Intended to provide temporary control or reduction of postpartum uterine bleeding with conservative management warranted
         (ii) While device in place or clinical status worsening, monitor closely for signs of:
            [a] Arterial bleeding
            [b] Atony bleeding
            [c] DIC
         (iii) Contraindications
            [a] Arterial bleeding requiring surgical exploration or angiographic embolization
            [b] Uterine atony bleeding
            [c] Cases indicating hysterectomy
         (iv) Follow manufacturer's instructions for insertion and inflation.
    (2) Hematoma
      (a) Evacuate.
      (b) Ligate areas of bleeding.
    (3) If patient unresponsive
      (a) Arterial ligation or embolization
      (b) Hysterectomy
      (c) Military antishock trousers (MAST)

10. General principles for management of hemorrhage
  a. Because of expanded blood volume in pregnancy, early signs and symptoms of hemorrhagic shock may be masked.
    (1) Earliest sign will be mild tachycardia with no change in BP.
    (2) COP reduced during pregnancy; further reduced with fluid resuscitation, therefore increased risk for pulmonary edema
  b. Must be alert for other causes of bleeding
    (1) Placenta previa
    (2) Abruptio placentae
    (3) Placenta accreta
    (4) Severe preeclampsia
    (5) HELLP syndrome
    (6) Eclampsia
    (7) Coagulopathies (chronic DIC)
    (8) Abdominal trauma
    (9) Amniotic fluid embolism
  c. Shock: emergency situation in which perfusion of body organs may become severely compromised and death may ensue
  d. Aggressive treatment necessary to prevent adverse sequelae
    (1) Initiate standing orders.
      (a) Start IV fluids.
      (b) Obtain CBC and coagulation studies.
      (c) Maintain airway.
    (2) If patient is still pregnant, maintain uterine displacement.
    (3) Trendelenburg position may interfere with cardiopulmonary functioning.
    (4) Anticipate need for invasive hemodynamic monitoring.
  e. Nursing implications
    (1) Assess and record respiratory rate, quality, and pattern.
    (2) Assess and record pulse rate and quality.
      (a) Rate increases and becomes irregular as shock progresses.
      (b) Immediate postpartum period: physiological bradycardia; may further mask mild tachycardia
    (3) Assess and record BP, capillary refill, pulse oximetry, skin color, and temperature.
    (4) Assess and record LOC and mentation.
    (5) Evaluate hemodynamic parameters if pulmonary artery catheter used.

G. DIC
  1. Pathophysiology
    a. Pathological form of clotting that is diffuse and consumes large amounts of clotting factors
    b. All aspects of coagulation system involved
    c. Pregnancy predisposes to DIC because of changes in coagulation system.
    d. Can be further defined as dilutional or consumptive DIC
      (1) Dilutional DIC
        (a) Secondary complication resulting from depletion of platelets and soluble clotting factors
        (b) Seen during hemorrhage when treated with aggressive fluid replacement only
        (c) Thrombocytopenia most common problem
      (2) Consumptive DIC
        (a) Secondary complication resulting from an identifiable, underlying process where there is an activation of procoagulants, leading to:
          (i)   Consumption of clotting factors
          (ii) Fibrin deposits
          (iii) Activation of plasminogen
        (b) Common obstetric conditions leading to consumptive DIC include:
          (i)   Abruption
          (ii) Preeclampsia
          (iii) Sepsis
  2. Pregnancy conditions that increase risk for DIC
    a. Abruptio placentae
    b. Preeclampsia
    c. HELLP syndrome
    d. Eclampsia
    e. Retained dead fetus syndrome
    f. Sepsis
    g. Anaphylactoid syndrome of pregnancy (amniotic fluid embolism)
    h. Saline induction of abortions
    i. Excessive hemorrhage
      (1) Be aware of maternal predisposing conditions.
      (2) Cardiovascular assessment
      (3) Respiratory assessment
      (4) Renal assessment
      (5) CNS assessment
  3. Fetal assessment
    a. Assess whether FHR baseline is appropriate for gestational age.
    b. Assess for changes in baseline rate.
    c. Assess for late decelerations.
  4. Monitor laboratory assessments for worsening condition or for signs of improvement.
  5. Assess for preterm labor.
  6. Institute supportive measures to correct acidosis, hypotension, and hypoperfusion.
  7. Initiate vigorous volume replacement.
    a. Start with isotonic crystalloids (normal saline or lactated Ringer's); blood component therapy as indicated.
    b. Isotonic crystalloids distribute evenly throughout extracellular space and do not promote an increase in intracellular fluid.
    c. At equivalent volumes, crystalloids less effective than colloids for expansion of intravascular volume
      (1) Two to 12 times volume of crystalloids necessary to achieve similar hemodynamic and volemic endpoints
      (2) Because of volume required, may increase risk for pulmonary edema

8. Initiate blood component replacement.
   a. Blood component replacement products include:
      (1) Packed RBCs (PRBCs)
      (2) Platelets
      (3) Fresh frozen plasma (FFP)
      (4) Fibrinogen
      (5) Cryoprecipitate
   b. PRBCs
      (1) Provide O_2 carrying and delivery capacity
      (2) Each unit PRBCs increases:
         (a) Total hemoglobin by 1 g
         (b) Hematocrit by 3%
      (3) Deficiency in factors (see Chapter 29)
         (a) V
         (b) VII
         (c) XI
         (d) Platelets
         (e) Soluble clotting factors
   c. Platelets
      (1) Can be either single-donor platelet or pooled platelet packs
      (2) Each unit of single-donor platelets increases total circulatory platelet count by 30,000 to 60,000/mm³ with less risk of infection; each unit of pooled platelets increases total circulatory platelet count by 7000 to 10,000/mm³.
      (3) Platelets should be replaced to 60,000/mm³.
      (4) Prophylactic transfusion indicated if total platelet count less than 10,000 to 20,000/mm³ or if preoperative platelet count <50,000/mm³
   d. FFP
      (1) Best source of soluble clotting factors, including fibrinogen
      (2) Must anticipate need for FFP because minimum of 30-minute preparation time required by blood bank
      (3) Each unit FFP increases total circulating fibrinogen by 5% to 10% mg.
9. Complications of aggressive fluid and blood replacement therapy
   a. Hypothermia: warm fluids if possible.
   b. Dysrhythmias: ECG monitoring indicated
   c. Acidosis: be aware of reperfusion injuries once perfusion reestablished.
   d. Electrolyte imbalances: monitor laboratory values.
   e. Coagulopathies: monitor coagulation studies and serum calcium levels (serum calcium an essential component of coagulation cascade).
H. Cardiac disease
   1. Significance
      a. Third leading cause of death in women 25 to 44 years of age
      b. Cardiac disease present in 1% to 3% of childbearing-age women
      c. Underlying cardiac disease responsible for 10% to 25% of maternal deaths (rate from congenital lesions has doubled; from acquired has halved)
      d. Congenital heart lesions more common today than rheumatic lesions; hypertensive and ischemic heart disease becoming more prevalent
      e. Adaptation of cardiovascular system in pregnancy may increase risk for cardiac decompensation, including congestive failure or worsening ischemia.
   2. Patient counseling and screening
      a. Ideally done before conception
      b. Pregnancy outcome depends on:
         (1) Functional capacity of heart
         (2) Underlying lesion
         (3) Likelihood of other complications that increase cardiac load during pregnancy and puerperium
         (4) Quality of medical care available
         (5) Psychosocial and economic capabilities of patient, her family, and community

3. Morbidity and mortality related to underlying maternal cardiac disease (see Chapter 32)
  a. Maternal mortality based on New York Heart Association (NYHA) functional classification
    (1) Class I: 1% mortality
    (2) Class II: 5% to 15% mortality
    (3) Class III: 25% to 50% mortality
    (4) Class IV: >50% mortality
    (5) Pregnancy increases NYHA class by at least one class; >50% of women with overt failure were class I early in pregnancy.
  b. Risk of maternal death by type of heart disease
    (1) Group 1 consists of the following diagnoses:
      (a) Atrial septal defect
      (b) Ventricular septal defect
      (c) Patent ductus arteriosus
      (d) Pulmonic or tricuspid disease
      (e) Corrected tetralogy of Fallot
      (f) Bioprosthetic valve
      (g) NYHA class I and II mitral stenosis
      (h) Mortality risk: <1%
    (2) Group 2 consists of the following diagnoses:
      (a) NYHA class III and IV mitral stenosis
      (b) Aortic stenosis
      (c) Aortic coarctation without valvar involvement
      (d) Uncorrected tetralogy of Fallot
      (e) Previous myocardial infarction
      (f) Marfan syndrome with normal aorta
      (g) Mortality risk: 5% to 15%
    (3) Group 3 consists of the following diagnoses:
      (a) Pulmonary hypertension
      (b) Aortic coarctation with valvular involvement
      (c) Marfan syndrome with aortic involvement
      (d) Mortality risk: 25% to 50%
  c. Predictability of cardiac event during current pregnancy
    (1) Identifies woman at greatest risk for a cardiac event occurring in current pregnancy
    (2) Cardiac event defined as onset of pulmonary edema, dysrhythmias, stroke, or death
    (3) Predictors of cardiac event can be remembered by mnemonic NOPE.
      (a) **N** = NYHA class III or IV
      (b) **O** = Obstruction of left side of the heart as indicated by a mitral valve diameter <2 cm, aortic valve diameter <1.5 cm, or peak gradient >30 mm Hg
      (c) **P** = Prior cardiac event before pregnancy such as:
        (i) Congestive heart failure (CHF)
        (ii) Dysrhythmias
        (iii) Transient ischemic attacks
        (iv) Stroke
      (d) **E** = Ejection fraction <40%
    (4) Number of predictors present indicates the risk of a cardiac event during current pregnancy.
      (a) No predictors present = 5% risk of cardiac event
      (b) One predictor present = 27% risk of cardiac event
      (c) More than one predictor present = 75% risk of cardiac event
  d. Fetal and neonatal risks
    (1) Increased risk of:
      (a) Spontaneous abortion
      (b) Intrauterine growth restriction (IUGR)
      (c) Intrauterine fetal death

(2) Maternal cardiac disease places fetus at risk for fetal heart disease.
  (a) Incidence: 5% to 10%
  (b) Fifty percent of fetuses will have concordant lesion.
(3) Greatest risks to fetus include (51% loss rate):
  (a) Maternal cardiac disease classified as NYHA class III or IV
  (b) Prepregnancy maternal arterial O_2 saturation <85%
  (c) Maternal hematocrit = 65%
  (d) Hemoglobin = 20 g/dL
  (e) Maternal partial pressure of O_2 in arterial blood (Pao_2) <70 mm Hg
4. General management
  a. Call obstetric unit for assistance and possible transfer or comanagement.
  b. Collaborative effort of:
    (1) Obstetrician
    (2) Cardiologist
    (3) Anesthesiologist
    (4) Nursing
    (5) Other needed disciplines
  c. Goals
    (1) To prevent CHF
    (2) To react promptly to early signs of CHF
    (3) To aggressively assess for and react to early signs of pregnancy complications
      (a) Preeclampsia
      (b) Diabetes
      (c) Infection
    (4) To prevent recurrence of acute rheumatic fever
    (5) To prevent infective endocarditis
  d. Avoid causes of tachycardia; treat when sustained HR >100 beats/min.
5. Management principles
  a. First stage
    (1) Labor and deliver in same room
    (2) Monitor vital signs.
      (a) Pulse rate
      (b) BP
      (c) Respiratory status
      (d) Lung bases
      (e) I&O
    (3) Keep HR <100 beats/min.
    (4) Prophylactic antibiotics for ventricular septal defect, aortic and mitral disease
    (5) Examine and reevaluate cardiac status of patient in labor.
    (6) Semi-Fowler's position or best position as determined with invasive or noninvasive monitoring for CO and oxygenation status
    (7) Never place in lithotomy position, even for delivery.
    (8) Adequate analgesia (narcotic epidural appropriate)
    (9) Digitalis if needed
    (10) Drugs and equipment to treat pulmonary edema
    (11) O_2 therapy and pulse oximetry
    (12) ECG monitoring as indicated
    (13) Cesarean birth for obstetric reasons only
    (14) Prevent fluid overload; use infusion pumps for all IVs and keep accurate I&O.
  b. Second stage of labor (delivery)
    (1) Recognize signs of decompensating heart.
    (2) Shorten second stage (episiotomy and forceps).
    (3) Avoid Valsalva's maneuver.
    (4) Cesarean birth
    (5) Atraumatic delivery
    (6) Do not put patient in lithotomy position.

        c. Third stage of labor (delivery of placenta)

            (1) Avoid postpartum hemorrhage.

            (2) Strict I&O

            (3) Beware of antidiuretic effect and cardiovascular effects of oxytocin.

            (4) Beware of cardiovascular effects of prostaglandin preparations; avoid methylergonovine (Methergine).

        d. Fourth stage (postpartum)

            (1) Observe for at least 24 hours after delivery.

            (2) Invasive hemodynamic monitoring as indicated

            (3) At least one third of maternal deaths occur in first 24 hours after delivery.

I. Pulmonary disease

    1. Pregnancy causes dramatic, predictable alterations in pulmonary function.

        a. Pao_2 must remain >60 mm Hg for adequate fetal oxygenation, providing all other factors influencing O_2 transfer across intervillous spaces remain optimum.

        b. Increased O_2 consumption associated with corresponding increase in CO_2 excretion

    2. Pulmonary edema

        a. A secondary disease process characterized by excess accumulation of fluid in pulmonary interstitial and alveolar spaces

            (1) Prevents adequate diffusion of both O_2 and CO_2

            (2) Quickly leads to pulmonary dysfunction that can lead to maternal and fetal hypoxemia

        b. Commonly associated with:

            (1) Preeclampsia

            (2) Preexisting cardiac disease

            (3) Tocolytic therapy

            (4) Infection

            (5) Fluid and blood replacement therapy

        c. Physiological adaptations of pregnancy increase risk for pulmonary edema.

            (1) Decreased intravascular COP

            (2) Maternal O_2 delivery dependent on maternal CO

            (3) Pregnancy a state of increased O_2 consumption

            (4) Pregnancy a state of chronic compensated respiratory alkalemia

            (5) Fetal oxygenation dependent on maternal cardiopulmonary system's ability to meet maternal needs

        d. Underlying mechanisms leading to development of pulmonary edema

            (1) Hydrostatic pulmonary edema

                (a) Results from imbalance of intravascular volume and intravascular/ interstitial pressures

                (b) Cardiogenic pulmonary edema

                    (i) Cardiac muscle in state of dysfunction; ventricular muscles are interdependent so if one ventricle fails, the other will fail.

                    (ii) Systolic dysfunction results from decreased myocardial squeeze and an ejection fraction <45%.

                    (iii) Diastolic dysfunction results from impaired ventricular muscle relaxation and high filling pressures.

                    (iv) Underlying valvular disease; most common is mitral stenosis.

                (c) Decreased COP

                    (i) COP is pressure resulting from ability of plasma proteins to hold water in intravascular space.

                    (ii) Opposes hydrostatic pressure

                    (iii) Pregnancy results in lowered COP.

                    (iv) Responds quickly to aggressive diuretic therapy

                (d) Increased negative interstitial pressure

            (2) Permeability edema

                (a) Results from increased pulmonary capillary permeability

                (b) A severe form of acute lung injury (ALI)

          (c) Characterized by an intense inflammatory response and fibrosis of lung tissue to infectious or noninfectious insults

          (d) Acute respiratory distress syndrome (ARDS) is an end stage of ALI.

          (e) Takes days to weeks to clear

          (f) Causes include:

             (i) Preeclampsia

             (ii) Aspiration

             (iii) Septic shock

             (iv) Pneumonia

             (v) Inhaled toxins

             (vi) Pancreatitis

      (3) Lymphatic insufficiency: rare in pregnancy

      (4) Unknown or poorly understood: includes causes that do not fit in above mechanisms

   e. Treatment

      (1) Same as for any patient with pulmonary edema taking fetal status into consideration

      (2) Call obstetric unit for assistance and possible transfer or comanagement.

3. Pulmonary embolism

   a. Incidence

      (1) Occurs in ~1 in every 2000 pregnancies

      (2) Untreated DVT correlates with 15% to 24% incidence of pulmonary embolism.

      (3) Mortality: 12% to 15%

   b. Predisposing conditions

      (1) Pregnancy

      (2) Prior history of DVT or pulmonary embolism

      (3) Surgical procedures, immobility

      (4) Obstetric complications

      (5) Inherited coagulopathies

      (6) Antiphospholipid antibody syndrome

      (7) Age

      (8) Race

      (9) Greatest risk in immediate postpartum period

   c. Treatment

      (1) Call obstetric unit for assistance and possible transfer or comanagement.

      (2) Anticoagulation with heparin

      (3) Antepartum management includes prophylactic anticoagulation.

      (4) If anticoagulation given during antepartum period, maintain anticoagulation during labor.

      (5) Low–molecular weight heparin preparations appropriate for use during pregnancy; however, be sure to switch to heparin at least 24 hours before delivery.

4. DVT (see Chapter 44)

   a. Leading cause of maternal morbidity and mortality during pregnancy and puerperium is thromboembolic disease caused by hypercoagulable state.

   b. DVT

      (1) Venous stasis in presence of hypercoagulability leads to development of DVT.

      (2) DVT predisposes to development of pulmonary embolism.

      (3) First sign of DVT may be pulmonary embolism.

   c. Women with DVT or pulmonary embolism in association with pregnancy may have no significant medical risk factors or problems.

      (1) Conditions with increased associated risk include:

          (a) Prior history of DVT or pulmonary embolism

          (b) Surgical procedures

   (c) Immobility

   (d) Obstetric complications

   (e) Hereditary deficiency of antithrombin III, protein C, or protein S

  (2) Time of greatest risk: immediate postpartum period, especially after cesarean birth

 d. Nursing implications

  (1) Primary goal is maintenance of pulmonary function.

  (2) Frequent assessments of respiratory status

  (3) O_2 exchange should be facilitated by positioning and supplemental O_2 administration.

  (4) Pulse oximetry should be used to monitor O_2 saturation in conjunction with arterial blood gases (ABGs).

  (5) Administer heparin to maintain:

   (a) Activated partial thromboplastin time of 1.5 to 2 times that of control levels

   (b) Plasma heparin level of 0.2 to 0.3 IU/mL antepartum (0.1 to 0.2 IU/mL intrapartum)

  (6) Anticipate need for protamine sulfate to reverse heparin effects (1 mg of protamine sulfate neutralizes 100 IU of heparin; maximum single dose, 50 mg).

  (7) Assess for signs of preterm labor if patient has not delivered (see Preterm Labor, section II.D).

5. Pneumonia

 a. Associated with several maternal and fetal complications

 b. Pregnancy predisposes to aspiration; immune system altered during pregnancy

 c. Varicella very dangerous to mother and fetus

 d. Mycoplasma common in pregnancy and is difficult to diagnose

 e. Bacterial infection often occurs as a secondary infection.

 f. Treatment

  (1) Call obstetric unit for assistance and possible transfer or comanagement.

  (2) Prompt diagnosis

  (3) Supportive therapy

  (4) O_2

  (5) Antibiotics

6. Asthma

 a. Incidence

  (1) Relatively common

  (2) Prognosis during pregnancy depends on:

   (a) Severity before pregnancy

   (b) Season of year

   (c) Presence of other respiratory infections

   (d) Patient's emotional state

 b. Effects of asthma during pregnancy

  (1) No consistent effect

  (2) Slightly higher risk for prematurity, IUGR because of decreased oxygenation

  (3) Must consider fetal risks of drug therapy

  (4) Exacerbations rare during labor

  (5) If severe, may require pregnancy termination

  (6) If prostaglandins used, should use prostaglandin E_2, a bronchodilator, instead of prostaglandin F_2-alpha, a bronchoconstrictor

 c. Treatment

  (1) Call obstetric unit for assistance and possible transfer or comanagement.

  (2) Supportive therapy

  (3) O_2 therapy

  (4) Bronchodilators

  (5) Antibiotics

7. Anaphylactoid syndrome of pregnancy (amniotic fluid embolism [AFE])
   a. Complex condition classically characterized by:
      (1) Hypotension or hemodynamic collapse
      (2) Hypoxia
      (3) Consumptive coagulopathy
   b. Incidence
      (1) Rare phenomenon, unique to pregnancy
      (2) From National Registry, mortality >60%; of those women who survive insult, most sustain neurological sequelae.
   c. Pathophysiology
      (1) Similar to both septic shock and anaphylactic shock
      (2) Entrance of a foreign substance into maternal circulation
      (3) Catecholamine release leads to hypertonic uterine activity.
      (4) Release of primary and secondary endogenous mediators, including arachidonic acid metabolites
         (a) Results in principal physiological derangements
         (b) Abnormalities include:
            (i) Profound myocardial depression
            (ii) Decreased CO
            (iii) Pulmonary hypertension
            (iv) DIC
         (c) Forty-one percent of patients in Amniotic Fluid Embolus Registry gave history of either drug allergy or atopy on hospital admission.
      (5) Syndrome appears to be initiated after maternal intravascular exposure to various types of fetal tissues.
      (6) Breaches of the immunological barrier between mother and antigenically different products of conception may, under certain circumstances and in susceptible maternal-fetal pairs, play role in AFE.
      (7) Clinical findings not consistent with embolic event
   d. Presentation
      (1) Initial episode is acute onset of profound hypoxia and hypotension followed by cardiopulmonary collapse.
         (a) Often complicated by consumptive coagulopathy, which may lead to exsanguination
         (b) In any patient, any of the three principal phases (hypoxia, hypotension, or coagulopathy) may either dominate or be entirely absent.
      (2) Clinical findings
         (a) Hypotension
         (b) Fetal distress
         (c) Pulmonary edema or ARDS
         (d) Cardiopulmonary arrest
         (e) Cyanosis
         (f) Coagulopathy
         (g) Dyspnea
         (h) Seizure
         (i) Uterine atony
         (j) Bronchospasm
         (k) Transient hypertension
         (l) Cough
         (m) Headache
         (n) Chest pain
      (3) Hemodynamic alterations
         (a) Initial transient phase involving systemic and pulmonary vasospasm
         (b) Secondary phase
            (i) Hypotension
            (ii) Depressed ventricular function
         (c) Mechanism of left ventricular (LV) failure uncertain

(i) Questionable coronary artery spasm and myocardial ischemia

(ii) Global hypoxia can lead to LV dysfunction.

(iii) Amniotic fluid decreases myometrial contractility (in vitro).

(4) Pulmonary manifestations

(a) Rapid and profound hypoxia

(b) Combination of initial pulmonary vasospasm and ventricular dysfunction

(c) Results in permanent neurological injury

(d) Lung injury can lead to ARDS and secondary oxygenation defects.

(5) Coagulopathy

(a) If survive initial hemodynamic insult, may succumb to secondary coagulopathy

(b) Amniotic fluid has been shown to:

(i) Shorten whole-blood clotting time

(ii) Have a thromboplastin-like effect

(iii) Induce platelet aggregation

(iv) Release platelet factor III

(v) Activate complement cascade

(vi) Contain a direct factor X–activating factor

(c) Coagulopathy may not always be present.

e. Significance

(1) Maternal outcome dismal

(2) Overall mortality rate: 60% to 80%

(3) Twenty-five percent die within first hour from cardiopulmonary collapse.

(4) If survive, 50% develop DIC within next 4 hours.

(5) Neurological impairment is the rule.

(a) Intact maternal survival rate

(i) If no cardiopulmonary arrest: 15%

(ii) If cardiopulmonary arrest: 8%

(b) No one therapy consistently associated with improved outcome

(6) Overall neonatal survival rate: 80%

(a) Of neonates who survive, 50% have residual neurological impairment.

(b) Relationship between neonatal outcome and event-to-delivery interval if maternal cardiopulmonary arrest

f. Treatment

(1) Rapidly lethal condition

(2) Supportive care initiated promptly and aggressively

(3) Maintain oxygenation with high concentrations of O_2; intubate early.

(4) Maintain CO and BP with volume expansion to optimize ventricular preload, and if needed inotropic agents.

(5) Treat coagulopathy.

(6) Initiate cardiopulmonary resuscitation (CPR) and call for appropriate personnel for resuscitation.

(7) Administration of corticosteroids may be considered.

8. Nursing implications for pulmonary disease during pregnancy

a. Call obstetric unit for assistance and possible transfer or comanagement.

b. Multifaceted care

c. Maintain adequate ventilatory function.

d. Optimize O_2 exchange.

e. ABG measurement

f. Monitor patient's response to therapy.

g. Emotional support

h. Avoid hypoxemia during suctioning or ventilatory tubing changes.

i. Hemodynamic monitoring as indicated

j. Adjust mechanical ventilation setting to reflect normal pregnancy pulmonary parameters and ABG values.

J. Multiple gestation
  1. Perinatal morbidity and mortality increase with multifetal gestation because of:
     a. Birth weight
     b. Gestational age
     c. Presentation of each fetus
     d. Mode of delivery
     e. Interval of time between deliveries
  2. Diagnosis
     a. Most important factor in successful outcome is early diagnosis.
     b. Most important clinical finding suggestive of multifetal gestation is fundal height or uterine size disproportionately greater than date.
     c. Ultrasonography for confirmation of diagnosis
  3. Maternal complications
     a. Hypertension complicates 14% to 20% of twin pregnancies versus 6% to 8% of singleton pregnancies.
     b. Sepsis with premature rupture of membranes three times more frequent
     c. Postpartum hemorrhage occurs in approximately 20% of all multifetal pregnancies.
     d. Anemia occurs two times more frequently.
  4. Fetal and neonatal complications
     a. Preterm labor and birth
     b. Congenital anomalies
     c. Discordant growth
  5. Nursing implications
     a. Assess for:
        (1) Anemia
        (2) Preeclampsia
        (3) Polyhydramnios
        (4) Preterm labor
     b. At risk for placenta previa
     c. After delivery, assess for postpartum hemorrhage.
K. Trauma in pregnancy
  1. Significance
     a. Leading cause of nonobstetric maternal death in women of childbearing age
     b. Motor vehicle accidents currently leading cause of injury
     c. Physical abuse may become leading cause (15%-20% of all pregnant women are battered).
     d. Maternal mortality most often from injuries sustained from motor vehicle accidents: head injuries, followed by multiple internal injuries, which lead to hypovolemic shock and exsanguination
  2. Abdominal trauma
     a. Significance
        (1) First-trimester fetus protected by bony pelvis and amniotic fluid buffer
        (2) Second-trimester pregnancy has become abdominal with minimum protection to fetus from pelvis.
        (3) Third trimester
           (a) With fetal engagement, increased risk for fetal skull fractures, intracranial bleeding
           (b) Increased risk for placental abruption; usually within first 48 hours
           (c) Complications unique to pregnancy
              (i)   Uterine trauma or rupture
              (ii) Bladder trauma or rupture
              (iii) Amniotic fluid embolus
              (iv) Placental abruption
              (v)   Trauma statistics in general population can be used to anticipate complications in pregnant trauma victim.

b. Blunt abdominal trauma
   (1) Motor vehicle accidents most common cause
   (2) Head injury and exsanguination from vessel rupture most common cause of maternal death
   (3) Leading cause of fetal death is maternal death.
   (4) Leading cause of fetal death when mother survives is abruptio placentae.
c. Penetrating abdominal trauma
   (1) Morbidity related to point of entry and number of organs penetrated
   (2) As pregnancy advances, abdominal organs displaced upward and laterally
   (3) Growing uterus may afford protection to abdominal organs located posterior to uterus, but fetus may be placed in position of greater risk.
   (4) All penetrating abdominal wounds may require laparotomy for full surgical exploration.
   (5) Gunshot wounds
      (a) Most common
      (b) Prognosis worse in that bullet path unpredictable and multiorgan involvement may occur
      (c) Greater damage to abdominal organs because of pregnancy displacement if bullet leaves uterine cavity
      (d) If bullet path limited to uterus, can have fetal, umbilical cord, or placenta damage
   (6) Stab wounds
      (a) Second most common
      (b) Prognosis better than with gunshot wounds
      (c) Upper abdomen wounds may be complicated by damage to:
         (i) Placenta
         (ii) Abdominal organs
         (iii) Lungs
         (iv) Heart
         (v) Fetus usually protected
      (d) Lower abdomen wounds may be complicated by damage to fetus, bladder.
3. Thermal trauma
   a. Skin integrity affected—body systems compromise
   b. Prognosis depends on extent and depth of burn.
   c. Especially vulnerable to intravascular volume deficit and hypoxia
   d. Increased risk for preterm labor resulting from maternal hypoxemia (maternal Pao_2 <60 mm Hg increases fetal compromise)
   e. Fetal survival depends on maternal stabilization and survival.
4. Pelvic trauma
   a. Bony ring fracture may cause fetal skull fracture or maternal bladder trauma or rupture.
   b. Retroperitoneal bleeding risk increases because of engorgement of pelvic veins.
   c. Genitourinary trauma results in greater blood loss related to increased vascularity.
   d. Bowel (small and large) trauma possible
5. Modifications of trauma care in pregnancy
   a. Cardiovascular system
      (1) Blood volume increase means greater blood loss needed to show signs and symptoms of shock.
      (2) Plasma volume expansion with greater RBC mass increase so there is physiological anemia during pregnancy.
      (3) Resting HR increases by 15 to 20 beats/min during pregnancy.
      (4) Decreased SVR and increased CO may delay development of cool, clammy skin with hypovolemic shock.
   b. Respiratory system
      (1) Normally in compensated respiratory alkalemia during pregnancy
      (2) Decreased O_2 reserve and less tolerant of hypoxia as a result of increased metabolic rate and O_2 consumption

        (3) Because chest wall is broadened and diaphragm elevated, thoracostomy will be performed above normal site.

        (4) Normal for pregnancy
            (a) Peripheral edema
            (b) Dyspnea
            (c) Third heart sound
            (d) May clinically mimic congestive ventricular failure

  c. Gastrointestinal system
      (1) Because abdominal viscera displaced and compressed:
            (a) Risk of liver or splenic rupture increased
            (b) Abdominal injury may be masked or mimicked.
            (c) Altered patterns for referred pain
            (d) Rebound tenderness may be present or absent.
      (2) Increased risk for aspiration because:
            (a) Decreased gastric motility
            (b) Prolonged gastric emptying time
            (c) Incompetent esophageal sphincter
      (3) Increased pelvic venous congestion: increased risk for hemorrhage
      (4) Protruding uterus or bladder: increased risk for trauma

  d. Hematological system in hypercoagulable state: increased risk for thrombosis

6. Nursing assessments and interventions

  a. Must remember that normal physiological and anatomical changes of pregnancy will mask serious alterations in maternal status

  b. Primary survey assessment
      (1) Airway
      (2) Breathing
      (3) Circulation
      (4) Neurological status
      (5) Interventions
            (a) Establish and maintain airway; nasal airway inappropriate because of increased vascularity of pregnancy.
            (b) Administer O_2 at 10 to 15 L/min through tight nonrebreather mask.
            (c) Place nasogastric tube to decrease risk of aspiration.
            (d) Anticipate need for mechanical ventilation if respiratory rate <12 or >25; obtain ABGs and avoid exacerbation of acidosis by keeping $Paco_2$ to normal pregnancy values.
            (e) Initiate CPR as indicated, maintaining uterine displacement.
            (f) Establish venous access.
            (g) Pneumatic antishock garment (MAST) may be indicated; abdominal compartment may be left uninflated once pregnancy becomes abdominal organ.
            (h) Control hemorrhage.

  c. Secondary survey assessment
      (1) Reassess neurological status.
            (a) **A** = alert, oriented
            (b) **V** = responds to verbal stimulus
            (c) **P** = responds to pain only
            (d) **U** = unresponsive
      (2) Examine for head injuries.
      (3) Reassess chest and circulation.
      (4) Anticipate laboratory and x-ray studies.
            (a) Kleihauer-Betke: maternal blood test to diagnose fetomaternal hemorrhage
            (b) Indirect Coombs' test to detect maternal Rh sensitization
            (c) Alum-precipitated toxoid test: blood test to determine whether specimen is maternal or fetal blood
      (5) Assess abdomen, noting pain, tenderness, distention.
      (6) Assess musculoskeletal status.

        (7) Reproductive assessment
           (a) Contraction frequency, duration, intensity, resting tone
           (b) Assess fundal height for approximate gestational age assessment.
           (c) Inspect perineum for bleeding, rupture of membranes.
           (d) If no bleeding, assess for cervical dilation.
           (e) Assess for signs and symptoms of abruptio placentae.
           (f) Assess for fetal status.

   d. Circulatory support essential; however, vasopressors should not be routinely used.
      (1) Peripheral vasoconstrictors will increase maternal MAP but decrease uterine blood flow.
      (2) Central vasoconstrictors will concomitantly increase uterine blood flow and MAP.
      (3) Assessment and treatment priorities for pregnant burn patient same as any other; call obstetric unit for assistance and possible transfer or comanagement.
        (a) Airway patency
        (b) Maintain normal intravascular volume.
        (c) Provide maximum oxygenation.

L. CPR in pregnancy
  1. Call obstetric unit for assistance and possible transfer or comanagement.
  2. Causes of cardiopulmonary arrest in pregnancy
    a. Maternal cardiac disease
    b. Severe preeclampsia, HELLP syndrome, eclampsia
    c. Preexisting medical conditions
    d. Acute complications
      (1) Pulmonary embolism or amniotic fluid embolism
      (2) Aspiration pneumonia
      (3) Hypermagnesemia
      (4) Anaphylaxis
      (5) Laryngeal edema
      (6) Bronchospasm
      (7) Anesthesia
      (8) Trauma
      (9) Sepsis
  3. Significance of pregnancy physiology on CPR
    a. Pregnancy a high-flow (CO), low-resistance (SVR) state
    b. Thorax less compliant, making mouth-to-mouth ventilation and chest compressions more difficult and less effective
    c. Decreased chest compliance impedes success of standard closed-chest CPR.
    d. Before 24 weeks' gestation, objective is maternal conservation; after 24 weeks' gestation, fetal well-being may influence management decisions, but primary patient is the mother.
    e. Prompt emergent delivery increases maternal survival; if no maternal response within 4 minutes, bedside cesarean delivery or open-chest massage recommended.
    f. After 12 weeks, uterus is abdominal organ.
      (1) Decreased thoracic compliance
      (2) Decreased venous return
      (3) Causes aortic or vena caval compression
      (4) Decreased forward flow of blood with compressions
      (5) Causes respiratory impedance
    g. If fetus of viable gestational age (>24 weeks):
      (1) Maternal hypoxia shunts blood from uteroplacental unit.
      (2) Fetal $Paco_2$ increases as maternal $Paco_2$ increases, resulting in fetal metabolic acidosis.
  4. Modifications of CPR in pregnancy
    a. Uterine displacement essential

    b. Correction of acidosis: rapid correction of maternal metabolic acidosis with sodium bicarbonate increases fetal $Paco_2$ levels.

    c. Rapid initiation of endotracheal intubation for ventilation with 100% O_2 a must

    d. Defibrillation as indicated for appropriate cardiac dysrhythmias

    e. Resuscitation drug therapy as indicated

    f. Pulseless electrical activity

        (1) Also known as electromechanical dissociation

        (2) Common cause of pulseless rhythms during pregnancy is hypovolemia.

    g. Be prepared to initiate neonatal resuscitation.

  5. If delivery fails to facilitate successful maternal resuscitation:

    a. Consider thoracotomy and open-chest cardiac massage.

    b. Consider use of cardiopulmonary bypass in the following situations:

        (1) Method of rewarming hypothermic patients, especially if result of rapid, massive volume infusion

        (2) Bupivacaine-induced cardiac toxicity (bupivacaine slowly dissociated from myocardial sodium channels)

        (3) Pulmonary embolectomy in presence of massive pulmonary embolus

III. OBSTETRIC ANESTHESIA

  A. General anesthesia

    1. Indications

      a. Rapid induction required for maternal or fetal compromise

      b. Failed regional anesthesia

    2. Pregnancy considerations

      a. Decreased anesthesia required because of physiological, anatomical, and hormonal changes of pregnancy

      b. More rapid loss of consciousness and protective airway reflexes at lower inspired concentrations of inhaled and IV anesthetics

      c. Airway changes may lead to difficulty in intubation.

      d. Magnesium sulfate therapy may cause prolonged neuromuscular blockade.

    3. Maternal effects

      a. Complications of endotracheal intubation and extubation

        (1) Increased risk of gastric regurgitation and aspiration

        (2) Failed intubation a leading cause of anesthesia-related maternal death

      b. Uterine activity

        (1) Ketamine increases uterine resting tone and muscular activity.

        (2) Nitrous oxide has no significant effect on uterine tone.

        (3) Halogenated gases decrease uterine resting tone, uterine muscle tension, and spontaneous uterine activity.

      c. Uterine blood flow

        (1) Decreased with ultrashort-acting barbiturate induction agents

        (2) Deep anesthesia leading to significant decrease in maternal CO and BP results in decreased uterine blood flow.

        (3) Endogenous catecholamine release from inadequate general anesthesia or airway manipulation can decrease uterine blood flow.

    4. Fetal effects

      a. Neonatal depression can result from placental transmission of depressant IV drugs or inhalation agents.

      b. Effects depend on length of time of exposure and agent used.

    5. Nursing implications

      a. Premedicate obstetric patients with Bicitra or H_2-receptor antagonist to decrease gastric acidity.

      b. Judicious use of narcotic analgesia before delivery of fetus and during immediate PACU period

      c. Maintain uterine displacement with hip wedge at all times if undelivered.

        (1) Aortocaval compression in supine position may cause profound hypotension.

    d. Hyperventilation should be avoided; hypocarbia and positive pressure ventilation decrease uterine blood flow.

    e. Be aware of potential for postpartum hemorrhage.

B. Neuraxial anesthesia

    1. Subarachnoid block (spinal)

        a. Anesthetic implications

            (1) Increased blood volume and inferior vena caval compression by uterus during pregnancy lead to engorgement of epidural veins.

                (a) Increased risk of intravascular injections

                (b) Increased risk of catheter migration into epidural veins

            (2) Epidural and subarachnoid spaces decrease in size and diameter.

            (3) Higher levels of sensorimotor blockade achieved during spinal anesthesia in pregnancy

            (4) Ability to generate expiratory airway pressure (cough) decreases by 50% with spinal, 10% with epidural.

            (5) Contraindications same as general population

        b. Maternal effects

            (1) Easier to perform than lumbar epidural

            (2) Rapid onset of action

            (3) Provides a solid sensory block and profound motor block

            (4) Intense blockade of sympathetic fibers results in higher incidence of hypotension.

            (5) Spinal headache may occur (<5%).

            (6) Total spinal is rare but can lead to paralysis of respiratory muscles.

            (7) Side effects

                (a) Nausea

                (b) Vomiting

                (c) Shivering

                (d) Urinary retention

            (8) Uterine hypertonicity or hypercontractility and uterine artery vasoconstriction may occur from unintentional IV administration of the "caine" drug.

        c. Fetal effects

            (1) Maternal hypotension may lead to decreased uteroplacental blood flow.

            (2) Hypoxia can occur because of decreased uteroplacental perfusion.

            (3) Fetal bradycardia (HR <100 beats/min) may occur.

        d. Nursing implications

            (1) Before administration, hydrate with minimum IV bolus of 500 to 1000 mL to compensate for vasodilation caused by sympathetic blockade.

            (2) Assist with positioning and provide emotional support during procedure.

            (3) Maintain uterine displacement intrapartum or intraoperatively.

            (4) Monitor maternal vital signs frequently.

            (5) Promptly treat hypotension (systolic BP <100 mm Hg) with:

                (a) Lateral positioning

                (b) Increase in IV fluids

                (c) Administration of IV ephedrine to maintain uteroplacental perfusion

                (d) Slight Trendelenburg position with lateral tilt, which prevents cranial spread of intrathecal anesthesia

                (e) Elevation of legs, which increases preload

                (f) MAP more reflective of hypotension status than systolic and diastolic BP

            (6) Assess dermatome levels bilaterally.

            (7) Assess for urinary retention.

            (8) Monitor fetal heart tones; fetal bradycardia precedes maternal hypotension.

            (9) Be alert for total spinal.

          (10) Physician's order may include lying flat after administration to avoid headache; however, this is controversial.

2. Lumbar epidural and caudal anesthesia
  a. Epidural catheter frequently used as continuous technique to provide analgesia and anesthesia
  b. Anesthetic implications
    (1) Epidural space decreased in diameter and size because of increased blood volume
    (2) Pain relief slower, and a higher volume of anesthetic agent required than for spinal
    (3) Continuous infusion of low concentrations of local anesthetics into epidural space versus intermittent epidural injections offers the following advantages:
      (a) Total volume of anesthetic less
      (b) Degree of motor blockade minimized; pelvic muscle tone maintained
      (c) Fewer hypotensive episodes
    (4) With continuous infusion, a potential complication is intravascular or subarachnoid migration of catheter during infusion or progressively increasing levels of anesthesia with resulting hypotension and respiratory distress.
    (5) Contraindications same as spinal
  c. Maternal effects
    (1) Produces good analgesia, which alters maternal physiological responses to pain and lowers maternal catecholamine levels
    (2) Hypotension may occur because of sympathetic blockade.
    (3) Woman awake and active participant in birth
    (4) Systemic toxic reactions after epidural are rare but may be caused by:
      (a) Unintentional placement of drug in subarachnoid space
      (b) Excessive amount of drug in epidural space
      (c) Accidental IV injection
  d. Fetal effects same as spinal
  e. Epidural opioids
    (1) Use of intrathecal and epidural routes for opiate-type agents
    (2) Common agents
      (a) Morphine (Duramorph)
      (b) Fentanyl (Sublimaze)
      (c) Hydromorphone (Dilaudid)
    (3) Mechanism of action involves specific opiate receptors in spinal cord.
    (4) Advantages
      (a) Decreased potential for toxic reaction
      (b) Long-lasting pain relief with minimal effects on voluntary muscle function or cardiovascular status
      (c) Minimal effects on fetus
    (5) Disadvantages
      (a) Pruritus
      (b) Nausea and vomiting
      (c) Urinary retention
      (d) Respiratory depression
  f. Nursing implications
    (1) Same as spinal
    (2) With epidural opioids, pruritus most common side effect; can be treated with:
      (a) Antihistamines
      (b) Naloxone
      (c) Opioid agonist–antagonist
    (3) Sedation sometimes seen; not always accompanied by respiratory depression
    (4) Respiratory depression can occur up to 24 hours after initial administration of opioid anesthesia.

   (5) Platelet count <100,000 or bleeding times >10 minutes require anesthesia consultation before removing epidural catheter.

   (6) Monitor for progression of profound block.

   (7) Observe for intravascular infusion.

    (a) Tinnitus

    (b) Light-headedness

    (c) Circumoral tingling or numbness

    (d) Metallic taste in mouth

    (e) Convulsions

    (f) Urinary retention

C. Local anesthesia and nerve blocks

 1. Indications and actions

  a. Pudendal block

   (1) Provides perineal anesthesia for second stage, delivery, episiotomy or laceration repair, forceps or vacuum extractor delivery

   (2) Relatively simple procedure but requires thorough knowledge of pelvic anatomy

  b. Local infiltration

   (1) Injection of anesthetic agent into intracutaneous, subcutaneous, and intramuscular area of perineum

   (2) Used at time of delivery for episiotomy

  c. Paracervical block

   (1) Anesthetizes inferior hypogastric plexus and ganglia to provide relief of pain from cervical dilation

   (2) Given during active labor

   (3) Does not give perineal pain relief

 2. Anesthetic implications

  a. Increased vascularity of perineal area, vagina, and cervix increases possibility of rapid absorption of agent, resulting in systemic toxic reactions.

  b. Relatively simple to administer

 3. Maternal effects

  a. Rapid onset of analgesia

  b. Hematomas may occur as result of vessel damage.

  c. Maternal hypotension rare

  d. No relief of uterine contractions

  e. Systemic toxic reaction can occur from IV injection.

 4. Fetal effects

  a. Fetal bradycardia frequently follows paracervical block because of systemic absorption of drug or accidental injection into fetal scalp.

  b. Usually few fetal effects with local infiltration

 5. Nursing implications

  a. Local anesthesia and nerve blocks usually do not alter maternal vital signs.

  b. After paracervical block, carefully monitor FHR for bradycardia.

   (1) If <110 beats/min:

    (a) Increase IV infusion rate.

    (b) Displace uterus.

    (c) Administer supplemental O_2.

  c. Observe for vaginal hematoma.

D. Alternative techniques for pain management

 1. Psychoprophylaxis

  a. Combines positive conditioning of mother with education on process of childbirth

  b. Basis is belief that pain of labor and birth can be suppressed by reorganization of cerebral cortical activity.

   (1) Conditioned pain responses replaced by newly created "positive" conditioned reflexes

   (2) Pain with purpose of delivering baby

    2. Hypnosis

       a. Hypnoidal trance provides maternal analgesia with no maternal or fetal compromise.

       b. Use not widespread

IV. ASSESSMENT OF FETAL WELL-BEING

    A. Call obstetric unit for consultation or comanagement of patient in a PACU requiring intermittent or continuous assessment of fetal status.

    B. Uterine activity

    C. FHR

       1. Characteristics of fetal heart baseline reflect a complex physiological process that occurs between mother and fetus.

       2. Mechanisms

         a. FHR is result of interaction between central and autonomic nervous systems and the fetal heart.

         b. Primary intrinsic factors

            (1) Autonomic nervous system

               (a) Parasympathetic response: cholinergic

               (b) Sympathetic response: adrenergic

            (2) Chemoreceptors

               (a) Respond to chemical changes (Pao_2, $Paco_2$) in blood and compensate accordingly

               (b) Decrease in Pao_2 results in increase in FHR.

            (3) Baroreceptors

               (a) Respond to changes in fetal BP to maintain a constant perfusion pressure

               (b) Increase in fetal SVR results in decrease in FHR.

               (c) Decrease in fetal SVR results in increase in FHR.

         c. Secondary intrinsic factors

            (1) Cerebral cortex

            (2) Hypothalamus

            (3) Medulla oblongata

            (4) Adrenal cortex

         d. Extrinsic factors

            (1) Placental pathology

            (2) Umbilical blood flow

            (3) Uterine blood flow

            (4) Uterine activity

            (5) Fetal reserve

            (6) Maternal cardiopulmonary function

            (7) Maternal environment

            (8) Maternal-fetal response to medication and interventions

       3. Baseline FHR

         a. Definition

            (1) Approximate mean FHR—rounded to increments of 5 beats/min during a 10-minute period excluding:

               (a) Periodic or episodic changes

               (b) Periods of increased FHR variability

               (c) Segments of the baseline that differ by ≥25 beats/min

            (2) Minimum baseline duration must be at least 2 minutes.

         b. Normal: 110 to 160 beats/min (related to gestational age)

         c. Tachycardia

            (1) Rate >160 beats/min for >10 minutes

            (2) Causes

               (a) Fetal hypoxemia (early sign)

               (b) Maternal fever

               (c) Infection (maternal, intra-amniotic, or fetal)

               (d) Drugs

               (e) Maternal hyperthyroidism

      (f) Fetal anemia

      (g) Fetal cardiac dysrhythmias

      (h) Maternal or fetal hypovolemia

  d. Bradycardia

    (1) Rate <110 beats/min for >10 minutes

      (a) Rate between 90 and 110 beats/min with stable baseline and variability benign

      (b) Hemodynamically significant bradycardia: rates sustained at <90 beats/min.

    (2) Causes

      (a) Hypoxemia (late sign)

      (b) Fetal cardiac dysrhythmias

      (c) Drugs

      (d) Maternal or fetal hypothermia

      (e) Reflex

4. Baseline FHR variability

  a. Determined in a 10-minute window, excluding accelerations and decelerations

  b. Defined as fluctuations in baseline FHR that are irregular in amplitude and frequency; visually quantitated as the amplitude of the peak to trough in beats per minute.

    (1) Absent FHR variability: amplitude range undetectable

    (2) Minimal FHR variability: amplitude range > undetectable and < 5 beats/min

    (3) Moderate FHR variability: amplitude range 6 to 25 beats/min

    (4) Marked FHR variability: amplitude range >25 beats/min

  c. Moderate FHR variability with normal baseline rate reliably predicts the absence of fetal metabolic acidemia at the time it is observed.

  d. Minimal or absent FHR variability alone does not reliably predict the presence of fetal hypoxemia or metabolic acidemia.

  e. Obtain obstetric consult for absent, minimal, or marked FHR variability.

5. Periodic FHR patterns

  a. Acceleration

    (1) Sign of fetal well-being

    (2) Defined as a visually apparent abrupt increase in FHR

      (a) Abrupt increase defined as an increase from the onset of acceleration to the peak in 15 seconds

      (b) Peak must be = 15 beats/min above the baseline, and the acceleration must last = 15 seconds from onset to return to baseline.

    (3) Prolonged acceleration is = 2 minutes but <10 minutes in duration.

    (4) Acceleration lasting = 10 minutes defined as a baseline change

    (5) Before 32 weeks' gestation, acceleration defined as having a peak = 10 beats/min and a duration of = 10 seconds

    (6) Presence of accelerations rules out metabolic acidosis.

    (7) No intervention required

  b. Early deceleration

    (1) Defined as visually apparent, usually symmetrical gradual decrease and return of FHR associated with a uterine contraction

    (2) Gradual FHR decrease defined as from the onset of FHR nadir (lowest point) of greater than or equal to 30 seconds

    (3) Decrease in FHR calculated from onset to nadir of deceleration

    (4) Nadir of deceleration occurs at same time as peak of contraction.

    (5) In most cases, the onset, nadir, and recovery of the deceleration are coincident with the beginning, peak, and ending of the contraction, respectively.

    (6) Benign pattern

    (7) Thought to be vagal response to head compression

    (8) No intervention required

    c. Variable deceleration
      (1) Defined as visually apparent abrupt decrease in FHR
      (2) Abrupt FHR decrease defined as from the onset of the deceleration to the beginning of FHR nadir of <30 seconds
      (3) Decrease in FHR calculated from onset to nadir of the deceleration
      (4) Decrease in FHR is greater than or equal to 15 beats/min, lasting greater than or equal to 15 seconds, and <2 minutes in duration.
      (5) When variable decelerations are associated with uterine contractions, their onset, depth, and duration commonly vary with successive uterine contractions.
      (6) Pattern reflects diminished blood flow to fetal heart and fetal hypoxemia, hypotension, or hypertension related to umbilical cord compression.
      (7) Treatment directed to relief of umbilical cord compression and improvement of umbilical blood flow
      (8) Obtain obstetric consultation.
    d. Late deceleration
      (1) Defined as visually apparent, usually symmetrical gradual decrease and return of FHR associated with a uterine contraction
      (2) Gradual FHR decrease defined as from the onset to FHR nadir of ≥30 seconds
      (3) Decrease in FHR calculated from onset to nadir of the contraction
      (4) Deceleration is delayed in timing, with nadir of deceleration occurring after peak of contraction.
      (5) In most cases, the onset, nadir, and recovery of the deceleration occur after the beginning, peak, and ending of the contraction, respectively.
      (6) Response to fetal hypoxemia secondary to uteroplacental insufficiency
      (7) In presence of abnormal baseline rate and baseline variability, pattern concerning
      (8) Interventions directed at measures to improve uteroplacental perfusion
      (9) Obtain obstetric consult.

V. POSTPARTUM CARE
  A. Vaginal birth without complications
    1. Postpartum observations
      a. Vital signs
        (1) BP consistent with baseline during pregnancy
          (a) Orthostatic hypotension may be present for 24 hours.
          (b) Increased BP may be caused by:
            (i) Preeclampsia
            (ii) Anxiety
            (iii) Essential hypertension
          (c) BP not reliable indicator of hypovolemia or shock
        (2) Temperature >100.4°F (38°C) after 24 hours may indicate infection.
        (3) Tachycardia (>100 beats/min) may indicate:
          (a) Hemorrhage
          (b) Pain
          (c) Fever
          (d) Dehydration
        (4) Tachypnea (>24 breaths/min) may indicate respiratory disease.
        (5) Lungs should be clear to auscultation.
      b. Condition of uterine fundus
        (1) Firm, midline, at level of umbilicus first 24 hours
        (2) Involution occurs at rate of 1 cm/day.
        (3) Boggy or higher-than-suggested normal level may indicate uterine atony related to overdistended uterus, structural anomalies, or overdistended bladder.
        (4) Overdistended bladder may cause lateral deviation of uterus.

    c. Lochia
       (1) Rubra
          (a) Bright red, bloody, may have small clots
          (b) Characteristic fleshy odor
          (c) Occurs 1 to 3 days postpartum
          (d) Heavy to moderate flow
       (2) Serosa
          (a) Pink to pink brown, serous, no clots
          (b) Usually no odor
          (c) Occurs 5 to 7 days after delivery
          (d) Decrease in flow
       (3) Alba
          (a) Cream to yellowish, may be brownish
          (b) Usually no odor
          (c) Occurs 1 to 3 weeks after delivery
          (d) Scant flow
       (4) Excessive lochia may be caused by:
          (a) Uterine atony
          (b) Laceration
          (c) Hematoma
          (d) Retained placental fragments
          (e) Infection
       (5) Malodorous lochia indicative of infection
   d. Perineum
       (1) Slight edema normal
       (2) Assessment of episiotomy
          (a) Redness
          (b) Edema
          (c) Ecchymosis
          (d) Discharge
          (e) Approximation
       (3) Rectal area free of hemorrhoids, hematoma
   e. Urinary system
       (1) Output up to 3000 mL/day
       (2) Distended bladder may cause uterine atony.
       (3) Burning on urination or inability to void may suggest infection.
       (4) Bladder atony may occur after instrument delivery or regional anesthesia.
   f. Intestinal elimination
       (1) Bowel movement by day 2 or 3 after delivery
       (2) Constipation may indicate sluggish bowel or pain (fear of pain also possible).
       (3) Diarrhea may be from multiple factors.
   g. Breasts
       (1) Assess feeding method.
       (2) Soft to palpation
       (3) Colostrum may be present; milk in 2 to 4 days.
       (4) Nipples intact, erect
       (5) Swollen, painful breasts may indicate infection.
   h. Rh status: is RhoGAM indicated?
2. Personal care and comfort
   a. Ambulation
   b. Shower or bathing
   c. Perineal care
   d. Sitz bath
   e. Breast support and comfort
   f. Nutrition
   g. Emotional adjustment

3. Family relations
   a. Visitors
   b. Children at home
   c. Sexuality and birth control
   d. Role transitions
   e. Adaptation of family routines
4. Infant care
B. Cesarean birth without complications
   1. Anesthesia (see Obstetric Anesthesia, section III)
   2. Potential complications same as for any patient undergoing abdominal surgery
   3. Postoperative assessments same as for any patient undergoing abdominal surgery
   4. Postpartum assessments same as for vaginal delivery
C. High-risk versus critical care
   1. About 1% of obstetric population requires critical care management.
   2. Pregnant-specific diseases and medical complications of pregnancy that often require critical care management
      a. Preeclampsia
      b. Cardiac disease
      c. Septic shock
      d. ARDS
      e. Diabetic ketoacidosis
      f. Thyroid storm
   3. Multidisciplinary care approach with collaboration between obstetric and critical care units
D. Emergency hysterectomy
   1. Cesarean hysterectomy usually emergency procedure
      a. Emergency indications requiring hysterectomy
         (1) Uterine atony (43%)
         (2) Placenta accreta (30%)
         (3) Uterine rupture (13%)
         (4) Extension (unplanned) of low transverse incision (10%)
      b. Complications
         (1) Increased blood loss
         (2) Occasional injury to bladder or ureters
         (3) Increased anesthesia exposure
   2. Nursing assessments and interventions same as for nonobstetric abdominal hysterectomy

BIBLIOGRAPHY

1. American Academy of Pediatrics, American College of Obstetricians and Gynecologists: *Guidelines for perinatal care*, ed 6, Elk Grove, IL, 2007, American Academy of Pediatrics.
2. American College of Obstetricians and Gynecologists Committee on Practice Bulletins—Obstetrics: ACOG practice bulletin. Diagnosis and management of preeclampsia and eclampsia. *Obstet Gynecol* 99(1): 159–167, 2002.
3. American College of Obstetricians and Gynecologists: ACOG practice bulletin. Obstetric analgesia and anesthesia. *Int J Gynaecol Obstet* 78(3):321–335, 2002.
4. Arafeh JM, Baird SM: Cardiac disease in pregnancy. *Crit Care Nurs Q* 29(1):32–52, 2006.
5. Blackburn ST: *Maternal, fetal, and neonatal physiology: A clinical perspective*, ed 3, WB Saunders, 2007, St Louis.

6. Briggs GG, Freeman RK, Yaffee SJ: *Drugs in pregnancy and lactation*, ed 8, Baltimore, 2008, Williams & Wilkins.
7. Burrow GN, Duffy TP, Copel JA, eds: *Medical complications during pregnancy*, ed 6, Philadelphia, 2004, WB Saunders.
8. Creasy R, Resnik R, Iams JD, et al, eds: *Creasy and Resnik's maternal-fetal medicine: Principles and practice*, ed 6, Philadelphia, 2009, Saunders.
9. Dildy GA, Belfort MA, Saade GR, et al, eds: *Critical care obstetrics*, ed 4, Malden, 2004, Blackwell Science.
10. Foley MR, Strong TH Jr, Garite TJ, eds: *Obstetric intensive care manual*, ed 2, New York, 2004, McGraw-Hill.
11. Gifford R, August P, Cunningham G, et al: *National High Blood Pressure Education Program Working Group National High Blood Pressure*

in Pregnancy. NIH Publication No. 00–3029, Bethesda, MD, 2000, National Institutes of Health, National Heart, Lung, Blood Institute.

12. Klein LL, Galan HL: Cardiac disease in pregnancy. *Obstet Gynecol Clin North Am* 31:429–459, 2004.

13. Martin JM Jr, Thigpen BD, Moore RC, et al: Stroke and severe preeclampsia and eclampsia: A paradigm shift focusing on systolic blood pressure. *Obstet Gynecol* 105(2): 246–254, 2005.

14. Poole JH, White D: *Obstetrical emergencies for the perinatal nurse.* ed 2, White Plains, NY, 2005, March of Dimes.

15. Raijmakers M, Dechend R, Poston L: Oxidative stress and preeclampsia: Rationale for antioxidant clinical trials. *Hypertension* 44(4):374–380, 2004.

16. Simpson KR, Creehan PA: *AWHONN perinatal nursing,* ed 3, Philadelphia, 2008, Lippincott Williams & Wilkins.

40 Ophthalmological Care

SEEMA HUSSAIN
KENNETH WICHTER

OBJECTIVES

At the conclusion of this chapter, the reader will be able to:

1. Identify the important functions of the eye.
2. Describe the structure of the eye.
3. Describe common ophthalmological surgical procedures.
4. List drugs frequently used for ophthalmological surgical procedures.
5. Identify possible complications of ophthalmological surgery.
6. Describe perianesthesia nursing care for the ophthalmological surgery patient.

I. ANATOMY AND PHYSIOLOGY OF THE EYE (Figure 40-1)
   A. Orbit
      1. Pyramid-shaped bony cavity that functions as protection for the eye
      2. Consists of seven fused bones
         a. Ethmoid
         b. Sphenoid
         c. Frontal
         d. Lacrimal
         e. Zygomatic
         f. Palatine
         g. Maxilla
      3. Orbit contains
         a. Eyeball
         b. Six extraocular muscles
         c. Ophthalmic artery veins
         d. Cranial nerves
            (1) The second (optic)
            (2) Third (oculomotor)
            (3) Fourth (trochlear)
            (4) Fifth (trigeminal)
            (5) Sixth (abducens)
         e. Lacrimal gland
         f. Lacrimal sac
         g. Orbital fascia, fat and ligaments
   B. Eyelids are continuous with the conjunctiva lining the inner aspect of the lid
      1. Act as protection for
         a. Anterior portion of the eyes
         b. Epithelium of the lids
      2. Spread lubricating solutions over globe
         a. Keep eyes moist
         b. Prevent evaporation of secretion
      3. Eyelashes situated along the margins and act as protective fibers

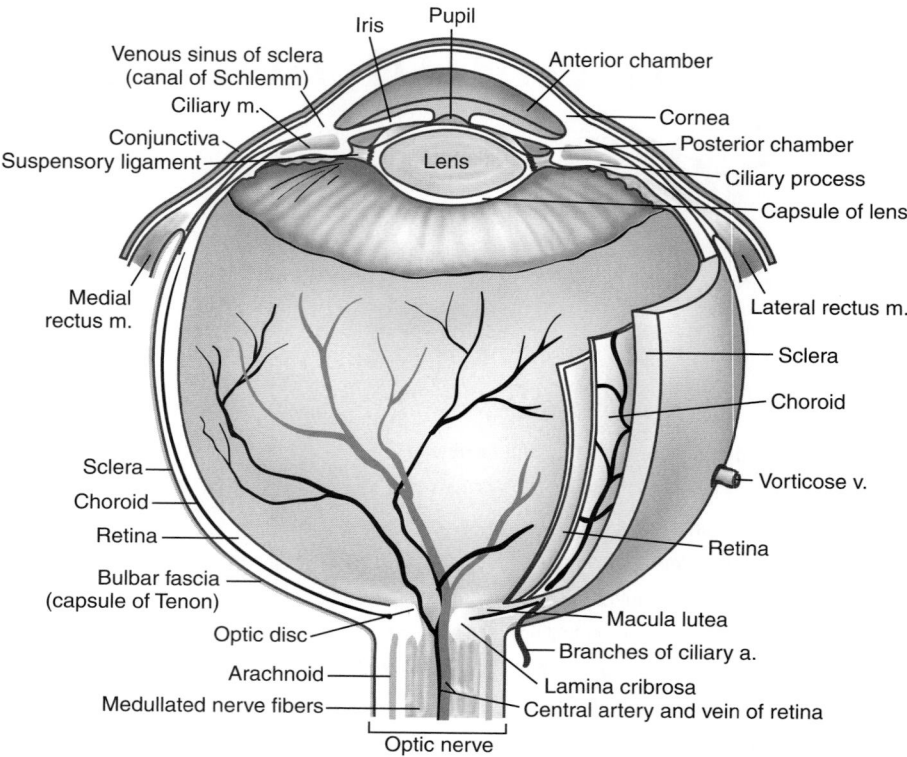

FIGURE 40-1 ■ Structure of the eyeball. (From Drain CB, ed: *Perianesthesia nursing: A critical care approach,* ed 4, St Louis, 2003, WB Saunders, p 453.)

4. Two muscle groups
   a. Orbicularis oculi sphincter responsible for closing eye
   b. Levator palpebrae responsible for raising eyelids
   c. Movements can be both involuntary and voluntary.
5. Function of the eyelids
   a. Cover eyes during sleep
   b. Protect eyes from excessive light
   c. Protect eye from injury
   d. Protect eye from foreign objects
   e. Lubricate the anterior surface of the eye
6. Lined with mucous membrane called palpebral conjunctiva

C. Conjunctiva
   1. Thin, transparent mucous membrane covering sclera and inner lids
   2. Lining upper and lower eyelids—palpebral conjunctiva
   3. Extends over sclera to corneal margin—bulbar conjunctiva
   4. Function of the conjunctiva
      a. Produces the mucin layer of the tear film, reducing the rate of tear evaporation
      b. Protects the eye against damage and infection
      c. Facilitates movement by moistening the surface of the eye and lids

D. Lacrimal apparatus: produces and drains tears
   1. Consists of:
      a. Lacrimal gland—located in upper outer aspect of each orbit and produces tears that:
         (1) Empty through lacrimal ducts onto conjunctiva of upper lid
         (2) Spread across eyeball by blinking
         (3) Enter lacrimal puncta

      b. Lacrimal puncta—two small openings located in the inner canthus of each upper and lower eyelid
         (1) Pass into lacrimal canals, lacrimal sac, nasolacrimal duct, and finally into inferior meatus of the turbinate bone of the nose
      c. Lacrimal sac—collects tears
      d. Nasolacrimal duct—drains tears from lacrimal sac to nose
   2. Tears
      a. Contains
         (1) Water
         (2) Protein
         (3) Glucose
         (4) Sodium
         (5) Potassium
         (6) Chloride
         (7) Urea
         (8) Lysozyme (bacterial enzyme)
      b. Purpose of tears
         (1) Aid refraction by providing an optically smooth corneal surface
         (2) Lubricate the anterior surface of the eye to aid movement
         (3) Clean dust particles from the eye
         (4) Protect against infection by the action of lysozymes
      c. Emotional stimulus of parasympathetic nervous system triggered
  E. Muscles controlling the eye (Figure 40-2)
   1. Extraocular muscles (six)
      a. Attached to outside of eyeball and to bones of the orbit
      b. Consist of voluntary skeletal muscle
         (1) Four rectus
            (a) Superior—oculomotor nerve
            (b) Inferior—oculomotor nerve
            (c) Medial—oculomotor nerve
            (d) Lateral—abducens nerve
         (2) Two oblique muscles
            (a) Superior—trochlear nerve
            (b) Inferior—oculomotor nerve
      c. Action
         (1) Muscles move eyeball through cranial nerves.
            (a) Third (oculomotor)—moves eyeball and upper eyelid
            (b) Size of iris (i.e., constriction and dilation of pupil to regulate amount of light admitted)
            (c) Control of ciliary muscle to regulate degree of refraction by lens
            (d) Fourth (trochlear)—movement of eyeball by superior oblique muscles
            (e) Sixth (abducens)—movement of eyeball by lateral rectus muscle
         (2) Muscles work in pairs.
         (3) Movement caused by:
            (a) Increase in tone of one set of muscles
            (b) Decrease in tone of antagonistic (opposite set) muscles
   2. Movement of upper eyelid
      a. Raised (opened) by levator palpebrae superioris muscle
         (1) Controlled by cranial nerve III and sympathetic nervous system
      b. Closed by orbicularis oculi muscle
         (1) Controlled by cranial nerve VII
   3. Iris and ciliary muscles
      a. Smooth, involuntary muscles
      b. Work inside eyeball
         (1) Regulate size of pupil
         (2) Control shape of lens during accommodation
         (3) Controlled through neural network

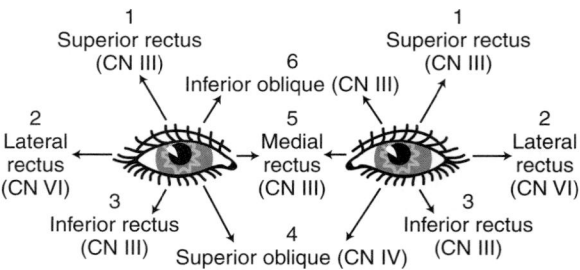

Cardinal Directions of Gaze	Muscles Working for Each Direction
Eyes up, right	Right superior rectus and left inferior oblique
Eyes right	Right lateral rectus and left medial rectus
Eyes down, right	Right inferior rectus and left superior oblique
Eyes down, left	Right superior oblique and left inferior rectus
Eyes left	Right medial rectus and left lateral rectus
Eyes up, left	Right inferior oblique and left superior rectus

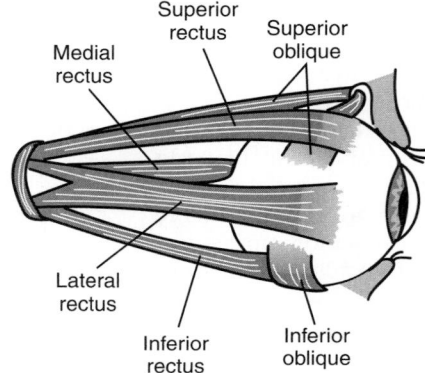

Muscles of Right Eye

FIGURE 40-2 ■ The six cardinal directions of gaze and the muscles responsible for each. The six cardinal directions are (1) right, (2) left, (3) up and right, (4) up and left, (5) down and right, and (6) down and left. (From Black JM, Matassarin-Jacobs E: *Medical-surgical nursing clinical management for continuity of care,* ed 5, Philadelphia, 1997, WB Saunders, p 936.)

      (a) Optic nerve (cranial nerve II)
      (b) Oculomotor nerve (cranial nerve III)
F. Globe (eyeball): supported in orbital cavity on a cushion of fat and fascia; composed of three layers
   1. External, corneal-scleral layer (fibrous, protects other two layers)
     a. Cornea
       (1) Anterior, transparent, avascular part of the external layer
       (2) Serves as a window through which light rays pass to retina
       (3) Supplied by branches of ophthalmic division of fifth cranial nerve
       (4) Composed of five layers
         (a) Epithelium
           (i)   Cell layers and nerve endings
           (ii) Account for corneal sensitivity
         (b) Bowman's membrane
           (i)   Composed of connective tissue fibers
           (ii) Forms a barrier between trauma and infection
           (iii) Does not regenerate if damaged
           (iv) Will leave a permanent scar

(c) Stroma
   (i)   Accounts for 90% of corneal thickening
   (ii) Composed of multiple lamellar fibers
(d) Descemet's membrane
   (i)   Thin layer between endothelial layer of cornea and substantia propria (fibrous, tough, and transparent main part of the cornea)
   (ii) If inflamed, called descemetitis
   (iii) If protrudes, called descemetocele
(e) Endothelium
   (i)   Single layer of hexagonal cells
   (ii) Does not regenerate
   (iii) Responsible for proper state of dehydration that keeps cornea clear
   (iv) Damage causes corneal edema and loss of transparency.

b. Sclera: posterior opaque part of the external layer; tough white outer coat of eyeball
   (1) Portion of sclera can be seen through the conjunctiva as the white of the eye.
   (2) Made up of collagenous fibers loosely connected with fascia, which receives the tendons of the muscles of the globe

2. Middle layer: middle covering of the eye comprises the choroid, ciliary body, and iris (referred to as uveal tract).
   a. Choroid
      (1) Most posterior portion of middle coat
      (2) Contains many blood vessels; highly vascular
      (3) Deeply pigmented
      (4) Purpose
         (a) Absorbs light rays
         (b) Prevents reflection within eyeball
         (c) Main source of nourishment to retina (through its blood supply)
   b. Ciliary body
      (1) Consists of an extension of the choroidal blood vessels, a mass of muscle tissue, and an extension of the neuroepithelium of the retina
      (2) Composed of ciliary muscle and ciliary processes
      (3) Ciliary muscle
         (a) Affects accommodation
         (b) Alters shape of lens as needed to focus light rays from near or distant objects on retina
      (4) Ciliary processes
         (a) Produce aqueous humor
   c. Iris
      (1) Colored area of eye
      (2) Anterior portion of the middle layer
         (a) Thin membrane situated in front of the lens
      (3) Peripheral border attached to ciliary body
      (4) Central border is free.
      (5) Divides the space between the cornea and the lens
         (a) Anterior and posterior chambers
         (b) Chambers filled with aqueous humor
      (6) Regulates the amount of light entering the eye
         (a) Muscles contract and relax.
         (b) Changes size of opening in center (pupil)
         (c) Assists in obtaining clear images

3. Internal layer: innermost layer of neural coat (retina)
   a. Retina
      (1) A thin transparent membrane extending from the ora serrata to the optic disc
      (2) Consists of network of nerve cells and fibers
         (a) Receives images of external objects
         (b) Transfers the impressions to the occipital lobe of cerebrum via

        (i)   Optic nerve
        (ii) Optic tracts
        (iii) Lateral geniculate body
        (iv) Optic radiations
    (c) Nerve fibers from retina converge to become optic nerve.
        (i)   Point at which optic nerve enters eyeball called optic disc (anatomic blind spot)
  (3) Covers choroid
  (4) Found only in back of eye
 b. Retina composed of layers
  (1) Outer pigment
    (a) Stores vitamin A; needed to produce photopigment rhodopsin
  (2) Inner neural
    (a) Consists of photoreceptor cells (rods and cones)
        (i)   Visual receptors that develop generator potentials
        (ii) Relays sensory information to ganglion cells of retina
    (b) Rods
        (i)   Located in peripheral retina
        (ii) Allow for vision in dim light
        (iii) Responsible for perception of different shades of light and dark, shapes, and movement
    (c) Cones
        (i)   Stimulated by bright light only
        (ii) Responsible for color vision and visual acuity

G. Refractive apparatus (cornea, aqueous humor, lens, and vitreous body)
 1. Cornea
  a. Has greatest refractive power of the ocular structures
  b. Variations in curvature of cornea change its refractive power.
 2. Aqueous humor
  a. Fluid responsible for maintaining intraocular pressure
  b. Produced by ciliary processes
  c. Secreted by ciliary body into posterior chamber
  d. Flows from posterior chamber through pupil into anterior chamber
  e. Flows into anterior chamber angle and is filtered out through the trabecular meshwork into Schlemm's canal
  f. Channeled into capillary network and into episcleral veins
  g. Maintenance of normal intraocular pressure
    (1) Occurs as long as there is a balance between:
      (a) Aqueous production
      (b) Aqueous humor outflow
 3. Lens
  a. Suspended behind the iris
  b. Anterior and posterior surfaces separated by rounded border
  c. Does not shed cells; as it grows, the cells compress and harden.
  d. Lens expands and retracts through zonular fibers (accommodation).
  e. Accommodation power lost with aging process
  f. Hardening eventually causes opacity of lens (cataract).
 4. Vitreous body
  a. Glasslike transparent gelatinous mass (vitreous humor)
  b. Composed of 99% water and 1% collagen and hyaluronic acid
  c. Fills the posterior four fifths of the eyeball
  d. Supports the posterior cavity
  e. Keeps the retina in place

H. Nerve and blood supply
 1. Optic nerve (second cranial nerve)
  a. Extends between posterior eyeball and optic chiasma
  b. Carries visual impulses and sensations of pain, touch, temperature from eye to brain

      2. Muscle innervation

         a. Oculomotor (third cranial nerve): primary motor nerve to all rectus muscles (except lateral rectus)

         b. Abducens (sixth cranial nerve) innervates lateral rectus.

         c. Trochlear (fourth cranial nerve) innervates superior oblique muscle.

      3. Ophthalmic artery

         a. Main arterial supply to orbit and globe

         b. Branch of internal carotid artery

II. COMMON OPHTHALMIC SURGICAL PROCEDURES

    A. Blepharoplasty—repair of the upper or lower eyelids to remove redundant skin; may be cosmetic or therapeutic when the eyelid interferes with vision

      1. Types

         a. Upper blepharoplasty (upper eyelid only)

         b. Lower blepharoplasty (lower eyelid only)

         c. Quadrilateral blepharoplasty (involving all four eyelids)

      2. Preoperative considerations

         a. Patient may be examined by ophthalmologist before procedure to rule out ocular symptomatology.

      3. Surgical procedure

         a. Excess skin and muscle resected; periorbital fat trimmed

         b. Requires meticulous hemostasis

         c. Closed using fine nonabsorbable or absorbable sutures

      4. Postoperative considerations

         a. Iced saline dressings applied immediately to control edema

    B. Removal of chalazion—granulomatous inflammation of a meibomian gland in eyelid, frequently caused by *Staphylococcus aureus*

      1. Surgical procedure

         a. Surgical incision and curettage

         b. Most commonly done under local anesthesia in physician's office

         c. Occasionally requires operating room (OR) setting

    C. Repair of entropion

      1. Entropion

         a. Eyelid margins turn in, especially the lower lid

         b. Caused by spasm of the orbicularis oculi muscle

         c. Scarring of the conjunctiva

         d. Lashes scrape across cornea with each eye blink, which is painful and results in

            (1) Corneal abrasions

            (2) Scarring

            (3) Ulcer

      2. Surgical procedure

         a. Surgical removal of excision of skin and/or muscle and/or the tarsal plate

            (1) Correction of the muscular fibers of the lid, everting the lid margins and eyelashes

            (2) Performed under local or general anesthesia

         b. Cryotherapy—may be used to freeze and remove lashes, which destroys lash follicle and prevents regrowth of lashes

            (1) Preferred method of treatment

    D. Repair of ectropion

      1. Ectropion—outward turning or eversion of eyelid, usually bilateral

         a. Caused by:

            (1) Relaxation of orbicularis oculi muscle

            (2) Scarring of the face near the eye

            (3) Normal aging process

            (4) Bell's palsy

            (5) Exposure of underlying conjunctiva

            (6) Congenital

         b. Can lead to keratitis (inflammation or infection of the cornea)

    2. Surgical procedure

      a. Shortening of lower lid in a horizontal direction

      b. Mild case can be treated with deep electrocautery 4 to 5 mm from the lid margins.

        (1) Resulting scar formation will draw lid to its normal position.

      c. Lateral tarsal strip procedure—lateral canthal tightening

        (1) Preferred method of treatment

        (2) Performed under local anesthesia

      d. Upper lid gold weight implantation for paralytic ectropion

E. Ptosis

    1. Drooping of the upper eyelid; can affect one or both eyes; caused by weakness of levator muscle, or less frequently, Muller's muscle

    2. Three types of ptosis

      a. Congenital—caused by failure of levator muscle to develop, weakness of superior rectal muscles

      b. Acquired—associated with loss of superior visual field in primary gaze

        (1) Causes

          (a) Mechanical failure—weight of eyelid neoplasms

          (b) Trauma—caused by laceration of third cranial nerve, the levator, or both

          (c) Myogenic, by disease—muscular dystrophy

          (d) Neurological disorders—myasthenia gravis

          (e) May be caused by a tumor

          (f) Aponeurotic ptosis—senescence, dehiscence, or chronic inflammation

        (2) Treatment based on cause and severity

      c. Senile

    3. Surgical procedure

      a. Objective is to create a good upper lid fold with elevation of the lid.

      b. Surgical procedures based on advancement of

        (1) Levator muscle

        (2) Frontalis muscle

        (3) Superior rectus muscle

F. Excision of pterygium

    1. Thick triangular growth of epithelial tissue

      a. Extends from corner of cornea to the inner canthus

      b. Appearances may be pale or white.

      c. May grow over the pupillary opening

      d. Cause thought to be exposure to constant irritant such as

        (1) Wind

        (2) Dust, including sand

        (3) Ultraviolet light

    2. Surgical procedure

      a. Growth dissected off the cornea and conjunctiva down to the sclera

      b. Low-dose radiation on surgical wound may be used to prevent regrowth.

        (1) Regrowth rate 20% to 40%

G. Lacrimal duct disorders

    1. Dacryocystorhinostomy (DCR)—establishment of a new tear passageway for drainage directly into the nasal cavity

      a. Dacryocystitis is an infection in the lacrimal sac and its mucous membranes that extends to the surrounding connective tissue, resulting in localized cellulitis.

      b. Surgical procedure

        (1) Nasal cavity anesthetized topically with cocaine preoperatively

        (2) Usually performed under general anesthesia

        (3) Lacrimal sac probed and opened

        (4) A stent is placed through lacrimal duct drainage system to keep system open until epithelium forms around it and creates a new opening.

        (5) Stent generally removed in 6 weeks

2. Conjunctivodacryocystorhinostomy
   a. Description
      (1) Variation of DCR
      (2) Necessary if lacrimal sac
         (a) Has been destroyed
         (b) Must be recreated
         (c) Canaliculi are absent.
   b. Surgical procedure
      (1) After completion of DCR, conjunctiva taken from lower lid and sutured to nasal mucosa to form lacrimal sac
      (2) If canaliculus cannot be kept open or is absent
         (a) Permanent stent (Pyrex tube) is placed.
         (b) Patient teaching includes:
            (i) How to place tube back in if it falls out
            (ii) How to clean tube
            (iii) How to hold tube in case of sneezing
3. Endoscopic DCR
   a. Uses endonasal laser to open pathway into lacrimal sac
   b. Uses endoscopic equipment
   c. Benefits
      (1) Eliminates external incision and scar
      (2) Decreases amount of postoperative discomfort
      (3) Provides hemostasis
      (4) Increases healing time
      (5) Decreased cost
H. Surgery for strabismus
   1. Description
      a. Inability to direct the two eyes at the same object because of lack of coordination of extraocular muscles
      b. Misalignment of axes of the eyes in which one or both eyes turned inward or outward
      c. Often accompanied by amblyopia (normal vision fails to develop despite absence of disease or refractive error)
      d. Normally done on children younger than 6 years
      e. May be done for cosmetic reasons for children older than 6 years
      f. Indications for performing procedure on adults
         (1) Bell's palsy
         (2) Muscular dystrophy
         (3) Traumatic injury
         (4) Untreated or unsatisfactory treatment of childhood strabismus
         (5) Muscular paralysis resulting from stroke
   2. Surgical procedure
      a. Corrective surgery performed to change the relative strength of individual muscles and therefore improve coordination
         (1) May require resection: the removal of a portion of muscle and attachment of cut ends
         (2) May require recession: severance of the muscle from its original insertion with reattachment more posteriorly on the sclera
         (3) May require transplanting a muscle to improve rotation of paralyzed muscle
      b. Intraoperative consideration
         (1) Manipulation of rectus muscle will cause transient bradycardia.
            (a) Treated with atropine
            (b) If severe, surgeon may have to stop manipulation of rectus muscle until heart rate returns to normal.
         (2) Bradycardia caused by innervation of branch of vagus nerve
I. Removal of globe
   1. Exenteration
      a. Entire contents of orbit removed
      b. Requires extensive plastic reconstruction

2. Evisceration
   a. Removal of contents of the globe
   b. Preserves sclera and muscular attachments
   c. Prosthesis inserted to maintain shape of eye
      (1) Sclera closed over prosthesis
      (2) Conjunctiva closed over sclera
      (3) Conformer placed under eyelids to maintain space until swelling subsides and artificial eye created
   d. Advantages
      (1) Natural attachment of eye muscles
      (2) Normal eye movement
3. Enucleation
   a. Removal of the diseased globe and a portion of the optic nerve
   b. General anesthesia usually administered
   c. Prosthesis may be inserted.
J. Corneal transplant (keratoplasty)
   1. Description
      a. Grafting of corneal tissue from one human eye to another
      b. Performed when patient's cornea thickened and opacified
      c. Transparency of cornea may be impaired from infection, burns, complications related to laser-assisted in situ keratomileusis (LASIK), or certain diseases.
      d. Corneal transplant performed to improve vision when basic visual structures of eye (optic nerve and retina) functioning properly
   2. Types
      a. Penetrating keratoplasty (full-thickness)
         (1) Most common
         (2) Performed with microscope
      b. Lamellar keratoplasty (partial thickness)
         (1) More difficult than penetrating keratoplasty, involving the removal and replacement of the anterior corneal stroma and Bowman's membrane with donor material
         (2) Higher success rate
            (a) Success because of layered cellular arrangement of corneal tissue and avascularity
            (b) Procedure preserves the host endothelium.
      c. Keratectomy (peeling of the cornea)
      d. Descemet's stripping automated endothelial keratoplasty
         (1) Procedure is a partial-thickness corneal transplant that replaces only the endothelial layer with donor cells.
      e. Tattooing (simulation of a pupil)
         (1) Rarely done
   3. Postoperative considerations
      a. Eye patch and shield remain in place until instructed to remove by surgeon.
      b. Activity is light to as tolerated.
      c. Resume preoperative diet.
      d. Healing of cornea is very slow.
         (1) Recovery of vision longer than after cataract surgery
   4. Potential complications
      a. Rejection of corneal transplant
         (1) Cornea becomes opaque.
         (2) Treated with steroids
         (3) May require repeated keratoplasty
K. Radial keratotomy
   1. Description
      a. Used to reduce myopia in adults
      b. Series of precise, partial-thickness radial incisions in the cornea
      c. Results in flattening the cornea, reducing refractive error

   2. Usually performed under topical anesthesia
   3. Potential complications
    a. Glaring from scars
    b. Permanent scarring
    c. Infection resulting in loss of vision
    d. Cataract formation caused by injury to lens
    e. Variations in level of correction
   4. Correction with excimer laser
    a. Ablates top of cornea
    b. Fewer complications
       (1) Minimal glare sensitivity problems
    c. Performed with topical anesthesia
    d. Complications
       (1) Overcorrection
       (2) Undercorrection
       (3) Haze, glare, or halos
       (4) Elevated intraocular pressure
    e. Postprocedure treatment
       (1) Instillation of
          (a) Tobramycin
          (b) Examethasone suspension drops
          (c) 5% homatropine hydrobromide antibiotic
          (d) Steroid drops
       (2) Pain management with analgesics
       (3) Placement of disposable soft contact lens for first 3 weeks
          (a) Promotes epithelial growth
       (4) Use of dark sunglasses
 L. Cataract extraction
  1. Description
    a. Cataract: gradual developing opacity of the lens of the eye
       (1) Can occur at any time
          (a) Etiology in infants
             (i)   Heredity
             (ii) Developmental abnormalities
             (iii) Infection
             (iv) Traumatic eye injury
             (v) Chemical imbalances (galactosemia and diabetes)
          (b) Etiology in adults
             (i)   Same as infant
             (ii) Prolonged exposure to ultraviolet light
             (iii) Medications (those used to treat glaucoma)
             (iv) Most common cause: normal part of aging process
    b. Cataract extraction is the removal of the opaque lens from the interior of the eye.
  2. Types of procedures
    a. Intracapsular cataract extraction (ICCE)
       (1) Removal of lens as well as anterior and posterior capsule, cortex, and nucleus
       (2) Method largely replaced by extracapsular cataract extraction
       (3) Risk of vitreous humor loss
    b. Extracapsular cataract extraction (ECCE)
       (1) Anterior portion of the capsule is first ruptured, then removed.
       (2) Lens cortex and nucleus are expressed from the eye, leaving the posterior capsule behind intact (posterior capsule is excellent support for intraocular lens implantation).
    c. Phacoemulsification
       (1) Lens removed by fragmenting it with ultrasonic vibrations
       (2) Simultaneously, fragments irrigated and aspirated without loss of lens capsule
       (3) Very small incision needed

3. Correction of aphakia (absence of lens)
   a. Patient sees objects larger than normal.
   b. Objects appear blurred and without detail.
   c. Options available for correction
      (1) Glasses
         (a) Aphakia spectacles
         (b) Fitted 6 to 8 weeks after lens extraction
         (c) Acceptable only for binocular aphakia
         (d) Distorts peripheral vision
         (e) Produces enlarged images
         (f) Clear image only in direct center of glasses
      (2) Contact lens
         (a) Better option for vision correction
         (b) Can be used for monocular aphakia
         (c) Patient has complete field of vision.
         (d) Less magnification of image required
      (3) Epikeratophakia
         (a) Procedure considered for patients with low endothelial cell counts
         (b) Form of refractive keratoplasty
         (c) Description of procedure
            (i) Piece of donor corneal tissue shaped to specific diopter on a cryolathe
            (ii) Tissue sutured to recipient's cornea
            (iii) Changes corneal curvature
            (iv) Results in change of refractive power of cornea
      (4) Placement of intraocular lens (IOL)
         (a) Most commonly used procedure today
         (b) Description of lens
            (i) Made of Plexiglas or polymethylmethacrylate, acrylic material, silicon
            (ii) Center can be either biconvex or convexoplano and two haptics (spring-hook appendages).
               [a] Polypropylene haptics break down over time.
               [b] Should not be used on young patients
            (iii) Lens cannot adjust anterior to posterior dimensions.
               [a] Provides only myopic (nearsighted) or hyperopic (farsighted) vision
               [b] Patient decides on need of glasses for distance or reading.
      (5) Advantages of IOL
         (a) Shorter rehabilitation period
         (b) Lens used for monocular aphakic correction
      (6) Lens placement
         (a) Anterior chamber
            (i) Used after ICCE
            (ii) Used for secondary lens implantation
         (b) Iris plane
         (c) Sulcus fixated
         (d) Posterior chamber
            (i) Only when cataract removed by ECCE or phacoemulsification
            (ii) Most physiological position for artificial lens
      (7) Sutureless cataract technique
         (a) Most common
         (b) Rapid visual rehabilitation
4. Preoperative considerations
   a. Inquire as to patient's use of anticoagulants, nonsteroidal, and anti-inflammatory drugs (Motrin or aspirin); can cause increase in bleeding intraoperatively.
   b. Identify adequate home support system; implement referrals if necessary.

      c. Review preoperative instructions with patient.
         (1) Provide instructions in large type.
         (2) Use off-white paper to reduce glare.
      d. Administer mydriatics and/or additional medications as ordered.

M. Procedures to treat glaucoma
    1. Iridectomy
      a. Description
         (1) Removal of a section of iris tissue
         (2) Peripheral iridectomy done in the treatment of acute, subacute, or chronic angle-closure glaucoma
           (a) Extensive peripheral anterior synechiae not yet formed
         (3) Reestablishes communication between posterior and anterior chambers
         (4) Relieves pupillary block
         (5) Facilitates movement of aqueous humor from posterior to anterior chamber
    2. Trabeculectomy
      a. Description
         (1) Creation of a fistula between anterior chamber of eye and subconjunctival space
         (2) Portion of the trabecular meshwork surgically excised
         (3) Facilitates drainage of aqueous humor from the posterior chamber to the anterior chamber for treatment of glaucoma
      b. Adjunctive medical therapy may be used to decrease postoperative fibrosis by applying 5-fluorouracil or mitomycin C under the conjunctival flap for 3 to 5 minutes.

N. Vitrectomy
    1. Description
      a. Removal of all or part of vitreous gel
    2. Indications (anterior segment)
      a. Vitreous loss during cataract extraction surgery
      b. Anterior segment opacities
      c. Miscellaneous causes
    3. Indications (posterior segment)
      a. Vitreous opacities
      b. Advanced diabetic eye disease
      c. Severe intraocular trauma
      d. Retained foreign bodies
      e. Endophthalmitis
    4. Procedural considerations
      a. Procedure varies according to location of pathological condition.
         (1) Anterior
         (2) Posterior
      b. Requires use of operating microscope, illuminations system, and cutting-suction-infusion system
    5. Intraoperative considerations
      a. Procedure time varies from 1 hour to 6 hours.
      b. Protect pressure area on patient.
      c. May use elastic stockings
    6. Postoperative considerations
      a. May experience more postoperative pain than is generally associated with ophthalmological surgeries
         (1) Strong analgesics may be necessary.
         (2) Ice packs may help reduce pain.

O. Retinal detachment
    1. Description
      a. Separation of portion of retina from choroid
      b. Goal of treatment aimed at repairing tears and returning retina to normal anatomical position

2. Causes
   a. Intraocular neoplasms
   b. Associated with injury (blow to head or previous ocular surgery)
   c. Normal aging process
   d. Severe myopia
   e. Congenital
   f. Inflammatory process
   g. Vascular disease
3. Signs and symptoms
   a. Patient may experience sudden onset of floaters (floating spots in front of eye).
   b. Loss of vision without pain
   c. Slow decrease in visual field (described as if someone were pulling a curtain in front of eye)
4. Types
   a. Primary detachment—(rhegmatogenous) hole in retina permits fluid to enter space between retina and choroid.
   b. Secondary detachment—fluid or tissue builds up between choroid and retina with no hole in retina.
5. Treatment
   a. Diathermy
      (1) Traditional method
         (a) Insertion of microneedles or needle tip of a probe into sclera
         (b) Shortwave radio frequency energy delivered through needles
         (c) Causes thermal changes in tissue
         (d) Results in scar formation and retinal reattachment at points of adhesion
         (e) Procedure rarely used anymore
   b. Cryotherapy
      (1) More popular method; less invasive than diathermy
      (2) Application of 80° C cryoprobe to scleral area of detachment
      (3) Inflammation causes adhesion and reattaches retina.
      (4) Fewer complications than diathermy
   c. Pneumoretinopexy
      (1) Injection of air or expansile gases into vitreous cavity
      (2) Usually done in physician's office
      (3) Cryotherapy may be used to close and seal hole before gas is injected.
      (4) Patient may be instructed to hold head in certain position until retina reattaches (usually 2 weeks).
   d. Laser therapy
      (1) Used to "spot weld" retina
      (2) Requires retina to be flat over retinal pigment epithelium before chorioretinal adhesion can be formed
      (3) Done in physician's office
      (4) Can be done in OR in conjunction with vitrectomy
   e. Scleral buckling
      (1) Description
      (2) Procedure developed to create indentation in retina so that adherence between detached area and underlying tissues will result in permanent reattachment
   f. Posterior vitrectomy
      (1) Description
         (a) Objective is to remove vitreous humor without pulling on retina; permits surgeon to work directly on retina
         (b) Can be performed with all techniques for reattaching retina
6. Preoperative considerations
   a. Instruct patient regarding activity limitations before surgery (reduces stress on area of detachment).
   b. Inform patient and family of potential for lengthy surgery (decrease anxiety level).

7. Postoperative considerations
   a. Patient usually on cycloplegic agents (atropine or cyclopentolate) to dilate pupil and rest muscles of accommodation
   b. May be on antibiotic and steroid eye drops
   c. Assess patient's ability to instill eye drops.
   d. Patients with an intraocular gas bubble should be instructed not to fly because gas bubble expands with changing atmospheric pressure.
P. Laser therapy
   1. Description
      a. Noninvasive ambulatory procedure in which a slit lamp is used to deliver the laser beam
      b. May eliminate the need for more invasive procedures
      c. Argon or yttrium aluminum garnet (YAG) lasers used in a procedure room
      d. Topical anesthetic drops instilled
   2. Procedures
      a. Laser trabeculoplasty
         (1) Treatment for open-angle glaucoma
      b. Laser iridotomy
         (1) Treatment for acute or chronic angle-closure glaucoma
      c. Laser posterior capsulotomy
         (1) May be required when patients experience decreased vision within 2 years after ECCE
         (2) YAG laser used to create a window in the posterior capsule
         (3) Patients may have pupils dilated.
         (4) Iopidine may be used to prevent increased intraocular pressure.
III. ANESTHETIC CONSIDERATIONS
   A. Types (overview)
      1. Topical
         a. Topical anesthetic eye drops used more frequently
         b. Rapid onset with moderate duration of action
         c. Decrease risk with retrobulba and infection
         d. Continue anticoagulation therapy
      2. Local anesthesia block
         a. Used frequently
         b. Contraindications
            (1) Patients who have difficulty lying still
            (2) Children
            (3) Patients who have frequent cough
      3. Moderate sedation and analgesia used in conjunction with block
      4. General anesthesia
   B. Topical anesthetic drops
      1. Used frequently
         a. Proparacaine hydrochloride 0.5%
         b. Tetracaine hydrochloride 0.5%
         c. Lidocaine hydrochloride 2%
   C. Eye block
      1. Types
         a. Retrobulbar block
            (1) Injection of anesthetic solution into base of eyelids at level of orbital margins or behind the eyeball to block the ciliary ganglion and nerves
         b. Peribulbar block
            (1) Local anesthetic deposited beside the globe instead of behind it
      2. Performed in two stages
      3. Stage I—blocks eyelid
         a. Three methods
            (1) Van Lint method—blocks peripheral branches of cranial nerve VII in the orbicularis oculi muscle

        (2) Atkinson method—blocks temporal arborization of cranial nerve VII to the orbicularis muscle

        (3) O'Brien method—blocks the main trunk of cranial nerve VII near the temporomandibular joint

    4. Stage II—retrobulbar block

      a. Provides anesthesia to globe and muscular attachments

      b. Blocks branches of cranial nerves III, IV, V, and VI

      c. Common medications used

        (1) Lidocaine hydrochloride 2% or 4%; mixed with equal parts of 0.75% bupivacaine hydrochloride with hyaluronidase (used for diffusing local anesthetic to surrounding tissue)

        (2) May add epinephrine hydrochloride to prolong effectiveness of agents

        (3) May use as much as 6 mL for retrobulbar block and 10 mL for peripheral tissue

      d. Nursing considerations

        (1) Inform patient of possible burning sensation.

        (2) Inform patient of possible feeling of pressure behind eye during injection of medication.

        (3) Inform patient that physician may massage eye after injection of medication.

          (a) Decreases intraocular pressure

          (b) Aids in diffusing agents

        (4) Patient frequently given intravenous sedation to decrease discomfort during the injection; administer medications per protocol.

        (5) Monitor vital signs per protocol.

        (6) Patient may be awake during procedure.

          (a) Monitor noise level.

          (b) Monitor patient's anxiety level.

      e. Nursing care after eye block

        (1) Patient will not have blink reflex; must keep eyelid closed to protect the cornea.

          (a) Tape the eyelid closed.

          (b) Reassure patient that it is normal to be unable to open the eyelid.

      f. Effectiveness of eye block

        (1) Generally very effective

        (2) Occasionally a block may be incomplete, and patient will experience pain.

        (3) Instruct patient to use hand signal during surgery if he or she experiences pain or discomfort.

      g. Potential complications—cancellation of surgical procedure strongly advised for any of the following complications:

        (1) Retinal detachment (caused by insertion of needle through globe)

        (2) Injection of anesthetic into optic nerve (irreparable damage)

        (3) Retrobulbar hemorrhage (most common)

          (a) Controlled by pressure to globe

  D. General anesthesia

    1. Indications

      a. Children

      b. Patients unable to tolerate local anesthetic with sedation

      c. Extremely anxious patients

      d. Patients with certain systemic diseases

      e. Patients undergoing prolonged operations

    2. Postanesthesia care

      a. Same as any patient who has undergone general anesthesia

IV. DRUGS FREQUENTLY USED FOR OPHTHALMOLOGICAL SURGERY

  A. Mydriatics

    1. Action

      a. Blocks cholinergic stimulation of sphincter muscle of iris (dilation of pupil)

      b. Blocks accommodative ciliary muscle of lens (paralysis of accommodation)

    2. Types

      a. Phenylephrine hydrochloride (Alconefrin, Neo-Synephrine, Prefrin)

      b. Hydroxyamphetamine (Paredrine)

B. Cycloplegics

    1. Action

      a. Dilate pupils and paralyze accommodation by acting on ciliary muscles (parasympatholytics)

    2. Types

      a. Atropine

      b. Homatropine (AK-Homatropine, Isopto Homatropine, Minims Homatropine)

      c. Cyclopentolate (Cyclogyl)

      d. Scopolamine (Isopto Hyoscine, Mydramide)

      e. Tropicamide (Mydriacyl)

C. Miotics

    1. Action

      a. Used to constrict the pupil (parasympathomimetics)

    2. Types

      a. Cholinergics

        (1) Pilocarpine hydrochloride

        (2) Carbachol (Miostat, Carbacel)

        (3) Acetylcholine chloride (Miochol)

      b. Anticholinesterase

        (1) Physostigmine (Eserine)

        (2) Isoflurophate (Floropryl)

        (3) Echothiophate iodide (Phospholine Iodide)

D. Osmotic agents

    1. Action

      a. Parenteral agents used to lower intraocular pressure through the blood-ocular gradient

    2. Types

      a. Mannitol (Osmitrol)

      b. Glycerin (glycerol, Glyrol, Osmoglyn)

E. Viscoelastic agents

    1. Action

      a. Used to maintain the intraocular chamber during surgery

    2. Types

      a. Sodium hyaluronate (Healon, Amvisc)

      b. Ocucoat

F. Carbonic anhydrase inhibitors

    1. Action

      a. Parenteral agent used to decrease intraocular pressure; used for glaucoma

    2. Types

      a. Acetazolamide (Diamox)

      b. Methazolamide (Neptazane)

G. Corticosteroids

    1. Action

      a. Anti-inflammatory agents

    2. Types

      a. Hydrocortisone (Solu-Cortef) ointment or eye drops

      b. Dexamethasone (Decadron) eye drops

      c. Prednisolone (Pred Forte, AK-Pred, Inflamase Mild, Inflamase Forte)

H. Topical antibiotics

    1. Action

      a. Used for prophylaxis of or treatment of infections; may be used in solutions or ointments

   2. Types
      a. Bacitracin, neomycin, erythromycin, tetracycline, gantrisin, tobramycin, gentamycin
      b. Chloramphenicol
V. PREOPERATIVE CONSIDERATIONS
   A. Assessment
      1. Patient's and family's understanding of:
         a. Eye disorder
         b. Goal of surgery
         c. What to expect before, during, and after surgery
         d. Postoperative care and support
      2. Assess in detail patient's understanding of intraoperative procedure, local anesthesia and sedation versus general.
      3. Identify patient's reaction to scheduled surgery.
         a. Unrealistic expectations regarding improved vision
         b. Anxiety over potential loss of vision
      4. Identify current visual status.
         a. May need additional safety precautions if severely impaired
         b. May need additional support postoperatively if visual status of unoperative eye is limited
   B. General health assessment per routine protocol
      1. Identify illnesses that can cause sneezing, coughing, history of postoperative nausea and vomiting, or increase in intraocular pressure.
         a. Patient may not be a candidate for local anesthesia with sedation.
         b. May require general anesthesia
      2. Consider co-morbidities of patients scheduled for surgery.
   C. Preoperative care
      1. Relieve anxiety related to impending surgery (the eyes are very sensitive to pain and pressure).
         a. Allow patient time to verbalize concerns.
            (1) Patient may have misconceptions regarding eye surgery.
            (2) Clarify misconceptions.
            (3) Some patients may think they will actually see the procedure through the operative eye.
         b. Involve the patient in the plan of care.
            (1) Provide clear written instructions in large type.
            (2) Reinforce physician's orders regarding preoperative and postoperative medications and eye drop schedules.
         c. Provide emotional support.
            (1) Convey positive realistic attitude.
            (2) Acknowledge validity of patient concerns.
      2. Verify correct surgical eye.
         a. Confirm with patient correct eye for surgery.
            (1) Initiate time-out procedure.
            (2) Document correct eye before preoperative sedation.
            (3) Keep in mind many patients may be unable to accurately identify the operative eye because of age or mental status.
         b. Document correct operative eye.
            (1) Verify the surgical consent and the history and physical with the scheduled procedure.
            (2) Investigate any discrepancy.
         c. Clearly identify surgical eye with skin marker (facility policy outlines process).
            (1) Visual marking should not be the sole way of identifying the correct surgical eye.
            (2) Every perianesthesia nurse caring for the patient should verify the patient's understanding, the consent, and the scheduled procedure before proceeding with care.

    3. What to expect
       a. Length of time (preoperatively, intraoperatively, postoperatively)
       b. Eye patch (depending on surgical procedure)
       c. Reinforcement that improved vision may require a period of time
    4. Demonstrate proper method of eye drop instillation.
       a. Explain ways to avoid contamination of eye medications.
       b. Reinforce need to follow prescription instructions accurately.
       c. Teach proper technique for instillation of eye drops.
          (1) Confirm on bottle that drops are for ophthalmic use.
          (2) Note the expiration date and discard if outdated.
          (3) Wash hands before using eye drops.
          (4) Confirm proper eye.
          (5) Tilt head back for instillation.
          (6) Keep eyes open, and look upward.
          (7) Gently pull down tissue below the lower lid.
          (8) Place correct number of eye drops into the conjunctival sac.
          (9) Close eyes, and try to avoid excessive blinking or squeezing for
             several minutes.
         (10) Gently blot any excess solution from beneath the eye.
         (11) Wait 5 minutes before instilling a different type of eye drop.
         (12) Do not touch tip of eye medication dispenser to the eyelid or with hands.
  D. Review postoperative routine.
    1. Include family and significant other as appropriate.
    2. Things to avoid postoperatively
       a. Quick movements
       b. Bending over from the waist
       c. Rubbing eyes
       d. Heavy lifting
    3. Moderation in activity
    4. Proper hand washing before caring for the eye
  E. Nursing considerations
    1. Visually impaired patient
       a. Approach from unaffected or least affected side.
       b. Identify self.
       c. Speak in normal tone.
       d. Provide method for patient to obtain immediate assistance (call bell in reach).
       e. Keep visual aids in close proximity.
       f. Allow patient to keep assistive devices as long as possible.
       g. Keep walking area clear of obstructions.
    2. Administer preoperative medications as ordered.
       a. Mydriatics to dilate pupil
       b. Notify physician if expected dilation does not occur.
    3. Encourage patient to void before procedure.
       a. Patient will become restless in OR if he or she has a full bladder.
  F. Overall assessment of patient's ability to tolerate anesthesia plan
    1. Procedure usually performed under local anesthesia with sedation (adults)
    2. Assess patient's ability to lie still under drapes for long period (1-3 hours).
    3. Factors influencing decision include:
       a. Chronic cough
       b. Airway difficulties
       c. Claustrophobia
       d. Involuntary motions
VI. POSTOPERATIVE CONSIDERATIONS
  A. Assessment
    1. Routine assessment per protocol
  B. Positioning
    1. Assist patient to chair or recliner.
       a. Avoid bumping or jarring.

    2. Orient patient to surroundings.

    3. Certain operations (vitreoretinal surgery) may require special positioning.

        a. Surgeon should provide specific instructions as to positioning.

        b. Patient may need to be on side or back.

    4. Patient may have decreased pain with head of bed elevated.

C. Drainage

    1. Type and amount; document.

    2. Notify physician per protocol.

D. Pain and discomfort level—assess and document.

    1. Varies with each procedure

        a. Usually uncommon after most eye surgeries

    2. Varies with type of anesthesia administered

    3. Patient may feel stiff and sore.

        a. Results from lying still and flat intraoperatively

    4. Pain usually relieved by acetaminophen, propoxyphene hydrochloride, or similar analgesics

    5. May experience significant pain after vitreoretinal surgery

        a. Administer narcotic analgesic as indicated.

        b. Apply ice pack.

        c. Notify ophthalmologist if pain not relieved by analgesics.

E. Nausea

    1. Caused by manipulation of eye and eye muscles during surgery

    2. May be caused by sedation

    3. Medicate immediately to prevent potential vomiting.

        a. Vomiting results in increased intraocular pressure.

        b. Instruct patient to notify nurse immediately if he or she begins to feel nauseous so that antiemetics may be given.

    4. To avoid potential for nausea and vomiting, oral fluids may be held for a while if patient underwent general anesthesia.

F. Visual impairment from surgery

    1. Ensure patient safety at all times.

    2. Requires assistance at home

    3. Verify arrangements before discharge.

G. Eye shields and dressings

    1. Dressing or eye shields may remain in place until the patient's first postoperative appointment at the physician's office.

        a. Instruct patient not to disturb or remove shield and dressing.

    2. Alteration in depth perception may be expected when one eye is bandaged.

        a. Evaluate patient for adequate balance before allowing him or her to ambulate unassisted.

    3. Provide clear written instructions for postoperative care at home.

        a. Wash hands before caring for eye.

        b. Do not rub eye.

        c. Surgeon will remove eye patch or shield during postoperative appointment.

        d. Wear glasses or shield at all times to protect the eye.

        e. Wear shield at night for sleeping.

        f. Do not bend at the waist.

        g. Avoid heavy lifting.

        h. Avoid reading (operative eye muscles will move together with unoperative eye, causing discomfort).

        i. Do not drive until after first postoperative appointment.

            (1) Do not drive at all if experiencing double vision.

        j. Take all eye medications as ordered.

        k. Notify physician if any of the following occur:

            (1) Pain not relieved by acetaminophen

            (2) Sudden loss of vision

            (3) Increasing double vision after surgery

(4) Temperature greater than 100° F

(5) Significant swelling or redness about the eye

(6) Unexpected drainage from the eye

H. Discharge instructions

    1. Inform patient to use strict aseptic technique when caring for eye and administering medications.

    2. Administer eye medications as directed by physician.

    3. Avoid activities that increase intraocular pressure.

        a. Bending

        b. Sneezing or coughing

        c. Sudden jarring or forceful movements

        d. Forceful nose blowing

        e. Sexual intercourse

        f. Straining during stools

    4. Wear sunglasses when outdoors.

    5. Avoid use of eye makeup.

    6. Responsible accompanying adult stays with patient for first 24 hours.

    7. Notify physician if any increase in pain, vision changes, or signs and symptoms of infection (redness, increased swelling, purulent drainage).

VII. POSSIBLE COMPLICATIONS OF OPHTHALMIC SURGERY

  A. Pain

    1. Minimal in most ophthalmic surgeries

    2. Causes: increased intraocular pressure, surgical manipulation, pressure from dressing

    3. Treatment: mild analgesic; be aware that need for stronger medication may indicate possible complications.

  B. Bleeding

    1. Minimal for all ophthalmic surgeries

    2. Cause: dressing too loose

    3. Treatment: apply or reinforce dressing; notify physician.

  C. Nausea and vomiting

    1. Usually minimal after ophthalmic surgery

    2. Causes: oculocardiac reflex, surgical manipulation, general anesthesia

    3. Treatment: antiemetic; avoid potential vomiting.

  D. Oculocardiac reflex (nervous response elicited by manipulation of extraocular muscles or surrounding ocular tissue)

    1. Causes: decreased heart rate, blood pressure, and level of consciousness

    2. Is seen immediately to 20 minutes postoperatively

    3. May be seen with all types of ophthalmic surgeries

        a. Risk increases with vitreoretinal and eye muscle surgeries.

        b. May be stimulated by retrobulbar block

    4. Treatment: intravenous atropine

BIBLIOGRAPHY

1. Burden N, ed: *Ambulatory surgical nursing,* ed 2, Philadelphia, 2004, WB Saunders.
2. Dirckx J, ed: *Stedman's concise medical dictionary for the health professions,* ed 4, Philadelphia, 2001, Lippincott Williams & Wilkins.
3. Drain C, Odom-Forren J: *Perianesthesia nursing: A critical care approach,* ed 5, St Louis, 2009, WB Saunders.
4. eMedicine from WebMD: *Otolaryngology and facial plastic surgery articles.* Available at: www.emedicine.com/ent. Accessed February 1, 2008.
5. Karch A, ed: *2006 Lippincott's nursing drug guide,* Philadelphia, 2006, Lippincott Williams & Wilkins.
6. Maloney W: Beveled blades have simplified clear corneal technique. *Ocul Surg News* 15(18):11, 1997.
7. Nettina S, ed: *The Lippincott manual of nursing practice,* ed 8, Philadelphia, 2000, Lippincott.
8. Phippen M, Wells M, eds: *Patient care during operative and invasive procedures,* Philadelphia, 2000, WB Saunders.
9. Pudner R, ed: *Nursing the surgical patient,* ed 2, Edinburgh, 2005, Elsevier.
10. Rothrock J: *Alexander's care of the patient in surgery,* ed 13, St Louis, 2007, Mosby.

41 Oral/Maxillofacial/ Dental Care

DENISE O'BRIEN

OBJECTIVES

At the conclusion of this chapter, the reader will be able to:

1. Describe anatomy and physiology of oral cavity pertinent to the patient undergoing oral and maxillofacial procedures.

2. Identify assessment parameters for patients undergoing oral and maxillofacial operative procedures.

3. Define nursing care priorities in each postanesthesia phase.

4. Describe patient education after oral and maxillofacial procedures related to diet, pain management, oral care, activity, and follow-up.

I. OVERVIEW
   A. Care of the oral or maxillofacial surgical patient presents many challenges.
      1. Patients may experience feelings of suffocation.
         a. Procedure may prevent normal breathing patterns (inability to breathe through mouth and/or nose).
      2. Continuous reassurance and explanations assist the patients in understanding they are not in any danger.
      3. Astute assessment skills are necessary.
         a. Compromise of the airway can occur at any time.
         b. Immediate corrective actions needed
   II. ANATOMY AND PHYSIOLOGY
   A. Mouth and oral cavity include the following structures:
      1. Lips, teeth, gums, buccal mucosa, tongue, palate (hard and soft), tonsils, pharynx, temporomandibular joints (TMJs) (Figure 41-1)
   B. Oral cavity is bounded by the jawbones and associated structures (muscles and mucosa) (Figures 41-2 and 41-3).
      1. Includes
         a. Cheek
         b. Palate
         c. Oral mucosa
         d. Glands whose ducts open into the cavity
         e. Teeth
         f. Tongue
      2. Except for the teeth, interior of mouth covered with mucous membrane, lined with salivary glands
         a. Secrete saliva
         b. Aid in first step of food digestion
   C. Oral cavity forms beginning of the digestive system
      1. Chewing occurs.
      2. Site of the organs of taste
      3. Mouth is entrance to the body for food, occasionally air.
      4. Major organ of speech and emotional expression

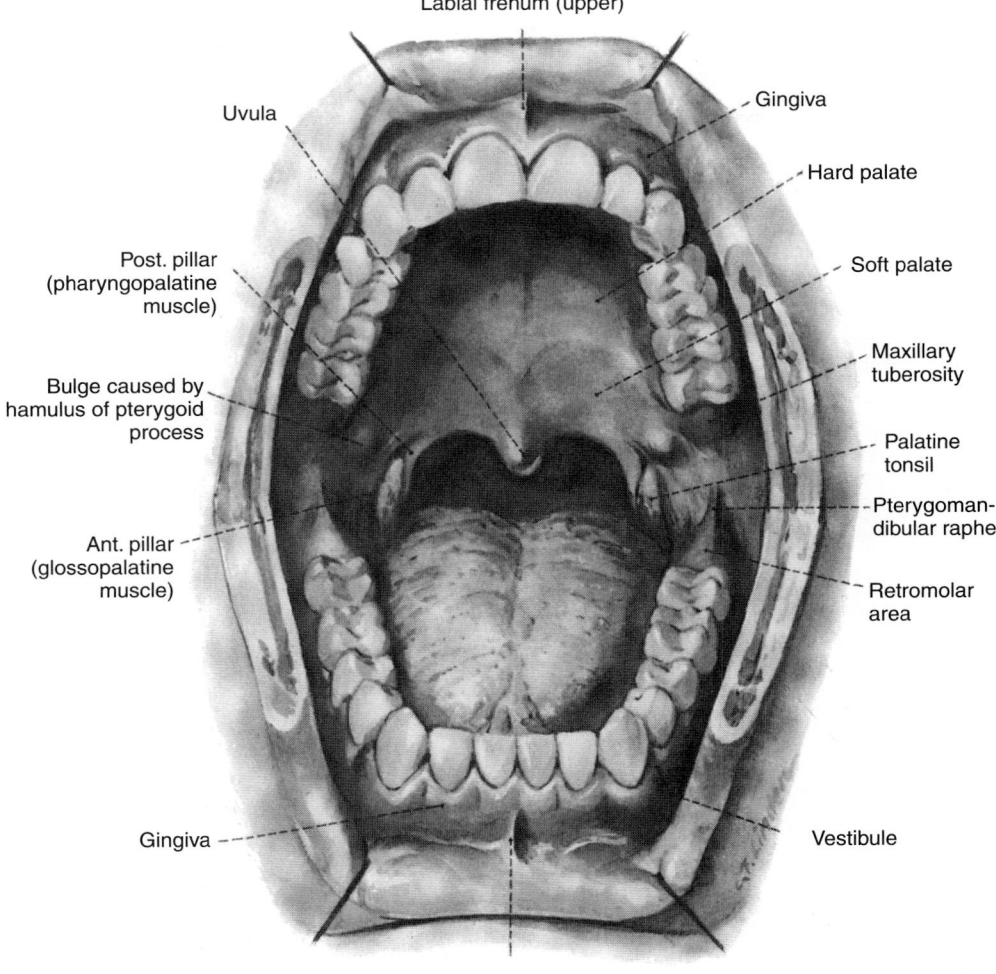

FIGURE 41-1 ■ The oral cavity. (From Massler M, Schour I: *Atlas of the mouth in health and disease,* 1958, by permission of the American Dental Association, Chicago.)

D. Associated structures
  1. Buccal: pertaining to or directed toward the cheek
  2. Tooth:
    a. Hard calcified structure set in the alveolar processes of the mandible and maxilla
    b. Mastication of food
  3. Gingiva: mucous membrane (the gum) surrounding the teeth
    a. Covers the tooth-bearing border of the jaw
    b. Overlies crowns of unerupted teeth
    c. Encircles the necks of erupted teeth
    d. Supporting structure for subjacent tissues
  4. Mandible:
    a. Horseshoe-shaped bone forming the lower jaw
    b. Largest and strongest bone of the face
    c. Articulates with skull at TMJs
  5. Maxilla
    a. Irregularly shaped bone that forms the upper jaw
    b. Two identically shaped bones that are considered one

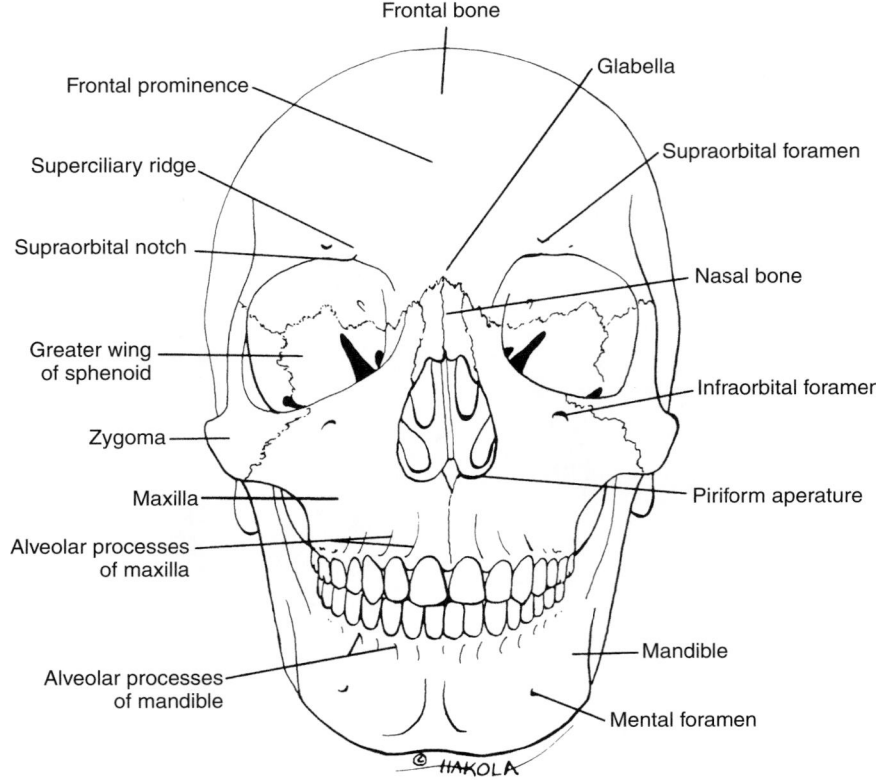

FIGURE 41-2 ■ The skull, anterior view. (From Ferraro JW: *Fundamentals of maxillofacial surgery,* New York, 1997, Springer-Verlag.)

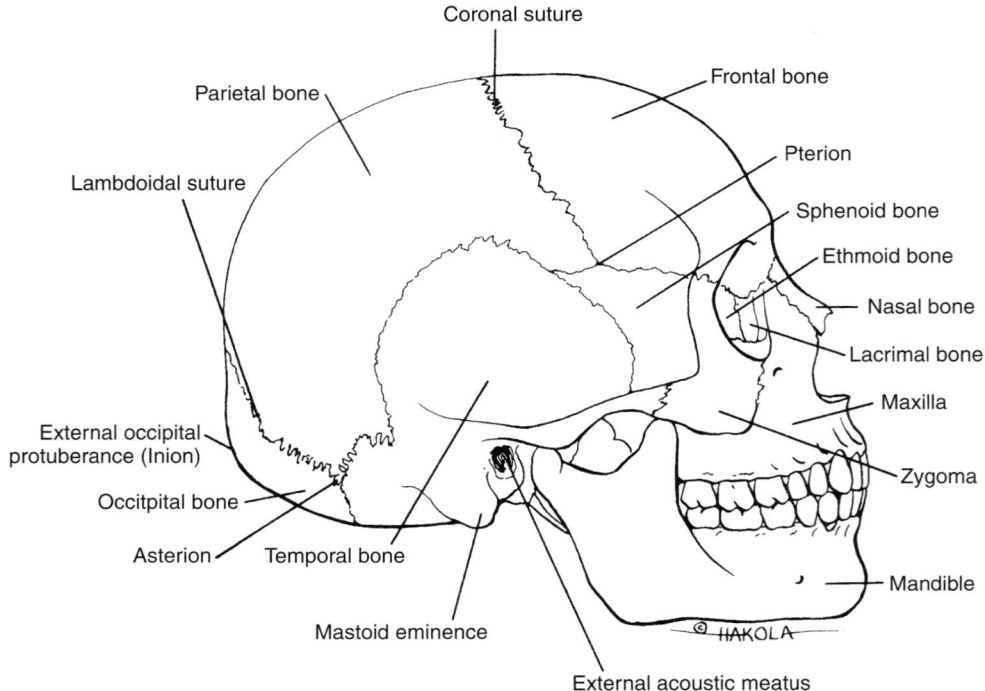

FIGURE 41-3 ■ Lateral view of the skull. (From Ferraro JW: *Fundamentals of maxillofacial surgery,* New York, 1997, Springer-Verlag.)

(1) Assists in the formation of the floor of the orbits, part of the lateral walls and floor of the nasal cavity, and the palate; contains the maxillary sinuses and tear ducts, which drain into the nasal cavity

(2) Supports the upper teeth

c. Described as the architectural key of the face; touches all facial bones, including the mandible, through the contact of upper and lower teeth

6. Palate—the roof of the mouth consists of:

a. Hard palate

(1) The rigid anterior portion

(2) Formed by the maxillae and the palatine bones

(3) Covered by mucous membrane

(4) Forms a bony partition between the oral and nasal cavities

(5) Hinged to the soft palate

b. Soft palate

(1) Posterior, fleshy part of the palate

(2) Arch-shaped muscular partition between the oropharynx and nasopharynx

(3) Lined by mucous membrane

(4) Flanked by tonsils

(5) Uvula is in the middle of the soft palate—a fleshy projection pointing down to the tongue.

(a) Forms seal posteriorly with the pharynx to help direct food to the esophagus and air to the trachea

(b) Critical to the development of normal speech patterns

7. Tongue

a. Movable muscular organ on the floor of the mouth

b. Accessory structure of the digestive system

c. Composed of skeletal muscle covered with mucous membrane

d. Location of organs of taste

e. Aids in chewing, swallowing (deglutition), cleansing tooth surfaces, and the articulation of sound (phonetics)

8. Nerves (Figure 41-4)

a. Sensation supplied to upper teeth and gingival by

(1) Maxillary division of the trigeminal nerve (cranial nerve V)

(a) Posterior superior alveolar

(b) Middle superior alveolar

(c) Anterior superior alveolar

b. Mandibular division gives off

(1) Lingual nerve (sensation of anterior two thirds of tongue, the floor of mouth, gums)

(2) Inferior alveolar nerve (sensation of premolar, molar teeth of mandible)

(3) Mental nerve (sensation of the lower lip and chin)

9. TMJ: bicondylar joint formed by

a. Head of the mandible

b. Mandibular fossa

c. Articular tubercle of the temporal bone

III. PREANESTHESIA ASSESSMENT AND PARAMETERS SPECIFIC TO PROCEDURES

A. Examination

1. Inspection and palpation of greatest use

a. Head and neck

(1) General appearance

(2) Facial appearance

(3) Trismus (limited degree of mouth opening)

(4) Neck lumps

(5) Gross facial swelling

(6) Skin color and texture

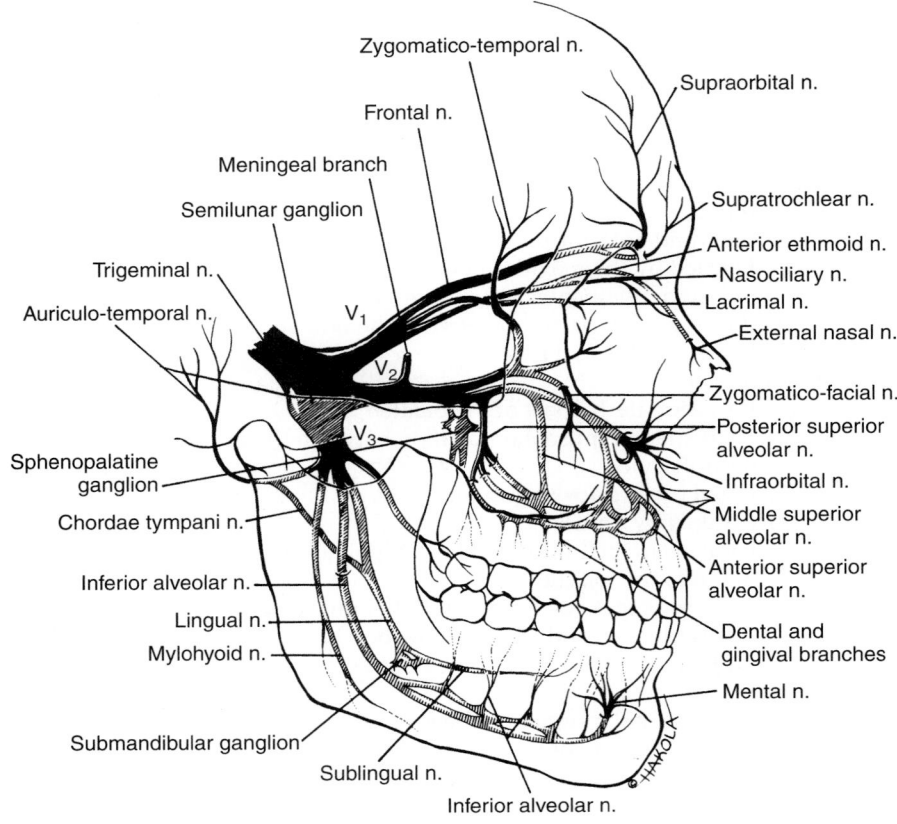

V₁ = ophthalmic division
V₂ = maxillary division
V₃ = mandibular division

FIGURE 41-4 ■ The trigeminal nerve (cranial nerve V). (From Ferraro JW: *Fundamentals of maxillofacial surgery*, New York, 1997, Springer-Verlag.)

    b. Intraoral
      (1) Tongue: size, mobility, color, and texture
      (2) Oral mucosa (palate, cheeks, labial mucosa, floor of mouth): examination for changes in color, texture, ulcers, lumps
      (3) Alveolar ridges and gingivae: color, texture, gingival recession, ulcers, and lumps
      (4) Teeth: number, position, restorations, crowns, caries, cracked, mobile and missing teeth, exposed structure
B. Increased risk associated with history or need to alter perioperative management
  1. Cardiac: may require antibiotic prophylaxis
    a. Endocarditis
    b. Heart transplant
    c. Valve implants
  2. Implants: antibiotic prophylaxis may be needed
    a. Joints (major replacements)
    b. Grafts of artificial materials
  3. Coagulation and bleeding disorders
    a. Factor VIII deficiency (hemophilia)

      b. Von Willebrand's disease: following may be given just before procedure begins:

         (1) Factor VIII

         (2) Synthetic factor VIII

         (3) Aminocaproic acid (EACA [Epsilon-aminocaproic acid] or Amicar)

         (4) DDVAP (desmopressin acetate)

      c. Anticoagulant therapy

         (1) Coagulation testing may be required (prothrombin, partial thromboplastin time, platelet count) to determine coagulation status before proceeding with elective surgery.

  4. Immunocompromised patient or immune disorders

      a. Human immunodeficiency virus, acquired immunodeficiency syndrome

      b. Patient with history of organ transplant

      c. Universal precautions should be used with every patient.

      d. Immunocompromised patient may require special care (isolation, scheduling, altered medication regimen).

  5. Patients with cancer receiving radiation therapy to the head and neck region

      a. Decreased salivary flow secondary to salivary gland atrophy requires saliva substitutes and aggressive anticaries management with

         (1) Custom trays

         (2) Topical fluoride applications

         (3) Immaculate oral hygiene

      b. Extractions usually completed before initiation of therapy to decrease the risk of development of osteoradionecrosis

         (1) Debilitating complication

            (a) Leaves a patient with painful exposed bone in the oral cavity

            (b) Can progress to

               (i)   Pathological fractures

               (ii) Recurrent infections

               (iii) Raining sinus tracks

      c. Hyperbaric oxygen treatment is indicated for surgical procedures if previous radiation dose totals >4500 cGy. (This is still used in some centers but has fallen out of favor because of poor efficacy and lack of literature supporting a benefit.)

  6. Trauma

      a. Edema present

         (1) Recent injury

         (2) May delay operative repair until edema diminishes

      b. Disfigurement: may be significant and emotionally disturbing to patient and others

  7. Chronic pain

      a. Pain tolerance alterations

      b. Chronic analgesic use may alter postoperative analgesic management.

  8. Nutritional status changes

      a. Difficulty chewing, swallowing

      b. Pain may interfere with ability to eat and meet caloric demands and nutritional requirements.

  9. Developmentally challenged

      a. Potential behavioral problems (combative, disruptive, abusive)

      b. Legal authorization appropriately obtained before treatment commences

C. Airway status evaluation

  1. Evaluation of airway for ease of intubation in oral or maxillofacial surgery

      a. Mobility of the neck—ability to touch chin to chest and each shoulder; flex and extend

      b. Position of the trachea relative to the mandible—distance from thyroid cartilage to anterior bony chin; at least 6.5 cm acceptable

      c. Ability of the patient to open the mouth—at least 3.6 cm in adults desirable

      d. Structures visualized when the patient opens the mouth and vocalizes "ahh…"—see the uvula and surrounding pharyngeal structures.

   D. Determine the educational needs of patient and caregiver.
      1. Oral care, analgesia, preoperative anxiety
      2. Discharge planning
 IV. INTRAOPERATIVE PRIORITIES
   A. Anesthesia choice: fit of the teeth is one of the best templates a surgeon can use to restore the original form of patient's face.
      1. General
         a. Nasal intubation desired for unobstructed visualization of orofacial structures
         b. Allows reconstruction of the upper and lower jaws to be guided by the patient's occlusion
      2. Sedation and analgesia with local anesthesia
         a. Midazolam, ketamine (glycopyrrolate to decrease oral secretions)
            (1) Less risk of respiratory depression
            (2) Reduced emergence delirium after ketamine with midazolam
         b. Benzodiazepine with fentanyl
            (1) Oxygen recommended when used with local anesthesia
            (2) May use methohexital or propofol for additional sedation
      3. Local anesthesia used alone for minor oral procedures or used as an adjunct during general anesthesia
         a. Minimizes immediate postoperative pain
         b. Minimizes bleeding in operative field
         c. Helps separate tissue planes to ease dissection
         d. Allows for less anesthetic agent because of reduced surgical stimulus
   B. Intraoperative concerns
      1. Hemostasis and intraoral bleeding
         a. Hemostatic agent may be used.
         b. Gelfoam, Surgicel, Avitene, topical thrombin, bone wax (for bone bleeders), Tisseel (fibrin sealant)
      2. Airway
         a. Loss of reflexes with excessive sedation
         b. Positioning of endotracheal tube, potential displacement
         c. Foreign body aspiration
 V. POSTANESTHESIA PRIORITIES
   A. Phase I
      1. Airway
         a. Spontaneous, unassisted breathing
         b. Adjunct in place: nasal trumpet, oropharyngeal airway
         c. Endotracheal tube: nasal insertion (most common)
         d. Observe for respiratory complications.
      2. Hemodynamic stability
         a. Vital signs stable, consistent with baseline
         b. Observe for cardiovascular complications.
      3. Bleeding
         a. Hemostasis may be difficult to obtain.
         b. Risk for hemorrhage
         c. Increases risk of nausea and vomiting
            (1) Swallowed blood may precipitate nausea and vomiting from irritating effect of blood in stomach.
      4. Report from anesthesia, oral surgeon, perioperative nurse (in addition to routine information)
         a. Implants and prostheses inserted
         b. Splints: location, type
         c. Oral packing: location, plan for removal
         d. Oral sutures: location, extreme care when suctioning
         e. Maxillomandibular fixation (MMF)/intermaxillary fixation (IMF)—wired jaws
            (1) Wire cutters and scissors immediately available

    (2) Clear instructions from surgeon when appropriate to cut fixation wires and what wires to cut

    (3) Usually cut for vomit and for respiratory distress (in extreme cases only)

5. Discomfort

  a. Maximum pain intensity occurs about 3 hours after surgery: begin analgesics intraoperatively or immediately postoperatively.

  b. Long-acting local anesthetic infiltrated into operative site; usually bupivacaine with epinephrine to provide 8 to 12 hours of analgesia

  c. Opioids: decreasing use in ambulatory oral and maxillofacial surgery because increased use of nonsteroidal anti-inflammatory drugs (NSAIDs; ketorolac)

  d. NSAIDs: ketorolac may provide superior analgesia after extractions.

6. Drainage from mouth

  a. Position to facilitate drainage of saliva, bloody secretions.

  b. Drooling or excessive salivation and unable to swallow (reflex absent or excessive pain)

  c. Suction as needed with soft catheter.

7. Dressing

  a. No dressing when incisions are intraoral

  b. Internal dressing may be moistened gauze sponge.

    (1) Best left with a "tail" hanging out of the patient's mouth when the patient is obtunded.

    (2) Tail facilitates removal and identification of potential airway obstruction in the early stages of emergence from anesthesia.

  c. External dressing

    (1) Pressure chin strap (Jobst type)

    (2) Foam tape

    (3) Head wrap with fluffs and cling wrap generally for 24 hours

8. Edema

  a. Can be significant, especially in longer procedures

  b. Position with head of bed elevated 30°.

  c. Administer steroid if ordered; continued controversy regarding effectiveness in reducing inflammatory reaction.

  d. Ice packs may help reduce blood flow to operative site and subsequent inflammatory response.

    (1) Check with surgeon before applying.

      (a) May actually increase blood flow (rebound effect after ice pack removed)

      (b) Can also be damaging to flaps through its vasoconstrictive effects

      (c) Apply for 20 minutes on, 20 minutes off.

9. Fluids and nutrition

  a. Clear to full liquid, high-caloric diet as tolerated and ordered

  b. Do not force fluids, especially when nausea and vomiting present.

  c. Causes of nausea and vomiting

    (1) Opioid analgesics

    (2) Blood in stomach

    (3) Starvation leading to weakness, low blood sugar levels

  d. Hydrate with intravenous fluids (replacement and maintenance).

    (1) Lactated Ringer's (Hartmann's)

    (2) Dextrose-containing solutions

  e. When nausea and vomiting present

    (1) Administer antiemetics as ordered; determine whether antiemetic prophylaxis given.

    (2) Commonly used (see Chapter 25 for discussion on antiemetics)

      (a) 5-hydroxytryptamine-3 (5-HT$_3$) serotonin antagonists

 (i) Ondansetron (Zofran)
 (ii) Dolasetron (Anzemet)
 (iii) Granisetron (Kytril)
 (b) Dexamethasone (Decadron)
 (c) Diphenhydramine (Benadryl)
 (d) Prochlorperazine (Compazine)
 (3) Important not to ignore vomiting, as the expelled material will be forced against suture lines and risk their rupture
10. Reaction to local anesthetics (LAs)
 a. What appears to be an allergic reaction to LA may actually be a reaction to preservative methylparaben or sulfite.
 b. Allergy to LA rare
 c. Traumatic penetration of a nerve (prolonged numbness), vein (hematoma), or artery (systemic toxic effects)
 d. Systemic (cardiac) reactions to epinephrine (used to minimize bleeding) in LA, rather than LA itself
 e. Toxicity caused by overdose leads to excitation of central nervous system (CNS) followed by
 (1) Profound CNS depression
 (2) Cardiovascular collapse
 (3) Possible death
11. Oral hygiene
 a. Take care not to disrupt clot.
 (1) Gently swab the oral cavity.
 (2) Hold saline rinse for 8 to 12 hours postprocedure.
 b. Lubricate lips with
 (1) Petroleum jelly or emollient cream
 (2) Steroid (0.5% hydrocortisone) lip cream—for long procedures
 (3) Expectance of significant edema of lips
12. Antibiotic as ordered
 a. Common after trauma
 b. Patients with cardiac valvular disease
 c. History of rheumatic fever
 d. Implants
 e. Oral cavity laden with bacteria
 (1) Bacteria enter the bloodstream through oral incisions
 (2) Traumatic lacerations
 f. Infections can lead to
 (1) Loss of bone and teeth
 (2) Distributive shock (septic)
 (3) Damage to heart valves
 (4) Endocarditis
 (5) Loss of implants
 (6) Scarring
 (7) Large vessel complications (carotid erosion or venous thrombosis)
13. Provide patient with means of communication while in PACU.
 a. Bell
 b. Writing tools
 (1) Pen or pencil, paper pad
 (2) Magic slate and stylet
 (3) Dry-erase board and marker
14. Reasons for admission after outpatient operative procedure
 a. Airway obstruction
 b. Unanticipated MMF/IMF
 c. Severe postoperative nausea and vomiting
 d. Excessive blood loss
 e. Severe pain
 f. Persistent bleeding from extraction sites
 g. Slow recovery from anesthesia

B. Phase II

    1. Operative site

        a. Continued bleeding: tamponade by biting saline-moistened gauze for approximately 30 minutes

        b. Epinephrine-soaked gauze or packs not recommended; rebound vasodilation can occur when a vasoconstrictor used, leading to increased bleeding.

        c. Pressure packs may need to be maintained for 2 hours or some specified time postprocedure—determine appropriate time for removal and discharge.

    2. Discomfort

        a. Oral analgesic medications initiated in preparation for discharge home

            (1) May have started in phase I

            (2) Determine effectiveness of medication before patient discharged home on same analgesic.

            (3) If ineffective, may need prescription changed or other follow-up (see Chapter 26 for more information on pain and comfort)

        b. Continue ice pack as ordered.

    3. Oral care

        a. Oral suctioning initiated by patient when appropriate and patient capable

        b. Begin oral fluids if desired and not already started in phase I.

        c. Avoid extremes of heat.

    4. Education (Box 41-1)

        a. Includes patient, family, responsible adult companion

        b. Instructions

            (1) Oral hygiene

            (2) Avoid temperature extremes in food and beverages.

            (3) Avoid sucking motion, which creates negative pressure (i.e., do not use a straw, do not spit).

■ **BOX 41-1**
■ **KEY PATIENT EDUCATIONAL OUTCOMES**

Phase I: Patient Will:
Express feelings of lessened anxiety.
Describe minimal to tolerable pain.
Request analgesic to manage pain.
Perform oral suctioning and handle oral secretions unassisted.
Be able to communicate with nurse without using verbal skills.

Phase II: Patient Will:
Tolerate discomfort following administration of oral analgesics.
Describe oral hygiene following instruction with caregiver.
Demonstrate use of gauze sponge for tamponade of bleeding.
Demonstrate safe, gentle, and effective oral suctioning.
Verbally describe wire cutting (patients with MMF/IMF) with caregiver.
Progress to upright position with minimal orthostatic effects: dizziness, lightheadedness, nausea.

Discharge: Patient, Family, and Responsible Accompanying Adult Will:
Describe follow-up required.
Identify risks associated with operative procedure: infection, hemorrhage, pain, vomiting.
Describe oral care, activity, medications, and diet.
Demonstrate knowledge of medications (analgesics, antibiotics, antiemetics, etc.) by describing purpose and administration of each medication prescribed.

IMF, Intermaxillary fixation; *MMF,* maxillomandibular fixation.

      (4) Care of bands and wires

      (5) For patient with MMF/IMF

         (a) How and when to cut wires

            (i) Airway distress

            (ii) Vomiting

      (6) Patients should keep wire cutters with them at all times.

         (a) Transport should not be permitted without wire cutters.

      (7) Pain-relief alternatives

         (a) Dental wax may be used to protect oral mucosa and decrease irritation and discomfort from protruding wires or metal bands.

C. After discharge

  1. Oral hygiene

    a. Brushing difficult if not impossible because of swelling and pain

      (1) Swelling reaches maximum in 2 to 3 days, subsides gradually.

      (2) Rinses may help in reducing swelling.

    b. Saline rinses (1 teaspoon table salt in one-half glass hot water) for 2 minutes, three to six times a day, especially after meals

      (1) No rinsing for at least 8 to 12 hours after procedure so as not to disturb clot (surgeon may order up to 24 hours before rinsing begins); disruption of the clot may lead to painful "dry socket" (localized osteitis).

         (a) Most often develops from second to fifth postoperative day

         (b) Chief complaint is pain; also may complain of odor or a bad taste.

         (c) Treatment is conservative.

            (i) Gentle warm saline irrigation of site

            (ii) Sedative

            (iii) Dressing over site until patient no longer symptomatic

      (2) Antiseptic mouthwashes may also be prescribed.

         (a) Most common is chlorhexidine 0.2%.

         (b) Held over surgical site for 1 minute, then expectorated

         (c) After a rinse, patients should have nothing by mouth for 30 minutes, as the chlorhexidine will bind to oral tissues if not rinsed away and continue to suppress bacterial regrowth.

    c. Continued bleeding

      (1) Instruct patient to replace gauze sponge over bleeding site and bite firmly for 20 to 30 minutes.

      (2) If a bleeding tooth socket, a moist tea bag over the socket may be helpful.

         (a) Tannic acid is a local vasoconstrictor.

      (3) If bleeding persists, patient needs to be evaluated by surgeon.

  2. Nutrition

    a. Instruct patient regarding alcohol and smoking avoidance for at least 2 weeks.

    b. Diet and food preparation

      (1) Avoid hot foods and liquids for first 48 hours (soft and cool diet choices).

      (2) Instruct patient to advance to soft foods or pureed diet (nutritional supplement) as tolerated or ordered by surgeon.

    c. Encourage fluid intake, especially during hot weather.

  3. Vomiting

    a. Prepare patient and family for possibility of vomiting swallowed blood; suggest adequately sized receptacle for ride home and at home in case of emesis.

    b. Caution patient and caregiver to call surgeon or facility:

      (1) If vomiting persists for >6 hours

      (2) If continuing to swallow blood: may require evaluation to determine source of bleeding

  4. Pain: peaks approximately 12 hours postoperatively

      a. Ice packs, heat application especially for TMJ procedures

      b. Oral analgesics

         (1) Suggest contacting surgeon if pain is not relieved by prescribed analgesics, intolerable, or increasing.

         (2) Unrelieved or increasing pain may indicate

            (a) Infection

            (b) Retained root

            (c) Bone

            (d) Foreign body

            (e) Maxillary sinus problems

      c. Alternatives

         (1) Dental wax may be applied to wires and bands to reduce mucosal irritation.

         (2) Explore with patient and caregiver other potential pain management techniques (see Chapter 26).

  5. Wound care

      a. See oral hygiene instructions for intraoral incisions.

      b. For external incisions

         (1) Keep wound clean and dry for minimum of 24 to 48 hours.

         (2) May be instructed to remove dressing after 24 to 48 hours

         (3) Clean incision with saline or half-strength hydrogen peroxide

         (4) Cover with antibiotic ointment.

         (5) Observe incision for signs of infection: redness, swelling, drainage.

  6. Activity

      a. Rest

         (1) Limit activity until pain and swelling subside.

         (2) Sleep with head elevated on several pillows to reduce swelling and minimize bleeding.

         (3) While taking opioid analgesics, avoid

            (a) Operating machinery

            (b) Driving automobiles

            (c) Using sharp or potentially injurious articles

            (d) Drinking alcohol

      b. Exercise

         (1) For first 24 hours, any exercise is discouraged.

         (2) Defer vigorous activity; restrict until surgeon allows; may be up to 4 weeks after surgery.

            (a) Aerobic activity may increase heart rate and blood pressure, leading to increased bleeding from operative site(s).

  7. Follow-up care

      a. Arrange for return visit with surgeon in specified time interval.

         (1) Patients with drains, MMF/IMF, extensive procedures may require return visit on first postoperative day.

         (2) Sutures removed in 5 to 7 days postoperatively

      b. Return to work dependent on procedure, patient work

      c. Risk for secondary hemorrhage

         (1) Seven to 10 days after surgery

         (2) Often caused by an infected wound and poor oral hygiene

      d. Fever: contact surgeon if temperature greater than 100.4° F (38° C) or as ordered by surgeon.

VI. COMMON OPERATIVE PROCEDURES (see also Chapters 43 and 45)

  A. Arch bars

    1. Purpose: used for treatment of avulsed teeth, fractures of the mandible, or maxilla

    2. Description: rigid metal bars used to splint and fix the teeth and/or maxilla or mandible; wire ligatures attach the bars to the teeth.

  B. Closed reduction of mandibular (jaw) fracture

    1. Purpose: used for alignment and stabilization of fractures to allow proper healing

      2. Description: Erich-type arch bars ligated to teeth most common method of fixation; MMF (which is synonymous with IMF) using stainless steel loops or elastics for 3 to 8 weeks considered best for providing reduction and fixation

      3. MMF/IMF acceptable for ambulatory surgery if there is no gross edema and/or bleeding

      4. Postanesthesia priorities

        a. Airway

        b. Nausea and vomiting

        c. Wire cutter at bedside, immediately available

      5. Psychosocial concerns

        a. Difficulty communicating

        b. Dietary modifications

      6. Complications

        a. Severe airway distress, epistaxis, or emesis requiring wires to be cut

  C. Dental examination

      1. Purpose: oral cavity inspected and teeth and supporting structures probed for defects, lesions, mobility, and infection

      2. Description: visual and instrument methods used for the examination

  D. Dental implant

      1. Purpose: replace a single missing tooth or multiple missing teeth, lost to injury or other reasons

      2. Description: a prosthetic tooth with an anchoring structure surgically implanted beneath the mucosal or periosteal layer or in the bone

  E. Dental prophylaxis

      1. Purpose: cleansing of teeth (stains, materia alba, calculus, removal of plaque)

      2. Description: dental instruments used to clean the teeth

  F. Dental restoration

      1. Purpose: replacing tooth structure by artificial means

      2. Description: reforming lost tooth structure, missing, damaged, or diseased teeth with alloy of silver, gold, or acrylic resin

  G. Genioplasty

      1. Purpose: operative repair of chin deformities (microgenia, macrogenia, asymmetric chin are a few of the defects)

      2. Description: repair done by open bone reduction, augmentation with synthetic or natural materials, or osteotomy with plate and screw fixation

  H. Gingivectomy

      1. Purpose: to eradicate periodontal infection and reduce the gingival sulcus depth

      2. Description: excision of all loose infected and diseased gingival tissue

  I. Implants

      1. Purpose: used to stabilize or totally support tooth replacements; prostheses may be fixed or fixed and removable.

      2. Description

        a. Osseointegration screw technique (Branemark)

          (1) Titanium screw inserted into jaw bone, grows into the bone (osseointegrates)

          (2) After 4 months (mandible) or 6 months (maxilla), attached to and loaded with a prosthesis

        b. Transmandibular implant/mandibular staple implant

          (1) Consists of a base plate, screws to fix the plate to the mandible, and posts that attach to a bar (Dolder) in the mouth

          (2) Lower prosthesis attached to the bar; prosthesis started 4 to 6 weeks after surgery

  J. Intraoral biopsy

      1. Purpose: removal of abnormal tissue for histopathological examination

      2. Description

        a. Excisional: complete removal of a lesion with primary closure

        b. Incisional: small representative portion of a lesion is removed if the lesion is large and the defect left from its removal could not be closed primarily.

K. Multiple dental extractions
  1. Purpose:
      a. May follow trauma
      b. Significant or recurring infection
      c. Nonrestorable teeth
      d. Preparation for prosthetic replacement
      e. Often done in preparation for
          (1) Solid organ transplant
          (2) Chemotherapy
          (3) Radiotherapy
          (4) Large joint replacement
  2. Description: surgical removal of teeth
L. Odontectomy: tooth extraction
M. Open reduction and internal fixation of zygomatic fracture
  1. Purpose: to realign fractured bone fragments and restore facial contour
  2. Description: by using a transconjunctival or lower eyelid subciliary incision with skin muscle flap and orbital floor exploration, the fracture reduced and fixated with wires or microplate system for the infraorbital rim and wires or miniplating fixation of the zygomaticomaxillary buttress
N. Osteotomy
  1. Purpose: correct maxillofacial deformities.
  2. Description
      a. Le Fort osteotomy: osteotomy performed along the classic lines of fracture as described by Le Fort to correct a maxillary skeletal deformity classified as
          (1) Le Fort osteotomy I, lower maxillary
          (2) Le Fort osteotomy II, pyramidal nasoorbitomaxillary
          (3) Le Fort osteotomy III, high maxillary/facial disarticulation (depending upon the location of the deformity)
          (4) Maxilla sectioned transversely and repositioned (see Chapter 43)
      b. Sagittal split mandibular osteotomy:
          (1) Intraoral surgical procedure for correction of retrognathism, prognathism or open bite
          (2) Mandibular rami and posterior body sectioned in the sagittal plane
      c. Segmental alveolar osteotomy
          (1) Intraoral surgical procedure in which segments of alveolar bone containing teeth are sectioned between, and apically to, the teeth for the repositioning of the alveolus and teeth
          (2) It may be maxillary or mandibular.
          (3) It may be combined with ostectomy.
      d. Sliding oblique osteotomy
          (1) Oral surgical procedure in which the mandibular ramus is cut vertically from the sigmoid notch to the angle; this facilitates posterior repositioning of the mandible in correction of mandibular prognathism.
          (2) May be performed extraorally or intraorally
          (3) Similar to vertical osteotomy
      e. Vertical osteotomy: oral surgical procedure similar to sliding oblique osteotomy
  3. Postanesthesia priorities
      a. Airway
      b. Bleeding
      c. Nausea and vomiting
      d. Swelling
      e. Pain management
  4. Psychosocial concerns
      a. Facial swelling distorting appearance
      b. Reason for procedure (trauma or cosmetic and functional appearance)

O. Splint
   1. Purpose:
      a. Stabilize the maxillomandibular position
         (1) Secured to the maxilla and mandible
         (2) Interlocked
         (3) Retain the desired position of the osteotomized units
      b. Reduce and stabilize maxillofacial fractures
      c. May be used in the interim before MMF/IMF or plate and screw (rigid) fixation
   2. Description:
      a. Made of acrylic resin or metal
      b. Used as space maintainer or fixator; to hold teeth in alignment
      c. Temporary, permanent, or removable
P. TMJ arthroscopy
   1. Purpose
      a. Diagnosis of internal joint pathology
      b. Lavage of joint
      c. Lysis of adhesions
      d. Biopsy of synovial tissue
   2. Description: direct visual inspection and examination of interior TMJ structures using an endoscopic instrument
   3. Postanesthesia priorities
      a. Trismus may be problem.
      b. TMJ physiotherapy initiated
      c. Provide information on jaw-opening exercises.
   4. Psychosocial concerns
      a. Chronic pain may be an issue; ongoing assessment and pain management essential.

BIBLIOGRAPHY

1. Booth PW, Schendel SA, Hausamen JE: *Maxillofacial surgery*, St Louis, 2007, Churchill Livingstone.
2. Chung WL, Sosovicka MF, Costello BJ: *Contemporary ambulatory anesthesia in oral and maxillofacial surgery*, Dallas, 2004, University of Texas Southwestern Medical Center at Dallas.
3. Dimitroulis G: *A synopsis of minor oral surgery*, Oxford, UK, 1997, Reed Educational and Professional Publishing.
4. Donoff RB: *Massachusetts General Hospital manual of oral and maxillofacial surgery*, ed 3, St Louis, 1997, Mosby.
5. *Dorland's illustrated medical dictionary*, ed 31, Philadelphia, 2007, WB Saunders.
6. Ferraro JW: *Fundamentals of maxillofacial surgery*, New York, 1997, Springer-Verlag.
7. Hupp JR, Ellis E, Tucker MR: *Contemporary oral and maxillofacial surgery*, St Louis, 2008, Mosby.
8. Kaban LB, Pogrel MA, Perrott DH: *Complications in oral and maxillofacial surgery*, Philadelphia, 1997, WB Saunders.
9. Kwon PH, Laskin DM: *Clinician's manual of oral and maxillofacial surgery*, ed 3, Chicago, 2001, Quintessence Publishing.
10. O'Toole MT: *Miller-Keane Encyclopedia and dictionary of medicine, nursing, and allied health*, ed 7, Philadelphia, 2003, WB Saunders.
11. Riden K: *Key topics in oral and maxillofacial surgery*, Oxford, UK, 1998, BIOS Scientific.
12. *Stedman's medical dictionary*, ed 28, Philadelphia, 2006, Lippincott Williams & Wilkins.
13. Yates C, ed: *A manual of oral and maxillofacial surgery for nurses*, Oxford, UK, 2000, Blackwell Science.

42 Orthopedic Care

NANCY SAUFL

OBJECTIVES

At the conclusion of this chapter, the reader will be able to:

1. Describe common orthopedic surgical procedures and their associated nursing interventions.
2. Describe the assessment and management of complications associated with orthopedic procedures.
3. Describe the pathophysiology and management of arthritic disorders.
4. Identify the various types of traction and the nursing care priorities for patients in traction.
5. Describe the treatment and nursing management of the patient with a fracture.
6. Identify the educational needs of the orthopedic patient.

I. ANATOMY AND PHYSIOLOGY
   A. Skeletal system
      1. System of living connective tissue, high in mineral content
         a. Haversian system
            (1) Nourishes bone tissue
            (2) Made up of blood vessels and lymphatics
            (3) Architectural unit of bone
         b. Types of bone
            (1) Cortical (compact) bone
               (a) Dense, hard outer layer of bone
               (b) Found in shafts of long bones
               (c) Poor blood supply
            (2) Trabecular (cancellous) bone
               (a) Spongy, porous bone
               (b) Found at ends of long bones and in vertebrae
               (c) Rich blood supply
         c. Types of cells
            (1) Osteoblasts: form new bone
            (2) Osteocytes: mature bone cell
            (3) Osteoclast: resorb bone
      2. Functions of the skeleton
         a. Provides framework for the body
         b. Provides attachment and leverage for muscles, facilitating movement
         c. Protects vital organs and soft tissue
         d. Manufactures red blood cells
         e. Provides storage for:
            (1) Minerals
            (2) Calcium
            (3) Phosphate ions
            (4) Lipids
            (5) Marrow elements
      3. Divisions of skeleton
         a. Axial: framework of head and trunk
         b. Appendicular: framework of arms and legs
      4. Classification of bones
         a. Long bones

(1) Diaphysis: shaft of bone
(2) Epiphysis
    (a) Ends of bone
    (b) Helps with bone development
    (c) Made of cancellous bone
(3) Metaphysis:
    (a) Flared portion between diaphysis and epiphysis
    (b) Growing part of bone
    (c) Has richest blood supply
(4) Physis or epiphyseal plate: growth plate between epiphysis and metaphysis of immature bone
(5) Periosteum: connective tissue that covers bone
b. Short bones
    (1) Sesamoid or accessory bones
        (a) Carpals
        (b) Tarsals
        (c) Patella
    (2) Primarily found in hands and feet
c. Flat bones
    (1) Skull
    (2) Ribs
    (3) Pelvic girdle
d. Irregular bones
    (1) Ossicles of ear
    (2) Vertebrae
B. Tissue of musculoskeletal system
  1. Connective tissue
    a. Development
      (1) Develops from mesenchymal cells
      (2) Later differentiates into specialized connective tissue cell types
    b. Types (three)
      (1) Collagenous tissue
        (a) Derived from dense fibrous connective tissue
        (b) Constructed primarily of collagen fibers
        (c) Tendons
          (i) Dense fibrous connective tissue strands at the ends of muscles that attach muscles to bone
          (ii) Characteristics: flexibility, strength, extensibility
        (d) Ligaments
          (i) Dense connective tissue bands that attach bone to bone and provide stability to joints
        (e) Tendons and ligaments can withstand pulling forces.
          (i) Activity
          (ii) Joint motion largely affects ligaments.
          (iii) Muscle contraction largely affects tendons.
        (f) Fascia
          (i) Made of connective tissue
          (ii) Has many proprioceptive endings
          (iii) Covers muscles; provides network of nerves, blood, and lymph vessels
      (2) Cartilage: nonvascular tissue composed of collagenous and elastic fibers
        (a) Hyaline cartilage—very elastic
          (i) Found in:
             [a] Trachea
             [b] Synovial joints
             [c] Larynx
             [d] Nasal septum
             [e] Ribs

          (ii)   Tends to get calcified in old age

      (b) White fibrocartilage—thick, shock absorbing

          (i)   Found in:

             [a] Symphysis pubis

             [b] Between vertebrae

             [c] Wrist and knee joints

             [d] Ends of clavicle

          (ii)   Interarticular fibrocartilage—flattened fibrocartilaginous plates between articular surfaces of joints, such as

             [a] Menisci of the knee

             [b] Temporomandibular

             [c] Sternoclavicular

             [d] Acromioclavicular

             [e] Wrist

             [f] Knee joints

         (iii) Connecting fibrocartilage—found in joints with limited mobility, such as the intervertebral disks

         (iv) Circumferential fibrocartilage—rims surrounding sockets of articular surfaces such as the glenoidal labrum of the hip and the shoulder

         (v) Stratiform fibrocartilage—forms a coating on osseous groove that tendons pass through

      (c) Yellow or elastic cartilage—dense, more flexible and pliant than hyaline cartilage; strong

          (i)   Found in outer ear, epiglottis, and eustachian tube

      (d) Synovial membrane—covers and lines joints; forms synovial fluid responsible for lubricating and nourishing articular cartilage

    (3) Bone

      (a) Osseous connective tissue

      (b) Predominantly made up of

          (i)   Fibrous component called collagen

          (ii)   An amorphous component called calcium phosphate

      (c) Highly porous and vascular

2. Muscular system

  a. Made up of muscle cell bundles

  b. Possess rich vascular supply

  c. Covered by fascia

  d. Attached to bone by tendons

  e. Produces bodily movement by contraction

  f. Controlled by complex interaction with the central nervous system

3. Joints: articulations where bones or two bone surfaces come together

  a. Diarthrosis—freely movable synovial joint

    (1) Uniaxial—move in one axis and only one plane

      (a) Hinge—knee, elbow, finger, toe

      (b) Pivot—radial head

    (2) Biaxial—moves around two perpendicular axes, in two perpendicular planes

      (a) Saddle—base of the thumb

      (b) Condyloid—distal radius and wrist bones

    (3) Multiaxial—moves in three or more planes and around three or more axes

      (a) Ball and socket—hip, shoulder

      (b) Gliding—vertebral joints

  b. Amphiarthrosis—limited movement

    (1) Symphysis pubis, intervertebral

  c. Synarthrosis—immovable

    (1) Sutures—fibrous tissue between skull bones

    (2) Syndesmosis—ligament connecting bones' distal radius and ulna, distal tibia and fibula

(3) Gomphosis—fibrous membrane connects to bone, tooth, and mandible or maxilla
(4) Range of motion—degree of movement of a joint (Figure 42-1)
    (a) Angular—changes the size of angles between articulating bones
        (i)   Flexion—shortens the angle by bending forward
        (ii) Extension—lengthens the angle by bending backward
        (iii) Abduction—movement away from the midline
        (iv) Adduction—movement toward the midline
        (v) Plantar flexion—increases the angle between the foot and the front of the leg by bending the foot and toes down and back

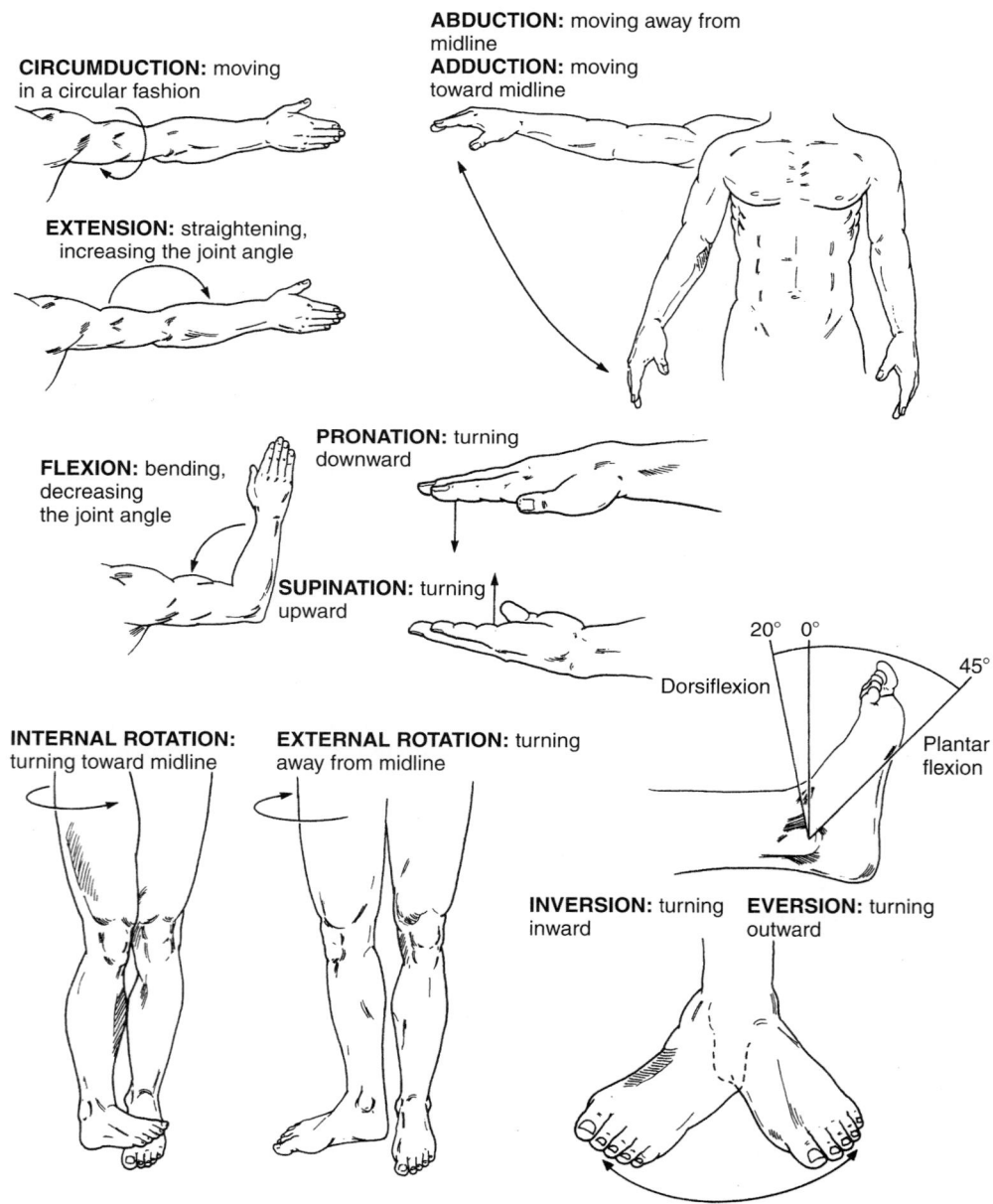

FIGURE 42-1 ■ Joint movements. (From Maher AB, Salmond SW, Pellino TA: *Orthopaedic nursing*, Philadelphia, 2002, WB Saunders.)

(vi) Dorsiflexion—decreases the angle between the foot and the back of the leg by bending the toes and foot upward

(vii) Hyperextension—stretching a part beyond its normal anatomical limits

(b) Circular—movement around an axis

(i) Rotation—moving or pivoting a bone around its axis (side to side of the head)

(ii) Circumduction—movement that resembles a cone shape; the distal part is a wider circle (winding up to throw).

(iii) Supination—palm turns upward while forearm rotates outward.

(iv) Pronation—palm turns downward while forearm rotates inward.

(c) Gliding—moving one joint surface over another with no circular or angular movement

(d) Miscellaneous movements

(i) Elevation—moving upward, lifting

(ii) Depression—moving downward, lowering

(iii) Inversion—sole of the foot turns inward.

(iv) Eversion—sole of the foot turns outward.

(v) Protraction—moving a part forward, such as the jaw or shoulder

(vi) Retraction—moving a part backward

(vii) Opposition—moving parts together (finger and thumb)

II. PATHOPHYSIOLOGY OF THE MUSCULOSKELETAL SYSTEM

A. Common congenital and developmental abnormalities

1. Joint dysplasia

a. Incomplete formation of diarthrodial joint

b. May lead to chronic subluxation or dislocation of joint

c. Developmental dysplastic hip, including congenital dislocated hip; may lead to early secondary osteoarthritis (OA)

2. Torsional problems of the long bones

a. Deformity related to abnormal development of bone

(1) Metatarsal adductus: metatarsal deviated medially

(2) Tibial torsion: tibia rotated externally or internally

(3) Femoral anteversion: leads to intoeing with internal or external rotation of leg

b. In extreme cases, may require surgical intervention

3. Clubfoot

a. Anomaly characterized by inversion of foot and forefoot, adduction, and equinus

b. Classified as fixed or rigid

4. Osteogenesis imperfecta ("brittle bone disease")

a. Genetic disease characterized by:

(1) Defect in collagen synthesis

(2) Generalized osteopenia

(3) Metabolical abnormalities

b. Classified according to severity: types I to III

5. Legg-Calve-Perthes disease

a. Idiopathic avascular necrosis of femoral head—flattening of femoral head

b. Seen in school-aged children

c. May lead to:

(1) Residual deformity of femoral head

(2) Fracture

(3) Early secondary OA

6. Slipped capital femoral epiphysis

a. Disruption of growth plate leading to posterior displacement of femoral head on the femoral neck

b. Seen in preteen and teenage children

c. May lead to avascular necrosis of the femoral head, limb shortening, or early secondary OA

    7. Scoliosis

      a. Lateral curvature of spine with vertebral rotation

      b. Classified according to causative factors

        (1) Idiopathic

          (a) Unknown origin: accounts for 90% of cases

          (b) Most frequent in children 10 to 12 years of age

          (c) Occurs 10 times more frequently in females

          (d) Familial pattern may be present.

        (2) Congenital

          (a) Develops in early embryonic life (6-8 weeks)

          (b) Malformation of spine occurs, resulting in hemivertebrae or failure of segmentation of vertebrae.

        (3) Neuromuscular

          (a) Neuropathic (paralytic): associated with spina bifida, poliomyelitis, or cerebral palsy

          (b) Myopathic: associated with muscular dystrophy

        (4) Additional types of scoliosis

          (a) Acquired—seen in:

            (i) Rheumatoid arthritis

            (ii) Rickets

            (iii) Spinal cord tumors

            (iv) Neurofibromatosis

          (b) Traumatic: resulting from vertebral fracture after radiation

  B. Metabolical bone disease

    1. Osteoporosis

      a. Common disorder characterized by a generalized reduction in the mass and strength of bone, leading to high risk for fracture

      b. Rate of bone resorption greater than rate of bone formation

      c. Multiple risk factors

        (1) Prevalent with Caucasian, Asian, or Hispanic/Latino people

        (2) Small skeletal frame

        (3) Estrogen deficiency or postmenopausal condition

        (4) Inactivity or immobility

        (5) High caffeine or alcohol consumption

        (6) Low-calcium or high-protein diet

        (7) Female

        (8) Older age

        (9) Family history

        (10) Certain medications (i.e., steroids, some anticonvulsants)

      d. Fractures common and may be induced by minor trauma

        (1) Wrists

        (2) Femoral head

        (3) Vertebrae

        (4) Pelvis

    2. Paget's disease (osteitis deformans): chronic disorder that typically results in enlarged and deformed bones

      a. Excessive breakdown and formation of bone tissue causes the bone to weaken.

      b. Slow, progressive disease caused by initial bone resorption, followed by period of reactive bone formation

      c. New bone is:

        (1) Thicker

        (2) Softer

        (3) Has reduced strength

        (4) Highly vascular

    3. Rickets

      a. Abnormal calcification of bone seen in childhood, leading to soft and deformed bones

　　　b. Related to deficiency in vitamin D caused by:
　　　　　(1) Nutritional deficit
　　　　　(2) Inability to absorb or use vitamin D
　　4. Osteomalacia
　　　a. Demineralization of bone in the adult leading to soft, deformed bones ("adult rickets")
　　　b. Related to inadequate supply of calcium or phosphorus caused by:
　　　　　(1) Nutritional deficit
　　　　　(2) Absorptive problem
C. Neoplastic disorders
　　1. Primary bone or soft tissue tumors
　　　a. Benign or malignant tumors
　　　　　(1) Bone
　　　　　(2) Cartilage
　　　　　(3) Connective tissue
　　　　　(4) Vascular tissue near bone
　　　b. May lead to local bone destruction and weakening of the tissue
　　　c. Relatively uncommon
　　2. Bone metastasis
　　　a. Spread of malignancy from a primary site of origin to bone
　　　b. Lytic or blastic lesions may lead to:
　　　　　(1) Bone destruction
　　　　　(2) Weakening
　　　　　(3) Impending or actual fracture
　　　c. Frequent sequelae of common malignancies
　　　　　(1) Breast
　　　　　(2) Prostate
　　　　　(3) Lung
　　　　　(4) Kidney
　　　　　(5) Thyroid
　　　　　(6) Bladder
D. Infection
　　1. Bone or joint tuberculosis
　　　a. Infection of bone or joint by *Mycobacterium tuberculosis,* leading to cartilage or bone destruction
　　　b. Weight-bearing joints and vertebral bodies most common sites
　　　c. May require surgical drainage of abscesses in addition to aggressive pharmacological treatment
　　2. Osteomyelitis
　　　a. Microbial invasion of bone leading to acute or chronic infection
　　　b. Classified according to method of microbial invasion
　　　　　(1) Hematological: acute or chronic infection spread to the bone through circulatory system
　　　　　　　(a) More common in children
　　　　　　　(b) More easily treated in children because of higher vascularity of their bones and supportive tissues
　　　　　(2) Contiguous: infection of the bone by direct extension of bacteria from infected soft tissue or surgical site
　　　　　　　(a) More common in adults older than 50 years
　　　　　　　(b) Risk factors include orthopedic surgeries or soft tissue trauma.
　　　　　(3) Traumatic: infection of the bone by direct contamination with environmental or bodily microbes
　　　　　　　(a) More common in young males and children
　　　　　　　(b) Risk factors include penetrating wounds, intramedullary rods, and open fractures.
　　3. Septic arthritis
　　　a. Microbial invasion of the synovial membrane, commonly bacterial in origin, leading to joint infection

        b. Joint infection usually accompanied by signs and symptoms of systemic infection

        c. May lead to destruction of articular cartilage and early secondary OA

   E. Arthritic disorders

     1. OA (degenerative joint disease or osteoarthrosis)

        a. Progressive noninflammatory disorder of diarthrodial joints characterized by loss of articular cartilage, marginal osteophytes (spurs), subchondral cysts, and sclerotic changes

          (1) Most common form of arthritis

          (2) Primarily affects weight-bearing joints: hips, knees, spine, shoulders, interphalanges

        b. Classified by causative factor

          (1) Primary OA

            (a) Cause unknown

            (b) Increased with:

              (i) Obesity

              (ii) History of repetitive trauma to joint

              (iii) Age

          (2) Secondary OA

            (a) Related to preexisting factors

            (b) Seen after trauma to:

              (i) Joint

              (ii) Dysplasia

              (iii) Other pediatric or congenital disorders of the joint

              (iv) Sepsis

              (v) As a result of a primary disease involving the joint such as hemophilia

        c. Clinical findings

          (1) Asymmetric distribution

          (2) Pain or stiffness in joint, especially with weight-bearing activities

          (3) Crepitation of joint

          (4) Deformity of joint or decrease in range of motion

          (5) Possible swelling and warmth of joint

          (6) Gait disturbance (limp)

        d. Conservative treatment

          (1) Reduction of risk factors

            (a) Weight loss if needed

            (b) Decrease in weight-bearing activities

          (2) Gait rest devices (cane, crutch)

          (3) Local application of heat or cold

          (4) Pharmacological therapy (Box 42-1)

        e. Nutritional supplements: glucosamine and chondroitin

          (1) Substances found naturally in the body and believed to play a role in:

            (a) Cartilage formation

            (b) Cartilage elasticity

          (2) Widely used as dietary supplement in the treatment of OA

          (3) Some studies have shown that some people with mild and moderate OA taking glucosamine/chondroitin have reported pain relief similar to that of nonsteroidal anti-inflammatory drugs (NSAIDs).

          (4) Some research has indicated that the supplements might slow down cartilage damage in patients with OA.

        f. Disease-modifying drugs

          (1) Current focus of pharmacological research

            (a) Pentosan

            (b) Enzyme inhibitors

              (i) Doxycycline

              (ii) Collagenase inhibitors

              (iii) Lipids

              (iv) Growth hormones

▪ BOX 42-1
▪ **PHARMACOLOGICAL THERAPY**

Nonsteroidal Anti-Inflammatory Drugs (NSAIDs)

Initial drug of choice for mild to moderate pain

NSAIDs inhibit prostaglandin formation through the cyclooxygenase (Cox) enzyme.

This enzyme exists in two isoforms, Cox-1 and Cox-2:

- Primary therapeutic effect of NSAIDs exhibited by blocking Cox-2.
- Celecoxib, (Celebrex)—100 to 200 mg orally twice per day
- Meloxicam, (Mobic)—7.5 to 15 mg orally daily (structurally related to piroxicam; selectively inhibits Cox-2 over Cox-1)
- Ketorolac, (Toradol)—10 mg orally every 4 to 6 hours or 30 mg IV or IM every 6 hours; if older than 65 years, 15 mg IV or IM every 6 hours
- Fenoprofen, (Nalfon, Fenopron)—300 to 600 mg orally three or four times per day to a maximum of 3.2 g daily
- Nabumetone, (Relafen, Relifex)—1000 mg orally daily or twice per day with maximum of 2000 mg per day
- Piroxicam, (Feldene, Pirox)—20 mg orally daily
- Sulindac, (Clinoril, Novo-Sundac)—150 to 200 mg orally twice per day with maximum daily dose of 400 mg
- Naproxen, (Anaprox, Aleve)—250 to 500 mg orally twice per day with maximum daily dose of 1.5 g
- Ketoprofen, (Orudis, Actron)—75 mg three times per day or 50 mg four times per day or 200 mg as extended-release form; maximum daily dose 300 mg, or 200 mg as extended-release form

Possible side effects:

- Abdominal pain
- Heartburn
- Ulcers
- Bleeding
- Renal failure
- Decreased liver function

Opioids

Added to NSAIDs for mild to moderate pain; adult dosage guidelines:

- Codeine—15 to 60 mg orally every 4 to 6 hours as needed with maximum daily dose of 360 mg
- Hydrocodone bitartrate, Lortab, Lorcet, or Roxicet combined in varying strengths with acetaminophen, 500 to 650 mg
- Oxycodone hydrochloride, Percodan, or Percocet combined in varying strengths with aspirin, 325 mg, or acetaminophen, 500 to 650 mg
- Propoxyphene hydrochloride, Darvon—65 mg orally every 4 hours, as needed with maximum daily dose of 390 mg

For persistent pain, stronger opioid added along with antidepressants or antianxiety drugs to increase tolerance for pain:

- Antidepressants helpful in reducing neuropathic pain
- Neurontin (Gabapentin)—originally developed for treatment of epilepsy; now widely used to relieve pain, especially neuropathic pain and postoperative chronic pain

---

IM, Intramuscular; *IV,* intravenous.

        g. Topical analgesics
           (1) Inexpensive, safe, effective
           (2) Application by massage releases endorphins.
           (3) NSAIDs
               (a) Salicylate
               (b) Benzydamine
               (c) Diclofenac
               (d) Ibuprofen
               (e) Indomethacin
               (f) Ketoprofen

        (g) Felbinac

        (h) Capsaicin

    h. Intra-articular injections

        (1) Corticosteroids

        (2) Local anesthetics

        (3) Viscosupplements (hyalgan products)

    i. Surgical options

        (1) Arthroscopy: diagnostic, for removal of loose bodies, and for treatment

        (2) Joint fusion (arthrodesis)

        (3) Osteotomy: option in early arthritis accompanied by deformity

        (4) Resection arthroplasty

        (5) Hemiarthroplasty: replaces one half of the joint with an artificial surface and leaves the other part in its natural (preoperative) state

            (a) Most commonly performed on the hip after fracture of neck of femur

            (b) Partial knee replacement (hemiarthroplasty, unicompartmental) may be performed on patient whose disease is limited to a single compartment (i.e., medial or lateral).

                (i) The unicompartmental knee replacement is less invasive.

                (ii) The small incision does not interfere with the main muscle control of the knee.

            (c) Shoulder hemiarthroplasty may be indicated in select patients with OA or posttraumatic disorders, providing pain relief and functional improvement.

        (6) Total joint replacement: arthritic or damaged joint removed and replaced with a prosthesis (artificial joint)

        (7) Hip resurfacing: type of hip replacement that replaces the two surfaces of the hip joint, conserving bone (head of femur preserved)

2. Rheumatoid arthritis

    a. Chronic systemic inflammatory disease potentially affecting multiple organs and joints; also considered an autoimmune disorder

        (1) Extra-articular manifestations

            (a) Cardiovascular changes: fibrinous pericarditis, cardiac myopathy, vasculitis

            (b) Pulmonary changes: pulmonary nodules, pleuritis, pulmonary fibrosis, pleural effusion

            (c) Neurological: peripheral neuropathy, carpal tunnel syndrome, nerve entrapment

            (d) Gastrointestinal: bowel and mesenteric vasculitis, malabsorption, enlarged spleen

            (e) Ocular: scleritis, episcleritis, Sjögren's syndrome

            (f) Integument: rheumatoid nodules, vasculitic skin lesions, purpura

            (g) Hematological: anemia, thrombocytopenia, granulocytopenia, increased sedimentation rate

            (h) Constitutional: fatigue, malaise, fever

        (2) Articular manifestations

            (a) Synovial proliferation

            (b) Pannus formation

            (c) Destruction of articular cartilage, with cartilage erosion, bone cysts, and osteophytes

            (d) Tendon and ligament scarring and shortening with ligamentous laxity, subluxation, and contracture

    b. Causative factors

        (1) Etiology unknown

            (a) Infectious

            (b) Traumatic

            (c) Stress related

         (2) Genetic predisposition exists.

        (3) Seen in all ages, affecting females to males 3:1

   c. Clinical manifestations (musculoskeletal)
      (1) Polyarticular symmetric joint distribution
         (a) Can affect any synovial joint
         (b) Most severe changes in weight-bearing joints
      (2) Joint swollen, erythematous, and warm to touch
      (3) Joint pain, stiffness, and possible contracture
      (4) Joint deformity, laxity, or subluxation
         (a) Deformities of knees, feet, phalanges possible
         (b) Subluxation of cervical vertebrae
      (5) Muscle atrophy
   d. Conservative treatment
      (1) Joint protection techniques
         (a) Weight loss if needed
         (b) Decrease in weight-bearing activities
         (c) Use of large, more proximal joints in more activities
      (2) Gait rest devices (cane, crutch)
      (3) Program of rest and exercise
      (4) Application of cold and heat
         (a) Use ice for first 48 to 72 hours postoperatively.
            (i) Specific duration of treatment for ice is 20 minutes "on" followed by one hour "off."
         (b) Next alternate ice with heat
         (c) Finally use strictly heat.
            (i) Duration of treatment for heat is 15 to 20 minutes "on" followed by a minimum of one hour "off."
      (5) Splinting or bracing of joint
      (6) Pharmacological therapy (see Box 42-1)
         (a) Oral NSAIDs (see OA)
         (b) Oral analgesics
         (c) Oral corticosteroids
         (d) Oral or parenteral gold therapy
         (e) Oral remittive agents: chloroquine phosphate
         (f) Oral immunosuppressives: methotrexate, cyclophosphamide, azathioprine
         (g) Intra-articular injection of steroid or local anesthetic
   e. Surgical options
      (1) Fusion of cervical spine or small joints (e.g., wrist)
      (2) Synovectomy
      (3) Osteotomy
      (4) Tendon repair or transfer
      (5) Hemiarthroplasty
      (6) Total joint replacement
F. Traumatic disorders
   1. Strain
      a. Musculotendinous injury caused by overstretching, repetitive stress, or misuse
      b. Classified according to degree of injury to musculotendinous unit
         (1) First degree: mild stretching or injury
         (2) Second degree: moderate stretching or tearing
         (3) Third degree: severe stretching, leading to rupture of the body or insertion site of the musculotendinous unit
   2. Sprain
      a. Ligamentous injury caused by overstretching or overuse
      b. Classified according to degree of injury to ligament
         (1) First degree: mild injury involving tear of few ligamentous fibers
         (2) Second degree: moderate injury with tearing of up to one half of ligamentous fibers

(3) Third degree: severe injury leading to rupture of the body of the ligament or from its bony attachment
3. Dislocation or subluxation
   a. Disruption of the contact of articulating surfaces of a joint caused by force to joint or development abnormality
      (1) Dislocation: complete disruption of joint
      (2) Subluxation: partial disruption of joint
   b. Most common in shoulder joint
   c. May be accompanied by soft tissue injury, including nerve palsy
   d. Recurrent dislocation may necessitate surgical repair of soft tissue or reconstruction of joint.
4. Fracture (Figure 42-2)
   a. Disruption of normal continuity of a bone, often accompanied by soft tissue trauma
   b. Classification of fractures
      (1) Severity of fracture
         (a) Compound (open): bone is broken with communication of the fracture site with an external wound.
         (b) Simple (closed): bone is broken with skin intact.
         (c) Complete: continuous fracture line through entire section of bone
         (d) Incomplete: break in continuity of one side of cortex only, as in the "greenstick" fracture
         (e) Displaced: edges of fractured bone not aligned, with higher risk for neurovascular damage
         (f) Nondisplaced: edges of fractured bone remain aligned.
         (g) Impacted: fractured bone fragment forcibly driven into an adjacent bone ("telescoped")
         (h) Avulsion: separation of small fragment of bone at site of a ligament or tendon attachment
      (2) Direction of line of fracture
         (a) Longitudinal (linear): fracture line runs parallel to axis of bone.
         (b) Oblique: fracture line runs at a 45° angle to axis of bone.
         (c) Spiral: fracture line encircles bone shaft.
         (d) Transverse: fracture line runs at a 90° angle to longitudinal axis of bone.
         (e) Comminuted: multiple fracture lines divide bone into multiple fragments.
      (3) Etiology of the fracture
         (a) Stress (fatigue): fracture occurs as result of repetitive microtrauma or an excessive musculotendinous pull that exceeds the strength of the bone.
         (b) Pathological (spontaneous): fracture through an area of disease-weakened bone, usually related to minor trauma
         (c) Compression: fracture resulting from compressive force
      (4) Fractures by name
         (a) Pott's fracture: fracture at distal fibula associated with severe tibiofibular disruption
         (b) Colles' fracture: fracture of distal radius within 1 inch of joint in a characteristic manner
   c. Etiology of fractures: fractures occur when bone subjected to more stress than it can absorb.
   d. Predisposing factors for fractures: factors that reduce bone strength or forces that exceed bone strength
      (1) Age: extremes in age
      (2) Nutritional deficiency: diet low in calcium, low in vitamin D, or high in protein
      (3) Metabolical diseases

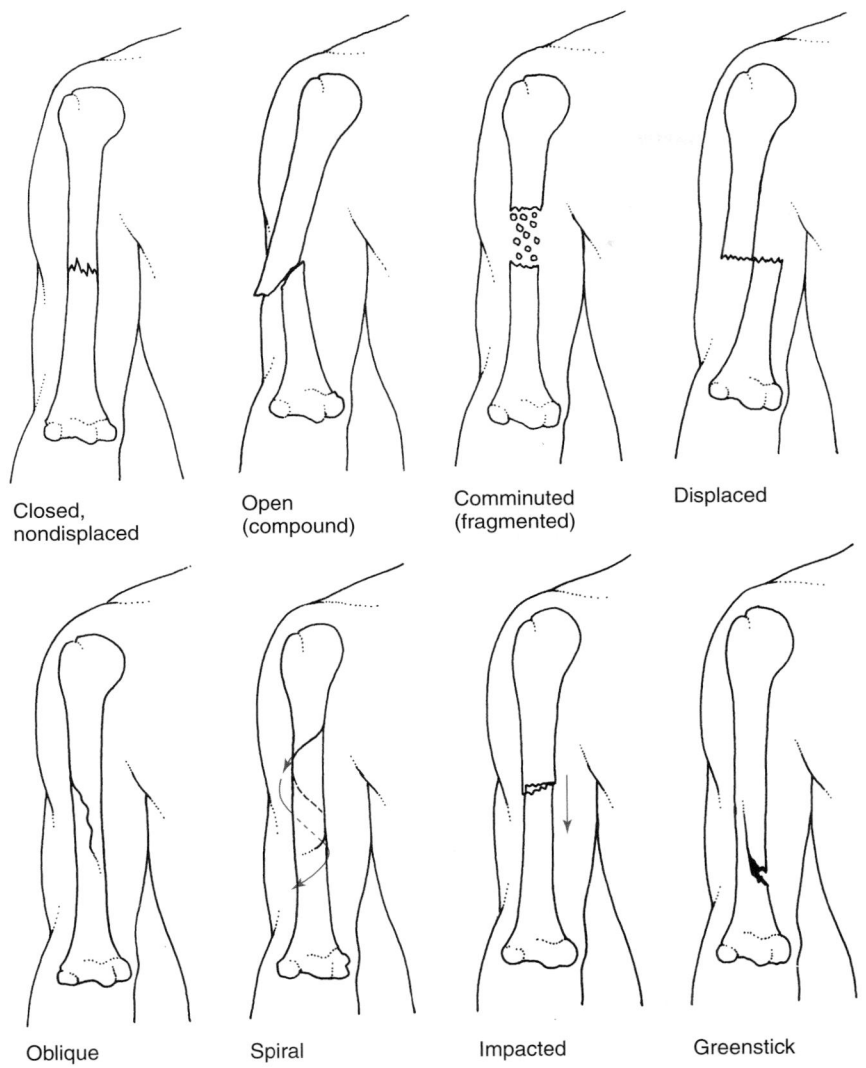

Closed, nondisplaced

Open (compound)

Comminuted (fragmented)

Displaced

Oblique

Spiral

Impacted

Greenstick

FIGURE 42-2 ■ Types of fractures. (From Ignatavicius DD, Workman ML: *Medical surgical nursing,* ed 4, Philadelphia, 2002, WB Saunders.)

       (4) Inactivity or immobility: bone remains strongest under stress ("Wolff's Law").

       (5) Physical abuse or trauma

   e. Fracture healing: healing maximized when bone edges approximated

       (1) Hematoma forms at site of fracture (first 24 hours).

       (2) Leukocytes infiltrate site, followed by macrophages.

       (3) Fibrous matrix of collagen proliferates at site.

       (4) Highly vascular "callus" forms.

       (5) Callus converts to loosely woven bone.

       (6) Callus calcifies and remodels (full fracture "union").

   f. Goals of fracture management

       (1) Reduce fracture to normal anatomical alignment.

       (2) Promote bone healing.

       (3) Maintain extremity function.

   g. Methods of fracture reduction

       (1) Closed reduction: reduction achieved without surgical intervention

        (a) Continuous traction: skin or skeletal
        (b) Manual traction
        (c) Splints or casts
        (d) External fixation
     (2) Open reduction and internal fixation
        (a) Allows visualization of fracture site
     (3) Repair with:
        (a) Pins
        (b) Rods
        (c) Nails
        (d) Wire
        (e) Screws
        (f) Plate and screw combinations

III. COMMON THERAPEUTIC DEVICES
  A. Casts
    1. Purpose
      a. Provide temporary immobilization.
      b. Prevent or correct deformities.
      c. Support bone and soft tissue during healing process.
      d. Promote early weight bearing.
    2. Types of casts
      a. Short extremity cast
        (1) Applied for stable fractures or tertiary sprains
        (2) May be weight bearing versus non–weight bearing
      b. Long extremity cast
        (1) Applied for stable or unstable fractures
        (2) Immobilizes joint to protect soft tissue injuries: Achilles tendon rupture
      c. Cylinder cast
        (1) Applied to treat stable fractures of long bones
      d. Body cast
        (1) Immobilizes spine (e.g., postoperative spinal fusion)
        (2) Corrects deformities (e.g., scoliosis)
      e. Spica cast
        (1) Immobilizes complex joint: shoulder, hip, thumb
        (2) Prevents dislocation of complex joint while promoting soft tissue healing
    3. Materials
      a. Plaster of Paris
        (1) Applied by wrapping wet plaster strips
        (2) Easily molded
        (3) Heavier weight
      b. Fiberglass—most common
        (1) Applied by wrapping wet plastic roll
        (2) More difficult to mold
        (3) Lightweight
      c. Fiberglass-free, latex-free polymer
        (1) Use in latex allergy or latex-sensitive patients.
      d. Hybrid
        (1) Combination of plaster of Paris and fiberglass
      e. Polyester and cotton knit
      f. Thermoplastic
        (1) Fabric tape composed of polyester polymer
    4. Early postcasting care
      a. Promote cast drying.
        (1) Plaster of Paris: may take 24 hours or greater to dry
          (a) Leave cast uncovered and open to air.
          (b) Use fans to aid drying of large casts.
          (c) Position casted part on pillow or smooth surface.

    (d) Move cast on pillow or with palms to avoid plaster indentation.

    (e) Advise patient to expect feeling of warmth as cast dries.

   (2) Fiberglass: dry within 30 minutes

    (a) Blot moisture from surface with paper towel.

    (b) Use blow dryer on cool or warm setting to aid drying of cast and skin.

  b. Potential complications

   (1) Skin breakdown

   (2) Neurovascular compromise

   (3) Compartment syndrome

   (4) Fracture misaligned

   (5) Superior mesenteric artery syndrome

    (a) Only seen in body spica casts

    (b) A decreased blood supply to bowel

     (i) Resulting from compression of mesenteric artery

     (ii) Causes necrosis to gastrointestinal tract and hemorrhage

    (c) Symptoms

     (i) Pain, distention, pressure in abdomen

     (ii) Bowel obstruction

     (iii) Nausea and vomiting

     (iv) Presenting symptoms may appear days or weeks after cast applied because of retroperitoneal fat loss after patient immobilized.

    (d) Postcasting care

     (i) Prevent complications related to ineffective breathing pattern with body or spica cast.

      [a] Note rate and quality of respirations.

      [b] Reposition patient in more upright position if possible.

      [c] Teach relaxation techniques, deep controlled breathing.

      [d] Cut a window in the cast, bivalve or remove cast.

      [e] Place nasogastric tube to decompress stomach.

      [f] Patient receives nothing by mouth (NPO), receiving intravenous (IV) fluids.

      [g] Prone position optimal

      [h] Ligament of Treitz released surgically

 c. Protect skin.

  (1) Remove loose particles of plaster or plastic from cast edges and skin.

  (2) Cover edges of cast to prevent skin irritation, especially important in personal area.

   (a) Turn edge of skin liner (stockinette) over cast edge and secure with tape.

   (b) If stockinette not used, "petal" edge with Transpore tape or moleskin.

   (c) Insert diaper at buttocks to prevent soiling in children with body or spica cast.

  (3) Instruct patient to avoid putting any object between cast and skin.

 d. Reduce postoperative or postinjury swelling.

  (1) Elevate extremity on pillow above level of heart.

  (2) When cast dry, apply ice to area of injury or fracture.

 e. Assess neurovascular status of extremity.

  (1) Perform integrated bedside assessment of extremity (Box 42-2).

  (2) Note amount and change in bloody drainage on cast and in dependent areas.

B. Traction

 1. Definition: application of pulling force in the presence of a counterforce

 2. Purpose

  a. Aligns fragments of displaced bones, preventing further soft tissue injury

  b. Reduces muscle spasm

  c. Maintains limb length

■ BOX 42-2
■ **INTEGRATED BEDSIDE ASSESSMENT OF EXTREMITY**

Assessment of Neurovascular Status	
Pain	Pulses
Edema	Temperature
Color	Sensation
Capillary refill	Motion

    d. Maintains alignment of limb while resting soft tissue
    e. Reduces contracture and deformity
  3. Types of traction
    a. Skin traction
      (1) Traction force applied via wraps, straps, or prefabricated boots secured to body (e.g., Russell's or Buck's traction)
      (2) Uses
        (a) Short-term immobilization of stable fractures (e.g., Buck's traction for proximal femoral fractures)
        (b) Intermittent traction (e.g., cervical neck traction)
      (3) Techniques of application
        (a) Traction applied at bedside by trained individual
        (b) "Customized" devices applied using Webril and moleskin
        (c) Prefabricated devices (e.g., boots)
        (d) Traction weight generally no more than 10 lb (4.5 kg)
    b. Skeletal traction
      (1) Traction applied directly to bone through transcortical or pericortical wires or screws (e.g., halo traction)
      (2) Uses
        (a) Long-term immobilization of fractures (commonly >1 week)
        (b) Short-term to long-term immobilization of unstable fractures of long bones or pelvis
      (3) Techniques of application
        (a) Traction applied at bedside or in operative suite
        (b) Local anesthetic applied to skin and injected into periosteum
        (c) Sedation and analgesia commonly used with pediatric patients
        (d) Amount of weight to traction according to patient's body weight and complexity of fracture, usually 15 to 40 lb
        (e) Use of portable x-ray to confirm fracture reduction
    c. Manual traction
      (1) Temporary traction applied by manual pull on extremity
      (2) Uses
        (a) Maintenance of alignment and position of extremity when skin or skeletal traction is being readjusted
        (b) Short transport of patient
        (c) Dislocation or relocation of joint, casting of extremity, and reduction of fracture
      (3) Techniques of application: firm manual pull placed on extremity while taking care to avoid pressure on bony prominences
  4. Nursing care of patient in traction
    a. Maintain traction apparatus to ensure proper alignment of body.
      (1) Reposition patient in neutral alignment, usually supine.
      (2) Obtain specific orders for:
        (a) Amount of traction pull
        (b) Position of extremity in bed
        (c) Head of bed—elevating head of bed decreases counterforce of body.

        (3) Readjust skin traction if device dislodged.

        (4) Apply manual traction to extremity whenever skeletal traction interrupted.

        (5) Avoid heavy coverings (blankets) over extremities, which may disrupt traction.

        (6) Inspect traction apparatus carefully every shift to ensure:

           (a) Bolts are tight on frame.

           (b) Knots are tight.

           (c) Weights are free hanging.

  b. Assess skin integrity.

        (1) Inspect pressure points between skin and apparatus.

        (2) Inspect bony prominences of body in bed.

        (3) Note redness, swelling, abrasion, pain caused by pressure.

  c. Assess for neurovascular compromise.

        (1) Perform integrated bedside assessment of extremity (see Box 42-2).

        (2) Compare affected with nonaffected side.

        (3) Note potential problems caused by disrupted traction or inappropriately sized devices (e.g., boots).

  d. Assess for complications related to skeletal pin.

        (1) Note:

           (a) Redness

           (b) Purulent drainage

           (c) "Tenting" of skin surrounding pin

           (d) Pain at insertion of skeletal pin

        (2) Note signs and symptoms of infection in patient with long-standing traction.

C. External fixator

  1. Definition: method of rigid fixation applied using percutaneous pins and wire in bone that attach to a portable external frame

  2. Purpose

    a. Reduces fractures, especially complex or open fractures

    b. Permits care of soft tissue wounds associated with fractures

    c. Corrects bony deformity

    d. Stabilizes fractures with delayed union or nonunion

    e. Stabilizes arthrodesis (fusion) of a joint

  3. Types of external fixators

    a. Simple

        (1) One or two bars on side(s) of limb (e.g., unilateral or bilateral frame)

        (2) Used to treat less complex fractures

    b. Complex

        (1) Multiple bars or semicircular rings placed in three-dimensional configuration around limb

           (a) Triangular

           (b) Quadrilateral

           (c) Semicircular

           (d) Circular frame

        (2) Used to treat more complex fractures, often accompanied by soft tissue trauma

  4. Nursing care of patient with external fixator

    a. Maintain external fixator.

        (1) Inspect device carefully every shift to ensure that bolts are tight on frame, with no movement of fixator pieces.

        (2) Move device and limb using pillow beneath extremity or by grasping longitudinal bars on each side of limb.

    b. Assess for neurovascular compromise.

        (1) Perform integrated bedside assessment of extremity (see Box 42-2).

        (2) Compare affected with nonaffected side.

     c. Assess for complications related to skeletal pin.
       (1) Note redness, purulent drainage, or pain at pin site.
       (2) Note signs and symptoms of infection in patient with long-standing device.
       (3) Note changes in sensorimotor status.
D. Assistive devices
   1. Definition: devices prescribed to assist in mobility by providing support to an injured or weakened lower extremity by redistributing weight to the upper extremities
   2. Purpose
     a. Promote healing of traumatically fractured bones.
     b. Promote healing of surgically osteotomized bones.
     c. Support weakened or injured soft tissue.
   3. Weight-bearing prescription
     a. Non–weight bearing (NWB): affected extremity should not touch floor.
     b. Touch-down weight bearing (TDWB): foot rests on floor with no weight.
     c. Partial weight bearing (PWB): 30% to 50% of body weight placed on affected extremity
     d. Weight bearing as tolerated: as much weight as patient can tolerate without extreme pain
     e. Full weight bearing: full weight should be placed on affected extremity.
   4. General instructions for patients
     a. Take small, controlled steps at all times.
     b. Wear sturdy walking shoes with nonskid soles.
     c. Avoid wet or snowy areas.
     d. Remove from path of walking:
       (1) Throw rugs
       (2) Electrical cords
       (3) Excess furniture
       (4) Other obstructions
     e. Stand erect, looking forward when walking.
     f. Lead with strong, unaffected leg.
   5. Types of assistive devices
     a. Crutches
       (1) Selection criteria: prescribed for persons with good coordination, balance, and upper body strength
       (2) Types of crutches
         (a) Axillary: most common crutch where
           (i)   Weight is placed on wrist and by tricep contraction.
           (ii) Consists of a central post, handgrip, and axillary pad
         (b) Platform: crutch used to distribute weight to forearm
           (i)   Consists of a central post and forearm platform
           (ii) Reduces stress on arthritic wrist or fingers
         (c) Canadian or Lofstrand: crutch used to distribute weight to wrist and hand; consists of a central post with a band that fits around the forearm
       (3) Proper fit of axillary crutches
         (a) Instruct patient to stand erect while wearing comfortable walking shoes.
         (b) Raise or lower central post so that two or three fingers can be inserted between the axilla and axillary pad.
         (c) Raise or lower handgrips so that elbows are bent 20° to 30°.
       (4) Crutch gaits
         (a) Two-point gait: patient advances one crutch at the same time as the contralateral leg in alternating fashion (common with PWB).
         (b) Three-point gait: patient advances both crutches along with affected leg (common in PWB, TDWB, and NWB).

    (c) Four-point gait: patient advances right crutch, left foot, left crutch, right foot, with three "points" on ground at all times (used only in patient with high disability).
  (5) Stair climbing
    (a) Climbing up stairs
      (i)   Patient holds banister on affected side and both crutches in contralateral hand.
      (ii) Patient steps up with unaffected leg.
      (iii) Patient follows with crutches and affected leg to same stair.
    (b) Climbing down stairs
      (i)   Patient holds banister on affected side and both crutches in contralateral hand.
      (ii) With weight on "good leg," patient steps down with affected leg and crutches.
      (iii) Patient brings unaffected leg down to same stair.
  b. Walkers
    (1) Selection criteria: prescribed for persons who require more stability than crutches can provide, such as those with impaired balance or coordination
    (2) Types of walkers
      (a) Simple walker: most common type of walker; consists of sturdy frame with handgrips
      (b) Platform walker: walker used to distribute weight to forearm; consists of a sturdy frame with forearm platform; reduces stress on arthritic wrist and fingers
    (3) Proper fit of simple walker
      (a) Instruct patient to stand erect while wearing comfortable walking shoes, heels even with back of walker.
      (b) Raise or lower all four legs of walker equally so that elbows are bent 20° to 30°.
    (4) Walker gait
      (a) Patient advances walker a short arm length forward, planting walker firmly on all four legs.
      (b) Patient advances affected foot, then advances body forward while supporting weight on arms.
    (5) Stairs: performed with folded walker in manner similar to stair climbing with crutches
  c. Canes
    (1) Selection criteria: prescribed for patients with minor disability and good balance, often after use of crutches or walker
    (2) Types of canes
      (a) Simple cane: central post with curved handle
      (b) Quad cane: central post with four distal legs and curved handle
    (3) Proper fit of cane
      (a) Instruct patient to stand erect while wearing comfortable walking shoes, cane 2 inches (5 cm) in front and 6 inches (15 cm) to the side of unaffected leg.
      (b) Raise or lower central post so that elbow is bent 20° to 30°.
    (4) Cane gait
      (a) Instruct patient to hold cane in hand opposite affected side.
      (b) Patient puts weight on "good leg," advancing affected leg and cane a comfortable distance.
      (c) Patient supports weight on both cane and affected leg, stepping through with "good leg."
    (5) Stairs: performed with cane hand opposite affected leg in manner similar to stair climbing with crutches

IV. ASSESSMENT PARAMETERS
  A. Vascular assessment (Box 42-2)
   1. Pulses
     a. Assess operative extremity first; compare finding with the opposite extremity.
        (1) Note rate, rhythm, quality.
        (2) Compare distal with proximal pulses and side to side.
     b. Diminished neurovascular function requires prompt intervention to prevent complications and/or permanent damage.
   2. Skin color
     a. Note pallor or blanching, suggestive of insufficient arterial blood flow.
     b. Note duskiness or cyanosis, suggestive of insufficient venous return.
     c. Compare side to side.
   3. Skin temperature
     a. Note increase or decrease in temperature.
        (1) Cold hand or foot may indicate diminished arterial blood supply to the area.
        (2) Extremity that is hot may indicate decreased venous return.
   4. Capillary refill
     a. Compress nail bed and quickly release; expect return of color in 3 seconds.
        (1) Rapid refill suggests venous congestion.
        (2) Slow refill suggests arterial insufficiency.
     b. Compare side to side.
   5. Edema
     a. Note location and severity.
     b. Note effect of elevating extremity above heart level on extent of edema.
     c. Compare side to side.
   6. Pain
     a. Assess level of pain.
        (1) Severe pain, particularly on passive motion, reliable sign of probable neurovascular compromise
        (2) If vascular status compromised, pain intensifies even with use of opioids and therapeutic measures.
  B. Peripheral nervous system assessment
   1. Sensory component
     a. Note patient's ability to detect sensory stimulation.
        (1) Pain
        (2) Light touch
        (3) Deep touch
        (4) Heat or cold
        (5) Vibratory sense
        (6) Proprioception
        (7) Two-point discrimination
     b. Note location and severity of any change.
     c. Compare side to side.
   2. Motor component
     a. Note patient's ability to move extremity actively through range of motion (ROM).
     b. Grade strength of major muscle groups.
        (1) Grade 5: active ROM against strong resistance (considered "normal" in well-functioning adult)
        (2) Grade 4: active ROM against moderate resistance
        (3) Grade 3: active ROM against gravity only
        (4) Grade 2: weak, incomplete ROM against gravity
        (5) Grade 1: no notable motion, but visible contractility of muscle group
        (6) Grade 0: no motion or visible contractility
     c. Compare side to side.

    C. Integrated peripheral nervous system assessment of extremities

        1. Upper extremity

            a. Radial nerve

                (1) Sensory: touch web space between thumb and index finger.

                (2) Motor: extend wrist, hyperextend thumb.

            b. Median nerve

                (1) Sensory: touch tip of index finger.

                (2) Motor: oppose thumb to small finger.

            c. Ulnar nerve

                (1) Sensory: touch tip of small finger.

                (2) Motor: abduct fingers.

        2. Lower extremity

            a. Peroneal nerve

                (1) Sensory: touch lateral side of great toe, medial side of second digit.

                (2) Motor: dorsiflex ankle, hyperextend great toe.

            b. Tibial nerve

                (1) Sensory: touch each lateral and medial aspect on sole of foot.

                (2) Motor: plantar flex ankle, flex great toe.

V. COMPLICATIONS COMMON TO ORTHOPEDICS

    A. Deep vein thrombosis (DVT)

        1. Definition: obstruction of deep venous circulation by a blood clot, usually distal to the cusp of a venous valve

        2. Etiology: Virchow's triad

            a. Venous stasis: immobilization, peripheral edema

            b. Vascular wall damage: trauma, traction of vessel during limb manipulation (dislocation), surgery

            c. Hypercoagulable state: clotting disorder, dehydration

        3. Incidence and risk factors

            a. Seen in 40% to 60% of patients with lower extremity surgery or injury

            b. Factors increasing risk for DVT

                (1) Increased age

                (2) Surgery

                    (a) Orthopedic

                    (b) Abdominal

                    (c) Gynecological

                (3) Immobility

                (4) Lower extremity trauma

                (5) Previous DVT

                (6) Obesity

                (7) Use of oral contraceptives

                (8) Coexistence of:

                    (a) Peripheral vascular disease

                    (b) Malignancy

                    (c) Stroke

                    (d) Pregnancy

                    (e) Cardiac disease

                    (f) Smoking

                    (g) IV drug abuse

                    (h) Inflammatory bowel disease

                    (i) Dehydration

                    (j) Sickle cell disease

            c. Factors decreasing risk for DVT

                (1) High mobility

                (2) Good hydration

                (3) Use of epidural anesthesia

                (4) Use of anticoagulants

        4. Postanesthesia care

            a. Assess for signs and symptoms of DVT: most common at least 48 to 72 hours after immobilization or surgery.

  (1) Unilateral edema of the lower extremity, unrelieved with elevation

  (2) Warmth, redness, tenderness, "fullness" of lower extremity

 b. Monitor results of diagnostic tests.

  (1) Noninvasive: Doppler ultrasonography

  (2) Invasive: ascending contrast venography (most diagnostic)

 c. Initiate interventions to prevent DVT.

  (1) Provide adequate hydration.

  (2) Encourage maximal mobility and early ambulation.

  (3) Apply mechanical devices per order in operating room or PACU to combat early DVT formation.

   (a) Antiembolic hose

   (b) Sequential compression devices to lower leg or calf

   (c) Plantar "foot pumps"

   (d) Inconclusive data exist comparing device effectiveness with or without anticoagulation.

  (4) Administer anticoagulants per order.

   (a) Oral warfarin: may be ordered day before, day of surgery, or in first 24 hours postoperatively

   (b) Low–molecular weight heparin: generally begun at least 12 hours postoperatively

   (c) Aspirin

   (d) Additional pharmacological agents for high-risk patients

    (i) Danaparoid

    (ii) Dextran

    (iii) Thrombin inhibitors

    (iv) Dermatan sulfate

 d. Initiate early interventions to treat patient with known DVT.

  (1) Administer anticoagulation per order: bolus heparin, then adjust to achieve recommended international normalized ratio (INR).

  (2) Decrease risk for clot embolization.

   (a) Maintain patient on bed rest per order: common with large proximal DVT.

   (b) Avoid aggressive massage of involved extremity.

   (c) Administer thrombolytic agent: uncommon therapy.

   (d) Prepare patient for surgical intervention: inferior vena cava filter inserted if multiple DVT.

   (e) Use noncemented prostheses if possible.

B. Pulmonary embolism (PE)

 1. Definition: complete or partial obstruction of the pulmonary artery or one of its branches by a systemically mobile thrombus or foreign body

 2. Causes: as listed for DVT

 3. Incidence and risk factors

  a. Seen clinically in 10% to 20% of patients undergoing major lower extremity surgery; fatal up to 10% of the time

  b. Factors increasing risk for PE: unrecognized DVT and all other risk factors for DVT

 4. Postanesthesia care

  a. Assess for signs and symptoms of PE: most common 48 to 72 hours after injury or surgery; vary with degree of vessel occlusion.

   (1) Dyspnea

   (2) Tachypnea

   (3) Restlessness

   (4) Pleuritic chest pain

   (5) Cough or hemoptysis

   (6) Rales

   (7) Pulmonary friction rub

   (8) Hypoxemia

   (9) Tachycardia

    b. Monitor results of diagnostic tests.
      (1) Noninvasive
        (a) Electrocardiogram (ECG) may show:
          (i)   T-wave inversion
          (ii) ST depression
        (b) Chest x-ray film may show:
          (i)   Wedge-shaped defect
          (ii) Accompanying diaphragmatic elevation
      (2) Invasive
        (a) Arterial blood gases: may be normal or show hypoxemia
        (b) Lung scan (ventilation/perfusion studies): not reliable in absence of signs and symptoms
        (c) Pulmonary angiography: highly diagnostic; usually performed only if lung scan nondiagnostic because of risk of examination
    c. Initiate interventions to prevent PE (see DVT).
    d. Initiate interventions to treat patient with known PE.
      (1) Promote adequate gas exchange.
        (a) Position patient in high Fowler's.
        (b) Instruct on slow deep breathing.
        (c) Provide oxygen: nonrebreathing mask common.
        (d) Prepare for intubation if necessary.
      (2) Administer anticoagulation per order: bolus heparin, then adjust to achieve recommended INR.
      (3) Decrease risk for clot embolization (see DVT).
C. Fat embolism syndrome (FES)
  1. Definition: mobilization of fat and free fatty acids that leads to acute pulmonary insufficiency
  2. Causes
    a. Mechanical theory: fat from marrow of broken bones embolized to lung and occludes small pulmonary vessels
    b. Biochemical theory
      (1) Stress response leads to release of catecholamines.
      (2) Free fatty acids mobilize.
      (3) Chylomicrons coalesce in lung.
      (4) Chylomicrons increase capillary permeability within alveoli.
  3. Incidence and risk factors
    a. Seen clinically:
      (1) In 1% to 10% of patients with fractures
      (2) In 5% to 10% of patients with multiple fractures or pelvic fractures
      (3) Up to 50% of patients with fractures may have subclinical FES.
      (4) Rarely with insertion of intramedullary rods or stemmed prostheses
    b. Possible at any age but most prevalent in:
      (1) Men aged 20 to 40
      (2) Elderly between ages 70 and 80
    c. Factors that increase the risk for FES
      (1) Invasion of intramedullary canal
      (2) Sepsis
      (3) Shock
  4. Postanesthesia care
    a. Assess for signs and symptoms of FES: often present 12 to 48 hours after causative event, often rapidly progressing.
      (1) Confusion, agitation, anxiety
      (2) Tachypnea, dyspnea, pulmonary edema
      (3) Hypoxemia, hypocarbia
      (4) Tachycardia, dysrhythmias, substernal chest pain
      (5) Hypotension
      (6) Petechiae of trunk or conjunctiva: occur 50% of time
      (7) Pyrexia

      b. Monitor results of diagnostic tests.
- (1) Noninvasive
  - (a) ECG: may show atrial fibrillation
  - (b) Chest x-ray film: may show diffuse pulmonary infiltrate
- (2) Invasive
  - (a) Arterial blood gases: may be normal or show hypoxemia
  - (b) Central venous pressure: elevated
  - (c) Pulmonary wedge pressure: initially reduced because of decreased perfusion of left atrium; later may rise
  - (d) Lung scan: may be performed in stable patient to rule out PE
  - (e) Pulmonary angiography: may be performed in stable patient to rule out PE
  - (f) Laboratory findings
    - (i) Elevated serum lipase
    - (ii) Elevated sedimentation rate
    - (iii) Elevated triglycerides
    - (iv) Elevated glomerular filtration rate
    - (v) Decreased hematocrit
    - (vi) Increased fat in urine

      c. Initiate interventions to prevent FES.
- (1) Maintain stability of fractured limbs.
- (2) Treat sepsis and shock aggressively.
- (3) Provide adequate hydration.
- (4) Controversial whether to administer methylprednisolone to maintain integrity of pulmonary vascular system

      d. Initiate interventions to treat patient with known FES: early diagnosis and aggressive treatment critical.
- (1) Promote adequate gas exchange.
  - (a) Position patient in high Fowler's.
  - (b) Instruct on slow deep breathing.
  - (c) Provide oxygen: nonrebreathing mask common.
  - (d) Prepare for intubation: common.
- (2) Administer corticosteroids: creates antiadhesive effect on platelets, decreases inflammation of vascular membranes.
- (3) Administer diuretics: reverses pulmonary edema.
- (4) Support cardiovascular system.
  - (a) Provide adequate fluid replacement.
  - (b) Administer blood products.
  - (c) Enhance blood pressure: dopamine.
  - (d) Enhance pulmonary arterial pressure and right ventricle afterload: nitroglycerin drip.

D. Compartment syndrome
1. Definition: condition in which increased pressure within a muscle compartment may lead to severe neurovascular compromise
   - a. In cases of massive muscle destruction, may also see myoglobinuric renal function
2. Cause: any event that leads to increased extracompartmental or intracompartmental pressure, leading to edema and ischemia
3. Pathophysiology: edema-ischemia cycle
   - a. Compromise of muscle compartment from:
     - (1) Overuse
     - (2) Extended compression of limb
     - (3) Fracture
     - (4) Bleeding produces profound, quick response by surrounding tissue.
   - b. As edema of muscles increases, capillary bed perfusion compromised and venous congestion ensues.
     - (1) Edema compresses nerves and vessels.
     - (2) Progressive edema causes muscle ischemia.

(3) Histamine release by ischemic muscles causes capillary dilation and enhanced capillary permeability.
(4) Edema increases, resulting in greater compromised tissue perfusion and tissue oxygenation.
(5) Lactic acid formation increases, causing anaerobic metabolism to accelerate.
(6) Blood flow increases, causing increase in tissue pressure, leading to greater compartmental pressures.
c. If edema-ischemia cycle not arrested:
(1) Irreversible muscle damage in 4 to 8 hours
(2) Permanent nerve damage in 8 hours
d. Three types
(1) Acute compartment syndrome
(a) Trauma related, limb threatening
(2) Chronic compartment syndrome
(a) Overuse of muscles (i.e., weekend exercise enthusiast)
(3) Crush syndrome
(a) Prolonged compression of limb
4. Incidence and risk factors
a. Uncommon in general population; most commonly associated with fractures or injuries of the lower extremities
b. Development within:
(1) Thirty minutes to 3 hours post injury
(2) Postoperatively during first 7 days
c. Factors that increase the risk for compartment syndrome
(1) Fracture
(2) Severe soft tissue injury (e.g., crush injury)
(3) Prolonged limb compression
(a) Restrictive wraps, cast, brace, or apparatus
(b) Prolonged compression of limb
(i) Unconscious victim lying on own limb
(ii) Prolonged pressure from positioning device during lengthy surgery
(c) Prolonged use of antishock trousers
(d) Tight fascial closure
(4) Internal bleeding
(5) Increased capillary permeability: related to histamine release
(a) Infiltrated IV fluids or medications
(b) Some poisonous snake bites
(c) Severe frostbite
d. Postanesthesia care
(1) Assess for signs and symptoms of compartment syndrome: perform comprehensive neurovascular assessment, noting deterioration as follows.
(a) Pain: most universal symptom related to muscle ischemia
(i) Pain extreme
(ii) Unrelieved
(iii) Aggravated by passive flexion or extension of digit or limb
(iv) Not well localized—involves entire compartment
(b) Pallor
(i) Seen in early stage; related to compression of artery
(ii) Later may be seen as cyanosis
(c) Paresthesias: commonly seen change related to compression of sensory nerve
(i) Burning
(ii) Searing
(iii) Electric sensations
(d) Pulselessness
(i) In early stage, pulse with decreased strength
(ii) Later, pulse nonpalpable but audible on Doppler ultrasonography

(iii) In later stages, no pulse found on Doppler ultrasonography
  [a] Muscle and nerve ischemia can be occurring without occluding an artery.
  [b] Pulses may be palpable in the patient with acute compartment syndrome.
(e) Paralysis
  (i) In early stage, may be motor weakness related to compression of motor nerve
  (ii) In later stage, may be complete paralysis
(f) Rigid or "tight" limb representing compartment engorgement
(g) Decreased urine output, with dark urine
(2) Monitor results of diagnostic tests.
  (a) Direct measurement of compartment pressures
    (i) Variety of methods in which catheter inserted into the compartment
      [a] Catheter purged with normal saline
      [b] Monitor intracompartmental pressure.
      [c] Pressures greater than 30 to 35 mm Hg considered diagnostic and warrant surgical intervention.
  (b) Laboratory findings of muscle destruction and renal insufficiency:
    (i) Elevated
      [a] Serum Creatine Kinase MM isoenzyme (CPK-MM)
      [b] White blood cell count
      [c] Serum potassium
      [d] Serum phosphate
      [e] Blood urea nitrogen (BUN)
      [f] Serum creatinine
    (ii) Reduced
      [a] Serum calcium
      [b] pH
    (iii) Elevated urine myoglobin
(3) Initiate interventions to prevent compartment syndrome.
  (a) Perform comprehensive neurovascular assessment on all patients at risk.
  (b) Provide early measures to decrease lower extremity edema.
    (i) Elevate limb above heart level.
    (ii) Ice limb at site of injury or surgery.
  (c) Decrease potential for further injury.
    (i) Carefully handle injured part.
    (ii) Maintain traction.
    (iii) Brace
    (iv) Cast
(4) Initiate interventions to treat patient with suspected or diagnosed compartment syndrome.
  (a) Perform comprehensive neurovascular assessment every 15 minutes with special attention to compartment at risk.
  (b) Maintain limb in neutral at level of heart.
    (i) Enhances arterial blood flow
    (ii) Reduces possible neurovascular impingement
  (c) Remove ice: reduce vasoconstriction.
  (d) Release or remove restrictive wraps, splints, or casts.
  (e) Assess pain and administer analgesics.
  (f) Maintain accurate input and output records.
  (g) Provide emotional support.
  (h) Assist with compartment pressure checks.
  (i) Prepare patient for fasciotomy per order.
    (i) Extensive surgical decompression of compartment
    (ii) High risk for infection as a result of ischemic conditions

VI. THE PERIANESTHESIA EXPERIENCE
- **A.** Preoperative phase—begins with patient's decision to have surgery and ends when he or she enters the operating room
  - **1.** Goals
    - **a.** Thorough assessment of patient's physical and psychosocial condition
    - **b.** Educating and preparing patient for surgery
  - **2.** Include the following:
    - **a.** Complete history including preexisting conditions
    - **b.** Medications
    - **c.** Allergies to foods, medications, or latex
    - **d.** Family history of anesthetic complications such as pseudocholinesterase deficiency and malignant hyperthermia
    - **e.** Social history—does the patient have assistance after surgery?
    - **f.** Lab work dependent on procedure and age of patient
    - **g.** Blood donation if replacement a possibility and time permits
    - **h.** Informed consent
    - **i.** NPO status
    - **j.** Preoperative education
      - (1) Begin discharge teaching.
        - (a) Use of assistive devices
        - (b) Pain management
        - (c) Signs of infection
        - (d) Dressing and incisional management
- **B.** Intraoperative phase—the time patient is in the operating room to the time patient admitted to phase I PACU
  - **1.** Goals
    - **a.** Appropriate surgical positioning
    - **b.** Prevent infection.
    - **c.** Prevent injury.
    - **d.** Maintain sterile field.
    - **e.** Perform accurate surgical counts.
    - **f.** Procure needed equipment (i.e., type of implant, traction, fixator, cast material).
    - **g.** Assess fluids and vital signs.
- **C.** Postoperative care, phase I—acute phase of recovery from anesthesia and surgical procedure
  - **1.** Routine phase I admission assessment and monitoring
  - **2.** Monitor surgical site.
    - **a.** Location of operative site
    - **b.** Neurovascular status
      - (1) Temperature
      - (2) Color
      - (3) Capillary refill
      - (4) Pulses
      - (5) Movement
      - (6) Sensation
  - **3.** Monitor patient's level of pain (Box 42-3).

■ BOX 42-3
■ **THE HIERARCHY OF IMPORTANCE OF THE BASIC MEASURES OF PAIN INTENSITY**

1. The patient's pain rating using a self-reported pain rating scale (e.g., 0-10 numerical rating scale)
2. The patient has experienced a procedure or condition that is thought to be painful (e.g., surgery).
3. Behavioral signs (e.g., facial expression, crying, restlessness, fidgeting)
4. Proxy pain rating provided by a family member or other person who knows the patient well
5. Physiological indicators (e.g., elevated vital signs)

From McCaffery M, Pasero C: *Pain clinical manual*, ed 2, St Louis, 1999, Mosby.

    4. Prevent/treat nausea and vomiting as indicated.

    5. Initiate physician orders.

    6. Discharge to phase II per criteria (see Chapters 30 and 51) when:

        a. Recovered from anesthesia

        b. Hemodynamically stable

        c. Pain managed

        d. Nausea and vomiting controlled

        e. Scoring criteria met

D. Postoperative care, phase II—observation period that includes preparing patient and support persons for home care (see Chapters 50 and 51)

    1. Routine phase II assessment

    2. Teaching postoperative care critical to successful recovery

        a. Medications (pain control, antibiotics, resuming routine home medications)

        b. Bowel management (stool softener)

        c. Assessing neurovascular status

        d. Care of dressings

           (1) Incision site

           (2) Wounds

           (3) Drains

           (4) Casts

           (5) Cryotherapy

           (6) Continuous passive motion (CPM)

           (7) Pin sites

        e. Signs of infection

        f. When to call physician

           (1) Increasing pain

           (2) Fever

           (3) Edema

           (4) Infection

           (5) Bleeding

           (6) Change in neurovascular status

        g. Diet

        h. Mobility guidelines

        i. Reinforce instructions on assistive devices.

        j. Postoperative appointment with surgeon

        k. Driving considerations

        l. Self-care (showering, bathing)

E. Postoperative care, extended observation (see Chapters 50-52)

    1. Extended stays

    2. Patient discharge goals (Box 42-4)

F. Nursing diagnosis for orthopedic patient

    1. Anxiety and fear related to surgical procedure, loss of control

    2. Knowledge deficit relating to surgical procedure and perianesthesia experience

---

■ BOX 42-4

■ **PATIENT DISCHARGE GOALS FOLLOWING AMBULATORY SURGERY AND ANESTHESIA**

  1. To promote patient satisfaction by minimizing disruptive influences associated with the patient's perioperative care

  2. To optimize quality patient care such that patients can be safely discharged from the facility

  3. To educate patients regarding the anticipated recovery process, thus facilitating patient participation and compliance with postoperative care plus early recognition of problems

  4. To proficiently manage patients to minimize cost to the patient, medical facility, and third-party payers

From Burden N, DeFazio Quinn DM, O'Brien D, et al (eds): *Ambulatory surgical nursing,* ed 2, Philadelphia, 2000, WB Saunders.

3. High risk for ineffective coping
4. Risk for neurovascular compromise from perioperative positioning
5. Pain management deficit
6. Impaired physical mobility secondary to surgical procedure and postoperative pain management
7. Knowledge deficits regarding mobility skills
8. Self-care deficits
9. Activity intolerance
10. Potential for constipation from immobility and use of opioids
11. High risk for skin breakdown
12. Potential for infection
13. Potential for neurovascular compromise related to cast or traction devices
14. Knowledge deficit relating to use of CPM, cryotherapy, and/or assistive devices
15. Potential for DVT

VII. COMMON OPERATIVE PROCEDURES
   A. Definitions
     1. Upper extremity
       a. Carpal tunnel release—decompression of the median nerve by dividing the transverse carpal ligament
       b. Finger amputation and revision—generally for:
         (1) Traumatic injuries
         (2) Infection
         (3) Vascular compromise
       c. Joint replacement—performed to improve function in patients with rheumatoid arthritis or other degenerative diseases
         (1) Shoulder
         (2) Small joints of the finger
         (3) Hand
         (4) Wrist
       d. Olecranon bursectomy—excision of bursal wall and calcifications
       e. Open reduction, internal fixation—surgical placement of hardware such as pins, screws, or plates to maintain position of bones for healing
       f. Release of de Quervain's hand—decompression of dorsal compartment of the hand to treat stenosing tenosynovitis of the wrist at the base of the thumb
       g. Release of Dupuytren's contracture—fasciotomy or fasciectomy to treat contracture in the palmar surface of the hand
       h. Rotator cuff repair—repair of muscles and tendons of the rotator cuff
       i. Synovectomy—removal of part or all of the synovial lining of a joint to retard progression of rheumatic destruction of the joint
     2. Lower extremity
       a. Anterior cruciate ligament (ACL) reconstruction—replacement of damaged ligament with autograft, allograft, or synthetic ligament to return stability to the knee after ligament tear
       b. Arthroscopic meniscectomy—removal of part of the meniscus (cartilage) of the knee using arthroscopic technique
       c. Osteotomy—cutting a bone to change its position for weight bearing or to correct an abnormal curvature
       d. Prepatellar bursectomy—excision of bursal wall and calcifications
     3. Miscellaneous
       a. Arthroscopy: shoulder, wrist, knee, ankle
         (1) Diagnostic arthroscopy can be performed in a variety of joints.
         (2) Involves insertion of fiberoptic instrument into a joint to visualize interior
         (3) Multiple procedures can be performed through a scope, including but not limited to:
           (a) Debridement
           (b) Biopsy
           (c) Meniscectomy

        (d) Ligament repair

        (e) Removal of loose bodies

  b. Bone biopsy—arthroscopic or open

  c. Cast change

  d. Closed reduction of fractures

  e. Cyst removal

  f. Debridement—arthroscopic or open

  g. Excision of bone spurs—commonly formed as a result of osteoarthritic changes

  h. Excision of ganglion—removal of cystic mass found over a joint or tendon sheath

  i. Excision of lesion

  j. Hardware removal

  k. Joint manipulation (e.g., after knee arthroplasty)

  l. Muscle biopsy

  m. Removal of foreign body

  n. Simple tendon repair

  o. Fasciotomy—surgical incision of fascia to relieve constriction and swelling in a muscle compartment

  p. Bone graft—transfer of autologous or homologous bone from one site to another to replace bone, stabilize an internal fixation, or promote a bony fusion

  q. Arthroplasty—surgical resection of a joint with placement of prosthesis; may be done as open repair or arthroscopically assisted repair

  r. Tendon transfer—transference of tendon insertion point to different position to improve muscle function

  s. Amputation—surgical removal of a body part

  t. Replantation—surgical reattachment of a body part (i.e., finger, hand, arm, toe) that has been completely cut from a person's body

        (1) Goal is to give the patient back as much use of the original area as possible.

VIII. TYPES OF ORTHOPEDIC SURGERY

  A. Rotator cuff repair

    1. Composed of four muscles and tendons

      a. Supraspinatus

      b. Subscapularis

      c. Infraspinatus

      d. Teres minor

    2. Areas of shoulder most easily seen arthroscopically

      a. Glenohumeral joint

        (1) Ball-and-socket joint at end of humerus

        (2) Most mobile joint in body

        (3) Muscles and ligaments of rotator cuff strengthen this joint

      b. Subacromial space

      c. Acromioclavicular joint

    3. Procedure: arthroscopically assisted repair; also done as open repair if large enough tear involving more than one tendon

    4. Purpose

      a. Pain relief

      b. Improvement of functional abilities of joint

    5. Types of tears

      a. Four muscles identified above and their tendons comprise rotator cuff.

        (1) Subscapularis most frequently torn muscle, responsible for internal rotation of humerus

      b. Tears occur more in women and are seen most frequently after age 40.

      c. Etiology

        (1) Degenerative weakened areas in cuff as a result of aging process

        (2) Severe tears may result from:

          (a) Heavy lifting

          (b) Throwing object

(c) Fall on shoulder

(d) Sudden adduction force applied to rotator cuff while arm is held in abduction

6. Postanesthesia care

a. Neurovascular assessment of affected arm

b. Support surgical arm in sling or sling and swathe with abductor pillow to maintain joint alignment and diminish tension from operative shoulder.

c. Ice packs or cryotherapy to decrease edema and pain

d. Monitor dressing; reinforcing or changing may be required because of multiple puncture sites and leaking of irrigation fluids used intraoperatively to visualize joint.

e. Pain management

(1) Intraoperative intra-articular injection of local anesthetic

(2) Interscalene block

(3) Opioids

(4) NSAIDs

f. Physical therapy and home mobility instructions reinforced

(1) Emphasize importance of following instructions to avoid exacerbation of condition.

(2) Rehabilitation usually takes 6 months to 1 year.

g. Complications

(1) Contractures of elbow and shoulder if patient noncompliant with rehabilitation program

(2) Potential damage to deltoid muscle

(3) Repair work to cuff not holding because of misuse or overuse by patient

B. Spinal fusion and stabilization (thoracolumbar spine)

1. Procedure: surgical stabilization of spine using mechanical instrumentation with or without bone graft augmentation

2. Purpose

a. Prevent progression of spinal deformity.

b. Correct spinal deformity: lateral curves greater than 40°.

c. Reduce actual or potential neurological or cardiopulmonary deficits.

3. Methods of spinal fusion

a. Posterior spinal fusion with instrumentation

(1) Cotrel-Dubousset instrumentation: most common

(2) Harrington distraction rods or spinous process wiring

(3) Luque rods: most common for paralytic scoliosis

b. Anterior spinal fusion

(1) Zielke instrumentation

(2) Harms instrumentation

c. Combined anterior and posterior surgery

(1) Recommended for adults or children with severe deformities

(2) Anterior approach performed first, posterior approach commonly staged 5 days or more later (but may be performed during the same surgery)

d. Bone graft

(1) Autograft: bone transplanted from one part of person's body to another part (i.e., from iliac crest)

(2) Allograft: donor bone or tissue

(3) Graft placed on decorticated spine to encourage osteoinduction

e. Minimally invasive spinal surgery

(1) Smaller incisions

(2) Microscopically assisted tissue dissection

(3) Conservative removal of only extruded or sequestered nucleus pulposus

        (4) Percutaneous techniques; microscopic diskectomy; endoscopically visualized methods

        (5) Less surgical morbidity

    4. Postanesthesia care

      a. Assess neurovascular status: perform comprehensive neurovascular assessment every 15 minutes for first 2 hours, then hourly.

        (1) Note bowel and bladder dysfunction.

        (2) Assist with somatosensory evoked potential monitoring as ordered.

        (3) Assess strength and sensation in extremities; notify surgeon of weakness and/or new paresthesias.

      b. Assess for headache, possibly related to spinal fluid leak.

      c. Assess for wound drainage.

        (1) Note dependent drainage on dressing and bed.

        (2) Note formation and extent of hematoma.

        (3) Maintain occlusive compression dressing to operative site.

        (4) Maintain drainage device if present.

      d. Position patient for safety.

        (1) Patient commonly positioned supine in regular hard bed

        (2) Maintain patient in neutral body alignment.

        (3) Log roll patient side to side with physician order.

        (4) Assist patient's movement with draw sheet.

        (5) Discourage patient use of trapeze or pulling under patient's axilla (to avoid rod displacement).

      e. Monitor for complications after spinal fusion (see Complications Common to Orthopedics, section V).

        (1) Reduced gas exchange and ineffective breathing patterns

          (a) Encourage coughing and deep breathing hourly.

          (b) Assess equality and clarity of breath sounds.

          (c) Obtain chest x-ray film after anterior fusion to determine lung expansion.

          (d) Monitor arterial blood gases.

          (e) Turn patient side to side every hour.

        (2) Gastric distention and decreased peristalsis

          (a) Auscultate for bowel sounds hourly.

          (b) Insert nasogastric tube if necessary.

          (c) Administer stool softener as needed.

C. Arthroplasty (joint reconstruction)

    1. Procedure: reconstruction of articulating surfaces of joint

    2. Purpose

      a. Relief of chronic disabling pain

      b. Improvement in joint function and activities of daily living

      c. Correction of deformity

      d. Prevention of further bone destruction

      e. Stabilization of joint

    3. Joints replaced

      a. Most common arthroplasties

        (1) Hip

        (2) Knee

        (3) Shoulder

      b. Other joints replaced

        (1) Elbows

        (2) Fingers (proximal interphalangeal joint, metacarpophalangeal joint)

        (3) Wrist and thumb

        (4) Ankle

        (5) Temporomandibular joint

    4. Common diagnosis prearthroplasty

      a. Degenerative arthritis (OA or osteoarthrosis)

      b. Rheumatoid arthritis

       c. Avascular necrosis (osteonecrosis or ischemic necrosis)

       d. Posttraumatic arthritis

  5. Types of arthroplasties

       a. Hemiarthroplasty (one joint surface reconstructed with artificial part)

          (1) Cup arthroplasty: placement of metal cup over femoral head (uncommon in modern arthroplasties)

          (2) Endoprosthesis: replacement of femoral head with stemmed prosthesis stabilized in proximal medullary canal

             (a) Austin Moore prosthesis: prosthetic femoral head articulates with natural acetabulum.

             (b) Bipolar prosthesis: prosthetic femoral head articulates with plastic liner of large metal "shell" placed against acetabulum (greatest motion is within prosthetic device).

          (3) Hip resurfacing: type of hip replacement that replaces the two surfaces of hip joint, conserving bone (head of femur preserved)

       b. Total joint arthroplasty: both joint surfaces reconstructed with artificial parts

  6. Materials commonly used

       a. Metals

          (1) Cobalt chromium

          (2) Titanium or titanium alloys

       b. Ceramics

       c. Plastics (high–molecular weight polymers)

       d. Polymethylmethacrylate ("bone cement")

  7. Methods of component fixation in bone

       a. Cement

          (1) "Gold standard" of fixation

          (2) Cement injected under pressure

          (3) Cement hardens in minutes, emits heat in process.

          (4) Allows for immediate full weight bearing on extremity

       b. Biological ingrowth

          (1) Microtextured surface of prosthesis allows bone to "grow into" and stabilize component.

          (2) Bone ingrowth optimized with tight fit of prosthesis into healthy dense bone

          (3) Attempts at "tight fit" can cause intraoperative fracture.

          (4) Postoperative weight-bearing restrictions generally continue for average of 2 months.

       c. Press fit

          (1) Used for stemmed components only

          (2) Stem impacted snugly into canal of bone with cement; stem mechanically supported by cortical bone

  8. Potential complications common to arthroplasties

       a. DVT

          (1) Single most common complication with lower extremity joint arthroplasty

          (2) Prophylaxis generally given to all patients

       b. PE

       c. Fat embolism: rare, possible during insertion of stemmed devices or in situations of acute traumatic injury

       d. Compartment syndrome: rare, may occur as a result of compression of contralateral limb during surgery or with large wound hematoma

       e. Peripheral neurovascular impairment

       f. Infection—number one causative organism, *Staphylococcus aureus*

          (1) Superficial wound infection

             (a) Generally limited

             (b) May be related to stitch abscess

             (c) Treated with topical or oral antibiotics or both

          (2) Deep wound infection

      (a) Acute: attributed to perioperative event

      (b) Late: attributed to hematological spread of infection in body from remote site

         (i) Urinary tract infection

         (ii) Abscessed tooth

      (c) Acute deep infection requires open irrigation of joint and possible exchange of liner and long-term antibiotics.

      (d) Late deep infection often requires:

         (i) Removal of prosthesis

         (ii) Debridement of bone or tissue

         (iii) Long-term antibiotics

9. Postanesthesia care of patient with hip arthroplasty

  a. Assess neurovascular status.

    (1) Perform comprehensive neurovascular assessment at least every hour for first 4 hours.

    (2) Note signs of peroneal nerve palsy, possibly resulting from stretch injury caused by intraoperative hip dislocation, limb lengthening, or hematoma.

      (a) Weak or absent dorsiflexion of foot and ankle against examiner resistance

      (b) Decreased sensation or numbness

         (i) Lateral aspect of great toe

         (ii) Medial aspect of second toe

  b. Assess for signs of wound drainage: blood loss should not exceed 500 mL in first 8 hours.

    (1) Note dependent drainage on dressing and bed.

    (2) Note formation and extent of hematoma.

      (a) May suggest active hemorrhage

      (b) May require surgical evacuation

    (3) Maintain occlusive compression dressing on operative site, reinforcing if necessary.

    (4) Maintain drainage device if present.

      (a) Closed suction device such as a hemovac commonly used

      (b) Gravity device: uncommon

      (c) Autotransfusion device: used to collect and reinfuse blood according to established guidelines

  c. Position lower extremity to reduce risk of dislocation.

    (1) Maintain operative extremity in neutral alignment.

    (2) Avoid hip adduction.

      (a) Place pillow or abduction device between legs at all times.

      (b) Turn patient carefully to unaffected side, maintaining abduction, if allowed.

    (3) Avoid hip flexion greater than 90°.

      (a) Avoid raising head of bed and foot of bed at same time.

      (b) Encourage use of overhead trapeze for support during position changes.

    (4) Avoid extremes in hip rotation using trochanteric roll to side(s) of affected leg, considering surgical approach.

      (a) Avoid internal rotation if posterior approach.

      (b) Avoid external rotation if anterolateral approach.

  d. Provide aids to enhance patient compliance to position restrictions.

    (1) Long-handled reacher

    (2) Long shoe horn

    (3) Sock aid

    (4) Elevated toilet seat

    (5) Chair cushions

  e. Provide for pain control.

    (1) Instruct patient regarding use of parenteral patient-controlled analgesia.

    (2) Expect IV, epidural, or intrathecal opioids postoperatively.

    f. Prevent infection.
       (1) Use strict aseptic technique for all invasive procedures.
       (2) Insert Foley catheter if signs of bladder distention.
       (3) Instruct patient in aggressive pulmonary hygiene.
10. Postanesthesia care of patient with knee arthroplasty
    a. Assess neurovascular status.
       (1) Perform comprehensive neurovascular assessment at least every hour for first 4 hours.
       (2) Note signs of tibial nerve palsy, possibly caused by stretch injury from:
          (a) Intraoperative knee dislocation
          (b) Extensive swelling
          (c) Hematoma
    b. Assess for signs of wound drainage: blood loss should not exceed 500 mL in first 8 hours.
    c. Position extremity to reduce edema and prevent constricture.
       (1) Maintain operated extremity in neutral alignment.
       (2) Elevate extremity on pillow or towel roll.
       (3) Avoid placement of pillow beneath popliteal fossa.
       (4) Avoid prolonged side lying with knee flexed.
    d. Provide assistive devices to enhance patient's independence.
       (1) Long-handled reacher
       (2) Long shoe horn
       (3) Sock aid
       (4) Elevated toilet seat
       (5) Chair cushions
    e. Encourage aggressive range of motion of knee.
       (1) Activate CPM machine as ordered.
          (a) Supplied and adjusted by trained personnel
          (b) Degrees of flexion and extension ordered by physician
          (c) Gradually increase knee flexion and extension per order according to patient tolerance.
    f. Provide for pain control.
    g. Prevent infection.
11. Postanesthesia care of patient with shoulder arthroplasty
    a. Assess neurovascular status.
       (1) Perform comprehensive assessment at least every hour for first 4 hours.
       (2) Note deficit in medial, radial, or ulnar nerve.
    b. Assess for wound drainage: blood loss should not exceed 150 mL in first 24 hours.
       (1) Note dependent drainage on dressing and bed.
       (2) Note formation and extent of hematoma.
       (3) Maintain occlusive compression dressing to operative site.
       (4) Maintain drainage device if present.
          (a) Suction device: most common
          (b) Gravity device: uncommon
    c. Positioning to reduce risk of dislocation
       (1) Maintain postoperative extremity positioning.
          (a) Shoulder adduction and internal rotation using sling and swathe dressing with affected arm at side: most common
          (b) Shoulder abduction with abduction frame or airplane splint: less common
    d. Assist with measures to reduce edema.
       (1) Encourage range of motion of upper extremity joints distal to shoulder.
          (a) Range of motion of fingers and wrist commonly encouraged at least every hour
          (b) Range of motion of elbow often allowed: patient lightly stabilizes upper arm with unaffected hand during elbow range of motion.

    e. Provide overhead trapeze and assistive devices to enhance patient ability to perform activities of daily living.

    f. Encourage range of motion of shoulder as soon as possible.

      (1) Activate CPM machine as ordered.

        (a) Supplied and adjusted by trained personnel

        (b) Used in supine position or in chair-sitting position

        (c) Degrees and direction of movement ordered by physician

        (d) Increase shoulder motion per order and according to patient tolerance.

    g. Provide for pain control.

    h. Prevent infection.

D. Open reduction internal fixation (ORIF) of femoral fracture

  1. Procedure: operative reduction of fracture of femur and stabilization with hardware

  2. Purpose

    a. Attains and maintains reduction of fracture

    b. Enhances fracture healing through stability

    c. Allows for early mobilization of patient

  3. Types of femoral fractures

    a. Femoral neck fracture

      (1) Basilar: fracture at distal neck of femur

      (2) Subcapital: fracture directly under femoral head

    b. Intertrochanteric fracture: fracture on a line through greater and lesser trochanter

    c. Subtrochanteric fracture: transverse fracture between lesser trochanter and a site 1 inch or more below greater trochanter

    d. Femoral shaft fracture: fracture between greater trochanter and knee

  4. Commonly used fixation devices

    a. Wires and pins

    b. Bone screws

    c. Plates with screws

    d. Compression (sliding) hip screw

    e. Intramedullary rods and nails

  5. Postanesthesia care

    a. Assess neurovascular status: perform comprehensive neurovascular assessment.

    b. Maintain proper positioning.

      (1) Place extremities in neutral position.

      (2) Use trochanter roll (rolled sheet or blanket) or sandbag to prevent rotation of lower extremities.

      (3) Turn patient only if physician order.

        (a) Usually approved to turn to unaffected side only

        (b) Maintain anatomical positioning by using pillows between legs and back for support.

      (4) Prevent dislocation after ORIF for femoral neck fracture (less stable because capsule of hip interrupted).

        (a) Avoid hip flexion greater than 90°.

        (b) Avoid hip adduction by placing abduction devices between legs.

        (c) Avoid extremes in rotation with trochanter roll.

        (d) Provide overhead trapeze to aid patient movement.

    c. Prevent extremity edema.

      (1) Elevate extremity above level of heart using pillows.

      (2) Avoid direct pressure in popliteal fossa.

    d. Monitor wound drainage.

      (1) Maintain patency of drainage device if present.

      (2) Expect pattern of decreasing drainage after first 2 to 4 hours postoperatively.

      (3) Assess for dependent drainage underneath operative site and for drainage on dressing or cast.

      (4) Maintain occlusive compression dressing, reinforcing if needed.

    e. Monitor for complications after femoral fracture.

      (1) Infection

        (a) Most common with open fracture

        (b) Assess for systemic signs or symptoms of infection.

        (c) Assess for local signs of infection (visibly reddened incision line).

        (d) Identify high-risk patient.

          (i) Malnourished

          (ii) Infirm

          (iii) Incontinent

          (iv) Urinary tract infection present

          (v) Tooth abscess present

      (2) DVT—high risk in patients who are:

        (a) Elderly

        (b) Dehydrated

        (c) Immobile

        (d) History of DVT

      (3) PE: high risk as for DVT

      (4) Compartment syndrome—high risk in patients with:

        (a) Prolonged limb compression

        (b) Extensive soft tissue trauma

        (c) Vascular trauma

        (d) Sepsis

      (5) FES—high risk in patients with:

        (a) Fracture of midshaft femur

        (b) Fractures associated with sepsis or shock

E. Arthroscopy

  1. Procedure: examination of interior of joint with small fiberoptic tube in effort to visualize accurately or treat joint cavity

  2. Purpose

    a. Diagnosis of pathological condition

      (1) Direct visualization

        (a) Articular surfaces

        (b) Synovium

        (c) Supportive tissue

        (d) Foreign tissue

      (2) Biopsy of synovium

    b. Treatment of pathological condition

      (1) Repair or resection of torn menisci

      (2) Debridement of cartilage

      (3) Removal of foreign body

      (4) Arthroscopic-assisted ligament repair

      (5) Fixation of minor damage to cartilage

  3. Joints amenable to arthroscopy

    a. Knee: most common

    b. Hip

    c. Ankle

    d. Shoulder

    e. Elbow

    f. Temporomandibular joint

  4. Postanesthesia care

    a. Assess neurovascular status: perform comprehensive neurovascular assessment.

    b. Assess multiple portal sites.

      (1) Monitor dressing for drainage.

      (2) Maintain original dressing, reinforce with additional bulky dressing, and Ace wrap if needed.

    c. Prevent extremity edema.
      (1) Elevate extremity above level of heart with pillows.
      (2) Avoid direct pressure in popliteal fossa.
    d. Monitor for postarthroscopy complications.
      (1) Infection
        (a) Monitor portal sites for:
          (i) Redness
          (ii) Swelling
          (iii) Pain
          (iv) Erythema
          (v) Most common complication: superficial infection
        (b) Instruct patient in manifestation of signs and symptoms of systemic and deep infection: uncommon, occurring more than 24 hours postoperatively.
      (2) Major complications: rare but may include DVT, PE, and compartment syndrome
    e. Instruct patient regarding use of crutches.
    f. Provide for pain control.
      (1) Oral opioids commonly used postoperatively
      (2) Parenteral patient-controlled analgesia may be used for 24 hours when more extensive joint repair performed (e.g., ACL repair).
    g. Position joint and allow for movement per order.
      (1) Avoid direct pressure under joint and on bony prominences.
      (2) Encourage active range of motion to all unaffected joints.
      (3) Provide CPM machine per order.
      (4) Provide for joint support with hinged brace or other device per order.
F. ACL repair
  1. Most frequently injured or torn ligament in knee joint
    a. Research supports increased ACL injury in female athletes.
      (1) ACL contains hormone receptor sites for:
        (a) Estrogen
        (b) Progesterone
        (c) Relaxin
      (2) Injuries seen more during menses, when estrogen causes ligament to relax
  2. Procedure: reconstruction may be arthroscopically assisted or as open arthrotomy. Graft choices for reconstruction include:
    a. Autogenous
      (1) Patellar tendon—graft of choice, most reliable
      (2) Semitendinous tendon
      (3) Iliotibial band
      (4) Gracilis muscle
      (5) Fascia lata
    b. Allograft—tissue from cadaver
      (1) Less painful for patient
      (2) Possibility of graft rejection
    c. Ligament substitutes
      (1) Scaffolds—protect soft tissue; allow ingrowth
      (2) Synthetic ligaments—prone to mechanical failure, usually used as last resource
        (a) Gore-Tex (polytetrafluoroethylene/Teflon), braided
        (b) Polyester—woven, mesh
  3. Purpose
    a. Improve joint stability by strengthening anterior-posterior control of knee.
  4. Complications of ACL repair
    a. Compartment syndrome
    b. Neurovascular impairment from inadvertent suturing of peroneal nerve, resulting in possible footdrop, decreased sensation to foot

      c. Prolonged tourniquet time could cause sciatic or femoral nerve palsy.

      d. Rare—fracture to femur or sprain to ligaments from leg brace used intraoperatively

      e. Pain from use of tourniquet and leg brace intraoperatively

      f. Rare—hemarthrosis and thromboembolism

  5. Postanesthesia care of patient with ACL repair

      a. Assess neurovascular status.

      b. Assess wound drainage; check dressing and drain.

      c. Position leg to decrease edema, pain.

      d. Begin cryotherapy, CPM as directed.

          (1) Cold from cryotherapy decreases:

              (a) Inflammation

              (b) Pain

              (c) Swelling

              (d) Potential for postoperative bleeding with hematoma formation and muscle spasm

      e. Keep knee immobilizer on to stabilize joint.

      f. Aggressively manage pain.

          (1) Multimodal, preemptive pharmacological approach most effective

              (a) Intra-articular injection of local anesthetics, opioids, NSAIDs, clonidine, and/or corticosteroids before incision made

              (b) Opioid receptors (mu, delta, kappa) found in peripheral nerves and play role in preventing and/or diminishing postoperative pain

              (c) Joint medication injection

                   (i) Local anesthetics (bupivacaine) manage pain approximately 2 to 4 hours.

                   (ii) Opioids such as morphine, 2 to 5 mg, injected into the joint may last up to 8 to 12 hours without systemic side effects.

                   (iii) Using a combination approach provides early onset and longer duration of analgesia.

                   (iv) Intra-articular meperidine has been shown to cause systemic side effects, but does appear to have an earlier onset than morphine.

              (d) Corticosteroids (methylprednisolone) and NSAIDs (ketorolac) provide analgesia by diminishing the inflammatory response after arthroscopic knee surgery.

              (e) Clonidine increases duration time of intra-articular morphine and local anesthetics.

              (f) Effective pain management promotes quicker healing and increased compliance with rehabilitation programs.

              (g) Use of preemptive analgesia reduces opioid use postoperatively.

          (2) Femoral block, no weight bearing until worn off

              (a) Average length of analgesia: 29 hours

          (3) Postoperative NSAIDs and opioids as directed

              (a) Controlled-release oxycodone (OxyContin): twice-per-day dosing schedule

                   (i) Provides extended pain relief

                   (ii) Promotes increased patient compliance

          (4) Epidural analgesia—allows for:

              (a) Earlier ambulation

               (b) More comfort during rehabilitation

              (c) Improved pulmonary function

G. Amputation

  1. Procedure: surgical (or traumatic) removal of a body part

  2. Purpose

      a. Reduce risk of systemic sepsis

      b. Control pain of ischemia

      c. Maximize mobility

3. Types of amputation
   a. Traumatic: results in extreme destruction of soft tissue and bone in presence of infectious microorganisms
   b. Elective
      (1) Closed (flap): performed in absence of infection
      (2) Open (guillotine): performed in presence of infection, allowing drainage of infectious material
4. Indications for elective amputation
   a. Peripheral vascular disease: most frequent indication for lower extremity amputation, often associated with diabetes mellitus
   b. Severe trauma: most frequent indication for upper extremity amputation
   c. Other indications (in order of frequency)
      (1) Acute or chronic infection: osteomyelitis or gangrene
      (2) Trophic ulcers
      (3) Severe crushing injuries
      (4) Malignancies
      (5) Frostbite
      (6) Congenital deformities
5. Postanesthesia care of patient after amputation
   a. Assess neurovascular status: perform comprehensive neurovascular assessment.
   b. Assess for signs of wound drainage.
      (1) Note dependent drainage on dressing and bed.
      (2) Note unusual odors or color of drainage (important in presence of infection).
   c. Maintain stump dressing.
      (1) Plaster cast: rigid dressing
         (a) Prevents swelling of stump
         (b) Protects stump from trauma
         (c) Used when patient will be fitted for immediate prosthesis (usually Pylon type)
      (2) Soft dressing: gauze with elastic wrap
         (a) Prevents swelling of stump
         (b) Used when use of prosthesis unlikely
   d. Position extremity to minimize complications.
      (1) Elevate stump to facilitate venous return first 24 to 48 hours.
      (2) After 48 hours, position to prevent hip flexion contractures.
         (a) Avoid stump elevation.
         (b) Instruct patient to lie intermittently prone (encourages hip extension).
   e. Provide for pain control.
      (1) Administer parenteral opioids as ordered for postoperative surgical pain.
      (2) Assess for phantom limb pain.
         (a) Pain sensation in area of absent, amputated limb
         (b) Common in first 24 to 48 hours postoperatively in traumatic amputation
         (c) Treated with opioids and phenytoin
         (d) Adequate treatment important to reduce risk of chronic phantom pain syndrome
   f. Instruct patient regarding phantom limb sensation: sensation that amputated limb present.
      (1) Inform patient that phenomenon is common in early postoperative period.
      (2) Instruct patient that sensation is normal phenomenon.
      (3) Treat with nonpharmacological methods.
   g. Provide emotional support.

H. Replantation of amputated digits or limbs
   1. Procedure: reattachment of totally or partially amputated part involving restoration of structures
      a. Vascular
      b. Nervous
      c. Bony
      d. Soft tissue
   2. Possible sites for replantation
      a. Upper extremity
         (1) Digits
            (a) Most common traumatic amputation
            (b) Replantation attempted in:
               (i) Proximal digit amputations
               (ii) Amputation of multiple digits
               (iii) Amputation of index finger or thumb
            (c) Viability after replantation: 80% to 90%
            (d) Functional return after replantation: 65%
         (2) Arms: less successful result
      b. Lower extremity
         (1) Digits: great toe
         (2) Leg
            (a) Amputation through tibia or fibula shows unfavorable results with high infection rate.
            (b) Leg length discrepancies common
   3. Factors influencing prognosis
      a. Positive factors
         (1) Clean-cut (guillotine) amputation
         (2) Young patient
         (3) Hemodynamically stable patient
         (4) Absence of systemic disease
         (5) No history of smoking, alcohol, or drug abuse
         (6) Absence of gross contamination of wound
         (7) Amputated part wrapped in gauze and placed in cool environment
         (8) Replantation attempted within 24 hours
      b. Negative factors
         (1) Crushing injury
         (2) Extremes of age
         (3) History of peripheral vascular disease, hypertension, or other chronic illness
         (4) History of smoking, alcohol, or drug abuse
         (5) Grossly contaminated wound
         (6) Delay in retrieval and care of amputated part
         (7) Delay in replantation
   4. Postanesthesia care of patient postreplantation
      a. Assess neurovascular status at least every 15 minutes.
         (1) Perform comprehensive bedside assessment.
         (2) Perform technical monitoring as ordered.
            (a) Doppler ultrasonography
            (b) Temperature probes
            (c) Muscle contraction monitoring (evoked M wave)
            (d) Fluorometry readings (determines venous return)
         (3) Promptly notify physician if negative change occurs.
      b. Promote circulation and prevent vasoconstriction.
         (1) Elevate extremity above heart level.
         (2) Administer thrombolytic agents to decrease clotting in peripheral vessels.
         (3) Maintain room temperature at 78° F to 90° F (26° C to 30° C).
         (4) Prevent patient exposure to nicotine and caffeine.
         (5) Maintain patient hydration.

    c. Prevent infection.
      (1) Administer antibiotics as ordered.
      (2) Assess for signs and symptoms of infection.
      (3) Provide for nutritional needs necessary for wound healing (high-protein diet).
    d. Provide for pain control.
      (1) Provide oral opioids as needed.
      (2) Assess pain, while noting that changes in pain pattern may be suggestive of ischemia.
    e. Provide emotional support.
    f. Complications
      (1) Venous congestion
        (a) Massage digit.
        (b) Leech therapy
        (c) Revision of replantation
      (2) Thrombosis
        (a) Anticoagulants
        (b) Revise surgically.
      (3) Sepsis
      (4) Renal failure
      (5) Contractures
      (6) Diminished or lost proprioception
I. Nursing interventions
  1. Upper extremity procedures
    a. Position the hand above heart.
    b. Provide a sling if ordered.
    c. Assess and protect cast and splint.
      (1) Cast should be kept dry.
      (2) Observe for cast defects that could lead to tissue compression damage.
    d. Apply ice packs as ordered.
    e. Check neurovascular status.
      (1) Nerve function
        (a) Radial
          (i)   Check sensation at thumb–index finger web.
          (ii) Have patient hyperextend thumb or wrist.
        (b) Median
          (i)   Check sensation on distal surface of index finger.
          (ii) Have patient oppose thumb and finger.
        (c) Ulnar
          (i)   Check sensation at distal end of small finger.
          (ii) Have patient abduct all fingers.
      (2) Vascular status—assess capillary refill.
        (a) Normal capillary refill: 3 seconds or less
        (b) Perform blanch test.
          (i)   Compress and release nail bed quickly.
        (c) Compare capillary refill with unaffected extremity.
        (d) Rapid filling may indicate venous congestion.
        (e) Sluggish filling is a sign of arterial insufficiency.
        (f) Note color, comparing with unaffected extremity.
          (i)   Blanching or pallor indicates arterial insufficiency.
        (g) Cyanosis indicates insufficient venous return.
      (3) Mobility
        (a) Within limitations of casts, splints, and so forth, have patient wiggle fingers.
          (i)   Should be easy
          (ii) Should not be painful
  2. Lower extremities
    a. Position extremity above heart.

   b. Assess and protect cast and splint.
     (1) Cast should be kept dry.
     (2) Observe for cast defects that could lead to tissue compression damage.
   c. Apply ice packs or cooling device as ordered.
   d. Check neurovascular status frequently.
     (1) Nerve function—peroneal
       (a) Check sensation at lateral surface of great toe and medial surface of second toe.
       (b) Have patient dorsiflex ankle and extend toes.
       (c) Peroneal nerve damage results in foot drop.
     (2) Nerve function—tibial
       (a) Check sensation at medial and lateral surfaces of sole of foot.
       (b) Have patient plantar flex ankle and flex toes.
       (c) Signs and symptoms of nerve damage
         (i) Pain that is:
           [a] Increasing
           [b] Persistent
           [c] Localized
         (ii) Paresthesia
         (iii) Hyperesthesia
         (iv) Numbness
         (v) Motor weakness
         (vi) Paralysis
     (3) Vascular status
       (a) Perform blanch test.
         (i) Compress and release nail bed quickly.
         (ii) Compare capillary refill with unaffected extremity.
         (iii) Rapid filling may indicate venous congestion.
         (iv) Sluggish filling is a sign of arterial insufficiency.
       (b) Note color, comparing with unaffected extremity.
         (i) Blanching or pallor indicates arterial insufficiency.
         (ii) Cyanosis indicates insufficient venous return.
       (c) Signs and symptoms of nerve damage
         (i) Loss of pulse
         (ii) Sluggish or absent capillary refill
         (iii) Pallor
         (iv) Cyanosis
         (v) Blanching
         (vi) Temperature decrease
         (vii) Paresthesia
         (viii) Hyperesthesia
     (4) Mobility
       (a) Within limitations of casts, splints, and so forth, have patient wiggle toes.
         (i) Should be easy
         (ii) Should not be painful
       (b) Severe pain on dorsiflexion of toes can indicate compartment syndrome.

BIBLIOGRAPHY

1. Baird C: First line treatment for osteoarthritis, part 1: Pathophysiology, assessment, and pharmacologic interventions. *Orthop Nurs* 20(5):17–24, 2001.
2. Bert JM: Unicompartmental knee replacement. *Orthop Clin North Am* 36(4):513–522, 2005.
3. Crovetti M, Tarno J: *Birmingham Hip Resurfacing System.* Available at: www.hipsurfacing.com. Accessed January 12, 2009.
4. Burden N: Care of the orthopedic patient in the ambulatory surgery setting. *J Perianesth Nurs* 22(3):207–210, 2007.

5. Cascio B, Wilckens J, Ain M, et al: Documentation of acute compartment syndrome at an academic health care center. *J Bone Joint Surg* 87(2):346–350, 2005.

6. Center Orthopedic & Neurosurgical Care & Research. Available at: www.neuro-ortho. com. Accessed January 12, 2009.

7. Cluett J: *ACL reconstruction-graft choices for ACL surgery.* Available at: About.com. Accessed 2006.

8. Drain CB, Odom-Forren J: Care of the orthopedic surgical patient. In Drain CB, Odom-Forren J, eds: *Perianesthesia nursing: A critical care approach,* ed 5, Philadelphia, 2009, Saunders.

9. Hodgson BB, Kizior RJ: *Saunders 2010 nursing drug handbook,* Philadelphia, 2010, Saunders.

10. Iacono MV: Osteoporosis: A national public health priority. *J Perianesth Nurs* 22(3): 175–183, 2007.

11. Mamaril EM, Childs SG, Sortman S: Care of the orthopaedic trauma patient. *J Perianesth Nurs* 22(3):184–194, 2007.

12. Nagelhout JJ, Plaus KL: *Handbook of nurse anesthesia,* ed 4, Philadelphia, 2010, Saunders.

13. Pasero C, McCaffery M: Orthopaedic postoperative pain management. *J Perianesth Nurs* 22(3):160–174, 2007.

14. Rothrock JC: *Alexander's care of the patient in surgery,* ed 13, St Louis, 2007, Mosby.

15. Worth MA, Tapscott RS, Southworth C, et al: Treatment of glenohumeral arthritis with hemiarthroplasty surgical technique. *J Bone Joint Surg* 89(2 Suppl 1):10–25, 2007.

16. Yeung AT, Yeung CA: Minimally invasive techniques for the management of lumbar disc herniation. *Orthop Clin North Am* 38(3):363–372, 2007.

DONNA R. McEWEN

OBJECTIVES

At the conclusion of this chapter, the reader will be able to:

1. Identify the pathophysiological ear, nose, throat, and head and neck conditions requiring surgical interventions.
2. Describe surgical procedures with the preanesthesia, perianesthesia, and postanesthesia problems encountered in the ear, nose, throat, and head and neck patient and the nursing interventions required in the management of these problems.
3. Identify possible complications that can arise after ear, nose, throat, and head and neck procedures.

I. ANATOMY AND PHYSIOLOGY
   A. Ear
     1. Structure and function
       a. Anatomy of ear (organ of hearing and equilibrium; Figure 43-1)
         (1) Outer ear
           (a) Visible portion consists of skin-covered flap of cartilage known as auricle or pinna.
             (i) Collects sound waves
             (ii) Directs sound waves to external acoustic meatus
           (b) Auditory canal—external acoustic meatus
             (i) Extends to tympanic membrane (eardrum)
           (c) Tympanic membrane
             (i) Thin, transparent, pearly gray, cone-shaped membrane
             (ii) Stretches across the ear canal
             (iii) Separates the middle ear (tympanic cavity) from the outer ear
           (d) Nerve supply
             (i) Auriculotemporal branch of the trigeminal nerve
               [a] General sensory
               [b] Innervates tympanic membrane, external acoustic meatus, anterior auricle
         (2) Middle ear
           (a) Structure
             (i) Ossicles
               [a] Malleus (hammer)
                  [1] Largest of the three ossicles
               [b] Incus (anvil)
                  [1] Middle ossicle
               [c] Stapes (stirrup)
                  [1] Innermost ossicle
             (ii) Eustachian tube
               [a] Channel connecting the tympanic cavity and the nasal part of the pharynx through which air reaches the middle ear

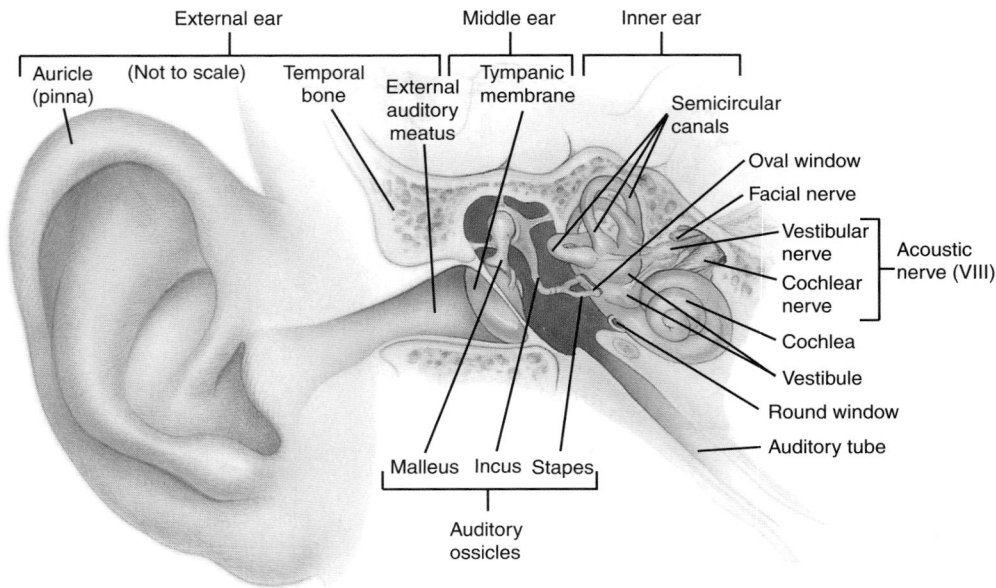

FIGURE 43-1 ■ The ear. (From Thibodeau GA, Patton KT: *Anatomy and physiology*, ed 7, St Louis, 2010, Mosby.)

(b) Function
- (i) Ossicles form a chain from tympanic membrane to the oval window.
- (ii) Transmits vibrations to inner ear, conducting sound to the inner ear

(3) Inner ear
- (a) Cochlea—spiral-shaped, forms the anterior part of the labyrinth of the inner ear; contains three compartments
  - (i) Scala vestibuli
    - [a] Part of the cochlea above the spiral lamina, which divides the canal
  - (ii) Scala tympani
    - [a] Part of the cochlea below the spiral lamina
  - (iii) Cochlear duct (scala media)
    - [a] Canal between the scala tympani and scala vestibuli
- (b) Organ of Corti
  - (i) Organ lying against the basilar membrane in the cochlear duct
  - (ii) Contains special sensory receptors for hearing
  - (iii) Consists of neuroepithelial hair cells that respond to vibration from the ossicles, converting mechanical energy to electrochemical impulses
- (c) Vestibular labyrinth—controls equilibrium
  - (i) Utricle
    - [a] Larger of the two divisions of the membranous labyrinth of the inner ear
  - (ii) Saccule
    - [a] Smaller of the two divisions of the membranous labyrinth of the vestibule
    - [b] Communicates with the cochlear duct by way of the ductus reuniens
  - (iii) Semicircular canals
    - [a] Description: three canals—anterior, lateral, and posterior
    - [b] Passages in the inner ear
    - [c] Located in the bony labyrinth
    - [d] Functions: control sense of balance

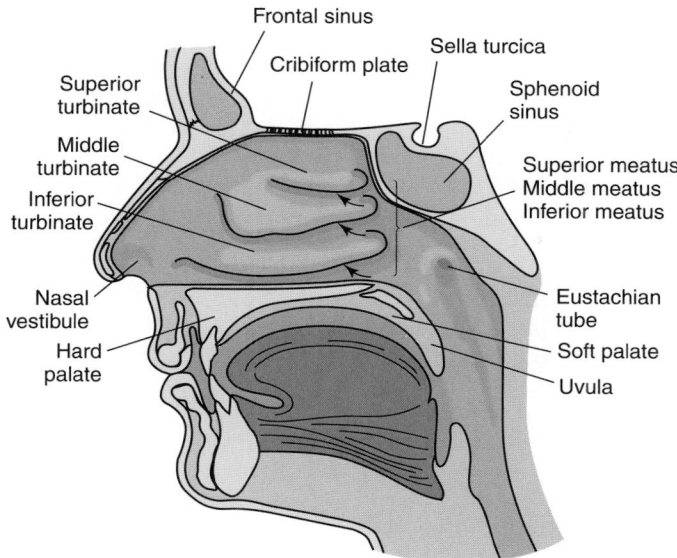

FIGURE 43-2 ■ Lateral wall of nose, showing superior, middle, and inferior turbinates. (From Monahan FD, Sands JK, Neighbors M, et al: *Phipps medical-surgical nursing*, ed 8, St Louis, 2007, Mosby.)

    [e] Respond to movement of head
    [f] Can cause feeling of dizziness or vertigo after spinning
    [g] Motion sickness results from unusual movements of the head that result in stimulation of the semicircular canals.
B. Nose
  1. Structure and function
    a. Anatomy of nose (organ of respiration and olfaction; Figure 43-2)
      (1) External
        (a) Upper—formed by nasal bones and maxilla
        (b) Lower—formed by connective tissue
        (c) Nares—separated by columella, formed from nasal cartilage
        (d) Nasal septum
          (i) Nasal cartilage
          (ii) Vomer bone
          (iii) Perpendicular plate of ethmoid bone
      (2) Internal—nasal cavity
        (a) Nares (nostrils)
          (i) External opening of the nasal cavity
        (b) Choanae
          (i) Paired openings between nasal cavity and oropharynx
        (c) Nasopharynx
          (i) Part of the pharynx above the soft palate
        (d) Eustachian tube
          (i) Narrow channel that connects tympanum with nasopharynx
        (e) Paranasal sinuses
          (i) Arranged in four pairs
            [a] Maxillary
            [b] Frontal
            [c] Sphenoid
            [d] Ethmoid
        (f) Nasal duct
          (i) Extends from the lower part of the lacrimal sac to the inferior meatus of the nose

(ii) Channel through which tear fluid is conveyed into the cavity of the nose
- (g) Turbinate bones
  - (i) Extend horizontally along the lateral wall of the nasal cavity
  - (ii) Separate the middle meatus of the nasal cavity from the inferior meatus
- (h) Nasal septum
  - (i) Separates the nasal cavity into two fossae
- (i) Nerve supply
  - (i) Trigeminal nerve
    - [a] Cranial nerve V
    - [b] General sensory, motor
    - [c] Face, teeth, mouth, nasal cavity
  - (ii) Cranial nerve I (olfactory)
    - [a] Special sensory
    - [b] Nerve of smell
- (j) Other nerves to consider
  - (i) Cranial nerve II (optic)
    - [a] Special sensory
    - [b] Nerve of sight
    - [c] Can be damaged in endoscopic sinus surgery
- (k) Arterial blood supply
  - (i) Internal maxillary
  - (ii) Anterior ethmoid
  - (iii) Sphenopalatine
  - (iv) Nasopalatine
  - (v) Pharyngeal
  - (vi) Posterior ethmoid

C. Throat
  1. Structure and function
  - **a.** Anatomy of oral cavity
    - (1) Mouth
      - (a) Lips
      - (b) Buccal cavity
      - (c) Lingual cavity
        - (i) Tongue
        - (ii) Hard palate
        - (iii) Soft palate
    - (2) Pharynx (Figure 43-3)
      - (a) Throat
        - (i) Nasopharynx
          - [a] Lies posterior to the nose and above the level of the soft palate
          - [b] Provides passageway for air
          - [c] Contains opening of the eustachian tubes
        - (ii) Oropharynx
          - [a] Extends from soft palate to the hyoid bone
          - [b] Provides passageway for both air and food
        - (iii) Laryngopharynx
          - [a] Extends from the hyoid bone to the lower border of the cricoid cartilage
          - [b] Continues with the esophagus
          - [c] Anterior entrance of the larynx is the epiglottis.
    - (3) Tonsils
      - (a) Types
        - (i) Palatine tonsils
          - [a] Pair of oval-shaped structures
          - [b] Size of almonds

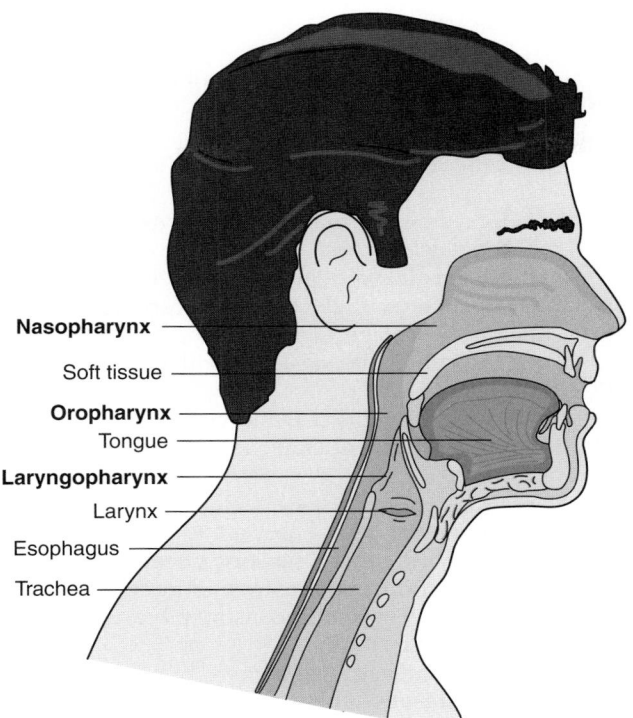

FIGURE 43-3 ■ Sagittal section of head showing pharynx and larynx. (From Monahan FD, Sands JK, Neighbors M, et al: *Phipps medical-surgical nursing,* ed 8, St Louis, 2007, Mosby.)

          [c] Partially imbedded in mucous membrane
          [d] One on each side of the throat
      (ii)   Lingual tonsils
          [a] Below palatine tonsils
          [b] At base of tongue
      (iii) Pharyngeal tonsils (adenoids)
          [a] Located in upper rear wall of oral cavity
          [b] Fair size in childhood, shrink after puberty
  (b) Functions
      (i)   Part of the lymphatic system
      (ii)   Assist in filtering the circulating lymph of bacteria and other foreign material that may enter body through mouth or nose
  (c) Nerve supply
      (i)   Middle and posterior branches of the maxillary and glossopharyngeal nerves
      (ii)   Cranial nerve X (vagus)
          [a] Parasympathetic, visceral, afferent, motor, general sensory
          [b] Supplies sensory fibers to ear, tongue, pharynx, and larynx
          [c] Supplies motor fibers to pharynx, larynx, and esophagus
  (d) Blood supply
      (i)   External carotid branch (ascending palatine branch of facial artery)
(4) Larynx
  (a) Thyroid cartilage
      (i)   Shield-shaped cartilage
      (ii)   Produces prominence on neck ("Adam's apple")
  (b) Hyoid bone
      (i)   Horse-shaped bone
      (ii)   Situated at the base of the tongue, just below the thyroid cartilage

          (c) Cricoid cartilage
             (i) Ringlike cartilage
             (ii) Forms lower and back part of larynx
          (d) Epiglottis
             (i) Lidlike cartilage structure
             (ii) Hangs over the entrance to the larynx
          (e) Arytenoid cartilages
             (i) Jug-shaped cartilage of the larynx
          (f) Corniculate cartilages
             (i) Two small conical nodules of yellow elastic cartilage
             (ii) Articulate with the arytenoid cartilages
          (g) Cuneiform cartilage
             (i) Elongated yellow elastic cartilage in the aryepiglottic fold
          (h) Glottis
             (i) Vocal apparatus of the larynx
             (ii) Consists of true vocal cords (vocal folds) and opening between them
          (i) Nerve supply
             (i) Superior laryngeal nerve
                [a] Motor, general sensory, visceral afferent, parasympathetic
                [b] Cricothyroid muscle and inferior constrictor muscles of the pharynx, mucous membrane of back of tongue and larynx
             (ii) Recurrent laryngeal nerve
                [a] Parasympathetic, visceral afferent, motor
                [b] Tracheal mucosa, esophagus, cardiac plexus
       (5) Thyroid gland
          (a) Located in anterior portion of the neck
          (b) Consists of right and left lobes united by isthmus
          (c) Vascular supply: superior and inferior thyroid arteries
          (d) Nerves in proximity
             (i) Recurrent laryngeal nerve
             (ii) Superior laryngeal nerve

II. GENERAL NURSING CONCERNS
   A. Preoperative concerns (see Chapter 15)
      1. Medical history assessment
      2. Nursing assessment
         a. Chief complaint
         b. Medications
            (1) Allergies
            (2) Current medications patient is taking, including over-the-counter and herbal medications
            (3) Use of aspirin, nonsteroidal anti-inflammatory medications, or medications containing aspirin (increased risk of bleeding)
            (4) Hormone therapy
            (5) Preoperative medications
         c. Patient's understanding of surgical procedure and expected outcomes
         d. Patient's psychosocial status
         e. Preexisting sensory deficits
      3. Usual laboratory and radiological evaluations
         a. Complete blood cell count
         b. Electrolytes based on patient history
         c. Urinalysis
         d. Coagulation studies
         e. Availability of designated blood products, type and crossmatch
         f. Electrocardiogram
         g. Chest radiograph
         h. Radiograph of sinuses, neck, mastoid

        i. Computed tomography
        j. Magnetic resonance imaging
        k. Pregnancy test for menstruating females
    4. Preoperative instructions
        a. Surgical procedure
        b. Operative site verification
        c. Expected outcomes
        d. Environment
        e. Alterations in lifestyle
        f. Self-care
        g. Suctioning
        h. Deep breathing
        i. Pain management
B. Intraoperative concerns
    1. Nursing assessment
        a. Assess respiratory status.
        b. Determine patient's comfort.
        c. Identify positioning needs.
        d. Establish priorities.
        e. Reinforce preoperative teaching.
            (1) Orient to perioperative environment.
            (2) Instruct patient in postoperative dressings.
        f. Determine patient's anxiety or apprehension.
        g. Operative site verification
    2. Aseptic technique
    3. Skin and tissue integrity
    4. Correct counts
    5. Medications given
    6. Intake and output
    7. Blood loss
    8. Patient's condition at time of transfer to post anesthesia care unit (PACU)
C. Postanesthesia concerns: phase I
    1. Nursing assessment
        a. Respiratory status
        b. Cardiovascular status
        c. Neurological status
        d. Psychosocial status
    2. Report from anesthesiologist or certified registered nurse anesthetist and/or operating room nurse
        a. Procedure, extent of surgery; complications
        b. Anesthetic agents and medications administered
        c. Blood loss and fluid replacement
        d. Placement of drains, packing
        e. Pertinent history, allergies
    3. Pain status
    4. Intake and output
    5. Patient's position
    6. Presence or absence of nausea
    7. Patient's ability to communicate
    8. Integrity of dressings and incision
    9. Patient's temperature
   10. Drainage from surgical site
D. Postanesthesia concerns: discharge from phase I
    1. Patient
        a. Conscious and able to maintain airway
        b. Able to maintain oxygen saturation greater than 92% after 15 minutes breathing room air without being stimulated

      c. Remains in this condition for 30 to 45 minutes after:

        (1) Extubation

        (2) Administration of narcotic or narcotic antagonist

    2. No active bleeding from operative site or drains

  E. Postanesthesia concerns: phase II

    1. Prepare for discharge (criteria and policies vary among facilities).

      a. Ensure adequate pain control.

      b. Validate ability to retain fluids and maintain hydration status.

      c. Validate patient's ability to urinate or return to previous level of urinary status.

      d. Assist patient with changing from hospital gown to personal clothing if necessary.

      e. Provide discharge instructions to patient and caregiver.

      f. Ensure that the patient is accompanied by responsible adult at discharge.

  F. Pediatric otolaryngology patients

    1. Special considerations

      a. Preoperative concerns (see Chapter 11)

        (1) Fear of separation, pain, injury, death: establish trust, reassure patient.

        (2) Child's feelings of "loss of control": allow child to choose flavoring for anesthetic induction mask.

        (3) Anxiety and fear of child and parents: prepare child and parents.

      b. Intraoperative concerns

        (1) Airway management: increased risk of laryngospasm and vomiting if anesthesia is induced while crying

        (2) Maintenance of body temperature (pediatric patient loses temperature faster than adult): keep patient covered with warm blankets, insulated drapes, convection or forced air warming blanket to prevent loss of body heat.

      c. Postoperative concerns

        (1) Maintenance of body temperature: use of warm blankets, insulated drapes, keep patient covered to prevent further heat loss and restore body temperature.

        (2) Increased risk for bleeding related to postoperative crying: administer pain medication as needed, provide reassurance to child and parents, allow family visitation postoperatively.

        (3) Fluid balance (pediatric patient dehydrates easier than adult): encourage fluid intake postoperatively, monitor intravenous (IV) fluids and output.

III. SURGICAL PROCEDURES

  A. Ear

    1. Myringotomy with or without tympanostomy tubes

      a. Purpose

        (1) Relieves pressure and allows for drainage of purulent or serous secretions from middle ear

        (2) Aerates middle ear

        (3) Relieves eustachian tube obstruction (thick, mucoid fluid)

        (4) May be short-term or long-term

      b. Description

        (1) Small incision made into posteroinferior aspect of tympanic membrane

        (2) Polyethylene tube can be inserted into eardrum.

      c. Indications

        (1) Acute otitis media unresponsive to antibiotics

        (2) Bulging tympanic membrane

        (3) Multiple episodes of acute otitis media along with chronic otitis media

      d. Preoperative concerns

        (1) Frequently performed on children

          (a) Preoperative medication provided in oral form

          (b) Usually performed under mask anesthesia; no IV access established

      e. Intraoperative concerns

(1) General anesthetic essential for children to ensure accurate incision of tympanic membrane and placement of tube

(2) Parents may be present in OR for induction of pediatric patients, depending on institutional policy and practice.

f. Postanesthesia priorities

(1) Phase I

(a) Standard phase I activities as previously described

(i) Nurse-to-patient ratio—1:1 until consciousness and reflexes return for pediatric patients

(ii) Children may struggle against face tent; provide humidified oxygen by placing tubing near mouth and nose.

(b) Depending on setting and institutional policy, patient may bypass phase I.

(2) Phase II

(a) Standard phase II activities as previously described

(b) Reunite parents with child as soon as possible to alleviate separation anxiety.

(c) Discharge instructions

(i) Avoid getting ears wet.

(ii) Change cotton balls as directed by physician.

(iii) Discuss pain management techniques.

(iv) Advise parents that tubes may fall out naturally.

g. Psychosocial concerns

(1) Children may experience separation anxiety.

(a) Allow for parent presence at induction if allowed by institutional policy.

(2) Allow child to assert control over situation when appropriate.

(a) Remain in pajamas or street clothes.

(b) Select flavor and scent of mask used for induction.

h. Complications

(1) Hearing loss

(2) Persistent otorrhea

(3) Chronic perforation

(4) Bleeding

(5) Premature tube extrusion

2. Tympanoplasty

a. Purpose

(1) Improve hearing.

(2) Prevent recurrent infection.

b. Description

(1) Refers to a variety of reconstructive surgical procedures performed on deformed or diseased middle ear components

(2) Some tympanoplasties carried out in two stages

(a) First procedure removes diseased tissue; second procedure involves reconstruction of hearing and middle ear function.

(3) Involves tissue grafts of cartilage, bone, fascia, skin, silicone, Teflon, or hydroxyapatite

(4) Types of tympanoplasty

(a) Type I (myringoplasty): repair of tympanic membrane

(b) Type II: graft rests on incus.

(c) Type III: graft attaches to head of stapes.

(d) Type IV: graft attaches to footplate of stapes.

c. Indications

(1) Defects in tympanic membrane

(2) Necrotic destruction of ossicles

(3) Cholesteatoma (epidermal pocket or cystlike sac filled with keratin debris)

(4) Chronic drainage from ear canal

(5) Conductive hearing loss

(6) Trauma

    d. Preoperative concerns

        (1) Hearing deficits may be present; adjust communication methods as appropriate.

        (2) Shampoo hair morning of surgery or night before surgery.

        (3) Advise patient that postoperative hearing may be diminished initially because of packing and dressing.

    e. Intraoperative concerns

        (1) Allow patient to wear hearing aids (if present) to the operating room (OR) to enhance communication.

        (2) Involves use of microscope for work on minute, delicate structures

        (3) Postauricular (behind ear) and/or endaural (through ear canal) approach used to expose structures of middle ear

        (4) Facial nerve monitoring may be used.

        (5) Positioning involves tilting OR bed at an angle to provide optimum exposure to operative ear; may cause pressure injury to dependent structures.

    f. Postanesthesia concerns

        (1) Phase I

            (a) Standard phase I activities as previously described

            (b) Elevate head of bed at least 30° to minimize eustachian tube edema; clarify positioning with surgeon for specific instructions.

            (c) Position with operative ear upward to prevent pressure and graft displacement.

            (d) Assess facial nerve function. Report any impairment to the surgeon. Assess facial symmetry by asking patient to:

                (i) Smile enough to show teeth.

                (ii) Wrinkle forehead.

                (iii) Pucker lips.

                (iv) Wrinkle nose.

                (v) Squeeze eyelids shut.

                (vi) Stick out tongue.

            (e) Prepare to treat nausea, vomiting, vertigo.

            (f) Avoid excess motion; transfer patient slowly and smoothly to minimize vertigo.

        (2) Phase II

            (a) Standard phase II activities as previously described if patient discharged to home

            (b) Discharge instructions

                (i) Avoid getting ears wet.

                (ii) Avoid sudden turning; encourage slow, smooth motion.

                (iii) Sneeze with mouth open to avoid pressure on eustachian tubes.

                (iv) Gentle nose blowing only

                (v) Noises such as popping and/or cracking may be heard in the ear by the patient and are considered normal.

    g. Psychosocial concerns

        (1) Anxiety related to hearing loss

    h. Complications

        (1) Facial nerve injury

        (2) Hearing loss caused by drill trauma to ossicles

3. Stapedectomy

    a. Purpose

        (1) Restoration of stapes bone function

    b. Description

        (1) Removal of diseased stapes and replacement with prosthetic graft

    c. Indications

        (1) Treatment of otosclerosis, a condition of unknown etiology characterized by the formation of spongy bone around the round window, which causes stiffening and hardness of the stapes

   d. Preoperative concerns
      (1) Hearing deficits may be present; adjust communication methods as
          appropriate.
      (2) Advise patient that postoperative hearing may be diminished initially
          because of packing and dressing.
   e. Intraoperative concerns
      (1) May be performed under local anesthesia with moderate sedation in
          adult patients
      (2) Involves use of microscope
      (3) May involve the use of the laser
      (4) Profound intraoperative vertigo may be noted in patients under local
          anesthesia.
      (5) Prosthesis fabricated from Teflon, stainless steel, or other synthetic
          material
   f. Postanesthesia priorities
      (1) Phase I
          (a) Standard phase I activities as previously described
          (b) Elevate head of bed at least 30° to minimize eustachian tube edema;
              clarify positioning with surgeon for specific instructions.
          (c) Position with operative ear upward to prevent pressure and graft
              displacement.
          (d) Nausea, vomiting, and vertigo should be anticipated.
      (2) Phase II
          (a) Standard phase II activities as previously described
          (b) Discharge instructions
              (i)   Avoid getting ears wet.
              (ii) Avoid sudden turning; encourage slow, smooth motion.
              (iii) Sneeze with mouth open to avoid pressure on eustachian
                    tubes.
              (iv) Gentle nose blowing only
   g. Psychosocial concerns
      (1) Patient may report immediate improvement in hearing, but hearing
          may decrease postoperatively because of accumulation of drainage.
   h. Complications
      (1) If chorda tympani is removed to expose stapes and footplate, loss of
          taste to anterior two thirds of tongue will occur on the affected side.
      (2) Facial nerve dehiscence
      (3) Ossicular chain dislocation
      (4) Perilymph leak
      (5) Dizziness
4. Mastoidectomy
   a. Purpose
      (1) To eradicate infected or diseased mastoid air cells
   b. Description
      (1) Simple mastoidectomy
          (a) Removal of mastoid air cells only
      (2) Modified radical mastoidectomy
          (a) Removal of mastoid cells, posterior and superior external bony
              canal walls
          (b) Conversion of mastoid and epitympanic space into one common
              cavity
      (3) Radical mastoidectomy
          (a) Removal of mastoid cells, posterior wall of external auditory canal,
              remnants of tympanic membrane, ossicles (except stapes), and
              middle ear mucosa
          (b) Removal of infected or diseased mucosa from middle ear orifice of
              the eustachian tube
          (c) Conversion of middle ear and mastoid space into one cavity

    c. Indications
        (1) Acute or chronic infection
        (2) Extension of cholesteatoma into mastoid cells
    d. Preoperative concerns
        (1) Hearing deficits may be present; adjust communication methods as appropriate.
        (2) Advise patient that postoperative hearing may be diminished initially because of packing and dressing.
    e. Intraoperative concerns
        (1) Involves use of microscope
        (2) Positioning involves tilting OR bed at an angle to provide optimum exposure to operative ear; may cause pressure injury to dependent structures.
    f. Postanesthesia concerns
        (1) Phase I
            (a) Standard phase I activities as previously described
            (b) Elevate head of bed at least 30°; clarify positioning with surgeon for specific instructions.
            (c) Position with operative ear upward to prevent pressure.
            (d) Assess facial nerve function. Report any impairment to the surgeon. Assess facial symmetry by asking patient to:
                (i)   Smile enough to show teeth.
                (ii) Wrinkle forehead.
                (iii) Pucker lips.
                (iv) Wrinkle nose.
                (v)   Squeeze eyelids shut.
                (vi) Stick out tongue.
            (e) Prepare to treat nausea, vomiting, vertigo.
            (f) Avoid excess motion; transfer patient slowly and smoothly to minimize vertigo.
        (2) Phase II
            (a) Standard phase II activities as previously described if patient discharged to home
            (b) Discharge instructions
                (i)   Avoid getting ears wet.
                (ii) Avoid sudden turning; encourage slow, smooth motion.
                (iii) Sneeze with mouth open to avoid pressure on eustachian tubes.
                (iv) Gentle nose blowing only
                (v)   Noises such as popping and/or cracking may be heard in the ear by the patient and are considered normal.
    g. Psychosocial concerns
        (1) Patient may report immediate improvement in hearing; hearing may decrease postoperatively from accumulation of drainage.
    h. Complications
        (1) Facial nerve dehiscence and damage
        (2) Dizziness
5. Endolymphatic shunt
    a. Purpose
        (1) To relieve pressure in endolymphatic sac
    b. Description
        (1) Placement of shunt (commercially prepared or fashioned by surgeon) into endolymphatic sac via a mastoidectomy to allow for drainage of excess endolymph
    c. Indications
        (1) Treatment of Meniere's disease
    d. Preoperative concerns
        (1) Vertigo may be present preoperatively; a quiet, dark environment is advised to minimize stimuli.

e. Intraoperative concerns
  (1) Transfer patient slowly to avoid exacerbation of vertigo.
  (2) See information on mastoidectomy (preceding section III.A.4.e).
f. Postanesthesia concerns
  (1) Phase I
    (a) Standard phase I activities as previously described
    (b) Elevate head of bed at least 30°; clarify positioning with surgeon for specific instructions.
    (c) Position with operative ear upward to prevent pressure.
    (d) Prepare to treat nausea, vomiting, vertigo.
    (e) Avoid excess motion; transfer patient slowly and smoothly to minimize vertigo.
  (2) Phase II
    (a) Standard phase II activities as previously described if patient discharged to home; patients may require 24-hour admission because of vertigo.
    (b) Discharge instructions
      (i)   Avoid getting ears wet.
      (ii) Avoid sudden turning; encourage slow, smooth motion.
      (iii) Sneeze with mouth open to avoid pressure on eustachian tubes.
      (iv) Gentle nose blowing only
      (v)   Noises such as pulsations, popping, and/or cracking may be heard in the ear by the patient and are considered normal.
g. Psychosocial concerns
  (1) Patients with Meniere's disease may experience feelings of
    (a) Loss of control
    (b) Depression
    (c) Powerlessness related to the unpredictability of the condition
  (2) Lifestyle modifications may be necessary to cope with vertigo and hearing deficits.
h. Complications
  (1) Deafness or profound hearing loss
  (2) Labyrinthitis
6. Vestibular neurectomy
  a. Purpose
    (1) To interrupt transmission of the vestibular branch of the acoustic nerve, reducing stimuli to the vestibule and alleviating vertigo
  b. Description
    (1) Resection of the vestibular portion of the acoustic nerve with preservation of the cochlear portion via transcochlear, translabyrinthine, middle fossa, retrolabyrinthine, or retrosigmoid approaches
  c. Indications
    (1) Meniere's disease
    (2) Traumatic labyrinthitis
    (3) Vestibular neuronitis
  d. Preoperative concerns
    (1) Vertigo may be present preoperatively; a quiet, dark environment is advised to minimize stimuli.
  e. Intraoperative concerns
    (1) A fat graft is obtained from either the abdomen or lateral thigh to obliterate the mastoid cavity at the end of the procedure.
  f. Postanesthesia concerns
    (1) Phase I
      (a) Standard phase I activities as previously described
      (b) Elevate head of bed at least 30°; clarify positioning with surgeon for specific instructions.

       (c) Position with operative ear upward to prevent pressure.

       (d) Prepare to treat nausea, vomiting, vertigo.

       (e) Avoid excess motion; transfer patient slowly and smoothly to minimize vertigo.

       (f) Assess facial nerve function. Report any impairment to the surgeon. Assess facial symmetry by asking patient to:

          (i) Smile enough to show teeth.

          (ii) Wrinkle forehead.

          (iii) Pucker lips.

          (iv) Wrinkle nose.

          (v) Squeeze eyelids shut.

          (vi) Stick out tongue.

    (2) Phase II

       (a) Patient may be transferred to intensive care unit (ICU) if middle fossa approach used.

       (b) Standard phase II activities as previously described if discharged home after transcochlear or translabyrinthine approaches; may require 24-hour admission

       (c) Discharge instructions

          (i) Avoid getting ears wet.

          (ii) Avoid sudden turning; encourage slow, smooth motion.

          (iii) Sneeze with mouth open to avoid pressure on eustachian tubes.

          (iv) Gentle nose blowing only

          (v) Noises such as pulsations, popping, and/or cracking may be heard in the ear by the patient and are considered normal.

g. Psychosocial concerns

    (1) Patients with vertigo may experience feelings of loss of control, depression, and powerlessness related to the unpredictability of the condition.

    (2) Lifestyle modifications may be necessary to cope with vertigo and hearing deficits.

h. Complications

    (1) Cerebrospinal fluid (CSF) leak

    (2) Dural herniation

7. Labyrinthectomy

a. Purpose

    (1) Alleviation of severe vertigo

b. Description

    (1) Destruction of the membranous labyrinth of the horizontal semicircular canal via transcanal or transmastoid approach

c. Indications

    (1) Refractive unilateral Meniere's disease in a deaf or near-deaf ear

d. Preoperative concerns

    (1) Causes total deafness in operative ear

    (2) Vertigo may be present preoperatively; a quiet, dark environment is advised to minimize stimuli.

e. Intraoperative concerns

    (1) Transfer patient slowly to avoid exacerbation of vertigo.

    (2) See information on tympanoplasty (preceding section III.A.2.e).

f. Postanesthesia priorities

    (1) Phase I

       (a) Standard phase I activities as previously described

       (b) Elevate head of bed at least 30°; clarify positioning with surgeon for specific instructions.

       (c) Position with operative ear upward to prevent pressure.

       (d) Prepare to treat nausea, vomiting, vertigo.

       (e) Avoid excess motion; transfer patient slowly and smoothly to minimize vertigo.

      (f) Assess facial nerve function. Report any impairment to the surgeon. Assess facial symmetry by asking patient to:

         (i) Smile enough to show teeth.

         (ii) Wrinkle forehead.

         (iii) Pucker lips.

         (iv) Wrinkle nose.

         (v) Squeeze eyelids shut.

         (vi) Stick out tongue.

   (2) Phase II

      (a) Standard phase II activities as previously described if discharged to home; may require 24-hour admission

      (b) Discharge instructions

         (i) Avoid getting ears wet.

         (ii) Avoid sudden turning; encourage slow, smooth motion.

         (iii) Sneeze with mouth open to avoid pressure on eustachian tubes.

         (iv) Gentle nose blowing only

         (v) Noises such as pulsations, popping, and/or cracking may be heard in the ear by the patient and are considered normal.

         (vi) Severe dizziness may be expected for several days as the brainstem must accommodate to labyrinth destruction and compensate.

         (vii) Temporary taste disturbances can occur, but normal functioning will generally return.

g. Psychosocial concerns

   (1) Patients with vertigo may experience feelings of loss of control, depression, and powerlessness related to the unpredictability of the condition.

   (2) Lifestyle modifications may be necessary to cope with vertigo and hearing deficits.

h. Complications

   (1) Meningitis

   (2) CSF leak

   (3) Tinnitus

   (4) Facial nerve paralysis

   (5) Taste disturbances

8. Facial nerve decompression and exploration

a. Purpose

   (1) To relieve facial nerve pressure caused by edema or other compromise

   (2) Repair of facial nerve transection

b. Description

   (1) Incision of facial nerve sheath at area of compromise via transmastoid, translabyrinthine, or middle cranial fossa approach

   (2) Repair of transected nerve with nerve graft

c. Indications

   (1) Bell's palsy: an idiopathic edema and inflammation of the facial nerve, possibly viral in origin

   (2) Trauma: skull or mandibular fractures, gunshot wounds

d. Preoperative concerns

   (1) Eye on affected side must be protected to guard against corneal dryness.

e. Intraoperative concerns

   (1) Eye on affected side protected with ointment or tarsorrhaphy

   (2) Nerve monitoring via electromyography

   (3) Auditory brainstem evoked potentials may also be used.

f. Postanesthesia priorities

   (1) Phase I

      (a) Standard phase I activities as previously described

        (b) Elevate head of bed at least 30°; clarify positioning with surgeon for specific instructions.

        (c) Place patient on side to prevent aspiration.

        (d) Assess facial nerve function. Report any impairment to the surgeon. Assess facial symmetry by asking patient to:

            (i) Smile enough to show teeth.

            (ii) Wrinkle forehead.

            (iii) Pucker lips.

            (iv) Wrinkle nose.

            (v) Squeeze eyelids shut.

            (vi) Stick out tongue.

    (2) Phase II

        (a) Patient may be transferred to ICU if middle fossa cranial approach is used.

        (b) Discharge instructions

            (i) Discuss aspiration risks and preventive measures.

            (ii) Review oral care procedures.

            (iii) Discuss importance of eye care and eye protection.

g. Psychosocial concerns

  (1) Body image disturbances related to appearance

  (2) Regeneration time of repaired nerves may be lengthy, resulting in slow changes to appearance and function.

h. Complications

  (1) Scarring of nerve after repair

  (2) CSF leak (if cranial approach used)

  (3) Infection

  (4) Dizziness

9. Removal of acoustic neuroma (vestibular schwannoma)

a. Purpose

  (1) To remove tumor mass while preserving nerve function

b. Description

  (1) Vestibular schwannomas are benign tumors arising from the Schwann cells of the vestibular portion of the acoustic nerve that may cause a myriad of symptoms including:

    (a) Hearing loss

    (b) Headache

    (c) Vertigo

    (d) Tinnitus

    (e) Gait disturbance

    (f) Ocular disorders

  (2) Procedure involves resection of tumors usually via a translabyrinthine or middle cranial approach.

c. Indications

  (1) Diagnosed vestibular schwannoma

  (2) Neurofibromatosis

d. Preoperative concerns

  (1) Hair removal may range from partial to complete head shave.

e. Intraoperative concerns

  (1) Middle cranial approach may be performed in sitting or prone position.

  (2) Risk for air embolism related to surgical positioning.

f. Postanesthesia priorities

  (1) Phase I

    (a) Standard phase I activities as previously described

    (b) Elevate head of bed at least 30°; clarify positioning with surgeon for specific instructions.

    (c) IV fluid infusion strictly monitored to prevent overload and possible cerebral edema

    (d) Patient will be transferred to ICU after phase I care.

      g. Psychosocial concerns

          (1) Partial or total hearing loss will necessitate lifestyle adjustments.

          (2) Possible body image disturbance related to hair removal

      h. Complications

          (1) CSF leak

          (2) Dural herniation

          (3) Air embolism

          (4) Tinnitus

          (5) Facial nerve paralysis

          (6) Vertigo

          (7) Hearing loss or dead ear

          (8) Meningitis

B. Nose

    1. Septoplasty, submucous resection

      a. Purpose

          (1) To repair acquired or congenital intranasal and septal defects that interferes with normal respiratory function

      b. Description

          (1) Excision of deviated septal cartilage and bone via intranasal incision

          (2) Removal of polypoid tissue, if present

          (3) May include turbinectomy (reduction of turbinate size)

          (4) Restoration of functional septal architecture

      c. Indications

          (1) Deviated nasal septum

          (2) Nasal polyps

          (3) Hypertrophied nasal turbinates

      d. Preoperative concerns

          (1) Discuss expected postoperative events.

             (a) Nasal packing may be in place and cause feeling of suffocation; patient will have to breathe through his or her mouth.

             (b) Drip pad (moustache) dressing will be in place; will be changed as necessary.

      e. Intraoperative concerns

          (1) May be performed under local anesthesia or monitored anesthesia care for adults

          (2) Nasal packing and/or nasal splints inserted

             (a) Nasal packing prevents hematoma.

             (b) Nasal splints help prevent synechiae (adhesions).

      f. Postanesthesia priorities

          (1) Phase I

             (a) Standard phase I activities as previously described

             (b) Progress from side lying to semi-Fowlers with head of bed elevated 30°.

             (c) Monitor patient closely for hypoventilation and hypoxia related to nasal packing and mouth breathing.

             (d) Apply ice packs as ordered to promote vasoconstriction and minimize edema.

             (e) Change moustache dressing as needed.

             (f) Observe for hemorrhage and/or septal hematoma.

                (i)   Frequent swallowing may indicate bleeding.

                (ii) Blood from septal hematoma dissects into cheeks, upper lip, and nose.

             (g) Excessive gagging may be indication that packing has dislodged and migrated to pharynx.

                (i)   Provide equipment for reinsertion.

                    [a] Bayonet forceps

                    [b] Nasal speculum

                    [c] Scissors

[d] Nasal packing

[e] Headlight

[f] Tongue depressor

(ii) Provide reassurance to patient.

(iii) Administer pain medications as necessary.

(2) Phase II

(a) Standard phase II activities as previously described

(b) Offer frequent mouth rinses to combat mouth dryness and rinse blood from oral cavity.

(c) Discharge instructions

(i) Change moustache dressing when soiled—maintain count of change frequency if excessively soiled.

(ii) Use a humidifier as ordered/needed to moisten the air.

(iii) No nose blowing; sniff secretions to the back of the nose; swallow or expectorate.

(iv) No bending, straining, or lifting

(v) Sneeze with the mouth open.

(vi) Bloody or tarry stools may be expected because of swallowed blood.

(vii) Nausea may be expected due to swallowed blood.

g. Psychosocial concerns

(1) Nasal packing may cause feelings of claustrophobia and anxiety.

h. Complications

(1) Bleeding

(2) Infection

(3) Edema

(4) Septal perforation

(5) Intranasal synechiae (adhesions)

(6) Septal hematoma

2. Rhinoplasty

a. Purpose

(1) Restoration and improvement of respiratory function

(2) Alteration of appearance of the nose

b. Description

(1) Nasal cartilage and bony structure reduced, realigned, or augmented via intranasal or small external skin incisions

(2) Surgical fracture of nasal bones

(3) May change appearance of sides, tip, or hump of nose

c. Indications

(1) Traumatic or congenital deformity

(2) Cosmetic appearance

d. Preoperative concerns

(1) Discuss expected postoperative events.

(a) Nasal packing may be in place and cause feeling of suffocation; patient will have to breathe through his or her mouth.

(b) Drip pad (moustache) dressing will be in place; will be changed as necessary.

(c) Facial edema and bruising may occur.

e. Intraoperative concerns

(1) May be combined with septoplasty to correct defects

(2) May be performed under local anesthesia or monitored anesthesia care in adult patients

(3) External nasal splint and dressing may be applied to maintain correction.

f. Postanesthesia priorities

(1) Phase I

(a) Standard phase I activities as previously described

(b) Progress from side lying to semi-Fowlers with head of bed elevated 30°.

     (c) Monitor patient closely for hypoventilation and hypoxia related to nasal packing and mouth breathing.

     (d) Apply ice packs as ordered to nose and eyes to promote vasoconstriction and minimize edema.

     (e) Change moustache dressing as needed.

     (f) Observe for hemorrhage.

         (i) Frequent swallowing may indicate bleeding.

     (g) Excessive gagging may be indication that packing has migrated to pharynx.

         (i) See information on septoplasty (preceding section III.B.1.f).

  (2) Phase II

     (a) Standard phase II activities as previously described

     (b) Offer frequent mouth rinses to combat mouth dryness and rinse blood from oral cavity.

     (c) Discharge instructions

         (i) Change moustache dressing when soiled. Maintain count of change frequency if excessively soiled.

         (ii) Use a humidifier as ordered/needed to moisten the air.

         (iii) No nose blowing; sniff secretions to the back of the nose; swallow or expectorate.

         (iv) No bending, straining, or lifting

         (v) Sneeze with the mouth open.

         (vi) Bloody or tarry stools may be expected because of swallowed blood.

         (vii) External splint should not be disturbed or removed by patient.

g. Psychosocial concerns

  (1) Initial cosmetic results may not meet patient's expectations.

  (2) Mild edema may persist for several months, obscuring final results of surgery.

h. Complications

  (1) CSF leak

  (2) Bleeding

  (3) Edema

  (4) Undesirable or unanticipated cosmetic appearance

3. Reduction of nasal fracture

a. Purpose

  (1) Restoration of nasal architecture

  (2) Prevention of nasal deformity

b. Description

  (1) Tactile manipulation of external nose to realign cartilaginous structures

  (2) Intranasal reduction of fracture with instrumentation

c. Indications

  (1) Nasal trauma

d. Preoperative concerns

  (1) Procedure may be delayed to allow swelling from injury to subside.

e. Intraoperative concerns

  (1) May be performed under local anesthesia or monitored anesthesia care in adult patients

  (2) Generally does not require postoperative nasal packing

f. Postanesthesia priorities

  (1) Phase I

     (a) Standard phase I activities as previously described

     (b) Progress from side lying to semi-Fowlers with head of bed elevated 30°.

     (c) Apply ice packs as ordered to nose and eyes to promote vasoconstriction and minimize edema.

  (2) Phase II

     (a) Standard phase II activities as previously described

        (b) Discharge instructions
           (i)   No nose blowing; sniff secretions to the back of the nose; swallow or expectorate.
           (ii) No bending, straining, or lifting
           (iii) Sneeze with the mouth open.
           (iv) Bloody or tarry stools may be expected because of swallowed blood.

g. Psychosocial concerns
   (1) Additional procedures may be necessary if acceptable cosmetic results not achieved.

h. Complications
   (1) Incomplete reduction of fracture
   (2) Septal hematoma
   (3) CSF leak

C. Paranasal sinuses
  1. Functional endoscopic sinus surgery
    a. Purpose
      (1) Removal of diseased sinus mucosa
      (2) Establishment or reestablishment of airflow, mucociliary clearance, and drainage from osteomeatal complex (channel that connects the nasal passage to the sinus cavity)

    b. Description
      (1) Nasal cavity examined via a rigid telescope inserted through the nares
      (2) Sinuses entered via fenestrations
      (3) Under direct vision, mucosa and/or polyps stripped and removed
      (4) Sinus osteomeatal complex enlarged as needed and bony structure altered to achieve functional drainage
      (5) Mucopurulent fluid drained

    c. Indications
      (1) Nasal polyps
      (2) Chronic sinusitis
      (3) Mucocele
      (4) Tumor masses

    d. Preoperative concerns
      (1) Discuss expected postoperative events.
         (a) Nasal packing may be in place and cause feeling of suffocation; patient will have to breathe through his or her mouth.
         (b) Drip pad (moustache) dressing will be in place; will be changed as necessary.

    e. Intraoperative concerns
      (1) May be performed under local anesthesia with sedation in adult patients
      (2) Uses telescopes and video equipment to visualize intranasal structures
      (3) Powered instrumentation may be used to remove diseased mucosa.
      (4) Care taken to maintain integrity of orbit to avoid ophthalmic injury
      (5) Packing may extend into sinus cavity.

    f. Postanesthesia priorities
      (1) Phase I
         (a) Standard phase I activities as previously described
         (b) Progress from side lying to semi-Fowlers with head of bed elevated 30°.
         (c) Monitor patient closely for hypoventilation and hypoxia related to nasal packing and mouth breathing.
         (d) Apply ice packs as ordered to nose and eyes to promote vasoconstriction and minimize edema.
         (e) Change moustache dressing when soiled. Maintain count of change frequency if excessively soiled.
         (f) Observe for hemorrhage.
            (i)   Frequent swallowing may indicate bleeding.

(g) Excessive gagging may be indication that packing has migrated to pharynx.

    (i)   See information on septoplasty (preceding section III.B.1.f).

(h) Observe for excessive orbital swelling, bruising, changes to visual acuity, impairment of extraocular movements.

(i) Observe for excessive clear rhinorrhea; could indicate possible CSF leak.

  (2) Phase II

    (a) Standard phase II activities as previously described

    (b) Discharge instructions

      (i)   No nose blowing; sniff secretions to the back of the nose; swallow or expectorate.

      (ii) No bending, straining, or lifting

      (iii) Sneeze with the mouth open.

      (iv) Change moustache dressing when soiled. Maintain count of change frequency if excessively soiled.

      (v) Bloody or tarry stools may be expected because of swallowed blood.

g. Psychosocial concerns

  (1) Patient may have altered postoperative appearance (orbital bruising ["raccoon eyes"]) if extensive surgery performed in ethmoid cavity.

h. Complications

  (1) Orbital hematoma

  (2) Optic nerve damage

  (3) CSF leak

  (4) Hemorrhage

  (5) Infection

  (6) Recurrence of nasal polyps

2. Caldwell Luc antrostomy

  a. Purpose

    (1) To access the maxillary sinus for removal of diseased sinus mucosa or polyps and/or to ligate the maxillary artery

    (2) Establishment or reestablishment of drainage from osteomeatal complex

  b. Description

    (1) Sublabial and nasal mucosal incisions created

    (2) Bone removed from antral wall to create opening for drainage

    (3) Mucosal material stripped from walls of maxillary sinus

    (4) Division and ligation of maxillary artery where indicated

    (5) Packing placed in maxillary sinus cavity and nasal cavity

  c. Indications

    (1) Chronic sinusitis unresponsive to medical therapy

    (2) Maxillary polyps

    (3) Maxillary tumors

    (4) Foreign bodies

    (5) Acute or chronic epistaxis

  d. Preoperative concerns

    (1) Discuss expected postoperative events.

      (a) Nasal packing may be in place and cause feeling of suffocation; patient will have to breathe through his or her mouth.

      (b) Drip pad (moustache) dressing will be in place; will be changed as necessary.

      (c) Facial edema may occur.

  e. Intraoperative concerns

    (1) May be performed under general or local anesthesia

  f. Postanesthesia priorities

    (1) Phase I

      (a) Standard phase I activities as previously described

      (b) Progress from side lying to semi-Fowlers with head of bed elevated 30°.

      (c) Monitor patient closely for hypoventilation and hypoxia related to nasal packing and mouth breathing.

      (d) Apply ice packs as ordered to face to promote vasoconstriction and minimize edema.

      (e) Change moustache dressing as needed.

      (f) Offer frequent mouth rinses to combat mouth dryness and eliminate bloody secretions from intraoral incisions.

      (g) Observe for hemorrhage.

         (i) Frequent swallowing may indicate bleeding.

      (h) Excessive gagging may be indication that packing has migrated to pharynx.

      (i) See information on septoplasty (preceding section III.B.1.f).

    (2) Phase II

      (a) Standard phase II activities as previously described

      (b) Discharge instructions

         (i) No nose blowing; sniff secretions to the back of the nose; swallow or expectorate.

         (ii) No bending, straining, or lifting

         (iii) Sneeze with the mouth open.

         (iv) Continue to brush teeth, but avoid intraoral incisions; avoid excessive brushing pressure to teeth and gums. Use a soft toothbrush.

         (v) Change moustache dressing when soiled. Maintain count of change frequency if excessively soiled.

         (vi) Bloody or tarry stools may be expected because of swallowed blood.

g. Psychosocial concerns

  (1) Numbness to lip may result in uneven smile or altered appearance to lip and mouth.

h. Complications

  (1) Persistent numbness to cheek, upper lip, gums, and teeth

  (2) Damage to maxillary division of the trigeminal nerve (cranial nerve V) will cause permanent loss of sensation to upper lip.

  (3) Oral antral fistula

3. Ethmoidectomy

  a. Purpose

    (1) Promotion of drainage of the ethmoid sinus

    (2) Used in conjunction with orbital decompression for exophthalmos

  b. Description

    (1) Intranasal or external medical canthal incision

    (2) Removal of bony walls between ethmoid air cells

    (3) Creation of common ethmoid cavity to promote drainage

  c. Indications

    (1) Chronic ethmoid sinusitis

    (2) Mucoceles

    (3) Polyps

  d. Preoperative concerns

    (1) Discuss expected postoperative events.

      (a) Nasal packing may be in place and cause feeling of suffocation; patient will have to breathe through his or her mouth.

      (b) Drip pad (moustache) dressing will be in place; will be changed as necessary.

      (c) Facial edema and bruising may occur.

  e. Intraoperative concerns

    (1) May use operating microscope

    (2) May use endoscopes

  f. Postanesthesia priorities

    (1) Phase I

(a) Standard phase I activities as previously described
(b) Progress from side lying to semi-Fowlers with head of bed elevated 30°.
(c) Monitor patient closely for hypoventilation and hypoxia related to nasal packing and mouth breathing.
(d) Apply ice packs as ordered to nose and eyes to promote vasoconstriction and minimize edema.
(e) Change moustache dressing as needed.
(f) Observe for hemorrhage.
  (i) Frequent swallowing may indicate bleeding.
(g) Excessive gagging may be indication that packing has migrated to pharynx.
  (i) See information on septoplasty (preceding section III.B.1.f).
(h) Observe for excessive orbital swelling, bruising, changes to visual acuity, impairment of extraocular movements.

(2) Phase II
  (a) Standard phase II activities as previously described.
  (b) Discharge instructions
    (i) No nose blowing; sniff secretions to the back of the nose; swallow or expectorate.
    (ii) No bending, straining, or lifting
    (iii) Sneeze with the mouth open.
    (iv) Sleep with head elevated to minimize edema.
    (v) Apply ice packs as ordered to face to minimize bruising.
    (vi) Bloody or tarry stools may be expected because of swallowed blood.

g. Psychosocial concerns
  (1) If eye pads and eye dressings are applied in the OR, patient may experience panic because of inability to see.
  (2) Patient will have altered postoperative appearance from edema and orbital bruising ("raccoon eyes").

h. Complications
  (1) CSF leak
  (2) Orbital injury
  (3) Optic nerve injury and loss of vision
  (4) Diplopia
  (5) Hemorrhage

4. Frontal sinusotomy and obliteration
  a. Purpose
    (1) To eradicate diseased mucosa from the frontal sinus and obliterate the space to prevent communication with the nasal cavity
    (2) Reduction and management of frontal sinus fractures
    (3) Removal of tumors
  b. Description
    (1) Approached through brow or scalp (bicoronal) incision
    (2) Periosteum elevated; bone cut superiorly and laterally
    (3) Fat graft removed from abdomen to pack sinus cavity
    (4) Pressure dressing applied
  c. Indications
    (1) Chronic frontal sinusitis
  d. Preoperative concerns
    (1) May require hair removal to accomplish bicoronal incision
    (2) Facial edema and bruising may occur.
  e. Intraoperative concerns
    (1) May require team approach from otorhinolaryngology and neurosurgery
  f. Postanesthesia priorities
    (1) Phase I
      (a) Standard phase I activities as previously described
      (b) Elevate head of bed at least 30°; clarify positioning with surgeon for specific instructions.

        (c) Place patient on side to prevent aspiration.

        (d) Monitor patient closely for hypoventilation and hypoxia related to nasal packing and mouth breathing.

        (e) Apply ice packs as ordered to face to promote vasoconstriction and minimize edema.

        (f) Observe for hemorrhage.

           (i) Frequent swallowing may indicate bleeding.

        (g) Excessive gagging may be indication that packing has migrated to pharynx.

           (i) See information on septoplasty (preceding section III.B.1.f).

    (2) Phase II

        (a) Standard phase II activities as previously described if patient discharged to home; may require 24-hour admission

        (b) Discharge instructions

           (i) No nose blowing; sniff secretions to the back of the nose; swallow or expectorate.

           (ii) No bending, straining, or lifting

           (iii) Sneeze with the mouth open.

           (iv) Sleep with head elevated to minimize edema.

           (v) Report signs and symptoms of infection to surgeon.

g. Psychosocial concerns

  (1) Unacceptable cosmetic appearance from hair removal, scarring, and/or prolonged edema

h. Complications

  (1) CSF leak

  (2) Meningitis

  (3) Brain abscess

  (4) Scalp hematoma

  (5) Fat necrosis

  (6) Infection to donor site

D. Oropharyngeal

1. Adenoidectomy

a. Purpose

  (1) To remove infected or hypertrophied adenoidal tissue

b. Description

  (1) Removal of adenoids with sharp and blunt dissection via intrapharyngeal incisions

c. Indications

  (1) Chronic infection (adenoiditis or otitis media)

  (2) Lymphoid hypertrophy

d. Preoperative concerns

  (1) Discuss expected postoperative events.

  (2) Frequently performed in pediatric population; use age-appropriate teaching techniques and interventions.

e. Intraoperative concerns

  (1) Performed under general anesthesia

  (2) Often performed in conjunction with tonsillectomy

  (3) Parents may be present in OR for induction of pediatric patients, depending on institutional policy and practice.

f. Postanesthesia priorities

  (1) Phase I

    (a) Standard phase I activities as previously described

    (b) Place patient on side to prevent aspiration; advance to semi-Fowlers with head of bed elevated 30° when patient awake.

    (c) Monitor closely for hemorrhage.

        (i) Bright red emesis

        (ii) Frequent and repeated swallowing

        (iii) Agitation and restlessness

        (d) Pediatric considerations
           (i)   Nurse-to-patient ratio 1:1 until consciousness and reflexes return for pediatric patients
           (ii)   Children may struggle against face tent; provide humidified oxygen by placing tubing near mouth and nose.
    (2) Phase II
        (a) Standard phase II activities as previously described
        (b) Discharge instructions
           (i)   Avoid throat clearing, coughing, vigorous nose blowing.
           (ii)   No bending, straining, or lifting
           (iii) Bland and soft diet
           (iv) Bloody or tarry stools may be expected because of swallowed blood
           (v)   Voice rest
           (vi) Throat discomfort increases between postoperative days 4 and 8 because of separation of eschar from pharyngeal bed.

g. Psychosocial concerns
  (1) Children may experience separation anxiety.
    (a) Allow for parent presence at anesthesia induction if allowed by institutional policy.
  (2) Allow child to assert control over situation when appropriate.
    (a) Remain in pajamas or street clothes.
    (b) Select flavor and scent of mask used for induction.

h. Complications
  (1) Otalgia
  (2) Velopharyngeal insufficiency
  (3) Hemorrhage
  (4) Hypernasality
  (5) Nasopharyngeal stenosis

2. Tonsillectomy
a. Purpose
  (1) To remove tonsillar tissue
b. Description
  (1) Removal of tonsils with sharp and blunt dissection via intrapharyngeal incisions
c. Indications
  (1) Chronic tonsillitis
  (2) Peritonsillar abscess
  (3) Tonsillar hypertrophy
  (4) Ulcerations, lesions, and masses
  (5) Obstructive sleep apnea
d. Preoperative concerns
  (1) Discuss expected postoperative events.
  (2) Frequently performed in pediatric population; use age-appropriate teaching techniques and interventions.
e. Intraoperative concerns
  (1) May be performed with local anesthetic and monitored anesthesia care in adults
f. Postanesthesia priorities
  (1) Phase I
    (a) See information on adenoidectomy (preceding section III.D.1.f.[1]).
  (2) Phase II
    (a) See information on adenoidectomy (preceding section III.D.1.f.[2]).
g. Psychosocial concerns
  (1) See information on adenoidectomy (preceding section III.D.1.g).
h. Complications
  (1) Hemorrhage
  (2) Postoperative airway obstruction secondary to edema

3. Uvulopalatopharyngoplasty
   a. Purpose
      (1) To reduce the amount of redundant pharyngopalatal mucosa
   b. Description
      (1) Removal of tissue, reduction of or removal of uvula via intrapharyngeal incisions; sharp and dull dissection
      (2) Tonsillectomy may also be performed.
   c. Indications
      (1) Obstructive sleep apnea
      (2) Snoring
   d. Preoperative concerns
      (1) Discuss expected postoperative events.
         (a) Possibility of tracheostomy if edema is excessive; reinforce physician information regarding tracheostomy.
   e. Intraoperative concerns
      (1) May be intubated awake if obstruction and amount of redundant tissue is severe
      (2) May be performed under local anesthesia with moderate sedation
      (3) Laser may be used.
      (4) Tracheostomy may be placed as temporary measure if extensive dissection performed or excessive airway edema is anticipated.
   f. Postanesthesia priorities
      (1) Phase I
         (a) Standard phase I activities as previously described
         (b) Progress from side lying to semi-Fowlers with head of bed elevated 30°.
         (c) Monitor patient closely for hypoventilation and hypoxia related to edema.
         (d) Perform intraoral suctioning with care to avoid trauma to mucosal incision lines.
      (2) Phase II
         (a) Often transferred to ICU for observation because of risk of airway edema and compromise
         (b) Generally will be admitted for minimum of 24 hours because of risk of airway edema
         (c) Discharge instructions
            (i) Avoid throat clearing and coughing.
            (ii) No bending, straining, or lifting
            (iii) Bland or soft diet
            (iv) Bloody or tarry stools may be expected because of swallowed blood.
            (v) Use humidifier to moisten the air.
            (vi) Maintain hydration.
            (vii) Voice rest
   g. Psychosocial concerns
      (1) Tracheostomy will temporarily affect verbal communication.
      (2) Patient and/or caregivers will require tracheostomy care instructions.
      (3) Procedure may alleviate snoring, but sleep apnea may still be present.
   h. Complications
      (1) Airway edema
      (2) Hemorrhage
      (3) Infection
4. Salivary gland surgery
   a. Purpose
      (1) To remove infected salivary glands, sialoliths, cysts, or neoplasms
      (2) Correction of ductal stenosis
   b. Description
      (1) Types

            (a) Submandibular gland excision
            (b) Parotidectomy
    c. Indications
        (1) Malignant and benign neoplasms
        (2) Diagnostic biopsy
        (3) Sialoliths and sialolithiasis
        (4) Trauma causing stenosis of the duct
        (5) Cysts
    d. Preoperative concerns
        (1) Discuss expected postoperative events.
    e. Intraoperative concerns
        (1) Facial nerve monitoring may be used.
    f. Postanesthesia priorities
        (1) Phase I
            (a) Standard phase I activities as previously described
            (b) Progress from side lying to semi-Fowlers with head of bed elevated 30°.
            (c) Monitor patient closely for hemorrhage.
            (d) Assess facial nerve function. Report any impairment to the surgeon. Assess facial symmetry by asking patient to:
                (i) Smile enough to show teeth.
                (ii) Wrinkle forehead.
                (iii) Pucker lips.
                (iv) Wrinkle nose.
                (v) Squeeze eyelids shut.
                (vi) Stick out tongue.
        (2) Phase II
            (a) Standard phase II activities as previously described if patient discharged to home; may require 24-hour admission
            (b) Discharge instructions
                (i) Avoid throat clearing and coughing.
                (ii) No bending, straining, or lifting
                (iii) Bland and soft diet
    g. Psychosocial concerns
        (1) Possible Frey's syndrome (manifested by flushing and sweating on the cheek area appearing when the patient eats, sees, or thinks about or talks about certain kinds of food that produce salivation)
    h. Complications
        (1) Hemorrhage
        (2) Facial nerve paralysis
        (3) Gustatory sweating (Frey's syndrome)
        (4) Salivary fistula
5. Esophagoscopy
    a. Purpose
        (1) To assess the structure and function of the esophagus and cardia (e.g., junction of esophagus and stomach) of the stomach
        (2) To obtain tissue biopsy to facilitate diagnoses
    b. Description
        (1) Direct visualization with a rigid or flexible scope
    c. Indications
        (1) Suspected carcinoma
        (2) Stricture and stenosis
        (3) Reflux
        (4) Bleeding
    d. Preoperative concerns
        (1) Discuss expected postoperative events.
    e. Intraoperative concerns
        (1) May occasionally be performed under topical anesthesia and moderate sedation

        f. Postanesthesia priorities
          (1) Phase I
            (a) Standard phase I activities as previously described
            (b) Progress from side lying to semi-Fowlers with head of bed elevated 30°.
            (c) Assess return of swallowing and gag reflex.
            (d) Observe for perforation and hemorrhage. Symptoms include:
               (i) Frank blood in emesis
               (ii) Agitation and restlessness
               (iii) Complaints of severe pain disproportionate to the procedure
          (2) Phase II
            (a) Standard phase II activities as previously described
            (b) Discharge instructions
               (i) Avoid throat clearing and coughing.
               (ii) Bland and soft diet when gag reflex returned
               (iii) Voice rest
               (iv) Avoid lifting and straining.
      g. Psychosocial concerns
        (1) Anxiety related to diagnostic findings
      h. Complications
        (1) Bleeding
        (2) Edema
        (3) Esophageal perforation
  E. Larynx
    1. Tracheostomy
      a. Purpose
        (1) To create a surgical opening in the trachea for airway maintenance
      b. Description
        (1) Incision over the trachea
        (2) Insertion of a catheter or cannula through tracheal rings
      c. Indications
        (1) Acute airway obstruction
        (2) Prolonged ventilator dependency
        (3) Prevention of aspiration
        (4) Bypass of upper airway obstruction because of tumor
      d. Preoperative concerns
        (1) May be emergent procedure
      e. Intraoperative concerns
        (1) Send obturator and ventilator adaptors to PACU with patient.
      f. Postanesthesia priorities
        (1) Phase I
          (a) Standard phase I activities as previously described
          (b) Elevate head of bed 30°.
          (c) Ensure that tracheostomy tube ties are secure.
          (d) Prepare to reinsert tracheostomy tube or obturator if tube is coughed out.
          (e) Observe for hemorrhage.
          (f) Assess for pneumothorax.
          (g) Provide alternate means of communication for patient (e.g., magic slate, pen and paper, communication board).
        (2) Phase II
          (a) May be transferred to ICU for observation; otherwise will require 24-hour admission at minimum
          (b) Discharge instructions
            (i) Discuss need for humidification.
            (ii) Teach tracheostomy care to patient, family, and/or caregivers.
            (iii) Discuss cardiopulmonary resuscitation needs with caregiver. Standard mouth-to-mouth rescue breathing will be ineffective.

g. Psychosocial concerns
   (1) Reduces ability to communicate verbally; alternate methods of communication must be used unless speaking valve is in place.
   (2) Body image disturbances
h. Complications
   (1) Hemorrhage
   (2) Dislodgement of tracheotomy tube
   (3) Tracheoesophageal fistula
   (4) Subcutaneous emphysema
   (5) Pneumothorax
   (6) Tracheostenosis
2. Laryngoscopy
   a. Purpose
      (1) To visualize the interior of the larynx
      (2) Obtain tissue biopsy for diagnosis
      (3) Removal of vocal cord lesions
   b. Description
      (1) Types
         (a) Direct laryngoscopy
            (i) Rigid
            (ii) Flexible
         (b) Microsuspension laryngoscopy
   c. Indications
      (1) Suspected carcinoma
      (2) Vocal cord polyps and nodules
   d. Preoperative concerns
      (1) Discuss expected postoperative events.
   e. Intraoperative concerns
      (1) Prepare for laryngospasm on extubation.
   f. Postanesthesia priorities
      (1) Phase I
         (a) Standard phase I activities as previously described
         (b) Progress from side lying to semi-Fowlers with head of bed elevated 30°.
         (c) Be alert to possibility of laryngospasm.
         (d) Assess for return of swallowing and gag reflexes.
         (e) Mild hemoptysis may be anticipated after vocal cord procedures or biopsies.
      (2) Phase II
         (a) Standard phase II activities as previously described
         (b) Discharge instructions
            (i)   Avoid throat clearing.
            (ii) Start bland and soft diet when gag reflex returned.
            (iii) Avoid straining or lifting.
            (iv) Voice rest as directed by physician
            (v)   Avoid whispering.
   g. Psychosocial concerns
      (1) Anxiety related to diagnostic findings
      (2) Anxiety related to vocalization changes
   h. Complications
      (1) Vocal cord trauma and paralysis
      (2) Laryngospasm
3. Phonosurgery
   a. Purpose
      (1) To improve voice quality and vocal cord mobility
   b. Description
      (1) Insertion of Silastic shim or prosthesis to maintain vocal cord position
         (a) Type I
            (i)   Improves or changes voice quality

              (b) Types II and III
                  (i)   Improves or changes pitch
                  (ii) Alters vocal cord tension

  c. Indications
     (1) Vocal cord paralysis caused by:
         (a) Trauma
         (b) Neoplasms
         (c) Thyroidectomy
         (d) Mechanical dysfunction

  d. Preoperative concerns
     (1) Discuss expected postoperative events.
     (2) Assess quality of patient's voice.

  e. Intraoperative concerns
     (1) Performed under local anesthesia with light sedation to allow patient to speak as a test of voice quality
     (2) Voice quality tested as shim or prosthesis manipulated to find best position to reapproximate vocal cords

  f. Postanesthesia priorities
     (1) Phase I
         (a) Most patients have minimal sedation; may bypass phase I.
     (2) Phase II
         (a) Standard phase II activities as previously described
         (b) Provide alternate means of communication for patient (e.g., magic slate, pen and paper, communication board) to allow patient to rest voice.
         (c) Observe for laryngeal edema.
         (d) Discharge instructions
            (i)   Voice rest as directed by physician
            (ii) Avoid whispering.

  g. Psychosocial concerns
     (1) Speech therapy may be needed to improve quality of voice.

  h. Complications
     (1) Airway edema
     (2) Infection
     (3) Need for revision surgery

4. Laryngectomy
  a. Purpose
     (1) Removal of larynx

  b. Description
     (1) Types
         (a) Hemilaryngectomy
            (i)   Removal of false vocal cord, arytenoids, and one side of thyroid cartilage
            (ii) Patient has hoarse voice postoperatively.
         (b) Supraglottic laryngectomy
            (i)   Removal of laryngeal tissues and structures above the epiglottis, hyoid bone, and false vocal cords
            (ii) Normal to near-normal voice postoperatively
         (c) Total laryngectomy
            (i)   Removal of larynx, hyoid bone, laryngeal muscles, and preepiglottic space
            (ii) Permanent stoma
            (iii) Loss of natural voice postoperatively

  c. Indications
     (1) Malignant neoplasm

  d. Preoperative concerns
     (1) Discuss expected postoperative events.
     (2) Discuss method to be used for communication in postoperative period.

        (3) Patients with the presenting disorder of laryngeal neoplasms may have other chronic health conditions (e.g., smoking, alcohol abuse, diabetes, pulmonary disease; adjust planned interventions accordingly).

   e. Intraoperative concerns

        (1) May be lengthy procedures; provide attention to patient positioning to avoid pressure injury.

        (2) May involve multiple specimens and frozen sections

        (3) May be combined with tracheoesophageal puncture to allow for postprocedure speech prosthesis

           (a) Creates small fistula from superior wall of trachea to proximal wall of esophagus

           (b) Postoperative catheter inserted to maintain integrity of passage; after healing, silicone voice prosthesis with one-way valve is inserted.

   f. Postanesthesia priorities

        (1) Phase I

           (a) Standard phase I activities as previously described

           (b) Elevate head of bed at least 30° to minimize edema; clarify positioning with surgeon for specific instructions.

           (c) Provide alternate means of communication for patient (e.g., magic slate, pen and paper, communication board).

           (d) Frequent oral care when patient awake and alert

           (e) Promote coughing and deep breathing.

        (2) Phase II

           (a) May be transferred to ICU if patient has concomitant health problems; otherwise may be transferred to medical-surgical nursing unit

           (b) Discharge instructions

               (i) Discuss need for humidification.

               (ii) Teach stoma care to patient, family, and/or caregivers.

   g. Psychosocial concerns

        (1) Depression related to alteration in body image and communication difficulties

        (2) Esophageal or electronic speech (i.e., from mechanical larynx) may be difficult to understand.

        (3) Patient will require speech rehabilitation.

        (4) Provide referral to support groups (American Cancer Society, Lost Cord Club, etc.).

   h. Complications

        (1) Hemorrhage

        (2) Pharyngocutaneous fistula

        (3) Pneumothorax

F. Neck

  1. Neck dissection

   a. Purpose

        (1) To remove cancerous and metastatic tissue and lymph nodes from the neck

   b. Description

        (1) Types

           (a) Radical: removal of lymph nodes, soft tissue, sternocleidomastoid muscle, eleventh cranial nerve, and internal jugular vein

           (b) Modified radical: removal of soft tissue of neck and lymph nodes with preservation of other structures

   c. Indications

        (1) Malignant neoplasms

        (2) Prophylaxis against metastasis

   d. Preoperative concerns

        (1) Discuss expected postoperative events.

        (2) Patients often have other preexisting health concerns (see Laryngectomy, section III.E.4.d).

    e. Intraoperative concerns
       (1) Usually combined with laryngectomy procedures
       (2) May be lengthy procedures; provide attention to patient positioning to avoid pressure injury.
       (3) May involve multiple specimens and frozen sections
    f. Postanesthesia priorities
       (1) Phase I
         (a) See information on laryngectomy (section III.E.4.f).
         (b) Support affected arm on pillow to minimize pain and edema.
       (2) Phase II
         (a) May be transferred to ICU for observation; otherwise will be transferred to general medical-surgical nursing unit
    g. Psychosocial concerns
       (1) Unacceptable cosmetic appearance (radical dissection)
       (2) Depression related to appearance, concern about prognosis
       (3) Physical therapy required to regain strength in remaining neck muscles
    h. Complications
       (1) Hemorrhage
       (2) Impaired circulation to tissue flaps
       (3) Pneumothorax
       (4) Chyle (e.g., fluid composed of lymph and small fat globules) leak
       (5) Infection
  2. Thyroidectomy
    a. Purpose
       (1) To remove a hypertrophied thyroid gland and/or parathyroid glands
       (2) Removal of thyroid tumors and nodules
    b. Description
       (1) Excision of thyroid gland and parathyroid gland via a neck incision
    c. Indications
       (1) Tumor and nodules
       (2) Hyperthyroidism (Graves' disease)
       (3) Hashimoto's thyroiditis
    d. Preoperative concerns
       (1) Discuss expected postoperative events.
       (2) Hypothyroidism may predispose patient to skin breakdown and edema.
    e. Intraoperative concerns
       (1) May be performed as video-assisted procedure using harmonic scalpel
       (2) Positioning is critical to expose gland. Neck is hyperextended with head resting on headrest.
       (3) Electrocautery not used in vicinity of recurrent laryngeal nerve to avoid thermal damage to nerve
    f. Postanesthesia priorities
       (1) Phase I
         (a) Standard phase I activities as previously described
         (b) Elevate head of bed at least 30° to minimize edema; clarify positioning with surgeon for specific instructions.
         (c) Obtain tracheostomy tray at bedside if signs and symptoms indicate respiratory distress.
         (d) Encourage deep breathing.
         (e) Observe for low calcium levels (have calcium gluconate at bedside).
           (i)   Cramping, tingling of extremities
           (ii) Numbness around lips
         (f) Monitor for thyroid storm.
           (i)   Rare if patient is euthyroid (normal) before surgery
           (ii) Characterized by increased heart rate, increased blood pressure, heat intolerance, high oxygen consumption, sweating
           (iii) Treated with beta-blockers, usually propranolol

    (2) Phase II

       (a) Standard phase II activities as previously described; will generally be admitted for 24-hour observation

       (b) Discharge instructions

          (i)   Discuss symptoms of hypocalcemia and instruct patient to notify surgeon if these occur.

          (ii) Keep all follow-up appointments; laboratory monitoring of thyroid levels and hypothyroidism imperative

          (iii) Encourage range-of-motion exercises for neck.

          (iv) Soft diet until dysphagia eases

          (v) Avoid heavy lifting and straining.

          (vi) Voice rest as directed by surgeon

g. Psychosocial concerns

    (1) Alteration in body image due to neck scar

h. Complications

    (1) Recurrent laryngeal nerve injury

    (2) Hemorrhage

    (3) Hypoparathyroidism

BIBLIOGRAPHY

1. Cummings CW, Flint PW, Haughey BH, et al: *Cummings: Otolaryngology: Head & neck surgery*, ed 4, Philadelphia, 2005, Mosby.

2. Drain C, Odom-Forren J: *Perianesthesia nursing: A critical care approach*, ed 5, St Louis, 2009, Saunders.

3. Ignatavicius D, Workman L: *Medical surgical nursing: Critical thinking for collaborative care*, ed 5, St Louis, 2006, Saunders.

4. Linton A: *Introduction to medical surgical nursing*, ed 4, St Louis, 2007, Saunders.

5. Rothrock JC: *Alexander's care of the patient in surgery*, ed 13, St Louis, 2007, Mosby.

6. Patton K, Thibodeau G: *Anatomy & physiology*, ed 7, St Louis, 2010, Mosby.

Peripheral Vascular Care

MAUREEN E. LISBERGER

OBJECTIVES

At the conclusion of this chapter, the reader will be able to:

1. Explain three factors that affect peripheral circulation.
2. Describe three causes of arteriosclerosis.
3. Compare the signs and symptoms of arterial and venous vascular disease.
4. Identify the risk factors that contribute to the development of peripheral vascular disease.
5. List three postarteriography assessment criteria.
6. Identify the most common sites of occurrence of peripheral vascular disease.
7. Describe operative and interventional radiology procedures performed on patients with peripheral vascular disease.
8. Describe the immediate postoperative nursing considerations for each operative procedure.
9. List postoperative complications of vascular surgery.
10. Describe complications of endovascular repair.
11. Describe the preoperative assessment, intraoperative, and postoperative care of the vascular patient.

I. ANATOMY AND PHYSIOLOGY
   A. Peripheral vascular anatomy
      1. Includes:
         a. Peripheral arterial
         b. Venous systems
      2. Excludes:
         a. Cardiac
         b. Pulmonary
         c. Cerebral systems
   B. Arterial and venous wall structure contains three layers (Figure 44-1).
      1. Adventitia—thin outer layer containing:
         a. Collagen
         b. Lymphatics
      2. Media: thick middle layer containing smooth muscle cells arranged into strong, intertwining sheets of elastin that constrict or dilate. Medial layer is thinner in veins.
      3. Intima: thin, inner, single endothelial layer; easily traumatized
   C. Circulatory path (Figure 44-2)
      1. Artery → Arteriole → Precapillary sphincter → Capillary (Figure 44-3)
         a. Artery: high pressure, low volume
         b. Arteriole (diameter <0.5 mm)
            (1) Offers resistance to blood flow
            (2) Regulates blood flow into capillary bed
         c. Precapillary sphincters
            (1) Rings of smooth muscle located at proximal end of a true capillary
            (2) Regulates flow of blood and oxygen (see Figure 44-1)
         d. Capillary: site of gas and nutrient exchange

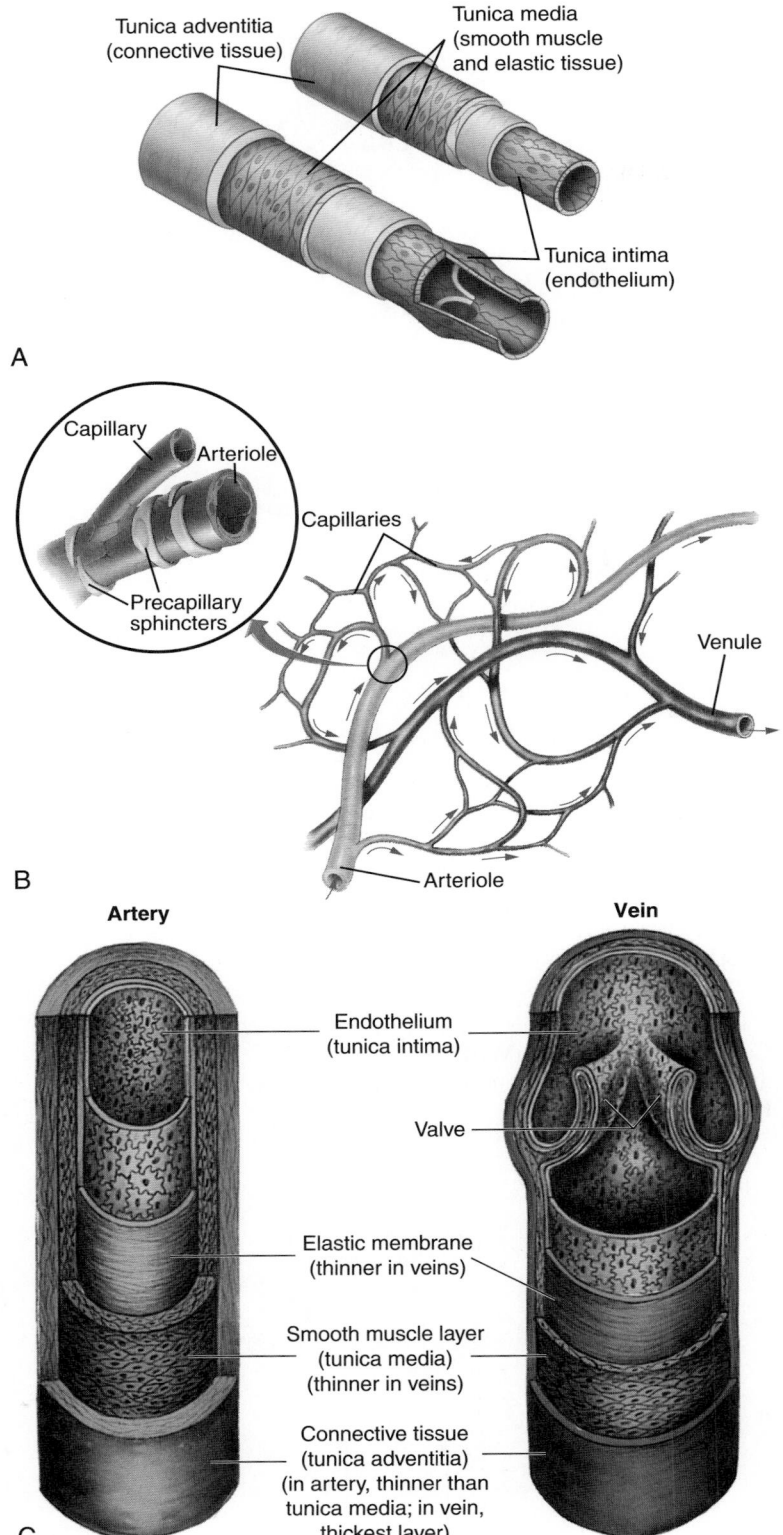

FIGURE 44-1 ■ **A,** Layers of artery and vein. **B,** Microcirculation. **C,** Cross section of an artery and vein showing the three layers: tunica intima, tunica media, and tunica adventia. Note the difference in wall thickness between the artery and the vein and the lack of valves within the artery. (**A** and **B** from Thibodeau GA, Patton KT: *Anatomy and physiology,* ed 5, St Louis, 2003, Mosby; **C** from Thompson JM, McFarland GK, Hirsh JE, et al: *Mosby's clinical nursing,* ed 5, St Louis, 2002, Mosby.)

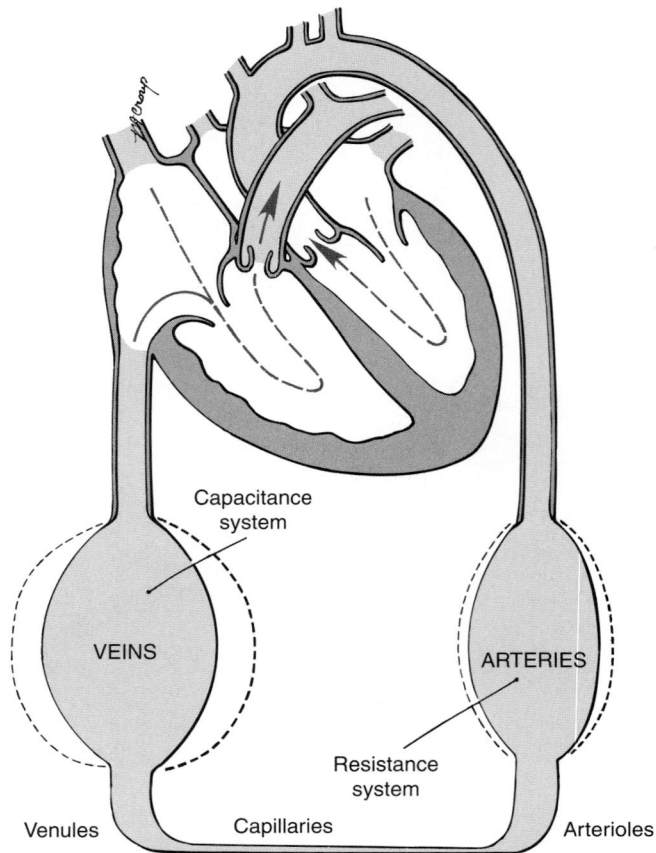

FIGURE 44-2 ■ Systemic circulation. (From Price SA, Wilson LM: *Pathophysiology: Clinical concepts of disease processes,* ed 6, St Louis, 2003, Mosby.)

2. Capillary → Venule → Vein (see Figure 44-3)
   a. Venule: as venules merge, rate of blood flow increases.
   b. Vein
      (1) Low pressure
      (2) High volume

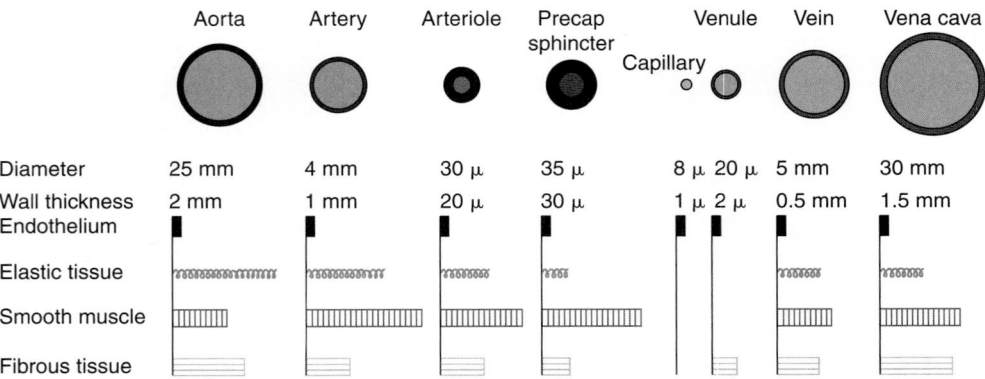

FIGURE 44-3 ■ Internal diameter, wall thickness, and relative amounts of the principal components of the vessel circulatory system. Cross sections of the vessels are not drawn to scale because of the huge range from aorta to vena cava to capillaries. (From Berne RM, Levy MN: *Cardiovascular physiology,* ed 8, St Louis, 2001, Mosby.)

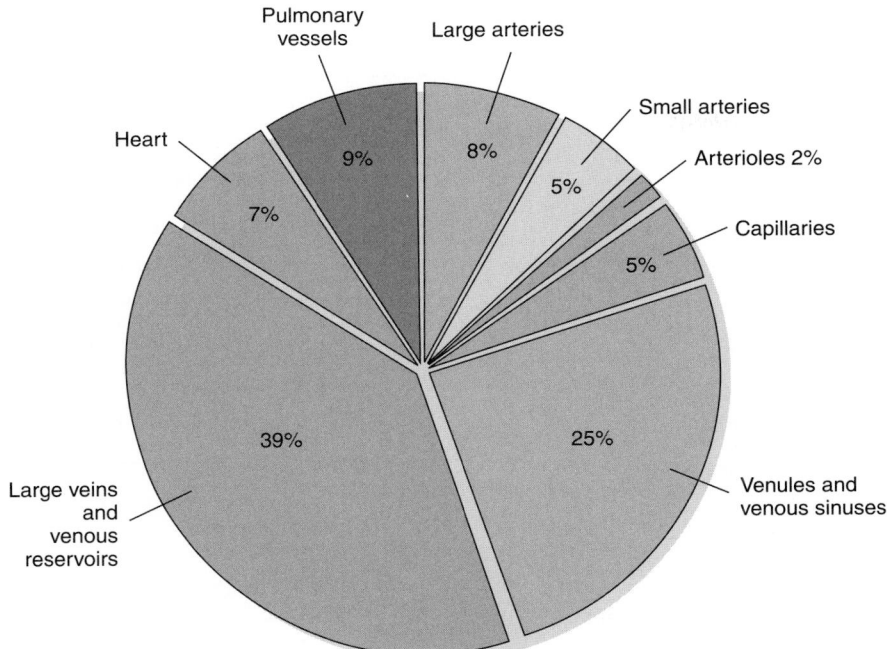

FIGURE 44-4 ■ Percentage of the total blood volume in each portion of the circulation system. (From Urden LD, Stacy KM, Lough ME: *Thelan's critical care nursing diagnosis and management,* ed 5, Philadelphia, 2006, Mosby.)

      (3) Veins are capacitance vessels because they accommodate large volumes of blood.

      (4) Unidirectional valves direct venous flow from feet toward heart and prevent reflux.

      (5) Approximately 70% of blood volume contained in venous circulation (Figure 44-4)

D. Arterial circulation (Figure 44-5)

  1. Aorta: largest peripheral vessel, which includes four sections (Figure 44-6)

    a. Ascending aorta: from aortic valve to arch

    b. Arch: where brachiocephalic and carotid vessels originate

    c. Descending thoracic aorta: from aortic arch to level of diaphragm

    d. Abdominal aorta: from thoracic to aortic bifurcation

  2. Aortic bifurcation: where aorta divides into common right and left iliac arteries

    a. Common iliac divides into:

      (1) Internal iliac (hypogastric)

      (2) External iliac: continuation of common iliac artery that becomes common femoral artery in thigh

    b. Common femoral (thigh) (Figure 44-7)

      (1) Lateral and medial femoral circumflex

      (2) Profunda (deep) femoral

    c. Popliteal: continuation of common femoral located posterior to knee surface divides into:

      (1) Anterior tibial

        (a) Dorsalis pedis

        (b) Posterior tibial

          (i) Medial and lateral plantar

          (ii) Peroneal

E. Venous circulation (Figure 44-8)

  1. Superficial system: in subcutaneous tissue

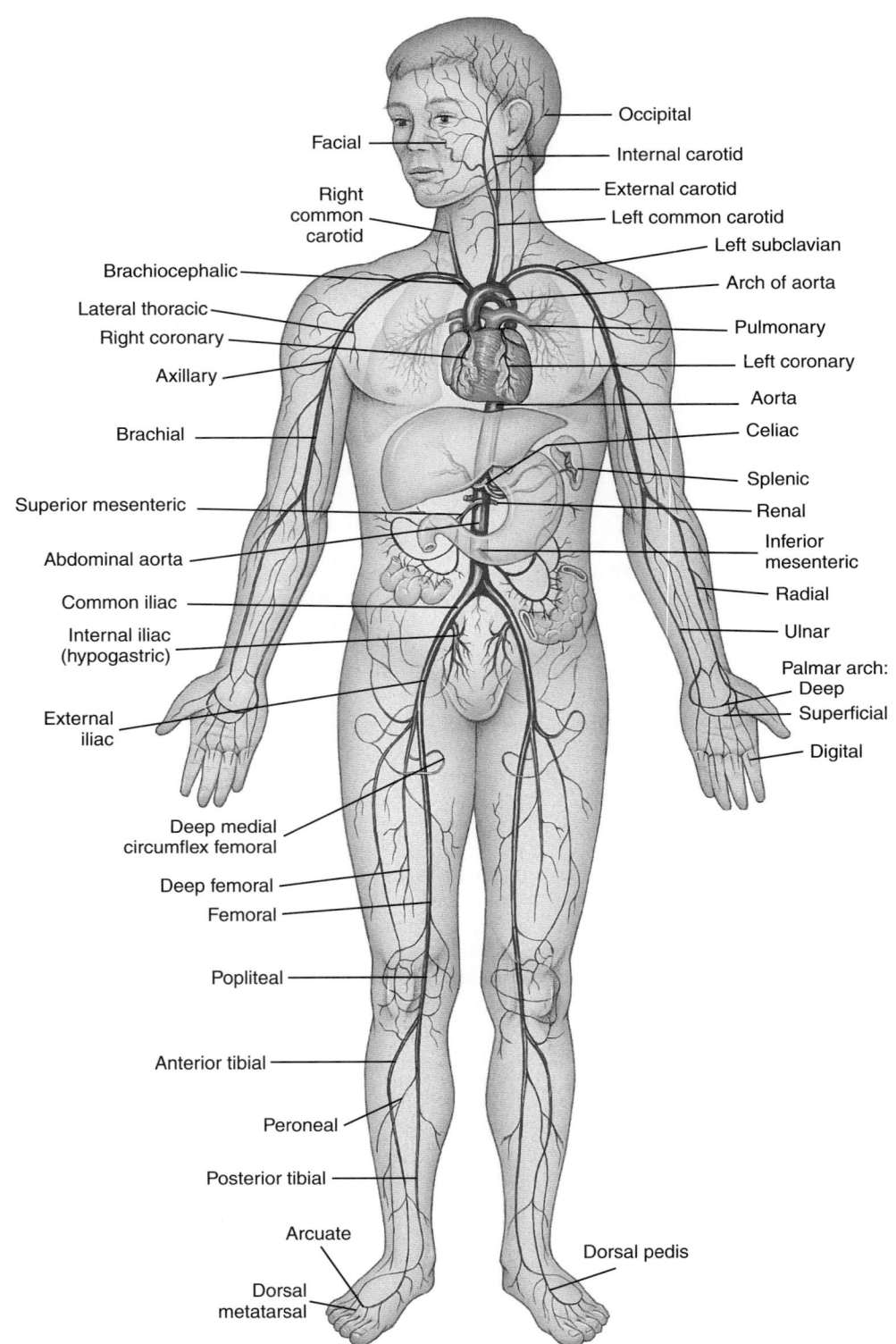

FIGURE 44-5 ■ Principal arteries of the body. (From Thibodeau GA, Patton KT: *Anatomy and physiology,* ed 6, St Louis, 2007, Mosby.)

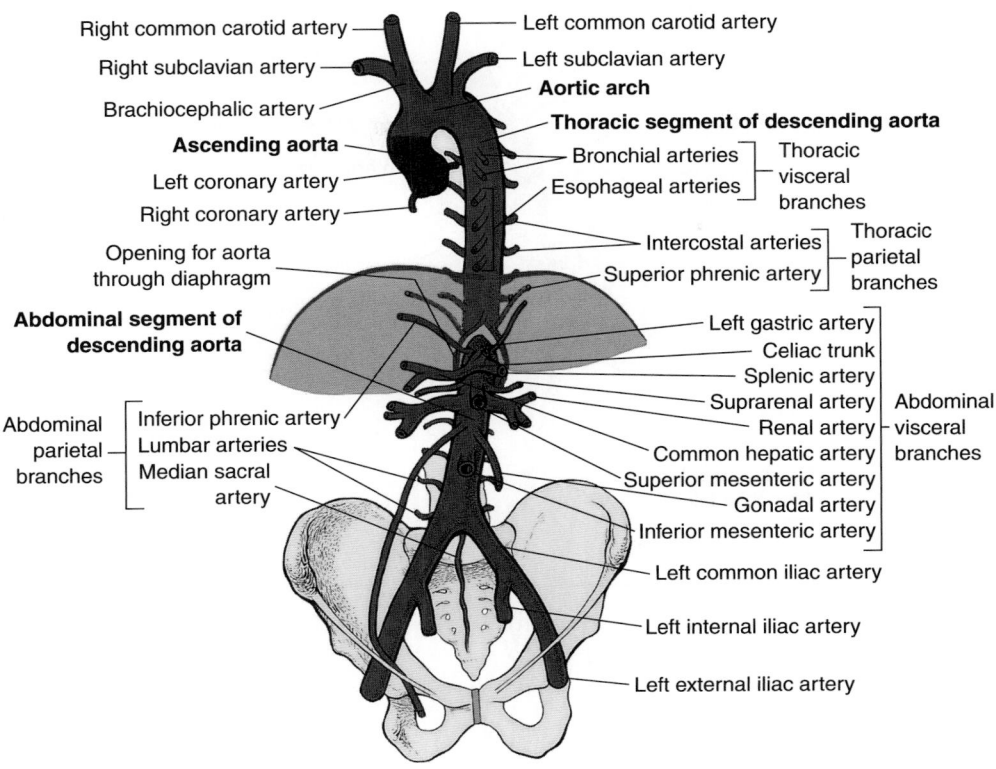

FIGURE 44-6 ■ The aorta. (From Rothrock J: *Alexander's care of the patient in surgery,* ed 12, St Louis, 2003, Mosby.)

    a. Greater saphenous: longest vein in body extending from malleolus of ankle to femoral vein (saphenous junction)

    b. Lesser saphenous: extends from ankle to popliteal vein in knee (saphenopopliteal junction)

  2. Deep veins: in muscular layers

    a. Anterior and posterior tibial

    b. Peroneal

    c. Popliteal

    d. Femoral, profunda femoris

    e. Iliac

  3. Perforating (communicating): vascular channels (Figure 44-9)

    a. Communicate between deep and superficial veins

    b. Flow shunted from superficial to deep system with help of unidirectional valves and finally to inferior vena cava

    c. Muscle contraction promotes forward flow; valves prevent backflow during muscular relaxation.

F. Factors affecting circulation

  1. Cardiac output (Cardiac output = Stroke volume × Heart rate): venous capacity will determine venous return that will affect stroke volume of heart.

  2. Arteriolar resistance: systemic vascular resistance (SVR) depends on:

    a. Degree of arteriolar constriction

    b. Resistance

      (1) Increases as vessels constrict

      (2) Decreases as vessels dilate

    c. High SVR will:

      (1) Decrease blood flow

      (2) Increase myocardial workload

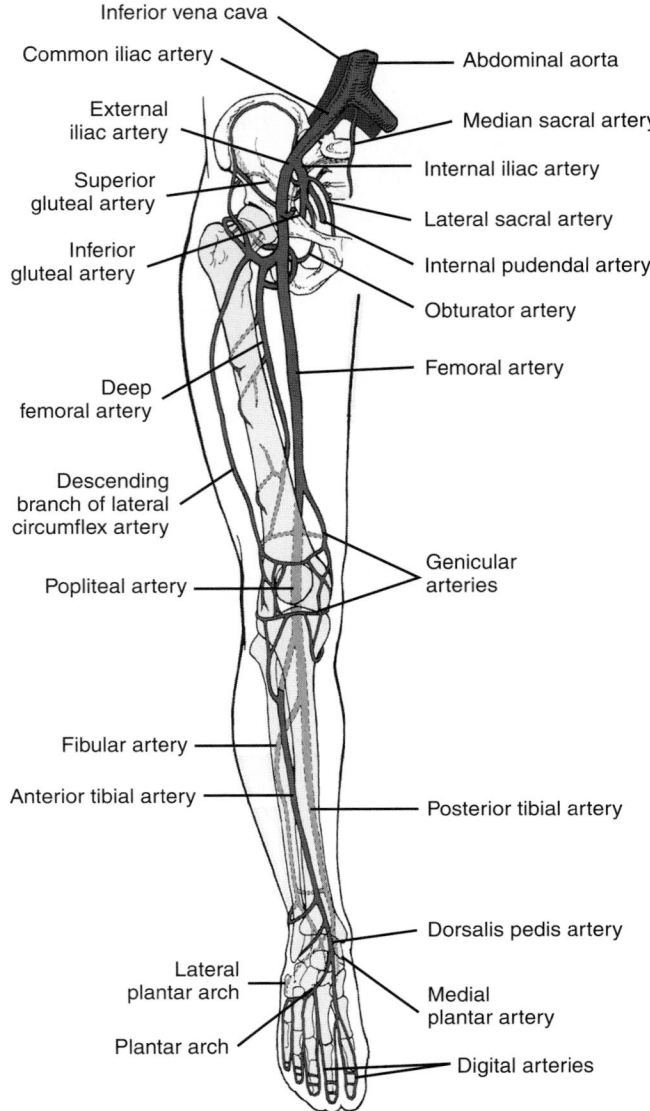

FIGURE 44-7 ■ Major arteries of the lower extremity. (From Rothrock J: *Alexander's care of the patient in surgery,* ed 12, St Louis, 2003, Mosby.)

    3. Vessel wall elasticity
       a. With low compliance, pressure is greater.
       b. Increased pressure will increase myocardial oxygen consumption.
    4. Fluid volume status: low fluid volume will reduce peripheral resistance.
    5. Diameter of vessel (arteriole diameter <0.5 mm)
       a. Vasoconstriction: exposure to cold, vasoconstrictive agents
       b. Vasodilation: exposure to heat, vasodilator agents
    6. Sympathetic nervous system: regulates amount of vasoconstriction
  G. Common sites of vascular disease (Figure 44-10)
    1. Internal carotid arteries
    2. Aorta above inguinal ligament inflow disease
    3. Aortoiliac: bifurcation of aorta and iliac arteries inflow disease

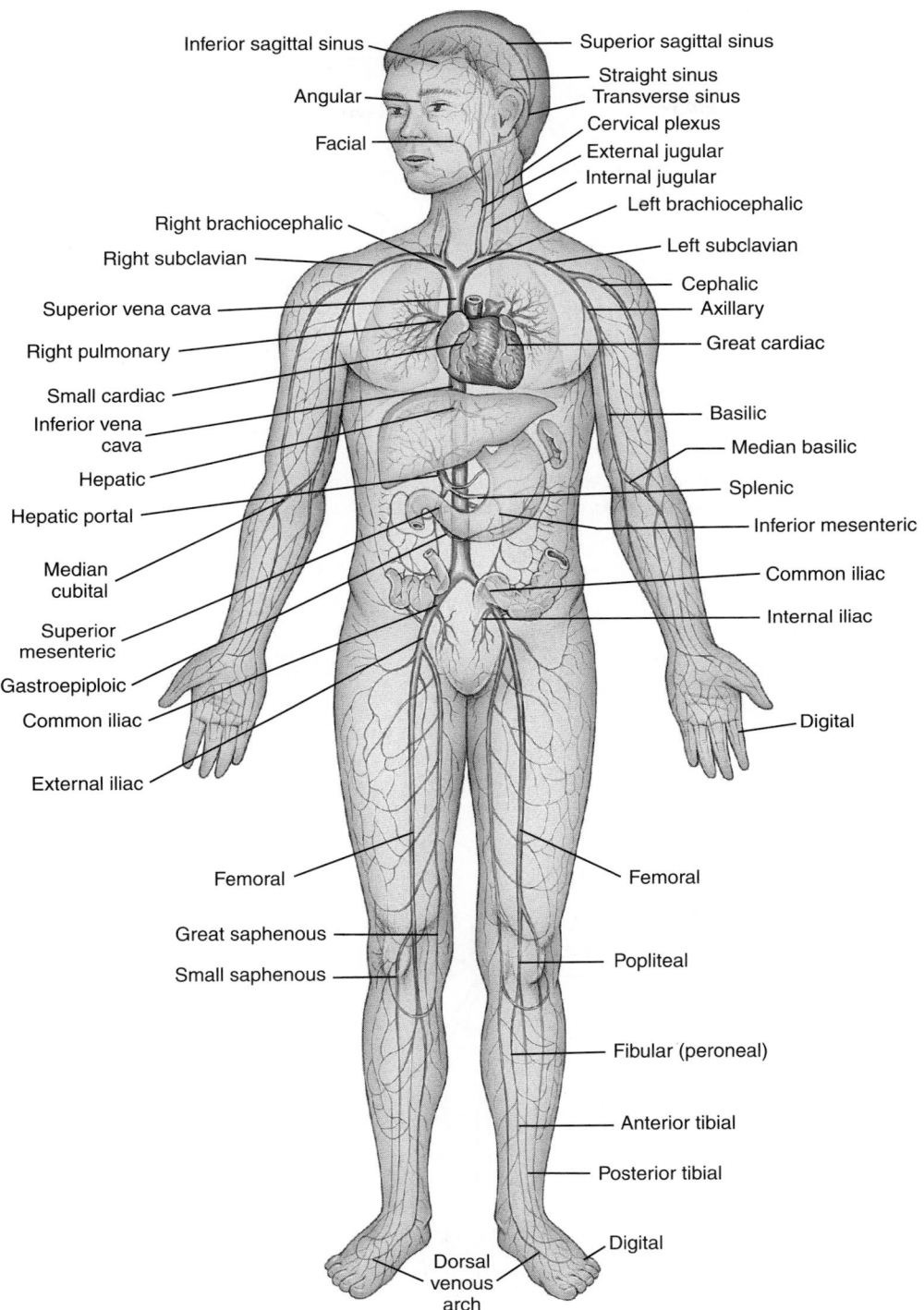

FIGURE 44-8 ■ Principal veins of the body. (From Thibodeau GA, Patton KT: *Anatomy and physiology,* ed 6, St Louis, 2007, Mosby.)

4. Superficial femoral: middle to distal thigh below inguinal ligament outflow disease
5. Popliteal artery outflow disease
6. Tibial arteries: common in patients with diabetes outflow disease

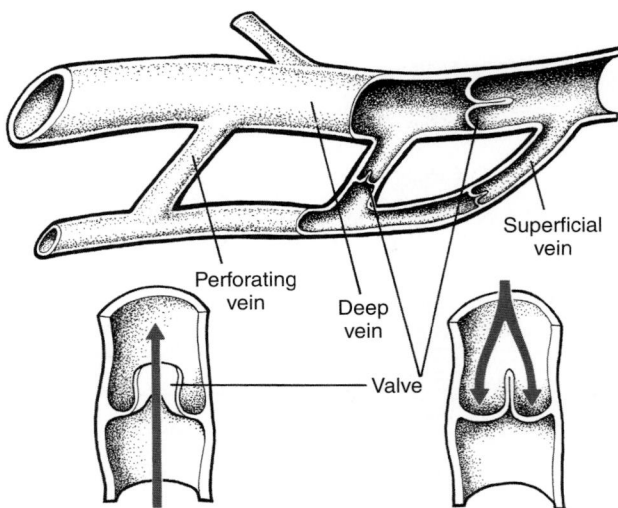

FIGURE 44-9 ■ Anatomy of the venous system of the leg. (From Price SA, Wilson LM: *Pathophysiology: Clinical concepts of disease processes,* ed 6, St Louis, 2003, Mosby.)

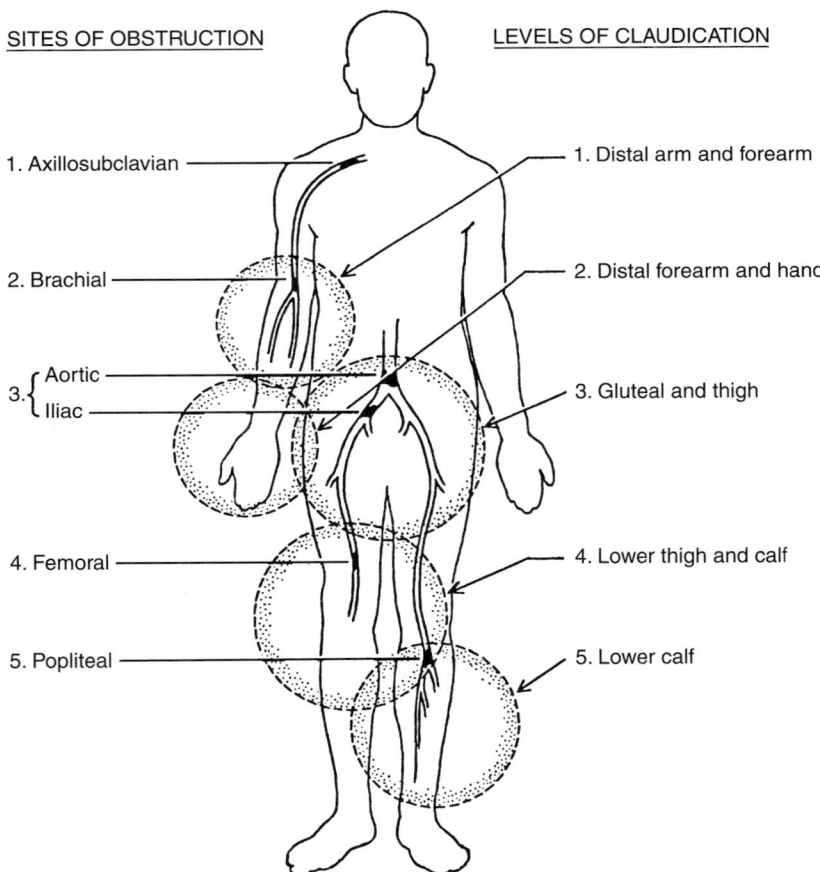

FIGURE 44-10 ■ Sites of arterial obstruction and corresponding levels of claudication. (From Fahey VA: *Vascular nursing,* ed 4, St Louis, 2004, Saunders.)

H. Incidence and risk factors associated with peripheral vascular disease
   1. Highest incidence among elderly, men, persons with diabetes, smokers
   2. Gender
      a. More common in men
      b. Earlier onset in men
      c. Postmenopausal women susceptible
   3. Age
      a. Occurs beyond 30 years of age
      b. Symptoms worsen after 65 years of age.
I. Risk factors of atherosclerosis
   1. Lifestyle habits
      a. Psychophysiologic stress triggers vasoconstriction.
      b. Sedentary; lack of exercise
      c. Smoking (major risk factor) for smokers and passive smoking (environmental tobacco smoke exposure)
         (1) Vasoconstrictive effect of nicotine
         (2) Inhalation of carbon monoxide in cigarette smoke
            (a) Increases carboxyhemoglobin levels (carbon monoxide binds with hemoglobin)
            (b) Impaired oxygen transport
            (c) Hypoxic injury to intimal lining of artery
            (d) Increased platelet aggregation caused by enhanced platelet adhesiveness
      d. Diet
         (1) Hyperlipidemia (hyperlipoproteinemia): accumulation of lipids in arterial wall
            (a) Elevated cholesterol: total serum levels
            (b) Elevated triglycerides
               (i) Low-density lipoproteins (LDL): high serum levels related to premature development of atherosclerotic process
               (ii) High-density lipoproteins (HDL): high serum levels demonstrate protective effect against atherosclerosis.
               (iii) Homocysteine: high serum levels block production of nitric oxide on vascular endothelium, making cell walls less elastic and permitting plaque to build up.
         (2) Obesity
   2. Positive family history
   3. Disease processes
      a. Diabetes mellitus
      b. Hypertension (major risk factor)
J. Indications for surgical intervention
   1. Ischemic pain at rest
   2. Significant limb ischemia
   3. Limiting claudication
II. PATHOPHYSIOLOGY
   A. Arterial occlusive disease
      1. Classified as inflow or outflow above or below inguinal ligament (Figure 44-11)
         a. Inflow obstruction involves distal end of aorta.
            (1) Common iliac arteries
            (2) Internal iliac arteries
            (3) External iliac arteries
         b. Outflow obstruction involves infrainguinal arteries below superficial femoral artery (SFA).
            (1) Femoral arteries
            (2) Popliteal arteries
            (3) Tibial arteries
      2. Obstruction or stenosis of vessel
         a. Decreased peripheral vessel blood flow
         b. Decreased vessel diameter

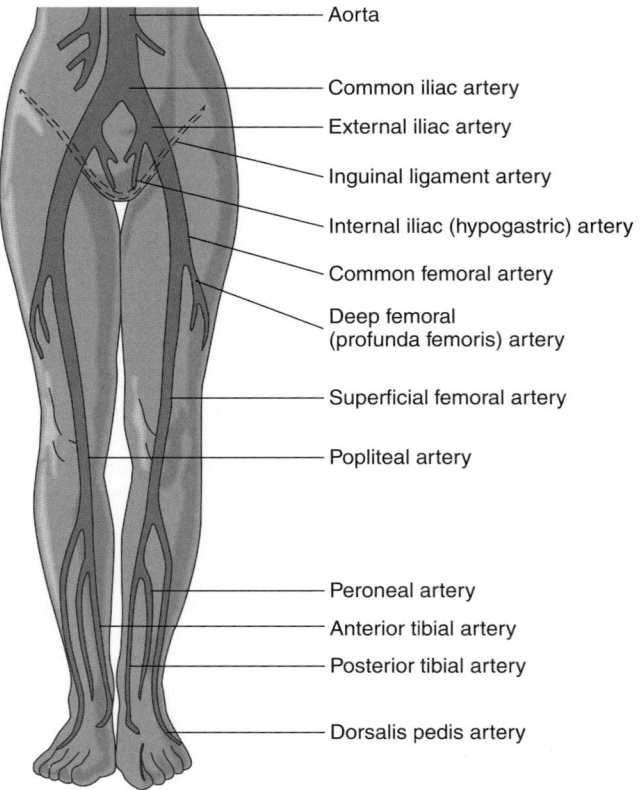

FIGURE 44-11 ■ Common locations of inflow and outflow lesions. (From Ignatavicius DD, Workman L: *Medical-surgical nursing: Critical thinking for collaborative care,* Philadelphia, 2006, Saunders.)

   c. Increased peripheral vascular resistance
   d. Decreased blood flow velocity
  3. Degenerative changes
   a. Reduced tissue oxygen and nutrient supply
    (1) Inadequate tissue integrity
    (2) Ischemic tissue
    (3) Destruction of muscle and elastic fibers
   b. Formation of calcium and/or cholesterol deposits
    (1) Thickening of arterioles
    (2) Loss of elasticity
 B. Venous disease
  1. Deep vein thrombosis (DVT): disease of deep veins of lower extremity, often accompanied by intraluminal clot
  2. Superficial thrombophlebitis: inflammation and clot in superficial veins
  3. Virchow's triad: three factors that increase incidence of venous thrombosis
   a. Hypercoagulability caused by alteration of platelet and clotting factors
   b. Venous stasis caused by incompetent venous valves
   c. Intimal damage caused by trauma, intravenous infusions, ischemia
  4. Pulmonary embolism: dislodged DVT with migration to pulmonary vasculature
  5. Varicose veins
   a. Structural weakness
   b. Vessel tortuosity
   c. Dilation
    (1) Incompetent venous valves
    (2) Reflux of blood results in venous pooling.

     6. Venous hypertension: hereditary

       a. Incompetent valves result in reduced blood return to heart.

       b. Venous stasis and pooling of blood results in venous hypertension.

   C. Arterial insufficiency: arterial occlusive disease

     1. Arteriosclerosis obliterans

       a. Atherosclerosis: most common form of arteriosclerosis obliterans

         (1) Accumulation of lipids and connective tissue

         (2) Intraluminal plaque formation

         (3) Platelet aggregation

         (4) Thrombus formation

         (5) Loss of elasticity

       b. Mönckeberg's arteriosclerosis: arteriosclerosis of peripheral arteries

         (1) Characterized by calcium deposits within medial layer

       c. Arteriolosclerosis: sclerosis of arterioles

     2. Aneurysm: abnormal dilation of vessel wall with high incidence of rupture and mortality when greater than 6 cm in diameter (Figures 44-12, 44-13, and 44-14)

       a. Fusiform: diffuse circumferential dilation of artery

       b. Saccular: area of pouching; affects localized part of arterial wall

       c. Dissecting: intimal layer torn; blood accumulates between layers.

       d. False aneurysm—when palpable hematoma often present, a complete tear of all three layers of arterial wall occurs caused by:

         (1) Trauma

         (2) Needle puncture

         (3) Suture failure at anastomosis site of prosthetic graft

       e. Pseudoaneurysm: dilated or tortuous segment of arterial wall without interruption of layers

       f. Theories of aneurysm pathogenesis (Table 44-1)

   D. Vascular diseases and conditions

     1. Acute

       a. Arterial embolism: sudden onset of symptoms of acute arterial insufficiency

         (1) Originates in myocardium or arterial aneurysm

         (2) May be secondary to external or iatrogenic trauma (catheter placement)

       b. Trauma: arterial wall tear or dissection

     2. Chronic

       a. Diabetes mellitus: medial layer calcification; arteries become noncompressible.

       b. Hypertension: increases permeability of intimal endothelium

       c. Polycythemia: increased blood viscosity caused by increase in red blood cell count

       d. Inflammatory processes: may cause occlusive lesions

         (1) Arteritis: inflammation of arterial wall

           (a) Polyarteritis nodosa (PAN): systemic disease causing arterial inflammation and aneurysm rupture in adults

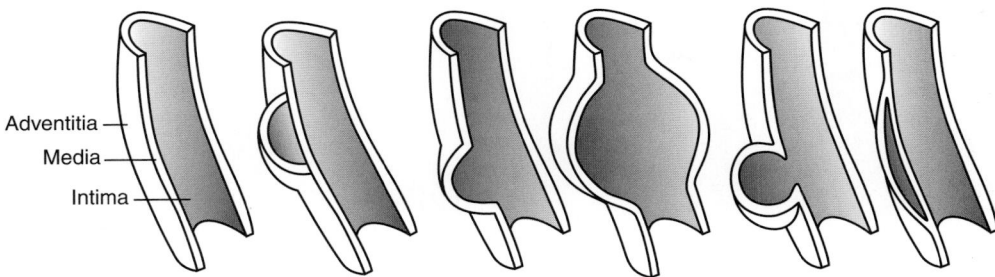

Adventitia
Media
Intima

FIGURE 44-12 ■ Aneurysm types. (From Smeltzer SC, Bare BG: *Brunner and Suddarth's textbook of medical-surgical nursing,* ed 10, Philadelphia, 2004, Lippincott Williams & Wilkins.)

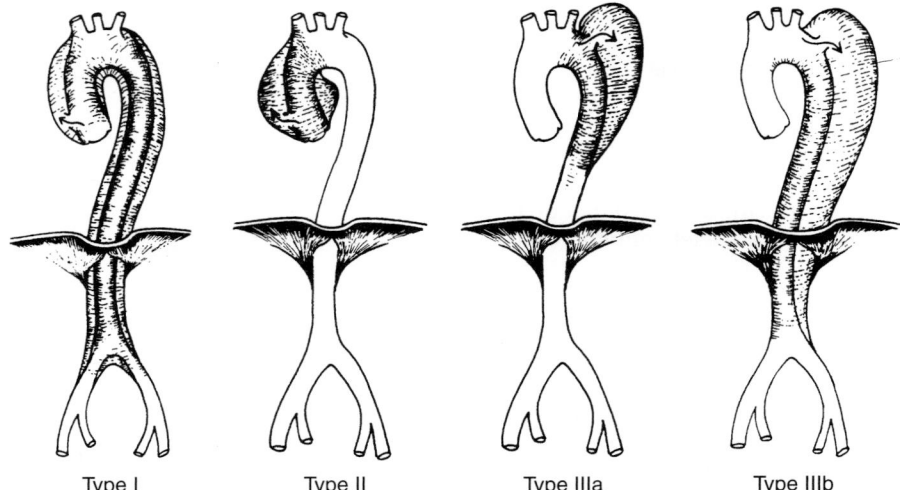

| Type I | Type II | Type IIIa | Type IIIb |

FIGURE 44-13 ■ Two popular classification schemes for aortic dissections. Diagnosis of involvement of ascending aorta has important prognostic and therapeutic implications. DeBakey types I and II are called type A in the Stanford classifications; DeBakey type III is equal to Stanford type B. (From Hamilton IN, Hollier LH: Thoracoabdominal aortic aneurysms. In Moore W, ed: *Vascular surgery: A comprehensive review,* ed 5, Philadelphia, 1998, W.B. Saunders.)

    (b) Kawasaki: similar to PAN; occurs in children
    (c) Cogan's: (rare condition) similar to PAN; inflammatory infiltration of large veins and muscular arteries
    (d) Behcet's: similar to PAN; affects both arteries and veins
    (e) Drug abusers: similar to PAN; necrotizing arteritis (intra-arterial injection of drugs)
  (2) Fibromuscular dysplasia: multiple areas of arterial stenosis and dilation
  (3) Buerger's disease: thromboangiitis obliterans, autoimmune disease
    (a) Inflammation of arterial walls
    (b) Thrombus formation caused by intimal thickening
    (c) Affects plantar and digital vessels
    (d) Pain at rest, extremity cold, cyanotic

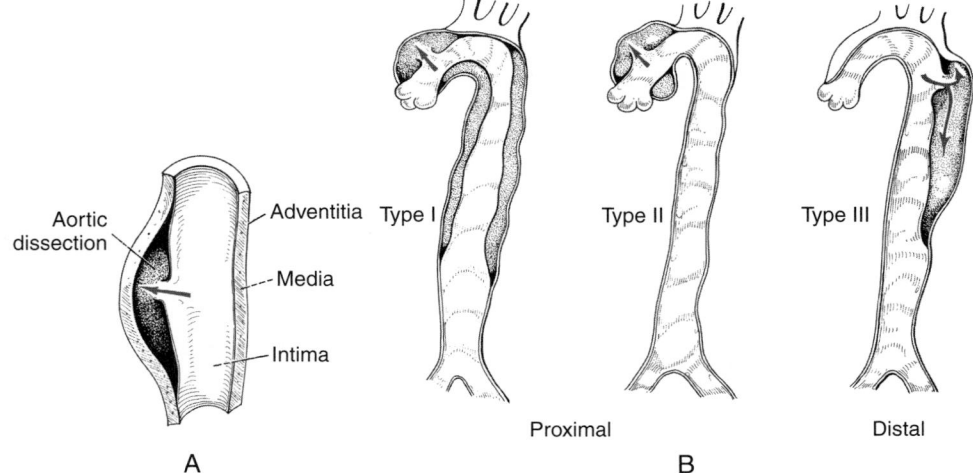

FIGURE 44-14 ■ Aortic dissection. **A,** Separation of vascular layers. **B,** Classification of aortic dissection. (From Price SA, Wilson LM: *Pathophysiology: Clinical concepts of disease processes,* ed 6, St Louis, 2003, Mosby.)

■ TABLE 44-1
■ ■ **Theories of Aneurysm Pathogenesis**

Etiology	Clinical Evidence	Theory
Genetic	Genetically linked enzyme deficiencies are associated with aneurysms. Familial clustering is observed. Male siblings have up to 25% lifetime risk of aneurysm.	X chromosome linked and autosomal dominant inheritance pattern Specific deficits in collagen
Atherosclerotic	Risk factors are similar to occlusive disease including smoking, hypertension, and aging. Aneurysm wall contains calcium and atherosclerotic lesions.	Compensatory dilation of the artery becomes uncontrolled.
Immunologic	A variant called inflammatory aneurysm is characterized by gross inflammation and microscopic leukocyte infiltrates.	Antigen, possibly through molecular mimicry, precipitates autoimmune response.
Degenerative	Disruption of normal aortic wall architecture Decreased amounts of elastin and collagen are found in aneurysms. Hernias are common in patients with aneurysms.	Elastin and collagen are aberrantly formed or digested.
Hemodynamic	Aneurysms typically occur proximal to bifurcations or distal to stenoses.	Wall tension, turbulence, vibration, and shear stress are increased dramatically in these areas.
Iatrogenic	Occur at graft anastomosis, after endarterectomy, angioplasty, or full-thickness traumatic disruption	Structural injury, end-to-side anastomosis
Infectious	*Salmonella, Chlamydia pneumoniae, Streptococcus* species, *Staphylococcus* species, *Treponema pallidum* are associated with aneurysms.	Microorganisms by direct extension, emboli, or infection from unknown primary may stimulate inflammation or degradation.

From Fahey VA: *Vascular nursing,* ed 4, St Louis, 2004, Saunders.

          (4) Granulomatous/giant cell arteritis
              (a) Takayasu's arteritis: transmural inflammatory process
                  (i)   Type I aortic arch and vessels originating from arch
                  (ii)   Type II abdominal aorta and visceral vessels
                  (iii) Type III both the arch and abdominal aorta
                  (iv)   Type IV pulmonary arteries
              (b) Temporal arteritis: thickening of intima, necrosis of media
          (5) Hypersensitivity angiitis: arterial damage from antigen-antibody complexes
       e. Raynaud's phenomenon and Raynaud's disease: vasospastic diseases that are related
          (1) Intense vasospasm of arteries and arterioles of extremities
          (2) Precipitated by exposure to cold
          (3) Ischemic changes: cyanosis, numbness, tingling
          (4) Occurs in 40% of patients with systemic lupus erythematosus, and 90% of patients with scleroderma
          (5) Raynaud's phenomenon occurs unilaterally in both men and women older than 30 years.
          (6) Raynaud's disease occurs bilaterally, mostly in females, between 17 and 50 years of age.
       f. Compartment syndrome: swelling within osteofascial compartments of leg or arm
          (1) Intracompartmental pressure increases from bleeding within the compartment, or external compression from dressings, cast, traumatic crush injury.

(2) Vascular perfusion decreases, compromising tissue.

(3) Ischemia affects nerves and muscles.

    (a) Pain

    (b) Tenseness of compartment

    (c) Paresthesia

    (d) Pulselessness

    (e) Paralysis

    (f) Pallor

III. CLINICAL SIGNS AND SYMPTOMS

  A. Arterial insufficiency

    1. Decreased blood flow may cause inadequate tissue oxygenation distal to lesion.

    2. A 70% to 90% occlusion of a large artery usually must occur before a decrease in blood flow or pressure causes symptoms at rest.

    3. A 60% obstruction may be sufficient to precipitate signs and symptoms during exercise.

    4. Acute

      a. Peripheral pulses diminished, weak, or absent

      b. Cold and pale extremity (sudden onset)

      c. Sudden, severe pain may occur during exercise or at rest: moderate to severe inflow disease.

        (1) Lower back and buttock pain: common iliac or abdominal aorta inflow disease (Figure 44-11)

        (2) Thigh pain at or above profunda femoris artery

      d. Limited sensory and motor function

        (1) Possible paresthesia

        (2) Atrophied skeletal muscle: restricted limb movement

      e. Minimal edema: usually unilateral

      f. Bruit present with partial occlusion; no bruit with total occlusion

    5. Chronic

      a. Diminished or weak distal pulses outflow disease (see Figure 44-11)

        (1) Below SFA

        (2) Popliteal artery

      b. Pain at rest related to severe ischemia: burning or cramping in calves, ankles, feet, toes

      c. Tissue necrosis: gangrene

      d. Intermittent claudication

      e. Skin

        (1) Skin ulceration

        (2) Delayed healing of skin lesions

        (3) Skin texture: thin, shiny, dry

        (4) Cool skin: poikilothermic

      f. Color: pale extremity

        (1) Increased pallor when elevated

        (2) Rubor or cyanosis or both when dependent

      g. Possible paresthesia of limb

      h. Edema: none or mild

        (1) Hair loss distal to occlusion

      i. Nails: thick, brittle

      j. Impotence: associated with aortoiliac disease

  B. Venous insufficiency

    1. Acute

      a. Moderate pain localized to area of inflammation

      b. Pulses present or diminished (absent in presence of concomitant disease)

      c. Skin warm, cyanotic, mottled, or pale

      d. Engorged veins when legs slightly dependent

      e. Moderate to severe peripheral edema

2. Chronic
   a. Minimal to moderate pain
   b. Moderate to severe edema, unilateral or bilateral
   c. Sensation of heaviness at site of occlusion
   d. Muscle cramps, aching
   e. Ulceration of ankle area
   f. Superficial veins may be prominent.
   g. Skin
      (1) Warm
      (2) Brawny (reddish brown) color
      (3) Pronounced lower leg pigmentation
      (4) Texture: thickening, scaling, and/or scarring

IV. DIAGNOSTIC ASSESSMENT
   A. Arterial tests
      1. Noninvasive laboratory studies
         a. Segmental pressure measurement: measurement of systolic blood pressure along selected segments of each extremity
            (1) Gradient >20 mm Hg: evidence of arterial stenosis in lower extremity
            (2) Gradient >10 mm Hg: evidence of arterial stenosis in upper extremity
         b. Ankle/brachial index (ABI): ratio of ankle to brachial pressure (normal ABI, ≥1.0)
            (1) One limitation is calcified vessels as in renal failure or diabetes.
         c. Toe pressure measurements: assess distal arterial flow.
            (1) Useful in diabetics with calcification of larger vessels
         d. Pulse volume recording: quantifies arterial flow to determine location of lesion and severity.
         e. Doppler ultrasound: determines blood flow and velocity
         f. B-mode ultrasonography: projects two-dimensional image in real time
         g. Duplex ultrasound imaging: assesses both anatomic characteristics and stenosis of peripheral arteries; combination of Doppler and B-mode ultrasonogram
         h. Air plethysmography (APG) and photoplethysmography: record volume changes in limb
         i. Treadmill exercise testing: objective evidence of walking capacity and evaluation of peripheral stenosis
         j. Computed tomography (CT): a tomograph is an image of a cross-sectional slice of a body part.
            (1) CT image is three dimensional: a camera rotates around selected body part taking two-dimensional images at multiple angles, which are converted to a composite three-dimensional image by a computer.
            (2) Contrast material (usually iodine) injected to heighten contrast between vessel wall and blood
            (3) Used for diagnosis of aortic aneurysms and aortic dissection
            (4) Able to detect hematomas or thrombi better with CT than with arteriography
         k. Magnetic resonance imaging: detailed and three-dimensional imaging of vessel lumen where contrast not needed; contraindicated in patients with pacemakers and cerebral aneurysm clips
         l. Magnetic resonance angiography: has replaced angiography for severe carotid stenosis and the lower extremities; uses intravenous gadolinium; no arterial puncture required
      2. Invasive laboratory studies
         a. Arteriography: invasive radiographic procedure in which radiopaque contrast injected into artery
         b. Transcatheter therapy: percutaneous transluminal angioplasty, stenting, lyse clot, therapeutic embolization
            (1) Purposes
               (a) Depict location of stenosis, occlusion, or view aneurysm

        (b) Visualize collateral, proximal, and distal arterial circulation to determine surgical treatment options

     (2) Complications

        (a) Intimal disruption

           (i) Hematoma formation at puncture site

           (ii) Plaque dislodgement

           (iii) Arterial occlusion: thrombosis

           (iv) Distal embolization

           (v) Arteriovenous (AV) fistula

           (vi) Arterial dissection

           (vii) Renal failure

        (b) Transient ischemic attack (TIA) or cerebrovascular accident (CVA)

        (c) Toxic reaction to contrast media: renal or cardiac

        (d) Allergic reaction

           (i) Rash

           (ii) Bronchospasm

           (iii) Altered consciousness

           (iv) Convulsions

           (v) Anaphylaxis

           (vi) Cardiac arrest

     (3) Postarteriography assessment and intervention

        (a) Assessment

           (i) Vital signs

           (ii) Hematoma and/or bleeding at puncture site

           (iii) Signs and symptoms of acute arterial insufficiency

              [a] Skin: color, temperature

              [b] Pulses distal to puncture site

              [c] Pain

              [d] Urinary output

              [e] Neurologic status

              [f] Signs of heart failure or respiratory distress

        (b) Intervention

           (i) Observe for rash.

           (ii) Maintain adequate hydration to flush contrast.

           (iii) Head of bed at 30° or less

           (iv) Keep affected extremity straight for 4 to 6 hours after procedure.

           (v) Wait a minimum of 4 hours to resume heparin if previously receiving heparin.

B. Venous tests

  1. Noninvasive laboratory studies

    a. Venous Doppler ultrasonography examinations: used to determine blood flow patterns and velocity

      (1) During inspiration, intrathoracic pressure decreases and venous return to heart increases.

      (2) During expiration, venous flow to lower extremities will increase.

    b. APG

      (1) Used to evaluate venous obstruction, reflux, and calf muscle pump function

      (2) Able to differentiate deep and superficial venous insufficiency

    c. Duplex imaging of valvular closing times indicates severity of venous reflux.

    d. Arm/foot pressure gradient measures outflow obstruction: normal difference between arm and foot is <4 mm Hg.

  2. Invasive testing

    a. Ascending phlebography: used to assess venous patency

    b. Descending phlebography: used to assess valvular function

V. GENERAL SYSTEMS ASSESSMENT OF VASCULAR PATIENTS
  A. Cardiovascular (see Chapter 32)
    1. Myocardial infarction remains leading cause of death after peripheral vascular procedures because of coexisting cardiovascular disease.
  B. Evaluation of cardiac status
    1. Hemodynamic profile: cardiac output, SVR
    2. Electrocardiogram: dysrhythmias
      a. Increased myocardial oxygen demands
      b. Increased cardiac ischemia: angina
    3. Signs and symptoms of myocardial infarction
      a. Chest pain
      b. Dysrhythmias
      c. Diaphoresis
      d. Nausea and vomiting
      e. Dyspnea
      f. Hypotension
    4. Chest x-ray film to assess heart size and fluid status
    5. Cardiac enzymes
      a. Creatine Kinase (CK)
      b. CK-MB isoenzyme
      c. Troponin T (cTnT) and troponin I (cTnI)
      d. Myoglobin never used alone but in conjunction with cardiac-specific markers
    6. Serum electrolytes
      a. Hyperkalemia
        (1) Oliguric renal failure
        (2) Volume depletion
        (3) Decreased effect of aldosterone: Addison's disease, chronic heparin administration
      b. Hypokalemia
        (1) Diuretic or digitalis therapy
        (2) Stress
        (3) Gastrointestinal disorders
          (a) Long-term steroid therapy: arthritis, chronic obstructive pulmonary disease (COPD)
          (b) Hypoaldosteronism
      c. Hypernatremia
        (1) Mechanical ventilation without humidification
        (2) Fever
      d. Hyponatremia
        (1) Diuretics
        (2) Gastrointestinal disorders
        (3) Hypotonic irrigating solutions
        (4) Hyperlipidemia
        (5) Hyperglycemia
      e. Hypermagnesemia
        (1) Renal failure
        (2) Adrenal insufficiency
        (3) Shock
        (4) Hypothermia
      f. Hypomagnesemia
        (1) Excessive loss of body fluids
        (2) Diuretics
        (3) Cardiac glycosides, aminoglycosides
        (4) Decreased intestinal absorption
        (5) Primary hyperaldosteronism
        (6) Hypercalcemia associated with hyperparathyroidism and hyperthyroidism
        (7) ECG reflects prolonged QT interval, decreased T-wave amplitude, shortened ST segment.

C. Accompanying cardiovascular disorders
   1. Hypertension
      a. High incidence (40%-60%) associated with peripheral vascular disease (PVD)
      b. Adds stress to anastomotic sites
      c. Precipitates postoperative incisional bleeding
   2. Hypotension
      a. Decreases cerebral, coronary, and renal artery perfusion
      b. Decreases stroke volume: decreased cardiac output
   3. Valvular disease: associated with decreased cardiac output and left ventricular failure
      a. Mitral valve stenosis: associated with pulmonary fibrosis and hypertension
      b. Aortic insufficiency: associated with circulatory collapse with sudden hypotension
D. Pulmonary status (see Chapter 41)
   1. Baseline parameters
      a. Respirations
         (1) Rate, quality
         (2) Pattern, excursion
      b. Auscultation of lungs
         (1) Wheezes
         (2) Rales
         (3) Rhonchi
         (4) Crackles
      c. Arterial blood gases (ABGs), mixed venous oxygen saturation (Svo_2) monitoring
      d. Pulmonary function studies
         (1) Forced vital capacity (FVC)
            (a) Measurement of volume of air expelled by fully inflated lung
            (b) Compromised FVC indicative of lung parenchymal restriction
         (2) Forced expiratory volume (FEV)
            (a) Decreased FEV indicative of impaired elastic recoil (emphysema)
            (b) Increased FEV indicative of airway resistance (chronic bronchitis or asthma)
         (3) Ventilation-to-perfusion ratio
      e. Chest x-ray film
         (1) Pulmonary infiltrate or lesion
         (2) Heart size
         (3) Congestive heart failure (CHF)
         (4) Fibrosis or effusion
   2. Pulmonary history
      a. Obstructive disorders (COPD, emphysema, asthma)
      b. Infections (bronchitis, tuberculosis)
      c. Presence of cough (lesions, smoking, bronchitis)
      d. Complaints of shortness of breath
      e. Orthopnea
E. Neurologic status (see Chapter 33)
   1. Postoperative assessment: compare with preoperative baseline.
      a. Level of consciousness
      b. Pupillary reactions
      c. Sensory and motor ability
      d. Evaluation of following cranial nerves
         (1) Facial (VIII): controls facial muscles; affects ability to smile, show teeth, wrinkle forehead, raise eyebrows
         (2) Hypoglossal (XII): most frequently traumatized; controls tongue; affects side-to-side motion of tongue
         (3) Glossopharyngeal (IX): controls posterior third of tongue, uvula; affects gag reflex
         (4) Vagus (X): controls pharynx, larynx, soft palate; affects gag reflex

          (5) Spinal accessory (XI): controls trapezius and sternocleidomastoid muscles; affects strength and tone of shoulder muscles
          (6) Phrenic nerve: controls diaphragm; affects diaphragmatic function in respiratory excursion
  2. Neurological history
    a. Vertigo
    b. Syncope
    c. TIA
    d. CVA
    e. Spinal cord ischemia with descending thoracic aorta repair

F. Renal status (see Chapter 37)
  1. Preoperative baseline studies
    a. Blood urea nitrogen
    b. Creatinine
    c. Electrolytes
    d. Calcium
    e. Phosphorus
    f. Urinalysis
  2. Specific renal function studies, if indicated
    a. Osmolar, free water, and sodium clearances
    b. Creatinine or insulin clearance to evaluate glomerular filtration
    c. Para-aminohippurate clearance to evaluate renal blood flow
    d. Postangiographic renal function to evaluate possibility of renal failure caused by radioactive dye
  3. Compromised renal system during vascular surgery caused by:
    a. Hemorrhage
    b. Trauma
    c. Renal vessel damage, tubular damage
    d. Anoxia
    e. Prolonged hypotension

G. Diabetes (see Chapter 34)
  1. Relationship to PVD
    a. High incidence of occurrence in patients with PVD
    b. Higher incidence of postoperative complications
    c. Altered fluid requirements
  2. Management of diabetes in a surgical patient (insulin regimen dependent on institutional policy)
    a. Preoperative dose: usually less than routine daily dose
    b. Stress of surgery with release of epinephrine and glucocorticoids increases need for insulin.
    c. Diet-controlled diabetics may require insulin in immediate postoperative period.
  3. Laboratory assessment
    a. Fasting glucose levels
    b. Electrolyte series
    c. Serum ketones and acetones
    d. Renal function studies
    e. ABGs

H. Hematologic evaluation (see Chapter 29)
  1. Laboratory studies
    a. Prothrombin time, partial thromboplastin time
    b. D-dimer assay
    c. Platelet count
    d. Bleeding time, clotting time
    e. Type and crossmatch
    f. Complete blood count
  2. Anticoagulant and antiplatelet aggregation medications
    a. Heparin (sodium warfarin, Coumadin)
    b. Aspirin

    c. Dipyridamole (Persantine)

    d. Ticlopidine (Ticlid)

    e. Clopidogrel (Plavix)

    f. Pentoxifylline (Trental) decreases blood viscosity and increases erythrocyte flexibility.

    g. Cilostazol (Pletal) inhibits platelet aggregation and increases vasodilation.

  3. Previous postoperative bleeding and clotting problems

    a. Disseminated intravascular coagulopathy

    b. Blood transfusion reactions

    c. Thrombophlebitis

    d. Pulmonary emboli

    e. History of any postoperative bleeding

VI. OPERATIVE PROCEDURES

  A. Endarterectomy (Figure 44-15)

    1. Opening of occluded portion of artery

    2. Removal of atheromatous material or plaque

    3. Excision of artery's intimal lining

    4. Performed on carotid, subclavian, iliac, or femoral artery

  B. Carotid-subclavian bypass

    1. Anastomosis of carotid and subclavian arteries to improve circulation

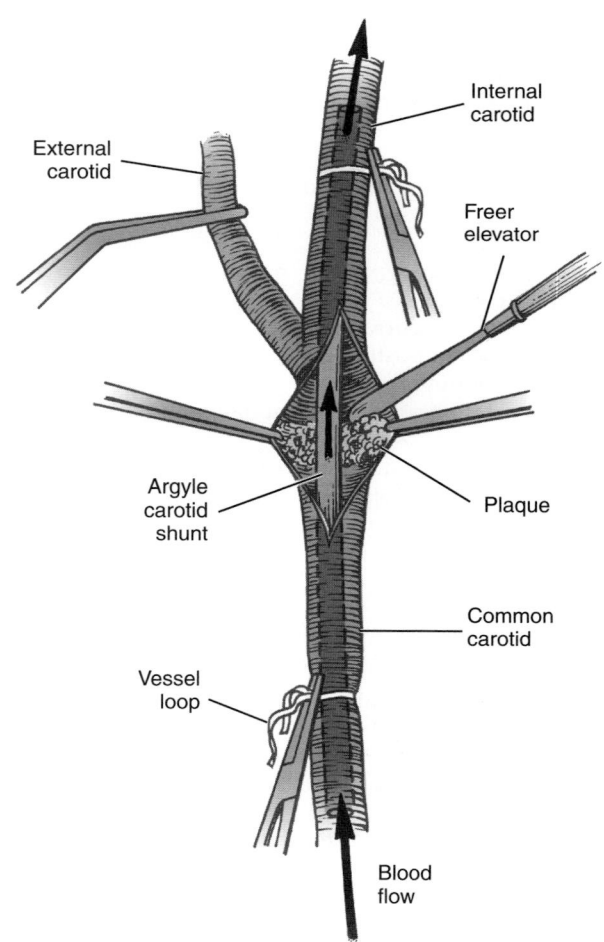

FIGURE 44-15 ■ Left carotid endarterectomy. Argyle carotid shunt in place to allow flow to the brain. Stenotic plaque being removed with Freer elevator. (From Rothrock JC, McEwen DR: *Alexander's care of the patient in surgery,* ed 13, St Louis, 2007, Mosby.)

   2. Common carotid used as donor for subclavian lesions
   3. Subclavian used to restore circulation for carotid lesions
C. Aortocarotid-subclavian bypass
   1. Insertion of bypass graft from ascending aorta into carotid or subclavian artery
   2. For occlusive lesions of both common carotid or innominate and subclavian arteries
D. Carotid artery ligation
   1. Surgical occlusion of carotid artery
   2. Temporary control of hemorrhaging during intracranial vessel surgery
   3. Permanent control of intracranial or nasal hemorrhaging
   4. Treatment of carotid-cavernous fistula
E. Aorto-innominate-subclavian bypass: thoracic aortic graft into innominate, subclavian arteries
F. Aneurysmectomy
   1. Excision of weakened dilated area of artery
   2. Insertion of synthetic prosthesis to reestablish circulatory continuity
   3. Usually occurring in abdominal aorta, thoracic aorta, or carotid, popliteal, or femoral artery
G. Thoracoabdominal aortic aneurysm repair
   1. Clots removed before anastomosis of Dacron graft
   2. Spinal catheter placed at L1 to L2 to allow for cerebrospinal fluid (CSF) drainage
   3. Spinal cord ischemia evaluated by monitoring CSF pressure
H. Bypass approaches for aortoiliac occlusions (Figure 44-16)
   1. Aortoiliac bypass: insertion of vascular graft from distal aorta into iliac artery or arteries
   2. Aortofemoral bypass (Figure 44-17)
   3. Anastomosis of distal aorta to femoral arteries
   4. Lesion bypassed with vascular graft
I. Axillofemoral bypass (Figure 44-18)
   1. Superficial flank placement
   2. Anastomosis of prosthetic graft from one axillary artery to one or both femoral arteries
   3. Restores blood flow beyond occlusive lesion
J. Femorofemoral bypass: femoral crossover graft (Figure 44-19)
   1. Extra-anatomic bypass procedure with subcutaneous placement across suprapubic area
   2. End-to-side anastomosis from patent femoral to stenotic femoral artery
   3. Diverts blood flow from one donor femoral artery to recipient stenotic artery
K. Aortorenal bypass: anastomosis of abdominal aorta to renal artery with vascular graft
L. Femoropopliteal bypass
   1. Establishes adequate circulation to leg and foot through popliteal artery and branches
   2. Graft used for superficial femoral artery occlusion
M. Femorotibial bypass
   1. Autogenous saphenous vein graft from common femoral artery to proximal anterior tibial artery
   2. Procedure indicated for superficial femoral and popliteal artery occlusion
N. Angioplasty: percutaneous insertion of balloon-tipped catheter to dilate areas of localized vessel stenosis has major limitations—recurrence restenosis within 1 year.
O. Vena cava ligation
   1. Partial or total surgical occlusion of vena cava to prevent emboli from entering pulmonary vasculature (Figure 44-20)
   2. Common ligation sites
      a. Superficial femoral
      b. Inferior vena cava below renal veins

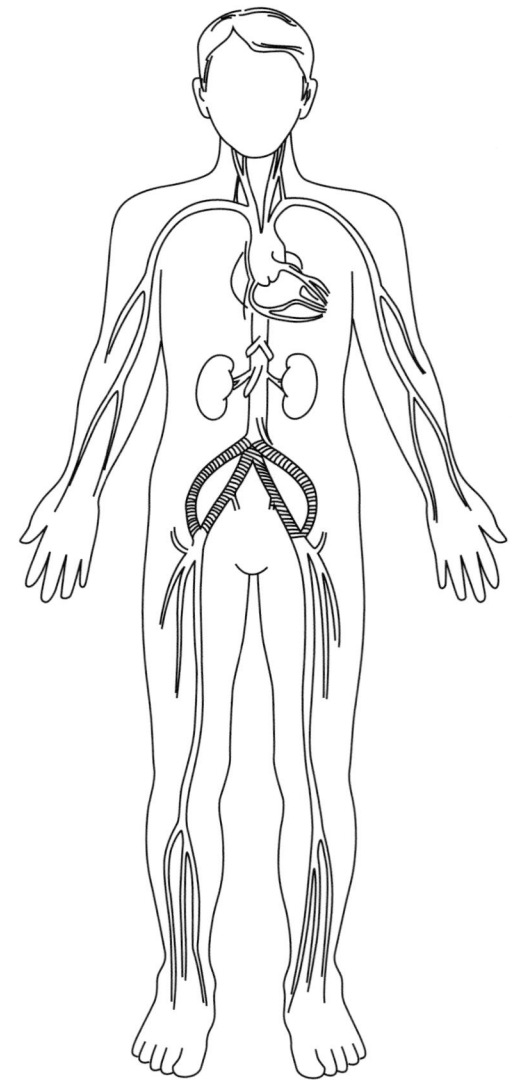

FIGURE 44-16 ■ Aortoiliac occlusion and graft: aortobifemoral bypass. (From Kinney MR, Dunbar SB, Brooks-Brunn JA, et al: *AACN's clinical reference for critical care nursing*, ed 4, St Louis, 1998, Mosby.)

P. Vena caval umbrella filter
   1. Insertion of intravascular device through jugular or femoral vein to occlude inferior vena cava (Figure 44-21)
   2. Prevents emboli from entering pulmonary vessels
   3. Risk of developing deep vein thrombosis
Q. Vein ligation and stripping: surgical ligation and removal of varicose vein(s) of leg(s)
R. Sympathectomy
   1. Interruption of some portion of sympathetic nervous system pathway
   2. Causes vasodilation, improvement in circulation to extremity
   3. Treatment of partial arterial obstruction with resultant distal trophic changes
S. Interventional radiology
   1. Catheter-directed thrombolysis
   2. Urokinase enzyme produced from human neonatal kidney tissue cells, lysis faster than streptokinase
   3. Streptokinase has a high rate of allergic reactions.

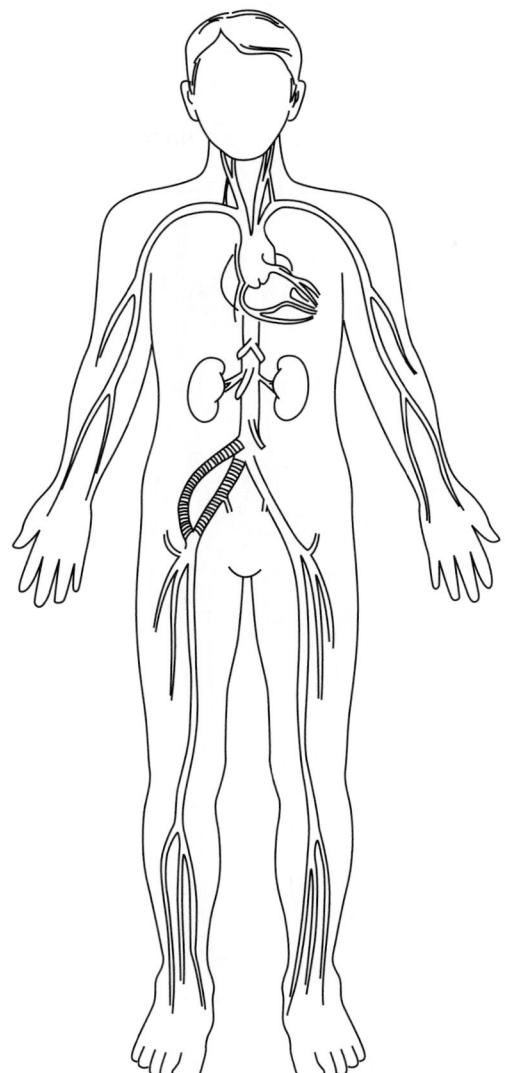

FIGURE 44-17 ■ Right iliac artery occlusion and graft: aortofemoral bypass. (From Kinney MR, Dunbar SB, Brooks-Brunn JA, et al: *AACN's clinical reference for critical care nursing,* ed 4, St Louis, 1998, Mosby.)

    4. Recombinant tissue plasminogen activator (rtPA)
    5. Alteplase weak plasminogen
    6. Reteplase plasminogen activator penetrates and destroys fiber in matrix.
    7. Platelet inhibitors: abciximab (ReoPro), tirofiban (Aggrastat), eptifibatide (Integrilin)
T. Percutaneous mechanical thrombectomy used in combination with thrombolytics
U. AV fistula
    1. Long-term vascular access for hemodialysis
    2. Primary AV fistula directly connects an artery and a vein via anastomosis (Figure 44-22).
        a. Endogenous connection of an artery and a vein via anastomosis (Figure 44-23)
            (1) Radial artery to cephalic vein (Figure 44-24)
            (2) Ulnar artery to basilic vein
            (3) Brachial artery to basilic or cephalic vein
        b. Graft fistula anastomosis of a conduit between an artery and a vein (Figure 44-25)

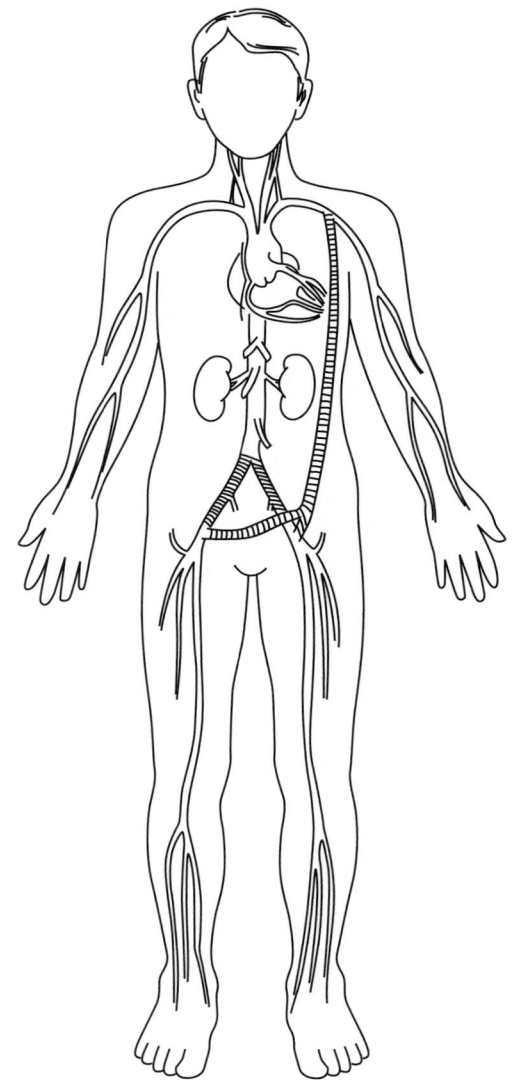

FIGURE 44-18 ■ Left iliac artery occlusion and graft: right-to-left femorofemoral prosthetic bypass graft. (From Kinney MR, Dunbar SB, Brooks-Brunn JA, et al: *AACN's clinical reference for critical care nursing,* ed 4, St Louis, 1998, Mosby.)

V. Endovascular surgery: minimally invasive treatment for vascular diseases
    1. Requires appropriate screening, of lesion type and location
    2. Percutaneous transluminal angioplasty: dilation of vessel with a balloon
    3. Transcatheter therapy endovascular graft, stent placement (Figures 44-26 and 44-27)
    4. Coronary, drug-eluting stents versus bare metal stents in lower extremity lesions are promising, but there needs to be more research and elimination of restenosis.
    5. Two other promising technologies
        a. Tiny razor (Silver Hawk) threaded through a catheter shaves off plaque.
        b. Cryoplasty is angioplasty with freezing nitrous oxide.
    6. Angiogenesis growth factors: intra-arterial infusions of vascular endothelial growth factor and fibroblast growth factor; much further study remains
W. Intrathoracic vascular procedures: thoracoabdominal aneurysm (Figure 44-28)
    1. Lung deflation during procedure
        a. To protect lung from injury
        b. For adequate exposure to operative site

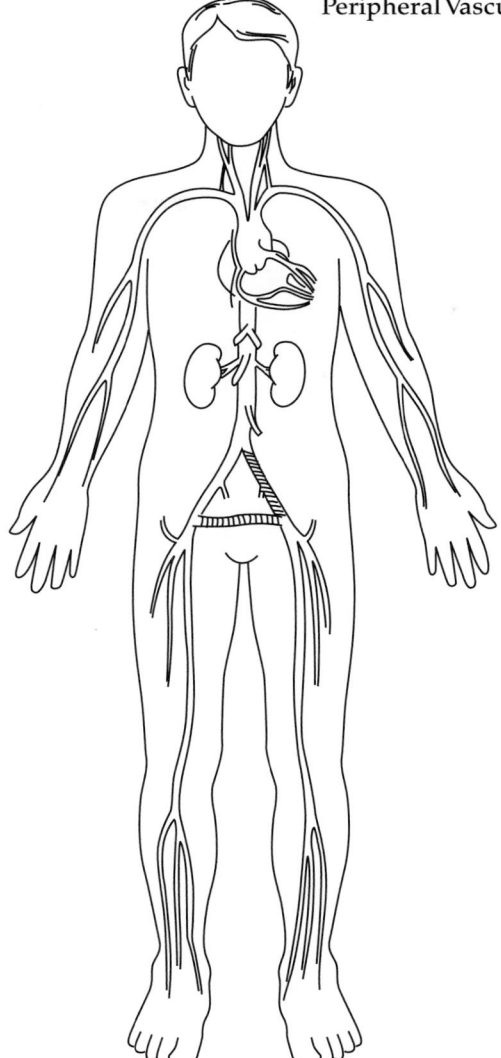

FIGURE 44-19 ■ Aortoiliac occlusion with extra-anatomic graft: left axillofemorofemoral bypass. (From Kinney MR, Dunbar SB, Brooks-Brunn JA, et al: *AACN's clinical reference for critical care nursing,* ed 4, St Louis, 1998, Mosby.)

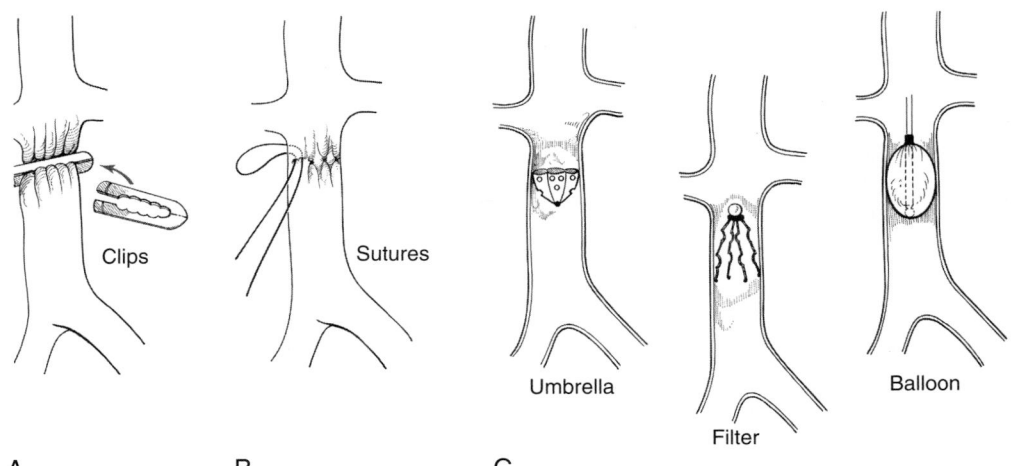

FIGURE 44-20 ■ Vena caval interruption techniques. **A,** Clipping. **B,** Suturing. **C,** Transvenous devices. (Modified from Moore WS: *Vascular surgery: A comprehensive review,* ed 3, Philadelphia, 1991, Saunders. In Price SA, Wilson LM: *Pathophysiology: Clinical concepts of disease processes,* ed 6, St Louis, 2003, Mosby.)

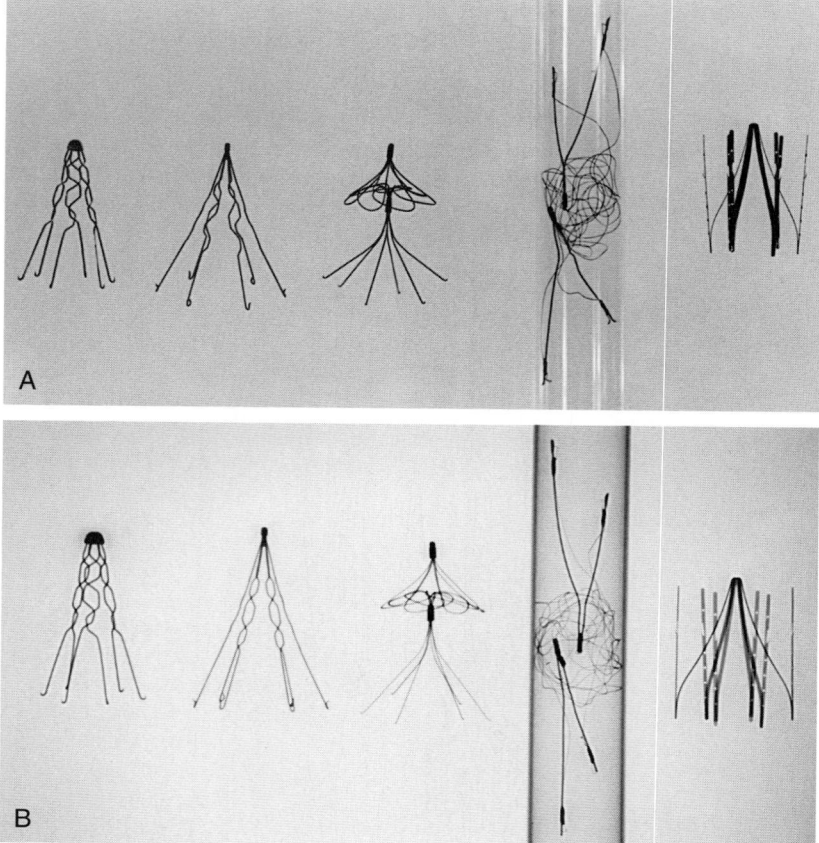

FIGURE 44-21 ■ Vena cava filters. **A,** Actual filters. **B,** Radiographic images. *Left to right,* Kimray-Greenfield, titanium Greenfield, Simon nitinol, Gianturco bird's nest, and Vena Tech. (From Ballinger PW: *Merrill's atlas of radiographic positions and radiologic procedures,* vol 2, ed 8, St Louis, 1995, Mosby.)

    2. Use of extracorporeal circulation, depending on location of lesion
    3. Use of hypothermia and/or temporary shunts to minimize organ ischemia
    4. Intraoperative complications
      a. CVA
      b. Pneumothorax, hemothorax
      c. Myocardial injury
      d. Severe hypotension
      e. Renal failure
      f. Spinal cord ischemia
X. Abdominal vessel procedures: abdominal aortic aneurysm repair
    1. Bowel preparation
      a. Decreases incidence of ischemic bowel injury
      b. Minimizes postoperative ileus
    2. Anesthesia choices
      a. Spinal and epidural for elective lower abdominal procedures
        (1) Advantages
          (a) Elimination of vasospasm
          (b) Reduction of respiratory complications

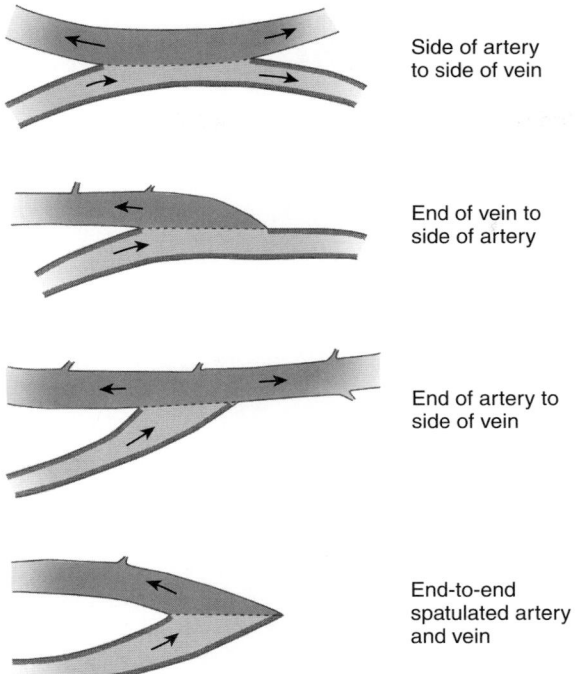

Side of artery
to side of vein

End of vein to
side of artery

End of artery to
side of vein

End-to-end
spatulated artery
and vein

FIGURE 44-22 ■ Four types of anastomoses between radial artery and cephalic vein. (From Wilson SE: *Vascular access: Principles and practice,* ed 3, St Louis, 1996, Mosby.)

(2) Disadvantages
    (a) Positional discomfort if procedure prolonged
    (b) Anxiety increases tachycardia, dysrhythmias.
    (c) Prolonged decreased sensory and motor function
b. General anesthesia (as previously outlined)

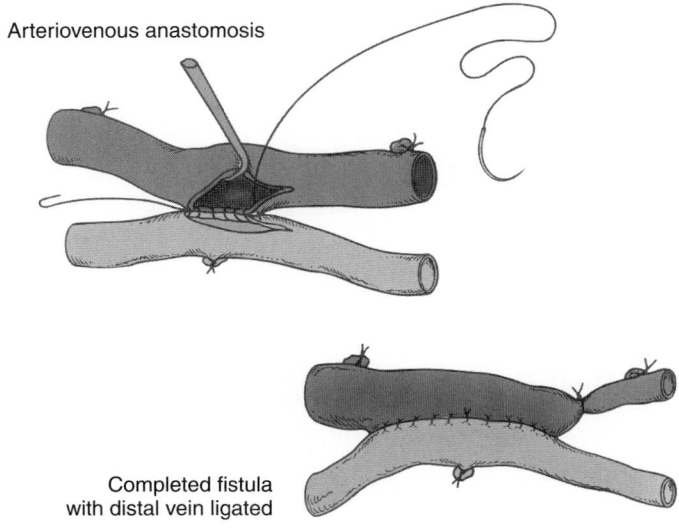

Arteriovenous anastomosis

Completed fistula
with distal vein ligated

FIGURE 44-23 ■ Arteriovenous anastomosis. The artery is anastomosed to the vein. (From Calne R, Pollard SG: *Operative surgery,* London, 1992, Gower.)

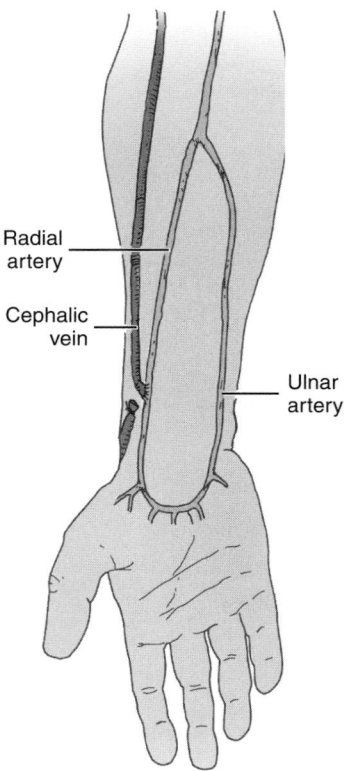

FIGURE 44-24 ■ End of the cephalic vein anastomosed to the side of the radial artery at a site superior to the usual location of the radiocephalic fistula. This technique can be useful if the distal radial artery is small or the cephalic vein at the wrist is thrombosed. (From Wilson SE: *Vascular access: Principles and practice,* ed 3, St Louis, 1996, Mosby.)

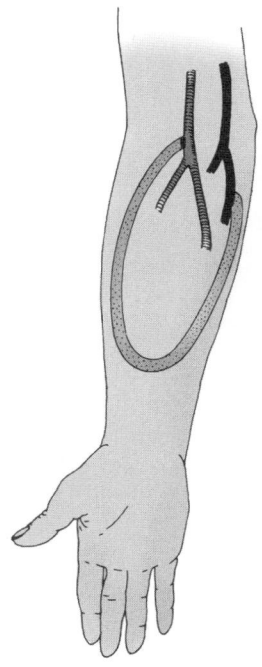

FIGURE 44-25 ■ An example of a loop fistula. A synthetic graft has been used to create a loop brachiocephalic fistula. (From Wilson SE: *Vascular access: Principles and practice,* ed 3, St Louis, 1996, Mosby.)

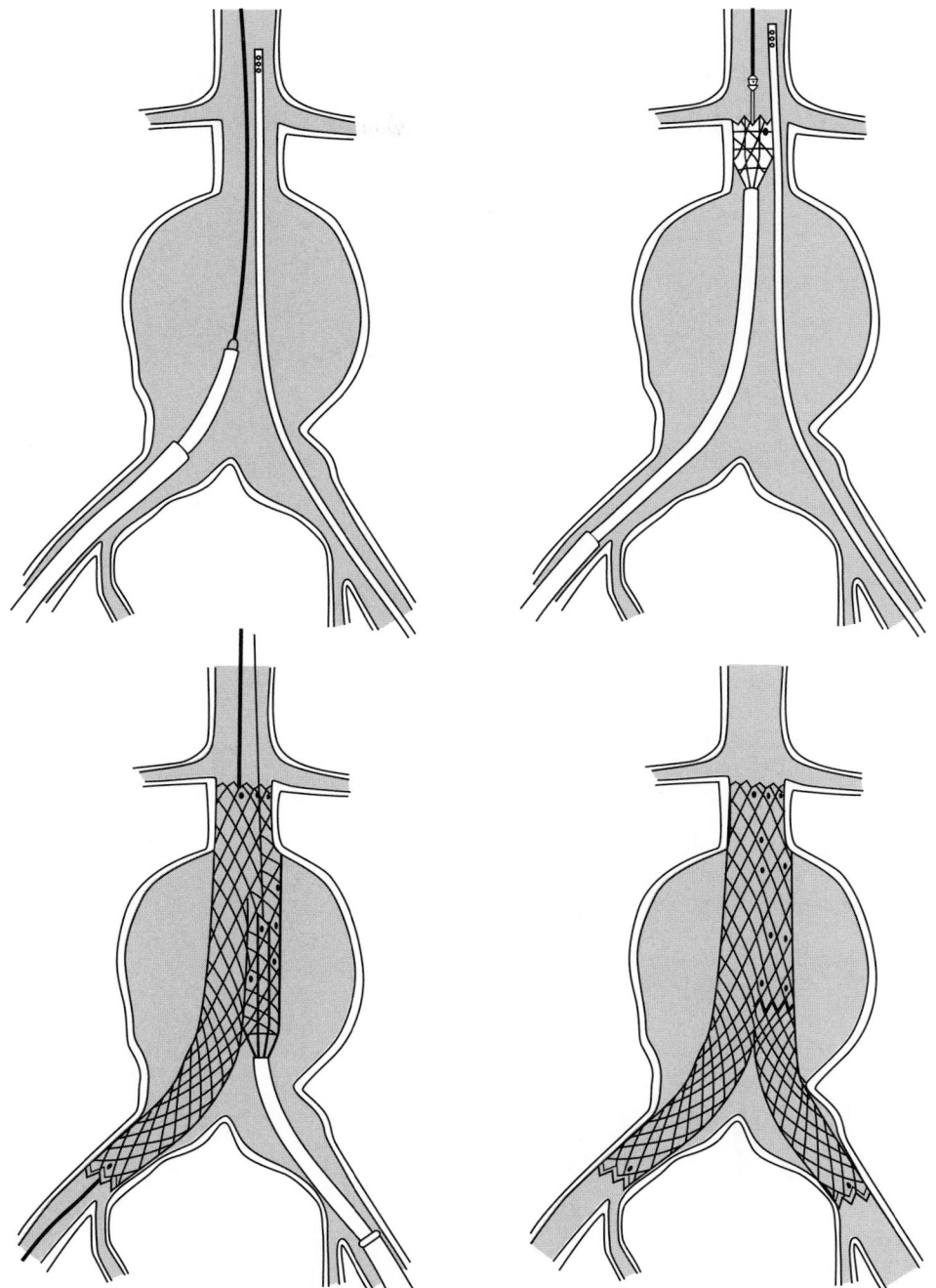

FIGURE 44-26 ■ Endovascular repair of infrarenal abdominal aortic aneurysms. (From Souba WW, Fink MP, Jurkovich GJ, et al (eds): *ACS surgery principles & practice,* New York, 2006, Web MD.)

3. Aortic cross-clamping
   a. Extreme hypertension can occur as aorta is clamped.
   b. Hypotension occurs after clamping released because of:
      (1) Vasodilation of lower extremities
      (2) Third-space fluid shifting
      (3) Metabolic acidosis: products of catabolism and ischemia released systemically

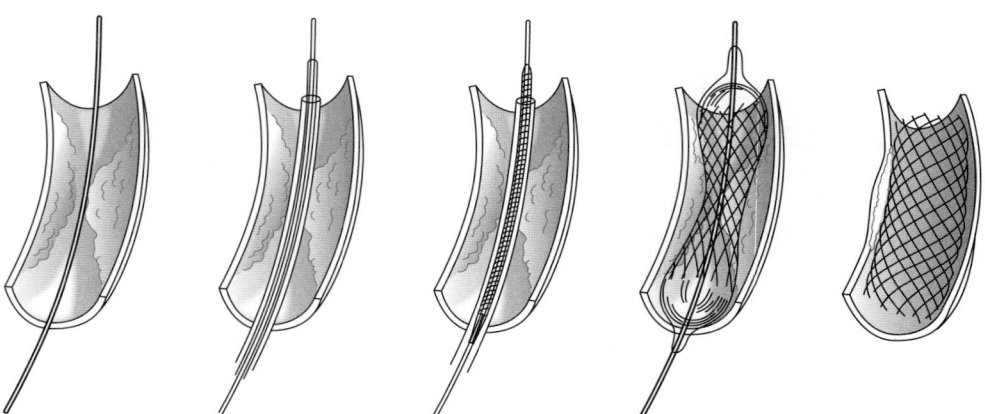

FIGURE 44-27 ■ Deployment of a balloon-expandable stent. (From Souba WW, Fink MP, Jurkovich GJ, et al (eds): *ACS surgery principles & practice,* New York, 2006, Web MD.)

4. Renal status changes
   a. Acute renal failure develops in approximately 20% of postoperative abdominal vessel patients.
   b. Transient oliguria if hypovolemia occurs
      (1) Fluid challenge
      (2) Mannitol: osmotic diuretic
      (3) Furosemide (Lasix): loop diuretic
   c. Hematuria
      (1) Possible reaction to transfusion
      (2) Ureteral damage
      (3) Dislodged microemboli in renal arteries (renal failure)
5. Decreased core temperature related to:
   a. Massive fluid replacement
   b. Length of procedure
   c. Extensive viscera exposure
   d. Cold irrigation fluid
   e. Rapid heat loss in elderly patients
   f. General anesthesia

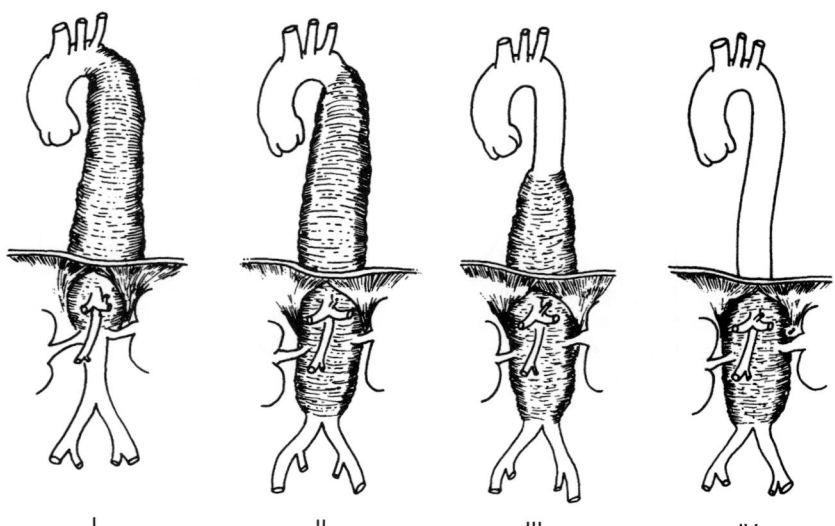

FIGURE 44-28 ■ Crawford classification of extent thoracoabdominal aneurysms. Extent I and extent II aneurysms are associated with higher risks for paraplegia. (From Hamilton IN, Hollier LH: Thoracoabdominal aortic aneurysms. In Moore W, ed: *Vascular surgery: A comprehensive review,* ed 5, Philadelphia, 1998, W.B. Saunders.)

 6. Intraoperative complications
   a. Hemorrhage: abdominal aorta, iliac vessels, inferior vena cava
   b. Injury to ureters
   c. Injury to duodenum, renal arteries and veins, kidney, or spleen
   d. Hemiplegia
   e. Ischemic bowel
 7. Anticoagulation and reversal
   a. Heparin administered during vessel clamping and anastomosis
   b. Protamine sulfate administered to reverse effects of heparinization before completion of procedure
Y. Sympathectomy: palliative surgical option for patients with PVD
 1. Peripheral blood vessels: under continuous control of sympathetic nervous system
   a. With normal vasculature, sympathetic system regulates amount of vasoconstriction.
     (1) To keep extremities warm, dry, and comfortable
     (2) To supply adequate amount of blood to periphery
   b. With compromised peripheral circulation
     (1) Surgical division of sympathetic chain (variable response in patients with PVD)
       (a) Permits permanent, maximal vasodilation
       (b) Allows for maximal blood supply to affected extremity
       (c) Not primary treatment for vascular obstructive disease
     (2) Benefits of sympathectomy
       (a) Increases warmth and comfort of extremity
       (b) Infection subsides; ulcers heal.
       (c) Small areas of gangrene or fibrosis improve.
       (d) Ischemic pain less severe
 2. Surgical approaches
   a. Lumbar sympathectomy: resection of ganglions L2, L3, L4
     (1) Indications for surgery
       (a) Vasospastic disease
       (b) Ischemic ulcers with pain at rest
       (c) Certain forms of causalgia (severe sensation of burning skin)
     (2) Specific surgical risks
       (a) Hemorrhage caused by lumbar arterial or venous damage
       (b) Impotence related to genitofemoral nerve damage
       (c) Ureteral damage: inadvertent ligation or clipping during excision of lumbar sympathetic chain
     (3) Nursing considerations
       (a) Supine, lateral recumbent position
       (b) Increased sensitivity to position change; turning, elevating of head must be performed slowly.
       (c) Flank dressing should remain dry.
       (d) Presence of urine on dressing: ureteral damage
       (e) Presence of blood on dressing: lumbar vessel damage
       (f) Nasogastric decompression to prevent paralytic ileus
       (g) Pain: usually moderate, relieved by analgesics; severe flank pain indicative of ureteral ligation, hydronephrosis; requires surgical reexploration
       (h) Urine output: bladder distention and acute retention associated with operative discomfort
     (4) Neurovascular assessment: both lower extremities
       (a) Increase in warmth and vasodilation: desired result
       (b) Neuralgia may occur from damaged nerve.
   b. Cervical sympathectomy: resection of thoracic ganglia T2 to T6 and half of stellate ganglia C8 to T1
     (1) Effectively denervates upper extremity of all extrinsic vasoconstrictor influences arising in sympathetic nervous system, permitting return of normal vasodilation

(2) Surgical approach: usually supraclavicular; may use thoracic, transaxillary, or transpleural approach

(3) Specific surgical risks

    (a) Hemothorax or pneumothorax

    (b) Phrenic nerve dysfunction: ipsilateral paralysis of diaphragm

    (c) Chylous leak caused by ligation of divided thoracic duct

(4) Nursing considerations: cervical sympathectomy

    (a) Elevation of head enhances respiratory exchange.

    (b) Position on side opposite chest tube; permits optimal lung inflation.

    (c) Chest tube drainage should be less than 200 mL in first 8 hours.

    (d) Vital signs: changes may indicate intrathoracic or intercostals bleeding.

(5) Cardiopulmonary assessment: includes care of mechanically ventilated patients and monitoring of cardiac parameters

(6) Neurovascular assessment

    (a) Palpable radial pulse: confirm with Doppler apparatus if necessary.

    (b) Circulation to affected extremity: warm, dry, pink

    (c) Observe for Horner's syndrome: common after cervical sympathectomy

        (i) Ptosis of upper eyelid

        (ii) Slight elevation of lower lid

        (iii) Constriction of affected pupil

        (iv) Increased salivation and drooping of mouth on affected side

(7) Pain management: per nursing diagnosis and intervention appropriate to unit policy

(8) Complications

    (a) Persistent pneumothorax: damage to underlying lung during thoracotomy

    (b) Intrathoracic bleeding: undetected intercostal vessel interruption

    (c) Radial nerve and artery damage

    (d) Pleural effusion

(9) Postanesthesia concerns—examples of related nursing diagnostic categories include:

    (a) Ineffective airway clearance

    (b) Pain

    (c) Ineffective breathing pattern

    (d) Altered peripheral tissue perfusion

    (e) Decreased cardiac output

    (f) Hypothermia

    (g) Paralysis

VII. INTRAOPERATIVE CONCERNS

  A. Carotid and other neck vessel procedures

    1. Anesthesia choices

      a. Local anesthesia

      (1) Advantages

        (a) Quick evaluation of level of consciousness and neurologic changes

        (b) Minimizes risk of cerebral ischemia

      (2) Disadvantages

        (a) Difficult to manage systemic complications (convulsions, dysrhythmias, hypotension, hypertension)

        (b) Positional discomfort

      b. General anesthesia

      (1) Advantages

        (a) Facilitates control of:

            (i) Hypertension

            (ii) Hypoxia

            (iii) Dysrhythmias

            (iv) Blood loss

        (b) Temperature control

      (2) Disadvantages
        (a) Inability to assess immediate neurologic status
        (b) May require postoperative ventilatory support
        (c) Anesthetic side effects
  2. Extubation as soon as possible allows for accurate neurologic evaluation.
  3. Maintenance of adequate cerebral blood flow: avoidance of hypotension
  4. Intraoperative complications of carotid surgery
    a. Hemorrhage
    b. Acute CVA: higher incidence when stenosis of opposite carotid and vertebral artery prevents adequate cerebral perfusion
    c. Facial and hypoglossal nerve damage (see Neurologic Status, section V.E.1)

VIII. GENERAL POST ANESTHESIA CARE UNIT (PACU) CARE OF VASCULAR PATIENT
  A. Postoperative report includes:
    1. Preoperative preparation
      a. Sedation: control of anxiety
      b. Anticholinergics for reduction of secretions
      c. Antibiotics
      d. Insulin: adjusted dose (according to regimen of institution)
      e. Heparin infusion rate
    2. Preoperative medications: often continued until time of surgery
      a. Nitroglycerin
        (1) Increases coronary perfusion
        (2) Decreases peripheral resistance
      b. Antihypertensives
        (1) Beta-blocker
        (2) Calcium channel blocker
        (3) Angiotensin-converting enzyme inhibitors
      c. Antidysrhythmics
    3. Background information
      a. Patient identification
      b. Baseline vital signs
      c. Procedure performed
      d. Anesthesia administered
      e. Drugs received
      f. Length of procedure
      g. Estimated blood loss
    4. Intraoperative vital signs and monitoring data
    5. Intraoperative problems encountered
    6. Anticipated problems
  B. Postoperative monitoring data: observe for compensatory mechanisms.
    1. ECG: rhythm, ST-segment changes
    2. Arterial line and/or noninvasive blood pressure
    3. Central venous pressure (CVP)
    4. Pulmonary artery pressures (Swan-Ganz catheter)
    5. Core temperature
    6. Ventilation and oxygen support
      a. Mechanical ventilation; parameters
        (1) Fraction of inspired oxygen (Fio_2)
        (2) Mode—continuous mechanical ventilation (CMV)
        (3) Synchronous intermittent mechanical ventilation (SIMV)
        (4) Continuous positive airway pressure (CPAP)
        (5) Tidal volume (TV)
        (6) Rate
        (7) Positive end-expiratory pressure (PEEP)
        (8) Pressure support
      b. Spontaneous ventilation: face mask
      c. Oxygen saturation (pulse oximetry)

      d. End-tidal carbon dioxide

      e. Svo_2

  C. Vascular assessment

    1. Skin

      a. Temperature: warm, cool, or cold

      b. Skin color: pink, ruddy, dusky, pale, or mottled

    2. Capillary refill

      a. Normal color return after nail bed blanching

      b. Color return should occur within 2 seconds.

    3. Peripheral pulses

      a. Head and neck arteries

      b. Carotid

      c. Temporal

      d. Upper extremity arterial pulses

        (1) Radial

        (2) Brachial

        (3) Axillary

      e. Lower extremity arterial pulses

        (1) Femoral artery

        (2) Popliteal artery

        (3) Posterior tibial artery

        (4) Dorsalis pedis artery

    4. Quality of pulse

      a. Reflection of cardiac output and peripheral vascular patency

      b. Use of objective pulse quality scale for charting purposes

        (1) 0: Absent pulse

        (2) 1+: Weak, thready pulse

        (3) 2+: Normal quality

        (4) 3+: Increased volume, strong and bounding

    5. Doppler ultrasound confirmation: device amplifies sound waves produced by pulsating blood flow in vessel and allows for detection of pulsatile flow in absence of palpable pulse.

    6. Marking of pulses: facilitates comparison of pulses and promotes continuity of care

    7. Extra-anatomic graft pulses: placed subcutaneously to improve recipient vessel circulation

  D. Neurologic assessment (see Chapter 33)

    1. Level of consciousness: orientation to person, place, time

    2. Motor and sensory function

      a. Motion and sensation of all extremities

      b. Bilateral and equal hand grasp

    3. Pupillary function: equal reaction and accommodation to light

    4. Abnormal findings

      a. Tics

      b. Tremors

      c. Gazing

      d. Seizures

  E. Neurovascular assessment: evaluate the six *p*'s.

    1. Pulses and pulselessness

    2. Pain

    3. Paresthesia

    4. Paralysis

    5. Pallor

    6. Poikilothermia (coldness)

  F. Fluid volume status

    1. CVP, pulmonary artery pressures

    2. Assessment of vital signs

    3. Laboratory data

      a. Hemoglobin, hematocrit

        b. Serum sodium, potassium

        c. Coagulation studies

    4. Replacement of blood and (third space) fluid loss

        a. Colloid

        b. Crystalloid

        c. Plasma expanders

G. Operative site observation

    1. Dressing site and condition

    2. Drains and drainage

    3. Presence of abnormalities

        a. Hematoma formation

        b. Discolorations

    4. Changes in abdominal girth, diameter

H. Limb protection

    1. Bed cradle

    2. Heel and elbow padding

    3. Lanolin for dry skin

    4. Lamb's wool between toes

    5. No pressure under knee

    6. Avoidance of joint (graft) flexion at hip or knee

IX. PACU CARE FOR SPECIFIC VASCULAR PROCEDURES

A. Carotid vessel procedures

    1. Neurological assessment

        a. Presence of swallow and gag reflexes

        b. Cranial nerve function: affected by intraoperative retraction and stretching of nerves

    2. Respiratory concerns

        a. Instruct patient to inhale deeply and minimize deep cough response to avoid elevation of venous pressure.

        b. Incentive spirometry encourages deep inhalation.

        c. Assess for possible respiratory obstruction.

            (1) Vocal cord edema and injury, surgical trauma

            (2) Tracheal deviation: hematoma development at operative site; may present with stridor

    3. Blood pressure concerns: maintain adequate blood pressure to maximize cerebral perfusion and minimize possible sequelae of hypertension or hypotension.

        a. Hypertension

            (1) Sequelae

                (a) Suture line disruption: tension at site of anastomosis may cause bleeding.

                (b) Hematoma formation: tracheal compression

                (c) Cerebral hemorrhage, edema

            (2) Nursing interventions

                (a) Elevate head of bed to decrease venous pressure.

                (b) Comfort measures to minimize pain and maintain desired blood pressure parameters

                (c) Ensure adequate ventilation.

        b. Hypotension

            (1) Sequelae resulting from hypersensitive carotid sinus

                (a) Sluggish blood flow through operative artery and graft

                (b) Difficult pulse assessment

                (c) Decreased cerebral or coronary artery perfusion

            (2) Nursing interventions

                (a) Increase fluids if indicated.

                (b) Reduce high Fowler's to more moderate position.

                (c) Titrate vasopressor.

        c. Pharmacologic intervention

            (1) Sodium nitroprusside (Nipride): vasodilator

                (a) Direct effect on arterial and venous smooth muscle

          (b) Used to treat severe acute hypertension: rapid onset

          (c) Reduces peripheral resistance and increases cardiac output

     (2) Nitroglycerin: vasodilator

          (a) Relaxes smooth muscle in small blood vessels

          (b) Causes venous and arterial dilation; increases coronary artery perfusion

          (c) Used for treatment of myocardial ischemia and hypertension

     (3) Trimethaphan (Arfonad): antihypertensive

          (a) Ganglionic blocking agent

          (b) Causes peripheral vasodilation; used to treat hypertension

     (4) Dopamine (Intropin): vasopressor

          (a) Directly stimulates beta-receptors and dopamine receptors

          (b) Low dose causes renal and mesenteric vasodilation and subsequently increases urine output.

          (c) Midrange dose produces a positive inotropic effect on myocardium.

          (d) High dose stimulates alpha-adrenergic receptors and causes renal vasoconstriction, increased peripheral resistance, and increased blood pressure.

     (5) Milrinone (Primacor)

          (a) Positive inotropic agent with vasodilator properties

          (b) Causes thrombocytopenia and may be contraindicated for some patients

     (6) Phenylephrine (Neo-Synephrine): vasopressor

          (a) Acts on alpha-adrenergic receptors

          (b) Produces vasoconstriction and increased peripheral resistance

          (c) Increases systolic and diastolic blood pressure

          (d) Reflex bradycardia occurs because of increased vagal activity.

     (7) Labetalol hydrochloride (Normodyne, Trandate): alpha-receptor and nonspecific beta-receptor blocking agent

          (a) Used for treatment of hypertension

          (b) Administer supine to avoid orthostatic hypotensive effect.

     (8) Esmolol (Brevibloc): beta-blocking agent used to treat supraventricular tachyarrhythmias

          (a) Rapid onset of action, short half-life

          (b) Hypotension most common side effect

     (9) Nifedipine (Procardia): calcium channel blocker used for treatment of chronic hypertension, acute hypertensive emergencies, and angina

          (a) Decreases systemic vascular resistance

          (b) Augments cardiac output

4. Bradycardia

  a. Causes

    (1) Altered baroreceptor responses

    (2) Vagal manipulation

    (3) Vagal pressure from hematoma formation

    (4) Myocardial infarction

  b. Interventions

    (1) Pharmacologic

        (a) Atropine (anticholinergic, parasympatholytic): inhibits action of acetylcholine; stimulates or depresses central nervous system depending on dose; used to treat bradycardia

        (b) Glycopyrrolate (Robinul; anticholinergic): inhibits action of acetylcholine; used to treat bradycardia

    (2) Surgical

        (a) Excision of hematoma

        (b) Reexploration of wound

5. Positioning: elevation of head

  a. Decreases venous pressure

  b. Facilitates respiratory excursion

6. Dressings and drains

      a. Dressings: light, nonconstricting

      b. Drains: Penrose, Jackson-Pratt, Hemovac

B. Intrathoracic vessel procedures

  1. Respiratory support

      a. Principles of care of intubated and mechanically ventilated patient

      b. Head elevation permits respiratory excursion and allows proper chest tube function.

      c. Turn, cough, deep breathe every 2 hours and as needed.

  2. Assess for complications.

      a. Atelectasis

      b. Pneumothorax, hemothorax

      c. Adult respiratory distress syndrome

      d. CHF and pulmonary edema

  3. Ensure proper chest tube functioning.

      a. Make sure connections are secure.

      b. Observe for air leaks.

      c. Measure drainage.

      d. Keep bottles below chest level.

      e. Auscultate lung sounds.

      f. Palpate for subcutaneous emphysema (crepitus).

  4. Neurovascular assessment (as previously outlined)

      a. Pulse assessment: upper and lower extremities

      b. Motor and sensory function

        (1) Spinal cord ischemia

          (a) Paraplegia can occur with prolonged thoracic and aortic occlusion.

          (b) Decreased perfusion pressure to spinal cord

        (2) Embolization to distal arteries, originating from aortic clot

  5. Monitor for cardiac, pulmonary, renal function (as previously outlined).

  6. Pain management (according to unit policy)

      a. Prevent splinting and permit lung expansion.

      b. Allay apprehension and fear.

      c. Decrease tachycardia and hypertension.

      d. Enhance mechanical ventilation compliance.

C. Abdominal vessel procedures

  1. Continuous cardiopulmonary assessment (as previously outlined)

  2. Observe for signs and symptoms of hypovolemic shock caused by hemorrhage.

  3. Gastrointestinal assessment

      a. Nasogastric tube: decompresses stomach, prevents paralytic ileus

      b. Complications

        (1) Ileus

        (2) Occlusion of inferior mesenteric artery, causing colon ischemia

        (3) Hemorrhage: measure and monitor abdominal girth.

  4. Renal assessment (as previously outlined)

      a. Hematuria: aortic cross-clamping, kidney and/or bladder trauma

      b. Oliguria: renal failure, tubular necrosis

  5. Neurovascular status (as previously outlined)

      a. Pedal pulses may be absent for 6 to 12 hours postoperatively.

        (1) Vascular spasm

        (2) Peripheral vasoconstriction

        (3) Vessel patency, verified by surgeon

        (4) Confirm absence with Doppler ultrasonography.

      b. Absence of previously palpable pulse

        (1) Signifies occlusion of vessel or graft

        (2) Requires immediate surgical reexploration

  6. Positioning

      a. Abdominal procedures: head elevation

        (1) Facilitates respiratory excursion

        (2) Decreases suture line stress

      b. Vena cava plication: supine to slight Trendelenburg

        (1) Prevents further reduction of venous return

        (2) Decreased venous return results in decreased cardiac output.

    7. Pain or vascular spasm

      a. Severe pain indicative of retroperitoneal bleeding

      b. Spasms

        (1) Usually after aortic surgery

        (2) Aggravated by:

          (a) Hypotension

          (b) Hypothermia

          (c) Pain

          (d) Carbon dioxide retention

    8. Hypothermia or shivering

      a. Sequelae

        (1) Increases oxygen requirement

        (2) ST-segment depression can occur with increased myocardial oxygen requirement.

        (3) Prolonged somnolence occurs with decreased cerebral perfusion.

        (4) Increases vasoconstriction and vasospasm

          (a) Increases difficulty in palpating pulses

          (b) Aggravates hypertension

        (5) Increases patient anxiety and discomfort

      b. Corrective nursing interventions

        (1) Heated blankets, automatic hyperthermia blanket

        (2) Warming lights

        (3) Heated aerosol nebulizers with oxygen delivery

    9. Complications

      a. Acute arterial occlusion

      b. Debris embolization: pulmonary, cerebral, peripheral

      c. Graft suture line hemorrhage

      d. Cardiopulmonary complications

        (1) Dysrhythmias

        (2) Myocardial infarction

        (3) CHF

      e. Third-space fluid accumulation

      f. Renal complications: failure, trauma

D. Extra-anatomic vessel bypasses (femoral crossover, axillofemoral bypass)

    1. Positioning: turn only to unoperated side.

      a. Avoid external pressure on graft.

      b. Avoid flexion of graft; careful pillow positioning.

    2. Pulse checks with femoral crossover

      a. Across symphysis pubis (femoral to femoral)

      b. Both lower extremities

    3. Pulse checks with axillofemoral bypass: monitor donor arm and revascularized limb.

      a. Avoid damage to donor artery; obtain blood pressure, draw blood from opposite arm.

      b. Specific complications of axillofemoral bypass

        (1) Brachial plexus injury

        (2) Subclavian or axillary artery injury

        (3) Upper extremity embolization

E. Extremity vessel procedures (arterial bypass grafts, embolectomies, vein stripping and ligation)

    1. Nursing concerns: arterial procedures

      a. Positioning: avoid severe joint flexion, crossing of legs, pillows under popliteal area.

      b. Nonrestrictive dressings

      c. Neurovascular assessment

        (1) Comparison of both extremities

(2) Doppler confirmation

(3) If no pulses expected by surgeon, successful revascularization assessed by dry, pink, warm legs and feet

 d. Limb protection (as previously outlined)

 e. Laboratory data

  (1) Monitor glucose level in diabetic patient: control of blood sugar can prevent infection.

  (2) Monitor potassium level: extracellular potassium increases with limb ischemia and infection.

  (3) Monitor for metabolic acidosis: causes increased serum potassium level.

 f. Administer low–molecular weight dextran (500 mL over 10-24 hours).

  (1) Anticoagulation effect: interrupts action of fibrinogen and clotting factors

  (2) Reduces platelet accumulation and adhesiveness

  (3) Increases tissue perfusion

  (4) Reduces blood viscosity

  (5) Increases colloid osmotic pressure

 g. Control of pain to prevent spasms

2. Complications of extremity vessel procedures

 a. Graft occlusion

 b. Vein, nerve injury

 c. Pulmonary or cerebral emboli

3. Nursing concerns: vein procedures

 a. Positioning

  (1) Supine to slight head elevation with leg elevation

  (2) Avoidance of knee bending or leg crossing

 b. Dressing: multiple wounds covered by ACE bandages

 c. Neurovascular assessment: bilateral comparison as previously outlined

 d. Pain assessment: incisional discomfort versus deep calf pain of thrombophlebitis

4. Complications of vein ligation, stripping procedures

 a. Hematoma and wound bleeding

 b. Femoral vein or femoral saphenous nerve damage

 c. Thrombophlebitis

 d. Edema

F. Endovascular repair stent grafts of abdominal aortic aneurysm

1. Selected by location of aneurysm and risk factor of open surgery

2. Graft inserted via catheter through skin

3. Stent deployed away from renal arteries and anchored in place with hooks

 a. Advantages of endovascular repair

  (1) Decreases length of stay

  (2) Minimally invasive

  (3) Shorter recovery time

 b. Disadvantages of endovascular repair

  (1) Aneurysm rupture

  (2) Peripheral embolization

  (3) Bleeding

  (4) Misdeployment of stent graft

  (5) Requiring open surgical procedure

BIBLIOGRAPHY

1. American Association of Critical Care Nurses: *Core curriculum for critical care nursing*, ed 6, Philadelphia, 2006, Saunders.

2. Arko FR, Zarins CK: Repair of infrarenal abdominal aortic aneurysms. In Souba WW, Fink MP, Jurkovich GJ, et al, eds: *ACS surgery principles & practice*, New York, 2006, Web MD.

3. Bartley MK: Keep venous thromboembolism at bay. *Nursing* 36(10):36–41, 2006.

4. Beese-Bjurstrom S: Hidden danger: Aortic aneurysms and dissections. *Nursing* 34(2): 36–41, 2004.

5. Bickley LS, Szilagyi PG: *Bate's guide to physical examination and history taking*, ed 8, Philadelphia, 2003, Lippincott Williams & Wilkins.

6. Blach DE, Ignatavic DD: Interventions for clients with vascular problems. In Ignatavic DD, Workman ML, eds: *Medical-surgical nursing: Critical thinking for collaborative care*, Philadelphia, 2006, Saunders.

7. Block PC: ACC/AHA guidelines for the management of patients with peripheral arterial disease (lower extremity, renal, mesenteric, and abdominal aortic). *ACC Cardiosource Rev J* 15(3):16–19, 2006.

8. Bussard ME: Reteplase. Nursing implications for catheter-directed thrombolytic therapy for peripheral vascular occlusion. *Crit Care Nurse* 22(3):57–63, 2003.

9. Casserly JS, Yadav S, Sachar R: *Manual of peripheral vascular intervention*, Philadelphia, 2005, Lippincott Williams & Wilkins.

10. Croft JA, Todd BA: Thoracoabdominal aneurysms. *Advance for Nurses* 7(20):16–17, 2005.

11. Crowther M, McCourt K: Get the edge on deep vein thrombosis. *Nurs Manage* 35(1):22–29, 2004.

12. Decousis H: Eight year follow-up of patients with permanent vena cava filters in the prevention of pulmonary embolism. *Circulation* 12:416–422, 2005.

13. Dilainas I, Nano G, Kashyap A, et al: Balloon angioplasty or nitinol balloon angioplasty versus implantation of nitinol stents in the superficial femoral artery. *N Engl J Med* 355(5):521–524, 2003.

14. Drain CB, Odom-Forren J: *Perianesthesia nursing: A critical care approach*, ed 5, Philadelphia, 2009, Saunders.

15. Fahey VA: *Vascular nursing*, ed 4, St Louis, 2004, Saunders.

16. Hirsch AT, Haskal ZJ, Hertzer NR, et al: ACC/AHA 2005 practice guidelines for the management of patients with peripheral arterial disease (lower extremity, renal, mesenteric, and abdominal aortic): A collaborative report from the American Association for Vascular Surgery/Society for Vascular Surgery, Society for Cardiovascular Angiography and Interventions, Society for Vascular Medicine and Biology, Society of Interventional Radiology, and the ACC/AHA Task Force on Practice Guidelines (Writing Committee to Develop Guidelines for the Management of Patents With Peripheral Arterial Disease): Endorsed by the American Association of Cardiovascular and Pulmonary Rehabilitation; National Heart, Lung and Blood Institute; Society for Vascular Nursing; TransAtlantic Inter-Society Consensus; and Vascular Disease Foundation. *Circulation* 113:e463–e465, 2006.

17. Horlander KT, Mannino DM, Leeper KV: Pulmonary embolism mortality in the United States, 1997–1998. *Arch Intern Med* 163(14):1711–1717, 2003.

18. Jarvis C: *Physical examination and health assessment*, ed 4, St Louis, 2004, Mosby.

19. Kinney MR, Packa DR, Dunbar SB: *AACN's clinical reference for critical-care nursing*, St Louis, 1998, Mosby.

20. Kuznar KA: Peripheral arterial disease. *Advance for Nurses* 6(13):19–24, 2004.

21. Lipsitz EC, Kim S: Antithrombotic therapy in peripheral arterial disease. *Clin Geriatr Med* 22(1):183–198, 2006.

22. Owings JT: Venous thromboembolism. In Souba WW, Fink MP, Jurkovich GJ, et al, eds: *ACS surgery principles & practice*, New York, 2006, Web MD.

23. Pamoukian VN, Shortell CK: Pulseless extremity and atheroembolism. Approach to the acutely ischemic limb. In Souba WW, Fink MP, Jurkovich GJ, et al, eds: *ACS surgery principles & practice*, New York, 2006, Web MD.

24. Price SA, Wilson LM: *Pathophysiology: Clinical concepts of disease processes*, ed 6, St Louis, 2001, Mosby.

25. Rice KL: How to measure ankle/brachial index. *Nursing* 35(1):56–57, 2005.

26. Rothrock JC: *Alexander's care of the patient in surgery*, ed 13, St Louis, 2007, Mosby.

27. Smeltzer SC, Bare BG: *Brunner & Suddarth's textbook of medical-surgical nursing*, ed 10, Philadelphia, 2004, Lippincott Williams & Wilkins.

28. Society of Interventional Radiology: *Peripheral vascular disease statistics*. Available at: www.sirweb.org. Accessed September 4, 2003.

29. Sontheimer DL: Peripheral vascular disease: Diagnosis and treatment. *Am Fam Physician* 73(11):1971–1976, 2006.

30. Souba WW, Fink MP, Jurkovich GJ, et al, eds: *ACS surgery principles & practice*, New York, 2006, WebMD.

31. Stoney RJ, Effeney DJ: *Wylie's atlas of vascular surgery: Thoracoabdominal aorta and its branches*, Philadelphia, 1992, Lippincott.

32. Patton KT, Thibodeau GA: *Anatomy & physiology*, ed 7, St. Louis, 2010, Mosby.

33. Tzou WS, Mohler ERIII: Peripheral arterial disease: Diagnosis and medical management. *Hosp Physician* 42(7):17–25, 54, 72, 2006.

34. Urden LD, Stacy KM, Lough ME: *Thelan's critical care nursing: Diagnosis and management*, ed 5, St Louis, 2006, Mosby.

35. Zelenock GB: *Mastery of vascular and endovascular surgery*, Philadelphia, 2006, Lippincott Williams & Wilkins.

45 Plastic and Reconstructive Care

THERESA L. CLIFFORD

OBJECTIVES

At the conclusion of this chapter, the reader will be able to:

1. Describe the clinical management of burn injuries.
2. Describe the anatomy of skin.
3. Describe the physiology of wound healing.
4. Describe preoperative preparation of the plastic surgery patient.
5. Describe common plastic and reconstructive surgeries.
6. Describe common medical conditions affecting surgical outcomes.
7. Identify anesthesia administration concerns for the plastic surgery patient.
8. List psychological factors that affect the plastic surgery patient.
9. Identify nursing care for individual surgical procedures.
10. Evaluate postoperative management and patient education concerns for the plastic surgery patient.

I. OVERVIEW
  A. Plastic and reconstructive surgery may be performed for a variety of reasons.
    1. Physical appearance
    2. Emotional well-being
    3. Body image
  B. Plastic surgery may be:
    1. Elective
    2. Cosmetic
    3. Reconstructive
       a. Correcting congenital or acquired abnormalities
       b. Restore normal function and appearance.
  C. Anesthetic needs vary on the basis of the complexity of the procedure.
    1. Local anesthesia for simple lesion removal
    2. Prolonged general anesthesia for complex reconstruction
  D. Perioperative needs of the plastic surgery and burn patient.
    1. Purpose
    2. Procedure
    3. Perianesthesia nursing care management
    4. Patient education for specific surgical interventions
II. OVERVIEW OF BURNS
  A. Determining severity of burn injury
    1. Initial area of burn should be reassessed frequently after admission.
    2. Size of percent of body surface involved (total body surface area [TBSA])
       a. Rule of 9s (Figure 45-1)
          (1) Body areas divided into equal multiples of 9
          (2) Head and each arm equal 9%.
          (3) Chest, back, and leg equal 18% each.
          (4) Perineum equals 1%.
       b. Berkow's method, or Lund and Browder chart
          (1) Used for children
          (2) Adjusts for differences in body part sizes between adults and children

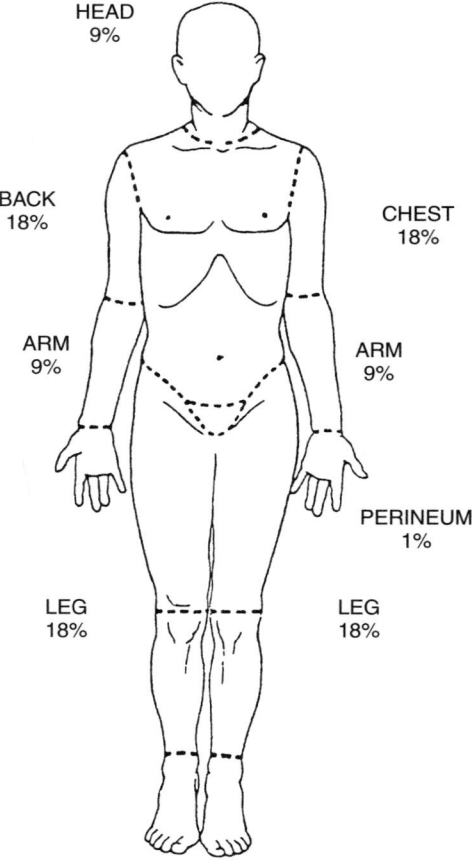

HEAD
9%

BACK
18%

CHEST
18%

ARM
9%

ARM
9%

PERINEUM
1%

LEG
18%

LEG
18%

FIGURE 45-1 ■ The rule of 9s.

      (a) Head in child younger than 2 years equals 18%.
      (b) Each leg in child younger than 2 years equals 13%.
  c. One percent method
    (1) Used for quick assessment
    (2) Palmar surface of patient's hand equals approximately 1% TBSA.
    (3) Not useful for large-area burns
  d. Major burn injury
    (1) Adults
      (a) Greater than 25% TBSA: partial-thickness burn, age <40 years
      (b) Greater than 20% TBSA: partial-thickness burn, age >40 years
      (c) Greater than 10% TBSA: full-thickness burn
    (2) Children
      (a) Greater than 20% TBSA: partial-thickness burn
      (b) Greater than 10% TBSA: full-thickness burn
    (3) Other factors
      (a) Burns of face, eyes, ears, hands, feet, and perineum
      (b) Electrical burns
      (c) Burns complicated by inhalation injury or major trauma
      (d) Patients' preexisting diseases may impact recovery (e.g., diabetes, congestive heart failure).
B. Depth of injury
  1. Superficial injury (first degree)
    a. Affects epidermis only
    b. Appearance: skin intact, red, blanches
    c. Painful

      d. Healing time: 2 to 10 days
      e. Causes: flash burns, sunburn
    2. Partial-thickness injury (second degree)
      a. Affects epidermis and part of dermis, leaving skin appendages intact
      b. Levels
        (1) Superficial partial-thickness: affects upper layers of dermis
        (2) Deep partial-thickness
          (a) Affects lower layers of dermis
          (b) May convert to full-thickness injury
      c. Appearance
        (1) Superficial partial-thickness: red, moist, blistered, blanches
        (2) Deep partial-thickness: deep red, moist, areas of white or yellow tissue, delayed capillary refill
      d. Very painful
      e. Healing time
        (1) If affecting outer layers of dermis, 5 to 21 days
        (2) If affecting deeper layers of dermis, 21 to 35 days
          (a) May convert to full-thickness burn in first few days after burn
          (b) May require skin grafting
      f. Causes: scald, flame, chemicals
    3. Full-thickness injury (third degree)
      a. Affects epidermis and entire dermis and may extend to subcutaneous tissue, muscle, or bone
      b. Appearance: hard, dry, leathery; color may be black, tan, white; nonblanching
      c. Minimal to no pain
      d. Healing time: requires excision and skin grafting
      e. Causes: flame, scald, chemicals, electrical, contact with hot surfaces
C. Part of body involved
    1. Specific areas of body have significant impact on healing, cosmetic appearance, and function.
    2. Head, face, and chest burns significantly related to respiratory function
    3. Hand, face, and feet burns significantly related to cosmetics and function
    4. Perineal burns significantly related to infection
    5. Circumferential burns significant because of compromised circulation
D. Burning agent
    1. Scald
      a. Most common type of burn, especially in children
      b. Caused by immersion, splash, or steam
    2. Flame and flash burns
      a. Second most common type of burn
      b. Commonly associated with smoke inhalation
      c. Frequently full thickness in nature
      d. From house fires, kerosene or gasoline ignition
    3. Contact burns
      a. Area burned is well defined in appearance in shape of item contacted.
      b. May occur from hot metal, asphalt, or sand
    4. Chemical burns
      a. Less than 10% of all injuries
      b. Acid or alkali
      c. May be topical or ingested
      d. More commonly from industrial accidents
    5. Electrical
      a. Least common
      b. May cause significant internal or external damage
      c. Direct current or alternating current
      d. Alternating current more dangerous than direct current because of increased risk for cardiopulmonary arrest

       e. Cataracts may occur 1 to 2 days to 3 years after burn.

       f. May require extensive reconstructive surgery (e.g., myocutaneous flaps)

  E. Age of burn patient

    1. Higher mortality in patients younger than 2 years or older than 60 years

    2. Thinness of skin in very young and very old makes injury more likely.

    3. Changes in immune status alter ability to heal.

  F. Preexisting medical conditions that impair healing process

    1. Cardiovascular disease

    2. Diabetes

    3. Pulmonary disease: asthma, chronic obstructive pulmonary diseases

  G. Other associated injuries at time of burn that might affect healing

    1. Smoke inhalation

    2. Traumatic injury (e.g., fractures, closed head injury)

    3. Need for tracheostomy significantly increases mortality risk.

III. ANATOMY AND PHYSIOLOGY

  A. Function of skin

    1. Largest organ of the body

    2. First line of defense against trauma and infection

    3. Retention of body fluids

    4. Regulation of body temperature

      a. Vasoconstriction and vasodilation

      b. Evaporation of water

    5. Secretion and excretion

      a. Secretion of oil from sebaceous glands to lubricate skin, preventing cracks and organism invasion

      b. Excretion of water, sodium chloride, cholesterol, and urea from sweat glands

    6. Metabolizes and produces vitamin D

    7. Sensation and communication

      a. Pressure, pain, touch, temperature

      b. Reaction to environmental stimuli

    8. Generates new skin

      a. Contributes to self-image

  B. Anatomy of skin

    1. Properties of the skin

      a. Accounts for one sixth of total body weight

      b. Receives one third of resting cardiac output

    2. Structure of skin

      a. Epidermis

        (1) Outermost layer—often tough and leathery

          (a) Made up of five layers of keratinocytes

            (i)   Stratum corneum

               [a] Layers of dead keratinized cells

               [b] Layers

                  [1] Provide vapor barrier

                  [2] Protect body from microorganisms and chemical irritants

               [c] A localized build-up of dead cells is a callus.

            (ii) Stratum lucidum

            (iii) Stratum granulosum

            (iv) Stratum spinosum

            (v) Stratum basale

               [a] Regenerates epithelial covering

               [b] Necessary for spontaneous healing

               [c] Journey from stratum basale to stratum corneum takes 14 to 21 days.

          (b) Surface and deepest layers most important in burn care

          (c) Blood supplied by dermis

          (d) Epidermis lines skin appendages

(i)   Sebaceous glands

(ii) Sweat glands

(iii) Hair follicles

(e) New skin can be generated from lining of skin appendages even if epidermis is destroyed.

(f) Varies in thickness from 0.05 to 1.5 mm.

(i)   Thickest at soles of feet, palms, scapula

(ii) Thinnest at eyelids

b. Additional epidermal cells

(1) Melanocytes

(a) Produce melanin, a pigment protecting skin from ultraviolet radiation

(b) Give skin its color depending on quantities of melanin

(2) Merkel cells

(a) Mechanoreceptors providing information on light touch sensation

(3) Langerhans' cells

(a) Help fight infection by engulfing foreign material

c. Epidermal appendages

(1) Hair

(a) Traps air between hair and skin to regulate body temperature

(2) Nails

(a) Protect the distal end of digits

(3) Sweat and sebaceous glands

(a) Help to cool the body as well as reduce infections

d. Dermis—the layer of skin lying immediately under the epidermis; the true skin.

(1) Five main functions of the dermis

(a) Support and nourish the epidermis

(b) Accommodate epidermal appendages

(c) Support infection control

(d) Support thermoregulation

(e) Provide sensation

(2) Two layers

(a) Papillary layer

(i)   Composed of fibrous connective tissue made of collagen and elastin

(ii) Contains numerous capillaries, lymphatics, and nerve endings

(b) Reticular layer

(i)   Densely arranged connective tissue increasing structural support for the skin

(3) Hypodermis—subcutaneous tissue

(a) Functions to:

(i)   Store fat for energy

(ii) Cushion

(iii) Insulate

(b) Contains fascia to facilitate structural movement

(c) Attached to dermis by collagen

e. Deeper tissues

(1) Muscles

(2) Tendons

(3) Ligaments

(4) Bones

C. Physiology of wound healing

1. An alteration in the integrity and function of tissues in the body

2. Intentional wounds from surgical procedure

3. Unintentional wounds include accidental trauma such as a motor vehicle crash or by persistent forces such as that which causes pressure ulcers

    4. Terms describing wounds include:
      a. Abrasion
      b. Avulsion
      c. Contusion
      d. Laceration
      e. Puncture
  D. Process of wound healing
    1. Inflammation
      a. Vascular response—hemostasis for bleeding control
        (1) Injury causes blood cells to enter wound and release coagulation factors to promote platelet aggregation and seal the vessel walls.
        (2) Thromboplastin is released from injured cells, activating the clotting cascade.
        (3) Platelets release growth factors required for tissue development during the subsequent phases of healing.
      b. Cellular response—combating infectious processes
        (1) Histamines are released from mast cells to cause vasodilation and increased capillary permeability to bring needed nutrients, chemical, and white blood cells (WBCs) to the injured area.
        (2) Epithelialization occurs; WBCs cleanse wound (phagocytosis).
        (3) Stage of exudate and wound drainage
        (4) Stage lasts from time of initial injury up to 4 days.
    2. Proliferation
      a. Four major events occur.
        (1) Neovascularization (angiogenesis)
          (a) Formation of new blood vessels in order to reestablish perfusion
        (2) Epithelialization
          (a) Migration of epithelial cells across the wound
        (3) Collagen formation
          (a) Collagen fibers add strength to the healing wound.
        (4) Granulation tissue formation and contracture
          (a) Temporary network of connective tissue formed to fill in wounds
          (b) Wound margins begin to move towards the center of the wound.
      b. Begins several days after an injury and lasts several weeks
    3. Remodeling and maturation
      a. Collagen fibers are remodeled, and scar matures.
        (1) Becomes flat, thin, silver in color
        (2) Stage lasts 1 to 2 years.
  E. Comorbidities affecting wound healing
    1. Local factors
      a. Healing affected by vascularity, tissue tension and motion relative to wound location
      b. Dimensions of wound (shape, size, depth)
      c. Temperature of wound (normothermic wounds heal better)
      d. Desiccation or dehydration of wound
      e. Presence of necrotic tissue, foreign bodies, or infection
      f. Incontinence or other chronic skin irritants
      g. Mechanical trauma such as prolonged or excessive pressure or friction to surface of wound
      h. Use of cytotoxic products near wound
      i. Dead space—accumulation of air or fluid slows healing, promotes infection.
    2. Age
      a. Children heal rapidly.
      b. Geriatric patients heal slower because of:
        (1) Decreased circulation
        (2) Higher incidence of chronic illnesses
    3. Activity limitations
      a. Increase risk of skin breakdown and delayed repair

4. Nutrition
   a. Malnutrition, dehydration, and vitamin deficiency slow healing process.
   b. Large healing demands require large nutritional reserves.
5. Behavioral risk taking
   a. Nicotine—causes poor healing because of:
      (1) Oxygen deprivation
      (2) Peripheral vasoconstriction
      (3) Increased platelet aggregation leading to "tough" clots
   b. Alcohol abuse can lead to poor nutrition.
6. Psychological stress
   a. Corticosteroids decrease inflammatory response.
   b. Catecholamines suppress microcirculation.
7. Medications
   a. Chronic use of:
      (1) Aspirin-containing products
      (2) Steroids
      (3) Nonsteroidal anti-inflammatory drugs (NSAIDs)
   b. Chemotherapy and other immunosuppressive drugs
8. Immunosuppression
   a. History of cancer, human immunodeficiency virus, hypothyroidism, etc.
9. Comorbidities
   a. Diabetes
      (1) Peripheral macrovascular and microvascular changes
      (2) Poor glycemic control
      (3) Loss of sensation and neuropathies
         (a) Impaired ability to recognize continued tissue damage
      (4) Impaired oxygenation and perfusion
      (5) Slowed epithelialization and wound contraction
      (6) Impaired phagocytosis
   b. Peripheral vascular disease
      (1) Impaired blood flow such as in venous stasis or anemia
   c. Pulmonary disease
      (1) Hypoxemia causes tissue hypoxia, which will divert necessary oxygen and nutrients from tissues.
   d. Obesity (>20% ideal body weight)
      (1) Increased incidence of wound dehiscence and infection
      (2) Poorly vascularized adipose increases risk of ischemia.
   e. History of bleeding disorders
F. Physiologic changes after burn injury
   1. Burn shock
      a. Massive fluid and protein shifts from intravascular space to interstitium
         (1) Vasodilation, increased capillary permeability, and altered cell membrane at injury site
         (2) Hypovolemic shock occurs because of volume loss.
         (3) Edema of tissues occurs from increased capillary permeability.
      b. Hypovolemia stage lasts for first 48 hours after injury.
      c. Sodium and protein lost from intravascular space into interstitium
   2. Hypothermia
      a. Loss of water and heat by evaporation
      b. Loss of skin's ability to vasoconstrict or vasodilate in response to environmental temperature
   3. Cardiovascular
      a. Decreased cardiac output related to hypothermia, uncompensated hypovolemia, and release of myocardial depressant factor
      b. Catecholamine release from stress response causes vasoconstriction and increases systemic vascular resistance.
      c. Potential for decreased organ perfusion exists.

4. Pulmonary
   a. Potential airway obstruction from edema of face and neck
   b. Decreased chest wall compliance if chest expansion is impaired by chest burns
   c. Bronchopulmonary mucosal damage from smoke inhalation
5. Metabolic
   a. Hypermetabolic state occurs as result of stress response.
   b. Patient develops catabolic state.
6. Immunologic
   a. Postburn immunosuppression occurs from changes in humoral and cell-mediated immunity.
   b. Loss of skin as first line of defense
7. Hematologic
   a. Potential red blood cell hemolysis from thermal injury
   b. Decreased coagulation ability from loss of clotting factors into interstitium
8. Gastrointestinal
   a. Development of paralytic ileus
   b. Prone to stress ulcer development
9. Renal failure
   a. Related to inadequate fluid resuscitation
   b. Related to myoglobinuria from muscle damage in electrical and severe flame burns

IV. ASSESSMENT
   A. Local procedures
      1. Complete blood cell count
      2. Prothrombin time (PT)/partial thromboplastin time (PTT) with a history of bleeding or easy bruising
      3. Additional tests as appropriate depending on the patient's medical history and physical exam
   B. General anesthesia
      1. Complete blood cell count
      2. Chemistry profile
      3. Electrocardiogram (ECG) in adults older than 45 years or with known cardiac condition
      4. Pulmonary function testing if necessary
      5. Chest x-ray film (in adults or in children with pulmonary pathologic findings)
      6. Bleeding profile:
         a. PT
         b. PTT
         c. International normalized ratio (INR)
      7. Pregnancy testing as indicated or desired
   C. Psychological considerations
      1. Body image—the mental picture we possess of our own body
         a. Body image is a changing dynamic entity influenced by internal and external factors.
         b. Body image is a component of how we feel about ourselves.
         c. Most patients undergo elective cosmetic surgery because of body image dissatisfaction.
      2. Motivation for plastic surgery
         a. Internal motivation—surgery to change physical appearance of oneself
         b. External motivation—surgery to change physical appearance at recommendation of others
         c. Patients who are internally motivated are most pleased with surgical outcomes.
         d. History of repeated surgeries
         e. Patients who are dissatisfied with results may:
            (1) Request or undergo repeat procedures
            (2) Experience

          (a) Depression

          (b) Isolation

          (c) Coping disturbances

          (d) Self-destructive behaviors

    f. Rule out body dysmorphic disorder—preoccupation with an aspect of one's appearance.

  3. Preoperative psychological assessment

    a. Determine mental status and mood.

      (1) Poor outcomes associated with history of depression and/or anxiety

      (2) Patients with personality disorders also have poor postoperative outcomes.

    b. Understand patient's perception of body deformity.

    c. Understand patient's expectation of surgical outcome.

    d. Explore significant other's feelings regarding procedure.

    e. Assess postoperative support and coping mechanisms.

  4. Integration of surgical changes into body image

    a. Patients may progress through the stages of grieving.

    b. Changed physical appearance slowly integrates into body image and then self-concept.

    c. Some patients never integrate changes into body image; may request more surgery or require counseling.

  5. Nursing care related to body image

    a. Encourage patient to verbalize feelings.

    b. Reassure patient that it is normal to desire physical attractiveness.

    c. Support the stages of grieving.

    d. Be nonjudgmental with verbal and nonverbal communication.

  6. Determine patient's expectations of surgery.

    a. Expectations realistic?

      (1) Poor outcomes associated with unrealistic expectations

    b. Motivation for surgery?

    c. Reinforce that immediate results may not meet patient's expectations because of swelling, color changes, and suture lines.

    d. Family expectations

    e. Reinforce that long-term results may not meet expectations.

  7. Impact of deformity on patient's self-perception

    a. How does patient view it as changing his or her life?

    b. How important is it to be attractive?

    c. Effect of others' reactions on patient

  8. Psychological evaluation and/or therapy may be appropriate before procedure.

V. PERIOPERATIVE CONCERNS

  A. Preprocedural teaching

    1. Preemptive medications should be reviewed with patient.

    2. NPO (nothing by mouth) instructions

    3. Review any over-the-counter medications and herbal remedies patient uses to determine whether any need to be stopped.

    4. Encourage patient to stop smoking before surgery.

    5. Encourage to wear loose, button-up clothing with preferably slip-on shoes for comfort.

    6. Have patient arrange for a ride and home care support.

  B. Procedural concerns

    1. Primary goals for plastic surgery procedures

      a. Provide cosmetically acceptable results.

      b. Restore function.

      c. Promote healing with minimal scarring.

      d. Prevent infection.

    2. Many procedures are carefully planned before surgery using photography, computerized imaging, and so forth.

3. Patient positioning requirements
   a. Provide comfortable access to surgical field.
      (1) Optimal position on table to allow for repositioning during procedure to evaluate results (e.g., mammoplasty)
   b. Prevent nerve compression from improper positioning.
      (2) Careful positioning
      (3) Padding of pressure points
4. Promote venous drainage.
   a. Use of sequential compression devices (SCDs) and thromboembolism deterrent stockings (TEDS), for example
5. Provide for greatest hypotensive advantages (reduction of bleeding) if deliberate hypotensive technique is used.
6. Incision placement
   a. Incisions placed so that scar lines lie parallel to existing skin lines or behind hairline
   b. Skin lines represent areas with minimal tension.
   c. Cosmetic effect better if tension is minimized
   d. Frequently found under long axis of muscle
7. Hemostasis
   a. Must be obtained and maintained to promote good cosmetic effect
   b. Bleeding under skin potentiates:
      (1) Inflammation
      (2) Infection
      (3) Pressure
      (4) Dehiscence
   c. Achieved with:
      (1) Ligation
      (2) Electrocautery
      (3) Pressure
8. Instrumentation
   a. Microinstrumentation for nontraumatic repair
   b. Use of operating microscope
      (1) Provides three-dimensional view (stereoscopic) that must be clearly seen by surgeon and assistants
      (2) Careful movements in vicinity of operating table
      (3) May require separate instrument tables for donor and recipient sites
   c. Lasers
      (1) LASER: acronym for light amplification by stimulated emission of radiation
      (2) Carbon dioxide (CO_2) laser, argon laser, and neodymium:yttrium-aluminum-garnet (Nd:YAG) laser may be used in aesthetic (cosmetic) surgery.
      (3) Uses
         (a) Removal of professional tattoos and traumatic scars
         (b) Obliteration of blood vessels
         (c) Removal of skin lesions and cancers
         (d) Alternative for skin resurfacing (CO_2 laser)
            (i) Laser blepharoplasty
      (4) Precautions
         (a) Warning signs should be posted indicating that a laser is being used.
         (b) Skin preparation solution may not contain combustible agents.
         (c) Surgical drapes around the site must be kept wet.
         (d) Proper eye protection for everyone must be provided.
   d. Endoscopy
      (1) Endoscope requires body cavity for insertion of scope and visualization.
         (a) No natural cavities in plastic surgery operative areas

(i) Cavity created by use of umbrella or balloonlike retractor on soft tissues

    (b) Uses

       (i) Endoscopic forehead lift

       (ii) Facelift

       (iii) Augmentation or reduction mammoplasty

       (iv) Abdominoplasty

C. Anesthesia concerns

   1. Selection of anesthetic routes and agent

     a. Local anesthesia

       (1) Suitable for minor plastic surgical procedures (e.g., skin lesions, rhinoplasty)

       (2) Often used for outpatients or office patients

       (3) Indicated for procedures that require patient participation (e.g., patients may need to open and close eyes during blepharoplasty)

       (4) Selection of agent that lasts 50 to 100 minutes longer than anticipated length of surgery

     b. Regional anesthesia

       (1) Suitable for procedures localized to extremity

         (a) Axillary, plexus blocks for upper extremities

         (b) Sciatic block for feet

         (c) Lumbar epidural or spinal for leg procedures

     c. General anesthesia

       (1) Suitable for long procedures, pediatrics, and anxious patients

       (2) Long plastic procedures generally require lighter general anesthesia.

       (3) Selection of inhalation agents

         (a) Agents that do not sensitize the heart to catecholamines because of large doses of epinephrine used in plastic procedures (e.g., isoflurane)

         (b) Agents that are less likely to precipitate coughing and laryngospasm, particularly in procedures of face and neck

         (c) Length of time required for elimination for short procedures (e.g., enflurane is rapidly eliminated if used in procedures that last less than 40 minutes)

         (d) Inducing deliberate hypotension

            (i) Selection of agents that induce hypotension

              [a] Reduces blood loss

              [b] Improves visibility at surgical field

            (ii) May be accomplished with volatile agents alone or in combination with:

              [a] Ganglionic blocking agents

              [b] Vasodilators

              [c] Alpha-blockers

              [d] Beta-blockers

            (iii) Used for reconstruction of head and neck

            (iv) Hypotension onset and reversal performed slowly to prevent rapid blood pressure fluctuations (e.g., perfusion to organ is maintained)

   2. Intraoperative management

     a. Airway management

       (1) Method of intubation (oral or nasal) depends on access to surgical field.

         (a) Nasal intubation for oral procedures

         (b) Use of oral or nasal Ring-Adair-Elwyn (RAE) tube for cleft lip and palate repair (endotracheal tubes with sharp curves that promote access to field by surgeon)

         (c) Intubation may be difficult and require fiberoptic bronchoscope in patients, particularly children, with maxillofacial deformities.

(2) Ensure vigorous spontaneous breathing before extubation in patients with maxillofacial surgery.

(3) Esophageal or precordial stethoscope to assess ventilation

(4) Monitor oxygenation.

    (a) Transcutaneous oxygen measurement

    (b) Direct arterial blood gas measurement

    (c) Pulse oximetry

(5) Carbon dioxide monitoring; end-tidal carbon dioxide

    (a) Elevated carbon dioxide levels result in vasodilation, which increases bleeding and intracranial pressure.

b. Cardiovascular management

(1) ECG monitoring (including ST-segment analysis) for patients at risk for coronary ischemia

    (a) From use of epinephrine

    (b) As result of deliberate hypotensive technique

(2) Direct or indirect blood pressure monitoring

    (a) Large blood loss common in plastic procedures

        (i) Crystalloids

        (ii) Colloids

        (iii) Blood products

    (b) Significant hypotension may result in graft or flap failure.

(3) Positioning and position change

    (a) Anesthetic agents affect vascular homeostasis and reflect pressure control mechanisms.

    (b) Position changes during procedure may be necessary.

        (i) To access donor and recipient sites

        (ii) To evaluate cosmetic result of procedure (e.g., mammoplasty)

    (c) Minimizing excessive hypotension

        (i) Slow, careful movement of patient

        (ii) Maintain light anesthesia.

(4) Emergence from anesthesia

    (a) Smooth emergence desired to prevent thrashing that may disrupt delicate suture lines

    (b) Prevent excessive coughing, particularly in head and neck procedures.

    (c) Minimize nausea and vomiting.

VI. COSMETIC BODY PROCEDURES

■ **TOP 5 SURGICAL COSMETIC PROCEDURES FOR 2006 ACCORDING TO AMERICAN SOCIETY OF PLASTIC SURGEONS**

Augmentation Mammoplasty Rhinoplasty Liposuction/Fat Transfer* Blepharoplasty Abdominoplasty	

*Most widely performed procedure worldwide.

Data from American Society of Plastic Surgeons: *2006 Quick facts: Cosmetic and reconstructive plastic surgery trends.* Available at: www.plasticsurgery.org/media/statistics/loader.cfm?url=/commonspot/security/getfile.cfm&PageID=23625. Accessed December 10, 2008.

A. Abdominoplasty

  1. Purpose

    a. Surgical correction of deformities of anterior abdominal wall

    b. Removal of apron deformities (panniculus)

    c. Repair of muscle wall from previous abdominal surgeries

    d. Improve body shape

    e. Also known as a "tummy tuck"

2. Procedure
   a. Surgical removal of loose and redundant tissue of the abdomen
   b. Involves skin, fascia, and adipose tissue
   c. May include closure of abdominal wall muscles
3. Perianesthesia care
   a. Anesthesia: general
   b. Patient selection important for ambulatory abdominoplasty
      (1) Must stay within close proximity to surgery center
      (2) Patient must be motivated.
      (3) Home support must be adequate.
   c. Maintain good pain control so patient can ambulate, cough, and deep breathe.
   d. Control nausea so pain medications will be tolerated.
   e. Maintain correct positioning.
      (1) Head of bed elevated
      (2) Pillow under knees
      (3) Use pillow splint for coughing and moving.
      (4) Walk in stooped position for 1 week.
   f. Empty drains as needed.
      (1) Two Jackson-Pratt drains not unusual
      (2) Empty and record drainage.
      (3) Maintain patency of drains.
         (a) Clots can be a sign of hematoma formation.
   g. Patient will wear a compression girdle for 2 to 3 weeks.
4. Patient education
   a. Review instructions with patient and caregiver.
      (1) Demonstration for positioning and moving
      (2) Activity restrictions: no straining, lifting, exercising for 4 to 6 weeks
      (3) Drain-emptying demonstration
      (4) Hematoma assessment
      (5) Pain management techniques
      (6) Keep compression garment on as directed.
      (7) Report signs and symptoms of infection.
B. Buttock, thigh, upper arm lifts
   1. Purpose
      a. Eliminate loose and sagging skin.
      b. Improve appearance and boost self-confidence.
   2. Procedure
      a. Excision of redundant skin and tissue
      b. Excisional surgery can be performed in conjunction with liposuction.
   3. Perianesthesia care
      a. Anesthesia: local or general
      b. Maintain good pain control so patient can ambulate, cough, and deep breathe.
      c. Monitor drains if used.
         (1) Maintain patency of drains.
         (2) Clots can be a sign of hematoma formation.
      d. Patient will wear a compression girdle for 2 to 3 weeks.
   4. Patient education
      a. Review instructions with patient and caregiver.
         (1) Demonstration for positioning and moving
         (2) Activity restrictions: no straining, lifting, exercising for 4 to 6 weeks
         (3) Drain-emptying demonstration
         (4) Hematoma assessment
         (5) Pain management techniques, including cold compress applications (avoid aspirin)
         (6) Keep compression garment on as directed.
         (7) Report signs and symptoms of infection.

    C. Liposuction and fat transfer

       1. Purpose

          a. To remove pockets of adipose tissue for body contouring

          b. Reimplantation of fat for tissue augmentation (liposhifting)

       2. Procedure

          a. Removal of adipose tissue with suction-assisted device from face, neck, abdomen, thighs, buttocks, flanks, and extremities

          b. Small (1-2 cm) incisions used to minimize scarring

          c. Adipose tissue aspirated using crisscross technique

          d. Compression dressing applied to collapse tunnels created

          e. Accurate volume loss recorded to monitor for hypovolemia and third spacing

       3. Perianesthesia care

          a. Anesthesia: general or local

            (1) More procedures being done with local anesthesia, allowing for better positioning and cooperation by awake patients

          b. Preprocedure, patient is marked in standing position.

          c. Often performed on outpatient basis unless more than 2500 mL of fat is removed

            (1) Admit for fluid replacement.

          d. Medicate for pain.

          e. Usually described as mild to moderate

          f. Maintain fluid balance.

          g. Observe for hypovolemia.

            (1) Replace fluids as indicated by clinical signs and symptoms.

            (2) Autologous blood should be available when high blood loss is expected.

            (3) Estimated blood loss will be decreased with the tumescent technique versus the nontumescent technique.

              (a) Tumescent technique

                (i) Involves infusion of saline, lidocaine, and epinephrine into area to be suctioned

                (ii) Lipolysis is improved and blood loss is decreased.

                (iii) Third spacing can occur with removal of large volumes of adipose tissue.

          h. Assess for hematoma and seroma formation.

          i. Compression applied with compression garment or ACE wraps

            (1) Keep dressings flat and smooth for even contouring.

       4. Patient education

          a. Instruct patient to push fluids to cover third-space fluid shifts.

          b. Patient should avoid aspirin-containing products.

          c. Compression garment will be worn for 24 hours to several weeks (physician preference).

          d. Activity

            (1) Rest; minimal activity for first week

            (2) Avoid strenuous activity for 1 month.

          e. Observe for hematoma and seroma formation.

          f. Bruising and swelling expected

          g. Female urinal can aid in elimination while compression garment is worn.

          h. Instruct patient to protect bedding the first 24 hours because copious serous-sanguineous drainage is not unusual.

          i. Sponge bathing may be required while patient is restricted to compression garment.

    D. Body contouring

       1. Purpose

          a. Increasing popularity of weight loss surgeries to remove excess skin primarily from the abdomen, back, upper arms, breasts, inner and outer thighs

      b. Excess skin can cause chafing, moisture retention, skin infections, musculoskeletal and postural strains.

      c. Improve sense of well-being and accomplishment

  2. Procedure

      a. Contouring will depend on the presence of excess and redundant tissue.

      b. Procedures often done in combination

         (1) Abdominoplasty

         (2) Mastopexy

         (3) Mammoplasty

         (4) Brachioplasty

         (5) Thigh lift

         (6) Mons reduction

         (7) Liposuction

         (8) Buttock augmentation

      c. Surgery usually planned once weight loss has plateaued for 12 to 24 months

  3. Perianesthesia care

      a. Anesthesia: general

      b. Surgery times can vary from 2 to 10 or more hours.

         (1) Increased risk for pressure ulcers in the operating room

         (2) Deep vein thrombosis

         (3) Pulmonary emboli

      c. Increased risks associated with weight loss surgery

         (1) Protein and/or vitamin deficiencies interfering with wound healing

         (2) Residual comorbidities such as diabetes, sleep apnea

         (3) Persistent or unhealed skin irritation and infections

         (4) Unresolved psychological component to weight management and eating disorders

         (5) Medication risks

            (a) Avoid because of increased risk for ulcers and bleeding

               (i)   NSAIDs

               (ii) Aspirin

               (iii) Cyclooxygenase-2 inhibitors

            (b) Avoid

               (i)   Tetracycline

               (ii) Macrolides

               (iii) Oxycodone

  4. Patient education

      a. Review instructions with patient and caregiver.

         (1) Demonstration for:

            (a) Positioning and moving

            (b) Early ambulation

         (2) Activity restrictions: no straining, lifting, exercising for 4 to 6 weeks

         (3) Drain-emptying demonstration

            (a) Hematoma assessment

            (b) Foley care if necessary

         (4) Pain and comfort management techniques, including cold compress applications, elevation of affected extremities, nausea control

         (5) Keep compression garment on as directed.

         (6) Report signs and symptoms of infection.

E. Spider vein therapy

  1. Purpose

      a. To treat spider veins (telangiectasia) and varicose veins

  2. Procedure

      a. Sclerotherapy

         (1) Injection of chemical agents to eliminate unsightly veins

         (2) Three categories of agents

            (a) Detergents

            (b) Osmotic agents

            (c) Chemical irritants

     b. Other treatment options include
       (1) Laser surgery
       (2) Electrodesiccation
  3. Perianesthesia care
     a. Anesthesia: local
     b. Observe for itching and burning at injection site.
  4. Patient education
     a. Keep compression bandages on as directed.
     b. Early return to walking regimens encouraged to promote aerobic circulation
     c. Mild analgesics may be required initially for cramplike discomfort.
     d. Reinforce with patient that area will "look and feel worse before it gets better."

VII. COSMETIC BREAST AND CHEST PROCEDURES
  A. Augmentation mammoplasty
    1. Purpose
      a. To improve body image and self-confidence
      b. To modify shape of breast to:
        (1) Increase breast size
        (2) Correct surgical defects with the use of a prosthesis
    2. Procedure
      a. Insertion of prosthetic devices (e.g., tissue expanders that are inflated with normal saline)
      b. Prosthesis placed under the pectoral muscle or mammary tissue through an inframammary, axillary, areolar incision, or endoscope
        (1) Submammary: beneath breast tissue on anterior surface of pectoralis muscle
        (2) Submuscular: beneath pectoralis major and serratus anterior muscles
    3. Perianesthesia care
      a. Anesthesia: general or local with monitored anesthesia care (MAC)
      b. Assess for hematoma.
        (1) Palpate superior aspect of pectoralis muscle over the third rib to the clavicle.
        (2) Breast size should remain equal.
      c. Assess for signs of pneumothorax.
        (1) More common with axillary incision
        (2) Have chest tube and drainage setup available.
        (3) Auscultate lung sounds.
      d. Provide pain relief.
        (1) Pain is moderate to severe.
        (2) Prosthesis beneath chest muscle is more painful.
        (3) Multimodal drug therapy effective
          (a) Preemptive oral narcotics
          (b) Toradol and narcotics intravenous (IV) or oral
          (c) Local anesthesia in wounds
          (d) Muscle relaxants for spasm
          (e) Ice may be helpful for pain control.
      e. Prevent and treat nausea so oral pain medications can be tolerated.
    4. Patient education
      a. Observe for hematoma.
      b. ACE wrap or soft-support bra may be worn for 1 week.
      c. Observe for capsule formation.
        (1) May occur months after surgery
      d. Massage instructions per physician preference
        (1) Massage usually begins within first 2 weeks.
        (2) Massage keeps prosthesis mobile in pocket.
        (3) Postmassage ice packs helpful
      e. Activity
        (1) Restrict arm activity for 3 to 4 weeks.

B. Pectoral implantation
  1. Purpose
   a. To provide an athletic chest contour for male patients
   b. To treat underdevelopment of muscles of one side of chest as a result of congenital defects or injury
  2. Procedure
   a. Small transaxillary incisions made
   b. Implants inserted under pectoralis muscles
   c. Can be done endoscopically to minimize risk of bleeding and infection
  3. Perianesthesia care
   a. Similar to breast augmentation surgery
   b. Usually no drains required
   c. Assess for hematoma formation.
  4. Education
   a. Pain is usually mild to moderate soreness.
   b. Normal activity can be resumed within a week, but strenuous exercise should be restricted for at least 6 weeks.
C. Gynecomastectomy
  1. Purpose
   a. To improve self-confidence and body image
  2. Procedure
   a. Removal of excessive breast tissue in male patient
   b. May combine excision of excess skin and tissue with liposuction
  3. Perianesthesia care
   a. Anesthesia: general or local (for small excision)
   b. Assess for hematoma formation.
   c. Maintain patency of drains (Jackson-Pratt not unusual).
   d. Pain usually described as moderate
  4. Education
   a. Observe for hematoma.
   b. Provide instruction and demonstration of drain care.
   c. Usually removed after 48 hours
   d. Arm activity limited for 1 month
   e. ACE wrap or compression vest usually worn for compression
D. Mastopexy
  1. Purpose
   a. Reshaping (uplifting) of redundant, sagging breast skin
   b. Generally less than 300 g of tissue removed
  2. Procedure
   a. Incisions usually placed in the inferior pedicle, maintaining nerve innervation to the nipple
  3. Perianesthesia care
   a. General anesthesia most common
   b. Usually same-day procedure
   c. Position supine or semi-Fowler's for comfort.
   d. Assess for hematoma formation.
   e. Maintain patency of drains if used (rarely).
   f. Pain usually described as mild
  4. Education
   a. Observe for hematoma.
   b. Surgical support bra may be worn.
   c. Inform patient about potential for scarring.
VIII. COSMETIC HEAD AND NECK PROCEDURES
  A. Blepharoplasty
   1. Purpose
    a. To repair or reconstruct upper or lower eyelid to correct "baggy" appearance
    b. To provide patient with a more youthful and less fatigued look
    c. To improve vision fields

2. Procedure
   a. Surgical removal of redundant skin and adipose tissue with shortening of muscles of upper and lower eyelids
   b. Incisions placed in the crease of the upper lid and in the lower lid below lash margin
   c. Surgical incisions may be done with laser or scalpel.
3. Perianesthesia care
   a. Anesthesia: local
   b. Assess for signs of retrobulbar hematoma formation.
      (1) Signs of medical emergency
         (a) Pressure behind eye
         (b) Loss of vision
      (2) Observe for:
         (a) Pallor, ecchymosis, firmness, or complaints of pain or tightness around eyes
         (b) Proptosis: forward displacement or bulging eye
   c. Maintain normal blood pressure.
      (1) Retards hematoma formation
      (2) Avoid straining, lifting, bending at least 1 week.
      (3) Elevate head of bed.
   d. Pain usually described as mild to moderate
      (1) Control with moderate strength narcotics (codeine or hydrocodone usually effective).
      (2) Ice packs provide pain control and decrease swelling.
4. Education
   a. Activity
      (1) Avoid activities that will increase blood pressure.
      (2) Keep head elevated.
      (3) Limit reading and television for 48 hours.
   b. Observe for hematoma formation.
   c. Use ice or cool, moist compresses as ordered.
      (1) Keep cloth between ice bag and skin.
      (2) Frozen peas in the bag work well.
   d. Eyes may be dry and lashes crusty with bloody drainage.
   e. Expect periorbital ecchymosis and swelling.
      (1) Mild blurring expected
      (2) Call immediately for loss of vision or pressure behind eye.
      (3) Use sterile saline drops to moisten eyes and separate lashes.
   f. Sutures usually removed in 5 days or surgeon preference
B. Genioplasty and mentoplasty
   1. Purpose
      a. Surgical reshaping of chin
      b. Modifications in mandible or insertion of prosthesis
      c. May be performed in conjunction with rhinoplasty to provide a balanced facial profile
   2. Procedure
      a. Incisions placed inside mouth or beneath chin
   3. Perianesthesia care
      a. Maintain dressing.
      b. Liquid or soft diet
      c. Meticulous oral hygiene if oral incisions placed
   4. Education
      a. Minimize facial movements.
      b. Offer suggestions for nutritional alternatives.
      c. Meticulous oral hygiene if oral incisions placed
C. Otoplasty
   1. Purpose
      a. Surgical reshaping or repositioning of ears

        b. To correct prominent or malformed ears (i.e., microtia)

        c. To improve body image and self-confidence

        d. May be performed on children after 6 years of age, when ears have reached most of their adult size

    2. Procedure

        a. Reshaping of cartilage and skin of the outer ear

        b. May require harvesting cartilage from ribs

    3. Perianesthesia care

        a. Anesthesia: local or general, depending on age of patient

        b. Frequently a procedure for school-age children

        c. Assess for hematoma formation.

          (1) Use severe pain as an indicator because of bulky head dressing.

        d. Maintain patency of any drains.

        e. Medicate for pain with oral narcotics.

          (1) Usually described as moderate pain

        f. Children have usually suffered teasing because of ears.

          (1) Assure them that surgical outcome is good.

    4. Education

        a. Activity

          (1) Elevate head with two pillows.

          (2) No strenuous activity for 2 to 4 weeks

        b. Ears will be sensitive to cold and swell in heat for 3 to 6 months.

        c. Observe for hematoma.

        d. Teach drain care.

        e. Bulky head dressing usually worn for 1 week

D. Rhytidoplasty, rhytidectomy, browlift

    1. Purpose

        a. To remove wrinkle and facial laxity giving a more rested, youthful appearance

        b. To tighten loose tissue in face

          (1) May involve skin, fat, subcutaneous tissue, and muscle

    2. Procedure

        a. Standard incisions placed in temporal area behind hairline

        b. Additional procedures may be performed in conjunction with rhytidectomy.

          (1) Tightening of underlying fascia in the superficial musculoaponeurotic system

          (2) Blepharoplasty, browlifting, chemical peel, suction-assisted lipectomy or lipolysis

        c. Rhytidectomy—facelift

          (1) Tightening of all tissue of the face and neck with excision of redundant tissue

        d. Coronal browlift

          (1) Tightening the tissue of the forehead and brow with excision of redundant tissue

        e. Endoscopic surgery of the head and neck

          (1) Face, neck, and browlift may be performed with the endoscopic technique when redundant tissue excision is not required.

          (2) Endoscopic techniques generally involve minimal bleeding.

    3. Perianesthesia care

        a. Anesthesia: MAC or general

        b. Assess for hematoma formation.

          (1) Palpate neck, forehead, and check frequently.

          (2) Bulky dressings common

            (a) Assess for absence of increasing tightness, difficulty breathing, or swallowing.

            (b) If any question of hematoma, notify surgeon so dressing can be taken down.

      c. Maintain patency of drains.
        (1) May have Jackson-Pratt or Penrose
      d. Maintain normal blood pressure.
        (1) To prevent hematoma formation
        (2) Manage pain before it increases blood pressure.
        (3) Treat uncontrolled hypertension with antihypertensives if pain management not the cause.
      e. Prevent nausea and vomiting.
      f. Provide calm, reassuring environment to decrease anxiety.
      g. Maintain comfort.
        (1) Pain can be considered moderate to severe for facelift.
        (2) Browlift pain usually described as severe headache
        (3) Begin medications before all local anesthesia has resolved.
        (4) Combination of oral and IV narcotics may be required.
        (5) Toradol very effective but contraindicated by some physicians because of bleeding potential
        (6) Cold compresses or ice can be effective.
      h. Positioning
        (1) Elevate head of bed to decrease swelling.
        (2) Avoid activities that increase blood pressure.
        (3) Avoid turning head side to side or nodding.
      i. Assess cranial nerve VII.
        (1) Temporary numbness of ears and cheeks are normal sequelae.
        (2) Ask patient to smile, frown, wrinkle forehead and nose.
        (3) Assess facial symmetry.
        (4) Assess sensation of earlobes.
          (a) If facial nerve damaged, it will regenerate with time.
    4. Education
      a. Activity
        (1) Avoid strenuous activity for 1 month.
      b. Elevate head and torso with two pillows at bedtime.
      c. Observe for hematoma formation.
        (1) Drain care demonstration
        (2) If drains present, usually removed in 24 hours
      d. Hair washing per physician
        (1) Usually after sutures are removed in 1 week
      e. Soft diet with little chewing
      f. Appropriate use of pain medications and ice for pain control
      g. Signs to report
        (1) Increased facial pain or unilateral numbness
        (2) Signs and symptoms of infection
  E. Rhinoplasty
    1. Purpose
      a. Surgical reshaping of nose
      b. To improve body image and self-confidence
    2. Procedure
      a. Excision of fat, cartilage, and skin with fracturing of nasal bones to reshape the nose
    3. Perianesthesia care
      a. Anesthesia: general or MAC with local anesthesia
      b. Provide comfort measures.
        (1) Pain usually described as moderate but may be severe
        (2) Medicate with oral or IV narcotics as needed.
          (a) NSAIDs can be helpful.
          (b) Begin medications before local anesthesia resolves.
          (c) Ice mask to reduce swelling and pain
      c. Provide calm, reassuring environment.
      d. Patient may have packing in both nares.

(1) Maintain nasal packing, and avoid removal of clots from nose.
(2) Change "drip pad" as needed.
(3) Avoid pressure to nose, including glasses.
(4) Sneeze through mouth.
(5) Inability to breathe through nose can be anxiety producing.
    (a) Provide reassurance.
(6) Mouth will be very dry.
    (a) Give frequent mouth care.
  e. Position patient with head of bed elevated.
  f. Prevent postoperative nausea and vomiting.
    (1) Encourage patient to expectorate any postnasal bloody secretions.
    (2) Medicate with antiemetics as needed.
4. Education
  a. Activity
    (1) No strenuous activity for 1 month
    (2) No flexing from waist
    (3) No flexing head
  b. Nasal packing usually removed in 24 to 72 hours
  c. Continue ice mask at home.
    (1) Swelling and bruising may be worse on second or third postoperative day.
  d. Use humidifier at home to prevent drying of mucous membranes.
  e. Force fluids.
F. Skin enhancement and minimally invasive procedures
  1. Purpose
    a. To remove signs of aging and give a youthful appearance
    b. Use of chemical agents to remove or destroy tissue to improve tone and texture of skin
    c. Removal of facial epidermis and part of superficial dermis to correct skin defects
      (1) Acne or depressed scarring
      (2) Wrinkles
      (3) Irregular skin pigmentation
  2. Procedures
    a. Chemical peels
      (1) Phenol: creates a controllable superficial thickness burn
      (2) Trichloroacetic acid: medium depth peel causing temporary blanching of skin
      (3) Alphahydroxy acid ("fruit peel"): better choice for "sensitive" skin because it causes less irritation and photosensitivity postapplication
      (4) Retin A: common topical treatment for acne
    b. Dermabrasion
      (1) Helpful for skin resurfacing: to make skin smoother, improve mild pigmentation problems, reduce pore size and treat acne, and give skin a smoother contour
      (2) Uses sanding with microparticles or rotating wire brushes on skin
    c. Collagen injections: injections of autologous or bovine collagen to enhance or remodel skin and tissue appearance
      (1) Scar revisions
      (2) Lip enhancement
      (3) Minor facial corrections
    d. Laser hair removal
    e. Soft tissue filling: hyaluronic acid
  3. Perianesthesia care
    a. Anesthesia: usually local, general if combined with total facial resurfacing
    b. Provide comfort measures.
      (1) NSAIDs helpful
      (2) Pain can be mild to moderate.
        (a) Ice to affected area or cold gel mask decreases discomfort and swelling.

      c. Elevate head of bed.

      d. Continue prophylactic antibiotics and antiviral agents as ordered.

      e. Skin care will vary according to physician preference.

  4. Education

  5. Activity

      a. Elevate head of bed.

      b. Minimize facial movement to decrease cracking of dead tissue.

  6. Skin and dressing care per physician's preference

      a. Avoid picking or scratching of skin.

      b. Expect erythema.

      c. Expect mild weeping serous fluid.

  7. Continue antiviral and antibiotic agents if ordered.

      a. Application of antibiotic or hydrocortisone ointments or powders if indicated

  8. Observe and report any signs of infection.

  9. Encourage patient to call office with any questions on skin care.

  10. Instruct patient to avoid sun while skin is healing.

      a. When healed, use at least a sun protection factor (SPF) 15 sunscreen.

  11. Instruct patient to notify physician if any hyperpigmentation changes are noted.

      a. Face will remain pink for 4 to 6 weeks.

      b. Camouflage makeup is helpful.

G. Laser resurfacing

  1. Purpose

      a. To remove signs of aging and give a youthful appearance

      b. Removal of facial epidermis and part of superficial dermis to correct skin defects

        (1) Acne or depressed scarring

        (2) Wrinkles and sun-damaged skin

        (3) Irregular skin pigmentation: freckles, liver spots, keratoses

  2. Procedure

      a. Short blasts of invisible light vaporize a thin layer of epidermis.

        (1) CO_2 and erbium:yttrium-aluminum-garnet (Er:YAG) lasers remove the epidermis.

        (2) Nd:YAG penetrates more deeply to dermis.

        (3) Pulsed-dye laser and intense pulse light both stimulate collagen growth and improve skin's appearance with less blanching.

      b. The deeper the laser penetrates, the more lines and wrinkles will be removed.

      c. Penetration that is too deep will cause scarring.

      d. Contraindicated in dark-skinned people

  3. Perianesthesia care

      a. Anesthesia: local or general

      b. Provide comfort measures.

        (1) Medicate with narcotics as needed.

          (a) NSAIDs helpful

        (2) Pain can be mild to severe.

          (a) Ice to affected area or cold gel mask decreases discomfort and swelling.

      c. Elevate head of bed.

      d. Continue prophylactic antibiotics and antiviral agents as ordered.

      e. Provide nourishment through a straw.

      f. Full face resurfacing will cause swelling around mouth.

      g. Child's toothbrush can assist with mouth care.

      h. Skin care will vary according to physician preference.

        (1) Open technique (no dressing)

          (a) Cool saline compresses on the face for first night

          (b) On day 1, four times per day, vinegar and water soaks with gentle removal of crusts

           (c) Frequent application of petroleum jelly or antibiotic based ointment

           (d) Goal is to keep skin soft, pink, and free of crusts.

           (e) Soaks continued until crusting ceases (7-10 days), then a moisturizer used

       (2) Closed technique

           (a) Flexan (biomembrane dressing) applied to the affected area

               (i) Any exposed areas treated with the open technique

               (ii) Flexan dressing changed according to physician's preference

           (b) N-terface dressing can be applied to affected areas.

               (i) Held in place with tube gauze and 4 × 4-inch bandages to absorb drainage

               (ii) Soaks may be done through the dressing, and application of petroleum jelly or other lubricant is put on over the dressing.

               (iii) Changed according to physician's preference

   4. Education

     a. Activity

       (1) Elevate head of bed.

     b. Skin and dressing care per physician's preference

       (1) Laser resurfacing patients require reassurance and reinforcement of skin care instructions.

       (2) Avoid picking or scratching of skin.

       (3) Expect erythema.

       (4) Expect weeping serous fluid.

     c. Continue antiviral and antibiotic agents as ordered.

       (1) Application of antibiotic or hydrocortisone ointments or powders if indicated

     d. Observe and report any signs of infection.

     e. Encourage patient to call office with any questions on skin care.

     f. Instruct patient to avoid sun while skin is healing.

       (1) When healed, use at least an SPF 15 sunscreen.

     g. Instruct patient to notify physician if any hyperpigmentation changes are noted.

       (1) Face will remain pink for 4 to 6 weeks.

       (2) Camouflage makeup is helpful.

     h. Pain management

IX. GENERAL RECONSTRUCTIVE PROCEDURES

■ **TOP 5 RECONSTRUCTIVE PROCEDURES FOR 2006 ACCORDING TO THE AMERICAN SOCIETY OF PLASTIC SURGEONS**

Skin Lesions/Tumor Removal
Laceration Repair
Scar Revisions
Hand Surgery
Reduction Mammoplasty

Data from American Society of Plastic Surgeons: *2006 Quick facts: Cosmetic and reconstructive plastic surgery trends.* Available at: www.plasticsurgery.org/Media/Statistics/2006_Statistics.html. Accessed April 13, 2009.

   A. Skin lesions/tumor removal

     1. Purpose

       a. Removal of skin lesions whether benign or malignant

       b. Benign skin lesions

         (1) Nevus

           (a) Most common skin lesion

              (i) Round

              (ii) Brown or black

              (iii) Flat or raised

              (iv) With or without hair

   (b) Three types
    (i) Intradermal
    (ii) Junctional
    (iii) Compound
     [a] Most need no treatment unless a change is noted or if there is constant irritation.
     [b] Junctional may convert to malignant melanoma.
  c. Malignant skin lesions
   (1) Basal cell carcinoma
    (a) Most common skin cancer
    (b) May be nodular with an ulcerated center or crusted, dermatitis-like
   (2) Squamous cell carcinoma
    (a) Begins as a red papule
    (b) Progresses to an area that ulcerates, then crusts
    (c) Invades underlying tissue
   (3) Malignant melanoma
    (a) Suspicious lesions with:
     (i) Change in size
     (ii) Change in color (brown to black)
     (iii) Change from smooth to rough
     (iv) Irregular borders
     (v) Change in sensation
     (vi) Satellite lesions

2. Procedure
 a. Simple excision
 b. Laser therapy
 c. Wide excision, possible flap graft, node dissection, radiation, topical chemotherapy, or cryosurgery

3. Perianesthesia care
 a. Anesthesia: local or general
 b. Provide reassurance, and allow patient to verbalize any fears or concerns regarding body image, diagnosis, and so forth.
 c. Elevate extremities.
 d. Monitor dressings and assess for hematoma.
 e. Position for comfort.

4. Education
 a. Teach patient proper dressing and wound care per physician preference.
 b. Protect healing incisions from sun.
 c. Minimize activity of affected areas for 1 to 2 weeks.
 d. Encourage proper follow-up care to monitor for new lesions.

B. Laceration repair and scar revisions (Z-plasty, V-plasty)

1. Purpose
 a. Repair skin lacerations (dog bites most common).
 b. Remove or reduce scar tissue.

2. Procedure
 a. Z-plasty
  (1) Use of Z-shaped incision to remove scar tissue
  (2) Requires tissue with elasticity
 b. V-plasty
  (1) Used to repair skin defects
  (2) Two triangular flaps of adjacent skin transposed
 c. Laser therapy can be used.
 d. All procedures can be offered in combination.

3. Perianesthesia care
 a. Anesthesia: local or general
 b. Wound and dressing assessments to observe for hematoma formation
 c. Analgesia as required
 d. Minimal activity involving operative site to reduce tension on operative sutures

    4. Education

        a. Signs and symptoms of infection

        b. Activity restrictions

        c. Pain management

C. Hand surgery

    1. Purpose

        a. To correct deformities of the hand

        b. To restore function

    2. Procedures

        a. Ganglionectomy: excision of painful fluid-filled cyst attached to a joint capsule or tendon

        b. Palmar fasciectomy: release of flexion contractures of metacarpophalangeal joints

        c. Carpal tunnel release: decompression of the carpal tunnel releasing pressure on the median nerve

            (1) May be done open or endoscopically

        d. Trauma repair: may involve open reduction with internal fixation of fractures or microvascular surgery

    3. Perianesthesia care

        a. Anesthesia: local, axillary or bier block, general

        b. Assess extremity for circulation and neurological status.

        c. Include sensory, motor, color, and capillary refill.

        d. Apply temporary sling after axillary block.

        e. Elevate extremity above level of heart using pillows.

        f. Provide adequate analgesia.

        g. Consider multimodal therapies.

        h. Maintain patency of drains.

    4. Education

        a. Activity restrictions as directed

        b. Maintain elevation of affected limb.

        c. Observe for changes in circulation and neurological status.

        d. Teach signs and symptoms of infection.

D. Cleft lip and palate

    1. Purpose

        a. Repair of congenital cleft lip or palate defects

        b. Repair of congenital defects from early closure of sutures (craniosynostosis)

        c. Repair of congenital maxillofacial deformities

        d. Obtain nostril symmetry and Cupid's bow of upper lip, and repair lip muscle.

            (1) Commonly performed when child (rule of 10s)

                (a) At least 10 weeks old

                (b) Weighs at least 10 lb (4500 g)

                (c) Has a hemoglobin of 10 g/dL

    2. Procedure

        a. May require extensive skeletal reconstruction

        b. May be performed in staged procedures

    3. Perianesthesia care

        a. Anesthesia: general

        b. Position side to side, never prone.

        c. Avoid crying and restlessness that strain suture lines.

            (1) Allow parents to hold the child.

            (2) Offer cool compresses to suture areas to reduce swelling and promote comfort.

        d. Monitor for bleeding.

            (1) Swelling or hematoma at lip

            (2) Excessive swallowing

        e. Maintain in elbow extension splints to protect incisions.

      f. Gentle oral suctioning with soft-tip catheter

      g. Provide mist humidifiers if possible to keep airway moist.

      h. Maintain elevation of head of bed to decrease intracranial pressure.

      i. Place on seizure precautions.

      j. Minimize activities that increase intracranial pressure.

        (1) Crying in children

        (2) Straining

      k. Medicate to provide comfort but not enough to mask neurologic symptoms.

    4. Education

      a. Feeding routines by physician preference

      b. Pain management

  E. Microvascular surgery

    1. Purpose

      a. Generally used to replant severed body parts

    2. Procedure

      a. Tedious anastomosis of severed blood vessels, nerves, and other injured structures

      b. Reconstruction of absent digits using transplanted body parts

      c. Example: reconstruction of absent finger using patient's toe

    3. Perianesthesia care

      a. Procedure-specific care

      b. Special attention given to observation of skin color at operative site

        (1) White indicates no blood is perfusing to area because of arterial obstruction.

        (2) Pink is normal.

        (3) Blue indicates hypoxemia in tissues.

        (4) Dark blue to black indicates impending tissue infarct from venous obstruction.

      c. Often require posttraumatic counseling

    4. Education

      a. Procedure-specific and site-specific patient education to include but not be limited to activity, pain management, and wound care

  F. Genitourinary/gender reassignment

    1. Purpose

      a. Surgical interventions for "intersex" children

      b. Most frequent disorder is genital ambiguity (congenital adrenal hyperplasia).

      c. Highly controversial circumstance concerning the appropriate developmental stage to pursue intervention

      d. Sex reassignment surgery for transsexual individuals

    2. Procedure

      a. Surgical restructuring of genitalia

      b. Feminizing genitalia involves clitoral reduction and/or vaginoplasty.

      c. Penile reconstruction

    3. Perianesthesia care

      a. Same as any major genitourinary procedure

    4. Education

      a. Patients and family require extensive counseling and education regarding treatment options and to address any underlying issues of self-esteem and psychological stress.

X. BREAST RECONSTRUCTIVE PROCEDURES

  A. Reduction mammoplasty

    1. Purpose

      a. Removal of excess breast mass to decrease neck, back, and shoulder pain

      b. To improve body image and self-confidence

      c. May be performed to correct severe asymmetry as in Poland's syndrome

 2. Procedure
   a. Surgical excision of redundant breast tissue and skin with recontouring of breast shape
   b. Areolar transplantation can be done through free tissue transfer to pedicle.
   c. On occasion, areola may be replaced as free graft, resulting in loss of breast-feeding abilities and sensation.
 3. Perianesthesia care
   a. Anesthesia: general
   b. Assess for hematoma.
     (1) Palpate superior aspect of pectoralis muscle over the third rib to the clavicle.
   c. Drains may be used postoperatively.
     (1) Monitor drainage.
     (2) Reinforce to keep clothing and bedding dry.
   d. Treat pain.
     (1) Usually described as moderate
     (2) May need IV narcotic on emergence
     (3) Control with strong narcotics at home (e.g., oxycodone for first day or two).
   e. Surgical bra or compression dressing applied postoperatively to maintain new breast contour and decrease fluid accumulation; compression bra
     (1) Tube gauze over bra assists in holding reinforcement ABD pads in place.
   f. Prevent and treat nausea and vomiting.
     (1) Vomiting can cause hematoma formation.
   g. Provide aggressive fluid replacement for blood loss.
     (1) Usual blood loss, 400 mL
     (2) Replace with crystalloid or colloid as needed.
     (3) Some patients may require hospitalization if symptomatic after blood loss and fluid replacement.
 4. Education
   a. Observe for hematoma formation.
   b. Activity
     (1) No heavy lifting or strenuous activity for 1 month
     (2) No pushing self up with arms
     (3) Instruct patient and caregiver on how to make position changes.
   c. Usually a return appointment in 24 hours for drain removal
   d. Steristrips or sutures may be removed in 1 week.
   e. Compression bra for 2 to 3 weeks
     (1) Demonstrate how to reinforce dressing.
B. Breast reconstruction
 1. Purpose
   a. Breast reconstruction after wide local excision and mastectomy for breast cancer to achieve breast symmetry
   b. Repair of traumatic injury
   c. Repair of defects from cancer treatment
 2. Procedure
   a. Insertion of breast implants
     (1) Creation of a pocket space under remaining breast tissues into which a soft prosthetic breast implant can be placed
     (2) Pocket can be created by means of inflatable tissue expander used to gradually increase the volume of pocket space to receive prosthesis.
   b. Transplantation of skin, muscle, and blood supply from autologous donor site to repair congenital or acquired tissue defects
     (1) Flaps or tissue transfer
       (a) At time of procedure, absence of infection required at recipient site
       (b) Donor muscle or skin for flap selected to appropriately fit defect and minimally impact patient's activity and function after removal
         (i) Muscle size will decrease at recipient site after denervation.

      (c) Pedicle flap (delayed) selected to reach defect comfortably
      (d) Preparation of recipient vessels
          (i) Devitalized tissue carefully removed
          (ii) Selection of recipient blood vessels that have been minimally impacted by trauma of defect
      (e) Anastomosis of vessels
          (i) Avoid twisting of vessels.
          (ii) Vessels must be delicately handled.
          (iii) Use of heparin-containing irrigating solutions
   (2) Types of flaps
      (a) Delayed flap
          (i) Donor tissue attached to recipient site without being separated from its blood supply
          (ii) Remains attached to donor site (by pedicle) until recipient circulation is established
      (b) Local flaps
          (i) Moved from location immediately adjacent to defect
          (ii) Maintains blood supply from original source
      (c) Free flap
          (i) Entire tissue and blood supply detached from donor site
          (ii) Requires prolonged microsurgery (6-12 hours)
   (3) Common sources of flaps
      (a) Skin flaps
          (i) Consists of skin and subcutaneous tissue
          (ii) May be placed to a remote area by means of pedicle
          (iii) May be advanced into a defect close to donor site or moved at a pivotal point and rotated into tissue defect
          (iv) Sources
             [a] Temporalis fascia: may be used to cover dorsum of hand or foot
             [b] Lateral forearm: skin and fascia used to cover areas requiring a thicker coverage
             [c] Omentum: for areas that require pliable tissue (e.g., frontal sinuses)
      (b) Muscle and myocutaneous flaps
          (i) Movement of muscle with or without skin to cover defect
             [a] Local transfer
             [b] Free transfer
          (ii) May require additional skin grafting at recipient site
          (iii) Sources
             [a] Latissimus dorsi
             [b] Pectoralis major
             [c] Tensor fascia lata
             [d] Rectus abdominus
             [e] Gluteus maximus
             [f] Gracilis
3. Perianesthesia care
  a. Anesthesia: general
  b. Monitor for and prevent factors that promote vasospasm and thrombosis.
   (1) Hypothermia
      (a) Results in vasoconstriction
      (b) Arterial flow compromised
      (c) Use warming blankets, lights, warmed fluids, increased room temperature.
   (2) Hypotension
   (3) Hypovolemia
      (a) Large blood loss may have occurred.

(b) Replacement with crystalloids and colloids

(c) Excessive red blood cell replacement may raise hematocrit, causing sluggish capillary flow.

(4) Agents that increase vasoconstriction and vasospasm (e.g., nicotine, caffeine)

c. Maintenance of normal body temperature

(1) Warmed IV and irrigating fluids

(2) Room temperature regulation

(3) Warming blankets

d. Assess condition of flap.

(1) Skin temperature

(a) Should be warm to touch

(b) Coolness reflects reduced blood flow.

(2) Capillary refill

(a) Blanching within 2 seconds

(b) Rapid blanching may indicate venous engorgement.

(c) Delayed blanching may indicate arterial insufficiency.

(d) Arterial and venous flow may be obtained by Doppler ultrasonography and are marked by surgeon with a marker or suture.

(e) Venous congestion frequently results in failure before arterial insufficiency.

(3) Color

(a) Normally white or gray immediately postoperatively

(b) Increasingly pale flaps suggest arterial insufficiency.

(c) Bluish color suggests venous congestion.

(d) Color of flap may be different from other skin in recipient area if obtained from tissue far removed.

(4) Edema

(a) Slight swelling expected

(b) Significant swelling may indicate hematoma or venous congestion.

(5) Monitor drainage from drains every 30 to 60 minutes.

(a) Gentle continuous suction

(b) Greater than 50 mL/hr is problematic.

(6) Monitor muscle donor site for bleeding.

(7) Antiplatelets or anticoagulants may be used to decrease platelet aggregation and thrombosis.

(a) Low–molecular weight dextran

(b) Heparin drip

(c) Aspirin

(8) Flap failure usually caused by inadequate circulation or infection

(a) Prevent patient from lying on operative site.

(b) Prevent compression of operative site by blankets.

(9) Patient care for patient with tissue expander or prosthetic implant same as augmentation mammoplasty

(a) When expansion complete:

(i) Prosthesis inserted

(ii) Nipple reconstruction done

(iii) Nipple tattoo or graft reconstruction

(b) Pain can be severe with initial insertion of expander.

(c) Anesthesia: general

(d) Psychological support crucial because patients have had multiple procedures and cancer diagnosis

4. Education

a. Observe for hematoma formation.

b. Report deflation of tissue expander.

(1) Could mean rupture

c. Limit arm activity for 1 month.

d. Frequent appointments required for inflation of expander with saline

XI. COMMON SURGICAL BURN PROCEDURES
  A. Escharotomy
    1. Indicated for circumferential full-thickness burns
      a. Burn eschar acts as tourniquet.
        (1) Decreases arterial flow
        (2) Causes venous congestion
      b. Common sites are extremities or trunk.
    2. Linear incisions placed extending through burn eschar down to superficial fascia, releasing constriction
    3. May be performed with or without anesthesia
      a. Nerve endings in eschar dead
      b. Premedication to relieve anxiety and discomfort
  B. Excision and skin grafting
    1. Goal is to restore function and maximize cosmetic appearance.
      a. Performed in burns with limited or inability to heal
      b. May require grafting months to years after injury to revise scar tissue
      c. Principles of grafting similar for burns and nonburn wounds requiring skin coverage
    2. Nonviable tissue removed
    3. Graft sources
      a. Autograft
        (1) Patient's own skin used
        (2) Permanent
      b. Cultured autologous human epithelium
        (1) Biopsy of patient's skin obtained
        (2) Skin grown in petri dish and then grafted to patient
      c. Homograft (allograft)
        (1) Skin obtained from another human
        (2) Fresh cadaver
          (a) Provides a temporary covering to excised tissue awaiting permanent grafting
          (b) May be placed over a widely meshed autograft to promote graft take
          (c) Patient will eventually reject.
        (3) Processed human dermis (AlloDerm)
          (a) Donated skin processed to remove components that cause rejection
            (i) Epidermis removed
            (ii) Cells that contain antigen targets for rejection removed
            (iii) Tissue (dermal matrix) freeze-dried for storage
          (b) Procedure
            (i) Wound excised
            (ii) AlloDerm applied to wound bed
            (iii) Thin autograft applied over AlloDerm
      d. Skin substitutes
        (1) Integra
          (a) Bilaminate skin substitute
            (i) Dermal analogue of collagen fibers
            (ii) Epidermal analogue is Silastic membrane.
          (b) Applied to excised wound
            (i) Dermal analogue develops vasculature.
            (ii) Silastic membrane removed after dermal vascularity established (approximately 2 weeks)
            (iii) Thin autograft applied after Silastic membrane removed
          (c) Requires a two-step process
            (i) Excision and application of Integra
            (ii) Removal of Silastic membrane and autograft
        (2) Biobrane
          (a) Synthetic polymer dressing
          (b) Porcine collagen base with nylon covering

          (c) Placed over excised tissue
          (d) Patient's dermis binds with collagen base.
          (e) Biobrane removed after dermal healing
          (f) Patient must have capacity for dermal regeneration.
          (g) May be placed over donor sites
     e. Heterograft (xenograft)
        (1) Tissue from another species, usually pigskin
        (2) Temporary covering over excised wounds

C. Primary closure
   1. May be used for small burns
   2. Burn tissue excised and closed primarily

XII. INTRAOPERATIVE CONSIDERATIONS FOR THE BURN PATIENT

A. Surgical concerns
   1. Minimize physiological stress experienced by patient.
     a. Limit operative time to 2-hour to 3-hour sessions.
     b. Limit excision to 20% of total body surface at any one operative session.
   2. Selection of donor sites
     a. Preferred sites: thighs, buttock, abdomen, back, scalp
     b. Best color match if skin obtained from area near burn
   3. Types of grafts
     a. Split-thickness skin graft
        (1) Donor skin contains epidermis and part of dermis.
        (2) Thickness: 0.012-inch
        (3) Graft "takes" as capillaries grow in from granulation bed into graft (begins to occur after 48 hours).
        (4) Donor site reepithelializes in 10 to 14 days and may be ready as donor site again in 21 days (scalp donor sites may heal in 7 days).
     b. Full-thickness graft
        (1) Entire epidermis and dermis used as donor
        (2) Used to cover deep defects, tendons, bone
        (3) Requires split-thickness skin graft on donor area from which full-thickness skin was removed
        (4) Less hyperpigmentation and contractures than with split-thickness skin graft
     c. Mesh graft
        (1) Split-thickness skin graft in which donor skin is passed through mesher to produce slits in skin
        (2) Allows for donor skin to be stretched covering large area
          (a) May be meshed 1.5 to 3 times original size
          (b) Useful in large burns
        (3) Meshing helps prevent fluid or blood from accumulating under graft, which prevents "take."
        (4) Less cosmetically perfect than sheet graft
     d. Sheet graft
        (1) Split-thickness skin graft placed on wound without meshing
        (2) Provides better cosmetic result, especially for hands, face, and neck
        (3) Fluid and blood can accumulate under graft, affecting "take."
   4. Burn wound excision
     a. Tangential (sequential) excision
        (1) Sequential removal of tissue until viable dermis reached
        (2) Provides optimal functional and cosmetic result
        (3) Large blood loss may occur.
        (4) May be difficult to determine endpoint of excision—too much or too little may be excised
     b. Fascial excision
        (1) Used in deep full-thickness burns that may extend into fat or underlying tissues
        (2) Tissue sharply dissected to fascia

          (3) Blood loss less than if tangentially excised

          (4) Easier to determine endpoint of excision

          (5) Risk of injury to nerves, joints, tendons

          (6) Results in cosmetic defects

5. Control of bleeding

    a. Patient may have considerable blood loss.

    b. Controlled with thrombin, epinephrine soaks, electrocautery

    c. Hemostasis must be obtained before graft is placed.

6. Factors promoting graft "take"

    a. Hemostasis

    b. Graft secured and immobilized

    c. Prevention of infection

    d. Good nutrition

B. Anesthesia concerns

  1. Anesthetic agents

    a. Pharmacokinetics may be altered because of physiological changes that occur after major burn injury.

    b. Serum protein levels decrease, making agents that bind to albumin more pharmacologically active.

    c. Narcotic anesthesia amounts may be high because of developed tolerance.

    d. Amount of cardiac depression must be weighed if inhalation agents are used.

    e. Increased sensitivity to depolarizing neuromuscular blocking agents occurs and may result in hyperkalemic response.

      (1) Succinylcholine use contraindicated because of hyperkalemic response

    f. Hyposensitivity to nondepolarizing neuromuscular blocking agents

  2. Ventilatory needs

    a. Intubation may be difficult because of burns of face and neck or limited oral mobility, requiring use of fiberoptic bronchoscope.

    b. Hypermetabolic response results in increased oxygen consumption and carbon dioxide production.

    c. Chest wall compliance may be decreased if chest burns are present.

    d. Ventilation-perfusion mismatches may occur with pulmonary injuries.

    e. Patient may need increased minute ventilation because of hypermetabolic state and positive end-expiratory pressure.

    f. Monitor oxygen saturation and end-tidal carbon dioxide.

  3. Prevention of hypothermia

    a. Room temperature maintained at 85° F

    b. Use of warming blankets and warmed fluids

    c. Temperature monitoring

    d. Warmed inspired gases

  4. Maintaining hemodynamic stability

    a. May be prone to hypotension because of position changes as donor skin is obtained and burn wound prepared

    b. Fluid loss through evaporation and bleeding

      (1) Replacement with red blood cells and fresh frozen plasma

      (2) Crystalloids to maintain adequate urine output without giving excess salt

  5. Fluid resuscitation criteria

    a. Calculated fluid requirements for first 24 to 48 hours after injury

    b. Thermal injuries uncommonly taken to operating room during burn shock period (first 24-48 hours)

      (1) Early excision after 24 hours to begin wound coverage to decrease metabolic rate and decrease wound infection

    c. Calculated requirements (Parkland formula)

      (1) Over first 24 hours: 4 mL/kg per TBSA percent of injury

        (a) One half of calculated requirements given over first 8 hours from time of injury

        (b) One half of calculated requirements given over next 16 hours

      (2) Fluids adjusted to maintain urinary output

    (a) Adult: 0.5 to 1 mL/kg per hour
    (b) Children: 1 to 2 mL/kg per hour
  d. Fluids used
   (1) Isotonic crystalloid
    (a) Normal saline
    (b) Lactated Ringer's
   (2) Hypertonic saline may be used.
    (a) Increases osmotic pull back to intravascular space
    (b) Decreases total fluid requirements and assists to minimize edema formation
   (3) Colloids rarely used in first 12 hours after burn injury because of increased capillary permeability
   (4) Care taken to avoid pulmonary edema and worsening of fluid shifts from overaggressive fluid resuscitation
  e. Electrical injury fluid requirements
   (1) More difficult to estimate fluid needs
   (2) Injury greater internally than what is seen externally
   (3) Calculate on basis of Parkland formula.
   (4) Adjust fluids to maintain urinary output of 75 to 100 mL/hr in adults or 2 to 3 mL/kg per hour in children.
   (5) Add sodium bicarbonate to alkalinize urine, promoting myoglobin excretion.
   (6) Administer mannitol to increase urinary flow, promoting myoglobin excretion.
  f. Inadequate fluid resuscitation is primary cause of death in first 24 to 48 hours after injury.

XIII. POSTOPERATIVE CONCERNS FOR THE BURN PATIENT
 A. Airway and ventilatory needs
  1. Upper airway injuries
   a. Caused by heat injury to oronasopharynx and vocal cords
   b. Swelling usually peaks 48 hours after injury.
   c. Edema may lead to obstruction.
   d. Intubation performed early, often prophylactically
   e. If patient is extubated postoperatively, observe for signs of obstruction (e.g., stridor, tachypnea, increased work of breathing, low arterial oxygen saturation [Sao_2], low mixed venous oxygen saturation [Svo_2]).
   f. Secure endotracheal tube.
    (1) Use ties in patients with face burns.
    (2) Tape will not adhere.
    (3) Avoid pressure on burned nose or ears.
    (4) Monitor ties for constriction as facial swelling increases.
  2. Lower airway injuries
   a. Injuries below glottis caused by chemical irritants released from smoke
   b. Lower airway damage results in:
    (1) Increased airway irritability, laryngospasm, bronchospasm
    (2) Bronchiolar edema and impaired airway flow
    (3) Increased mucus production caused by chemical irritants
    (4) Damage to epithelial lining of bronchial tree and alveolar cells
   c. Management considerations
    (1) Frequent assessment of respiratory function and airway patency
     (a) Respiratory effort
     (b) Chest wall expansion and symmetry
     (c) Monitor oxygenation with pulse oximeter and arterial blood gases.
     (d) Monitor end-tidal CO_2
    (2) Assess need for bronchodilator therapy.
    (3) Assess chest expansion.
     (a) Constriction of nonexcised chest burns
     (b) Constriction of chest dressings

(4) Deep breathing and coughing to facilitate mucus mobilization

(5) Provide for oxygen and ventilatory needs.

    (a) May need increased minute ventilation (rate or tidal volume or both) because of hypermetabolic state

    (b) Humidified oxygen

    (c) Prevent oxygen administration device from applying pressure if grafts have been placed on face or neck.

B. Circulatory function

  1. Blood and fluid loss may be significant.

  2. Monitor for signs of hypovolemia.

    a. Tachycardia

    b. Decreased blood pressure and presence of pulsus paradoxus

    c. Delayed capillary refill

    d. Monitor urinary output.

      (1) Maintain 30 to 50 mL/hr in adults.

      (2) Maintain 1 to 2 mL/kg per hour in children.

  3. Provide fluid replacement.

    a. Isotonic or hypertonic crystalloids

    b. Colloids: red blood cells, fresh frozen plasma, albumin

  4. Monitor circulatory function distal to burn.

    a. Distal to escharotomy sites every 15 to 30 minutes

    b. Assess circulatory compromise caused by constricting dressings or splints.

    c. Assessment

      (1) Pulses

      (2) Capillary refill

      (3) Movement and sensation

      (4) Color

C. Infection

  1. Thorough hand washing and gloves are essential.

  2. Prevent cross-contamination with other patients.

  3. Isolation precautions, including gown, mask, and gloves, may be necessary in large burns.

  4. Aseptic wound technique

  5. Frequent change of invasive catheters

D. Temperature control

  1. Assess body temperature every 30 minutes.

  2. Warm fluids and blood products before infusion.

  3. Use heat shields or warming blankets.

  4. Adjust room temperature to 75° F to 85° F.

  5. Monitor for ST-segment changes caused by myocardial ischemia.

E. Wound care

  1. Monitor graft and donor sites for bleeding.

    a. Grafts will fail if blood collects beneath them.

    b. Dressings usually not changed for first few days

  2. Monitor status of sheet grafts that do not have dressing.

    a. Assess for fluid and blood collection under graft.

      (1) Aspiration of fluid using syringe and small-gauge needle

      (2) Removal of fluid by "rolling" fluid to edges of graft with cotton-tipped applicator

    b. Avoid pressure or shearing.

    c. Antimicrobial ointment may be applied to edges and seams of graft.

  3. Maintain joint immobility if graft is over joint.

  4. Elevate grafted extremities to minimize edema and promote venous return.

F. Pain control

  1. Pain usually more severe at donor site than at grafted areas

  2. May have high analgesic needs because of previous narcotic needs during wound care

   3. IV administration preferred over intramuscular in large burns because of poor absorption

   4. Avoid aspirin-containing products.

 G. Emotional support for patient and family

   1. Patient and family must deal with change in physical appearance from first day after injury.

   2. Ongoing emotional support required

    a. Change in physical appearance

     (1) Long-term results may be uncertain.

     (2) Must begin to adjust to fact that even with the best cosmetic results, patient will never look the same again

    b. Possible changes in function if severe burns of extremities, hands, feet, face

   3. Surgical procedure may be the first or one of many.

    a. Expectations of each may differ.

    b. May view regrafting as a setback because of graft failure or poor cosmetic result

   4. Provide support appropriate to stage of adjustment that patient or family is experiencing.

   5. Use additional health care workers to assist in support (e.g., child life specialists, clergy, mental health practitioners, social worker).

   6. Priorities of care: life, limbs, looks (in that order)

 H. Discharge instructions for the ambulatory skin graft patient

   1. Maintain dressing dry and intact.

    a. Donor site dressing may exhibit some bloody drainage.

    b. Avoid getting dressings wet.

   2. Keep grafted area immobile.

    a. Avoid activities that would cause sheer.

    b. Grafts over joint must remain immobile—may have splints in place.

    c. Reinforce weight-bearing status or crutch walking for lower extremity grafts.

    d. Elevate grafted extremity to limit edema.

   3. Pain management

    a. Reinforce that donor site may be more painful.

    b. Instruct on use of prescribed analgesia.

   4. Notify physician of:

    a. Temperature >38.5° C (101.3° F)

    b. Numbness, paresthesia of grafted extremity

    c. Pain that is not controlled by analgesia

    d. Bleeding of graft or donor site

   5. Reinforce follow-up instructions.

    a. Dressing usually changed and graft evaluated 3 to 5 days after grafting

BIBLIOGRAPHY

1. American Society of Plastic Surgeons: *2006 Quick facts: Cosmetic and reconstructive plastic surgery trends.* Available at: www.plasticsurgery.org/media/statistics/loader.cfm?url = /commonspot/security/getfile.cfm&PageID = 23625. Accessed December 10, 2008.

2. Bosch JA, Engeland CG, Cacioppo JT, et al: Depressive symptoms predict mucosal wound healing. *Psychosom Med* 69(7):597–605, 2007.

3. Bowser A: Lipo innovations: Female breast reduction, 'plasty' alternatives expand. *Dermatology Times* 26(2):84, 2005.

4. Bryant R: Early pioneer describes autologous fat transfers. *Dermatology Times* 26(2):85–86, 2005.

5. Dell DD, Weaver C, Kozempel J, et al: Recovery after transverse rectus abdominis myocutaneous flap breast reconstruction surgery. *Oncol Nurs Forum* 35(2):189–196, 2008.

6. Dittmann M: Plastic surgery: Beauty or beast? *Monitor on Psychology* 36(8):30, 2005.

7. Dugas B: Choosing the right peel for your patient. *Plast Surg Nurs* 27(2):80–84, 2007.

8. Figueroa-Haas CL: Effect of breast augmentation mammoplasty on self-esteem and sexuality. *Plast Surg Nurs* 27(1):16–36, 2007.

9. Guttman C: Survey: Chemical peels remain mainstay in dermatologic surgery armamentarium. *Dermatology Times* 29(1):72, 2008.

10. Hackenschmidt A: Burn trauma priorities for a patient with 80% total body surface area burns. *J Emerg Nurs* 33(4):405–408, 2007.

11. Hainsworth T: Risks and benefits associated with cosmetic procedures. *Nurs Times* 102(11):23–24, 2006.

12. Hill O, White K: Exploring women's experiences of TRAM flap breast reconstruction after mastectomy for breast cancer. *Oncol Nurs Forum* 35(1):81–88, 2008.

13. Hilton L: In search of the perfect filler. *Dermatology Times* 25(8):39–48, 2004.

14. Iverson RE, Lynch DJ, ASPS Task Force on Patient Safety in Office-based Surgery Facilities: Patient safety in office-based surgery facilities: II. Patient selection. *Plast Reconstr Surg* 110(7):1785–1790, 2002.

15. Myers BA: *Wound management: Principles and practice*, ed 2, Upper Saddle River, New Jersey, 2008, Prentice Hall.

16. Nash K: Liposuction: Safety paramount; not every patient a candidate. *Dermatology Times* 28(2):10–11, 2007.

17. Rasberry CN: Battling body image: Confessions of a health educator. *J Am Coll Health* 56(4):423–426, 2008.

18. Robles TF: Stress, social support, and delayed skin barrier recovery. *Psycosom Med* 69(8):807–815, 2007.

19. Sattler G: Advances in liposuction and fat transfer. *Dermatol Nurs* 17(2):133–139, 2005.

20. Sicoutris CP, Homes JH: Fire and smoke injuries. *Crit Care Nurs Clin North Am* 18(3):403–417, 2006.

21. Sobralske M: Primary care needs of patients who have undergone gender reassignment. *J Am Acad Nurse Pract* 17(4):133–138, 2005.

22. Venes D: *Taber's cyclopedic medical dictionary*, ed 20, Philadelphia, 2005, FA Davis.

23. Wagner KD, Johnson KL, Kidd PS: *High acuity nursing*, ed 4, Upper Saddle River, New Jersey, 2005, Prentice Hall.

24. Warner DO: Perioperative abstinence from cigarettes: Physiologic and clinical consequences. *Anesthesiology* 104(2):356–367, 2006.

25. Zuelzer HB, Baugh NG: Bariatric and body-contouring surgery: A continuum of care for excess and lax skin. *Plast Surg Nurs* 27(1):3–13, 2007.

46 Podiatric Care

LYNDA MARKS

OBJECTIVES

At the conclusion of this chapter, the reader will be able to:

1. Identify the skeletal structure of the foot.
2. Describe specific physical and psychosocial assessment for podiatric patients.
3. Describe operative procedures of the foot.
4. Describe perianesthesia care to be provided to patients having surgical procedures on the foot.

I. ANATOMY AND PHYSIOLOGY
   A. Bony structure—7 tarsal, 5 metatarsal, 14 phalanges (Figure 46-1)
      1. Tarsals—seven bones of the ankle, hindfoot, and midfoot
         a. Talus—irregularly shaped bone
            (1) Located between bimalleolar fork and tarsus
            (2) Ligament attachments, no tendons
         b. Calcaneus—largest bone in foot
         c. Cuboid—wedge shaped
         d. Scaphoid (navicular)—bound with ligaments
         e. Three cuneiforms
            (1) Interposed between scaphoid, first three metatarsals, and cuboid
            (2) Wedge shaped
      2. Metatarsals—five
         a. First toe (great toe)
         b. Four lesser toes
         c. Articulates with three cuneiforms
         d. Form tarsometatarsal or Lisfranc's joint
      3. Phalanges
         a. Great toe—proximal and distal
         b. Lesser toes (2, 3, 4, 5)—proximal, middle, distal
      4. Sesamoids
         a. Small, round bones
         b. Embedded (partially or totally) in substance of corresponding tendon
         c. Pressure-absorbing mechanism
   B. Arches
      1. Formed by bony structure
      2. Longitudinal (lengthwise) arches
         a. Medial longitudinal arch—formed by calcaneus, talus, navicular, three cuneiforms, and first three metatarsals
         b. Lateral longitudinal arch—formed by calcaneus, cuboid, and fourth and fifth metatarsals
      3. Transverse—across the ball (top) of the foot
   C. Muscles, ligaments, and tendons; nerves (multiple structures)
  II. ASSESSMENT PARAMETERS (PROCEDURE SPECIFIC)
   A. Structural disorders—causes
      1. Weakness of muscles, ligaments, and tendons
      2. Imbalance between bone support and supporting structure
      3. Constant wear, rub

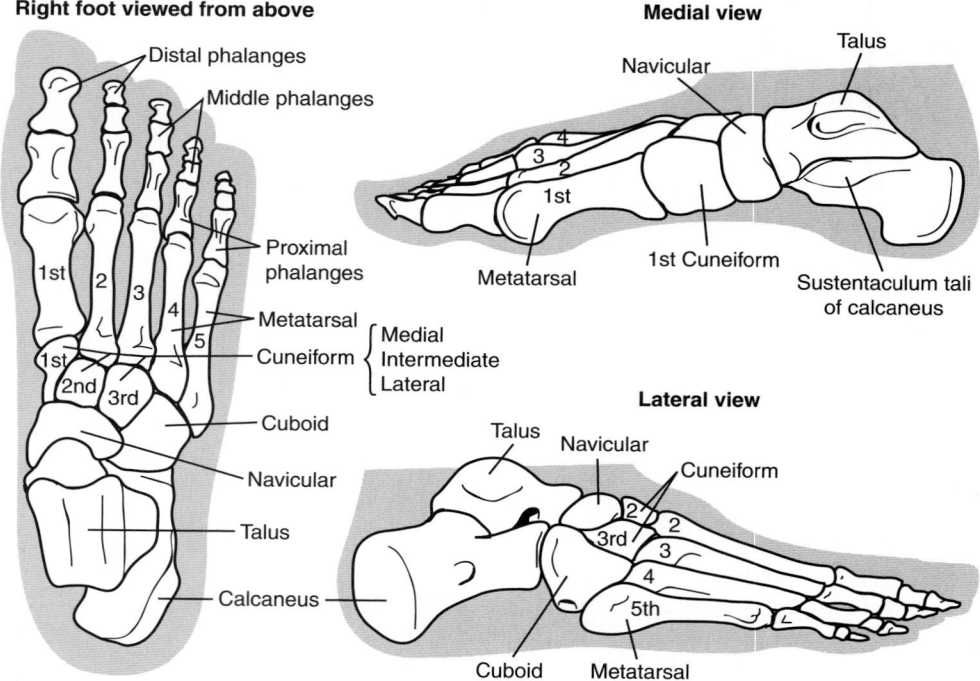

Right foot viewed from above

Distal phalanges
Middle phalanges
Proximal phalanges
1st
2
3
4
5
Metatarsal
Cuneiform
1st
2nd
3rd
Cuboid
Navicular
Talus
Calcaneus
Medial
Intermediate
Lateral

Medial view

Talus
Navicular
4
3
2
1st
Metatarsal
1st Cuneiform
Sustentaculum tali
of calcaneus

Lateral view

Talus
Navicular
Cuneiform
2
2
3rd
3
4
5th
Cuboid
Metatarsal

FIGURE 46-1 ■ Bones of the right foot. (Redrawn from Jacob S, Francone C: *Elements of anatomy and physiology,* ed 2, Philadelphia, 1989, WB Saunders.)

B. Identified disorders (Table 46-1 for podiatric definitions)
1. Hallux valgus (also called bunion): deformity of the foot involving the first metatarsal and great toe (hallux)
   a. Lateral angulation of great toe
   b. Progresses, resulting in medial deviation of first metatarsal
   c. Often accompanied by multiple disorders and symptoms; commonly affects lesser toes
   d. Occurs in females nine times more often than males; may be congenital or as a result of rapid growth
   e. Symptoms
      (1) Adults—pain or dull ache over metatarsal head
      (2) Adolescents—chief complaints are unrelenting pain, altered body image; may have family history.
   f. Radiographs show exostosis with subluxation or dislocation of first metatarsal head.
2. Hallux varus
   a. First metatarsal deviates medially, and the great toe deviates laterally.
   b. Condition may start in late childhood or early adult life.
   c. More common in females
   d. May be agitated by improperly fitting footwear
3. Hallux rigidus—"stiff big toe"
   a. Painful stiffness of first metatarsophalangeal joint of the toes when walking; toe becomes rigid.
   b. Caused by arthritis
4. Corns—conical thickening of skin in areas of constant irritation
5. Bursal hypertrophy—inflammation of the joint
6. Digital deformity

■ TABLE 46-1
■ ■ **Podiatric Definitions**

Arthrodesis	Surgical immobilization or fusion of a joint
Arthrolysis	Surgical procedure in which mobility is restored to an ankylosed (fused/immobile) joint
Arthroplasty	Surgical repair or reformation of a joint
Arthrotomy	Incision into a joint
Bunion	Enlargement and inflammation of the joint bursa at the base of the great toe, usually causing the toe to displace laterally; usual etiology is long-term wearing of tight-fitting shoes.
Capsulotomy	Incision into the joint capsule
Exostosis	A bony growth on the surface of a bone, also called "osteoma" or "hyperostosis"
Hallux	The great toe
Hallux valgus	Displacement of the great toe laterally toward the other toes; often coexists with a bunion, but often the two terms are inaccurately used synonymously.
Hammer toe	A deformity in which there is dorsiflexion of the metatarsophalangeal joint (joint between the foot and the toe) or plantar flexion of interphalangeal (IP) joints.
Mallet toe	A deformity in which the most distal IP joint is involved.
Morton's neuroma	Interdigital nerve entrapment within a metatarsal interspace that causes pain, particularly with weight-bearing
Osteotomy	Incision into a bone
Plantar	Regarding the sole of the foot
Tenotomy	Incision of a tendon, often used to correct hammer toe

From Burden N, Dawes B, O'Brien D, et al: *Ambulatory surgical nursing*, ed 2, Philadelphia, 2000, WB Saunders.

    a. Mallet toe—congenital abnormality of the distal interphalangeal joint, usually genetic
       (1) Flexion posture of the distal interphalangeal joint
       (2) Most commonly affects second toe
       (3) Associated with a long digit
       (4) Caused by pressure at tip of toes
       (5) Occurs in persons with peripheral neuropathy; no known reason
    b. Varus toes
       (1) Curly or overlapping toes
       (2) Flexion and varus rotation
       (3) Commonly affects third, fourth, and fifth toes
    c. Hammer toe deformity
       (1) Affects one of the lesser four toes (commonly second toe)
       (2) Hyperextension at metatarsophalangeal joint, flexion at proximal interphalangeal joint
       (3) Etiology unknown
    d. Clawtoe
       (1) Hyperextension of metatarsophalangeal joint with flexion of the proximal interphalangeal joint
       (2) Associated with cavus foot deformity and neuromuscular conditions
  7. Interdigital deformity (Morton's neuroma)
    a. Benign enlargement of third common digital branch at site of bifurcation of interdigital nerves (medial plantar nerve)
    b. Frequently between and distal to third and fourth metatarsal heads
    c. Symptoms and common findings
       (1) Pain in plantar forefoot area (sharp, dull, throbbing, or burning sensation)
       (2) Swelling of plantar metatarsal
       (3) Affects females more than males
       (4) Overweight person

8. Pes planus (flatfoot)
   a. Loss of normal medial longitudinal arch
   b. Initial treatment is conservative therapy with shoes, arch supports.
   c. Surgical treatment with onset of disabling pain
   d. Correction procedures include Miller, Durham flatfoot plasty, triple arthrodesis, calcaneal displacement osteotomy.
9. Pes cavus (hollow foot, clawfoot)
   a. Occurs with neuromuscular conditions such as spina bifida, cerebral palsy, muscular dystrophy, congenital clubfoot
   b. Muscular weakness in foot
   c. Several procedures required for repair
      (1) Soft tissue release, decrease contracture
      (2) Tendon transfer to correct muscle imbalance
      (3) Osteotomy—incision into a bone
      (4) Arthrodesis—surgical immobilization or fusion of a joint

III. ELECTIVE OPERATIVE PROCEDURES
   A. Treatment of disorders
      1. Determined by the degree of involvement
      2. Goals toward alignment, shortening, stabilization
      3. Multiple procedures may be indicated.
   B. General intraoperative care
      1. Tourniquet application
      2. Operative site cleansing (including clipping of hair and cleaning toenails)
      3. Provision of sterile instruments, supplies
      4. Availability of implants including joint replacement, K-wire (pins), screws
   C. Procedures
      1. Arthrodesis
         a. Excision of bone wedges with fusion
         b. Indicated for severe compromise of muscle function; digital and metatarsophalangeal joint stability inadequate
         c. Treatment for hallux valgus
            (1) Method: divide tendon, resect cartilage, provide stability to joint with K-wire or other means.
         d. Triple arthrodesis—subtalar joint, talonavicular joint, tarsometatarsal joint
            (1) Treatment for equinus deformity, cavus deformity, flatfoot, or forefoot cavus
      2. Arthroplasty
         a. Resection or replacement of bony structure of joint
         b. Indicated for alleviation of pain and correction of digits with flexor to rigid deformity caused by:
            (1) Inflammatory arthritis
            (2) Degenerative arthrosis
            (3) Congenital deformity
            (4) Flail toes
            (5) Revision of previous surgery
         c. Keller resection arthroplasty:
            (1) Tissues released around the joint
            (2) Articular surface exposed
            (3) Medial eminence resected
            (4) Implant (K-wire) seated
            (5) Capsulorrhaphy completed
      3. Bunion procedures
         a. Revision of soft tissue structures and/or bone to correct deformity
         b. Soft tissue procedures correct muscle imbalance: McBride, DuVries, Mann, Silver.
         c. Soft tissue and bone procedure: Keller resection arthroplasty, Chevron osteotomy, Akin procedure

   d. Purpose: simple treatment of hallux valgus causing impaired function and/or pain; cosmetic improvement
4. Capsulotomy
   a. Incision of capsule
   b. Treatment of equinovarus foot
   c. Performed in conjunction with other procedures
   d. Method: incision through superficial fascia, expose joint, incise capsule
5. Endoscopic plantar fasciotomy
   a. Operative tissue repair using a less invasive procedure
   b. Completed using fluoroscopy
   c. Procedure: stab incision, blunt dissection to create a channel, pass a trocar, release the plantar fascia
   d. Open procedure more invasive; appropriate procedure for fascia release
6. Exostectomy
   a. Resection of lateral prominences (callus) of toes
   b. Commonly fifth toe
7. Hammer toe repair
   a. Abnormal flexion posture of the proximal interphalangeal joint of one of the lesser four toes
   b. Second toe most frequently affected
   c. Metatarsophalangeal joint
   d. Stage of deformity depends on joint involvement and degree of contracture.
   e. Treatment
      (1) Soft tissue procedures: Girdlestone, Taylor, Parrish, Mann, Coughlin
      (2) Soft tissue and bone procedures
8. Mallet toe repair
   a. Flexion posture of the distal interphalangeal joint
   b. Second toe most frequently affected
   c. Etiology
      (1) Pressure at tip of toes, possibly caused by shoes
      (2) Persons with peripheral neuropathy; no known reason
   d. Treatment
      (1) Flexor tenotomy at distal interphalangeal flexion crease
      (2) Subtotal or total resection of middle phalanx
9. Osteotomy
   a. Removal or addition of a bone wedge
   b. Extra-articular or intra-articular
   c. Extra-articular most commonly in the calcaneus for cavovarus heel
   d. Metatarsal osteotomy for plantar calluses, hallux valgus: many types including wedge resection, Chevron, "Z," Reverdin, Mitchell
   e. Mitchell osteotomy: capsular incision, medial eminence removed, drill holes offset, and suture passed; double osteotomy completed with excision of bone between, capital fragment displaced, and suture tied; medial capsulorrhaphy completed
10. Tenotomy
   a. Incision of tendon: eliminates tendon function, relieves contracture
   b. Completed in conjunction with other procedures

IV. PERIANESTHESIA PRIORITIES
   A. Preoperative (Box 46-1)
      1. Support system
         a. Available assistance
         b. Impaired mobility related to other disease processes
      2. Awareness of procedure and expected outcomes
         a. Procedure to be performed
         b. Anesthetic type
            (1) General anesthetic

■ BOX 46-1
■ **KEY PATIENT EDUCATIONAL OUTCOMES**

Patient Will:
Demonstrate proper use of supportive devices (crutches, walker, walking shoe).
Describe proper dosing procedure for prescribed analgesic medication(s) and report uncontrolled pain.
Report excessive drainage on dressings.
Describe signs and symptoms of infection and report findings to physician immediately.
Report any neurological or circulatory impairment.
Describe understanding of need for limited mobility for 6 to 8 weeks.

(2) Ankle block with intravenous conscious sedation
  (a) Procedure for block
  (b) Sensory deficit—length and precautions
c. Complications
  (1) Loss of function, muscular imbalance
  (2) Neurovascular compromise, swelling
B. Phase I
  1. Predisposing factors
    a. Congenital, acquired, or traumatic
    b. Older adults and children included in the spectrum
    c. Existing conditions
      (1) Neuromuscular disease
      (2) Neuropathy
      (3) Diabetes
      (4) Arthritis
    d. Previous procedures or anticipated future procedures (bilateral treatment needs)
  2. Condition of foot: appearance and sensation
    a. Soreness, tenderness, edema
    b. Temperature equal on each foot
    c. Note presence of pins.
  3. Color
    a. Blanching of nail beds
    b. Capillary refill
  4. Vascular status
    a. Presence of dorsalis pedis pulse on dorsal center of metatarsal area of each foot
    b. Poor vascularity may impede healing.
  5. Goals of procedure
    a. Pain relief
    b. Return or improvement of mobility
    c. Cosmetic improvement
    d. Extent of procedure influences outcome.
C. Phase II
  1. Neurovascular status
    a. Sensation in affected and opposite extremity
    b. Pulses
    c. Coloration, blanching of nail beds, capillary refill
  2. Preventive measures
    a. Elevation of extremity
    b. Ice therapy if ordered by physician, being careful not to place ice over the toes
D. Extended observation/discharge home
  1. Ambulation and mobility
    a. Home care availability

    b. Sensory deficit with use of ankle block up to 8 hours

    c. Support devices—crutches, walker, walking shoe, boot

       (1) Proper fit

          (a) Walking shoe long enough to protect toe, short enough to prevent tripping

       (2) Return demonstration of use

    d. Non–weight-bearing ambulation 3 to 5 days

    e. Limited mobility 6 to 8 weeks (longer depending upon procedure)

2. Wound care

    a. Incision site clean, dry

       (1) Report bleeding, discharge.

       (2) Protect K-wire(s) if used.

          (a) Clean around site with alcohol daily.

          (b) Removal time depends on procedure; possibly 6 to 8 weeks.

    b. Dressings remain intact, clean, dry (use protective waterproof cover for showering).

    c. Soft tissue procedures

       (1) Bulky, soft dressing for support

       (2) Three to 6 weeks with bandages in place (more involved procedures, longer bandage remains)

       (3) Compression dressing after 2 to 4 weeks

    d. Soft tissue and bone procedures

       (1) Six to 8 weeks with bandages in place, guarded ambulation

       (2) External support several additional weeks

       (3) If bone graft used, may immobilize 3 to 6 months

    e. Skin care beneath cast, dressing

3. Return of function

    a. Pain management

       (1) Nonsteroidal anti-inflammatory medications

          (a) Pain after foot surgery intense

          (b) Evaluate medication interactions.

       (2) Elevation of extremity

       (3) Ice therapy if ordered by physician, being careful not to place ice over the toes

    b. Ambulation to tolerance

    c. Preventive measures

       (1) Eliminate pressure, rub on toes from footwear.

BIBLIOGRAPHY

1. Black J, Hokanson Hawks J: *Medical-surgical nursing: Clinical management for positive outcomes*, ed 7, St Louis, 2004, Saunders.
2. Burden N, Dawes B, O'Brien D, et al: *Ambulatory surgical nursing*, ed 2, Philadelphia, 2000, WB Saunders.
3. *Lippincott manual of nursing practice*, ed 8, Ambler, 2006, Lippincott Williams & Wilkins.
4. McGlamery ED, Banks AS, Downey MS: *Comprehensive textbook of foot surgery*, ed 2, Baltimore, 2001, Lippincott Williams & Wilkins.
5. Pudner R: *Nursing the surgical patient*, ed 2, Edinburgh, Scotland, 2005, Bailliere Tindall.
6. Rothrock JC: *Alexander's care of the patient in surgery*, ed 13, St Louis, 2007, Mosby.

Trauma Care

JUDY STEVENSON

OBJECTIVES

At the conclusion of this chapter, the reader will be able to:

1. Identify the impact that the mechanism of injury has on the actual injury.
2. Describe the continuum of trauma care from prehospital to post anesthesia care unit (PACU).
3. List elements of primary and secondary assessments in the PACU as they relate to trauma care.
4. Describe total body systems management of the trauma patient.
5. Identify potential complications as they relate to trauma care and appropriate interventions to treat and/or prevent them.
6. Describe the value of a collaborative approach to care and communication.
7. Identify the types of shock and how they impact the trauma patient.

I. OVERVIEW
   A. Trauma care is complex.
      1. Many pathophysiological responses
      2. May be single surgical intervention
      3. May need repetitive surgical interventions
      4. Consider multiple disciplines.
   B. PACU nurse
      1. Focus on vigilant continuous assessment.
      2. Anticipate problems.
      3. Identify subtle changes.
         a. Remember medications can alter expected responses.
      4. Intervene appropriately and promptly.
      5. Prevent complications.
      6. Offers challenge in caring
      7. Requires knowledge of current research and treatment
      8. Expect the unexpected since trauma happens to:
         a. Children
         b. Pregnant women
         c. The elderly
         d. The sick
         e. The wealthy
         f. The impoverished
         g. Families
II. PREHOSPITAL
   A. Goal of emergency medical services (EMS)
      1. Improve field stabilization
      2. Resuscitation
      3. Transportation to the appropriate level trauma center
   B. The Golden Hour
      1. Introduced by R. Adams Crowley, MD
      2. Emphasizes the importance of time in resuscitation
      3. Goal is to achieve maximal survival.
      4. Represents the window of opportunity to institute lifesaving and limb-saving measures

C. Prehospital phase
    1. Vital information
       a. Condition at the scene
          (1) Age of victim
          (2) Sex of victim
          (3) Mechanism of injury
          (4) Obvious injuries
          (5) Questionable injuries
          (6) Potential injuries
          (7) Vital signs
          (8) Intervention at the scene
          (9) Intravenous (IV) fluids
          (10) Response to interventions
          (11) Stabilization
          (12) Presence of drugs or alcohol
          (13) Pertinent past medical history
             (a) AMPLE
                (i)   **A**llergies
                (ii) **M**edications
                (iii) **P**ast medical history
                (iv) **L**ast meal
                (v)   **E**vents
           (14) Transport time
          (15) Any other pertinent information
       b. Mechanism of injury (factors that can influence outcome)
          (1) Motor vehicle
             (a) Restraint devices
             (b) Air bag deployment
             (c) Patient ejection
             (d) Car rolling
             (e) Windshield star or shatter
             (f) Speed of vehicle
             (g) Where impact occurred on vehicle
             (h) Other fatalities at the scene
          (2) Motorcycle
             (a) Speed of cycle
             (b) Object with impact
             (c) Front, rear, or side impact
             (d) Ejection from cycle (front, rear, or side)
             (e) Helmet usage
             (f) Protective covering (e.g., leather jacket, gloves)
             (g) Burns in addition to other injuries
             (h) Other fatalities at the scene
          (3) Strike with blunt object (e.g., fist, ball bat, ball)
             (a) Object that struck
             (b) Place struck
             (c) Speed at which struck
             (d) Presence of protective covering
             (e) One strike or multiple strikes
             (f) Injury after initial injury (e.g., fall to the ground)
          (4) Strike with penetrating object (e.g., gunshot, knife, screwdriver)
             (a) Object penetrated
             (b) Depth of object
             (c) Diameter of object
             (d) Twisting or stationary
             (e) Direction of penetration
             (f) Location of penetration
             (g) One wound or multiple wounds

      (h) Entrance or exit wound
      (i) Object stabilized and secure or removed
      (j) Injury after initial injury (e.g., fall to the ground)
    (5) Fall
      (a) Height from fall
      (b) Body position upon landing (e.g., feet, buttock)
      (c) Incident before landing (e.g., hit head, slipped)
      (d) Protective equipment (e.g., hard hat)
    (6) Crush injury
      (a) Weight of object
      (b) Area compressed
      (c) Other injuries
      (d) Protective equipment
  c. Victim assistance
    (1) Bystanders before EMS
      (a) Movement of victim before treatment
    (2) EMS providers
      (a) Dressings
      (b) Stabilization of possible fractures
      (c) Cervical collar
      (d) Spine board
      (e) Safety straps
      (f) Airway confirmation
      (g) Lifesaving interventions
      (h) Vascular access

III. MECHANISM OF INJURY
  A. Basic understanding
    1. Related to the type of injuring forces and subsequent tissue response
    2. Helps to determine the extent of potential injuries
  B. Factors that influence injury
    1. Amount of force: energy is unloaded onto the body.
    2. Mass of the object
    3. Mass of the body
    4. Velocity at which the object is moving
    5. Deceleration forces
      a. Stop or decrease velocity of moving object
      b. Examples: falls, person striking dashboard
    6. Acceleration forces
      a. Stationary person struck by object
      b. Example: pedestrian struck by car
    7. Multiple forces
      a. Both deceleration and acceleration forces together
      b. Example: pedestrian struck by car pushing into another vehicle
      c. Three impacts involved in auto crash
        (1) Automobile to object
        (2) Body into automobile
        (3) Organs within body
    8. Blunt injury
      a. Direct impact
      b. Acceleration or deceleration
      c. Continuous pressure, shearing, or rotary forces
      d. May be less obvious and therefore more serious
      e. Can leave little outward evidence of internal damage
      f. Underlying tearing by rotary and shearing forces
      g. Disrupts blood vessels and nerves
      h. Can cause widespread epithelial and endothelial damage
      i. Stimulates cells to release their constituents activating the complement
      j. Coagulation cascade can begin.
      k. Masks more serious complications

9. Penetrating injury
    a. Definition: that which cuts or pierces
    b. Multiple objects can be impaled (e.g., knife, firearms, handlebars).
    c. Causes penetrating and crushing of underlying tissue
    d. Produces capillary injury and destruction of tissue
    e. Bullets (important factors affecting injury)
        (1) Size and type of gun
        (2) Velocity
        (3) Range
        (4) Mass
        (5) Trajectory
        (6) Entrance and exit wound
    f. Stab wounds
        (1) Length of object
        (2) Force applied
        (3) Angle of entry
        (4) Twisting or stationary
        (5) Penetrating object left in place or removed
    g. Firearms
        (1) More than bullets
        (2) Include explosives such as bottle rockets, missiles, bombs
        (3) Occurs many times more than penetrating injury occurs
    h. Wounds cause disruption of tissue and cellular function.
    i. Introduces debris and foreign bodies into wounds
    j. May occur as local ischemia or may extend to fulminate hemorrhage
10. Compression injury
    a. Blunt trauma significant to produce capillary injury and destruction
    b. Contusion of tissue occurs.
    c. Extravasation of blood causes discoloration, pain, and swelling.
    d. Massive hematoma increases myofascial pressure.
    e. Significant myofascial pressure can result in compartment syndrome.
        (1) Increased pressure inside an osteofascial compartment
        (2) Impedes circulation and causes cellular ischemia
        (3) Results in alteration in neurovascular function
        (4) Damaged muscular vessels dilate in response to histamine.
        (5) Dilated vessels leak fluid into tissue; loss of capillary integrity
        (6) Microvascular perfusion is impeded, and edema increases.
        (7) Tissue pressure occurs.
        (8) Most commonly occurs in lower leg or forearm
        (9) Compartment pressure can be measured.
            (a) Normal is <10 mm Hg.
            (b) Greater than 30 mm Hg is significant.
        (10) Fasciotomy is treatment to prevent muscle or neurovascular damage.
11. Chemical
    a. Can be topical, ingested, or inhaled
    b. Caustic agent
        (1) Alkaline
        (2) Acids
        (3) Petroleum-based products
    c. Damage often limited to localized area
    d. Factors to include
        (1) Route
        (2) Amount
        (3) Concentration of substance
        (4) Type of substance
        (5) Time lapse after exposure
        (6) Prehospital treatment

    12. Electrical

      a. Always think of safety of rescuer.

      b. Internal burn not obviously seen

      c. Presents in unusual ways

        (1) Burned hair on affected extremity

        (2) Chest pain

        (3) Thermal burn

        (4) Enter and exit wounds (often hands or feet)

      d. Factors that influence

        (1) Voltage

        (2) Time of exposure

        (3) Area affected

        (4) Systemic symptoms

    13. Radiant

      a. Events generating heat and/or flames

      b. Topical or inhalation

      c. Can occur in combination with other injuries

      d. Burn can occur to skin and underlying structures.

      e. Vasoactive chemicals released from mast cells

      f. Intravascular volume lost because of tissue disruption and protein leakage

      g. Hyperemia increases blood flow and increases fluid loss.

      h. Seriousness of injury dependent on:

        (1) Surface area

        (2) Degree of burn: percent calculated on the amount of second- and third-degree burns only

        (3) Presence of systemic problems

        (4) Prehospital treatment

      i. Inhalation reaction from radiant event

        (1) Damage to respiratory vasculature can occur.

        (2) Low inhaled oxygen and increased inhaled carbon dioxide can cause hypoxia.

        (3) Carboxyhemoglobin levels

        (4) Smoke inhalation causes:

          (a) Edema of small airways

          (b) Atelectasis

    14. Predicable injuries

      a. Can be based on specific mechanism of injury

      b. All injuries cannot be predicted based on mechanism of injury.

C. Scoring systems

    1. Numerous scoring mechanisms can be used.

      a. Anatomic

        (1) Abbreviated Injury Score (AIS)

        (2) Injury Severity Score (ISS)

        (3) New Injury Severity Score (NISS)

      b. Physiological

        (1) Glasgow Coma Scale (GCS)

        (2) Revised Trauma Score (RTS)

        (3) Trauma and Injury Severity Score (TRISS)

      c. Injuries assigned to body parts

        (1) General

        (2) Head and neck

        (3) Chest

        (4) Abdomen

        (5) Extremities and pelvis

    2. Assists in determining severity of injuries

    3. Assists in determining likelihood of outcome

    4. Accuracy limitations can occur despite score used.

IV. STABILIZATION PHASE
  A. Initial assessment, resuscitation, and stabilization
    1. Initiated in emergency department (ED) or trauma center
    2. Extend into operating room (OR)
    3. Continue into PACU
    4. Will further continue in the critical area or the surgical floor
    5. Can extend even beyond discharge
      a. Significance of discharge instructions cannot be overstressed.
  B. Hypovolemia in trauma patient
    1. Most common cause of shock
      a. Result of acute blood loss
      b. Result of fluid redistribution
    2. Fluid resuscitation necessary
      a. Prompt fluid replacement
        (1) Assists in tissue perfusion
        (2) Assists in delivery of oxygen to the tissues
        (3) Often requires use of rapid-volume fluid infuser
          (a) Can deliver IV fluids at rate of 500 to 700 mL/min
        (4) Beneficial to give warm IV fluids
          (a) Prevents hypothermia
      b. Fluid selection
        (1) Crystalloids
          (a) Electrolyte solution
            (i) Lactated Ringer's (LR) closely resembles electrolyte composition of blood serum.
            (ii) LR may decrease bleeding when compared with normal saline.
          (b) Diffuses through capillary endothelium
          (c) Distributed throughout extracellular compartment
            (i) Only one fourth stays in vascular space.
          (d) Common selections are LR and normal saline.
          (e) Recommended first line for replacement
          (f) Administration should be three to four times blood loss.
          (g) Use LR in caution with suspected liver injury.
          (h) Cheaper than colloids
        (2) Colloids
          (a) Contain protein or starch molecules
          (b) Molecules remain in intravascular space.
          (c) Increase osmotic pressure gradient within vascular compartment
          (d) Administration is volume per volume.
          (e) Half-life longer than crystalloids
          (f) Common selections are:
            (i) Plasma protein fraction
            (ii) Dextran
            (iii) Albumin
            (iv) Hetastarch
        (3) Hypertonic solutions
          (a) Controversial in treatment
          (b) Resuscitative in shock
            (i) Volume expander (from extracellular source)
          (c) Common selections are hypertonic or isotonic saline.
          (d) Pulls fluids from extracellular space to support blood pressure (BP)
          (e) Can be helpful in head injury patients
            (i) Decreases brain edema
            (ii) Decreases intracranial pressure
            (iii) Increases cerebral pulse pressure
          (f) May protect gut and inhibit acute lung injury

(g) Cautions
  (i) Renal insufficiency
  (ii) Hypernatremia
(4) Blood products
  (a) Only blood can replace blood.
  (b) Restores capacity to carry oxygen
  (c) Given after fluid administration
  (d) Packed red blood cells most common
  (e) Universal donor is O negative.
  (f) O positive can be given to nonchildbearing females and males.
  (g) Type-specific blood preferred when waiting is an option
  (h) Platelets may be indicated if coagulopathy suspected.
  (i) Massive transfusion
    (i) More than 10 to 50 units in first 12 to 24 hours
(5) Hemoglobin-based oxygen carriers/blood substitutes
  (a) Modified hemoglobin molecule able to carry oxygen to tissue
  (b) Longer shelf life
  (c) Absence of ABO antigens
  (d) No incompatible reactions
  (e) Currently only available through research protocols
c. Delayed fluid administration (permissive hypotension)
  (1) Can be useful in hemorrhagic patients
  (2) Fluids delayed until the start of surgery
  (3) Early fluid administration may delay transport.
  (4) Restoration of volume can have adverse complications.
    (a) Hemodilutes/disrupts body's hemostatic mechanisms and clot formation
  (5) Exacerbation of blood loss can occur from increased BP.
    (a) Radial pulse is guideline.
  (6) Controversial among trauma surgeons
d. Volume replacement guidelines
  (1) Hemorrhage
    (a) 3:1 Rule
      (i) Administer 3 mL electrolyte solution to 1 mL blood loss.
  (2) Burns
    (a) Parkland burn formula employs LR alone for first 24 hours.
      (i) Adults: LR 2 to 4 mL × Body Weight (kg) × Percent of Burn
      (ii) Pediatrics: LR 3 to 4 mL × Body Weight (kg) × Percent of Burn
      (iii) Add maintenance fluids with 5% dextrose in water (D_5W) to prevent hypoglycemia and to maintain adequate urine output of 1 mL/kg/hr.
  (3) Combination patients (burns and hemorrhaging)
    (a) Receive volume calculated for burns.
    (b) Also receive volume estimates for hemorrhage loss.
e. Monitoring effective resuscitation
  (1) BP goal: Systolic >90 mm Hg
  (2) Hourly urine output
    (a) Adults: 0.5 mL/kg per hour (30-50 mL/hr)
    (b) Peds: 1 mL/kg per hour
  (3) Lactate levels
  (4) Base excess
3. Other causes of shock in trauma patient
  a. Cardiogenic shock can result from:
    (1) Cardiac tamponade
    (2) Tension pneumothorax
  b. Neurogenic shock
    (1) Related to spinal cord injury
    (2) Spinal anesthesia

       c. Septic shock
         (1) Usually late
         (2) Caused by infectious process
V. DIAGNOSTIC STUDIES AND PROTOCOLS
  A. Diagnostic tests
    1. Vital role in establishing injury
    2. Necessary for accurate diagnosis
    3. Assists in planning effective treatment
    4. X-rays
      a. Lateral cervical spine
      b. Upright chest anteroposterior (CXR)
         (1) Repeat if initial CXR done flat (on backboard).
      c. Anteroposterior pelvis
      d. Any extremity with questionable injury
      e. Thoracic and lumbar spine
      f. Any other identified injured area
      g. Soft tissue films can be helpful if impaled object suspected.
    5. Computed tomography (CT) scan
      a. Head (without contrast)
      b. Chest
      c. Abdomen
      d. Pelvis
    6. Ultrasound (FAST exam)
      a. FAST
         (1) **F**ocused
         (2) **A**ssessment
         (3) **S**onography
         (4) **T**rauma
      b. Rapid, accurate, and inexpensive
      c. Blunt trauma
      d. Reveals presence of hemoperitoneum
      e. To be positive, 200 to 500 mL fluid must be present.
      f. Four areas to evaluate
         (1) Hepatorenal fossa
         (2) Splenorenal fossa
         (3) Pericardial sac
         (4) Pelvis
      g. Cannot diagnose hollow visceral and retroperitoneal injuries or injuries not associated with hemoperitoneum
    7. Twelve-lead electrocardiogram
      a. Useful with chest injury
      b. May be needed if after chest pain, additional trauma occured
    8. Diagnostic peritoneal lavage
      a. Controversial
      b. Used only with suspected abdominal injury and severe hypotension
      c. Abdominal CT scan more useful with specific injury information
      d. Accuracy rate for presence of blood: 98%
      e. Not useful for retroperitoneal blood
      f. Before performing lavage, must place nasogastric (NG)/orogastric tube and Foley catheter to decompress bladder and stomach so that inadvertent puncture avoided
    9. Arteriogram: perform if vascular injury suspected
  B. Laboratory studies
    1. Vital role in establishing current status
    2. Common laboratory studies
      a. Arterial blood gases
      b. Electrolytes
      c. Glucose

         d. Lactate level
         e. Renal function studies
         f. Liver function studies
         g. Coagulation studies
         h. Complete blood cell count
         i. Type and crossmatch
         j. Urinalysis
         k. Pregnancy test (childbearing females)
         l. Alcohol and drug testing are controversial.
      3. Assist in planning effective treatment.
 VI. COLLABORATIVE APPROACH
    A. Essentials
      1. Begins with prehospital personnel
         a. Witnesses at scene
         b. First responder
         c. Paramedic
         d. Police
         e. Fire department
         f. Air ambulance personnel if activated
      2. ED or trauma center
         a. Emergency physician
         b. Registered trained trauma nurse
         c. Emergency technician and paramedic
         d. Respiratory therapist
         e. X-ray personnel
         f. Trauma surgeon
         g. Anesthesiologist
         h. OR personnel
         i. Chaplain
      3. OR
         a. OR nurse
         b. Scrub technicians
         c. Anesthesia provider
      4. After the OR
         a. PACU
         b. Critical care
         c. Surgical floor
         d. Discharge nurse
    B. Communication
      1. Vital communication initiated prehospital
      2. Continues throughout hospital stay
      3. Comprehensive in approach
         a. Physician to physician
         b. ED nurse to OR nurse
         c. OR nurse to PACU nurse
         d. PACU nurse to floor nurse
         e. Physician to family
         f. Nurse to family
      4. Systematic reports
         a. Situation
         b. Background
           (1) Mechanism of injury
           (2) Past medical history
         c. Assessment
           (1) Airway, breathing, circulation
           (2) Vital signs
           (3) Include diagnostic findings
           (4) Treatments
           (5) Suspected injuries

       (6) Abnormal assessment
       (7) Vital nursing information
       (8) Fluids and/or blood products
    d. Recommendations
       (1) Pending orders
VII. POSTANESTHESIA CARE
  A. Anesthesia report
    1. Valuable information
      a. Presenting status
        (1) Name
        (2) Age
        (3) Surgeon
        (4) Anesthesiologist
        (5) Level of consciousness preoperatively
      b. Significant facts pertaining to mechanism of injury
      c. Prehospital phase
      d. ED course
        (1) Cervical spine (C spine) clearance documentation
          (a) MUST be done by ED physician, trauma surgeon, or neurosurgeon
      e. Operative procedure
        (1) Single procedure
        (2) More than one procedure
        (3) More than one surgeon
      f. Intubation
        (1) Routine intubation
        (2) Difficult intubation
        (3) Rapid sequence intubation
        (4) Full stomach
        (5) Airway stability
        (6) Intubation time and tolerance
      g. Anesthetic agents
        (1) Rapid sequence intubation
        (2) Inhalation agents
        (3) IV agents
        (4) Balanced anesthesia
        (5) Narcotic usage (with time of last dose)
        (6) Muscle relaxants (with time of last dose)
        (7) Reversal agents (with time of last dose)
        (8) Antibiotics
      h. Estimated blood loss
        (1) Prehospital
        (2) ED
        (3) OR
      i. Fluid resuscitation
        (1) Prehospital
        (2) ED
        (3) OR
        (4) Crystalloids
        (5) Blood products
        (6) Chest drains
        (7) Cell saver usage
        (8) Ortho refuser (orthopedic refuser system)
        (9) Other drains
      j. Cardiopulmonary status
        (1) Vital signs
        (2) Pulse oximetry
        (3) Vasopressors
        (4) Antidysrhythmics
        (5) Arterial line

(6) Thermodilation catheter
(7) Urine output (to ensure end-organ perfusion)
  k. Other identified injuries
    (1) Surgical interventions
    (2) Nonsurgical interventions
  l. Treatment abnormalities
    (1) Hypothermia
    (2) Abnormal laboratory values
    (3) Abnormal x-ray results
    (4) Volume replacement
    (5) Tetanus status
  m. Treatment plans
B. Nursing assessment, primary survey
  1. Airway
    a. Patency
    b. Proper head position
    c. Ensure cervical spine protection until cleared.
      (1) Do not remove cervical collar if not cleared.
    d. Suctioning as needed for removal of secretions
    e. Airway management as indicated
      (1) Nasopharyngeal
      (2) Oropharyngeal
      (3) Oral or nasal endotracheal tube (ETT)
    f. Continual reassessment
  2. Breathing
    a. Consider mechanism of injury.
      (1) Blunt
      (2) Penetrating
      (3) Acceleration
      (4) Deceleration
      (5) Acceleration and deceleration
    b. Location of injury
      (1) Chest injury may indicate pulmonary injury.
      (2) Rib fractures
      (3) Pulmonary contusion
      (4) Pneumothorax
      (5) Tension pneumothorax
      (6) Neurological event affecting respiratory status
    c. Spontaneous respirations
      (1) Absence of respiratory effort
        (a) NOT a result of thoracic trauma
        (b) Result of head trauma or drugs
        (c) Respiratory rate and pattern is the most sensitive vital sign in the patient with a neurologic deficit.
    d. Chest wall movement
      (1) Chest wall can move without air going in or out.
    e. Respiratory accessory muscle use
    f. Work of breathing
    g. Palpation
      (1) Subcutaneous emphysema
      (2) Trachea position
    h. Auscultation
      (1) Bilateral breath sounds
      (2) Adventitious breath sounds
    i. Pulse oximetry continuous
    j. End-tidal carbon dioxide
    k. Arterial blood gases
    l. Carboxyhemoglobin level (if indicated)

    m. Oxygen delivery
        (1) 100% mask for spontaneous respiratory efforts
        (2) Bag valve mask with assisted respiration or mechanical ventilation
  3. Circulation
    a. Pulses
        (1) Carotid: ≥60 beats/min
        (2) Radial: ≥80 beats/min
        (3) Femoral: ≥70 beats/min
        (4) Popliteal and dorsalis pedis pulses
        (5) Bilateral
        (6) Quality
        (7) Rate
        (8) Upper extremities to lower extremities
        (9) Pulseless electrical activity (PEA) can occur in trauma patient.
            (a) Tension pneumothorax
            (b) Cardiac tamponade
            (c) Hypovolemia
            (d) Hypothermia
            (e) Hypoxia
            (f) Hypoglycemia
            (g) Head injury
            (h) Acidosis
            (i) Hypokalemia
            (j) Hyperkalemia
            (k) Thrombosis
                (i) Pulmonary
                (ii) Coronary
        (10) Start cardiopulmonary resuscitation if heart rate (HR) <60 beats/min in a child.
    b. Cardiac monitor
        (1) Rate
        (2) Rhythm
        (3) Dysrhythmia presence
        (4) Continual cardiac monitor observance
    c. BP
        (1) Hypertension
        (2) Hypotension
        (3) Normal BP range for patient
        (4) Vasopressors
        (5) Monitor every 10 minutes if stable.
        (6) Monitor every minute if unstable.
        (7) Noninvasive cuff
        (8) Arterial line
        (9) Capillary refill may be more beneficial in pediatric patient.
    d. Vascular access
        (1) Number of sites
        (2) Location of sites
        (3) Type of fluids presently hanging
        (4) Intake
    e. Dressings
        (1) Surgical dressings for drainage
        (2) Drainage from nonsurgical wounds
        (3) Surgical drain placement and volume of drainage
        (4) Bloody drainage versus nonbloody drainage
        (5) Total output
    f. Urine output
        (1) Ensures end-organ perfusion
        (2) Essential for input and output (I&O) balance

C. Nursing assessment, secondary survey
  1. General information
     a. Done only after primary assessment
     b. High degree of suspicion concerning mechanism of injury
     c. Note any injuries not previously addressed.
        (1) Swelling and bruising can take time to develop.
     d. Life-threatening injuries may limit time for secondary survey in ED.
        (1) Immediate surgery may be needed for life-threatening injuries.
  2. Head-to-toe assessment
     a. Neurological evaluation
        (1) Level of consciousness (AVPU)
           (a) **A**wake
           (b) **V**erbal
           (c) **P**ain response
           (d) **U**nresponsive
        (2) Appropriate verbal response
        (3) Pupil reactivity and symmetry
        (4) Following commands
        (5) Movement of all four extremities
        (6) Compare results with preoperative assessment.
        (7) May need head CT if taken to OR immediately on arrival
     b. Examination of head and face
        (1) Abrasions
        (2) Lacerations
        (3) Puncture wounds
        (4) Ecchymosis: raccoon eyes (periorbital bruising)
        (5) Edema: facial edema can result in potential airway compromise.
        (6) Gross vision exam
        (7) Check for presence of contact lens.
     c. Ears
        (1) Ecchymosis: Battle's sign (bruising behind ear)
        (2) Drainage from nose
           (a) Bloody
           (b) Clear fluid (potential for cerebrospinal fluid [CSF] leak)
              (i) Check for presence of glucose.
        (3) Never pack or suction nose if CSF leak suspected.
        (4) If CSF leak suspected and/or Battle's sign, never insert NG tube;
            consider orogastric tube if needed.
     d. Evaluate neck.
        (1) Edema
        (2) Ecchymosis
        (3) Tracheal deviation
        (4) Pulsating or distended neck veins
        (5) Subcutaneous emphysema
     e. Chest assessment
        (1) Anterior, lateral, and axilla examination
        (2) Lacerations
        (3) Abrasions
        (4) Contusions
           (a) Seat belt bruising can be seen on the chest.
        (5) Puncture wounds
        (6) Edema
        (7) Subcutaneous emphysema
        (8) Chest wall symmetry
        (9) Depth of respirations
        (10) Reevaluation of breathing
        (11) Auscultation of breath and heart sounds
           (a) Adventitious sounds

        (b) Murmurs
        (c) Bruits
        (d) Muffled heart sounds
     (12) Chest pain that may indicate:
        (a) Pulmonary contusion
        (b) Rib fractures
        (c) Cardiac contusion

  f. Abdomen, pelvis, and genitalia evaluation
     (1) Abrasions
     (2) Contusions
     (3) Edema
     (4) Ecchymosis
        (a) Seat belt bruising often seen across abdomen
     (5) Tenderness
     (6) Presence of bowel sounds
     (7) Abdominal girth
     (8) Pelvis examined for stability over crests and pubis
     (9) Presence of priapism could indicate spinal cord injury.
     (10) Urinary catheter
        (a) Should be in place for all multiple trauma patients
        (b) Examine urine.
        (c) I&O documented
        (d) Ensure adequate output to prevent rhabdomyolysis.
     (11) Rectal exam
        (a) Presence of blood
        (b) Rectal tone
           (i) Lack of rectal tone suggestive of spinal injury
        (c) Trauma surgeon or ED physician

  g. Extremity assessment
     (1) Circulatory
     (2) Sensory
     (3) Motor function
     (4) Range of motion
     (5) Edema
     (6) Ecchymosis
     (7) Lacerations
     (8) Abrasions
     (9) Reexamine if intervention activated.

  h. Back evaluation
     (1) Log roll with cervical spine support.
     (2) Inspect and palpate back, flanks, and buttocks.
     (3) Lacerations
     (4) Abrasions
     (5) Ecchymosis
     (6) Edema
     (7) Pain
     (8) Rectal exam

  i. ED intervention assessment
     (1) Open wounds need tetanus booster.
     (2) Antibiotics often started preoperatively
     (3) Pain medication
     (4) Antianxiety medication
     (5) Nausea medication
     (6) Wound cleansing and dressings

D. Nursing interventions
  1. Pain control (trauma considerations)
    a. Note preoperative medications given in ED.
      (1) Intramuscular medications can have long half-life.

    b. Pain may be inclusive of more than the surgical site.
       (1) Musculoskeletal injuries
       (2) Sutured lacerations
       (3) Extremity fractures
       (4) Rib fractures
       (5) Contusions and bruising
    c. Pain evaluation (see Chapter 26)
       (1) Subjective
       (2) Verbal
       (3) Nonverbal
       (4) Hemodynamic changes (increased HR and BP)
       (5) Splinting
       (6) Nausea
       (7) Crying
       (8) Guarding
       (9) Use standard pain scale to assess.
    d. Pain management
       (1) IV injection
       (2) Patient-controlled analgesia
       (3) Epidural catheter
       (4) Major plexus block
       (5) Music therapy
       (6) Guided imagery
       (7) Relaxation techniques
       (8) Visitors
    e. Pain goals
       (1) Minimize cardiovascular depression.
       (2) Minimize intracranial hypertension.
       (3) Substance abusers may require higher pain doses (includes smokers).
       (4) Pain management is vital to optimal care.
2. Nausea management (trauma considerations)
    a. Can be of great concern for the trauma patient
    b. Seldom are trauma patients prepared with nothing by mouth (NPO).
    c. Consider trauma patient having anesthesia as having potentially full stomach
    d. Vomiting can lead to aspiration.
    e. Extubation may be delayed until gag reflex returns.
    f. NG tube does not always function if food particles are large.
    g. Nausea has higher incidence in trauma patient.
    h. Nausea can be indication of increased intracranial pressure.
3. Psychological management
    a. Emotional consideration increases postoperatively.
    b. Life-threatening interventions have been implemented.
    c. May be challenging postoperatively
       (1) Initial shock may have worn off.
       (2) Questions concerning others involved
       (3) Fear of consequences
       (4) Life-changing injuries
       (5) Pre-event drug or alcohol use can complicate.
    d. Emergence from anesthesia
       (1) Orient to place and time.
       (2) Brief explanation of the event
       (3) Acknowledges fears
         (a) Death
         (b) Mutilation
         (c) Change in body image
         (d) Loss of control
         (e) Loss of family members and friends

         (4) Same information may need to be repeated several times.

         (5) Be honest with information.

         (6) Encourage appropriate coping skills.

         (7) Psychological concepts of trauma

            (a) Need for information

            (b) Need for compassion

            (c) Need for hope

    4. Infection risks (related to trauma care)

       a. May have limited past medical history

       b. Large amount of unknown information may exist.

       c. High risk for:

         (1) Tetanus

         (2) Wound infection

         (3) Sepsis

         (4) Communicable diseases

         (5) Human immunodeficiency virus

         (6) Hepatitis

         (7) Sexually transmitted diseases

         (8) Chicken pox

       d. Universal precautions should be observed.

       e. Hand washing is the best defense.

    5. Nursing diagnosis: potential for:

       a. Ineffective airway clearance

       b. Ineffective gas exchange

       c. Alterations in cardiac output

       d. Alteration in tissue perfusion

       e. Fluid volume deficit

       f. Hypothermia

       g. Risk of injury

       h. Altered comfort

       i. Altered thought process

       j. Altered communication

       k. Anxiety

       l. Ineffective coping

       m. Disturbance in self-concept

       n. Posttraumatic stress

       o. Surgical interventions and injuries dependent on circumstances

    6. Nursing care

       a. Vigilant continuous reassessment

       b. Treatment priorities

       c. Recognition of complex pathophysiological responses

       d. Anticipation of subtle or overt signs of shock

       e. Prevention of complications

         (1) Acute respiratory distress syndrome

         (2) Sepsis

         (3) Acute renal failure

         (4) Hypoxic liver

         (5) Multisystem organ failure

VIII. SHOCK IN THE MULTITRAUMA PATIENT

  A. Shock as a complication

    1. Most common complication associated with traumatic injury

    2. Different types of shock all exhibit problems with:

       a. Delivery of oxygen to the cell

       b. Delivery of nutrients to the cell

       c. Inadequate tissue perfusion (cellular hypoxia)

       d. Increased lactic acid level (caused by oxygen debt)

         (1) Degree of rise correlates with severity and prognosis.

       e. Functional impairment of cells

        f. Functional impairment of organs

        g. Functional impairment of body systems

        h. Heart, brain, liver, kidneys, and lungs require increased oxygen.

        i. Ischemia initiates complex events.

           (1) Energy-dependent functions cease.

           (2) Protein synthesis depleted

           (3) Loss of intracellular potassium

           (4) Production of lactic acid

           (5) Death of vital tissue

    3. Clinical manifestations of shock

        a. Cool, clammy skin

        b. Cyanosis

        c. Restlessness

        d. Altered level of consciousness

        e. Altered skin temperature

        f. Tachycardia

        g. Dysrhythmias

        h. Tachypnea

        i. Pulmonary edema

        j. Decreased urine output

        k. Decreased end-organ perfusion

        l. Increased platelet, leukocyte, and erythrocyte counts

        m. Sludging of the blood

        n. Metabolic acidosis

  B. Types of shock

    1. Hypovolemic

        a. Most common type

        b. Results from acute hemorrhagic loss

        c. Volume shift in burn patients

    2. Cardiogenic

        a. Rare in trauma patients

        b. Inadequate contractility of cardiac muscle

        c. May be secondary to:

           (1) Blunt cardiac injury

           (2) Myocardial infarction (MI)

    3. Distributive

        a. Includes:

           (1) Neurogenic

           (2) Anaphylactic

           (3) Septic

        b. Abnormality in vascular system and maldistribution of blood volume

           (1) Loss of vasomotor tone regulated by sympathetic nervous system

        c. Neurogenic most common in trauma patient from spinal cord injury

    4. Obstructive

        a. Compression of great vessels or heart from:

           (1) Tension pneumothorax

           (2) Cardiac tamponade

  C. Hypovolemic shock

    1. Definition

        a. Decrease in intravascular volume

        b. Decrease in filling the intravascular compartment

    2. Causes

        a. Internal hemorrhage

        b. External hemorrhage

        c. Plasma volume loss

        d. Third spacing of fluids

        e. Decreased venous return

    3. Classification of hemorrhage

        a. Characteristic clinical manifestations according to approximate loss

    b. American College of Surgeons' Advanced Trauma Life Support Course

    c. Class I

        (1) Early phase

        (2) Loss of as much as 750 mL

        (3) Approximately 1% to 15% total blood volume loss

        (4) Minimal physiological changes in:

            (a) HR (<100 beats/min)

            (b) BP (normal)

            (c) Capillary refill (normal)

            (d) Respiratory rate (14-20 breaths/min)

            (e) Urine output (>30 mL/hr)

        (5) Mild anxiety in response to sympathetic nervous system

        (6) Treatment

            (a) Rapid infusion of 1 or 2 L of balanced salt solution

            (b) Maintain renal output of more than 0.5 mL/kg per hour.

    d. Class II

        (1) Moderate phase

        (2) Loss of 750 to 1500 mL blood

        (3) Approximately 15% to 30% total blood volume loss

        (4) Multiple incremental physiological changes

            (a) Increased anxiety

            (b) Restlessness

            (c) Catecholamine release

            (d) HR >100 beats/min

            (e) Minimal BP changes

                (i) Rise in diastolic BP

                (ii) Decreasing pulse pressure

            (f) Slight capillary refill delay

            (g) Cool, pale skin

            (h) Slight depression in urine output

        (5) Treatment

            (a) Rapid infusion of 1 or 2 L of balanced salt solution

            (b) Maintain renal output of more than 0.5 mL/kg per hour.

    e. Class III

        (1) Progressive phase

        (2) Loss of 1500 to 2000 mL blood

        (3) Approximately 30% to 40% total blood volume loss

        (4) Obvious physiological changes

            (a) Cerebral hypoperfusion—decreased level of consciousness

            (b) Confusion

            (c) Agitation

            (d) Anxiety

            (e) HR >120 beats/min

            (f) Hypotension

            (g) Capillary refill >4 seconds

            (h) Deep, rapid respirations

            (i) Metabolic acidosis

            (j) Decreased urine output (approximately 5-15 mL/hr)

        (5) Treatment

            (a) Fluid administration

            (b) Consider blood transfusion.

    f. Class IV

        (1) Hemorrhage

        (2) More than 2000 mL blood loss

        (3) Approximately 40% total blood volume loss

        (4) Profound impact

            (a) Lethargic

            (b) Stuporous

            (c) Unresponsive

          (d) HR ≥140 beats/min
          (e) Peripheral pulses weak and difficult to palpate
          (f) Capillary refill >10 seconds
          (g) Severe hypotension, BP difficult to obtain
          (h) Cold, clammy, diaphoretic, or cyanotic skin
          (i) Shallow, irregular respirations with respiratory rate >35 breaths/min
          (j) No renal end-organ perfusion, resulting in anuria
      (5) Treatment
          (a) Fluid administration
          (b) Blood administration
   g. The Golden Hour
      (1) Treatment within the first hour associated with lower mortality
      (2) Filling the vascular tank allows:
          (a) Adequate cardiac output
          (b) Perfusion of tissues

D. Cardiogenic shock

  1. Definition

    a. Inadequate cardiac output

    b. Circulatory failure

    c. Impaired contractility

    d. Shock secondary to acute myocardial dysfunction
      (1) Systolic BP less than 80 mm Hg (<30% baseline)
      (2) Cardiac index less than 2.1 L/min

    e. Mortality rate: 80% to 100%

  2. Causes in trauma

    a. Secondary to blunt injury to heart muscle

    b. Occasionally MI occurs preceding trauma event.

    c. History of heart disease in association with trauma and/or anesthesia can increase likelihood of intraoperative MI.

    d. Rapid fluid administration and ensuing cardiac failure

    e. Disruption in normal conduction sequence (heart block, dysrhythmias)

  3. Classifications of cardiogenic shock

    a. Coronary
      (1) Obstructive coronary artery disease interrupting blood flow
      (2) Interruption of blood flow causing ischemic heart muscle
      (3) Ischemic heart muscle results in decreased contraction.
      (4) Decreased contraction results in inadequate cardiac output.
      (5) Incidence rises with compromise of 40% left ventricular function.
      (6) Increased left atrial pressure
      (7) Increased pulmonary venous pressure
      (8) Increased pulmonary capillary pressure
      (9) Pulmonary edema

    b. Noncoronary
      (1) Absence of coronary artery disease
      (2) Cardiac muscle damage
          (a) Cardiomyopathy
          (b) Valvular heart abnormalities
          (c) Cardiac dysrhythmias

  4. Clinical indicators

    a. Systolic BP less than 80 mm Hg (<30% baseline)

    b. Cardiac index less than 2.1 L/min

    c. Urine output less than 20 mL/hr

    d. Diminished cerebral perfusion evidenced by confusion

    e. Cold, clammy, cyanotic skin

    f. Classic signs and symptoms
      (1) May not be seen in the hypovolemic trauma patient
      (2) Pulmonary edema
      (3) Jugular vein distention
      (4) Hepatic congestion

   g. Decreased cardiac, stroke, and left ventricular stroke work index
   h. Increased pulmonary capillary wedge pressure
   i. Increased pulmonary artery pressure
   j. Increased systemic vascular resistance
   k. Decreased systemic venous oxygen saturation
   l. Decreased cardiac output
   m. Respiratory and metabolic acidosis
 5. Treatment
   a. Early recognition
   b. Improvement of myocardial oxygen supply
   c. Improvement of tissue perfusion
   d. Airway management, ventilation, and oxygenation
   e. Correct acidosis
   f. Pain relief
   g. Pharmacological support to improve or correct rhythm
   h. Increasing cardiac output by increasing intravascular volume
   i. Vasoactive medications
      (1) Dobutamine
      (2) Dopamine
      (3) Epinephrine
   j. Decrease afterload (systemic vascular resistance)
   k. When pharmacological support fails
      (1) Intra-aortic balloon pump
      (2) Ventricular assist device
 E. Distributive shock
  1. Definition
   a. Also called vasogenic shock
   b. Abnormal placement of the vascular volume
   c. Heart pump and blood volume are normal.
   d. Alteration exists within the vascular circulatory network.
   e. Three types
      (1) Neurogenic
      (2) Anaphylactic
      (3) Septic
  2. Neurogenic shock
   a. Definition
      (1) Tremendous increase in vascular capacity
      (2) Normal amount of blood incapable of adequately filling vasculature
      (3) Loss of sympathetic vasomotor tone causes massive vasodilation.
      (4) Venous pooling and decreased return to right side of the heart
      (5) Frequently transitory
      (6) Not common in occurrence except in spinal cord–injured patients
   b. Causes
      (1) Deep general or spinal anesthesia
      (2) Loss of sympathetic vasomotor tone in the trauma patient
         (a) Brain concussion or contusion of basal regions
         (b) Spinal cord injury above level of T6
   c. Clinical symptoms
      (1) Decreased peripheral vascular resistance
      (2) Decreased stroke volume
      (3) Decreased cardiac output
      (4) Hypotension
      (5) Decreased tissue perfusion
      (6) Differs from hypovolemic shock
         (a) Bradycardia
         (b) Warm, dry, flushed skin
   d. Treatment
      (1) Extensive volume expansion

      (2) Vasopressors
        (a) Ephedrine
        (b) Neosynephrine
      (3) Spinal anesthesia as causative event
        (a) Head of bed flat
        (b) Supine position
        (c) Elevate legs if possible.

3. Anaphylactic shock
  a. Definition
    (1) Severe antigen-antibody reaction
    (2) Relates to inflammatory process
    (3) Activation of complement and arachidonic cascade
      (a) Immunoglobulin E produced and binds to mast cells and basophils
      (b) Mast cells trigger vasoactive contents.
      (c) Histamine and vasoactive mediators released by mast cells
      (d) Vasoactive mediators cause massive vasodilation.
      (e) Vasoactive mediators cause increased capillary permeability.
    (4) Rarely occurs in the trauma patient but should be of concern if no past medical history
  b. Causes
    (1) Antigen-antibody reaction
    (2) Can occur with exposure to any allergen; in the trauma patient consider:
      (a) Antibiotics
      (b) Contrast medium
      (c) Blood transfusions
  c. Clinical symptoms
    (1) Vary with severity
    (2) Conjunctivitis
    (3) Angioedema
    (4) Hypotension
    (5) Laryngeal edema
    (6) Urticaria
    (7) Bronchoconstriction
    (8) Dysrhythmias
    (9) Cardiac arrest
    (10) One or any combinations of the preceding signs can occur.
    (11) Repeat exposures can increase symptoms.
  d. Treatment
    (1) Removal of causative agent
    (2) Discontinue blood transfusion.
    (3) Oxygen
    (4) Epinephrine
      (a) Bronchodilator
      (b) Helps restore vascular tone
      (c) Increases arterial BP
    (5) Aminophylline, if wheezing
    (6) Diphenhydramine (Benadryl), antihistamine
    (7) Steroids: decrease inflammatory process
    (8) Gastric acid blocker
      (a) Famotidine (Pepcid)
      (b) Cimetidine (Tagamet)
      (c) Nizatidine (Axid)
      (d) Ranitidine (Zantac)

4. Septic shock
  a. Definition
    (1) Acute systemic response to invading blood-borne microorganisms
    (2) Clinical syndrome on a continuum

(3) Begins with sepsis and ends with multisystem organ failure
(4) Complex cellular disease
(5) Loss of autoregulation and tissue dysfunction despite increased cardiac output
(6) Activation of kinins, complement, arachidonic, and coagulation cascades
(7) Hemodynamic instability
    (a) Initial phase
        (i) High cardiac output
        (ii) Low systemic vascular resistance
    (b) Later phase
        (i) Low cardiac output
        (ii) Extremely high systemic vascular resistance
(8) Myocardial depression related to severity of sepsis
(9) Release of vasoactive chemical mediators and endotoxins
(10) Decreased ventricular preload
(11) Increased capillary permeability
    (a) Augments myocardial depression
    (b) Produces decreased vascular volume
(12) Endotoxin stimulates complement split products.
(13) Neutrophil and platelet aggregation to the lungs
(14) Fluid collects within the pulmonary interstitium.
(15) Pulmonary compliance decreased
(16) Acute respiratory distress syndrome ensues.
(17) Profound alteration in metabolism
(18) Increased oxygen debt
(19) Rising blood lactate levels
(20) Trauma patient is predisposed because of:
    (a) Contaminated wounds
    (b) Poor nutritional status
    (c) Preexisting disease states
    (d) Altered integrity of body's defense mechanism
(21) Principal cause of death in trauma patient surviving first 3 days

b. Causes
(1) Gram-positive microorganisms less common
(2) Gram-negative microorganisms most common
(3) Viruses
(4) Fungi
(5) Parasites

c. Clinical symptoms
(1) Warm, flushed, and dry skin
(2) Rapid respiratory rate
(3) Confusion
(4) Increased HR
(5) Hypotension
(6) High cardiac output
(7) Low systemic vascular resistance
(8) Late clinical signs: skin changes to cold and clammy.

d. Treatment
(1) Identification and elimination of infection
(2) Cultures
(3) Proper definitive antimicrobial therapy
(4) Hemodynamic monitoring
(5) Oxygenation and ventilation support
(6) Fluid administration
(7) Pharmacological support
    (a) Positive inotropes
    (b) Vasopressors

5. Obstructive shock
   a. Definition
      (1) Myocardium normal
      (2) Compression to the atria
      (3) Obstruction in venous return
      (4) Prevents atrial filling
      (5) Decrease in stroke volume
   b. Causes
      (1) Obstructive source
      (2) Pulmonary embolism
      (3) Dissecting aortic aneurysm
      (4) Vena cava obstruction
      (5) Cardiac tamponade
      (6) Tension pneumothorax
   c. Clinical symptoms dependent on causative mechanism and can include:
      (1) Muffled heart sounds
      (2) Jugular vein distention
      (3) Tracheal deviation
      (4) Diminished or absent lung sounds
      (5) Hypotension
      (6) Pulseless electrical activity (PEA)
   d. Treatment
      (1) Correct the cause.
      (2) Dissecting aneurysm: surgical intervention
      (3) Vena cava obstruction: surgical intervention
      (4) Cardiac tamponade: cardiocentesis until surgical intervention
      (5) Tension pneumothorax: needle decompression, chest tube

BIBLIOGRAPHY

1. *Advanced cardiac life support provider manual*, ed 5, Dallas, 2006, American Heart Association.
2. *Advanced trauma life support course*, ed 7, Chicago, 2004, Committee on Trauma of the American College of Surgeons.
3. Alam HB, Rhee P: New developments in fluid resuscitation. *Surg Clin North Am* 87(1):55–72, 2007.
4. Alspach J, Epgang T, editors: *Core curriculum for critical care nursing*, ed 6, Philadelphia, 2006, Saunders.
5. Cocchi MN, Kimlin E, Walsh M, et al: Identification and resuscitation of the trauma patient in shock. *Emerg Med Clin North Am* 25(3):623–642, 2007.
6. *Course in advanced trauma nursing: A conceptual approach*, Park Ridge, IL, 2006, Emergency Nurses Association.
7. Davidson J, Griffin R, Higgs S: Introducing a clinical pathway in fluid management. *J Perioper Pract* 17(6):248–250, 255–256, 2007.
8. Drain CB, Odom-Forren J: *Perianesthesia nursing: A critical care approach*, ed 5, St. Louis, MO, 2009, Saunders.
9. *Emergency nurse pediatric course*, ed 3, Park Ridge, IL, 2007, Emergency Nurses Association.
10. Jacob M, Chappell D: Saline or albumin for fluid resuscitation in traumatic brain injury. *N Engl J Med* 357(25):2634–2635, 2007.
11. Mizushima Y, Tohira H, Mizobata Y, et al: Fluid resuscitation of trauma patients: How fast is the optimal rate? *Am J Emerg Med* 23(7):833–837, 2005.
12. Moore KM: Controversies in fluid resuscitation. *J Trauma Nurs* 13(4):168–172, 2006.
13. Pascual JL, Maloney-Wilensky E, Reilly PM, et al: Resuscitation of hypotensive head-injured patients: Is hypertonic saline the answer? *Am Surg* 74(3):253–259, 2008.
14. Pepe PE, Dutton RP, Fowler RL: Preoperative resuscitation of the trauma patient. *Curr Opin Anaesthesiol* 21(2):216–221, 2008.
15. Schweer L: Pediatric trauma resuscitation: Initial fluid management. *J Infus Nurs* 31(2):104–111, 2008.
16. Sperry JL, Minei JP, Frankel HL, et al: Early use of vasopressors after injury: Caution before constriction. *J Trauma* 64(1):9–14, 2008.
17. *Trauma nursing core course*, ed 6, Park Ridge, IL, 2006, Emergency Nurses Association.
18. Yanagawa Y, Sakamoto T, Okada Y: Hypovolemic shock evaluated by sonographic measurement of the inferior vena cava during resuscitation in trauma patients. *J Trauma* 63(6):1245–1248, 2007.

48 Bariatric Care

KIM A. NOBLE

OBJECTIVES

At the conclusion of this chapter, the reader will be able to:

1. Describe the normal anatomy and physiology of the gastrointestinal (GI) tract.
2. Describe the incidence and physiological impact of obesity.
3. Compare and contrast surgical options for weight loss with bariatric surgery.
4. Describe important considerations for patient selection for bariatric surgery.
5. List the potential complications and their physiological rationale(s) for bariatric surgery.
6. Describe the implications for the perianesthesia care of the bariatric surgical patient.

I. OVERVIEW
    A. Parallel to the pandemic occurrence of obesity is the incidence of bariatric surgery (Table 48-1).
    B. Obesity is defined as a body mass index (BMI) >30.
        1. Associated with an increased comorbidity risk (Box 48-1)
        2. Approximately 30% of the adult population in the United States and more than 300 million people worldwide considered obese
            a. Crosses all demographic classifications
    C. Morbid obesity is approximately twice ideal body weight with BMI >40.
    D. Bariatric surgery has been shown to be the best weight loss option for obese patients.
    E. Caring for patients undergoing bariatric surgery is challenging because they frequently have derangements leading to challenges for their perianesthetic management.
        1. Respiratory
        2. Metabolic
        3. Endocrine
    F. A comprehensive understanding of bariatric surgery and the physiological challenges of caring for obese patients can lead to potential surgical complication:
        1. Prevention
        2. Earlier identification
        3. Treatment
II. ANATOMY AND PHYSIOLOGY OF DIGESTION AND ABSORPTION
    A. Stomach
        1. Gastric anatomy (Figure 48-1)
            a. Pouchlike reservoir for ingested food located in the upper abdomen
            b. Has three anatomic areas
                (1) Fundus
                    (a) The upper arching area immediately distal to the cardiac sphincter
                    (b) Location of the gastric crypts containing secretory cells
                    (c) Responsible for the chemical digestion of ingested food
                    (d) Primary area for the accommodation of the ingested meal
                (2) Body
                    (a) Central, thick walled muscular central area of the stomach
                    (b) Responsible for the mechanical digestion of ingested food

■ TABLE 48-1
■ ■ **Bariatric Surgery Worldwide**

Country	No. of Bariatric Procedures	No. of Bariatric Surgeons	Year Bariatrics Began
Argentina	200	30	1988
Australia (New Zealand)	2750	68	1960
Austria	1396	38	1973
Belgium	6000	200	1970
Brazil	4000	510	1973
Czech Republic	400	6	1983
Egypt	2750	12	1996
France	12,000	200	1984
Germany	1100	54	1975
Greece	500	8	1978
Hungary	30	1	1999
Israel	1000	50	1978
Italy	3000	200	1973
Japan	20	20	1982
Mexico	2500	200	1971
Netherlands	800	40	1973
Panama	60	5	2002
Poland	145	14	1974
Russia	350	35	1969
Spain	2000	160	1977
Sweden	600	20	1970
Switzerland	800	90	1970
Turkey	150	5	1990
Ukraine	150	10	1978
United Kingdom	600	13	1955
USA/Canada	103,000	850	1953
Totals	**146,301**	**2,839**	

Data from Buchwald H, Williams SE: Bariatric surgery worldwide. *Obes Surg* 14:1157–1164, 2004.

(3) Antrum
    (a) Funnel-like portion of the stomach between the body and pyloric sphincter
  c. Contains two sphincters
    (1) Cardiac sphincter at the junction of the esophagus and stomach
    (2) Pyloric sphincter at the junction of the stomach and duodenum
  d. Gastric wall structure
    (1) Has four layers consistent with entire GI tract
      (a) Gastric mucosal layer
        (i) Innermost layer
          [a] Made up of epithelial cells that produce the mucous barrier
          [b] Rapid cellular turnover; complete replacement every 4 to 5 days
        (ii) Provides protective mucous barrier
          [a] A prostaglandin grid work containing mucus and bicarbonate
          [b] Protects gastric cells from acid digestion and provides lubrication
      (b) Gastric submucosal layer
        (i) Connective tissue
        (ii) Contains blood vessels, nerves, and secretory structures

■ BOX 48-1
■ **COMORBIDITY ASSOCIATED WITH BMI >25**

Cardiovascular Comorbidity
Hypertension
Dyslipidemia
Coronary artery disease
Atherosclerosis
Angina
Sudden cardiac death
Congestive heart failure

Endocrine Comorbidity
Type 2 diabetes
Insulin resistance
Glucose intolerance

Neurological Comorbidity
Stroke

Gastrointestinal Comorbidity
Cholecystitis
Cholelithiasis
Gastroesophageal reflux disease

Respiratory Comorbidity
Obstructive sleep apnea
Asthma

Musculoskeletal Comorbidity
Osteoarthritis
Gout

Reproductive Comorbidity
Complications of pregnancy
Poor female reproductive health
Endometrial, breast, prostate cancers

Urological Comorbidity
Stress incontinence
Bladder infection
Renal calculi

Miscellaneous Comorbidity
Colon cancer
Depression
Eating disorders
Distorted body image

BMI, Body mass index.

    (c) Gastric muscular layer
        (i)   Thick muscular layer arranged in longitudinal, circular, and oblique direction
        (ii) Provides grinding contractions involved in the mechanical digestion
    (d) Gastric serosal layer
        (i)   Outermost protective layer continuous with the lesser omentum
        (ii) Made up of fibrous connective tissue

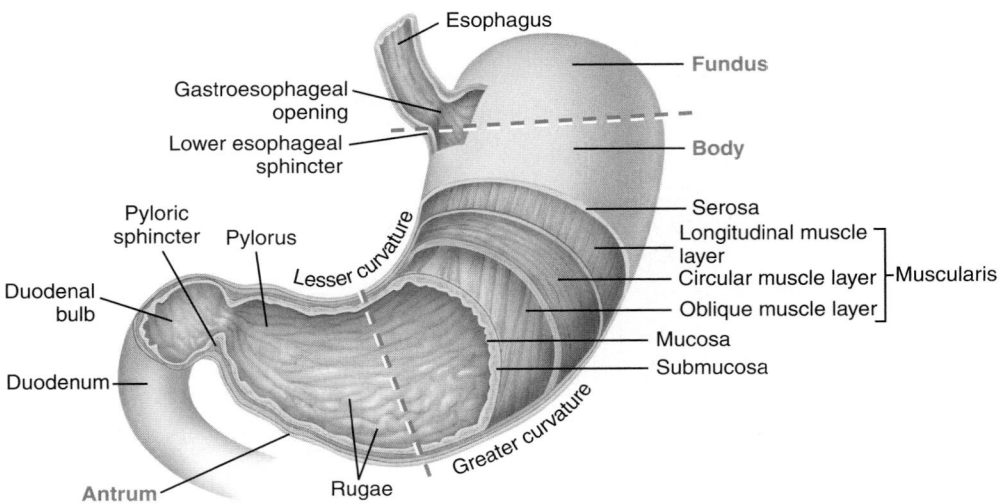

FIGURE 48-1 ■ Stomach. (From McCance KL, Huether SE: *Pathophysiology: The biologic basis for diseases in adults and children*, ed 5, St Louis, 2006, Mosby.)

    e. High degree of gastric accommodation (enlargement) with ingested meals
        (1) Empty stomach contains approximately 50 mL of acid with a significantly low pH.
        (2) Stomach can expand to almost 1000 mL without an increase in intraluminal pressure.
  2. Gastric physiology
    a. Stomach receives ingested food from the esophagus via the cardiac sphincter.
    b. Chemical digestion begins in the stomach.
        (1) Gastric acid secretion amounts to 2 L of fluid daily.
            (a) Control of gastric acid secretion
                (i) Endocrine secretion: blood-borne hormonal control of acid secretion
                    [a] GI tract is the largest endocrine organ in the body.
                    [b] Direct hydrochloric acid (HCl) release occurs when gastrin is released by:
                        [1] Parasympathetic nervous system
                        [2] Presence of alcohol
                        [3] Calcium-containing foods
                        [4] Protein in the stomach
                    [c] Secretin released from duodenum upon entry of chyme with pH <4.5, causes the release of large amounts of bicarbonate and water from the pancreas and liver into the common bile duct (CBD), and enters the duodenum via the sphincter of Oddi
                    [d] Cholecystokinin released from duodenum upon entry of protein and fat, leading to the release of pancreatic enzymes via the CBD and contraction of the gallbladder, leading to emptying of bile into the CBD and duodenum via the sphincter of Oddi.
                (ii) Paracrine secretion: local control of acid secretion
                    [a] Histamine secretion from cells adjacent to parietal cells (local) stimulated by the endocrine release of gastrin. Histamine causes:
                        [1] Parietal cell stimulation
                        [2] Increased release of HCl

[b] Somatostatin released locally during times of fasting (decreasing pH) and leads to inhibition of gastrin and HCl release from the parietal cells
  (b) Structures responsible for chemical digestion in the stomach
    (i) Parietal cells
      [a] Approximately 1 billion parietal cells located in the fundus
      [b] Produce HCl
      [c] Produce intrinsic factor necessary for vitamin B_{12} absorption
    (ii) Chief cells
      [a] Produce pepsinogen, an inactive substance
      [b] Rapidly converted to pepsin in an acidic environment
      [c] Pepsin chemically digests protein.
    (iii) Gastric lipase enzymatically degrades dietary fats into fatty acids.
  (2) Chemical digestion is the process of chemically dividing food items into smaller parts.
    (a) Starch and fibers degraded by gastric acid
    (b) Protein degraded into small particle through the action of pepsin
    (c) Fats delivered to the small intestine in a nondigested state
  (3) Combination of the food derivative and gastric secretions called chyme
c. Mechanical digestion begins in the mouth (teeth) and continues in the stomach.
  (1) Mechanical digestion (gastric motility) grinds food into chemically digestible particles.
  (2) Gastric motility
    (a) Peristaltic mixing and churning contractions begin in the body of the stomach and move toward the antrum, propelling the chyme toward the antrum.
    (b) Large particles return to the body of the stomach for additional mechanical digestion.
    (c) Opening of the pylorus and gastric empting into the duodenum is regulated by:
      (i) pH of the chyme: pH is sensed by receptors on the duodenal wall, and a low pH delays gastric empting, allowing time for buffered secretions from the liver and pancreas to normalize pH before movement into the portal circulation.
      (ii) Fat content of the chyme: fat delays gastric empting.
      (iii) Osmolarity of the chyme: either hyperosmotic (caloric-dense foods or high protein content) or hypoosmotic chyme will delay gastric empting.
      (iv) Volume of chyme in the stomach: an increase in the volume and gastric intraluminal pressure will accelerate empting.
    (d) With each peristaltic contraction, a small amount of digested chyme is propelled through the pyloric sphincter.
  (3) Neural control of gastric motility
    (a) Enteric nervous system
      (i) Local neural control in the muscular layer of the wall of GI tract
        [a] Responsible for muscular contraction along the length of GI tract
    (b) Autonomic nervous control of gastric motility
      (i) Sympathetic nervous system stimulation
        [a] Directly decreases GI motility and secretion
      (ii) Parasympathetic nervous system stimulation
        [a] Directly increases motility and acid secretion
    (c) Endocrine control of gastric motility

(i) Gastric inhibitory peptide is released from the duodenal mucosa in response to increased concentration of glucose and/ or fat in the duodenum; this causes the inhibition of
[a] Gastric acid secretion
[b] Gastric motility
[c] Gastric emptying
B. Small intestine (Figure 48-2)
1. Anatomy
a. Contains same layers as found in the stomach; anatomical variation in layers based on function
b. Muscle fibers thin compared with gastric muscle and have a longitudinal and circular arrangement allowing for coordinated peristalsis
c. Small intestine has plica, or wrinkles, that slow chyme movement to allow additional time for absorption.
(1) Plica are most numerous in:
(a) Jejunum
(b) Ileum
d. Small intestine consists of three segments:
(1) Duodenum
(a) U-shaped connection with the pylorus; entry into the small intestine
(b) Approximately 22 cm (10 inches) long
(c) Entry point for CBD via sphincter of Oddi

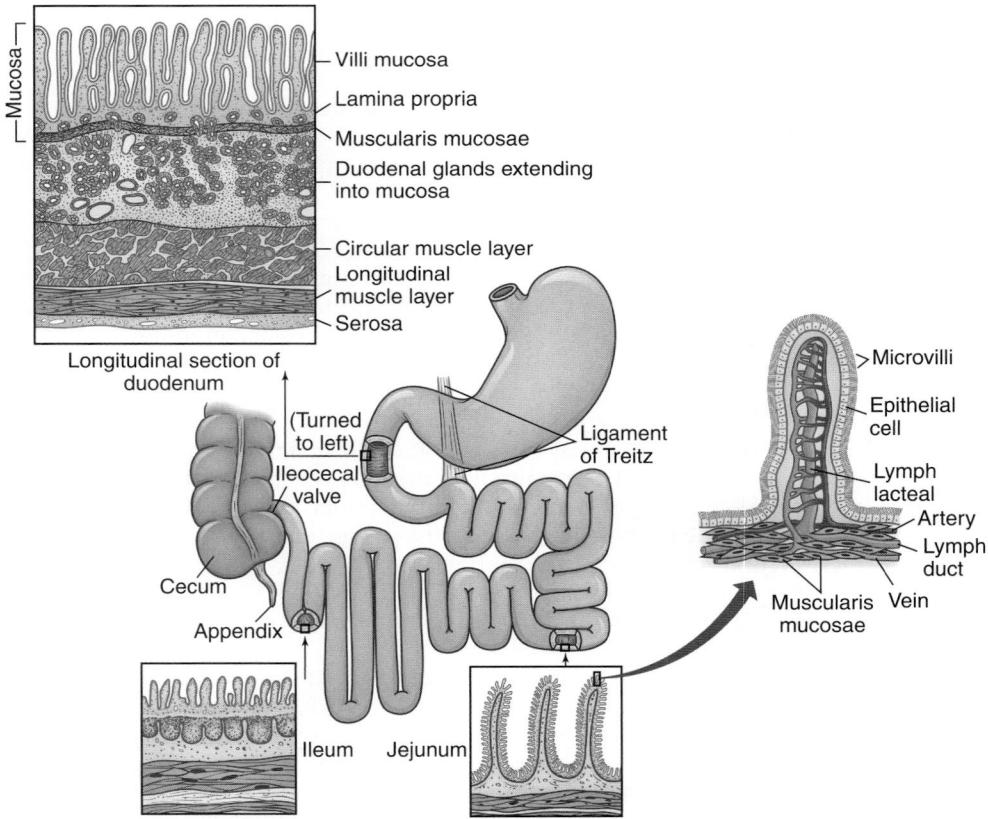

FIGURE 48-2 ■ Intestine. (From McCance KL, Huether SE: *Pathophysiology: The biologic basis for diseases in adults and children,* ed 5, St Louis, 2006, Mosby.)

   (i) Entry point for pancreatic enzymes and bicarbonate from the pancreas and liver after the endocrine release of secretin

   (ii) Entry point for bile stored in the gallbladder after the endocrine release of cholecystokinin

  (d) Large surface area for absorption related to villi and microvilli; projections of enterocyte-covered portal capillaries

   (i) Villi and microvilli decrease the distance required for the diffusion of nutrients from the GI lumen into the portal blood supply, increasing absorption.

 (2) Jejunum

  (a) Together with the ileum approximately 7 m (23 feet) long

  (b) No clear separation from duodenum or ileum

 (3) Ileum

  (a) Terminates into the large intestine

  (b) Separated from the large intestine by the ileocecal valve

  (c) Location of the appendix

2. Physiology

 a. Chyme propelled through the pylorus as a liquid containing small, undigested food particles

 b. Chemical digestion continues in the segments of the small intestine.

  (1) Carbohydrates break down into disaccharides and monosaccharides (single sugars).

  (2) Protein breaks down into amino acids and peptides.

  (3) Fats emulsified into monoglycerides and fatty acids

 c. Digestive role of small intestine

  (1) Duodenum

   (a) Digestive role for fat with entry of bile

   (b) Protein digestive role with pancreatic enzymes, which activate due to acidic pH

   (c) Continued digestion of carbohydrates through the secretion of digestive enzymes from the intestinal enterocytes

   (d) Intestinal secretion amounts to approximately 4 L of fluid daily.

  (2) Jejunum

   (a) Additional intestinal length for digestion and absorption as needed

  (3) Ileum

   (a) Additional intestinal length for digestion and absorption as needed

 d. Small intestine nutrient absorption based on anatomic location

  (1) Duodenum

   (a) Primary site of absorption of iron, calcium, sugars, and proteins

   (b) Primary site of absorption of water and water-soluble vitamins

   (c) Primary site of energy-dependent absorption of magnesium and sodium

  (2) Jejunum

   (a) Upper jejunum is the major site of absorption of:

    (i) Bile salts

    (ii) Fatty acids

    (iii) Fat-soluble vitamins (A, D, E, K)

   (b) Additional surface area for sugar and protein absorption

  (3) Ileum

   (a) Primary site for absorption of:

    (i) Bile salts

    (ii) Vitamin B_{12} (intrinsic factor)

    (iii) Chloride

 e. Intestinal motility

  (1) Stimulated by the arrival of chyme to mix secretions

   (a) Pancreatic

   (b) Gallbladder

   (c) Hepatic

    (2) Segmentation
      (a) Produced by the contraction of circular muscle fibers
      (b) More common in proximal small intestine (duodenum)
      (c) Divides and mixes chyme and increases contact with absorptive surfaces
    (3) Peristalsis
      (a) Produced by the contraction of longitudinal muscle fibers
      (b) Slow wave of contraction to propel chyme through the small intestine

III. OBESITY

  A. Overview

    1. Obesity is a syndrome of increased percentage of body fat that is correlated with increased comorbidities and decreased life expectancy (see Box 48-1).

    2. Definition of obesity

      a. BMI in kilograms per meter squared (kg/m^2) (Table 48-2)

        (1) A ratio of weight, adjusted for height, expressed as weight in kilograms (kg) divided by height in meters squared (m^2)

        (2) Important to incorporate age- and gender-related differences, especially in children (Figure 48-3)

        (3) Abdominal circumference should also be measured, since athletes with increased muscle mass would have high BMI without obesity.

  B. Epidemiology

    1. World Health Organization estimates 300 million people are obese worldwide.

    2. Adult obesity

      a. In the United States, the incidence of obesity nearly doubled over the past 25 years.

        (1) 12.8% in 1962

        (2) 22.5% in 1994

        (3) 27% in 2000

      b. Obesity at higher incidence in racial and ethnic minority populations (African Americans and Hispanic Americans) as compared with white ethnic groups

    3. Childhood obesity

      a. Reached when child's weight exceeds the 95th percentile

      b. Almost a 400% increase in incidence of obesity in children aged 6 to 11 years between 1963 and 2000 (from 4% to 15%)

      c. For adolescents (12–19 years of age) during the same time frame (from 1963 to 2000), incidence increased 300% (from 5% to 15%)

  C. Pathophysiology

    1. Overview

      a. Obesity is complex and multifactorial in nature.

      b. Obesity follows a positive energy balance, where energy expenditure exceeds energy output.

      c. Obesity carries a strong genetic predisposition with a familial pattern for excess weight.

    2. Theory of ectopic fat deposition

      a. When adipose tissue can no longer expand to store excess calories, fat is deposited in body tissues.

        (1) Liver

        (2) Skeletal muscle

        (3) Pancreas

        (4) Heart

      b. Excess circulating fatty acids promote insulin resistance and type 2 diabetes mellitus.

      c. Adipose tissue is an endocrine tissue and secretes:

        (1) Hormones

        (2) Inflammatory substances

TABLE 48-2
Body Mass Index (BMI)

Height (inches)	19	20	21	22	23	24	25	26	27	28	29	30	31	32	33	34	35
									Body Weight (lb)								
58	91	96	100	105	110	115	119	124	129	134	138	143	148	153	158	162	167
59	94	99	104	109	114	119	124	128	133	138	143	148	153	158	163	168	173
60	97	102	107	112	118	123	128	133	138	143	148	153	158	163	168	174	179
61	100	106	111	116	122	127	132	137	143	148	153	158	164	169	174	180	185
62	104	109	115	120	126	131	136	142	147	153	158	164	169	175	180	186	191
63	107	113	118	124	130	135	141	146	152	158	163	169	175	180	186	191	197
64	110	116	122	128	134	140	145	151	157	163	169	174	180	186	192	197	204
65	114	120	126	132	138	144	150	156	162	168	174	180	186	192	198	204	210
66	118	124	130	136	142	148	155	161	167	173	179	186	192	198	204	210	216
67	121	127	134	140	146	153	159	166	172	178	185	191	198	204	211	217	223
68	125	131	138	144	151	158	164	171	177	184	190	197	203	210	216	223	230
69	128	135	142	149	155	162	169	176	182	189	196	203	209	216	223	230	236
70	132	139	146	153	160	167	174	181	188	195	202	209	216	222	229	236	243
71	136	143	150	157	165	172	179	186	193	200	208	215	222	229	236	243	250
72	140	147	154	162	169	177	184	191	199	206	213	221	228	235	242	250	258
73	144	151	159	166	174	182	189	197	204	212	219	227	235	242	250	257	265
74	148	155	163	171	179	186	194	202	210	218	225	233	241	249	256	264	272
75	152	160	168	176	184	192	200	208	216	224	232	240	248	256	264	272	279
76	156	164	172	180	189	197	205	213	221	230	238	246	254	263	271	279	287

Data from the National Institutes of Health.

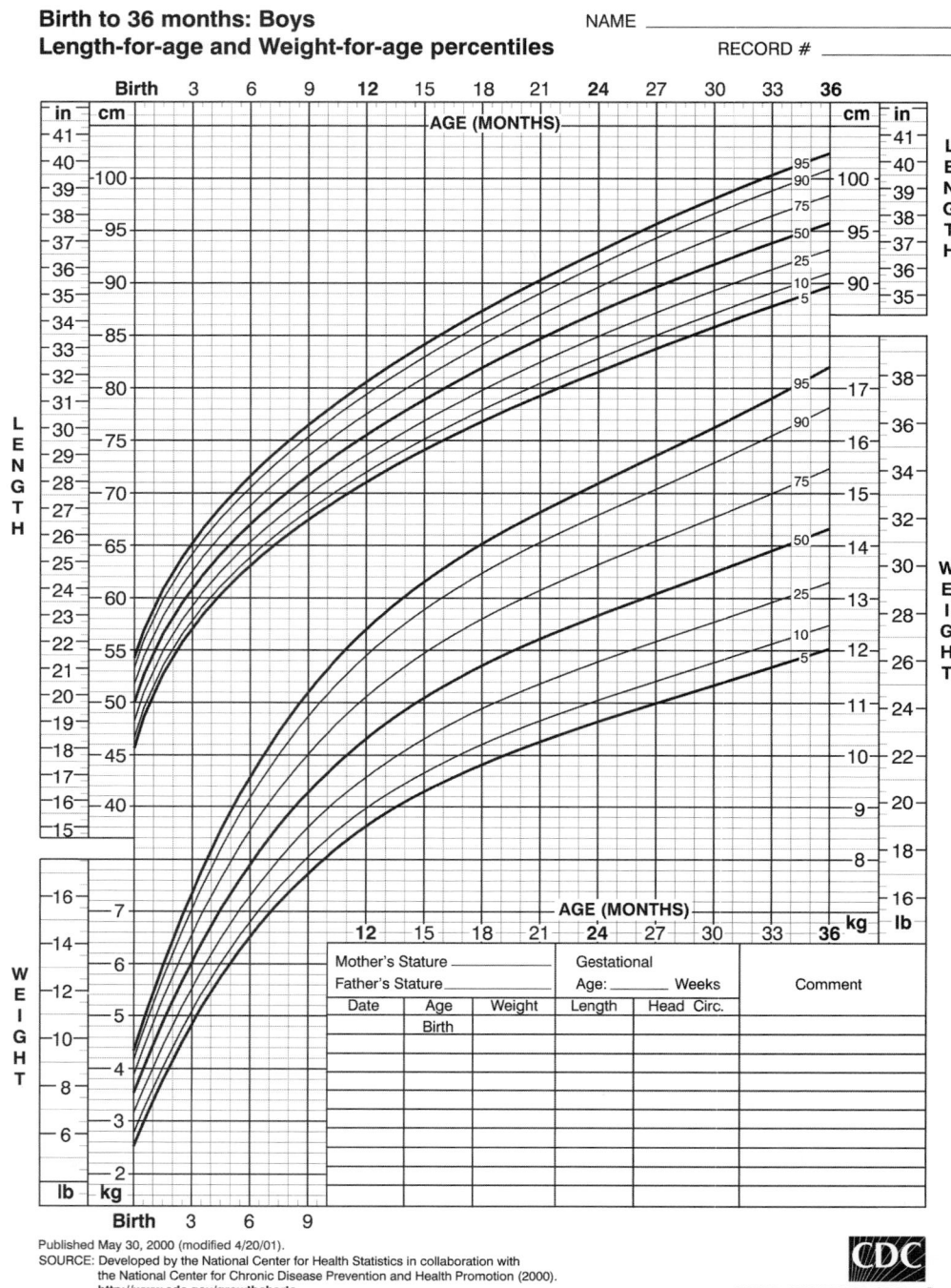

Birth to 36 months: Boys
Length-for-age and Weight-for-age percentiles

NAME _____

RECORD # _____

Published May 30, 2000 (modified 4/20/01).
SOURCE: Developed by the National Center for Health Statistics in collaboration with
the National Center for Chronic Disease Prevention and Health Promotion (2000).
http://www.cdc.gov/growthcharts

FIGURE 48-3 ■ Sample growth chart for boys up to 36 months of age. (From the Centers for Disease Control and Prevention.)

3. Comorbidities of obesity affect virtually every organ system (see Box 48-1).
  a. Hypertension
    (1) Approximately 50% of obese individuals (BMI >30 kg/m²) have hypertension.
    (2) Hypertension is seen in overweight individuals across all demographics.

(3) Hypertension is a primary risk factor for the development of atherosclerosis.

(4) Surgical treatment of obesity improves both hypertension and cardiac function.

b. Dyslipidemia

(1) Forty percent to 50% of obese individuals have dyslipidemia with:

(a) Increased low-density lipoprotein (LDL: "bad cholesterol")

(b) Decreased high-density lipoprotein (HDL: "good cholesterol")

(2) Hyperlipidemia is a primary risk factor for the development of atherosclerosis.

(3) Gastric bypass has been shown to be very effective in:

(a) Lowering triglycerides and LDL

(b) Increasing HDL

c. Diabetes and impaired glucose tolerance

(1) Obesity is the primary risk factor for diabetes and 90% of type 2 diabetics are obese.

(2) Thirty-six percent of individuals with impaired glucose tolerance will progress to type 2 diabetes within 10 years.

(3) Diabetes is a risk factor for the development of:

(a) Atherosclerosis

(b) Vascular disease

(c) Obesity

(d) Combined risk factors predict lethal health consequences.

(4) Weight loss in obese type 2 diabetic patients can restore blood glucose and insulin sensitivity to near-normal levels.

d. Cardiac and peripheral vascular disease

(1) Obesity is a primary risk factor for the development of atherosclerotic cardiac and peripheral vascular disease.

(2) Obesity leads to large vessel disease.

(a) Coronary artery disease

(b) Cerebrovascular accident

(c) Carotid occlusive disease

(d) Subclavian steal syndrome

(e) Aneurysmal disease

(f) Vascular occlusive disease

(g) Vascular insufficiency

(3) Obesity and diabetes lead to small vessel disease.

(a) Retinopathy

(b) Nephropathy

e. Obstructive sleep apnea (OSA)

(1) Approximately 50% of obese individuals have OSA, with increased abdominal girth the single most important risk factor for OSA.

(2) Diagnosis of OSA is made when there are the following three findings:

(a) Individuals have breathing cessation exceeding 10 seconds during sleep.

(b) Apneic episodes occur more than five times per hour.

(c) Apneic episodes have a concurrent 4% decrease in oxygen saturation.

(3) Nocturnal OSA has been associated with cardiac dysrhythmias and sudden cardiac death.

(4) OSA may carry over into the daylight hours, leading to:

(a) Drowsiness

(b) Inattentiveness

(c) Impaired job performance

(d) Decrease in cognitive functioning

(5) OSA is categorized as:

(a) Central

(b) Oropharyngeal obstructive

(c) Combined form

  (6) Marked weight loss (secondary to bariatric surgery) has been nearly 100% effective in managing OSA.

 f. Asthma

  (1) Asthma is a prevalent comorbidity for obesity, thought to be due to decreased lung volumes (from increased abdominal girth) sensitizing the airway and leading to reactive airways.

  (2) The following contribute to asthma:

   (a) OSA

   (b) Respiratory stasis

   (c) Gastroesophageal reflux disease (GERD)

  (3) Obese children have three times greater risk for asthma (30%).

  (4) Obese adults have a 25% increased risk for the development of asthma.

 g. Obesity hypoventilation syndrome (OHS) or Pickwickian syndrome

  (1) OHS present in 30% of patients with morbid obesity, but less common than OSA

  (2) OHS caused by decreased lung volumes (increased abdominal pressure), which causes:

   (a) Chronic shortness of breath

   (b) Decreased expiratory reserve volume

   (c) Increased oxygen consumption

   (d) Increased circulating partial pressure of carbon dioxide (Pco_2)

  (3) Long-term effects of obesity are:

   (a) Pulmonary hypertension

   (b) Right-sided heart failure

   (c) Polycythemia

   (d) Ultimately death

  (4) The following is seen after bariatric surgery:

   (a) Marked improvement in symptoms associated with pulmonary hypertension

   (b) Improved blood oxygenation

   (c) Reduced hypercarbia

 h. Peripheral osteoarthritis

  (1) Weight-bearing destruction (osteoarthritis) found at an accelerated rate in the obese patient's:

   (a) Knees

   (b) Hips

   (c) Ankles

   (d) Feet

  (2) Obesity increases the necessity of surgical intervention.

 i. Gastroesophageal Reflux Disease (GERD)

  (1) GERD is a relatively common finding in the general population.

   (a) Incidence in general population: 20%

   (b) Incidence in obese patients: up to 50%

  (2) GERD is the retrograde movement of acidic chyme into the esophagus, leading to a chronic inflammation and the potential for precancerous lesions (Barrett esophagus).

  (3) Correlation of GERD and obesity most probably related to increased abdominal pressure

 j. Back and disk disease

  (1) Chronic lower back pain is the most common orthopedic complaint of obese persons.

  (2) With increasing age, the incidence of lower back pain in obese individuals is 100%.

  (3) Decreased mobility and the use of assistive devices are common findings with obesity.

 k. Nonalcoholic steatohepatitis (NASH)

  (1) Fatty infiltration of the liver, or NASH, present in 100% of the morbidly obese population

(2) Severity of NASH increases linearly with increasing BMI.

(3) Over time, fatty infiltration of the liver leads to fibrosis, leading to cirrhosis and possible hepatocellular carcinoma.

l. Female endocrine and reproductive disorders

(1) Estrogen released from adipose tissue, and obese females have increased levels of estrogen

(2) Increased estrogen can cause menstrual abnormalities, dysfunctional bleeding, early menopause, and infertility.

(3) Polycystic ovarian syndrome three times more common in obese patients

(4) Obesity during pregnancy increases the risk for:

(a) Preeclampsia

(b) Urinary tract infections

(c) Gestational hypertension and/or diabetes

(d) Overdue birth

(e) Prolonged labor

(f) Increased blood loss during labor and cesarean delivery

(5) Chronically increased estrogen levels increase the risk for endometrial (3-4 times higher), ovarian (3-4 times higher), and breast (2 times higher) cancers.

m. Depression

(1) Depression related to the social and economic consequences of obesity

(2) Estimated that 50% of obese females are taking antidepressant agents

(3) Adolescent and young females at high risk for the development of depression

4. Mortality and obesity

a. BMI >35 kg/m² approximately doubles all causes of mortality.

b. Coronary artery disease is the major killer in both overweight and obese subjects.

c. Mortality secondary to diabetes and cancer much more common in the obese patient

IV. BARIATRIC SURGERY

A. Overview

1. Rationales for the use of bariatric surgery (Table 48-3)

a. Although traditional medical treatment for obesity has been unsuccessful, bariatric surgery has been found to lead to a significant, sustained loss of weight.

b. Obese individuals who lose significant weight can reverse:

(1) Glucose intolerance

(2) Diabetes mellitus

(3) OSA

(4) OHS

(5) Hypertension

(6) Serum lipid abnormalities

c. Patients undergoing bariatric surgery rarely achieve their ideal body weight.

2. Indications for bariatric surgery

a. Multidisciplinary evaluation and treatment guides patient selection and surgical care.

b. 1991 National Institutes of Health (NIH) Consensus Conference established bariatric surgical indications. Indications reviewed and endorsed by 2004 American Society of Metabolic and Bariatric Surgery (ASBS) Consensus Conference

(1) Patient must be:

(a) Adult (specifically not an adolescent)

(b) Motivated

(c) Well informed of acceptable operative risks with effective informed consent

■ TABLE 48-3
■ ■ **Evidence-Based Practice Findings for Bariatric Surgery**

Author	Year	Question	Sample	Findings
Buchwald et al. Systematic review; meta-analysis (Level I)	2004	Evaluate the effect of bariatric surgery on weight loss, mortality, diabetes, hyperlipemia, hypertension, and OSA	136 studies $N = 22,094$	1. Substantial weight losses: 47.5% for gastric banding; 61.6% for gastric bypass; 68.2% for gastroplasty; 70.1% for BIP/DS 2. Mortality at 30 days: 0.1% banding + gastroplasty; 0.5% gastric bypass; 1.1% BIP/DS 3. Improvement in type 2 diabetes seen with all surgery types 4. Significant improvement in hyperlipemia seen with all surgery types 5. Significant improvement in hypertension seen with all surgery types 6. Significant improvement in OSA seen with all surgery types
Chalhoub et al. Experimental design (Level II)	2006	Study the effects of increased tidal volume and PEEP on oxygenation	$N = 52$	1. PEEP alone moderately and slowly increased Po_2, and saturation 2. PEEP + vital capacity maneuver significantly magnified the positive effects of PEEP
Madan et al. Retrospective case review (Level V)	2007	Looked at outcomes of morbidly obese teenagers treated in an adult program	$N = 5$	1. Five morbidly obese adolescents having laparoscopic Roux-en-Y procedures; no complications; good weight loss 2 years out 2. Difficulty maintaining follow-up noted
McCullough et al. Retrospective case review (Level V)	2006	Evaluate the relationship between CV fitness and complications after laparoscopic Roux-en-Y	$N = 109$	1. A critical inverse relationship exists between CV fitness and complications after bariatric surgery
Livingston et al. Retrospective case review (Level V)	2006	Evaluate the rate of surgical outcomes in patients undergoing all types of bariatric surgery in the Veterans Administration system	$N = 575$	1. 30-day mortality rate: 1.4%; 3% for males and 0.8% for females 2. 2-year mortality rate: 3.1%; 70% to 80% lacked complete follow-up 3. Postoperative complication rate: 19.7%; cardiac arrest (#1); renal failure (#2)

Study	Year	Purpose	Sample	Findings
Hooper et al. Longitudinal observation (Level V)	2007	Determination of prevalence of MSK diseases in patients before and after bariatric surgery	N = 48	1. Higher incidence of MSK disease in obese population; with upper extremity disease 2. Significant improvement in MSK in 6–12 months after bariatric surgery
Haines et al. Longitudinal observation (Level V)	2007	Determination of prevalence of OSA disease in patients before and after bariatric surgery	N = 348	1. OSA found in 45% of patients having bariatric surgery 2. Weight loss in this patient population (high rate of dropout) significantly improved OSA and quality of sleep
Livingston et al. Case report (Level V)	2006 (Reprint)	Compared the rate of adverse effects after bariatric surgery as a function of age (patients <65 years of age and >65)	Record review DRG #288; pt. >65 years of age	1. Adverse events after bariatric surgery increase with age 2. Adverse event rate non-Medicare patients <65 years: 8%; 21.6% for Medicare patients <65; 32.3% >65

BIP/DS, Biliopancreatic diversion/duodenal switch; *CV*, cardiovascular; *MSK*, musculoskeletal; *OSA*, obstructive sleep apnea; *PEEP*, positive end-expiratory pressure; Po_2, partial pressure of oxygen.

        (2) Willing to undergo lifelong medical surveillance

        (3) BMI >40 kg/m^2

        (4) Some cases with BMI >35 kg/m^2 acceptable if high-risk comorbid conditions present

           (a) Cardiopulmonary comorbidity

           (b) Severe OSA

           (c) Pickwickian syndrome (OHS)

           (d) Obesity-related cardiomyopathy

           (e) Severe diabetes mellitus

           (f) Joint disease

           (g) Social effects on employment, family function, or ambulation

3. Contraindications to bariatric surgery

    a. Consider risk-to-benefit ratio

        (1) Active malignancy

        (2) Human immunodeficiency virus infection

        (3) High risk

    b. High risk not prohibitive to anesthesia

        (1) Cardiac ischemia

        (2) Esophageal varices

        (3) Active peptic ulcer

    c. Absolute contraindications to surgery

        (1) Active substance abuse or alcoholism diagnosed on psychological assessment

        (2) Active anorexia or bulimia

    d. Mild eating disorders: closely consider ability to comply with postoperative dietary requirements.

4. Other criteria for bariatric surgery according to 1991 NIH Consensus Conference

    a. Age criteria: for patients younger than 18 years of age or older than 55, consider overall health status.

    b. Weight criteria

        (1) BMI used; excess body weight (45 kg or 100 lb) over ideal weight as a secondary indication for surgical appropriateness

        (2) A maximum weight for surgical selection not identified

    c. Psychological or psychiatric criteria

        (1) Well-controlled major depression, bipolar disorder, and schizophrenia do not preclude surgery and may continue to improve with surgical weight loss.

        (2) Prior abuse, especially sexual abuse, may lead to obesity and should be carefully evaluated on an individual basis.

    d. Behavioral criteria

        (1) Intelligence

           (a) No intelligence limit

           (b) Patient needs to be able to communicate with a multidisciplinary team.

           (c) Informed consent imperative

        (2) Social support

           (a) Individually determined

           (b) Better success adapting to the postsurgical lifestyle with adequate support system

        (3) Motivation

           (a) Motivation highly desirable with better surgical outcome

           (b) Subjective characteristics considered individually

        (4) Socioeconomic status

           (a) In United States, 20 million bariatric candidates

           (b) Patients with the highest BMIs have lowest socioeconomic status.

           (c) Patients with lowest socioeconomic status at highest risk of disease because of:

               (i) Poor medical resources

(ii) Physical environment

(iii) Social support systems

(d) All patients provided equal access regardless of socioeconomic status

(5) Pregnancy

(a) Maximal weight loss 18 to 24 months after bariatric surgery may lead to:

(i)   Electrolyte imbalance

(ii) Metabolic derangement

(b) Pregnancy during the 2 years after surgery discouraged

(c) After the risk period, obesity-related derangements with pregnancy resolve.

e. Nutritional criteria

(1) Dietitian evaluation necessary and completed preoperatively

(2) Early provision of educational materials provided for adequate postoperative nutrition

(3) Eating habits may affect surgical procedure selection.

(a) Grazer eating occurs when patients eat small amounts continuously; restrictive procedures less effective.

(b) Sweeter eating occurs with the ingestion of calories mostly from sweet foods; may have side effects with malabsorptive procedures.

(c) Bloater eating occurs with the ingestion of huge meals at one sitting; successfully treated with restrictive procedures.

(d) Rarely do individuals have single eating habits; most often a combination.

B. Bariatric surgical procedures

1. Overview

a. Traditional weight loss methods ineffective; bariatric surgery is treatment of choice for long-term, significant weight loss.

b. Bariatric surgical classifications

(1) Malabsorptive procedures

(a) Lead to incomplete digestion and absorption of nutrients

(b) Degree of malabsorption controlled by length of small intestine segment

(c) May be combined with gastric resection to prolong weight loss

(d) Generally result in 10% to 20% greater loss of weight than restrictive procedures

(2) Restrictive procedures

(a) Reduce the size of the stomach to:

(i)   Limit the intake of food.

(ii) Create a rapid feeling of fullness.

(b) Variety of surgical approaches and surgical procedures.

(c) Reversible only with adjustable gastric banding systems.

(3) Combined procedures (malabsorptive and restrictive)

(a) Decrease adverse effects on the GI tract

(b) Consistent long-term weight loss

2. Bariatric surgical procedures

a. Laparoscopic adjustable gastric banding (Figure 48-4)

(1) Restrictive procedure

(2) Laparoscopic technique

(a) Less invasive

(b) Small incisions

(c) Reduced pain

(d) Reduced length of stay.

(3) Completely adjustable and reversible with the addition or removal of saline in the subcutaneous reservoir

(4) Good weight loss but takes longer than with other procedures

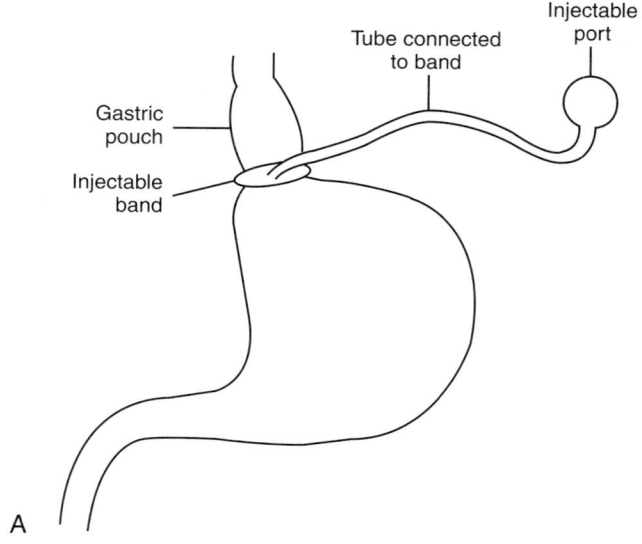

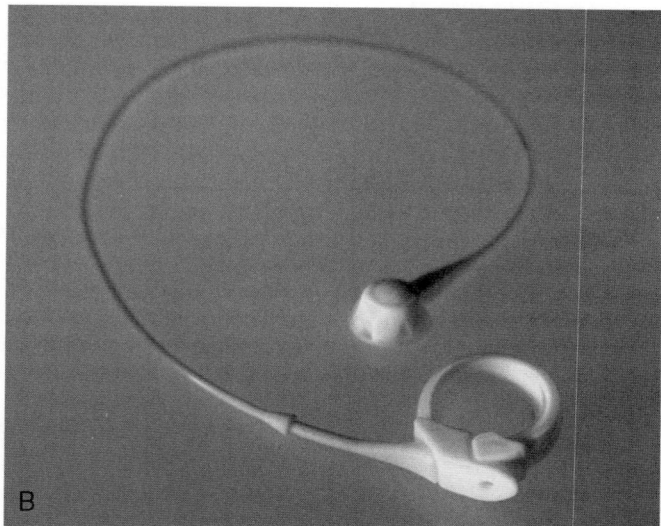

FIGURE 48-4 ■ **A,** Laparoscopic adjustable gastric banding. **B,** Adjustable gastric band. (**A** from Ellison SR, Ellison SD: Bariatric surgery: A review of the available surgical procedures and complications for the emergency physician. *J Emerg Med* 34[1]:21–32, 2008; **B** from Buchwald H, Cowan GS, Pories WJ: *Surgical management of obesity,* Philadelphia, 2007, Saunders.)

    (5) Critical need for follow-up with frequent band size adjustments
        (slippage rate 23%) to prevent potential esophageal complications
    (6) Significantly lower rate of complications as compared with other
        bariatric surgical procedures
    (7) Vomiting should be avoided because it may cause band slippage.
  b. Vertical banded gastroplasty (Figure 48-5)
    (1) Restrictive procedure
    (2) Can be performed either laparoscopically or as open procedure
    (3) Early band position was horizontal; currently using vertical banding.
    (4) Gastric pouch 20 mL and reinforced to prevent dilation over time
    (5) Noncompliance with dietary restrictions leads to decreased weight
        gain over time.
    (6) Surgical complications

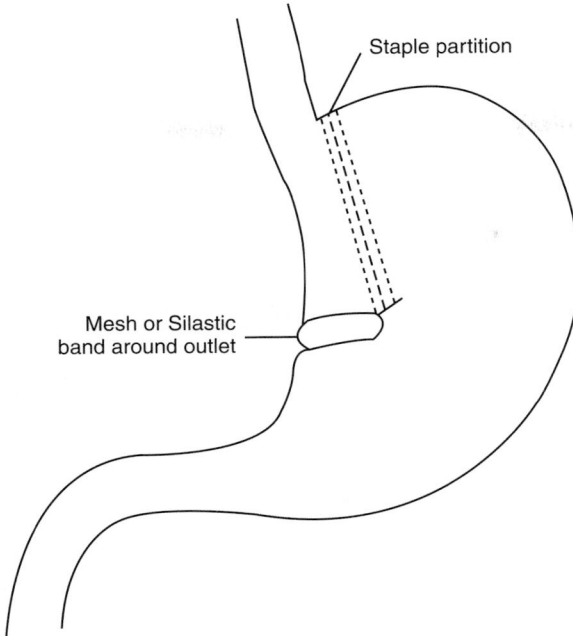

Staple partition

Mesh or Silastic
band around outlet

FIGURE 48-5 ■ Vertical banded gastroplasty. (From Ellison SR, Ellison SD: Bariatric surgery: A review of the available surgical procedures and complications for the emergency physician. *J Emerg Med* 34[1]:21–32, 2008.)

　　　(a) Bleeding
　　　(b) Leakage from stomach
　　　(c) Deep vein thrombosis/pulmonary embolism
　　　(d) Gastroplasty failure necessitating revisional surgery
　c. Roux-en-Y gastric bypass (RYGBP) (Figure 48-6)
　　(1) Combined procedure
　　(2) Most frequently performed bariatric surgery in North America
　　(3) Surgical procedure
　　　(a) Stomach horizontally transected leaving a 30-mL pouch
　　　(b) Distal jejunal "Roux" limb between 50 and 150 cm in length (to ileocecal valve) brought up and attached to the gastric pouch
　　　(c) Jejunojejunostomy created attaching the stomach stump to the Roux limb
　　　(d) Gastric and intestinal digestive secretions (bile, pancreatic, and hepatic contribution) from stomach stump move to the jejunojejunostomy and then the distal small intestine for absorption.
　　(4) Can be performed either laparoscopically or as open procedure
　　(5) Long-limb derivation increases weight loss without altering complication rate.
　　(6) Optimal, long-term weight loss
　　(7) Nutritional deficiency risk from loss of duodenum (calcium, iron, vitamins A, D, E, and K)
　　(8) Surgical complications
　　　(a) Anastomosis leak and hemorrhage
　　　(b) Bowel obstruction
　　　(c) Marginal ulceration
　　　(d) Deep vein thrombosis/pulmonary embolism
　　　(e) Hernia
　d. Banded gastric bypass (banded RYGBP)
　　(1) Combined procedure

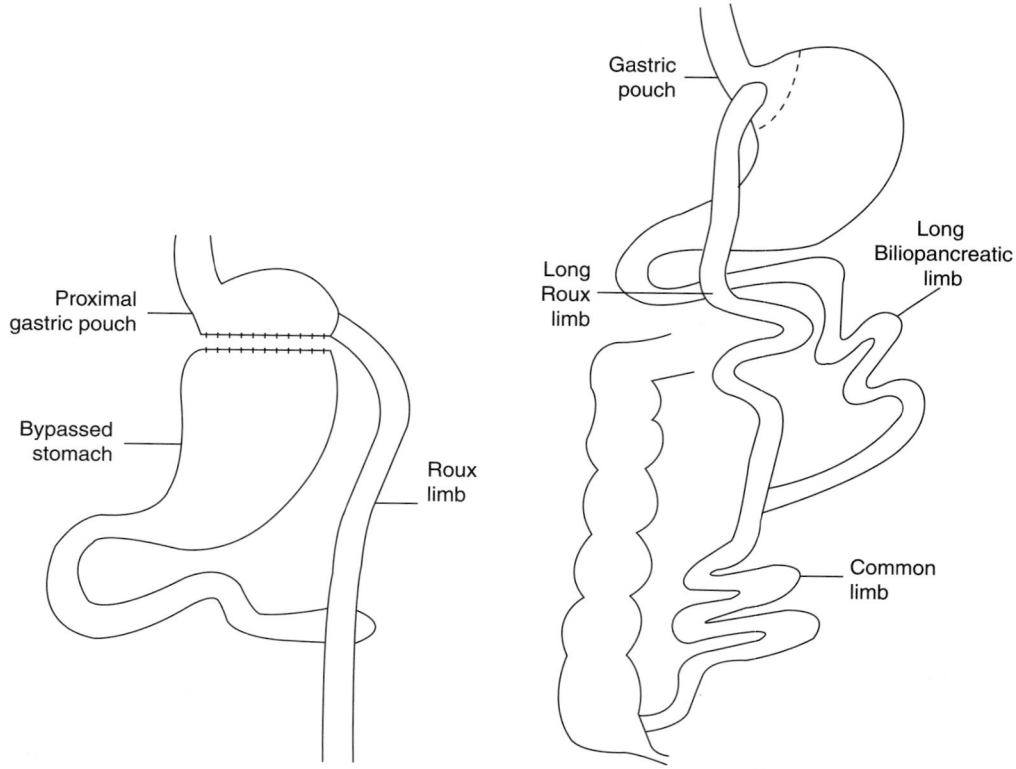

FIGURE 48-6 ■ Roux-en-Y gastric bypass. (From Ellison SR, Ellison SD: Bariatric surgery: A review of the available surgical procedures and complications for the emergency physician. *J Emerg Med* 34[1]:21–32, 2008.)

    (2) Surgical procedure similar to RYGBP except:
       (a) Gastric resection is vertical.
       (b) Gastric pouch reinforced with a Silastic ring or polypropylene mesh bands
       (c) Both segments of small intestine are relatively short (60 cm).
    (3) Can be performed either laparoscopically or as open procedure
    (4) Surgical complications similar to RYGBP
  e. Biliopancreatic diversion
    (1) Combined procedure
    (2) Surgical procedure
       (a) Distal vertical gastrectomy with 200- to 500-mL gastric pouch remaining
       (b) Long Roux-en-Y reconstruction with jejunojejunostomy 50 cm from ileocecal valve
    (3) Can be performed either laparoscopically or as open procedure; longer surgical time
    (4) Lifetime malabsorption of:
       (a) Fat
       (b) Starch
       (c) Protein
       (d) Monosaccharides and disaccharides
       (e) Alcohol
       (f) Sweets
       (g) Soft drinks
       (h) Milk

          (i) Creates negative reinforcement for eating restricted foods and liquids

     (5) Lifetime soft stools high in fat; two to four stools and flatulence daily

     (6) Larger stomach pouch allows return of "normal" eating habits as weight loss stabilizes.

     (7) Extraordinarily good weight loss maintenance

     (8) Surgical complications

          (a) Anemia

          (b) Stomal ulcer

          (c) Bone demineralization

          (d) Protein malnutrition

     (9) Duodenal switch may be added (leaving a short portion of the duodenum attached to the pylorus); reduces the incidence of stomal ulcers.

   f. Laparoscopic duodenal switch and sleeve gastrectomy procedure

     (1) Combined procedure

     (2) Surgical procedure

          (a) Same as biliopancreatic duodenal switch

          (b) Gastric resection is long and horizontal.

     (3) Can be performed either laparoscopically or as open procedure

     (4) Used in the super obese because of sustained large weight losses (>200 lb first year)

     (5) Technically demanding especially when performed laparoscopically

     (6) Surgical complications similar to those for biliopancreatic duodenal switch

   g. Implantable gastric stimulator

     (1) An exciting new approach to the treatment of morbid obesity

     (2) Surgery less invasive than bariatric surgery

     (3) Used since the 1990s and has the lowest rate of complications

     (4) Pacing used to disrupt normal gastric contractions and alter digestion

     (5) Patients experience meaningful weight loss.

     (6) Pacemaker apparatus similar to cardiac pacemaker with a bipolar lead

     (7) No reported incidence of major complications

     (8) Preoperative screening tool improves weight loss by improving accurate patient selection. Only approximately 25% of all morbidly obese patients are appropriate for gastric pacing.

C. Preoperative patient preparation

  1. Overview

   a. Bariatric surgery unique as a surgical subspecialty

     (1) Bariatric surgery is a behavior modification tool that can lead to a complete change of life for the involved patient.

     (2) Bariatric surgery success is strongly related to:

          (a) Skill of the surgeon

          (b) Preoperative risk assessment

          (c) Patient education

  2. Preoperative educational priorities

   a. Full informed consent

     (1) Description of significant health risks and poor quality of life with morbid obesity

     (2) Details of surgical GI alterations

          (a) Description of surgical procedure

          (b) Risks and benefits of laparoscopic versus open procedures

          (c) Description of anesthesia and patient implications

          (d) Description of hospital length of stay and inpatient expectations

          (e) Description of early and late complications

             (i) Prophylaxis for complication prevention

            (ii) Anticipated implication for complication prevention while inpatient

[a] Patients with OSA using continuous positive airway pressure (CPAP)

[b] Instruct to bring their equipment to the hospital with them.

(iii) Educational points for complication prevention after hospital discharge

[a] Include description of continued prophylaxis for deep vein thrombosis.

(iv) Importance of long-term follow-up care

[a] Anticipated schedule of postoperative physician and specialist office visits for the first year

(f) Estimation of surgical outcomes and anticipated physiological implications of large weight loss

(i) Possible need for body contour procedures after stabilization of weight loss

(3) Importance of multidisciplinary evaluation and follow-up throughout the surgical experience

b. Nutritional education

(1) Implication of gastric resection and malabsorption on weight loss

(2) Details of concepts of energy balance and its application to health and weight loss

(3) Clear description of postoperative eating patterns and anticipated lifestyle changes

(4) Importance of increasing activity to facilitate weight loss

(5) Importance of careful follow-up and routine serum analysis for the prevention of nutritional deficiencies

3. Perioperative risk assessment

a. Medical history

(1) Current medication schedule

(a) Prescription medications and schedule

(b) Over-the-counter medication schedule

(c) Schedule of herbal supplements and non-Western weight loss treatments

b. Meticulous physical examination

(1) Pulmonary examination and screening

(a) Pulmonary abnormalities associated with obesity

(i) Reduction in lung and chest wall compliance

(ii) Increase in respiratory system resistance

(iii) Reduction in lung volumes

(iv) Increased effort required for the work of breathing

(b) Pulmonary function testing should be obtained for:

(i) Morbidly obese patients

(ii) Patients with self-reported respiratory illness or shortness of breath

(iii) All patients with a history of OSA

(c) Baseline arterial blood gas analysis while breathing room air

(i) Screen for perioperative hypercarbia.

(d) Planned cessation of smoking 8 weeks before surgery

(e) Detailed assessment on patients reporting OSA

(i) Careful screening and sleep studies for patients reporting:

[a] Heavy snoring

[b] Apneic episodes witnessed by bed partner

[c] Daytime somnolence

[d] Lack of restful sleep

(ii) Patients with suspected OSA need careful preoperative identification and stabilization.

(f) Thorough assessment of patient's airway to rule in or out a difficult intubation

(i) Airway assessment using the Mallampati classification

(ii) Assessment completed by the anesthesia care provider

(iii) Assessment of mandibular opening and relative size of tongue and oral cavity opening

(g) Concerns/abnormalities discovered in the preoperative pulmonary exam must be communicated to the anesthesia team.

(2) Cardiovascular examination and screening

(a) Cardiovascular abnormalities associated with obesity

(i) Cardiac hypertrophy

[a] Left-sided secondary to hypertension

[b] Right-sided secondary to pulmonary hypertension

(ii) Increased preload

(iii) Diastolic dysfunction

(iv) Rarely systolic dysfunction associated with cardiomyopathy

(v) Cardiac dysrhythmias

(vi) Ischemic heart disease

(b) Meticulous screening of cardiovascular status including exercise tolerance

(c) Baseline electrocardiogram

(i) Identified abnormalities referred for cardiologist surgical clearance

(ii) Interventional cardiac procedures as indicated

(d) Skin and peripheral vascular assessment

(3) Endocrine examination and screening

(a) Type 2 diabetes

(i) At risk for infection and poor wound healing

(ii) Blood glucose increases substantially with physiological stress response.

(iii) Current medication schedule

(iv) Baseline blood glucose

(b) Rule out thyroid disease as detailed by history.

(i) Thyroid function testing baseline as indicated by history

(c) Rule out adrenal disease as detailed by history.

(i) Symptoms that may indicate Cushing's syndrome

[a] Hypertension

[b] Diabetes

[c] Central obesity

[d] Weakness

[e] Muscle atrophy

[f] Hirsutism

[g] Striae

[h] Osteoporosis

[i] Acne

D. Bariatric surgical complications (Table 48-4)

1. Overview

a. Obesity increases risk of complications since there is a decreased physiological reserve.

2. Obesity-related complications

a. Pulmonary derangements

(1) Physiological overview

(a) Respiratory complications the most frequent postoperative complication, occurring in 5% of all bariatric procedures

(b) Obesity

(i) Increases the work of breathing related to an increase in the elastic work and a decrease in the efficiency of the respiratory muscles

(ii) Obese patients:

[a] Have higher metabolical demands

[b] Produce more carbon dioxide

[c] Require a higher amount of oxygen

■ TABLE 48-4
■ ■ **Historical Development of Bariatric Surgery**

Decade	Procedure	Classification	Comments
1950s	Jejunoileal (JI) bypass	Combined	Significant weight loss associated with electrolyte imbalance, diarrhea, liver failure
1960s	JI bypass; less radical	Combined	Series of procedures; continued side effects
1960s	Gastric bypass	Restrictive	Stomach divided horizontally; pouch 150 mL
1960s	Biliopancreatic diversion	Malabsorptive	Distal horizontal gastrectomy; Roux-en-Y limb of small intestine
1970s	Roux-en-Y gastric bypass (RYGB)	Combined	Stomach divided vertically; good results; short and long versions of small intestine
1970s	Gastroplasty	Restrictive	Partial gastric transection (vertical)
1980s	Vertical band gastroplasty	Restrictive	Partial gastric transection (horizontal); Silastic ring used to close lower end
1980s	Gastric banding	Restrictive	Small pouch created by band around upper stomach; no staples so reversible; in 1986 a port added to allow manipulation of ring
1990s	Laparoscopic procedures: RYGB and banding	Combined	Shorter surgery; smaller incisional lines; reduced rates of complications; surgeon experience very important
1990s	Implantable gastric stimulator	Nonbariatric surgery	Safe; less invasive; improving efficacy

     (iii) Obesity decreases the functional reserve capacity, and when obese patients are placed supine, this is greatly increased.

     (iv) Chest wall of obese patients less compliant because of fat deposition in the chest wall

  (2) Potential postoperative pulmonary complications

    (a) OSA

    (b) OHS

    (c) Atelectasis

    (d) Pneumonia

      (i) Patients who weighed >250 lb were found in one study to be at an almost 40% greater risk for developing pneumonia.

  b. Thromboembolic derangements

  c. Fluid and electrolyte derangements

3. Surgical complications

  a. Early surgical complications

    (1) Anastomotic leaking

      (a) Caused by:

        (i) Failure of anastomotic staple or suture line

        (ii) Leakage of digestive juices

      (b) Screened during procedure with injection of diluted methylene blue and observation

      (c) Postoperative symptoms

        (i) Unexplained tachycardia (>120 beats/min)

        (ii) Abdominal pain not responsive to analgesia

        (iii) Fever as a late sign

      (d) Dependent on severity of the leak, operative exploration and correction of defect

(2) GERD
   (a) Conflicting reports with gastric banding; may indicate need of band evaluation for malplacement and readjustment
   (b) No effect in GERD seen with vertical gastric banding
   (c) Reduction in GERD seen with Roux-en-Y surgery
b. Late surgical complications
   (1) Anastomotic stricture/stenosis
      (a) Relatively common occurrence with:
         (i) RYGBP
         (ii) Vertical gastric banding (VGB)
      (b) Typically seen in first 6 months after surgery
      (c) Symptoms include:
         (i)   Postprandial epigastric pain
         (ii) Vomiting
         (iii) Dysphagia
      (d) Diagnosis with upper endoscopy
      (e) Treatment with endoscopic dilation; rare need of surgical revision
   (2) Anastomotic ulceration
      (a) Most often develops at gastrojejunal anastomosis site
      (b) Present in up to 16% of RYGBP procedures
      (c) Contributing factors
         (i)   Gastric acidity
         (ii) Nonsteroidal anti-inflammatory use
         (iii) *Helicobacter pylori* infection
         (iv) Local ischemia or tension at anastomosis site
      (d) Symptoms consistent with peptic ulcer
      (e) Diagnosis with upper endoscopy
      (f) Treatment is empirical based on cause of ulcer.
   (3) Anastomotic rupture or dehiscence
      (a) Potential complication of RYGBP and VGB procedures
      (b) May be asymptomatic or present similar to ulceration
      (c) Diagnosis with upper endoscopy
      (d) Treatment most often with surgical revision; however, may be successfully treated with endoscopic manipulation
   (4) Band erosion
      (a) Present in 1% to 2% of patients having VGB procedures
      (b) Symptoms include pain or weight gain from reduction of gastric restriction.
      (c) Diagnosis with upper endoscopy
      (d) Treatment includes removal of band and bariatric operation.
   (5) Bowel or Roux limb obstruction
      (a) Small bowel obstruction
         (i)   Incidence of 3% with a laparoscopic RYGBP
         (ii) Incidence of 2% in open procedures
         (iii) May follow the development of an internal hernia
      (b) Symptoms may include:
         (i)   Abdominal pain
         (ii) Nausea/vomiting
         (iii) Fever
      (c) Surgical evaluation necessary if correction is warranted
   (6) Hernia
      (a) Several gaps created by RYGBP (incidence, 18%-20%) and VGB procedures, necessitating gap closure for both open and laparoscopic procedures
      (b) Incidence of hernia also increased with rapid weight loss
      (c) Symptoms may include a palpable mass or abdominal pain but would increase in severity with incarceration.
      (d) Surgical evaluation necessary if correction is warranted

(7) Cholelithiasis
  (a) Related to rapid weight loss
  (b) Seen in up to 32% of patients after Roux-en-Y procedures; 40% of those patients symptomatic
  (c) May be prevented by incidental cholecystectomy at time of bariatric surgery
  (d) Symptoms consistent with nonbariatric cholelithiasis
  (e) Diagnosis with abdominal ultrasonography
  (f) Treatment
    (i) Elective cholecystectomy easier after weight loss
(8) Dumping syndrome
  (a) Caused by the rapid transit of high-caloric, high-osmolar (concentrated) foods into the small intestine
  (b) Portal fluid into the lumen of the GI tract, decreasing preload
  (c) Symptoms
    (i) Nausea/vomiting
    (ii) Diaphoresis
    (iii) Palpitations/tachycardia
    (iv) Abdominal cramping
    (v) Dizziness
    (vi) Syncope
  (d) Negatively reinforces the restriction of highly concentrated sweets or alcoholic beverages and milk from the diet
4. Nutritional deficiency
  a. Iron deficiency
    (1) Common after RYGBP or biliopancreatic diversion (20%-49% of patients)
    (2) Premenopausal patients at higher risk because of menstrual losses
    (3) Mechanism for deficiency:
      (a) Decreased iron intake due to intolerance of red meat
      (b) Primary site of iron absorption is the duodenum, which is bypassed in RYGBP.
    (4) Patients need to receive iron replacement.
    (5) Concurrent supplementation with vitamin C improves iron absorption.
  b. Vitamin B_{12} deficiency
    (1) Common in RYGBP (25%-75% of patients)
    (2) Mechanism for deficiency
      (a) Decreased B_{12} intake due to intolerance of meat and milk
      (b) Loss of intrinsic factor secretion by the parietal cells (fundus of the stomach)
    (3) Leads to the development of pernicious anemia
    (4) Replacement necessary with intramuscular B_{12} injections or oral crystalline B_{12}
  c. Folate deficiency
    (1) Common in RYGBP
    (2) Mechanism for deficiency
      (a) Decreased folate intake
      (b) B_{12} action as a coenzyme for folate metabolism
    (3) Replacement necessary with daily folate
  d. Thiamine deficiency
    (1) Mechanism for deficiency
      (a) Decreased thiamine intake or protracted vomiting
      (b) Malabsorption from surgical bypass of the duodenum
    (2) Prevention, early recognition and immediate treatment necessary to prevent Wernicke's encephalopathy
    (3) Replacement necessary with daily thiamine
  e. Vitamin D and calcium deficiency

(1) Fat-soluble vitamin D deficiency common in malabsorptive or combined procedures

(2) Calcium deficiency common from malabsorption secondary to bypass of duodenum

(3) Vitamin D and calcium necessary for prevention of metabolic bone disease

(4) Replacement necessary with daily 1200 to 1500 mg calcium citrate with vitamin D

f. Protein deficiency

(1) Protein deficiency common in bariatric procedures where the duodenum (site of primary absorption of protein) is bypassed

(2) Although poorly understood, protein deficiency also thought to be related to the physiological response to the starvation associated with bariatric surgery

(3) Average time for the appearance of protein deficiency is 18 months after bariatric surgery; however, may be present 3 months after surgery

(4) Protein malnutrition should be associated with any patient with pitting edema or a low serum albumin level.

(5) Severe protein wasting will affect coagulation (plasma protein based) and immune function.

(6) Nitrogen replacement is paramount with:

(a) Oral supplementation if tolerated

(b) Use of enteral feedings

5. Body contouring after massive weight loss

a. Skin of obese individuals not able to retract after large weight losses

b. Body contouring

(1) May be medically necessary

(a) Abdominal and thigh skin folds are subject to:

(i) Rashes

(ii) Fungal infections

(iii) Irritation

(iv) Ulceration

(v) Resistance to topical medical therapy

(2) Excess skin surgically removed by several staged, plastic procedures

V. NURSING PROCESS

A. Receive report from anesthesia care provider

1. Preoperative data

a. Past medical history including medication history

b. Allergies

c. Preoperative diagnostic data

2. Intraoperative data

a. Surgical procedure performed; intraoperative surgical complications

b. Anesthetic

(1) Type(s) of anesthetic used for surgery

(2) Agents and dosages administered; patient response

(3) Vital signs throughout procedure

(4) Anesthetic complications or difficulties

c. Airway status

(1) Intubation history

(a) Paralytic agent used

(b) Presence of difficult airway

(c) Number of intubation attempts

(d) Assistive equipment if used

(2) Extubation history

(a) Reversal agents timing

(b) Neuromuscular response at time of reversal

(i) Peripheral nerve stimulator

(ii) Train of four: number of twitches present at reversal

      (c) Patient response before extubation
         (i)   Presence of adventitious sounds, if any
         (ii) Strength and ability to follow commands
         (iii) Additional medications given (i.e., bronchodilators, narcotics)
    (3) Presence of any artificial airway devices
  d. Fluid balance
    (1) Fluid intake
      (a) Crystalloids: type and amount
      (b) Colloids: type and amount
      (c) Irrigations if used: type and amount
    (2) Fluid output
      (a) Estimated blood loss
      (b) Urine output
      (c) Additional losses
  e. Blood glucose response
    (1) Perioperative blood glucose
    (2) Intraoperative blood glucose
    (3) Any blood glucose regulation during anesthetic
  f. Additional medications administered
    (1) Antibiotics
    (2) Narcotics
    (3) Antiemetics
    (4) Local anesthetic infiltration
B. Admission assessment
  1. Complete a head-to-toe admission assessment.
    a. Neurological assessment
      (1) Assess level of consciousness and orientation status.
      (2) Assess extremity movement and strength in response to verbal command.
      (3) Assess patient's pain level using the pain scale included in patient's preoperative educational plan.
    b. Pulmonary assessment
      (1) Apply supplemental oxygen as ordered or per protocol.
      (2) Evaluate the effectiveness of gas exchange.
        (a) Observe ventilatory rate, depth, and pattern.
      (3) Elevate head of bed as soon as stable blood pressure obtained.
        (a) Uses gravity to remove redundant abdominal fat from the chest
        (b) Eases pressure on diaphragm to decrease the work of breathing
        (c) Increases tidal volume and reduces tendency toward atelectasis and intrapulmonary shunting
      (4) Apply CPAP as ordered in patients with preoperative history of OSA.
      (5) Monitor continuous pulse oximetry.
      (6) Encourage deep breathing and coughing exercises included in patient's preoperative educational plan.
    c. Cardiovascular assessment
      (1) Initiate frequent vital sign and continuous cardiac monitoring.
      (2) Obtain 12-lead electrocardiogram as ordered. Report results to anesthesia care provider.
      (3) Assess skin and nail bed color and timing of capillary refill.
      (4) Assess extremity circulation.
        (a) Presence of peripheral pulses
        (b) Presence and location of edema
        (c) Application of compression boots/compressive stockings as ordered
    d. Gastrointestinal assessment
      (1) Assess surgical dressings.
        (a) Location and number of dressings
        (b) Presence of drainage

          (i)   Note location, character, and color.

          (ii) Reinforce dressing as ordered.

          (iii) Report excessive drainage to surgical team and anesthesia care provider as indicated.

    (2) Assess drainage tubes.

       (a) Location, type, and number of drainage tubes

       (b) Presence of drainage

          (i)   Note location, character, and color.

          (ii) Report excessive drainage to surgical team and anesthesia care provider as indicated.

    (3) Assess for presence of postoperative nausea/vomiting.

       (a) Report occurrence of nausea/vomiting to anesthesia care provider.

       (b) Obtain orders for pharmacological management of nausea/vomiting.

       (c) Administer ordered pharmacological interventions.

       (d) Assess and record patient response to pharmacological agent.

       (e) Continue communication with anesthesia care provider as needed.

e. Pain assessment

    (1) Assess patient's pain level at admission using the pain scale discussed in patient's preoperative educational classes.

       (a) Note characteristics of the pain.

          (i)   Location, character, quality, aggravating and alleviating factors

          (ii) Visually inspect pain loci for swelling, drainage, discoloration, or redness as a cause of the pain.

       (b) Report occurrence of pain to anesthesia care provider.

       (c) Obtain orders for pharmacological management of pain.

       (d) Administer ordered pharmacological interventions.

       (e) Assess and record patient's response to pharmacological agent.

       (f) Continue communication with anesthesia care provider as needed.

       (g) Begin patient-controlled analgesia (PCA) as soon as patient's condition warrants its use.

          (i)   Describe the use/purpose of PCA to patient.

          (ii) Monitor patient's use of PCA and success of pain management.

          (iii) Document and communicate the effectiveness of PCA use to surgeon.

f. Fluid balance assessment

    (1) Reassess perioperative fluid management.

    (2) Measure the volume of urinary output on admission and as per protocol.

       (a) Report any abnormal findings to the anesthesia care provider.

       (b) Initiate physician orders as received.

    (3) Obtain ordered postoperative lab work.

       (a) Communicate results to ordering physician and anesthesia care provider.

       (b) Initiate physician orders as received.

g. Skin assessment

    (1) Assess skin integrity, especially at pressure points.

       (a) Ensure arms not resting on side rails because that may place pressure on the median nerve and lead to potential peripheral nerve injury

          (i)   Place patient in size-appropriate bed as available.

          (ii) Pad side rails and reposition arms frequently to prevent the development of pressure.

    (2) Assess bilateral lower extremities for circulatory compromise.

       (a) Pad and reposition as indicated.

h. Musculoskeletal assessment

    (1) Assess for musculoskeletal pain.

       (a) Position of comfort (as long as adequate gas exchange is maintained) for lower back pain

(b) Patients in supine position; may place pillow under knees to remove lower back pressure
  (2) Assess for extremity strength.
    (a) Encourage foot and leg movement as per preoperative teaching.
  i. Thermal balance assessment
    (1) Admission temperature measurement as per protocol
      (a) Apply warming blankets as indicated.
      (b) Report occurrence of postanesthetic shivering to anesthesia care provider.
      (c) Obtain orders for pharmacologic management of postanesthetic shivering.
      (d) Administer ordered pharmacologic interventions.
      (e) Assess and record patient response to pharmacologic agent.
      (f) Continue communication with anesthesia care provider as needed.
  j. Psychosocial assessment
    (1) Complete an assessment of patient's anxiety and emotional well-being.
    (2) Reassure patient as appropriate.
      (a) Place patient in calm, quiet environment.
      (b) Provide patient reassurance of nurse's presence and touch.
      (c) Question source of anxiety and use factual statements to relieve anxiety.
    (3) Reorient patient as to completion of procedure and current location.
    (4) Initiate visitation of family or significant other as per protocol.
  k. Additional data collection
    (1) Obtain postoperative blood glucose reading.
    (2) Report results to anesthesia care provider.
    (3) Obtain orders for pharmacologic management of blood glucose as indicated.
    (4) Administer ordered pharmacologic interventions.
    (5) Assess and record patient response to pharmacologic agent.
    (6) Continue communication with anesthesia care provider as needed.
2. Admission auscultation
  a. Pulmonary auscultation
    (1) Auscultate patient's regular breathing for adventitious sounds.
      (a) Wheezing indicative of:
        (i) Increased airway resistance
        (ii) Bronchospasm
      (b) Snoring may indicate a partial obstruction of the upper airway from redundant tissue of the neck or mouth.
        (i) Remove pillow and reposition head using chin lift maneuver to clear snoring.
        (ii) If snoring is from retained secretions, ask patient to cough and clear airway.
        (iii) Suction secretions as needed for patients with ineffective airway clearance.
        (iv) Insert artificial airway as indicated.
        (v) Report any abnormality to anesthesia care provider.
      (c) Stridor or crowing may indicate a partial laryngospasm from mechanical manipulation of the larynx with intubation.
        (i) Notify anesthesia care provider immediately.
        (ii) Stridor can be broken by using positive pressure ventilation with 100% oxygen and an Ambu bag.
        (iii) Nebulized racemic epinephrine or the administration of corticosteroids may also be used to reduce swelling of the vocal cords.
        (iv) Have intubation equipment available.
    (2) Auscultate all lung fields bilaterally, asking patient to take deep, slow breaths.

(a) As above, listen for adventitious breath sounds.

(b) Ask patient to take additional deep breaths and cough to clear abnormal sounds.

(c) Record and report any abnormality to anesthesia care provider.

b. Auscultate gastrointestinal function.

(1) Auscultate gently, all four abdominal quadrants.

(a) Absence of bowel sounds a normal finding, especially in open surgical procedures

(b) Presence of hypoactive bowel sounds also a normal finding in laparoscopic procedures

(c) Presence of subcutaneous emphysema common after laparoscopic surgery and placement of pneumoperitoneum

3. Develop perianesthesia plan of care.

a. Interact with anesthesia care provider.

(1) Report elicited physiological abnormalities.

(2) Receive medical orders for interventions as indicated by patient status.

b. Perform ongoing assessment for current status and response to interventions.

c. Evaluate and revise plan of care based on patient response as needed.

d. Upon anesthesia care provider order, follow established nursing protocol and medical orders for patient transfer of care to admitting unit.

(1) Patient care hand-off as per hospital policy via written or oral report

(2) Assemble needed equipment and personnel for safe transfer of care.

4. Evaluation of outcomes

a. Ongoing evaluation of patient response to treatment plan conducted throughout length of stay

(1) Physiological indicators

(a) Adequate gas exchange

(b) Stable vital signs (including oxygen saturation)

(c) Absence of cardiac dysrhythmias

(d) Adequate fluid administration to maintain perfusion and sufficient urinary output

(e) Blood glucose within normal range

(f) Abdominal dressings clean, dry, and intact; minimal drainage from tubes

(g) Absence of nausea/vomiting

(h) Control of surgical pain

(i) Intact distal nervous function

(j) Prophylactic measures implemented for prevention of thromboembolism

(2) Cognitive indicators

(a) Follows instructions correctly

(b) Institutes postoperative behaviors per preoperative teaching plan

(i) PCA

(ii) Deep breathe and cough

(iii) Foot movement

(iv) Foley

(c) Appropriate use of pain scale for adequate pain relief

(3) Affective indicators

(a) Verbalizes individual needs

(b) Verbalizes and demonstrates compliance with treatment plan

(4) Supportive resources

(a) Family members involved in patient plan of care

(b) Identification of appropriate support groups and community resources

(5) Patient satisfaction

BIBLIOGRAPHY

1. Ali MR, Maguire MB, Wolfe BM: Assessment of obesity-related comorbidities: A novel scheme for evaluating bariatric surgical patients. *J Am Coll Surg* 202(1):70–77, 2006.

2. AORN bariatric surgery guideline, *AORN J* 79(5):1026–1052, 2004.

3. Apovian CM, Lenders CM, eds: *A clinical guide for management of overweight and obese children and adults*, Boca Raton, FL, 2007, CRC Press.

4. Bagchi D, Preuss HG, eds: *Obesity: Epidemiology, pathophysiology and prevention*, Boca Raton, FL, 2007, CRC Press.

5. Barrow C: Roux-en-Y gastric bypass for morbid obesity. *AORN J* 76(4):590–604, 2002.

6. Blouw EL, Rudolph AD, Narr BJ, et al: The frequency of respiratory failure in patients with morbid obesity undergoing gastric bypass. *AANA J* 71(1):45–50, 2003.

7. Buchwald H: Consensus conference statement for bariatric surgery for morbid obesity: Health implications for patients, health professionals, and third-party payers. *J Am Coll Surg* 200:593–604, 2005.

8. Buchwald H, Avidor Y, Braunwald E, et al: Bariatric surgery: A systematic review and meta-analysis. *JAMA* 292(14):1724–1737, 2004.

9. Buchwald H, Cowan GS, Pories WJ: *Surgical management of obesity*, Philadelphia, 2007, Saunders.

10. Buchwald H, Williams SE: Bariatric surgery worldwide. *Obes Surg* 14:1157–1164, 2004.

11. Chaloub V, Yazigi A, Sleilaty G, et al: Effect of vital capacity manoeuvres on arterial oxygenation in morbidly obese patients undergoing open bariatric surgery. *Eur J Anaesthesiol* 24:283–288, 2006.

12. Daniels J: Obesity: America's epidemic: What goes up does not always come down. Is there a solution? *Am J Nurs* 106(1):40–49, 2006.

13. Decker GA, Swain JM, Crowell MD, et al: Gastrointestinal and nutritional complications after bariatric surgery. *Am J Gastroenterol* 102:2571–2580, 2007.

14. DeMaria EJ, Latifi R, Sugerman HJ, eds: *Laparoscopic bariatric surgery: Techniques and outcomes*, Georgetown, TX, 2002, Landes Bioscience Vademecum.

15. Ellison SR, Ellison SD: Bariatric surgery: A review of the available surgical procedures and complications for the emergency physician. *J Emerg Med* 34(1):21–32, 2008.

16. Ezri T, Muzikant G, Medalion B, et al: Anesthesia for restrictive bariatric surgery (gastric bypass not included): Laparoscopic vs open procedures. *Int J Obes* 28:1157–1162, 2004.

17. Fatima J, Houghton SG, Iqbal CW, et al: Bariatric surgery at the extremes of age. *J Gastrointest Surg* 10(10):1392–1396, 2006.

18. Goldberg S, Rivers P, Smith K, Homan W: Vertical banded gastroplasty: A treatment for morbid obesity. *AORN J* 72(6):987–1010, 2000.

19. Gould JC, Garren MJ, Gutowski KA: Bariatric surgery. *Clin Obstet Gynecol* 49(2):375–388, 2006.

20. Haines KL, Nelson LG, Gonzalez R, et al: Objective evidence that bariatric surgery improves obesity-related obstructive sleep apnea. *Surgery* 141(3):354–358, 2007.

21. Han SH, Gracia C, Mehran A, et al: Improved outcomes using a systematic and evidence-based approach to laparoscopic Roux-en-Y gastric bypass in a single academic institution. *Am Surg* 73(10):955–958, 2007.

22. Hooper MM, Hallowell PT, Seitz BA, et al: Musculoskeletal findings in obese subjects before and after weight loss following bariatric surgery. *Int J Obes* 31:114–120, 2007.

23. Hydock CM: A brief overview of bariatric surgical procedures currently being used to treat the obese patient. *Crit Care Nurs Q* 28(3):217–226, 2005.

24. Jazet IM, Groot GH, Tuijnebreyer WE, et al: Cardiovascular risk factors after bariatric surgery: Do patients gain more than expected from their substantial weight loss? *Eur J Intern Med* 18:39–43, 2007.

25. Livingston EH: Obesity and its surgical management. *Am J Surg* 184:103–113, 2002.

26. Livingston EH, Arterburn D, Schifftner TL, et al: National Surgical Quality Improvement Program analysis of bariatric operations: Modifiable risk factors contribute to bariatric surgical adverse outcomes. *J Am Coll Surg* 203(5):625–633, 2006.

27. Livingston EH, Langert J: The impact of age and Medicare status on bariatric surgery outcomes. *Arch Surg* 141:1115–1120, 2006.

28. Madan AK, Dickson PV, Ternovits CA, et al: Results of teenaged bariatric patients performed in an adult program. *J Laparoendosc Adv Surg Tech* 17(4):473–477, 2007.

29. Marley RA, Hoyle B, Ries C: Perianesthesia respiratory care of the bariatric patient. *J Perianesth Nurs* 20(6):404–431, 2005.

30. McCance KL, Huether SE: *Pathophysiology: The biologic basis for disease in adults and children*, ed 6, St Louis, 2010, Mosby.

31. McCullough PA, Gallagher MJ, deJong AT, et al: Cardiovascular fitness and short-term complications after bariatric surgery. *Chest* 130(2):517–525, 2006.

32. McGlinch BP, Que FG, Nelson JL, et al: Perioperative care of patients undergoing bariatric surgery. *Mayo Clin Proc* 81(10):S25–S33, 2006.

33. McNatt SS, Longhi JJ, Goldman CD, et al: Surgery for obesity: A review of the current state of the art and future directions. *J Gastrointest Surg* 11:382–402, 2007.

34. Moos DD, Cuddelford JD: Implications of obstructive sleep apnea syndrome for the perianesthesia nurse. *J Perianesth Nurs* 21(2):103–118, 2006.

35. Murray D: Morbid obesity-psychosocial aspects and surgical interventions. *AORN J* 78(6):990–995, 2003.

36. Nguyen NT, Ho HS, Palmer LS, et al: A comparison study of laparoscopic versus open gastric bypass for morbid obesity. *J Am Coll Surg* 191(2):149–155, 2000.

37. Pinkney J, Kerrigan D: Current status of bariatric surgery in the treatment of type 2 diabetes. *Obes Rev* 5:69–78, 2004.

38. Porth CM: *Pathophysiology: Concepts of altered health states*, ed 8, Philadelphia, 2009, Lippincott Williams & Wilkins.

39. Rea JD, Yarbrough DE, Leeth RR, et al: Influence of complications and extent of weight loss on quality of life after laparoscopic Roux-en-Y gastric bypass. *Surg Endosc* 21:1095–1100, 2007.

40. Steinbrook R: Surgery for severe obesity. *N Engl J Med* 350(11):1075–1079, 2004.

41. Venable HD, Schlink CL: Anesthesia for bariatric surgery. *Plast Surg Nurs* 24(3):99–101, 2004.

42. Voelker M: Assessing quality of life in gastric bypass clients. *J Perianesth Nurs* 19(2):89–104, 2004.

43. Voelker M, Foster TG: Nursing challenges in the administration of oral antidepressant medications in gastric bypass patients. *J Perianesth Nurs* 22(2):108–124, 2007.

44. Woodard CB: Pregnancy following bariatric surgery. *J Perinat Neonatal Nurs* 18(4):329–340, 2004.

49 Special Procedures

THERESA L. CLIFFORD

OBJECTIVES

At the conclusion of this chapter, the reader will be able to:

1. List common ambulatory nonsurgical diagnostic or interventional procedures.

2. Describe assessment parameters pertinent to the patient undergoing special procedures.

3. Identify nursing interventions appropriate to the care of the patient undergoing select nonsurgical diagnostic or interventional procedures.

4. Describe six types of reactions that can occur as a result of a blood transfusion.

5. Identify three potential complications for the patient undergoing electroconvulsive therapy (ECT).

I. OVERVIEW
   A. Definition
      1. Variety of procedures performed throughout facility may be termed "special procedures."
         a. Endoscopic procedures
         b. Diagnostic procedures
         c. Interventional procedures
         d. Electroconvulsive therapy
         e. Infusion therapies
      2. May be performed in:
         a. Endoscopy
         b. Radiology
         c. Vascular or catheterization lab
         d. Operating room/minor surgery suite
         e. Nursing unit
         f. Post anesthesia care unit (PACU)
         g. Ambulatory care unit
   B. Responsibilities of perianesthesia staff
      1. May or may not include:
         a. Preprocedure preparation of patient
         b. Intraprocedure assessment and monitoring
         c. Postprocedure recovery and discharge
      2. Varies according to facility protocols
      3. Varies according to patient workflow processes
II. ANATOMY AND PHYSIOLOGY
   A. Gastrointestinal (GI) procedures (see Chapter 35)
      1. Anatomy of GI tract
         a. Mouth (oral or buccal cavity)
            (1) Teeth, tongue, hard and soft palates, cheeks, lips, pharynx
            (2) Salivary glands
               (a) Parotid
               (b) Sublingual
               (c) Submandibular
         b. Esophagus
            (1) Hollow muscular tube

    (2) Approximately 23 to 25 cm (10 inches) long
    (3) Approximately 2 to 3 cm (1 inch) in diameter
    (4) Extends from pharynx to stomach
        (a) Passes through diaphragm into the abdomen opening called diaphragmatic hiatus
    (5) Positioned posterior to trachea and anterior to vertebral column
    (6) Wall made up of three layers
        (a) Mucosa
        (b) Submucosa
        (c) Muscularis
    (7) Sphincters
        (a) Upper pharyngoesophageal
        (b) Lower esophagogastric (cardiac)
    (8) Disorders
        (a) Gastroesophageal reflux disease
        (b) Esophageal varices
        (c) Tumors
        (d) Diverticula
        (e) Motility disorders
        (f) Foreign bodies
        (g) Strictures, rings, and webs
        (h) Infectious disease
  c. Stomach
    (1) J-shaped distensible organ
    (2) Located in left upper quadrant of abdomen (just below diaphragm, between esophagus and duodenum)
    (3) Approximately 25 to 30 cm (10-12 inches) long
    (4) Approximately 10 to 15 cm (4-6 inches) wide at widest point
    (5) Function
        (a) Digests food and prepares nutrients for absorption
        (b) Serves as reservoir for swallowed food, drink, and digested secretions
        (c) Mixes and delivers chyme to the small intestine for further digestion and absorption
        (d) Originates signals for hunger and satiety
    (6) Consists of:
        (a) Fundus
        (b) Body
        (c) Pylorus (antrum)
        (d) Cardiac region
    (7) Sphincters
        (a) Esophagogastric (cardiac)
            (i) Prevents backward reflux of stomach contents
        (b) Pyloric
            (i) Works with duodenum to create pressure gradient, which allows emptying of stomach
    (8) Disorders
        (a) Acid-peptic disorders
        (b) *Helicobacter pylori*
        (c) Polyps
        (d) Gastritis
        (e) Gastric cancer
        (f) Gastric varices
        (g) Hiatal hernia
        (h) Gastric outlet obstruction
        (i) Stress ulcers
        (j) Motor dysfunction—swallowing disorders
        (k) Bezoars (concretions of foreign material found in stomach)

d. Small intestine
    (1) Tube-shaped structure
    (2) Approximately 18 feet long, 1 inch in diameter
    (3) Three sections
        (a) Duodenum
            (i)   C shaped
            (ii) First section
            (iii) Begins at pyloric sphincter
            (iv) Ends at ligament of Treitz
        (b) Jejunum
            (i)   Middle section (proximal two fifths)
        (c) Ileum
            (i)   Last section
            (ii) Distal three fifths of small bowel
    (4) Properties
        (a) Circular folds increase absorptive surfaces of small intestine.
    (5) Disorders
        (a) Duodenal ulcer
        (b) Bacterial and viral infections
        (c) Parasitic disease
        (d) Crohn's disease
        (e) Meckel's diverticulum
        (f) Malabsorption syndromes
        (g) Celiac spruce (poor food absorption and gluten intolerance)
        (h) Tropical sprue (chronic disorder acquired in endemic tropical areas)
        (i) Whipple disease
            (i)   Rare disorder characterized by chronic diarrhea and progressive wasting
        (j) Short bowel syndrome
        (k) Lactase deficiency
        (l) Small bowel tumors
        (m) Motility disorders
e. Large intestine
    (1) Tube-shaped structure
        (a) Approximately 4 to 6 cm (2 inches) in diameter
        (b) Approximately 90 to 150 cm (4-5 feet) long
        (c) Extends from ileocecal value to the anus
    (2) Consists of:
        (a) Cecum
            (i)   Positioned at junction of ileum and colon
            (ii) Contains ileocecal valve and appendix
        (b) Ascending colon
            (i)   Portion from cecum to hepatic flexure
        (c) Transverse colon
            (i)   Segment from hepatic flexure to splenic flexure
            (ii) Transverses abdominal cavity
        (d) Descending colon
            (i)   Segment from splenic flexure to iliac crest
            (ii) Located on left side of abdomen
        (e) Sigmoid colon
            (i)   S-shaped segment
            (ii) Ends at rectum
        (f) Rectum
            (i)   Last portion of large intestine
            (ii) Approximately 5 inches long
            (iii) Segment after sigmoid colon
            (iv) Connects to anal canal

        (3) Disorders
          (a) Polyps
          (b) Angiodysplasia (vascular dilations in the submucosa)
          (c) Colitis
          (d) Necrotizing enterocolitis
          (e) Ulcerative colitis
          (f) Pseudomembranous colitis
          (g) Crohn's colitis
          (h) Irritable bowel syndrome
          (i) Diverticular disease
          (j) Diverticulosis
          (k) Colorectal cancer
          (l) Hemorrhoids
          (m) Anorectal disorders
          (n) Encopresis (chronic constipation that results in involuntary leaking of feces)
          (o) Anal fissure
          (p) Rectal prolapse
          (q) Anorectal abscess
          (r) Anorectal fistula
          (s) Anorectal fissure

2. Nerve supply—occurs two ways

  a. Neural transmission to smooth muscle

    (1) Stimulates movement of food through GI tract

    (2) Occurs as a result of distention of myenteric plexus or submucosal plexus

  b. Autonomic nervous system

    (1) Sympathetic

      (a) Thoracic and lumbar splenic nerves

      (b) Inhibit secretions and movement

      (c) Cause contraction of sphincters

    (2) Parasympathetic

      (a) Vagus nerve: causes increase in motor activity

      (b) Causes increase in secretions

      (c) Causes sphincters to relax

      (d) Results in peristalsis

3. Function of GI system

  a. Ingestion

  b. Transport

  c. Digestion

  d. Absorption

  e. Elimination

B. Pulmonary procedures

  1. Pulmonary anatomy (see Chapter 31)

    a. Nose and sinuses

      (1) Upper airway cleans, humidifies, and warms air.

      (2) Sinuses lighten the skull, assist in speech, and produce mucus.

    b. Pharynx

      (1) Divided into three regions

        (a) Nasopharynx

          (i) Area where tonsils and adenoids (masses of lymphoid tissue in the back wall of nasopharynx) trap and destroy infectious agents

        (b) Oropharynx

          (i) Carries both air and food

          (ii) During swallowing, the soft palate rises to prevent food from entering the nasopharynx.

          (iii) The lining of the oropharynx protects it from damage by friction and from chemicals in food and fluids.

(c) Laryngopharynx
[i] Passageway for both food and air; connects oropharynx to larynx
  c. Larynx
    (1) Contains vocal cords to produce speech
    (2) Protected by cartilages to keep it open
  d. Lungs
    (1) Soft and spongy, composed of elastic connective tissue
    (2) Apex of each lung just below the clavicle
    (3) Base of each lung rests on the diaphragm.
    (4) Right lung has three lobes.
    (5) Left lung is smaller, with only two lobes.
  e. Bronchi and alveoli
    (1) Trachea divides into right and left mainstem bronchi.
    (2) Mainstem bronchi enter lungs at the hilus.
    (3) Bronchi branch into smaller bronchi.
    (4) Smaller bronchi branch into smaller bronchioles.
    (5) Bronchioles end in the tiny alveoli.
      (a) Where gas exchange occurs
      (b) Extremely thin walls, made of a single layer of cells over a very thin connective tissue (basement) membrane
      (c) Oxygen and carbon dioxide easily diffuse across the walls of the alveoli and capillaries.
      (d) Alveoli contain cells that secrete surfactant, a detergent-like substance that helps keep them open.
C. Vascular procedures
  1. Vascular anatomy (see Chapter 44)
    a. Peripheral vascular system
      (1) Network of blood vessels that carries blood to peripheral tissues and then returns it to the heart; network includes arteries, veins, and capillaries.
    b. Arteries
      (1) Arteries carry blood away from the heart.
      (2) Oxygenated blood leaves the left ventricle via the *aorta.*
      (3) Major arteries branch off the aorta and into successively smaller arteries. These eventually divide into arterioles.
      (4) Arterioles feed into beds of hairlike capillaries within the organs and tissues.
        (a) In capillary beds, oxygen and nutrients are exchanged for metabolic wastes, and deoxygenated blood begins its journey back to the heart through venules.
      (5) Venules join onto veins, which in turn join larger veins.
    c. Veins
      (1) Carry blood toward the heart
      (2) Peripheral veins empty into the superior and inferior vena cava, and then into the right atrium.
    d. Three layers of blood vessel walls
      (1) Tunica intima
        (a) Endothelium; has a slick surface to assist blood flow
      (2) Tunica media
        (a) Contains smooth muscle
        (b) Layer is thicker and more elastic in arteries than it is in veins.
        (c) Allows arteries to expand and contract, maintaining blood flow to the capillaries between heartbeats
      (3) Tunica adventitia
        (a) Outermost layer
        (b) Connective tissue that protects and anchors the vessel
III. GENERAL CARE
  A. Preprocedure education
    1. General
      a. Nothing-by-mouth (NPO) instructions as appropriate

     b. Hygiene

     c. Environment

     d. Facility protocols

     e. Aftercare arrangements

     f. Amnesic effects of sedation and analgesia

     g. Medication—discontinue or dose as usual

B. Perianesthesia priorities

  1. Preprocedure

     a. Objectives

       (1) Assess and prepare patient for procedure.

       (2) Obtain baseline data.

       (3) Allow for development and implementation of nursing care.

       (4) Initiate educational process.

         (a) Continues throughout continuum of care

     b. Nursing process

       (1) Assessment parameters

         (a) Physical assessment as noted previously

         (b) Assess for educational needs.

         (c) Assess for psychosocial needs related to developmental age including:

           (i) Availability of family member or responsible adult companion

           (ii) Community resources needed

     c. Plan of care

       (1) Include patient, family, responsible adult companion in developing plan of care appropriate to patient's age.

       (2) Nursing diagnosis might include:

         (a) Anxiety and fear related to:

           (i) Knowledge deficit

           (ii) Unfamiliar environment

           (iii) Separation from family

           (iv) Lack of control

         (b) Pain related to procedural intervention

         (c) Potential for injury

         (d) Potential for infection

     d. Interventions

       (1) Nursing interventions might include:

         (a) Ensure that all laboratory studies completed as ordered and indicated.

         (b) Provide information on preprocedure preparation.

           (i) NPO status

           (ii) Medications

           (iii) Hygiene

           (iv) Discharge arrangements

             [a] Ride

             [b] Aftercare

         (c) Obtain baseline vital signs.

         (d) Ensure legal authorization is appropriate (informed consent).

         (e) Provide orientation to surroundings.

  2. Evaluation

     a. Evaluation of interventions and patient response might include:

       (1) Laboratory results reviewed, and follow-up completed as indicated

       (2) Patient, family, responsible adult companion questioned to determine understanding of preoperative instructions

       (3) Determine that patient has arranged for aftercare as appropriate.

C. Nursing interventions

  1. General

     a. Monitor vital signs per protocol.

     b. Administer medications for pain and nausea as ordered.

          c. Observe for bleeding and other complications.

          d. Ensure a safe environment.

D. Postprocedure

  1. Objectives

     a. Ensure that patient safely recovers from immediate effects of procedure and anesthesia.

     b. Provide care in PACU, depending on facility policy.

     c. Transport directly to PACU phase II, depending on facility policy.

  2. Nursing process

     a. Assessment parameters

       (1) General

         (a) Routine PACU protocol

         (b) Airway status—patient is at high risk for airway compromise.

         (c) Vital signs monitored frequently during and after procedure

         (d) Effects of medications administered

         (e) Intravenous (IV) sedation and analgesia protocol

  3. Plan of care

     a. Include patient, family, responsible adult companion in developing a plan of care appropriate to patient's age.

     b. Nursing diagnoses might include those listed previously.

     c. Provide for patient safety.

     d. Be alert for potential complications.

  4. Nursing interventions

     a. Monitor vital signs per protocol.

     b. Administer medications as ordered.

     c. Observe for potential complications.

     d. Ensure a safe environment.

  5. Evaluation

     a. Respond to interventions continually throughout patient's stay.

     b. Alter plan of care.

E. Preparation for discharge

  1. Objective

     a. Ready the patient to return home.

     b. Prepare patient and caregiver to successfully manage postprocedure care.

     c. Educate patient and caregiver.

  2. Nursing process

     a. Assessment parameters

       (1) Airway and respiratory status

       (2) Vital signs

       (3) Level of consciousness

       (4) Postoperative nausea and vomiting

       (5) Bleeding

       (6) Reactions to local anesthetics

       (7) Discomfort

  3. Plan of care

     a. Include patient, family, responsible adult companion.

     b. Plan should be appropriate for patient's age.

     c. Nursing diagnoses might include:

       (1) Anxiety and fear related to:

         (a) Knowledge deficit

         (b) Unfamiliar environment

         (c) Separation from family

         (d) Lack of control

       (2) Alteration in comfort level

       (3) Ineffective breathing patterns related to sedation

       (4) Potential for infection

  4. Educational interventions

     a. Discussion, demonstration, written materials

      b. Copies of all materials given to patient should be maintained in medical record.

  F. Evaluation

    1. Evaluation of clinical interventions is ongoing until patient is stable and ready for discharge.

    2. Evaluation of learning

      a. Patient and caregiver verbalize understanding.

      b. Patient and caregiver able to demonstrate skill

        (1) Patient and responsible adult companion should sign that they have been instructed and had the opportunity to have questions answered.

IV. GI PROCEDURES

  A. Abdominal paracentesis

    1. Removal and drainage of ascitic fluid in the peritoneal cavity

    2. Diagnostic tool to examine ascitic fluid

    3. Palliative measure to relieve abdominal pressure that may be interfering with respiratory function

    4. Fluid withdrawn with a large-bore needle or a trocar and cannula inserted in the abdominal wall

    5. Before paracentesis, important to have patient void to reduce risk of accidental injury to the bladder

  B. Endoscopy—overview

    1. Direct visual examination of lumen of GI tract

    2. Usually performed with lighted flexible fiberoptic scope or videoscope

    3. Provides undistorted image of body cavity

    4. Illumination provided by external light source

    5. Scope designed to allow for passage of instruments

      a. Allows for:

        (1) Pictures to be taken

        (2) Biopsies to be obtained

        (3) Polyps to be removed

        (4) Foreign objects to be removed

        (5) Bleeding areas to be cauterized

  C. Anoscopy

    1. Anoscope: a clear plastic or metal speculum designed to examine the anus and lower rectum

  D. Anal manometry

    1. Used to assess:

      a. Anal and rectal muscles

      b. Sphincter problems

        (1) Can be associated with several disorders, especially fecal incontinence

      c. Chronic constipation

  E. Colonoscopy

    1. Direct visualization of lower GI tract from rectum to ileocecal valve using a long, flexible endoscope (length, 120-180 cm)

    2. Used to evaluate for:

      a. Malignancy

      b. Polyps

      c. Inflammatory bowel disease

      d. Diverticulitis

      e. Strictures

      f. Bleeding

  F. Endoscopic retrograde cholangiopancreatography (ERCP)

    1. Invasive exam using both endoscopic and radiological techniques to visualize pancreatic ducts, hepatic ducts, and common bile ducts

    2. Uses a flexible fiberoptic duodenoscope

    3. Contrast material injected

    4. May include removal of stones, sphincterotomies, or dilation

    G. Esophageal dilation
        1. Enlargement of lumen of esophagus
        2. Accomplished by forcing a series of increasingly larger dilators through a narrowed area (axial force)
        3. May use a balloon dilator to accomplish opening of a narrowed area (radial force)
    H. Esophagogastroduodenoscopy (EGD)
        1. Direct visualization of esophagus, stomach, and proximal duodenum
        2. Flexible fiberoptic endoscope (<10 mm in diameter) passed through mouth allows for direct vision with still and video photography.
        3. Used to assess, diagnose and/or treat:
            a. Esophageal or gastric lesions
            b. Hiatal hernia
            c. Esophageal varices
            d. Esophagitis
            e. Ulcer disease
            f. Polyps
            g. Strictures (achalasia)
            h. Bleeding
            i. Motility disorders
            j. Preoperative evaluations
    I. Liver biopsy
        1. Use of sterile technique to excise or needle punch a small sample of liver
            a. Tissue examined microscopically for cell morphology and tissue anomalies
            b. May also be done using ultrasound or computed tomographic guidance
        2. Performed to diagnose or confirm the cause of chronic liver disease and liver tumors
        3. After liver transplants performed to determine
            a. Cause of elevated liver function test values
            b. Whether rejection is occurring
    J. Paracentesis
        1. Sterile procedure using a needle inserted through the abdominal wall to obtain a sample of any fluid that is present
        2. Purpose: to obtain fluid for diagnostic purposes or to drain a larger volume of fluid to relieve pressure
    K. Percutaneous endoscopic gastrostomy (PEG)
        1. Placement of feeding tube via endoscopy for enteral nutrition
        2. Procedure
            a. Lighted endoscope inserted into stomach
            b. Light shines against abdominal wall.
                (1) Allows visualization of tube placement site
            c. Large-gauge needle and suture passed through abdominal wall and stomach wall
                (1) Snare or biopsy forceps used to bring inner end of suture up through patient's mouth (via endoscope)
            d. PEG tube tied to suture
                (1) Pulled through mouth into stomach
                (2) Pulled out abdominal wall
            e. Tube anchored using internal and external rubber bumpers or internal retention balloon and outer disk
        3. Advantages
            a. Less risk than surgical gastrostomy
            b. Procedure done under sedation rather than general anesthesia
            c. Faster recovery
            d. Feedings can begin within 24 hours.
            e. Can be performed in endoscopy suite or at bedside
            f. Less costly

L. Percutaneous endoscopic jejunostomy (PEJ)
   1. Tube passed into jejunum through opening in abdominal wall
   2. Approach can be surgical or percutaneous.
   3. Procedure
      a. Small tube passed through percutaneous endoscopic gastrostomy tube
      b. Guided via endoscope into duodenum
      c. Tube propelled by peristalsis into jejunum
      d. Placement confirmed by x-ray
         (1) Contrast medium injected
   4. Considerations
      a. Small diameter of tube predisposes it to clogging.
      b. Tube can migrate back to stomach as a result of vomiting.
      c. Feedings are continuous because jejunum is not a normal reservoir for nutrients.
M. Polypectomy
   1. Removal of a protruding growth or mass of tissue that protrudes from a mucous membrane; usually performed via endoscope
      a. Pedunculated—attached to mucous membrane by a slender stalk or pedicle
      b. Sessile—broad-based polyp
N. Proctosigmoidoscopy (also called rectosigmoidoscopy)
   1. Endoscopic exam of distal sigmoid colon, rectum, and anal canal using a small, hollow, stainless steel tube approximately 1.5 cm in diameter
   2. Performed to evaluate:
      a. Rectal bleeding
      b. Polyps
      c. Tumors
      d. Persistent diarrhea
      e. Fissures
      f. Fistulas
      g. Abscesses
      h. Inflammatory bowel disease
   3. Performed as an initial colorectal cancer screen
   4. Advantages
      a. Better tolerated than rigid proctosigmoidoscopy
      b. Allows for examining more of colon than possible with proctoscope
O. GI procedures education
   1. Bowel preparation as appropriate
   2. Course of procedure
   3. Expectations
   4. Recovery period
P. GI procedures assessment parameters
   1. Preprocedure
      a. Preprocedure emphasis on screening for:
         (1) Bleeding disorders in patient or family
         (2) Medications affecting clotting
         (3) Bowel activity
         (4) Swallowing ability
      b. Ensure understanding of preprocedure preparation.
         (1) Nothing per orum (NPO) status
         (2) Diet
         (3) Enema
   2. Postprocedure
      a. General
         (1) Airway and respiratory status
         (2) Vital signs
         (3) Level of consciousness

       3. Procedure specific

         a. Upper GI tract

           (1) Swallowing ability

           (2) Pain

           (3) Bleeding

           (4) Reaction to local anesthetic

           (5) Temperature

         b. Lower GI tract

           (1) Pain

           (2) Flatus

           (3) Bleeding

  Q. Nursing interventions

       1. Withhold fluid until gag reflex intact.

       2. Observe for complications.

       3. Activity restriction per physician orders

  R. Potential complications

       1. GI

         a. Bleeding

         b. Perforated viscus

           (1) Signs include:

             (a) Increased temperature

             (b) Abdominal distention

             (c) Pain

             (d) Shortness of breath

             (e) Subcutaneous emphysema

         c. Respiratory depression

         d. Vasovagal reaction

       2. Liver biopsy

         a. Hemorrhage

         b. Fluid leakage

         c. Subcutaneous emphysema

         d. Perforation of viscus

  S. Key patient educational outcomes

       1. Patients undergoing a GI procedure will be able to identify the signs and symptoms of a perforation

         a. Abdominal/chest pain

         b. Dyspnea

         c. Fever

         d. Light-headedness

         e. Distended abdomen

V. Electroconvulsive Therapy (ECT)

  A. Application of brief electrical stimulus to induce a cerebral seizure

       1. Used to treat major psychiatric disorders (e.g., severe depression)

       2. Procedure may be performed in PACU setting.

  B. Education

       1. Preprocedure emphasis includes screening for:

         a. Baseline mental status

         b. Confusion

         c. Disorientation

         d. Cardiovascular disease

         e. Cerebral pathology and/or suspected increased intracranial pressure

       2. Instruct patient to wash hair night before procedure to remove hair products that may interfere with conduction.

  C. Assessment parameters

       1. Preprocedure assessment per routine protocol

         a. Assess for hypotension and bradycardia.

           (1) Orientation to time, place, and person

  b. Preprocedure parameters
   (1) Have patient void immediately before procedure.
    (a) Prevents incontinence
    (b) Prevents bladder distention
   (2) Apply monitoring devices as indicated.
    (a) Electrocardiogram
    (b) Pulse oximetry
    (c) EEG according to facility policy
    (d) Nerve stimulator
 2. Postprocedure assessment parameters
  a. Airway status
   (1) Patient is at high risk for airway compromise.
  b. Vital signs monitored frequently (per protocol) during and after ECT procedure
  c. Effects of medications
  d. IV sedation and analgesia protocol
 3. Plan of care
  a. Include patient, family, responsible adult companion in developing a plan of care appropriate to patient's age.
  b. Nursing diagnoses might include those listed previously.
  c. Provide for safety.
  d. Be alert for potential complications.
 4. Nursing interventions
  a. Monitor vital signs per protocol.
  b. Administer medications as ordered.
  c. Observe for complications.
   (1) Dysrhythmias
   (2) Aspiration
   (3) Hypotension
   (4) Prolonged seizure
  d. Ensure a safe environment.
   (1) Bite block to prevent damage to teeth and oral cavity during seizure
 5. Evaluation
  a. Response to interventions evaluated continually throughout patient's stay
  b. Alterations to plan of care made as indicated
 D. Potential complications
  1. Bradycardia
  2. Tachycardia
  3. Hypotension
  4. Hypertension
  5. Airway management problems
VI. PULMONARY PROCEDURES
 A. Bronchoscopy
  1. Direct visualization of walls of trachea, mainstem bronchus, and major subdivisions of the bronchial tubes through a bronchoscope
   a. Rigid bronchoscopy—performed under general anesthesia
   b. Fiberoptic (flexible) bronchoscopy
  2. Indications
   a. Diagnosis
    (1) Lesions, bleeding sites
    (2) Obtain biopsies, bronchial brushing, bronchial washing.
   b. Treatment
    (1) Destroy or remove lesions.
    (2) Clear airway of retained secretions.
    (3) Foreign body
   c. Evaluation of disease progression
   d. Evaluation of effectiveness of therapy
   e. May be combined with laser (yttrium-aluminum-garnet [YAG]) therapy for ablation of tracheal and bronchial obstructions

    B. Thoracentesis
- **1.** Withdrawal of fluid or air from the pleural space
  - **a.** Amount of removal limited to 1 to 2 L at one time to avoid mediastinal shift and impaired venous return
- **2.** Indications
  - **a.** Diagnostic
    - (1) Obtain specimen—fluid evaluated for chemical, bacteriologic, and cellular composition.
  - **b.** Therapeutic
    - (1) Relieve respiratory distress.
    - (2) Instill medication into pleural space.

C. PT education and teaching
- **1.** Bronchoscopy
  - **a.** Maintain NPO at least 4 to 6 hours prior.
  - **b.** Instruct not to drive self.
  - **c.** Review nonverbal communication signals when unable to talk.
  - **d.** Report any unusual shortness of breath or prolonged hemoptysis.
  - **e.** Maintain NPO at least 2 hours after procedure.
- **2.** Thoracentesis
  - **a.** Review necessary positioning for procedure.
  - **b.** Instruct not to move suddenly during procedure.
  - **c.** Instruct to report any unexplained dyspnea, chest pain, fever, or cough.

D. Assessment parameters
- **1.** Bronchoscopy
  - **a.** Preprocedure
    - (1) NPO for 4 to 6 hours before procedure
      - (a) Decrease risk of aspiration.
      - (b) Remove dentures.
  - **b.** Postprocedure
    - (1) Assess for return of swallow and gag reflex.
    - (2) Blood-streaked sputum expected for several hours postprocedure
    - (3) Frank bleeding indicative of hemorrhage

E. Potential complications
- **1.** Bronchoscopy
  - **a.** Bronchospasm
  - **b.** Laryngospasm
  - **c.** Hypoxia
  - **d.** Bleeding
  - **e.** Pneumothorax
  - **f.** Perforation
  - **g.** Aspiration
  - **h.** Cardiac dysrhythmias
  - **i.** Reaction to local anesthetic
- **2.** Thoracentesis
  - **a.** Hemothorax
  - **b.** Pneumothorax
  - **c.** Air embolism
  - **d.** Subcutaneous emphysema
  - **e.** Bleeding

F. Key patient educational outcomes
- **1.** Report any of the following:
  - **a.** Shortness of breath
  - **b.** Prolonged hemoptysis
  - **c.** Unexplained dyspnea
  - **d.** Chest pain
  - **e.** Fever
  - **f.** Cough

VII. Infusion therapy
    A. Therapy types
        1. Blood transfusion
            a. Types
                (1) Whole blood
                (2) Packed red blood cells
                (3) Frozen red blood cells
                (4) Platelets
                (5) Granulocytes
                (6) Plasma
                (7) Albumin
                (8) Coagulation factor concentrates
                (9) Prothrombin complex
                (10) Cryoprecipitate
                (11) Immune serum globulins
            b. Collected from:
                (1) Donor (homologous)
                (2) Recipient (autologous)
                (3) Donor designated by recipient (designated direct blood)
        2. Medical infusion therapy
            a. Treat illness.
            b. Provide for patients who need:
                (1) Medication for chronic illnesses such as Crohn's disease, asthma, multiple sclerosis, diabetes
                (2) Pain management
                (3) IV hydration
                (4) Low-dose chemotherapy
                (5) Long-term antibiotic therapy
                (6) Immunomodulators
                (7) Therapeutic phlebotomy
    B. Education
        1. Patient's level of understanding regarding procedure
        2. History of transfusion reactions
        3. Prepare for any preinfusion requirements.
    C. Assessment parameters
        1. Blood transfusion
            a. Preprocedure
                (1) Ensure informed consent and/or specific transfusion consent form is complete.
                (2) Obtain baseline vital signs, including temperature.
                (3) Assess patient history of transfusion reactions.
                (4) Educate patient to signs and symptoms of potential reactions.
            b. Administration
                (1) Ensure blood has been typed and crossmatched and that ABO group and Rh factor match patient's type.
                (2) Check blood for abnormal color or cloudiness (indicates hemolysis).
                (3) Check for presence of gas bubbles (indicates bacterial growth).
                (4) Check expiration date on blood bag.
                (5) Confirm information with another professional.
                (6) Document confirmation.
                (7) Administration of unrefrigerated blood should begin within 1 hour.
                (8) Total administration time should generally not exceed 4 hours.
            c. Nursing interventions during procedure
                (1) Assess vital signs per protocol.
                (2) Be alert for signs of transfusion reaction.
                (3) Types of reactions
                    (a) Acute hemolytic
                        (i) Caused by infusion of ABO-incompatible blood
                        (ii) May cause most severe symptoms

    (b) Febrile, nonhemolytic
        (i)   Most common
        (ii) Treat symptomatically.
    (c) Mild allergic
        (i)   Rash, itching, low-grade fever
        (ii) May administer antihistamines
    (d) Anaphylactic
        (i)   Mild to severe symptoms
    (e) Circulatory overload
        (i)   Rare
        (ii) Caused by rapid infusion in patient unable to accommodate volume
        (iii) Patient may have history of cardiac disease.
    (f) Septic reaction
        (i)   Caused by contaminated blood
        (ii) Symptoms are immediate.
        (iii) Fever, chills, hypotension, shock
        (iv) Treat with IV antibiotics.
    (g) Delayed
        (i)   Can occur several days to 2 weeks after transfusion
(4) Blood transfusion potential complications
    (a) Transfusion reaction signs and symptoms
        (i)   Integumentary
            [a] Itching
            [b] Rashes
            [c] Swelling
            [d] Cyanosis
            [e] Excessive perspiration
        (ii) Respiratory
            [a] Tachypnea
            [b] Dyspnea
            [c] Apnea
            [d] Wheezing
            [e] Cyanosis
            [f] Rales
        (iii) Urinary
            [a] Pain on or during urination
            [b] Oliguria
            [c] Changes in urine color
                [1] Dark, concentrated
                [2] Shades of red, brown, amber
        (iv) Circulatory
            [a] Chest pain
            [b] Increased heart rate
            [c] Palpitations
            [d] Hypotension
            [e] Hypertension
            [f] Bleeding
        (v)   General
            [a] Muscle aches, pain
            [b] Back pain
            [c] Chest pain
            [d] Headache
            [e] Fever
            [f] Chills
        (vi) Nervous system
            [a] Tingling
            [b] Numbness
            [c] Apprehension, impending doom

2. Medical infusion assessments
   a. Vital signs per protocol
   b. Confirm known patient allergies.
   c. Assess for infusion reactions.
   d. Monitor infusion sites.
D. Key patient educational outcomes
   1. Patient undergoing a blood transfusion will be able to accurately relate information regarding the transfusion and the signs and symptoms of a latent reaction.
   2. Patients undergoing infusion therapy must report signs of site irritation or infection, reactions to medications, etc.

BIBLIOGRAPHY

1. Altman GB: *Delmar's fundamental & advanced nursing skills*, ed 2, Clifton Park, NY, 2004, Delmar.
2. British Committee for Standards in Haematology Writing Group, Baglin TP, Brush J, et al: Guidelines on use of vena cava filters. *Br J Haematol* 134(6):590–595, 2006.
3. Burke KM, LeMone P, Mohn-Brown EL, et al: *Medical-surgical nursing care*, ed 2, Upper Saddle River, NJ, 2007, Prentice-Hall.
4. McDaniel C: Uterine fibroid embolization: The less invasive alternative. *Nursing* 37(7):26–27, 2007.
5. Rosenthal K: Are you up-to-date with the infusion nursing standards? *Nursing* 37(7):15, 2007.
6. Saastamoinen P, Piispa M, Niskanen MM: Use of postanesthesia care unit for purposes other than postanesthesia observation. *J Perianesth Nurs* 22(2):102–107, 2007.
7. Segal JB, Streiff MB, Hoffman LV, et al: Management of venous thromboembolism: A systematic review for a practice guideline. *Ann Intern Med* 146(3):211–215, 2007.
8. Venes D: *Taber's cyclopedic medical dictionary*, ed 20, Philadelphia, 2005, FA Davis.
9. Wagner KD, Johnson KL, Kidd PS: *High acuity nursing*, ed 4, Upper Saddle River, NJ, 2006, Pearson Education.

AMBULATORY SURGICAL NURSING COMPETENCIES

50 Immediate Postoperative Assessment and Postanesthesia Assessment Phase II

MARY C. REDMOND

Acknowledgment: I thank Hope Brown, Kenny Oyer, and Anna and Don Siner for their patient and persistent technical support.

OBJECTIVES
At the conclusion of this chapter, the reader will be able to:

1. Describe components of patient transfer reports for postanesthesia/postsedation and postoperative care.
2. Interpret holistic assessment criteria systematically in phase I and phase II post anesthesia care unit (PACU).
3. Develop patient care plans to support uneventful recovery throughout the surgical continuum of care.
4. Identify three concepts of postoperative/postprocedure and postanesthesia/postsedation care.
5. Describe postoperative assessment care provided in a safe environment.

I. DEFINITIONS
    A. Postoperative/postprocedure nursing care
        1. Involves distinct levels of patient care to meet holistic patient care needs
            a. Physical
            b. Mental
            c. Emotional
            d. Spiritual
        2. Provisions
            a. Provided to patients who have received anesthesia and/or sedation during:
                (1) Surgical procedures
                (2) Other procedures
            b. Provided in a manner that meets patients' varying needs
            c. Not limited to care provided at a specific physical location
    B. Levels of postoperative care
        1. Phase I PACU involves the most intense care after surgery/anesthesia in preparation for a patient's transfer to:
            a. Phase II PACU

        b. Nursing unit

        c. Acute care area

   2. Phase II PACU involves progressive care in preparation for a patient's transfer to:

        a. Home

        b. Extended care facility

        c. Extended observation

II. POSTOPERATIVE CARE SETTINGS

  A. Practice settings

    1. Hospitals

    2. Ambulatory surgery units within hospital settings or hospital outpatient departments

    3. Freestanding ambulatory surgery centers

    4. Surgical hospitals

    5. Various procedure areas, cardiovascular lab

        a. Electroconvulsive therapy

        b. Gastroenterology/endoscopy

        c. Diagnostic and interventional radiology

        d. Oncology

        e. Pain management

    6. Clinics

    7. Physicians' offices

  B. Design

    1. Should be efficient, functional, and aesthetically pleasing to:

        a. Patients and visitors

        b. Professional care providers and staff

    2. Preoperative patients are separated from patients:

        a. Undergoing procedures

        b. Recovering from anesthesia/sedation

    3. Layout varies by facility

        a. Phase I PACU

            (1) Located in close proximity to where anesthesia is administered

                (a) Allows visibility of all patients through direct observation and monitoring

                (b) Allows space for visiting family members according to policy

            (2) Design may include:

                (a) One large room sectioned with curtains for patient privacy

                (b) One large room sectioned according to patient specialty needs

                (c) Isolation room for patients with communicable diseases or in need of protective isolation

                (d) Procedure area

                (e) Exit to lobby for visiting family members

        b. Phase II PACU

            (1) Provides a friendly, family-oriented atmosphere with sufficient space for each patient and several visitors

            (2) May be located in:

                (a) Another area of PACU

                (b) Another multipurpose area

            (3) Design may include:

                (a) One large room with recliners and curtains to maintain patient privacy

                (b) Series of private rooms with beds or recliners

                    (i) Provides maximum privacy during patient care, teaching, and observing return demonstrations as appropriate

                    (ii) Provides private and confidential area conducive to patient/family willingness to ask questions

                (c) Isolation room for patients with communicable diseases

    (d) Area for procedures

    (e) Separate room for children and families to interact without disturbing adult patients

    (f) Diversionary material: soothing music, magazines, television

    (g) Clerical area for documentation

    (h) Security system for managing valuables

    (i) Area for personal articles

      (i) Closet or lockers for patients' clothing and other personal articles

      (ii) Clothing and personal articles may remain on beds, accompanying patients as they move from one area to another, dependent on institution policy.

    (j) Dressing rooms

  c. Both phase I and phase II PACU

    (1) Emergency preparedness

     (a) Emergency alarm system to obtain help when needed

     (b) Emergency equipment and medications

    (2) Interdepartmental/intradepartmental communication system

     (a) To obtain or convey vital information

     (b) To summon help when needed

    (3) Bathrooms

     (a) Call mechanisms available in case of emergency or to obtain help

     (b) Doors that can be opened from the outside, if locked, in case of emergency

    (4) Tracking system to keep visitors informed of patients' status and location

    (5) Efficient documentation system: computer and paper forms

    (6) Nourishment center

    (7) Medication center

    (8) Areas for storage of supplies and equipment

C. Furniture, equipment and supplies

 1. Phase I PACU (Box 50-1)

  a. For each operating room (OR): 1.5 beds

  b. Two beds for each OR for short procedures and/or pediatric cases

  c. Chairs for visitors

 2. Phase II PACU (Box 50-2)

  a. Beds, carts, or recliners

  b. Chairs for visitors

  c. Wheelchairs for patient transport

D. Policies and procedures

 1. Should be evidence-based

 2. Staff reviews policies and procedures per institutional guidelines.

E. Documentation of care

 1. Charting via forms or computer should include:

  a. Vital signs

  b. Scoring parameters if used, for example:

   (1) Modified Aldrete Scoring System

   (2) Post Anesthetic Discharge Scoring System

  c. Unit-specific clinical criteria checklists

  d. Narrative notes

 2. Characteristics of acceptable documentation

  a. Accurate

  b. Comprehensive

  c. Factual

  d. Objective

  e. Timely

 3. Chart

  a. Legal document

  b. Source of information for multiple professional purposes

■ BOX 50-1
■ **EQUIPMENT FOR PHASE I PACU LEVEL OF CARE**

The following list of equipment for phase I PACU level of care includes, but is not limited to:
- Each patient bedside will be equipped with the following:
  - Various types and sizes of artificial airways
  - Various means of oxygen delivery
  - Constant and intermittent suction
  - Means to monitor blood pressure
  - Adjustable lighting
  - Capacity to ensure patient privacy
  - ECG monitor
  - Pulse oximeter
- Equipment will be available to assess:
  - Hemodynamic status
  - Blood glucose
  - Arterial blood gases
  - End-tidal CO_2
  - Pulses (e.g., bedside portable ultrasound)
  - Urine volume (e.g., bladder scanner)
- A means to monitor patient temperature and a method to warm the hypothermic patient will be available.
- Supplies as recommended by the Malignant Hyperthermia Association of the United States*
- Available and easily accessible ventilators and bag-valve-masks of assorted sizes for the patient population
- Emergency call system
- Adult and pediatric emergency cart with:
  - Supplies for insertion of arterial lines, central venous lines, and pulmonary artery catheters
  - IV pole
  - Emergency drugs and equipment
- Defibrillator with adult and pediatric pads/paddles and cardiac pacing capability readily available
- Stock or readily available medications include but are not limit to:
  - Antibiotics
  - Medications to control blood pressure and heart rate
  - Medications to treat respiratory insufficiency
  - Antiemetics
  - Reversal agents
  - Analgesics: opioid and nonopioid
  - Muscle relaxants
  - Steroids
  - Anxiolytic agents
- Latex-free intravenous supplies
- Patient-protective devices available to use per facility policy
- Flashlights and emergency lighting system
- Latex-free stock supplies including:
  - Dressings
  - Facial tissues
  - Gloves
  - Bedpans and urinals
  - Syringes, needles, and protective needle devices
  - Emesis basins
  - Patient linens
  - Alcohol swabs
  - Ice bags
  - Tongue blades
  - Irrigation trays

■ BOX 50-1
■ **EQUIPMENT FOR PHASE I PACU LEVEL OF CARE—cont'd**

- Urinary catheterization supplies
- Personal protective equipment
- Nasogastric tube supplies
- Assorted tapes
- Equipment for safe transport of patients from phase I PACU as appropriate (e.g., portable oxygen, pulse oximetry, suction, cardiac monitoring equipment)

*See www.MHAUS.org or call 1-800-MHHYPER.
CO₂, Carbon dioxide; *ECG*, electrocardiogram; *IV*, intravenous; *PACU*, post anesthesia care unit.
Modified from American Society of PeriAnesthesia Nurses: *Standards of perianesthesia nursing practice 2008-2010,* Cherry Hill, NJ, 2008, American Society of PeriAnesthesia Nurses.

■ BOX 50-2
■ **EQUIPMENT FOR PHASE II PACU LEVEL OF CARE**

The following list of equipment for phase II PACU level of care includes, but is not limited to:
- The unit will be equipped with the following:
    - Means to deliver oxygen
    - Means to provide constant and intermittent suction
    - Means to monitor blood pressure
    - Means of monitoring patient temperatures
    - Adjustable lighting
    - Capacity to ensure patient privacy
- ECG monitor and pulse oximeter readily available
- Bag-valve-masks of assorted sizes
- Blood glucose monitor
    - Bladder scanner for urine volumes
    - Portable ultrasound for pulse checks
    - Supplies as recommended by the Malignant Hyperthermia Association of the United States*
- Emergency call system
- Emergency cart available at all times
- Defibrillator with adult and pediatric pads/paddles and cardiac pacing readily available
- Warming measures
- Stock medications include but are not limited to the following:
    - Antibiotics
    - Antiemetics
    - Anesthesia reversal agents
    - Analgesics: opioids and nonopioids
    - Ammonia ampules
- Intravenous supplies
- Flashlights and emergency lighting system
- Latex-free stock supplies include:
    - Dressings
    - Facial tissues
    - Gloves
    - Bedpans and urinals
    - Syringes, needles, and protective needle devices
    - Emesis basins
    - Patient linens
    - Alcohol wipes
    - Ice bags

*See www.MHAUS.org or call 1-800-MHHYPER.

Continued

■ BOX 50-2
■ **EQUIPMENT FOR PHASE II PACU LEVEL OF CARE—cont'd**

- Tongue blades
- Urinary catheterization supplies
- Personal protective equipment
- Variety of tapes
- Access to other latex-free patient supplies
  - Slings in various sizes
  - Arm/shoulder, leg immobilizers
  - Orthopedic shoes and boots
  - Crutches in various lengths
- Equipment for safe transport of patients from phase II PACU as appropriate
  - Wheelchairs of various sizes
  - Cart
  - Portable oxygen, pulse oximetry, suction
  - Cardiac monitoring equipment

ECG, Electrocardiogram; *PACU*, post anesthesia care unit.
Modified from American Society of PeriAnesthesia Nurses: *Standards of perianesthesia nursing practice 2008-2010*, Cherry Hill, NJ, 2008, American Society of PeriAnesthesia Nurses.

      (1) To communicate patient condition to other health professionals
      (2) For risk management and quality-of-care management
      (3) For research data
      (4) For reimbursement from the government and insurance

  F. Staffing
    1. Requirements vary throughout the day based on a variety of patient factors (Box 50-3):
      a. Procedures
      b. Type of anesthesia
      c. Patient acuity
      d. Phase I and phase II PACU patient flow process
    2. If departmentally feasible, the staff may cross-train to one or more areas.
      a. Preoperative
      b. OR or procedure area
      c. Phase I PACU
      d. Phase II PACU
      e. Extended observation
    3. Considerations in cross-training the staff
      a. Uses staff wherever needed throughout the patient flow process
      b. Offers nurses the opportunity to increase their knowledge
      c. May help avoid "burnout" for nurses desiring more diversity
      d. Limiting specialization to a specific area leads to mastery of skills, technical knowledge, and efficiency.
      e. Nurses may specialize in a particular area by choice or preference.
    4. Perianesthesia nurses strive to ensure:
      a. Competency by integrating knowledge, attitudes, skills, and behaviors
      b. Responsibility to patients
        (1) Preserve human dignity, autonomy, confidentiality, and worth.
        (2) Protect patient rights and support patient well-being.
      c. Professional responsibility
        (1) Accountable for care provided
        (2) Maintain compliance with regulatory and professional agencies.
      d. Collegiality with members of the multidisciplinary health care team
      e. Participating in and conducting research to improve practice and education

■ BOX 50-3

■ **PATIENT CLASSIFICATION/RECOMMENDED PHASE I AND PHASE II PACU STAFFING GUIDELINES**

Phase I PACU Level of Care

- The perianesthesia registered nursing roles during this phase focus on providing postanesthesia nursing care to the patient in the immediate postanesthesia period, and transitioning them to phase II level of care, the inpatient setting, or to an intensive care setting for continued care.
- *Two registered nurses, one of whom is an RN competent in phase I postanesthesia nursing, are in the same unit where the patient is receiving phase I level of care.*

Class 1:2—**One nurse to two patients**

- One patient is unconscious, stable, without artificial airway, and over the age of eight (8) years; and one conscious, stable and free of complications.
- Two conscious, stable, and free of complications.
- Two conscious, stable, eight (8) years of age and under with family or competent support staff present.

Class 1:1—**One nurse to one patient**

- At the time of admission, until the critical elements* are met
- Unstable airway**
- Any unconscious patient eight (8) years of age and under
- A second nurse must be available to assist as necessary.

Class 2:1—**Two nurses to one patient**

- One critically ill, unstable, complicated patient
- Critical elements can be defined as:
  - Report has been received from the anesthesia care provider, questions answered, and the transfer of care has taken place.
  - Patient has a secure airway.
  - Initial assessment is complete.
  - Patient is hemodynamically stable.
- Examples of an unstable airway include, but are not limited to, the following:
  - Requiring active interventions to maintain patency such as manual jaw lift or chin lift
  - Evidence of obstruction, active or probable, such as gasping, choking, crowing, wheezing, etc.
  - Symptoms of respiratory distress including dyspnea, tachypnea, panic, agitation, cyanosis, etc.

Phase II PACU Level of Care

The professional perianesthesia nursing roles during this phase focus on preparing the patient/family/significant other for care in the home, extended observation level of care, or the extended care environment.

- *Two competent personnel, one of whom is an RN competent in phase II postanesthesia nursing, are in the same unit where the patient is receiving phase II level of care. An RN must be in the phase II PACU at all times while a patient is present.*

Class 1:3—**One nurse to three patients**

- Over eight (8) years of age
- Eight (8) years of age and under with family present

Class 1:2—**One nurse to two patients**

- Eight (8) years of age and under without family or support staff present
- Initial admission of patient postprocedure

Class 1:1—**One nurse to one patient**

- Unstable patient of any age requiring transfer

PACU, Post anesthesia care unit; *RN,* registered nurse.
Modified from American Society of PeriAnesthesia Nurses: *Standards of perianesthesia nursing practice 2008-2010,* Cherry Hill, NJ, 2008, American Society of PeriAnesthesia Nurses.

5. Staff characteristics and educational background
   a. Organized, energetic, versatile, independent thinkers
   b. Possess common sense and a caring attitude
   c. Work efficiently, independently, and collaboratively
   d. Exhibit a positive attitude and are physically and emotionally supportive
   e. Previous medical-surgical and/or critical care nursing experience advantageous
   f. Use strong clinical assessment and critical thinking skills
   g. Demonstrate strong teaching skills
   h. Have a basic understanding of anesthetic agents and side effects
   i. Maintain certification as appropriate to the patient population served
      (1) Basic life support (BLS)
      (2) Advanced cardiac life support (ACLS)
      (3) Pediatric advanced life support (PALS)
   j. Certification in perianesthesia nursing encouraged
      (1) Certified PeriAnesthesia Nurse (CPAN)
      (2) Certified Ambulatory PeriAnesthesia Nurse (CAPA)

III. PHASE I PACU CARE
   A. Focus of care
      1. Providing nursing care to the patient in the immediate postanesthesia period
         a. Basic life-sustaining needs are of the highest priority.
         b. Constant vigilance required during this period
      2. Transitioning the patient for continued care to phase II PACU, an inpatient nursing unit, or critical care/special care unit
   B. Transfer of the patient to phase I PACU
      1. PACU receives advance notice of transfer of patient from OR to PACU.
         a. To have necessary equipment available and ready for use
         b. To assign the patient to an appropriately experienced PACU practitioner
      2. Admission of the patient to phase I PACU is a joint effort shared by:
         a. Anesthesia provider
         b. OR circulating nurse
         c. Phase I PACU nurse
      3. OR transporting team responsibilities
         a. Help settle the patient safely in phase I PACU.
         b. Report information to the phase I PACU nurse.
            (1) Report components may be shared by anesthesia provider and circulating nurse.
            (2) Report contains essential patient care information.
         c. Defer verbal report if the patient's condition becomes unstable, requiring emergent interventions.
         d. Remain with the patient until the phase I PACU nurse accepts responsibility.
   C. Initial assessment
      1. Initial patient assessment is multifaceted.
         a. Begins immediately upon the patient's arrival in phase I PACU
         b. Continues concurrently with the report of the transfer team
      2. Phase I PACU nurses will:
         a. Apply oxygen.
         b. Assess the respiratory status.
            (1) Patent airway
            (2) Presence and type of airway
            (3) Breath sounds
         c. Apply appropriate monitoring equipment to the patient.
         d. Report current vital signs to the anesthesia provider.
            (1) Respirations
            (2) Arterial oxygen saturation (Sao_2), end-tidal carbon dioxide ($ETCO_2$) levels as appropriate

       (3) Blood pressure: cuff or arterial line
       (4) Heart rate, rhythm
  3. Essential contents of transfer report to phase I PACU nurse
    a. Patient's name and age
    b. Surgeon's name
    c. Procedure
    d. Anesthetic
       (1) Type (Box 50-4)
       (2) Type and time of reversal agents if applicable
       (3) Unplanned responses
         (a) Treatment
         (b) Outcome
    e. Pain and comfort management interventions and plan
    f. Allergies
    g. Medications administered preoperatively and intraoperatively
       (1) Analgesics
       (2) Antiemetics
       (3) Antibiotics
       (4) Others
    h. Relevant history
       (1) Comorbidities
       (2) Level of severity and management
    i. Vital signs
       (1) Blood pressure: cuff or arterial
       (2) Temperature, route
       (3) Heart rate, rhythm
       (4) Respirations
         (a) Breath sounds

■ BOX 50-4
■ **ANESTHESIA/SEDATION TECHNIQUES**

- General
- Regional
  - IV regional block: Bier block (arm or leg procedures)
  - Peripheral nerve block
    - Brachial plexus block
      - Interscalene (shoulder procedures)
      - Supraclavicular (shoulder/upper extremity procedures)
      - Axillary (procedures distal to elbow)
    - Cervical plexus block (carotid endarterectomy)
    - Digital nerve block (finger or toe procedures)
    - Intercostal block (postoperative abdominal or thoracic pain control)
    - Lower extremity block (postoperative lower extremity pain control)
  - Regional block (abdominal or lower extremity procedures)
    - Caudal (pediatric surgery and for labor and delivery)
    - Epidural (abdominal or lower extremity procedures)
      - Single injection
      - Repetitive bolus via catheter
      - Continuous injection via catheter
    - Spinal (abdominal or lower extremity procedures)
      - Intrathecal
      - Subarachnoid
- Sedation (minor surgical procedures)
  - Intravenous (IV)
  - Gaseous inhalation
- Local infiltration (simple surgical procedures, postoperative pain control)
- Topical (to start IVs)

   (b) Type of airway
   (c) Sao$_2$
   (d) Mechanical ventilator settings if applicable
  (5) Hemodynamic pressure readings if applicable
   (a) Central venous
   (b) Pulmonary artery
   (c) Pulmonary artery occlusive/pulmonary artery wedge
   (d) Intracranial
 j. Intake
  (1) Crystalloid fluids
  (2) Colloid fluids
  (3) Blood/blood products
 k. Output
  (1) Blood loss
  (2) Urine output
  (3) Others (e.g., nasogastric tube, chest tube)
 l. Laboratory tests
 m. Radiology diagnostic tests
 n. Emotional status on arrival in OR/procedure room
 o. Medical record is a resource for information not included in the verbal report.

4. Anesthesia provider and phase I PACU nurse assess the patient for stability.
 a. Intervene if necessary.
 b. Reassess until the patient is stable.

5. Transfer team answers any questions before departing phase I PACU.

6. Phase I PACU nurse continues the complete initial patient assessment (Box 50-5).
 a. Initial assessment identifies the patient's physiological status at phase I PACU arrival.
 b. Assessment must be rapid, efficient, and thorough.
 c. Any assessment manner is acceptable as long as it:
  (1) Meets standards
  (2) Incorporates information from the OR/procedure transfer team
  (3) Head-to-toe systems assessment is comprehensive and easy to learn.
   (a) Neurological
   (b) Respiratory
   (c) Cardiovascular
   (d) Gastrointestinal
   (e) Genitourinary
   (f) Neurovascular
   (g) Comfort
  (4) Assessment in order of major body systems most affected by anesthesia prioritizes information.
   (a) Airway patency
   (b) Breathing
    (i) Rate and rhythm
    (ii) Breath sounds
    (iii) Sao$_2$, ETCO$_2$ as appropriate
   (c) Cardiovascular
    (i) Heart rate and rhythm
    (ii) Electrocardiogram (ECG) strip
    (iii) Blood pressure
    (iv) Temperature
    (v) Skin condition
   (d) Age- and condition-appropriate neurological function
    (i) Responsiveness to stimulation
    (ii) Orientation

■ BOX 50-5
■ **INITIAL ASSESSMENT: PHASE I PACU**

Initial assessment and documentation include, but are not limited to:
1. Integration of data received at transfer of care
   - Relevant preoperative status
   - Anesthesia/sedation technique and agents
   - Length of time anesthesia/sedation administered, time reversal agents given
   - Pain and comfort management interventions and plan
   - Medications administered
   - Type of procedure
   - Estimated fluid/blood loss and replacement
   - Complications occurring during anesthesia course, treatment initiated, response
   - Emotional status on arrival to the operating/procedure room
2. Vital signs
   - Airway patency, respiratory status, breath sounds, type of artificial airway, mechanical ventilator settings, Sao_2; $ETCO_2$ if available and indicated
   - Blood pressure: cuff or arterial line
   - Pulse: apical, peripheral
   - Cardiac monitor rhythm documented
   - Temperature/route
   - Hemodynamic pressure readings: central venous, pulmonary artery and wedge, intracranial pressure if indicated
3. Pain and comfort level
4. Level of emotional comfort
5. Neurological function including level of consciousness
6. Pupillary response as indicated
7. Sensory and motor function as appropriate
8. Position of patient
9. Condition and color of skin
10. Patient safety needs
11. Neurovascular: peripheral pulses, sensation of extremities as applicable
12. Condition of dressings, visible incisions, procedural site
13. Type, patency, and securement of drainage tubes, receptacles, catheters
14. Amount and type of drainage
15. Location and condition of IV site(s), type and amount of solution(s) infusing
16. Procedure-specific assessment (e.g., abdominal firmness)
17. Postanesthesia scoring system if used

$ETCO_2$, End-tidal carbon dioxide; *IV*, intravenous; *PACU*, post anesthesia care unit; Sao_2, arterial oxygen saturation.
Modified from American Society of PeriAnesthesia Nurses: *Standards of perianesthesia nursing practice 2008-2010*, Cherry Hill, NJ, 2008, American Society of PeriAnesthesia Nurses.

          (iii) Ability to follow commands appropriately
          (iv) Ability to move extremities purposefully and equally unless affected preoperatively by anesthesia, or by surgery
      (e) Renal
          (i)   Intake and output
          (ii) Patency of intravenous (IV) lines
          (iii) Patency of drains/tubes
  D. Ongoing patient assessment and care planning
      1. Initial assessment establishes the patient's baseline level so the effect of anesthesia and surgery can be assessed and predicted as they affect current physiology.
      2. Ongoing assessment of the patient (Box 50-6)
          a. Identifies progress in recovery from anesthesia, noting residual effects

■ BOX 50-6
■ **ONGOING ASSESSMENT AND MANAGEMENT: PHASE I PACU**

Ongoing assessment and management include, but are not limited to the following:
1. Monitor, maintain, and/or improve respiratory function.
2. Monitor, maintain, and/or improve circulatory function.
3. Monitor, maintain, and/or improve neurological function, including level of consciousness.
4. Assess sensory and motor function as appropriate.
5. Monitor temperature and promote normothermia.
6. Promote and maintain effective pain and comfort management.
7. Promote and maintain emotional comfort.
8. Monitor surgical/procedural site; continue procedure-specific care.
9. Document nursing action/interventions with outcome.
10. Notify patient care unit of needed equipment, if appropriate, before transfer.
11. Include family/care provider in patient care as indicated.
12. Notify patient care unit when patient is ready for phase I discharge; provide report of all significant events in the OR and PACU.
13. Postanesthesia scoring system if used

OR, Operating room; *PACU*, post anesthesia care unit.
Modified from American Society of PeriAnesthesia Nurses: *Standards of perianesthesia nursing practice 2008-2010,* Cherry Hill, NJ, 2008, American Society of PeriAnesthesia Nurses.

    b. Allows periodic reexamination of the patient so physiological and emotional trends become obvious
    c. Assesses ongoing status of the surgical site and its effect on any preexisting conditions and recovery
    d. Allows compilation and trending of patient-specific characteristics
  3. Phase I PACU nurse develops patient care plan for ongoing care as a result of:
    a. Initial assessment findings
    b. Based on the ongoing cyclical nursing process
      (1) Assess the patient's condition and note special needs, deficits, challenges, and preferences.
        (a) Sensory deficits and aids
        (b) Developmental deficits
        (c) Prosthetic devices
        (d) Language barrier
        (e) Cultural influences
        (f) Religious preferences
      (2) Diagnose actual or potential problems.
      (3) Plan the appropriate intervention.
        (a) May include, but is not limited to:
          (i) Clinical protocols based on evidence-based practice
          (ii) Physicians' orders
          (iii) Standards of care
          (iv) Clinical pathways
        (b) Prioritize the plan of care.
      (4) Implement the interventions.
      (5) Evaluate and reevaluate the patient's outcome.
    c. Perform ongoing comprehensive nursing assessments.
      (1) At intervals defined by policy
      (2) As indicated by the patient's condition
        (a) Identify actual or potential problems (Table 50-1).
        (b) Continually upgrade the care plan according to patient needs.

■ TABLE 50-1

■ Phase I PACU Patient Outcomes*

Potential and Actual Problems (Nursing Diagnoses)	Outcome Goals (The Patient Will be Able to:)	Nursing Interventions	Resources
Ineffective airway clearance Potential for aspiration Ineffective breathing patterns, respiratory depression related to: sedation, anesthesia, positioning, pain Increased secretions Nausea/vomiting	Maintain normal respiratory parameters (rate, depth, ease, clarity of breath sounds). Maintain clear airway. Avoid aspiration. Maintain adequate oxygenation of tissues. Avoid symptoms of hypoxia. Perform effective cough and deep breathing exercises.	Know effects of anesthetics, analgesics, sedatives, and muscle relaxants and associated drug interactions Know airway maintenance techniques. Continuously assess abnormal symptoms. Administer oxygen per protocol. Identify preexisting respiratory disease and individualize care appropriately. Request patient to deep breathe frequently. Position patient to provide optimal respiratory function. Report abnormal symptoms to anesthesiologist/surgeon.	Physiological monitoring equipment at each bedside Adequate staffing patterns to ensure proper nurse-to-patient ratio Immediate access to anesthesia provider Comprehensive anesthesia report before transfer of patient ASPAN *Standards of Perianesthesia Nursing Practice* Facility policies regarding interventions for cardiovascular/respiratory problems Oxygen and suction at each bedside Immediate access to emergency equipment: crash cart, resuscitator bag-valve-mask, ventilator, airway maintenance supplies Medications
Cardiovascular instability Potential for altered mental status Potential alterations in tissue perfusion	Maintain normal cardiovascular parameters, avoiding hypertension and hypotension. Demonstrate expected postoperative arousal and mental status. Demonstrate normal parameters of peripheral circulation.	Assess all parameters of vital signs in ongoing fashion, including heart rate BP and rhythm. Assess mental status. Assess peripheral pulses, color, and sensory adequacy frequently. Maintain adequate fluid balance and hydration. Report abnormal symptoms to anesthesiologist/surgeon.	Physiological monitoring equipment Preoperative assessment documentation

Continued

*This type of table can replace writing traditional nursing care plans. The phase I PACU nurse need only select applicable nursing diagnoses and follow-through for the individual patient.

■ TABLE 50-1

■ Phase I PACU Patient Outcomes—cont'd

Potential and Actual Problems (Nursing Diagnoses)	Outcome Goals (The Patient Will be Able to:)	Nursing Interventions	Resources
Altered skin integrity related to surgical wound Potential for infection at surgical site	Experience appropriate and uncomplicated wound healing.	Assess surgical site throughout phase I PACU stay. Use aseptic technique when changing bandages. Avoid constricting bandages at surgical site.	Standard precautions Personal protective equipment and sterile dressing supplies Antibiotics if ordered
Altered skin integrity related to pressure points, positioning	Avoid skin breakdown related to pressure, tape, constricting bandages.	Position patient using appropriate padding to avoid pressure points. Assess full body for pressure areas.	Nonallergic tape Padding, pillows, foam, for protection
Anxiety related to unfamiliar surroundings, isolation from family or responsible adult, potential diagnosis or surgical outcome	Express reduced anxiety. Display calm demeanor. Verbalize needs related to family, emotional support.	Block sights/sounds or other areas of phase I PACU whenever possible. Encourage/allow family presence in phase I PACU as appropriate. Provide emotional support and answers to patient's questions within boundaries of nursing. Monitor and oversee patient care while patient is vulnerable to environment.	Separation of phase I PACU critical care patients and patients undergoing treatments from preoperative and phase II PACU patients Cubicle curtains to reduce view of phase I PACU Policy allowing families/ responsible adult to visit in phase I PACU ASPAN *Standards of Perianesthesia Nursing Practice*
Altered thought process and/or memory loss related to sedation/anesthesia	Display/verbalize appropriate orientation to surroundings and situation. Avoid self-injury related to altered thought patterns.	Provide frequent affirmation of orientation to time, place, and events. Assess patient's orientation.	Pharmaceutical literature outlining effects of anesthesia and sedative medications Predetermined phase I PACU discharge criteria that include assessment of mental status ASPAN *Standards of Perianesthesia Nursing Practice*

Alteration in comfort: pain	Express acceptable comfort level.	Assess and administer appropriate analgesics; evaluate effectiveness. Position patient for comfort. Apply cold therapy as ordered. Provide positive reinforcement and encourage philosophy of wellness throughout process. Encourage appropriate pace for increased activity.	Analgesic medications. Knowledge of nursing interventions for comfort: "ASPAN Pain and Comfort Clinical Guideline". Positioning and support of body areas. Breathing exercises. Positive reinforcement of comfort.
Alterations in comfort: nausea and vomiting	Express acceptable comfort level. Avoid vomiting and retching.	Assess for presence of protective reflexes: cough, gag, swallow. Encourage appropriate pace for oral intake of fluids. Administer antiemetics as needed. Provide positive reinforcement and encourage philosophy of wellness throughout process. Use complementary therapies if acceptable to patient.	Antiemetic medications. Intravenous fluids. Literature related to reducing GI symptoms. Appropriate food and beverages; avoid acid-producing juices, spicy or difficult-to-digest foods.
Self-care deficit	Display sufficient level of alertness and self-care for discharge to phase II or to a nursing unit.	Provide comprehensive nursing care modified to patient's abilities. Assess patient for ability to turn, move, and call for assistance before transfer.	Level of consciousness scale. Phase I PACU discharge criteria.
Actual or perceived loss of privacy, confidentiality, or dignity	Express satisfaction with level of privacy and confidentiality provided. Maintain dignity and sense of self-esteem.	Support patient's right to privacy, confidentiality, and dignity. Provide privacy and ensure confidentiality. Provide curtains, blankets, and clothing that covers the patient. Allow patient as much decision-making as is possible in the phase I PACU setting.	Surroundings that are friendly, family-focused, private, and apart from the view of other patients and staff.

Continued

■ TABLE 50-1
■ **Phase I PACU Patient Outcomes—cont'd**

Potential and Actual Problems (Nursing Diagnoses)	Outcome Goals (The Patient Will be Able to:)	Nursing Interventions	Resources
Risk of hemorrhage	Maintain blood volume at normal level. Avoid hypertension.	Ensure availability of intravenous solutions. Observe surgical site for signs of bleeding and report to physician. Administer anxiolytic and/or antihypertensive medications as ordered.	Blood bank contract and policies for rapid availability of blood products for freestanding ambulatory surgery unit Antihypertensive agents Anxiolytic medications IV fluids and supplies
Alterations in health that can complicate postanesthesia care	Provide honest preoperative information about any existing medical factors. Comply with instructions to optimize medical status before the day of surgery. Experience no complications related to prior medical status.	Encourage patient to provide complete and accurate information regarding health status and practices before surgery that may have a perianesthesia influence. Assess patient's physical status frequently. Use active listening and observe for clues to patient's health status. Review record and receive comprehensive report from anesthesia provider. Individualize patient care related to prior health status.	Structured preoperative time frame for physical and historical assessment Books and literature on patient assessment and various medical conditions Primary care physician available to assist in optimizing patient's health status before and after surgery
Risk of injury related to environment, equipment, positioning, medications, emergence delirium	Remain free from allergic reactions, burns, skin breakdown or pressure points, falls, or nerve or joint injuries. Complete phase I PACU experience without complications or injury.	Observe patient at all times. Reinforce patient's orientation to time. Identify symptoms of emergence delirium and intervene appropriately. Position patient according to acceptable standards of care and individual needs using proper body mechanics for staff and patient. Ensure that side rails remain in up position. Lock bed/stretcher wheels at all times while patient is on it. Keep only the current chart at the bedside. Check the emergency alarm system and emergency equipment regularly.	Patient record Competency-based nursing practice ASPAN *Standards of PeriAnesthesia Nursing Practice* Manufacturer's instructions for proper use of equipment Appropriate positioning supplies: pillows, padding, foam sheeting Ongoing program of preventive maintenance of equipment Ongoing safety programs for employees Policy on enacting Safe Medical Devices Act Soft restraint policy

Hypothermia Discomfort related to cold	Maintain normal body temperature. Avoid shivering. Verbalize comfort with temperature.	Assess and document patient's temperature on admission and periodically in phase I PACU. Keep patient covered as fully as possible, including head and neck areas. Apply warm blankets or use forced air warming equipment, especially on patients at high risk for hypothermia (infants and frail elderly).	ASPAN *Standards of PeriAnesthesia Nursing Practice* Cabinets for warming blankets and solutions Forced warmed air heating blankets Thermometers
Discomfort related to thirst	Express comfort.	Moisten the mouth if the patient is NPO. Give ice chips or sips of water initially if the patient is not NPO.	Physician's orders

ASPAN, American Society of PeriAnesthesia Nurses; *BP*, blood pressure; *GI*, gastrointestinal; *NPO*, nothing by mouth; *PACU*, post anesthesia care unit; *IV* intravenous.
Modified from Burden N, Quinn DMD, O'Brien D, et al: Ambulatory surgical nursing, ed 2, Philadelphia, 2000, Saunders.

E. Respiratory adequacy (see Chapter 31)
  1. Assessment
    a. Auscultation of bilateral breath sounds
    b. Assessment of bilateral chest expansion
      (1) Ease and depth of respirations
      (2) Use of accessory muscles
      (3) Skin and mucous membrane color
    c. Administration of oxygen
      (1) Considered standard treatment:
        (a) After heavy sedation or general anesthesia
        (b) According to patient needs
      (2) Usual means of delivery
        (a) Nasal cannula
        (b) Face mask
          (i) Simple
          (ii) Nonrebreather
          (iii) Aerosol
    d. Body's oxygen demand increases with:
      (1) Shivering, up to 400%
      (2) Pain
      (3) Anxiety
      (4) Fever
      (5) Hypotension/hypertension
      (6) Cardiac events
        (a) Tachydysrhythmias
        (b) Bradydysrhythmias
        (c) Left ventricular failure
      (7) Rapid fluctuations in intravascular volume
      (8) Thromboembolic event
      (9) Catecholamine release
  2. Monitoring methods
    a. Primary—registered nurse (RN)
      (1) Observation
      (2) Auscultation
      (3) Palpation
    b. Mechanical
      (1) Pulse oximetry
        (a) Considered a standard of care in anesthesia and PACU
        (b) Measurement of oxygenated hemoglobin to total hemoglobin; expressed as a percent
        (c) Sensitive to changes in oxygen content of blood; identifies hypoxic event before clinical signs become evident
        (d) Advantages
          (i) Ease of use
          (ii) Noninvasive
          (iii) Continuous display
          (iv) Applicable for all ages
          (v) Relatively low expense
        (e) Disadvantage in patients with:
          (i) Motion at sensor site
          (ii) Low perfusion of the arterial bed being monitored because of:
            [a] Hypothermia
            [b] Hypotension
            [c] Large doses of vasopressors/vasoconstriction
          (iii) Significant dysrhythmias
          (iv) Carbon monoxide or methemoglobin in the blood
          (v) Severe anemia with hemoglobin <5 g/dL
          (vi) Venous pulsation; sensor too tight

        (vii) Electrical interference

        (viii) Interference from ambient or extrinsic light source, IV dyes

   (f) Complications

        (i)   Burns/blisters usually involving infants/children

        (ii) Pressure ulcer from sensor

  (2) ETCO$_2$ (capnography)

   (a) Monitors adequacy of mechanical ventilation

   (b) Assesses intubation of trachea versus esophagus

   (c) Monitors integrity of the mechanical ventilator circuit and artificial airway

   (d) Rapid indicator of possible apnea

  (3) Arterial blood gas analysis

  (4) Respirometer

   (a) Used to determine readiness for extubation

   (b) Lung volume parameters

        (i)   Tidal volume

        (ii) Vital capacity

   (c) Negative inspiratory force (NIF)

3. Respiratory complications

  a. Hypoxemia from hypoventilation or apnea

  (1) Clinical signs

   (a) Unresponsiveness

   (b) Lethargy

   (c) Confusion

   (d) Restlessness

   (e) Anxiety

   (f) Dysrhythmias

   (g) Cyanosis

   (h) Decreased partial pressure of carbon dioxide in arterial blood (Paco$_2$) possibly leading to respiratory acidosis

   (i) Hypertension followed by hypotension

  (2) Determine exact cause for appropriate treatment.

  b. Treatment of hypoxia due to pharmacological causes

  (1) Opioids

   (a) Narcotic antagonist naloxone (Narcan)

        (i)   Adults

            [a] For respiratory depression: 1 mcg/kg (0.01 mcg/kg) IV and repeat in 5 to 10 minutes as needed

            [b] For apnea and pulselessness: 1 mg IV

        (ii) Infants and children: consult with anesthesiologist.

   (b) Side effects

        (i)   Cessation of analgesia

        (ii) Agitation

        (iii) Hypertension

        (iv) Noncardiogenic pulmonary edema

        (v) Atrial and ventricular dysrhythmias

        (vi) Cardiac arrest

        (vii) Resedation if circulating opioid remains after naloxone metabolized

  (2) Muscle relaxants

   (a) Depolarizing muscle relaxant: succinylcholine (Anectine)

        (i)   Short acting: 90 to 120 seconds

        (ii) Effects usually dissipate before admission to phase I PACU.

        (iii) Not pharmacologically reversible

        (iv) Metabolized by pseudocholinesterase

        (v) May develop a phase II block: mimics characteristics of nondepolarizing blockade in doses >3 mg/kg

   (b) Nondepolarizing muscle relaxants

(i) Reversed by anticholinesterase agents (neostigmine, pyridostigmine, or edrophonium)

(ii) Can cause vagal reactions (bradycardia)

(iii) Usually administered in combination with vagolytic agent (atropine or glycopyrrolate)

(c) Reparalysis (recurarization)

(i) Major cause of respiratory depression

(ii) Primarily due to inadequate pharmacological reversal

(iii) Other factors influencing effects of neuromuscular blockers

[a] General anesthetics

[b] Hypothermia

[c] Antidysrhythmics: quinidine, procainamide, calcium channel blockers

[d] Respiratory acidosis

[e] Metabolic alkalosis

[f] Hypokalemia

[g] Hypocalcemia

[h] Local anesthetic agents (including lidocaine given as an antidysrhythmic by IV drip or bolus postoperatively)

[i] Furosemide IV in doses of 1 mg/kg

[j] Dehydration

[k] Hyponatremia

[l] Antibiotics, particularly mycins, and aminoglycosides

(3) Benzodiazepines: diazepam (Valium), midazolam (Versed), lorazepam (Ativan)

(a) May cause dose-related respiratory depression

(b) Monitor airway patency, respiratory rate and depth.

(c) Use pulse oximetry and oxygen as appropriate.

4. Intubated patient not requiring artificial ventilator support

a. Nursing care

(1) Provide constant nursing observation.

(2) Administer humidified oxygen.

(a) Compensates for bypassed upper airway

(b) Provides moisture to artificially inspired air

(3) Protect patient from aspiration by maintaining cuff inflation.

(a) Position properly.

(b) Suction as appropriate.

(4) Ensure proper position of endotracheal tube.

(a) Auscultate breath sounds.

(b) Observe symmetrical chest expansion.

(c) Secure tube appropriately.

b. Extubation criteria

(1) Return of muscle strength after muscle relaxants have worn off

(a) Sustained equal hand grasps

(b) Sustained head lift from pillow for at least 5 seconds

(2) Respiratory parameters via respirometer if used

(a) Tidal volume at least 10 mL/kg

(b) Vital capacity at least 15 to 20 mL/kg

(c) NIF of 20 to 25 cm water pressure

(3) Ability to respond to requests as appropriate to age and condition

(a) Performs "yes" or "no" head movements appropriate for questions

(b) Indicates responses on a sign or picture board if appropriate

(c) Writes if able

(d) Protrudes tongue

(e) Opens eyes widely

(f) Swallows and coughs

(g) Regular respiratory rate >10 breaths/min

    c. Precautions after extubation

        (1) Observe closely for hypoventilation.

        (2) Presence of endotracheal tube (ETT) may have stimulated the patient to remain awake, breathing adequately.

F. Circulatory adequacy

  1. Cardiac status

    a. Constant assessment of pulse for rate, rhythm, amplitude

      (1) Causes of a weak, absent, or irregular pulses

        (a) Hypovolemia

        (b) Decreased cardiac output

        (c) Myocardial ischemia

          (i) Prior cardiac compromise increases risk of cardiac complications from anesthesia.

          (ii) Observe for clinical signs of myocardial ischemia.

            [a] Chest pain

            [b] Change in skin color

            [c] Diaphoresis

            [d] Gastrointestinal (GI) sequelae

            [e] ECG changes

        (d) Acute myocardial infarction (MI)

          (i) Previous MI is the single most important risk factor.

            [a] Nonurgent surgery should be delayed at least 6 months post-MI to reduce perioperative morbidity.

            [b] Patients receiving beta-blocker therapy should continue on regular regimen during perioperative period.

          (ii) Most often seen in elderly, diabetic, and hypertensive patients

          (iii) Early ECG signs of perioperative acute infarction or ischemia

            [a] T-wave inversion or ST-segment depression of 1 mm or more below baseline is indicative of ischemia.

            [b] ST elevation indicates actual myocardial injury.

            [c] ST and T-wave changes may be caused by digitalis therapy, hypothermia, electrolyte abnormalities, or dysrhythmias.

            [d] Cardiac dysrhythmias

          (iv) Clinical signs and symptoms

            [a] Subjective changes described by patient

            [b] Anginal pain (often constant); only 25% of patients who have MIs in the postoperative period experience typical angina pain.

            [c] Feeling of impending doom or dying

            [d] Nausea, vomiting

            [e] Diaphoresis

      (2) Causes of a bounding pulse include:

        (a) Excitement

        (b) Hypertension

        (c) Fluid overload

        (d) Assess the elderly especially for:

          (i) Uncompensated congestive heart failure

          (ii) Pulmonary edema

  2. Peripheral circulation assessment

    a. Peripheral pulses as indicated based on location of surgery

    b. Changes indicate impaired peripheral circulation.

      (1) Color

      (2) Temperature

      (3) Sensation

      (4) Movement

      (5) Pain

G. Fluid and electrolyte balance

  1. Most patients can compensate for fasting and intraoperative fluid losses by adequate and appropriate fluid replacement.

2. Assess daily fluid requirements.
   a. Children's fluid replacement based on weight
      (1) <10 kg: 100 mL/kg
      (2) 10 to 20 kg: 1000 mL + 50 mL/kg for each additional kilogram between 10 and 20 kg
      (3) ≥20 kg: 1500 mL + 20 mL/kg for each additional kilogram over 20 kg
   b. Adults' fluid replacement based on:
      (1) Deficit: time patient has nothing by mouth (NPO) to time surgery begins
      (2) Maintenance: depends on type and length of surgical procedure
      (3) Blood loss
      (4) Invasive tube drainage
3. Patients at risk for homeostatic imbalance
   a. Small children
   b. Adults with disease processes involving the following systems:
      (1) Renal
      (2) GI
      (3) Endocrine
      (4) Cardiovascular
   c. Elderly
4. Other factors related to fluid and electrolyte disturbances
   a. Stress
      (1) Fear
      (2) Anxiety
   b. GI disturbances
      (1) Nausea and vomiting
      (2) Nasogastric suctioning
      (3) Bowel preparation causing loss of sodium and potassium
      (4) Poor nutrition
   c. Excessive bleeding
5. Blood and blood products
   a. May be required if patient experiences any of the following conditions:
      (1) Excessive preoperative or intraoperative blood loss
      (2) Development of blood-related problems
         (a) Idiopathic thrombocytopenia
         (b) Disseminated intravascular coagulation
         (c) Preexisting coagulation disorder
   b. Types of donated blood
      (1) Nondirected donated blood
      (2) Autologous blood
      (3) Directed donor blood (donated by others for a specific patient)
      (4) Specific blood products may be donated for specific disorders.
   c. Other options for transfusion
      (1) Intraoperative blood salvage
         (a) Blood lost by a patient processed by centrifuge, then returned to the patient
         (b) Often approved by a Jehovah's Witness patient if the blood not processed outside the OR
      (2) Autotransfusion devices
         (a) Patient's lost blood collected for transfusion into the same patient
         (b) Blood collection takes place over 2 to 4 hours and is transfused over 2 hours.
         (c) Often used during joint replacements and cardiac surgery
6. Transfusion precaution
   a. No difference in procedures for autologous or allogeneic transfusions
      (1) Secure blood from blood bank.
      (2) Identify patient.
      (3) Identify blood bag.

       (a) Two nurses identify patient and blood bag.
       (b) One RN and another professional may substitute for identification.
           (i) Certified Registered Nurse Anesthetist (CRNA)
           (ii) Physician
    (4) Initiate transfusion.
       (a) Monitor patient throughout the transfusion including temperature.
       (b) Observe for untoward reactions.
           (i) Volume overload
           (ii) Bacterial contamination causing sepsis
           (iii) Air emboli
           (iv) Venous emboli
           (v) Hypotension
           (vi) Hypocalcemia; citrate intoxication
           (vii) Hypersensitivity to plastics or stabilizers in tubing and bag
           (viii) Anaphylaxis, hemolytic reactions, urticaria
           (ix) Chest tightness or pain
           (x) Dyspnea
           (xi) Hyperthermia
           (xii) Wheezing

b. In the event of an untoward reaction:
  (1) Discontinue the infusion immediately.
  (2) Maintain a patent IV line with new tubing and solution.
  (3) Notify physician.
  (4) Monitor vital signs.
  (5) Administer oxygen.
  (6) Diphenhydramine (Benadryl) is the antihistamine of choice.
  (7) Policies may require urine and blood specimens be sent to the blood bank with tubing and remaining blood in bag for analysis.

7. Nonblood volume expanders
  a. Dextran: synthetic plasma substitute
    (1) Advantages
       (a) Administered through standard IV tubing
       (b) Relatively inexpensive
       (c) Readily available
       (d) No risk of communicable disease
    (2) Disadvantages
       (a) Hypersensitivity reactions, usually in first 30 minutes of infusion
       (b) Interference with platelet function causing transient, prolonged bleeding time
       (c) Affects some methods of typing and crossmatching
  b. Hetastarch (Hespan): artificial colloid
    (1) Inexpensive
    (2) Derived from cornstarch; closely resembles human glycogen
    (3) Available in 6% in 0.9% sodium chloride solution
    (4) Minimal coagulation effects
    (5) Less likely to produce allergic reactions

8. Oral intake
  a. Observe physician's orders regarding NPO status.
  b. Assess patient's readiness to drink fluids.
    (1) Awake and sufficiently alert
    (2) All protective reflexes present: cough, gag, swallowing
    (3) No nausea
  c. Elevate head of bed to facilitate swallowing without choking.
  d. Offer water or ginger ale in small amount.
    (1) Discourage rapid ingestion.
    (2) Citrus juice and coffee may cause nausea.
  e. Continue IV fluids until oral intake well tolerated

  H. Urinary status

    1. Adequate urinary output is necessary to excrete waste products.

      a. Optimal amounts to ensure kidney function and adequate hydration

        (1) Infant to 2 years: >2 to 3 mL/kg per hour

        (2) 3 to 6 years: >1 to 2 mL/kg per hour

        (3) 7 to 12 years: 0.5 to 1 mL/kg per hour

        (4) Adults: 30 mL/hr

      b. Urine production can decrease as a result of:

        (1) Hypovolemia

        (2) Hypothermia

        (3) Body's reaction to stress

    2. Urinary retention

      a. Assess bladder for distention after any of the following:

        (1) Urinary procedures

        (2) Inguinal herniorrhaphy

        (3) Gynecological procedures

        (4) Spinal and epidural anesthesia

        (5) Use of local anesthesia surrounding pelvic structures

        (6) Surgical manipulation

        (7) Spinal cord surgery

      b. Symptoms of bladder distention

        (1) Restlessness

        (2) Lower abdominal pain

        (3) Hypertension

        (4) Tachycardia

        (5) Anxiety

        (6) Tachypnea

        (7) Diaphoresis

      c. May require catheterization

      d. Urination may be required for home discharge per physician's order or policy.

        (1) Transfer patient from phase I PACU if not distended or uncomfortable.

        (2) Allow patient to use bathroom if sufficiently alert, and assess adequacy of output.

 I. Temperature regulation (see Chapter 24)

    1. Normothermia

      a. Hypothalamus is the regulatory center.

        (1) Normal core temperature: 36° C to 38° C (96.8° F to 100.4° F)

        (2) Conversion formulas

          (a) $F = (C \times 9/5) + 32$

          (b) $C = (F - 32) \times 5/9$

      b. Major sites of body heat production

        (1) Muscles: 25%

        (2) Liver: 50%

        (3) Glands: 15%

    2. Hypothermia

      a. Heat loss mechanisms in surgery

        (1) Conduction

          (a) Heat transferred from body to cold surfaces

          (b) Accounts for up to 10% of heat loss

        (2) Convection

          (a) Heat loss to air current

          (b) Accounts for 25% to 35% heat loss

        (3) Radiation

          (a) Electromagnetic energy loss to colder objects in room

          (b) Accounts for 40% to 60% heat loss

        (4) Evaporation

          (a) From skin and through respiratory system

          (b) May account for up to 25% heat loss

    b. Nearly all patients become hypothermic unless actively warmed intraoperatively.
        (1) Mild hypothermia: core temperature <36° C (<96.8° F)
        (2) Significant hypothermia: core temperature <35° C (<95° F)
            (a) Planned
            (b) Unplanned
    c. Factors affecting body temperature in surgery
        (1) Patient weight: thin patients lose more heat than heavier patients.
        (2) Length of surgery and exposure of skin and internal structures
        (3) Surgical site, especially peritoneal exposure
        (4) IV infusion of fluids at room temperature
        (5) Cool irrigation and skin preparation solutions
        (6) Ambient room temperature
            (a) Constant air circulation creates cooling effect on room temperature.
                (i)   Children aged 6 months to 2 years have a greater degree of heat loss because of larger body surface area compared with muscle mass.
                (ii) Elderly generally have shrinking muscle mass and decreasing subcutaneous fat layers.
            (b) OR temperature normally 24° C (68° F)
    d. Anesthesia-related factors affecting heat loss
        (1) Depressed thermoregulatory center
        (2) Neuromuscular relaxants stop muscle activity, preventing shivering.
        (3) Inhalation agents
            (a) Respiratory heat loss from unwarmed oxygen and inhalation gas delivery
            (b) Vasodilating effects
    e. Prevention of heat loss in surgery
        (1) Raise room temperature, especially for newborns and premature babies.
        (2) Heated blankets/forced air heat
        (3) Head covering; more than 50% of body heat may be lost as radiation from scalp.
        (4) Foil blankets to prevent radiation of patient's body heat
        (5) Warmed preparation fluids, IV fluids, and irrigation fluids
        (6) Warmed oxygen delivery system
    f. Effects of hypothermia
        (1) Slows metabolic rate so effects of medications greatly enhanced
        (2) Active medication remains in the body longer.
        (3) Less medication needed to produce desired effect
    g. Treatment of hypothermia in PACU
        (1) Observe for cyanosis of extremities.
            (a) Distant vessels vasoconstrict to conserve heat.
            (b) Dysrhythmias may be secondary to hypothermia.
            (c) Reparalysis (recurarization): dose of reversal agents in hypothermic patients is no longer effective when metabolic rate increases in response to a warmer temperature.
        (2) Warming measures
            (a) Increase ambient room temperature: minimum of 20° C to 24° C (68° F to 75° F).
            (b) Radiant heat
            (c) Heated blankets/forced air heat; cover head and torso.
            (d) Warmed oxygen as appropriate
            (e) IV fluids at room temperature or warmed
3. Shivering
    a. Major mechanism of heat production
    b. Can occur spontaneously without known cause in normothermic and hypothermic patients
    c. Uncomfortable and unpleasant for the awakening patient

      d. Untoward effects
        (1) Hypertension
        (2) Injury to operative site or teeth
        (3) Increased oxygen demand up to 400%
        (4) Prolonged phase I PACU time, additional supplies and medications
        (5) Diffuse muscle aches
          (a) Determine intensity of involvement.
          (b) Patient may require analgesia unrelated to surgical site/procedure.
      e. Treatment
        (1) Oxygen therapy
        (2) Medications
          (a) Narcotic: meperidine (Demerol)—80% effectiveness with 12.5 to 25-mg IV dose
          (b) Opiate agonist-antagonist analgesic: butorphanol tartrate (Stadol)—95% effective within 5 minutes
        (3) Warming devices if shivering related to low temperature
          (a) Infants burn brown fat to increase body temperature without shivering.
    4. Malignant hyperthermia
      a. Serious hypermetabolic state
        (1) Genetic origin
        (2) Triggered by certain inhalational anesthetic agents and the depolarizing muscle relaxant, succinylcholine (Anectine)
      b. Treatment as outlined by the Malignant Hyperthermia Association of the United States (MHAUS)
  J. Level of consciousness
    1. Unconscious patient should never be left alone.
      a. Protective reflexes and cognitive abilities absent
      b. Patient totally dependent on phase I PACU nurse for environmental protection
    2. Hearing is the first sense to return upon awakening.
      a. Speak in calm, low tones to arouse and orient the semiconscious patient.
      b. Continue periodic attempts until patient responds except in case of upper airway obstruction.
        (1) Signs include gagging, coughing.
        (2) Treatment
          (a) Administer oxygen.
          (b) Position to avoid aspiration.
          (c) Allow slow awakening without intervention to decrease risk of laryngospasm.
    3. Use of ketamine (Ketalar)
      a. May cause severe delirium/hallucinations
      b. Treatment
        (1) Medication per order of anesthesia provider
          (a) Diazepam (Valium): 5 to 10 mg IV
          (b) Thiopental (Sodium Pentothal): 50 to 75 mg IV
        (2) Protective environment
          (a) Raised side rails
          (b) Monitor, but avoid unnecessary stimulation (e.g., bright lights, laughter, personal conversations).
    4. Emergence delirium (emergence excitement)
      a. Symptoms
        (1) Restlessness, thrashing of extremities
        (2) Combativeness
        (3) Crying, moaning, screaming
        (4) Irrational talking, disorientation
      b. Causes
        (1) Preoperative medications
        (2) Pain

        (3) Bladder distention

        (4) Feelings of suffocation during awakening

        (5) Possible cerebral hypoxia

        (6) Preoperative psychological status

            (a) Fear of surgery or of a surgical diagnosis

            (b) Fear of body disfigurement, particularly in children and adolescents

  c. Untoward effects

        (1) Injury to limbs, tongue

        (2) Straining, opening suture lines

        (3) Dislodging IV lines

        (4) Self-extubation

  d. Treatment

        (1) Monitor, but avoid unnecessary stimulation (e.g., bright lights, laughter, personal conversations).

        (2) Have one person speak softly to patient.

        (3) Provide safe environment.

            (a) Gentle physical restraint as necessary; total physical restraint may increase agitation.

            (b) Pad side rails to prevent patient injury.

        (4) Medication per order of anesthesia provider

            (a) Benzodiazepines

                (i) Midazolam (Versed)

                (ii) Lorazepam (Ativan)

            (b) Opioids if indicated

            (c) Physostigmine (Antilirium)

                (i) Use is controversial as reversal agent to end emergence delirium.

                (ii) May be used to reverse effects of scopolamine or other anticholinergic drugs

                    [a] Give incremental 1-mg IV doses slowly.

                    [b] Do not exceed total of 3 mg.

                (iii) Can cause bradycardia

5. Delayed awakening

  a. Causes—impaired metabolism, ventilation, or circulation as a result of:

        (1) Type and amount of preoperative medication

            (a) Benzodiazepines

            (b) Neuroleptic agents

            (c) Opioids

            (d) Barbiturates

        (2) Intraoperative medications

            (a) Inhalation agents

            (b) Opioids

            (c) Barbiturates

        (3) Other preoperative medications and herbal supplements

        (4) Hypothermia

        (5) Hyperthermia/malignant hyperthermia

        (6) Metabolic diseases

        (7) Pseudocholinesterase deficiency

        (8) Cardiovascular pathology

            (a) Hypertension

            (b) Hypovolemia

            (c) Myocardial ischemia

        (9) Respiratory inadequacy

            (a) Opioid induced

            (b) Pathological in nature

        (10) Increased intracranial pressure

        (11) Undiagnosed intraoperative seizure

  b. Treatment: according to cause

K. Positioning
    1. Ensure proper body alignment.
    2. Provide comfort and safety.
        a. Prevent aspiration; position laterally if appropriate.
        b. Support patient's head and neck.
        c. Position extremities to avoid damage to nerves, tendons, and muscles.
        d. Avoid hyperextension of joints.
        e. Separate opposing skin surfaces with padding.
        f. In the event of prolonged unconsciousness:
            (1) Provide gentle passive range-of-motion exercises.
            (2) Reposition frequently.
    3. Promote cardiovascular and respiratory homeostasis.
        a. Reposition slowly to avoid compromise.
        b. Reassess after repositioning.
    4. Special surgery-specific positioning
        a. Extremities
            (1) Elevate above heart level to reduce risk of bleeding and edema.
            (2) Decreases pain
        b. Plastic surgery
            (1) Fowler's position generally ordered for head, face, neck, breast, and abdominal surgery to reduce risk of bleeding and edema
            (2) Surgeon may order special positioning to reduce strain on suture line.
        c. Eye and ear surgery: usually surgeon specific
L. Operative site
    1. Assess wounds/dressings.
        a. General bleeding
            (1) Obvious bloody drainage
            (2) Rapid filling of collection system
            (3) Bruising/abnormal skin discoloration
            (4) Swelling or unanticipated firmness without obvious bruising or bleeding
            (5) Excessive swallowing after ear, nose, or throat procedures; subjective complaints of drainage in back of throat
            (6) Heavy vaginal flow
            (7) Excessive hematuria
        b. Intra-abdominal bleeding
            (1) May not appear until blood loss is significant
            (2) Signs and symptoms
                (a) Apprehension
                (b) Hypotension
                (c) Increased abdominal girth
                (d) Tachycardia
                (e) Splinting
                (f) Abdominal pain
                (g) Tenderness and rigidity
                (h) Pallor
                (i) Diaphoresis
                (j) Frequent urination of small amounts or sense of urgency without voiding
                (k) Depressed level of consciousness
                (l) In neurological procedures: unexpected loss of sense or movement
        c. Laparoscopic procedures
            (1) Particularly at risk for occult bleeding
            (2) Potential for laceration or inadvertent burning of abdominal vessels or organs
            (3) Cold laparoscopic gas may vasoconstrict initially, resulting in delayed bleeding after warming.

2. Treatment
   a. Assure and reassure patient.
   b. Initiate measures to reduce or stop any excessive bleeding.
   c. Notify anesthesiology department.
      (1) Manual pressure if possible
      (2) Elevate site if possible.
      (3) Specific protocols
         (a) Ice or cool compresses to affected area
         (b) Increase IV rate; may need a second IV line
         (c) Vasopressor agents
         (d) Blood replacement with colloids or blood products
         (e) Oxygen
         (f) Sedation if needed
      (4) Airway involvement
         (a) Position appropriately.
         (b) Suction mouth gently for oral bleeding.
   d. Notify surgeon to return if unable to control bleeding.
   e. Patient may return to surgery to control bleeding.
      (1) Consent must be obtained from family member if not included in original consent.
      (2) Sedated patients cannot sign a legal document.
M. Peripheral circulation
   1. Assess surgically involved extremities for circulatory adequacy.
   2. Considerations
      a. Constriction causing circulatory compromise may be due to:
         (1) Tight encircling wraps: ACE bandage or cast
         (2) Thrombus
         (3) Embolus
         (4) Internal pressure
         (5) Hemorrhage
      b. Peripheral pulses
         (1) Palpate bilaterally for presence, strength, symmetry.
         (2) Numerical description
            (a) Absent = 0
            (b) Weak and thready = 1+
            (c) Normal = 2+
            (d) Full and bounding = 3+
         (3) If not palpable:
            (a) Reposition extremity and palpate pulse site again.
            (b) Use Doppler ultrasound stethoscope if necessary.
               (i) Noninvasive
               (ii) Uses sound-wave frequency to detect blood movement in underlying vessels
      c. Pulse oximeter gives a visual indication of pulse strength in the affected extremity.
      d. Color of skin and nail bed
         (1) Vasoconstriction in a hypothermic patient may mimic cyanosis resulting from more severe causes.
         (2) Blanching or redness from an intraoperative tourniquet in phase I PACU
      e. Capillary refill
         (1) When blanched by pressure, color normally returns to nail bed or distal area of skin in 3 seconds.
         (2) Helpful when dressings on an extremity permit only visual evaluation of digit tips
N. Analgesia (see Chapter 26)
   1. Pain is a complex phenomenon.
      a. Types of pain

     (1) Visceral
       (a) Poorly localized and distant quality
       (b) Nociceptors activated in visceral tissues
     (2) Somatic
       (a) Well localized with familiar quality
       (b) Nociceptors activated in somatic tissue
     (3) Neuropathic
       (a) Localized in distribution of central nervous system or peripheral nerve tract
       (b) Experienced as burning, squeezing, or sensory loss, numbness
       (c) Multiple mechanisms including peripheral nerve compression, sensory ganglion inflammatory changes, demyelization of sensory tracts

b. Requirements for pain production
     (1) Transduction
       (a) Mediators released at tissue injury site
       (b) Mediators stimulate peripheral sensory afferent nerves extending to dorsal horn of spinal cord.
     (2) Transmission: peripheral sensory afferents stimulate ascending nerves running from dorsal horn of spinal cord to brain.
     (3) Modulation
       (a) Descending pathways from brain to dorsal horn modulate activity of peripheral nerves.
       (b) Enkephalins and endorphins released
     (4) Perception of pain: occurs in brain reflecting whether pain is amplified or suppressed

c. Pain is a personal experience for each individual.
     (1) Varies for the same person at different times; varies among people
     (2) Patient's self-report of pain is most reliable assessment tool.

d. Emotional impact of pain may be affected by preoperative education.
     (1) General description of reasonable expectations for pain
     (2) Direct relationship exists between preoperative education and decreased analgesic needs.
       (a) Less fear
       (b) Decreased feeling of powerlessness
       (c) Earlier ambulation
     (3) Analgesia must be balanced with sedation.
       (a) Multimodal approach provides better pain relief than would be possible with any single agent.
       (b) Side effects are dose related.
     (4) Reassure patient that PACU discharge will not be attempted without adequate pain relief.

2. Factors influencing postoperative pain
  a. Patient's perception and expectations
  b. Patient's preoperative medical condition
  c. Social issues
     (1) Cultural influences
       (a) Expressions of pain
       (b) Acceptance of pain management techniques
     (2) Family/significant others' interaction may affect pain expression and management.
  d. Psychosocial factors
  e. Surgical site
  f. Surgical procedure and techniques
  g. Anesthesia and adjuncts
  h. Other sources
     (1) Bladder distention
     (2) Gastric distention

(3) Uncomfortable positioning
(4) IV and hemodynamic monitoring sites
(5) Drainage tubes
 (a) Chest tubes
 (b) Jackson-Pratt
 (c) Autotransfusion devices
(6) Postoperative complications
 (a) Embolic events
 (b) Myocardial ischemia or infarction
 (c) Pulmonary ischemia
 (d) Hemorrhage
 (e) Ruptured viscus

3. Pain is subjective.
 a. Only patients are aware of the amount of pain they are experiencing.
 b. Objective observations are only clues.
  (1) Changes in vital signs
   (a) Hypertension
   (b) Tachycardia
   (c) Tachypnea
  (2) Restlessness
  (3) Facial expression
  (4) Splinting
  (5) Posturing
  (6) Mood
  (7) Voice
  (8) Refusal to be repositioned
 c. Nursing responsibilities
  (1) Assess pain thoroughly.
   (a) Location
   (b) Intensity using pain scale appropriate for age and cognitive level
    (i) Numerical (0-10)
    (ii) Wong-Baker FACES (smiling-crying)
    (iii) Colors (blue-red)
    (iv) VAS (Visual Analogue Scale: no pain to pain as bad as it could possibly be)
    (v) FLACC (Face, Legs, Activity, Cry, Consolation)
     [a] Each area rated 0 to 2 for total score of 0 to 10 with 0 = best, 10 = worst
     [b] Particularly useful for preverbal or nonverbal child
    (vi) CRIES score (Crying, Requires O_2 for Sao_2 >95%, Increased vital signs from preoperative values, Expression, Sleepless)
     [a] For neonates through infants 6 months of age
     [b] Each consideration rated 0 to 2 with 0 = best, 10 = worst
     [c] Intervention recommended when a baby's score = 4
   (c) Description, if patient is able to provide
    (i) Sharp or dull
    (ii) Aching, throbbing, or burning
    (iii) Piercing or stabbing
   (d) Duration
   (e) Aggravating influences
   (f) Alleviating influences
  (2) Take appropriate action.

4. Postoperative expectations of patient/family
 a. Patient's analgesic needs will be met.
 b. Plan for pain management is in place before discharge from PACU.

5. Nonpharmacological techniques to relieve pain in PACU
 a. Proper body alignment and positioning
 b. Ice to affected area if indicated

    c. Soothing reassurance

    d. Hand-holding and gently touching patient's shoulder

        (1) Pain often exacerbated by fear and anxiety

        (2) Ask patient's preference and get permission to touch.

        (3) Consider cultural norms.

        (4) Awake patients: incorporate positive encouragement of relaxation.

            (a) Distraction techniques

                (i)   Rhythmic deep breathing

                (ii) Counting slowly

                (iii) Guided imagery: pleasant visions, sounds, smells

                (iv) Music

                (v) Visiting with family/friends

            (b) Requires:

                (i)   Patient acceptance

                (ii) Nursing skills

                (iii) Preoperative discussion and practice

6. Types of analgesia

    a. Types used are jointly determined by anesthesiologist and surgeon based on:

        (1) Patient's general condition

        (2) Type and length of procedure

        (3) Anticipated short- and long-term course/analgesic needs

        (4) Patient's desired level and means of comfort

    b. Multimodal balanced analgesia may be most effective approach.

        (1) Nonsteroidal anti-inflammatory drugs

        (2) Oral, IV opioids

        (3) Epidural and intrathecal opioids

        (4) Transdermal, transmucosal, opioids

        (5) Local infiltration and regional anesthesia

        (6) Transcutaneous electrical nerve stimulators

7. Nursing care relative to analgesic administration

    a. Observe proper precautions.

        (1) Correct patient

        (2) Correct medication

        (3) Correct dose based on:

            (a) Weight

            (b) Medication history relative to analgesics/sedatives

            (c) Heavy alcohol, tobacco, or drug use

        (4) Correct route of administration at correct site

        (5) Correct time

        (6) Check for allergies/sensitivities, contraindications, and incompatibilities.

        (7) Adhere to anesthesia/departmental policy.

    b. Consider preoperative and intraoperative medications and time administered.

    c. Relieve pain but avoid oversedation.

    d. Follow anesthesia protocol.

    e. Monitor closely; take appropriate action for adverse effects.

        (1) Respiratory depression/hypoxia

        (2) Hypotension

        (3) Increased level of sedation/inability to arouse readily

        (4) Postoperative nausea and vomiting (PONV)

        (5) Sensitivity/allergic reactions

        (6) Pruritus, especially with intrathecally administered opioids

        (7) Urinary retention/bladder distention

        (8) Skin irritation at pressure points

        (9) Spinal hematoma after epidural anesthesia

      (10) Nerve damage after a peripheral nerve block

8. Untoward effects of inadequate analgesia

       a. Gaps in epidural opioid administration/pain relief
         (1) Causes
            (a) Improper catheter placement
            (b) Catheter kinks
            (c) Medication leaks
            (d) Inadvertent catheter removal
            (e) Malfunction of pump
         (2) Notify anesthesiologist immediately if following symptoms occur:
            (a) Increased pain
            (b) Redness, swelling, pain, or discharge at catheter site
            (c) Dizziness or lightheadedness
            (d) Blurred vision
            (e) Ringing or buzzing in ears
            (f) Metal taste in mouth
            (g) Numbness or tingling around mouth, fingers, or toes
            (h) Nausea or vomiting
            (i) Drowsiness or confusion
       b. Respiratory dysfunction
         (1) Secondary to wound splinting
         (2) Shallow respirations leading to respiratory acidosis
       c. Tachycardia
       d. Hypertension
       e. Increased peripheral resistance
       f. Increased cardiac output
       g. Increased myocardial oxygen demand
       h. Gastric stasis
         (1) Paralytic ileus
         (2) Increased incidence of PONV
         (3) Risk of aspiration
       i. Endocrine and metabolical changes
     9. Advantages of adequate pain relief
       a. Patient comfort
       b. Patient/family satisfaction
       c. Reduced patient stress, a major cause of postoperative morbidity
       d. Timely discharge from hospital/ambulatory care facility
       e. Facilitates patient convalescence
       f. Can positively impact a patient's long-term prognosis
O. PONV (see Chapter 25)
     1. Disadvantages
       a. Major source of patient discomfort, fear, and dissatisfaction
       b. Incidence
         (1) For patients undergoing anesthesia: 20% to 30%
         (2) For patients at high risk: 80%
       c. Contributes to postoperative complications: aspiration, electrolyte imbalance
       d. Increases cost of care: medications, time, professional intervention
       e. Delays patient recovery and return to work
     2. Risk factors
       a. Patient-specific
         (1) Female gender
         (2) Nonsmoking status
         (3) History of PONV
         (4) Motion sickness
         (5) Obesity, presence of hiatal hernia
       b. Anesthetic-related
         (1) Use of volatile anesthetics
         (2) Use of nitrous oxide
            (a) Gravitates to any air-filled area of stomach and bowel
            (b) Collects in middle ear affecting the vestibular system
         (3) Administration of postoperative opioids

    c. Surgery-related
      (1) Duration of surgery and anesthesia
      (2) Type of surgery
        (a) Laparoscopy
        (b) Ovum retrieval
        (c) Abdominal procedures
        (d) Orchiopexy
        (e) Ear, nose, and throat: results from blood entering stomach
  3. Sequence of events and signs
    a. Nausea: unpleasant sensation usually preceding vomiting
      (1) Excessive salivation and swallowing
      (2) Dilated pupils
      (3) Tachypnea
      (4) Pallor and sweating
      (5) Tachycardia
    b. Retching: involuntary attempt to vomit
      (1) Nausea worsens.
      (2) Tachycardia may change to bradycardia.
    c. Vomiting: oral ejection of gastric contents
  4. Nursing interventions
    a. Nonpharmacological
      (1) Allow patient to awaken slowly.
        (a) Avoid aggressive stimulation.
        (b) Move patient slowly.
      (2) Position to prevent aspiration: head down, lateral unless otherwise ordered.
        (a) Apply oxygen to prevent respiratory compromise.
        (b) Provide emesis basin.
        (c) Have suction equipment available for gentle oral suctioning.
      (3) Maintain ETT cuff, removing the tube and oral airway when safe to limit upper airway irritation.
      (4) Continue to monitor.
        (a) Provide privacy if vomiting.
        (b) Assess, especially by auscultating the chest bilaterally.
        (c) Report any possible aspiration of vomitus to the physician.
      (5) Place cool washcloth on forehead.
      (6) Encourage to deep breathe when responding.
      (7) Eliminate noxious odors; offer aromatherapy—isopropyl alcohol, peppermint oil.
      (8) Place in a calm environment and offer words of encouragement.
      (9) Ensure adequate hydration with IV fluids.
    b. Pharmacological interventions
      (1) American Society of PeriAnesthesia Nurses (ASPAN), in conjunction with the American Society of Anesthesiologists (ASA), has developed evidence-based protocol for:
        (a) Preoperative patient management—PONV easier to prevent than treat
        (b) Postoperative management of PONV—phase I PACU/phase II PACU
      (2) Adhere to department protocol.
P. Special needs of patients after select anesthetic techniques
  1. Patients undergoing certain blocks may bypass phase I PACU as long as they meet phase I PACU assessment and phase I discharge criteria.
    a. Brachial plexus
    b. Intravenous
    c. Periorbital
  2. Patients undergoing regional anesthesia
    a. Admitted to phase I PACU:
      (1) Until their condition is stable
      (2) Until effects of anesthesia have passed

b. Types of regional anesthesia
- (1) Spinal anesthesia
  - (a) Technically easier and less time-consuming
  - (b) Appropriate for ambulatory surgery patients
- (2) Epidural anesthesia
  - (a) Ability to control titration of medication through a continuous catheter
  - (b) Low incidence of foreign/infectious material into cerebrospinal fluid

3. Complications after spinal or epidural anesthesia

a. Hypotension
- (1) Vasodilation of a large portion of vasculature
  - (a) Arteries and arterioles unable to constrict because of sympathetic block
  - (b) Compensatory mechanism lost
  - (c) Blood pools in lower extremities.
- (2) Maintain IV fluids until full motor and sensory function return.
- (3) Aggressive therapy includes ephedrine, 10 to 25 mg IV, diluted and given slowly.

b. Tachycardia

c. Bradycardia

d. Hypothermia
- (1) Due to peripheral dilation
- (2) Warm slowly to decrease risk of hypotension.

e. Pressure injury
- (1) Maintain proper body alignment, repositioning occasionally.
- (2) Elevate heels from mattress to avoid tissue trauma.
- (3) Provide gentle passive range-of-motion movement.

f. Epidural hematoma
- (1) Hemorrhage at injection site a rare complication
- (2) Internal pressure from hematoma can result in permanent neurological damage.
- (3) Symptoms
  - (a) Rapid onset of neurological deficits after block has begun resolving
  - (b) Severe back pain
- (4) Surgical intervention must occur within 12 hours to prevent permanent damage.

g. High or total spinal
- (1) Involves cardiac and/or respiratory function and upper extremities
  - (a) Incidence is rare.
  - (b) May be caused by:
    - (i) Increased intrathecal pressure from coughing or straining
    - (ii) Too rapid injection or too large a volume injected
    - (iii) Patient placed in head-down position before anesthetic agent has set at intended spinal level
- (2) Treatment initiated in OR and continues in phase I PACU
  - (a) Mechanical ventilation
  - (b) IV fluids
  - (c) Vasopressors for hypotension
  - (d) Atropine or glycopyrrolate (Robinul) for bradycardia
  - (e) Emotional support

h. Postdural puncture (spinal) headache (PDPH)
- (1) Initially, fluids and caffeine may help.
- (2) May require epidural blood patch for unrelieved headache

i. Bladder distention
- (1) Signs/symptoms
  - (a) Restlessness
  - (b) Hypotension

(c) Bradycardia

(d) May or may not feel suprapubic pain depending on level of sensory block

(2) Treatment

(a) Have patient void if possible.

(b) Catheterize if necessary.

(c) Provide specific follow-up instructions.

4. The order of regional block takes effect as follows:

a. Sympathetic functions

(1) Vasomotor

(2) Bladder control

b. Temperature

c. Pain

d. Touch

e. Movement

f. Pressure

g. Proprioception

5. Resolution of regional anesthetic effect

a. The return of the regional block functions is the reverse of how it took effect, i.e., proprioception →→ sympathetic function as identified above.

b. Major dermatome levels

(1) T4 – nipple line

(2) T10 – umbilicus

(3) L1 – groin

(4) L4 – knees

Q. Emotional and psychological support

1. Should begin preoperatively

2. Must continue throughout patient's surgical experience

a. PACU nurse is the first line of security after surgery/anesthesia.

(1) Use positive language to promote a sense of wellness.

(2) Read the patient's body language.

(3) Anticipate and verify patient's needs.

(4) Address the patient's concerns.

(a) Pathology or surgical outcome

(b) Family or friends who are waiting: follow facility policy for visitation in phase I PACU (Box 50-7).

(c) Ability to manage pain satisfactorily after PACU discharge

(d) Home care plans

b. Contact necessary support staff for patient during stay as appropriate.

(1) Interpreter

■ BOX 50-7
■ **VISITATION IN PHASE I PACU**

A growing body of nursing research supports family visitation and presence at the bedside. ASPAN supports family visitation in phase I PACU with guidelines for development:

- Appropriate education for patients and families regarding visitation to maintain a safe and beneficial experience
- The confidentiality and privacy of all patients shall be maintained.
- The visit will take place at an appropriate time for the patient, visitor, and clinical staff.
- Perianesthesia nurses should work together with hospital administration to establish a well-organized family visitation program supported by appropriate personnel to meet needs of families in this unique setting.

ASPAN, American Society of PeriAnesthesia Nurses; *PACU,* post anesthesia care unit.
Modified from American Society of PeriAnesthesia Nurses: *Standards of perianesthesia nursing practice 2008-2010,* Cherry Hill, NJ, 2008, American Society of PeriAnesthesia Nurses.

    (2) Pastoral care

    (3) Social worker

   c. Enforce privacy and reassure the patient of confidentiality.

 R. Concepts of care

  1. Accelerated postoperative recovery program

   a. Total concept of care involving accelerated recovery from surgery

    (1) Current standard of care appropriate to patient's needs

    (2) Evidence-based: improves patient outcome

    (3) Favored by patients, professional care providers, third-party payers

    (4) Has long been successful with orthopedic patients in "joint (replacement) camps"

   b. Surgical stress response

    (1) All surgical patients experience it in varying degrees postoperatively.

    (2) It involves:

     (a) Alterations in organ function

     (b) Erosion of cell mass and physiological reserve

    (3) Subsequent adverse effects may include:

     (a) GI dysfunction and ileus

     (b) Hypoxemia

     (c) Fatigue and muscle wasting

     (d) Impaired cognition

     (e) Cardiopulmonary, infectious, thromboembolic complications

    (4) May result in:

     (a) Delayed hospital discharge

     (b) Extended convalescence

     (c) Negative impact on patient's long-term prognosis

   c. Key factors in accelerated recovery programs

    (1) Multidisciplinary, concentrated, coordinated efforts involving:

     (a) Patient and family

     (b) Primary care physician, surgeon, anesthesia provider

     (c) Nurses in various locations/roles

      (i) Office

      (ii) Preadmission/preoperative

      (iii) Perioperative (OR) and perianesthesia

      (iv) Nursing unit/critical care unit

      (v) Case manager

      (vi) Home health services

     (d) Pharmacists

     (e) Nutritionists

     (f) Respiratory, physical, occupational, speech therapists as appropriate

     (g) Social workers as appropriate

     (h) Pastoral care

    (2) Primary goal: reduce patient morbidity and mortality

     (a) Patient has an active role in achieving interrelated short- and long-term goals.

     (b) All other participants help the patient achieve those goals.

   d. Components of accelerated recovery programs

    (1) Preoperative patient education

     (a) "Perioperative optimization"

      (i) Patient undergoes thorough preoperative evaluation to identify postoperative morbidity and mortality risk factors.

      (ii) Measures taken to achieve optimal health status preoperatively

     (b) Nurses teach the patient pathway contents.

      (i) Nature of progressive care

      (ii) Associated time frame

      (iii) Rationale

      (c) Benefits
         (i) Better compliance
         (ii) Improved prognosis
         (iii) Timely discharge
         (iv) Cost-effectiveness
   (2) New anesthetic, analgesic, and surgical techniques aimed at reducing surgical stress responses and discomfort
      (a) Less invasive surgical techniques cause less extensive tissue damage.
      (b) Rapid-onset, short-acting anesthetics, opioids, muscle relaxants allow:
         (i) Faster recovery from anesthesia
         (ii) More rapid patient participation in the recovery process
      (c) Multimodal balanced analgesia
         (i) Provides superior pain relief
         (ii) Accelerates recovery
   (3) Aggressive postoperative rehabilitation includes early enteral nutrition and ambulation.
      (a) Early enteral nutrition builds tissue.
      (b) Aggressive ambulation, given the nature of surgery/procedure, prevents muscle wasting and fatigue.
   (4) Physician's evidence-based decision-making regarding use of catheters, tubes, drains, monitoring, and general rehabilitation
      (a) Various tubes can affect mobility when used for extended periods.
      (b) Physicians must consider selective rather than routine use.

2. Rapid postanesthesia progression (RPP)
  a. Concept of rapid progression of a patient through phase I PACU in preparation for safe transfer to phase II PACU, then discharge to home
  b. Progression based on patient's condition versus time
   (1) Phase I PACU nurse provides quality aggressive care.
      (a) Assesses the patient more frequently
      (b) Develops and continually revises a patient care plan, especially regarding:
         (i) Respiratory and cardiac status
         (ii) Comfort: prevention or control of pain, PONV to patient's satisfaction
         (iii) Provides holistic biopsychosocial, emotional, and spiritual nursing care based on patient needs
      (c) Conducts a thorough phase I PACU discharge assessment
      (d) Determines whether a patient meets phase I PACU discharge criteria
   (2) When a patient meets discharge criteria, the nurse transfers the patient to phase II PACU for less acute progressive care.
  c. Conditions for success
   (1) Appropriate patient selection
   (2) Highly motivated patients and staff
   (3) Appropriate selection and management of anesthetic agents, antiemetics, and multimodal analgesics
   (4) Sufficient number of skilled nurses who:
      (a) Efficiently deliver appropriate nursing care
      (b) Promote the wellness concept
   (5) Competent support staff
  d. Pros
   (1) May reduce total length of stay
   (2) Earlier phase I PACU discharge may reduce total expenses.
   (3) Has been safely implemented in both inpatient and outpatient settings
  e. Cons
   (1) Not every patient suited for RPP
   (2) Patient may feel rushed.
   (3) Patient still spends some time in phase I PACU, incurring the associated expenses.

■ BOX 50-8
■ **PHASE I PACU BYPASS/FAST-TRACKING**

Wherever fast-tracking (phase I bypass) is practiced, a collaborative plan of care is developed between the anesthesiology department and perianesthesia services. The plan should include written guidelines addressing the following:
- Appropriate patient selection
- Preoperative education of the patient and family
- Appropriate selection and management of anesthetic agents
- Assessment criteria used to evaluate patient readiness in bypassing phase I PACU at the end of the surgical procedure
- Discharge criteria
- Monitoring and reporting patient outcomes

PACU, Post anesthesia care unit.
Modified from American Society of PeriAnesthesia Nurses: *Standards of perianesthesia nursing practice 2008-2010*, Cherry Hill, NJ, 2008, American Society of PeriAnesthesia Nurses.

3. Phase I PACU bypass/fast-tracking
   a. Involves direct transfer of patients having received general, regional, monitored anesthesia care (MAC), or local anesthesia from OR to phase II PACU
      (1) Perianesthesia nurses have identified concerns with this practice as it relates to the delivery of care in a safe, appropriate, and cost-effective manner.
      (2) ASPAN has taken a position on fast-tracking (Box 50-8).
   b. Conditions for success
      (1) Patient considerations
         (a) Appropriate patient selection
         (b) Patient is a candidate for same-day surgery.
         (c) Physical health status is ASA I or II.
            (i) Some children ≥8 years may qualify.
               [a] If they meet established age-specific criteria
               [b] If surgery lasts <90 minutes
            (ii) Advantages
               [a] Reduces child-parent separation time and anxiety
               [b] Improves satisfaction
         (d) Patient motivated for the progressive continuum of care
         (e) Patient's condition deemed physiologically and psychosocially appropriate
         (f) Competent caregiver available after discharge as appropriate
      (2) Preoperative education of the patient and family
         (a) Begins in surgeon's office and continues through preadmission visit and preoperative phone call
         (b) Presents realistic expectations about:
            (i) Phase I PACU bypass/fast-tracking process
            (ii) Perception of the patient being rushed out
            (iii) Postoperative comfort level before discharge
      (3) Appropriate selection and management of anesthetic agents
         (a) Agents with rapid onset, short half-life, and relatively few side effects
         (b) Preemptive multimodal analgesic and antiemetic administration
         (c) Bispectral index of electroencephalogram
            (i) Allows anesthesia to be maintained at a lighter plane, resulting in faster response and recovery
            (ii) Results in fewer postanesthesia side effects

(4) Postoperative nursing care considerations
    (a) Phase I PACU bypass/fast-track patients deserve and receive same quality of care that all phase II PACU patients receive.
    (b) Care based on same criteria for all phase II PACU patients
(5) Monitoring and reporting patient outcomes
    (a) Incorporate patient outcomes into PACU performance improvement process.
    (b) Monitoring should include:
        (i) Patient satisfaction with medical and nursing care
        (ii) Readmission to phase I PACU or to the hospital

  c. Patients requiring continuous monitoring are not appropriate candidates for phase I PACU bypass/fast-tracking; reasons include:
    (1) Safety needs: physical, emotional, or environmental
    (2) Stabilizing preexisting or new health conditions
    (3) Intraoperative/perianesthesia complications
    (4) Acute unresolved management of pain, PONV
    (5) Extremes of age
        (a) Infants routinely transferred to phase I PACU (see Chapter 11)
            (i) Unstable condition can occur quickly.
            (ii) Response time critical
        (b) Elderly at greater risk for untoward events after general/regional anesthesia
            (i) They have more comorbidities.
            (ii) They have many physiological changes affecting all systems.
  d. Pros of phase I PACU bypass/fast-tracking:
    (1) Cost-effective: economic issues should never be the determining factor for utilizing this concept.
    (2) Overall decreased length of stay
  e. Cons of phase I PACU bypass/fast-tracking:
    (1) Potential for unexpected problems exists.
    (2) Resolution results in additional time and resources.

S. Patient discharge from phase I PACU
  1. Assessment considerations (Box 50-9)
    a. Should address patient's physical, cognitive, and emotional status
    b. Should be appropriate for:
      (1) Patient's condition
      (2) Surgery/procedure and anesthetic/sedation
      (3) Intended destination: hospital room, critical care unit/special care unit, phase II PACU
    c. Phase I PACU bypass/fast-track patients
      (1) Anesthesia provider, circulating nurse, and/or surgeon conduct phase I PACU assessment at conclusion of surgery/procedure.
      (2) Meeting phase I PACU discharge criteria in the OR at the end of surgery/procedure qualifies the patient to transfer directly to phase II PACU.
  2. Phase I PACU discharge criteria
    a. Discharge criteria
      (1) Developed collaboratively with nursing, medical staff, and department of anesthesiology
      (2) Use specific assessment parameters.
      (3) Must be approved by department of anesthesiology and medical staff
    b. A physician is responsible for the discharge of a patient from phase I PACU.
      (1) Internal policy may require a physician's attendance for discharge.
      (2) In the absence of the physician responsible for discharge, predetermined criteria may allow the phase I PACU nurse to discharge patients when criteria are met.

■ BOX 50-9
■ **DISCHARGE ASSESSMENT: PHASE I PACU**

Data collected and documented to evaluate the patient's status for discharge include, but are not limited to:
- Airway patency, respiratory function, Sao_2
- Cardiac and hemodynamic status
- Thermoregulation
- Level of consciousness
- Pain and comfort control
- Sensory/motor function
- Patency of tubes, drains, catheters, IV lines
- Skin color and condition
- Condition of dressing, surgical site, procedure site
- Intake and output
- Emotional status
- Child-parent/significant others interactions
- Postanesthesia scoring system if used

  Discharge criteria should be developed in consultation with the anesthesia department using the above assessment parameters. Discharge criteria must be approved by the department of anesthesiology and the medical staff.

IV, Intravenous; *PACU,* post anesthesia care unit; *Sao₂,* arterial oxygen saturation.
Modified from American Society of PeriAnesthesia Nurses: *Standards of perianesthesia nursing practice 2008-2010,* Cherry Hill, NJ, 2008, American Society of PeriAnesthesia Nurses.

3. Safe transfer of patient care
   a. Notify receiving unit of impending patient transfer to determine appropriate patient placement and staff assignment.
   b. Give a complete report to a licensed nurse responsible for patient's care before or at the time of transfer (Box 50-10).
   c. Answer all questions.
   d. Professional nurse arranges safe transportation of the patient to the receiving area.
      (1) Determine mode, number, and competency level of accompanying personnel based on patient's condition/needs.
      (2) Accompany patient as appropriate.
         (a) Requires continuous cardiac monitoring
         (b) Requires evaluation and/or treatment during transport (i.e., vasopressor infusions or pulse oximeter)
   e. Transport personnel
      (1) Notify the receiving area personnel of the patient's arrival.
      (2) Help move and settle the patient in the receiving area and place the call signal within easy reach of the patient.
      (3) Remain with the patient until the receiving unit personnel are with the patient to assume responsibility for care.
IV. POSTANESTHESIA ASSESSMENT PHASE II
   A. Focus of care
      1. Meet patient's immediate postanesthetic/postsedation and postoperative/postprocedure needs in a progressive care method.
         a. Patients generally require less acute level of care; nurses trained to anticipate and respond appropriately to any changes in a patient's condition.
         b. Length of stay based on patient's condition/needs versus time
         c. Facilitate adequate recovery from anesthesia/sedation rather than from surgery/procedure.
      2. Prepare the patient and family/caregiver for care in the home, extended observation, or an extended care environment.

■ BOX 50-10
■ **SAFE TRANSFER OF CARE**

When the postanesthesia/postprocedural patient meets phase I or phase II PACU level of care discharge criteria, or has been discharged by the anesthesiologist/surgeon, the perianesthesia nurse should include the following information in the transfer report as appropriate to the patient's surgery/procedure, anesthesia/sedation, condition, and destination:

- Name and age of patient
- Pertinent patient history including allergies, medical history, physical limitations
- Name of surgeon and procedure performed
- Type of anesthesia/sedation
- Pertinent information regarding unusual events during the procedure
- Estimated blood loss and fluid replacement
- Postanesthetic/postprocedural course including, but not limited to:
  - Level of consciousness/orientation
  - Vital signs, including temperature
  - Status of dressings/surgical site, drainage tubes
  - Amount and type of IV fluids infusing and credit in present bag
  - Medications given and effects if appropriate
  - Pain management interventions, effects, present pain score, patient goal
  - Comfort status/PONV
  - Tests and treatments performed
  - Results of physical assessment
  - Review of postoperative orders as applicable
  - Disposition of valuables/sensory aids
  - Social support present/coming

IV, Intravenous; *PACU*, post anesthesia care unit; *PONV*, postoperative nausea and vomiting.
Modified from American Society of PeriAnesthesia Nurses: *Standards of perianesthesia nursing practice 2008-2010*, Cherry Hill, NJ, 2008, American Society of PeriAnesthesia Nurses.

  B. Transfer of a patient to phase II PACU
    1. Having received transfer notice, a patient may arrive from either of two sources:
      a. Phase I PACU
        (1) Accelerated recovery program
        (2) RPP
      b. Directly from OR/procedure area: phase I bypass/fast-tracking
    2. Patients arrive by cart/bed, wheelchair, or ambulatory as appropriate.
    3. Admission of a patient to phase II PACU is a joint effort shared by:
      a. Phase I PACU nurse and/or support staff if the patient is from phase I PACU
      b. Circulating nurse if the patient is from surgery/procedure area
      c. Transporters are responsible for:
        (1) Helping the patient settle safely, placing the call signal within easy reach (if used)
        (2) Remaining with the patient until the phase II PACU nurse assumes responsibility for the patient's care
      d. If the patient's condition becomes unstable on arrival in phase II PACU:
        (1) Measures must be taken to stabilize the patient
        (2) Verbal report may need to be delayed as appropriate
    4. Transfer report
      a. Responsible person verbally reports to the phase II PACU nurse who will care for patient.
        (1) Professional person transferring the patient from phase I PACU
        (2) Anesthesia provider/circulating nurse transferring the phase I PACU bypass/fast-track patient from OR

        b. Content includes all relevant information.
            (1) Patient's name
            (2) Type of surgery/procedure
            (3) Anesthesia/sedation, level of consciousness
            (4) Comfort levels: pain, PONV, emotional
            (5) Allergies, medications administered before phase II PACU admission
            (6) Location and condition of dressings
            (7) Location and output of drains, tubing, catheter/voiding
            (8) IV intake, oral intake and tolerance
            (9) Neurovascular and muscular strength as appropriate
            (10) Comorbidities
            (11) Physician's orders completed
            (12) Sensory deficits/special needs
            (13) Numeric score if used by facility
        c. Answer questions.
        d. Patient's medical record available for additional information
    C. Initial patient care: phase II PACU
        1. Complete initial assessment of the patient (Box 50-11)
        2. Tend to any immediate needs/changes in patient's condition as appropriate.
        3. Reunite the patient with the family/caregiver as soon as stable and possible.

■ BOX 50-11
■ **INITIAL ASSESSMENT: PHASE II PACU**

Initial assessment and documentation include, but are not limited to:

1. Integration of data received at transfer of care
   - Relevant preoperative status
   - Anesthesia/sedation technique and agents
   - Length of time anesthesia/sedation administered, time reversal agents given
   - Pain and comfort management interventions and plan
   - Medications administered
   - Type of procedure
   - Estimated fluid/blood loss and replacement
   - Complications occurring during anesthesia course, treatment initiated, response
   - Emotional status
2. Vital signs
   - Respiratory rate and status
   - Blood pressure
   - Pulse rate
   - Temperature/route
   - Sao_2
3. Pain and comfort level
4. Level of emotional comfort
5. Level of consciousness
6. Position of patient
7. Patient safety needs
8. Condition and color of skin
9. Neurovascular assessment as applicable
10. Condition of dressings, visible incisions, drains and tubes as applicable
11. Muscular response and strength/mobility status as applicable
12. Location and condition of IV site, type and amount of solution infusing
13. Postanesthesia scoring system if used

IV, Intravenous; *PACU*, post anesthesia care unit; *Sao₂*, arterial oxygen saturation.
Modified from American Society of PeriAnesthesia Nurses: *Standards of perianesthesia nursing practice 2008-2010*, Cherry Hill, NJ, 2008, American Society of PeriAnesthesia Nurses.

    a. Especially important for:

        (1) Infants and children

        (2) Patients who are mentally or sensory challenged

        (3) Interpreter for patients/families who speak no English

    b. Relieves mutual anxiety of patient and family/caregiver

    c. Fosters communication and facilitates recovery

D. Ongoing assessment and management: phase II PACU

  1. Continue to monitor vital signs according to patient's condition and department policy.

  2. Perform ongoing assessments and reassessments as determined by patient's condition and department policy (Box 50-12).

  3. Integrate all information.

    a. Results of initial assessment

    b. Results of a scoring system if used

    c. Information received during transfer report

  4. Develop care plan to optimize the patient's progression of care physically, emotionally, and environmentally (Table 50-2).

  5. Implement appropriate general care in addition to surgery/procedure-specific care based on:

    a. Patient assessments and needs

    b. Desired patient goals and outcomes

    c. Patient/caregiver expectations

  6. Depending on surgery/procedure, anesthesia/sedation, and patient's condition, ongoing care generally focuses on:

    a. Cardiovascular and respiratory concerns

        (1) Check vital signs according to patient's condition/trends, facility policy.

        (2) Patient's/family's concerns, nursing observations

            (a) Postural hypotension after patient's change in position (after sitting up, standing): fainting

                (i) Place in supine position, elevate legs.

                (ii) Increase IV rate.

                (iii) Oxygen if appropriate

                (iv) Medications as ordered by anesthesia provider

                    [a] Ephedrine

                    [b] Atropine for hypotension with bradycardia

                (v) Resume activity gradually under supervision.

■ BOX 50-12

■ **ONGOING ASSESSMENT AND MANAGEMENT: PHASE II PACU**

Ongoing assessment and management include, but are not limited to the following:

1. Monitor, maintain, and/or improve respiratory function.
2. Monitor, maintain, and/or improve circulatory function.
3. Promote and maintain effective pain and comfort management.
4. Promote and maintain emotional comfort.
5. Monitor surgical/procedural site and continue procedure-specific care.
6. Administer medication as ordered; document results.
7. Promote patient safety.
8. Encourage fluids by mouth as indicated.
9. Progress to preprocedure level of mobility as appropriate.
10. Review discharge instructions with patient, family/accompanying responsible adult as appropriate; provide written discharge instructions.
11. Provide follow-up for extended care as indicated.

PACU, Post anesthesia care unit.

Modified from American Society of PeriAnesthesia Nurses: *Standards of perianesthesia nursing practice 2008-2010,* Cherry Hill, NJ, 2008, American Society of PeriAnesthesia Nurses.

■ TABLE 50-2
■ Phase II PACU Patient Outcomes*

Potential and Actual Problems (Nursing Diagnoses)	Outcome Goals (The Patient Will be Able to:)	Nursing Interventions	Resources
Ineffective airway clearance Potential for aspiration Ineffective breathing patterns, respiratory depression related to sedation, anesthesia, positioning, pain, increased respiratory secretions, vomiting Untoward reactions to medications or local anesthetics	Maintain normal respiratory parameters: rate, depth, ease, clarity of breath sounds. Maintain clear airway. Avoid aspiration. Maintain adequate oxygenation of tissues. Avoid symptoms of hypoxia. Perform effective coughing and deep breathing exercises.	Know effects of anesthetics, analgesics, sedatives, and muscle relaxants and associated drug interactions Know airway maintenance techniques. Continuously assess respiratory status. Administer oxygen per protocol. Apply stir-up regimen and encourage deep breathing. Identify preexisting respiratory disease and individualize care appropriately.	Physiological monitoring equipment, oxygen, suction available in unit Adequate staffing patterns to ensure proper nurse-to-patient ratio Immediate access to anesthesia provider Comprehensive anesthesia and/or nursing report of patient care ASPAN *Standards of Perianesthesia Nursing Practice* Facility policies regarding interventions for cardiovascular/respiratory problems Spirits of ammonia ampules available, especially in bathrooms Functional emergency call system Immediate access to emergency equipment: crash cart, resuscitator bag-valve-mask, ventilator, airway maintenance supplies Medications
Cardiovascular instability Potential alteration in tissue perfusion	Maintain normal cardiovascular parameters, avoiding hypertension and hypotension. Demonstrate expected postoperative arousal and mental status. Demonstrate normal parameters of peripheral circulation. Ambulate as appropriate without faintness or hypotension.	Assess all parameters of vital signs in ongoing fashion including heart rate and BP rhythm. Assess peripheral pulses, color, and sensory adequacy. Maintain adequate fluid balance and hydration. Report untoward symptoms to anesthesiologist/surgeon. Assist patient in progressive ambulation within individual patient's abilities.	Physiological monitoring equipment

*This type of table can replace writing traditional nursing care plans. The phase II PACU nurse need only select applicable nursing diagnoses and follow-through for the individual patient.

Continued

■ TABLE 50-2
■ ■ **Phase II PACU Patient Outcomes—cont'd**

Potential and Actual Problems (Nursing Diagnoses)	Outcome Goals (The Patient Will be Able to:)	Nursing Interventions	Resources
Altered skin integrity related to surgical wound Potential for infection at surgical site	Experience appropriate and uncomplicated wound healing.	Assess surgical site throughout phase II PACU stay. Use aseptic technique and teach to family and patient. Avoid constricting bandages at surgical site.	Standard Universal precautions Personal protective equipment and sterile dressing supplies Antibiotics if ordered
Altered thought processes and/or memory loss related to sedation/anesthesia	Demonstrate thought processes consistent with the pre-sedation/pre-anesthesia status Display/verbalize appropriate orientation to surroundings and situations. Avoid self-injury related to altered thought patterns. Assume self-care activities within parameters of surgical restrictions. Rely on RA who understands nature of patient's temporarily altered thought patterns and responsibility for patient care.	Provide frequent affirmation of orientation to time, place, and events. Assess patient's orientation. Monitor and oversee patient care while patient is vulnerable to environment. Provide appropriate time for drug clearance before patient discharge. Administer medications with caution to avoid further sedation that would alter patient's mental status.	Comprehensive report from prior care provider regarding sedative medications and prior mental status Predetermined phase II PACU discharge criteria that include assessment; consider mental status and availability of RA to drive and provide home support. ASPAN *Standards of Perianesthesia Nursing Practice*
Alterations in comfort: pain	Express acceptable comfort level.	Administer appropriate analgesics. Apply cold therapy as ordered. Position patient for comfort. Provide positive reinforcement and encourage philosophy of wellness throughout process. Encourage appropriate pace for increased activities.Distraction as appropriate	Analgesic medications Knowledge of nursing interventions for comfort: "ASPAN Pain and Comfort Clinical Guideline" Positioning and support of body areas Breathing exercises Positive reinforcement of comfort

Alteration in comfort: nausea and vomiting	Express acceptable comfort level. Avoid vomiting and retching.	Encourage appropriate pace for oral intake of fluids. Administer antiemetics as needed. Administer IV fluids for hydration as ordered. Provide positive reinforcement and encourage philosophy of wellness throughout process. Utilize complementary therapies if acceptable to patient.	Antiemetic medications IV fluids Literature related to reducing GI symptoms Appropriate food and beverages (avoid acidic juice, spicy or difficult-to-digest foods)
Self-care deficit	Display sufficient level of alertness and self-care for safe phase II PACU discharge to home with RA, extended observation, or extended care facility.	Provide nursing care modified to patient's abilities. Assess patient for ability to ambulate if appropriate, and call for assistance before discharge. Ensure availability of a care provider before discharge.	Phase II PACU discharge criteria
Risk of hemorrhage	Maintain blood volume at normal level. Maintain BP at normal level; avoid hypertension.	Ensure availability of IV solutions. Observe surgical site for signs of bleeding and report to physician. Administer anxiolytic and/or antihypertensive medications as ordered. Instruct patient on appropriate support of surgical site.	Blood bank contract and policies for rapid availability of blood products for freestanding ambulatory care facilities Antihypertensive agents Anxiolytic medications IV fluids and supplies
Potential for injury related to faintness, weakness, fatigue, prolonged regional block, altered sensory perception	Remain free from injury. Ambulate as appropriate, without faintness or injury.	Encourage appropriate pace for progression of activity/ambulation. Monitor vital signs in relationship to activity/ambulation. Provide ongoing assessments for potential complications related to activity/ambulation. Reduce obstacles to safe ambulation: wet floors, slippery shoes, improper fit of slings, braces, surgical shoes, crutches, etc. Suggest appropriate modification of the home setting for safety.	Safe environment Nursing attendance during activity/ambulation attempts and while the patient uses the bathroom RA in home setting Preoperative interview with patient or RA

Continued

TABLE 50-2

Phase II PACU Patient Outcomes—cont'd

Potential and Actual Problems (Nursing Diagnoses)	Outcome Goals (The Patient Will be Able to:)	Nursing Interventions	Resources
Actual or perceived loss of privacy, dignity, or confidentiality	Express satisfaction with the level of privacy and confidentiality provided. Maintain dignity and self- esteem.	Support patient's right to privacy, dignity, and confidentiality. Respect patient's request about the amount and nature of personal information that may be shared and with whom. Provide privacy: curtains, blankets, and clothing that covers patient. Allow patient as much decision-making as is possible and encourage the RA to do the same.	Surroundings that are friendly, family-focused, private, and apart from the view of other patients and staff Patient linens that provide adequate cover Cubicle curtains or a private room Patient Bill or Rights
Alterations in health that can complicate extended recovery	Express the effects of surgery/anesthesia/ sedation on preexisting medical conditions. Comply with instruction to optimize medical status postoperatively. Experience no complications related to prior medical status.	Assess patient's health status frequently. Use active listening skills and observe for clues related to health status. Individualize patient care related to prior health status. Encourage questions from patient/ RA and provide honest answers.	Books and literature on surgery, anesthesia, and various medical conditions PCP available to assist in optimizing patient's health status postoperatively

| Anxiety related to fear of incomplete/inappropriate home care without nursing presence | Express lingering fears and questions about home care or other topics. Display calm demeanor. Verbalize reduced anxiety. Remain free from injury. Ambulate if appropriate without faintness or injury. | Provide written and verbal instructions and ongoing explanations regarding care issues within limits of nursing practice. Ensure home support before discharge. Encourage questions from patient and RA. Provide names and phone numbers of contacts should questions or problems arise. Assure of a nurse's follow-up contact and provide approximate time frame. | Verbal and written instructions that include emergency contact information RA willing and able to provide appropriate home support |

ASPAN, American Society of PeriAnesthesia Nurses; *BP*, blood pressure; *GI*, gastrointestinal; *IV*, intravenous; *PACU*, post anesthesia care unit; *PCP*, primary care physician; *RA*, responsible adult.
Modified from Burden N, Quinn DMD, O'Brien D, et al: *Ambulatory surgical nursing*, ed 2, Philadelphia, 2000, Saunders.

      (b) Vagal reaction after anesthetic agents or sympathetic blockade/ major regional anesthesia, breath-holding, vomiting, or straining
          (i) Dangerous to patients with primary heart disease if prolonged
          (ii) Atropine for bradycardia with hypotension
      (c) Hypertension
          (i) Patient should be treated and monitored in phase I PACU before transfer to phase II PACU when stable.
          (ii) Resume ambulation slowly as appropriate to prevent hypotension.
      (d) Patients in respiratory distress not appropriate candidates for phase II PACU care
          (i) Chronically O_2-dependent patients may be admitted if not in acute respiratory distress.
          (ii) Patient experiencing respiratory compromise while in phase II PACU must be treated immediately and vigorously.
             [a] Apply O_2 and monitor Sao_2.
             [b] Notify anesthesiologist.
             [c] Return patient to phase I PACU for acute care as appropriate.
             [d] Treatment may include:
                [1] Bronchodilators for asthma
                [2] Antihistamines for allergic reactions
                [3] Diuretics for cardiac complications
                [4] Chest tube insertion for pneumothorax related to surgery or regional anesthesia technique

b. Level of consciousness
  (1) Patients requiring constant, close observation not appropriate candidates for phase II PACU area
  (2) Determine preoperative level of responsiveness; compare with current condition.
  (3) Determine possible cause of decreased level of consciousness.
      (a) Preoperative medications
      (b) Residual effects of anesthesia
      (c) Residual effects of analgesics
      (d) Preoperative medical condition
      (e) Normal preanesthesia/presedation patient condition
  (4) Treatment
      (a) Administer O_2 and monitor Sao_2 as appropriate.
      (b) Cautious stimulation to avoid disorientation
      (c) Stir-up regimen, coughing and deep breathing as appropriate
      (d) Avoid oversedation from additional medication administration.
      (e) Caution caregiver about measures to maintain patient's safety.
          (i) Positioning to maintain airway
          (ii) Caregiver in attendance to avoid falls
          (iii) Administer medications only as ordered.
          (iv) Avoid making legal commitments, driving, working with hazardous equipment until alert and responding normally.

c. Comfort level
  (1) Pain
      (a) Manage/improve physical pain to a level acceptable to the patient.
      (b) Assess current level and determine acceptable level.
      (c) Review measures already implemented: pharmacological, anesthetic techniques.
      (d) Determine whether additional pharmacological approach is appropriate; if so, administer medication and monitor patient.
      (e) Implement/continue nonpharmacological interventions.
      (f) Notify anesthesiology department as appropriate.

 (2) PONV
  (a) Manage/improve PONV to a level acceptable to the patient.
  (b) Assess current level and determine acceptable level.
  (c) Review pharmacological measures already implemented.
  (d) If unresolved PONV continues, notify anesthesiologist.
  (e) Administer medications as ordered and monitor patient.
  (f) Implement/continue nonpharmacological interventions.
 (3) Emotional
  (a) Attend to special needs/sensory needs.
  (b) Provide respect and honesty.
  (c) Maintain privacy and confidentiality.
  (d) Reinforce progressive care and concept of wellness; give positive reinforcement.
  (e) Promote a comfortable, family-oriented atmosphere.
   (i) Reunite with family/caregiver.
   (ii) Observe patient's body language.
   (iii) Observe patient's interaction/comfort with family/caregiver.
d. Surgery/procedure site
 (1) Observations
  (a) Observe for possible changes evidenced by specific parameters.
   (i) Excessive bleeding, hematoma formation, wound dehiscence
   (ii) Circulatory impairment, nerve compression
  (b) Anesthesia-related problems
   (i) Convulsions, serious dysrhythmias, pneumothorax, aspiration
   (ii) Residual motor and sensory effects due to blocks
  (c) Procedure-related problems
   (i) Nerve injury caused by intraoperative/procedural positioning
   (ii) Skin injury caused by allergic reactions to prep solutions, removal of electrocautery pads or cardiac monitoring pads, tape burns
 (2) Notify physician as appropriate and complete associated orders.
 (3) Treat minor problems symptomatically as appropriate.
 (4) Offer emotional support and reassurance.
e. Progressive activity
 (1) As appropriate regarding surgery/procedure, anesthesia/sedation, and postoperative orders
 (2) Ensure patient safety.
  (a) Eliminate obstacles.
  (b) Dangle before standing.
  (c) Provide sufficient help to support/assist as necessary.
 (3) Provide appropriate assistive devices unless other arrangements have been made.
  (a) According to orders: weight-bearing status, restricted use, amount of sensation
  (b) Teach appropriate use of equipment: crutches/walkers, slings/immobilizers, braces, shoes/boots, appliances.
 (4) Determine patient's tolerance of activity.
  (a) Determine appropriate use through return demonstration.
  (b) Progress at appropriate rate to maintain stability of vital signs and comfort.
f. Intake and output
 (1) Oral intake as permitted and tolerated to prevent/control PONV
  (a) Check for return of gag and cough reflexes, ability to swallow.
  (b) Sit up to swallow safely.
  (c) Begin with water; causes less danger if accidentally aspirated.
   (i) Initially avoid very hot or cold liquid temperatures.
   (ii) Progress gradually as tolerated.
  (d) Avoid dairy products, coffee, citrus juice; may provoke nausea.
  (e) Progress to crackers or dry toast, then bland food as tolerated.

(2) Voiding
    (a) Assist to bathroom as appropriate.
    (b) Remain available to assist patient.
    (c) Follow department policy regarding voiding before discharge.
g. Address diverse problems.
  (1) Examples
    (a) Sore throat after intubation
    (b) Headache after spinal anesthesia or caffeine deprivation
    (c) Sore muscles resulting from intraoperative positioning or shivering
    (d) Sore lip from biting or if caught between lip and airway
    (e) Cold or sore extremity after use of intraoperative tourniquet
    (f) Blurred vision after intraoperative use of eye ointment
  (2) Offer explanations to patient.
  (3) Treat symptomatically unless contraindicated.
7. Evaluate and reevaluate patient outcomes to:
a. Meet patient's changing condition and progressive needs.
b. Anticipate/avoid potential problems.
c. Notify anesthesiology department or surgeon, as appropriate, of any adverse situations, problems, or questions.
  (1) Complete new orders.
  (2) Evaluate outcome.

E. Postoperative/postprocedure education
1. Provide to patient/caregiver as appropriate before discharge.
2. Discharge instructions based on postoperative/postprocedure orders and patient needs
3. Encourage and answer all questions.
4. Provide verbal and written instructions in a manner suited to patient's/caregiver's needs.
5. Include contact and emergency information.
6. Confirm receipt with signature of unsedated patient or caregiver and chart documentation.

F. Discharge from phase II PACU.
1. Destination: home, extended observation, or extended care facility
2. Determine patient readiness.
a. Complete phase II PACU discharge assessment (Box 50-13).
b. Sleepiness is not necessarily a deterrent to discharge as long as:
  (1) Patient's condition is stable.
  (2) Patient will be in a safe location and monitored by a responsible adult.
  (3) Patient meets discharge criteria or discharge is approved by anesthesia provider.
c. Determine whether patient meets established discharge criteria of facility.
  (1) Guidelines established by national accrediting organizations and professional organizations
  (2) Discharge criteria
    (a) Developed collaboratively with nursing, medical staff, and the department of anesthesiology
    (b) Using specific assessment parameters
    (c) Discharge criteria must be approved by the department of anesthesiology and the medical staff.
  (3) Licensed independent practitioner, usually an anesthesiologist, responsible for discharge decisions
  (4) Alternatives, with the anesthesiologist's name recorded, include:
    (a) Policy, protocol, standing orders, or collaborative practice
    (b) Type of scoring system, if used
d. Patient meeting all established criteria may be discharged from phase II PACU.
e. Perianesthesia nurses must adhere to institutional policy for patient reassessment postdischarge.

■ BOX 50-13
■ **DISCHARGE ASSESSMENT: PHASE II PACU**

Data collected and documented to evaluate the patient's status for discharge include, but are not limited to:
- Airway patency, respiratory function, and Sao_2
- Vital signs
- Thermoregulation
- Level of consciousness
- Swallowing
- Pain and comfort level
- Level of emotional comfort
- Ambulation if applicable
- Skin color and condition
- Condition of dressing/surgical or procedural site
- Voiding
- Child-parent/significant others interactions
- Patient and home care provider knowledge of discharge instructions
- Written discharge instructions given to patient/accompanying responsible adult
- Arrangements for safe transportation from the facility
- Provision of additional resources to contact if any problems arise
- Postanesthesia scoring system if used
- Patient reassessment after discharge per institutional policy

Discharge criteria should be developed in consultation with the anesthesia department using the above assessment parameters. Discharge criteria must be approved by the department of anesthesiology and the medical staff.

PACU, Post anesthesia care unit; *Sao₂,* arterial oxygen saturation.
Modified from American Society of PeriAnesthesia Nurses: *Standards of perianesthesia nursing practice 2008-2010,* Cherry Hill, NJ, 2008, American Society of PeriAnesthesia Nurses.

    3. Discharge process
        a. May be discharged to home, extended observation, or extended care facility
        b. Caregiver or staff may assist patient to dress as appropriate.
        c. Verify receipt of:
            (1) Personal valuables
            (2) Discharge instructions, medications/prescriptions
            (3) Supplies, equipment provided at facility
        d. Verify means of safe transport.
        e. If the patient is going home:
            (1) Arrange transport to exit by appropriate method.
            (2) Accompany to exit and assist into vehicle.
            (3) Coordinate postoperative follow-up phone call after 24 hours.
        f. If the patient is going to another department for treatment before discharge, to extended observation, or to an extended care facility:
            (1) Verify destination and anticipated transfer time; notify family if present.
            (2) Call report to:
                (a) Next department for treatment
                (b) Extended observation or extended care facility as appropriate
            (3) Send chart, discharge instructions, medications/prescriptions, supplies and equipment, personal valuables with patient.
            (4) Confirm safe transport as appropriate.
    G. Care of patient with unsupplemented local anesthesia
        1. If stable, patient usually allowed to walk from surgery to phase II PACU, accompanied by OR circulating nurse

2. Discharge requirements may vary by facility but usually include:
   a. Minimum of one set of vital signs
   b. General assessment including evaluation of surgical site, pain level, and emotional status
   c. Completion of postoperative orders
   d. Receipt of prescriptions and discharge instructions that may include:
      (1) Protect the insensitive area from injury.
      (2) May drive unless prohibited by surgical procedure
   e. Need not be accompanied unless condition prohibits
3. May discharge when patient meets discharge criteria (numerical scoring system)

BIBLIOGRAPHY

1. American Society of PeriAnesthesia Nurses: *Standards of perianesthesia nursing practice 2008–2010*, Cherry Hill, NJ, 2008, American Society of PeriAnesthesia Nurses.
2. Bond LM, Flickinger D, Aytes L, et al: Effects of preoperative teaching on the use of a pain scale with patients in the PACU, *J Perianesth Nurs* 20(5):333–340, 2005.
3. Burden N: Some is not a number, soon is not a time: Saving lives in America's health care facilities, *J Perianesth Nurs* 21(3):200–203, 2006.
4. Burden N, Quinn DMD, O'Brien D, et al: *Ambulatory surgical nursing*, ed 2, Philadelphia, 2000, Saunders.
5. Dewar A, Scott J, Muir J: Telephone follow-up for day surgery patients: Patient perceptions and nurses' experiences, *J Perianesth Nurs* 19(4):234–241, 2004.
6. Ead H: From Aldrete to PADSS: Reviewing discharge criteria after ambulatory surgery, *J Perianesth Nurs* 21(4):259–267, 2006.
7. Geisz-Everson M, Wren KA: Awareness under anesthesia, *J Perianesth Nurs* 22(2):85–90, 2007.
8. Golembiewski J, Torrecer S, Katke J: The use of opioids in the postoperative setting: Focus on morphine, hydromorphone, and fentanyl, *J Perianesth Nurs* 20(2):141–143, 2005.
9. Iacono MV: Perianesthesia staffing: Thinking beyond numbers, *J Perianesth Nurs* 21(5):346–352, 2006.
10. Litwack K: *Core curriculum for perianesthesia nursing practice*, ed 4, Philadelphia, 1999, Saunders.
11. McCamant KL: Peripheral nerve blocks: Understanding the nurses' role, *J Perianesth Nurs* 21(1):16–23, 2006.
12. Noble KA: Chill can kill, *J Perianesth Nurs* 21(3):204–207, 2006.
13. Passero C, Belden J: Evidence-based perianesthesia care: Accelerated postoperative recovery program, *J Perianesth Nurs* 21(3):168–176, 2006.
14. Sandlin D: Anesthesia awareness, *J Perianesth Nurs* 21(2):135–137, 2006.
15. Stanhope N: Temperature management in the phase I PACU, *Anesth Analg* 78(5):836–841, 1994.
16. Sullivan EE: The safe transfer of care, *J Perianesth Nurs* 19(2):108–110, 2004.
17. Voepel-Lewis T: Pain assessment for the PACU nurse: Science or art? *J Perianesth Nurs* 19(4):257–260, 2004.

51 Patient Discharge Education in the Phase II Setting

NANCY SAUFL

OBJECTIVES

At the conclusion of this chapter, the reader will be able to:

1. Utilize the nursing process in providing patient, family, and/or accompanying responsible adult appropriate education (assessment, nursing diagnosis, planning, intervention, and evaluation).

2. Review The Joint Commission's patient education standards.

3. Identify postoperative education needs for the patient, family, and/or accompanying responsible adult.

4. Identify learning deficits of the patient, family, and/or accompanying responsible adult.

5. Develop the education plan for the patient, family, and/or accompanying responsible adult based on learning deficits and needs.

6. Define the postoperative education needed for patient, family, and/or accompanying responsible adult.

7. Define documentation standards for education of patient, family, and/or accompanying responsible adult.

I. REVIEW OF THE JOINT COMMISSION'S (TJC) PATIENT EDUCATION STANDARDS
   A. "The goal of patient and family education is to improve patient health by promoting healthy behavior and involving the patient in care and care decisions."
   B. Expectations
      1. Provide the patient and family or accompanying responsible adult with information that will enhance their knowledge and the skills necessary to promote recovery and improve function.
      2. Provide the patient with education and training as appropriate.
         a. Assessed needs
         b. Abilities and learning preferences
         c. Readiness to learn
      3. Consider barriers in education assessment.
         a. Cultural
         b. Religious
         c. Physical
         d. Cognitive limitations
         e. Language
         f. Financial
      4. Educate patients about:
         a. Their medications according to their needs
         b. Equipment and supplies and means of obtaining them
      5. Teach patients regarding foods and diets appropriate to illness as well as possible food-drug interactions.

      6. Provide patients with information on obtaining follow-up care and accessing community resources.

      7. Provide patients with education about pain management as part of treatment.

      8. Provide patients with information about their rights and responsibilities.

        a. Patient's Bill of Rights acknowledges the patient's right to participate in his or her own health care.

        b. TJC "Speak Up" initiative: urges patients to take a role in preventing health care errors by becoming active, involved, and informed participants

      9. Provide discharge instructions that contain information about:

        a. Diet

        b. Activity

        c. Medications

        d. Follow-up care

        e. Contact number if the patient has questions

     10. Document patient education provided to patient and family in:

        a. Verbal form

        b. Written form

     11. Promote the education process among the multidisciplinary health care team members.

        a. Include the opportunity for health care providers to ask questions.

  C. Patient's rights information emphasizes the importance of educating patients regarding ongoing health care requirements after discharge.

  D. When the nurse evaluates the patient's discharge status, the American Society of PeriAnesthesia Nurses (ASPAN) states that the nurse must:

     1. Review the discharge instructions with the patient, family, and accompanying responsible adult as appropriate.

     2. Assess the patient and home care provider's knowledge of the discharge instructions.

     3. Ensure that written discharge instructions have been given to the patient/accompanying responsible adult.

 II. EDUCATION ASSESSMENT

  A. Use information collected through:

     1. Needs assessment (see Chapter 15)

     2. Health history

     3. Interview with patient, family, and/or responsible accompanying adult

  B. Determine patient's preferred methods of learning (see Chapter 3).

  C. Consider the patient's, family's, and/or responsible accompanying adult's understanding of the surgical or invasive procedure and the process.

  D. Evaluate

     1. Health beliefs

     2. Practices

     3. Economic factors

     4. Cultural factors

  E. Ascertain the patient's support system.

  F. Determine:

     1. Readiness to learn

     2. Motivation

     3. Reading level (see Chapter 3)

  G. Determine home care and postoperative education needs based on:

     1. Patient learning and knowledge deficits

     2. Method/type of anesthesia

     3. Procedure

       a. Learning needs and deficits are determined by:

         (1) Anticipated diet

         (2) Activity

(3) Potential emergency conditions

(4) Dressing and wound care

(5) Medication reconciliation

    (a) Medications prescribed for postoperative period

    (b) Routine home medications

(6) Follow-up care

(7) Home care requirements

(8) Typical recovery progression

III. NURSING DIAGNOSIS

  A. Identify patient's, family's, and/or responsible accompanying adult's learning deficits.

    1. Learning needs can be designated in two ways.

      a. Primary concerns or problems

      b. As the etiology of a nursing diagnosis associated response to health alterations or dysfunction

      c. Nursing diagnosis from North American Nursing Diagnostic Association (NANDA) and ASPAN's Perianesthesia Data Elements (PDE) may be used.

        (1) Knowledge deficit: deficiency in cognitive knowledge or psychomotor skills concerning the condition or treatment plan, or information-seeking behaviors

        (2) Health-seeking behavior: the state in which an individual in stable health actively seeks ways to alter personal health habits and/or the environment in order to move toward a higher level of wellness

        (3) If the knowledge deficit is considered the etiology, then the nursing diagnosis will be identified as the "risk for …" (risk for infection …).

      d. Examples of nursing diagnosis may include the following:

        (1) Altered skin integrity related to (R/T) surgical wound

        (2) Potential for infection at surgical site

        (3) Alterations in comfort—pain

        (4) Alterations in comfort—nausea and vomiting

        (5) Self-care deficit

        (6) Actual or perceived loss of privacy or dignity

        (7) Risk of hemorrhage

        (8) Anxiety R/T fear of home care without nursing support, separation from family

        (9) Potential for injury R/T faintness, weakness, fatigue, prolonged regional block, altered sensory perception

       (10) Altered thought processes and/or memory loss R/T sedation and analgesia

       (11) Ineffective airway clearance

       (12) Potential for aspiration

       (13) Ineffective breathing patterns, respiratory depression R/T sedation, anesthesia, positioning, pain, increased respiratory secretions, vomiting, or untoward reactions to medications or local anesthetics

       (14) Potential alteration in tissue perfusion, cardiovascular instability

      e. Outcome goals, nursing interventions, and resources determined as part of the patient discharge education plan may be R/T the preceding examples or other identified problems.

        (1) Education provided must address the outcome goals and nursing interventions to provide consistency and safe care.

IV. PLANNING

  A. Develop the patient's, family's, and responsible accompanying adult's education plans based on learning deficits and needs.

    1. Formulate the teaching plan and modify as needed.

      a. Be conscious of sensory or language barriers.

      b. Discharge planning begins with initial contacts, preoperative assessment, and evaluation.

  2. Identify patient discharge education materials.

      a. Base planning of materials on "need to know versus nice to know."

      b. Generic information and procedure-specific information

      c. Large print size—12-point font or larger

         (1) Sans serif or serif fonts (Arial, Tahoma, etc.)

      d. Readability

         (1) Should be at fifth grade level or less

            (a) Various readability programs: Simple Measure of Gobbledygook (SMOG) index, RIGHTwriter, Grammatique, Suitability Assessment of Materials (SAM); readability formulas are also available in at least 12 languages.

            (b) Allows information to be more easily understood

         (2) Most individuals will read at four to five grade levels less than last formally completed grade level, unless they are reading technical journal type materials routinely.

  3. Develop educational materials

      a. Evaluate color contrast between ink and paper—avoid blues and greens for geriatric patients.

      b. Simple sentences instead of complex sentence structures—short sentences

      c. Limit number of three syllable words—increases reading level.

      d. Use familiar words, not medical terminology.

      e. Use active voice, not passive voice.

      f. Limit number of components and facts in each paragraph.

      g. Limit to two pages or less.

      h. Layout should be easy to read—pleasant format that provides adequate "white space."

  4. Review and/or revise education materials on a predetermined schedule.

      a. Every 1 to 2 years

      b. Avoid duplication and distribution of copy—keep a master.

  5. Develop content for education material by using data from:

      a. Physician interviews

      b. Current literature

      c. Standards of practice—regulatory agencies, medical associations, nursing and medical textbooks, etc.

  6. Personalize instructions.

V. INTERVENTIONS

  A. Define education needed for the postoperative patient, family, and/or responsible accompanying adult.

  1. Education can be formal or informal.

      a. Encourage and facilitate learning—assess patient's understanding of process, information, etc.

      b. Assist in verbalization of concerns, questions, etc.

      c. Build on knowledge that is available at the point in time.

      d. Use questions to reveal knowledge and deficits.

      e. Provide education based on information obtained in planning section.

  2. Methods

      a. Written instructions

      b. Pamphlets

      c. Brochures

      d. Verbal discussion

      e. Classes with return demonstration

      f. Television

      g. Video

      h. Internet

   3. Successful teaching techniques
      a. Maintaining eye contact
      b. Providing a quiet, distraction-free environment
      c. Providing only necessary information
      d. Requesting feedback
      e. Using short sentences, simple words, and a conversational voice tone
      f. Using visual aids
      g. Progressing in the order that the information will be used
      h. Using familiar words and phrases
      i. Showing respect for the learner
B. Postoperative education—key points for standard discharge instructions
   1. Patient must be in the care of a responsible adult for 24 hours.
   2. Patients should not drive and make any important personal or business decisions for 24 hours.
   3. Medication reconciliation—prescribed medications and over-the-counter medications
      a. Name, purpose, dosage schedule for each medication; emphasize importance of following directions on label.
      b. Resume medications taken before surgery per physician's order and instructions.
      c. Pain medication as prescribed
         (1) Purpose and limitations of the medication must be clearly understood.
         (2) Patient should realize surgery is not a continual pain-free situation.
         (3) Patient should be advised to take a prophylactic approach to pain control and not wait until the pain is significantly pronounced before taking pain medication (but must understand dosage limitations).
         (4) Patient should clearly understand to contact physician for any questions or concerns or if pain medication is not effective.
      d. Caregiver needs to clearly communicate the possibility of medication interactions with food and other drugs.
      e. Common side effects of medication should be reviewed.
      f. Taking medications alone or in combination with other medications should be discussed.
      g. Patients should be cautioned against taking additional acetaminophen if indicated.
      h. If the patient received a medication (pain medication, antibiotics, etc.) at the facility that will be continued at home, the time the next dose is due must be documented on the patient's written discharge instruction sheet.
   4. Activity
      a. Patient, family, and/or responsible accompanying adult should be informed of the minor discomforts that may be experienced in the recovery process.
         (1) Minor headache, muscle aches, sore throat that are relieved by mild over-the-counter analgesics (unless contraindicated)
      b. Patient should be advised to rest the remainder of the day or for the next 24 hours—fatigue, dizziness, and drowsiness are to be expected.
         (1) Plan a gradual return to normal activities.
         (2) Plan periods of rest during the day's activities.
      c. In general, there is no driving for 24 hours postoperatively or as long as regularly taking opioids or sedatives.
         (1) Surgeon may restrict for longer period.
         (2) Dependent on procedure
      d. Specifics about lifting or performing strenuous activities require clearance from the surgeon.
      e. Unless contraindicated by the patient's procedure, sexual activity may be resumed when patient comfort permits.
      f. Limited activity instructions (i.e., weight bearing) may be related to the patient's procedure.

    g. Patients should also be cautioned against the lack of activity.
        (1) Importance of ambulation (as allowed)
        (2) Frequent change of position (as allowed)
        (3) Deep breathing

5. Diet and elimination
    a. Any specific restrictions; for example, start with liquids, progress as tolerated.
    b. If no restrictions needed, instruct to progress to a regular diet as tolerated.
    c. Foods to avoid—spicy, fatty, heavy foods on day of surgery
    d. Precautions if history of reflux or gastroesophageal reflux disease
    e. Avoidance of foods or liquids that might increase or potentiate nausea and vomiting
    f. Use of laxatives, stool softeners based on opioids and/or procedure
    g. Voiding—by when and what to do if unable to urinate
    h. Patient should be advised not to consume any alcoholic beverages, including beer and wine, for 24 hours or while taking pain medications.

6. Anesthesia precautions
    a. Typically determined by anesthesia type used
    b. Possibility of sleepiness, drowsiness, and fatigue
    c. Possibility of impaired cognitive and psychomotor skills
        (1) Impaired judgment
        (2) Slower reaction times
    d. Potential for postoperative nausea and vomiting
    e. Potential for postoperative myalgia or sore throat
    f. Sensory blocks
        (1) Instruct patient that he or she won't have normal response to painful stimuli until block subsides.
        (2) Advise patient to be mindful of positioning and protecting extremity until block has subsided.
    g. Signs and symptoms that should be reported

7. Hygiene
    a. Importance of hand washing by patient and caregivers
    b. When patient can shower or bathe will be dependent on type of procedure, dressings, drains, etc.
    c. How to protect dressings or incision
    d. Keeping casts clean and dry

8. Surgical considerations
    a. Postoperative pain expectations—report pain not relieved by prescribed pain medication.
    b. Expected postoperative bleeding—be procedure specific.
    c. Pertinent signs and symptoms that could indicate postoperative complications and should be reported
        (1) Fever with a temperature >38.3° C [101° F]
        (2) Breathing problems
        (3) Bleeding problems—dressing saturated with continually increasing amount of blood
        (4) Pain not relieved by pain medication
        (5) Urinary retention or inability to urinate within defined time frame
        (6) Continual nausea and vomiting
        (7) Extreme swelling or redness around surgical wound, drainage that has changed to yellow or green
        (8) Persistent, atypical pain or increased pain
        (9) Intravenous catheter site observation and care if needed

9. Treatments and tests
    a. Procedures that the patient or responsible adult is expected to perform (dressing changes, warm compresses, ice packs, etc.)

        b. Complete list of supplies needed
        c. Date, time, and location of follow-up tests if ordered
        d. Postoperative follow-up care (i.e., time, physician phone number, necessity of calling to make appointment)
        e. Crutches, incentive spirometer, antiembolic stockings, emptying of drains, catheters, etc.

   10. Operative site and wound care
        a. Instructions for appropriate care
        b. Incision care
        c. Preventing infection
        d. Dressing changes
        e. Drains
        f. Swelling, numbness, or tingling of affected extremity
        g. Ice, elevation as appropriate or ordered

   11. Emergency care
        a. Patient and caregiver must have a clear understanding of what to do in the event of an emergency or an unexpected problem.
        b. Patient and caregiver should be advised to contact emergency services for serious problems such as respiratory distress or postoperative hemorrhage (dial 911 or report to nearest emergency department).

C. Transcultural considerations (see Chapter 20)
   1. Obtain teaching materials in language of patient and family if possible.
        a. Required by law to provide materials for cultural group that is 5% or greater of the general population
   2. Use visual aids to communicate meaning.
        a. Pictures, charts, or diagrams
   3. Use concrete instead of abstract words.
        a. Simple language
        b. Present only one idea at a time.
   4. Allow time for questions.
   5. Avoid the use of medical terminology or health care language.
   6. Validate brief information in writing if having difficulty understanding patient's, family's, or accompanying responsible adult's pronunciations.
   7. Use humor cautiously.
   8. Do not use slang words or colloquialisms.
   9. Do not assume that a patient and family who nod, use eye contact, or smile are communicating an understanding of what is being taught.
   10. Invite and encourage questions during teaching.
        a. Avoid asking negative questions.
        b. In some cultures, expressing a need or confusion may be perceived as inappropriate or rude.
   11. Be cautious when explaining procedures or functions R/T personal areas of the body.
        a. May be appropriate to have a nurse of the same sex do the teaching
        b. Be aware of need to have family member or interpreter of same sex present when giving instructions.
   12. Include the family in planning and teaching.
   13. Ask the patient or family member, the patient's nickname or what the patient prefers to be called.
   14. Identify cultural health practices and beliefs.
   15. Provide interpreter if needed.

VI. EVALUATION
  A. Determine effectiveness of education provided to patient, family, and/or accompanying responsible adult.
   1. Evaluation is an ongoing and final process when determining what has been learned.
   2. Learning is measured against the predetermined learning objectives.

3. Evaluation can occur using a variety of methods.
   a. Direct observation of behavior—return demonstration
   b. Oral questioning
   c. Self-reports and self-monitoring
   d. Postoperative phone call
   e. Patient satisfaction surveys
   f. Feedback from physicians
4. Evaluate teaching.
   a. It is important for nurses to evaluate own teaching and content of teaching programs.
      (1) Consider timing, teaching strategies, amount of information, and whether teaching was helpful.
   b. Patients, families, and accompanying responsible adults should be given opportunity to evaluate learning experiences.
      (1) Feedback questionnaires
      (2) Patient satisfaction surveys
      (3) Postoperative phone call contacts
   c. Forgetting is normal and should be anticipated.
      (1) Increases with level of anxiety
VII. DOCUMENTATION
   A. Define documentation standards for patient's, family's, and accompanying responsible adult's education.
      1. Document information provided.
         a. Preoperative instructions
         b. Postoperative instructions
            (1) Procedure-specific information—what to expect, activity R/T procedure, pain, general care, and when to call the doctor
            (2) Information R/T anesthesia, diet, medications, activity, special instructions
            (3) Indicate to whom education was given (who will be caring for patient).
            (4) Follow-up contact information—phone number and who will be receiving information (Adhere to Health Insurance Portability and Accountability Act [HIPAA] guidelines).
            (5) Discharge orders for treatments, medications, nutrition, and activity
            (6) How and whom to contact in case of emergency
            (7) Procedure-specific instruction sheets provided as indicated
            (8) Method of discharge instruction—verbal, written, return demonstration, for example
            (9) Time of follow-up medical appointments
            (10) Provide copy of written instructions—follow facility policy.
         c. Physician's specific verbal instructions that vary from routine
         d. Patient's response to instructions documented
         e. Nurse's assessment of understanding of postoperative instructions
         f. Any specific instructions and requests from the patient for confidentiality that vary from the norm
         g. Instructions should be signed by nurse and person to whom they were delivered—family or accompanying responsible adult.
            (1) If instructions given preoperatively, patient can sign if necessary—should only be for procedure-specific information.
            (2) Anesthesia and medication information should be given to family member or accompanying responsible adult and signed for by this individual.

BIBLIOGRAPHY

1. American Society of PeriAnesthesia Nurses: *Standards of perianesthesia nursing practice 2008–2010*, Cherry Hill, NJ, 2008, American Society of PeriAnesthesia Nurses.

2. Assai J, Golay A, Visser A: *New trends in patient education: A trans-cultural and inter-disease approach*, St Louis, 1995, Excerpta Medica.

3. Berman A, Snyder S, Kozier B: *Kozier & Erb's fundamentals of nursing: Concepts, process, and practice*, ed 8, Upper Saddle River, NJ, 2008, Pearson Hall Books.

4. Burden N: *Ambulatory surgical nursing*, ed 2, Philadelphia, 2000, WB Saunders.

5. Canobbio MM: *Mosby's handbook of patient teaching*, ed 2, St Louis, 2006, Mosby.

6. *Chart-smart: The A to Z guide to documentation*, ed 2, Philadelphia, 2007, Lippincott Williams & Wilkins.

7. Doak CC, Doak LG, Root JH: *Teaching patients with low literacy skills*, ed 2, Philadelphia, 1996, Lippincott.

8. Drain C, Odom-Forren J: *Perianesthesia nursing*, ed 5, St Louis, 2009, Mosby.

9. Intermountain Health Care, Urban Central Region Hospitals Education Department: *Patient family education: Process for creating a patient education handout*, Salt Lake City, 2003, Intermountain Health Care.

10. Intermountain Health Care, Urban Central Region Hospitals Quality Resource Department: Commitments: *Assessment of patients*, Salt Lake City, 2002, Intermountain Health Care.

11. Intermountain Health Care, Urban Central Region Hospitals Quality Resource Department: *Fact sheets: Patient education*, Salt Lake City, 2003, Intermountain Health Care.

12. *Joint Commission Resources*. Available at: www.jcrinc.com. Accessed January 12, 2009.

13. Mulroy M: *Regional anesthesia*, ed 3, Philadelphia, 2002, Lippincott Williams & Wilkins.

14. Redman B: *The practice of patient education*, ed 10, St Louis, 2007, Mosby.

15. The Joint Commission: *Speak up initiatives*. Available at: www.jointcommission.org/generalpublic/speak+up/. Accessed January 12, 2009.

16. Ziolkowski L, Strzyzerski N: Perianesthesia assessment: Foundation of care. *J Perianesth Nurs* 16(6):359–370, 2001.

Discharge Planning: Extended Observation, Home and Follow-Up Care

SUSAN FOSSUM

OBJECTIVES

At the conclusion of this chapter, the reader will be able to:

1. Describe guidelines for extended care and observation.
2. Describe the best times for planning patient discharge.
3. Identify appropriate discharge instructions that should be provided to the patient and family/caregiver.
4. Describe guidelines for discharging the ambulatory surgical patient.
5. List postdischarge follow-up techniques.

I. DISCHARGE PLANNING
   A. Definition
      1. Discharge plan individualized to meet specific patient needs; involving patient and family as active participants along with interdisciplinary team
         a. Ambulatory surgical patient needs
         b. Extended care/observation patient needs
         c. Patient transferred to long-term care facility
         d. Postdischarge follow-up.
      2. To ensure safe and efficient discharge process
      3. Assessment findings will guide interventions.
      4. Ensure implementation of cost containment strategies.
      5. Implement measures to improve patient outcomes and satisfaction.
   B. Process includes:
      1. Identification
      2. Assessment
      3. Goal setting
      4. Planning
      5. Coordination
      6. Implementation
      7. Evaluation
   C. Initially takes the form of patient assessment
   D. Primary goal for ambulatory patient—in a minimal period, patient will be:
      1. Clinically stable, "home ready," "fit for discharge"
         a. Hemodynamically stable
         b. Mental status returned to baseline
         c. Pain at a manageable level
         d. Minimal nausea/vomiting
      2. Safely discharged
      3. Returned to "preprocedure" level of function

E. Extended observation level of care
  1. Admission criteria
      a. Clinically stable but needing extended care
      b. Awaiting transportation home
      c. Patients with no caregiver
      d. Patients having procedures requiring extended observation/interventions
          (1) Risk for bleeding
          (2) Pain management
          (3) Postoperative nausea and vomiting
          (4) Dizziness
  2. Provide follow-up for extended care as indicated.
      a. Ongoing assessment and management
      b. Medication management
      c. Review of discharge instructions as appropriate
      d. Safe transfer of care including structured handoff process
  3. Extended observation staffing
      a. Two competent personnel, one of whom is an RN possessing competence appropriate to the patient population
      b. One RN to 3 to 5 patients
      c. Additional registered nurse and support staff as dependent on:
          (1) Patient acuity
          (2) Patient census
          (3) Physical facility
F. Discharge planning should begin as soon as possible.
  1. Individualized to patient-specific identified needs
      a. Cognitive ability
      b. Pain assessment
      c. Medication history
      d. Laboratory and diagnostic testing
      e. Cultural and language preferences
      f. Advanced directive
  2. Starts at the time patient is scheduled for the procedure or hospital admission
  3. Discussed at the time of the preadmission visit
      a. Comprehensive history is key tool in discharge planning.
      b. Type/duration of surgery/anesthesia taken into consideration
      c. Available support systems conducive to home management discussed
      d. Identification and resolution of physiological home care problems
          (1) Fall risk assessment
          (2) Physical barriers that impede normal activities of daily living
              (a) Ability to shower
              (b) Mobility in home environment (stairs, tub, etc.)
          (3) Equipment needed (crutches, canes, wheelchair, continuous passive machine, wound vac, etc.)
          (4) Supplies needed (dressings, medications, etc.)
  4. Review and reinforce plan in preoperative holding unit.
      a. Obtain comprehensive nursing history (if not done previously) to include:
          (1) Personal coping deficits
          (2) Family and community support available
          (3) Geographic isolation
          (4) Physical limitations
  5. Planning discussed in phase II/extended observation with patient/next caregiver before discharge
G. Discharge planning addresses:
  1. Safe home environment
  2. Availability of responsible adult caregiver
  3. Safe transportation home
      a. Two responsible persons when transporting infant or child, one to attend to child while other drives vehicle
      b. Place child in appropriate-sized car seat or with seat belt.

    4. Safe transfer of care to next responsible caregiver

    5. Access to medical care after discharge

    6. Postsurgical issues: pain management, complications, resuming of daily activities, work, school, etc.

H. Guidelines for discharge of ambulatory surgical patients include:

    1. Organizational guidelines

        a. The Joint Commission

        b. Accreditation Association for Ambulatory Health Care

        c. Ambulatory Surgery Center Association

        d. American Society of PeriAnesthesia Nurses

        e. American Society of Anesthesiologists

        f. American College of Surgeons

    2. Institutional guidelines

        a. Detailed process developed in consultation with and approved by:

           (1) Nursing

           (2) Anesthesia

           (3) Medical Staff

    3. Process includes:

        a. Protocols

        b. Policies

        c. Collaborative practices

        d. Patient evaluated before discharge

        e. Established discharge criteria (Box 52-1; see Chapters 30 and 51)

        f. Postprocedure follow-up within 24 to 48 hours after discharge

           (1) Phone call

           (2) Post cards/letters

 I. Responsible adult available to:

    1. Assist patient with activities of daily living.

    2. Ensure patient complies with postoperative instructions.

    3. Ensure medications and specific supplies are available.

    4. Monitor patient progress.

 J. Postoperative and follow-up care instructions provided to patient/next caregiver

    1. Reviewed with patient and caregiver

        a. Reviewed verbally with written instructions provided for home care

        b. Reviewed verbally with structured transfer-of-care handoff for extended observation

        c. Nurse validates patient's and caregiver's ability to reiterate instructions to ensure that they understand.

        d. Interpreter used to ensure appropriate level of understanding when applicable

           (1) Give instructions in patient's native language to ensure understanding.

           (2) Discharge instructions should be printed in the patient's language.

■ BOX 52-1
■ **DISCHARGE ASSESSMENT CRITERIA**

Vital signs (circulation; blood pressure, pulse, respirations, oxygen saturation, temperature)
Comfort level (pain, nausea, oral analgesics)
Surgical site (dressings)
Nourishment
Hydration
Level of consciousness
Activity level (ambulation)
Instructions
Support of responsible adult
Ability to urinate if appropriate

(3) Because of confidentiality, patient's family member is not a preferred translator.

(4) Ideally, interpreters should be of the same sex as the patient.

(5) Interpreter services may be obtained through ATT Language Line Services (1-800-752-6096) if no other available.

2. Written copy provided

a. Written level of instructions at fifth grade

b. Large print available for visually impaired

c. Instructions available in multiple languages for culturally diverse patient population

d. Emergency contact information provided in writing (physician's office, clinic, emergency contact numbers)

3. Place copy of instructions in patient medical record.

4. Box 52-2 includes education topics to cover on discharge instruction sheets.

5. Document education provided to patient/next caregiver.

6. Postprocedure/discharge follow-up

a. Telephone calls

(1) Sample questions for follow-up phone call (Box 52-3)

b. Written survey

■ BOX 52-2
■ **EDUCATION POINTS FOR DISCHARGE INSTRUCTIONS**

Medications
- Note the name, purpose, and dosage schedule for each medication; emphasize the importance of following the directions on the label.
- The patient should resume medications taken before surgery per physician's order.
- If pain medication is not prescribed, nonprescription, nonaspirin analgesics (e.g., acetaminophen, ibuprofen) may be effective for mild aches and pains.
- Additional pain medication may be ordered by the physician after surgery. The patient should take these medications as directed, preferably with food to prevent gastrointestinal upset.
- Nonpharmacological alternative therapies/adjuncts to pain relief (e.g., ice, relaxation techniques)

Activity Restrictions
- Advise the patient to take it easy for the remainder of the day after surgery. Dizziness or drowsiness is not unusual following surgery or anesthesia.
- Emphasize care to affected limb if regional block performed (e.g., femoral, scalene).
- For the next 24 hours, the patient should not:
  - Drive a vehicle or operate machinery or power tools
  - Consume alcohol, including beer and wine
  - Make important personal or business decisions or sign important documents
- Activity level: In specific behavioral terms (e.g., do not lift objects heavier than 20 lb), describe any limitation of activities.

Diet
- Explain any dietary restrictions or instructions.
- If no dietary restriction exists, instruct the patient to progress as tolerated to a regular diet.

Surgical and Anesthesia Side Effects
- Anticipated sequelae of surgery (e.g., bleeding and pain) should be delineated.
- Common side effects associated with anesthesia include dizziness, drowsiness, myalgia, nausea and vomiting, or sore throat.

Possible Complications and Symptoms
- Instruct the patient and responsible adult in pertinent signs and symptoms that could be indicative of postoperative complications.

Continued

■ BOX 52-2
■ **EDUCATION POINTS FOR DISCHARGE INSTRUCTIONS—cont'd**

Possible Complications and Symptoms—cont'd
- The patient should call the responsible physician if he or she develops:
  - Fever >38.3° C (101° F)
  - Persistent, atypical pain
  - Pain not relieved by medication
  - Bleeding or unexpected drainage from the wound that does not stop
  - Extreme redness or swelling around the incision site or drainage of pus
  - Urinary retention
  - Continual nausea or vomiting

Treatment and Tests
- Procedures that the patient or responsible adult is expected to perform (e.g., dressing changes or the application of warm, moist compresses) should be described in detail.
- A complete list of necessary supplies should be included.
- If any postoperative tests are to be conducted, instructions as to the date, time, test location, and any preop visit preparation should be listed.

Access to Postdischarge Care
- Note the telephone number of the responsible and available physician.
- Include the telephone number of the ambulatory center and the hours of operation.
- Note also the name, address, and the telephone number of the appropriate emergency care facility.

Follow-Up Care
- Identify the date, time, and location of the patient's scheduled return visit to the clinic or surgeon.

From Burden N, Quinn D, O'Brien D, et al (eds): *Ambulatory surgical nursing,* Philadelphia, 2000, WB Saunders.

    K. Freestanding facilities to have written transfer agreements with nearby hospitals in the event hospitalization for more definitive care or prolonged care becomes necessary
        1. Unplanned medical emergencies (cardiac, respiratory, etc.)
        2. More extensive surgery required
        3. Surgical complications (hemorrhage, dehiscence, etc.)
        4. Uncontrolled pain
        5. Persistent nausea and vomiting

■ BOX 52-3
■ **SAMPLE QUESTIONS FOR FOLLOW-UP PHONE CALL**

- Do you have any questions?
- Do you have any problems relating to your procedure?
- Is your pain controlled?
- What level of pain are you experiencing (scale of 0-10)?
- Have you taken any pain medications? Has it helped?
- Do you or have you had any nausea or vomiting?
- Did you receive verbal and written instructions?
- Did you understand the instructions given?
- How did you find your stay on the unit?
- How could we improve the service we provide?
- Is there anything we could have done to make your stay better?
  Allow questions to arise naturally in the conversation and respond accordingly.
  Refer to physician if patient has further questions.

L. Special needs populations that may require more sophisticated discharge planning (may require extended observation or admission to rehabilitation facility)
   1. Elderly patient with limited ability to care for self
   2. Patient with significant disabilities and functional impairment
      a. Hearing impaired—written and sign language instructions
      b. Sight impaired—Braille standardized instructions and audiotapes
   3. Patient with advanced malignancy
   4. Patient with one or more significant socioeconomic difficulties
      a. Homeless
      b. History of substance abuse
      c. History of violence/abuse in the home
M. Checklist for patient to discuss with health care provider
   1. Diet: special dietary restrictions (i.e., diabetic diet)
   2. Activities of daily living
      a. How soon before ability to resume:
         (1) Bathing
         (2) Driving
         (3) Work/school
         (4) Housework/lawn care
         (5) Sexual activity
         (6) Exercise/rigorous activity
      b. Responsible person will be available to assist until normal activities can be resumed.
   3. Procedure specific
      a. Instructions regarding wound care
      b. Specific positioning requirements
   4. Pain management
      a. Length of time pain is expected to last
      b. Medications available
         (1) Prescription
         (2) Over the counter
      c. What to do if medication not effective
      d. Alternative therapies
   5. Follow-up
      a. Postprocedure therapy (physical, occupational, etc.)
      b. Next scheduled clinic visit with surgeon
   6. Legal considerations
      a. Recurrent excuses for not seeking treatment postoperatively because patient did not know:
         (1) What to look for
         (2) The significance of the symptoms experienced
         (3) What to do or whom to contact
      b. Medication instructions need to be explicit.
         (1) Reasons for noncompliance
            (a) Patient did not know when to take the medication.
            (b) Patient did not know when not to take the medication.
            (c) Patient did not know when to stop taking the medication.
         (2) Nurse should reinforce physician's teachings.
         (3) Medication reconciliation forms should be reviewed with patient and family.
   7. Emergency contact
      a. Under what circumstances physician or nurse should be contacted
      b. Emergency contact numbers patient should have
N. Research studies on discharge planning
   1. Show mixed results
      a. Reduction in hospital length of stay was seen.

    b. Reduction in readmission to hospitals
    c. Increase in patient satisfaction
    d. No evidence that health care costs reduced
  2. Discharge planning programs implemented in different ways

BIBLIOGRAPHY

1. Aldrete J: Modifications to the postanesthesia score for use in ambulatory surgery. *J Perianesth Nurs* 13(3):148–155, 1998.
2. American Society of Anesthesiologists: *Standards for postanesthesia care. ASA standards, guidelines and statements*, 2005, American Society of Anesthesiologists.
3. American Society of PeriAnesthesia Nurses: *Standards of perianesthesia nursing practice 2008–2010*, Cherry Hill, NJ, 2008, American Society of PeriAnesthesia Nurses.
4. Burden N, Quinn D, O'Brien D, et al, eds: *Ambulatory surgical nursing*, Philadelphia, 2000, WB Saunders.
5. Dewar A, Scott J, Muir J: Telephone follow up for day surgery patients: Patient perceptions and nurses' experience. *J Perianesth Nurs* 19(4):234–241, 2004.
6. *Discharge planning for the older adult*. National Guideline Clearinghouse. www.guideline.gov. John A. Hartford Foundation Institute for Geriatric Nursing.
7. Drain C, Odem-Forren J: *PeriAnesthesia nursing: A critical care approach*, ed 5, St Louis, 2009, Saunders.
8. Mamaril M: Fast-tracking the postanesthetic patient: The pros and cons. *J Perianesth Nurs* 15(2):89–93, 2000.
9. Marley R, Moline B: Patient discharge from the ambulatory setting. *J Post Anesth Nurs* 11(1):39–49, 1996.
10. National Alliance for Caregiving, United Hospital Fund of New York: *Hospital discharge planning: Helping family caregivers through the process*. Available at: www.caregiving.org/pubs/brochures/DischargePlanner.pdf. Accessed March 3, 2008.
11. *WebMD: Surgery: What to expect*. Available at: www.webmd.com/a-to-z-guides/surgery-what-to-expect-topic-overview. Accessed March 3, 2008.

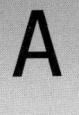

A Certification of Perianesthesia Nurses: The CPAN® and CAPA® Certification Programs

BONNIE NIEBUHR

Please note: For the most up-to-date information about the Certified Post Anesthesia Nurse (CPAN®) and the Certified Ambulatory Perianesthesia Nurse (CAPA®) certification programs, contact the American Board of Perianesthesia Nursing Certification (ABPANC) directly at 800-6ABPANC, e-mail abpanc@proexam.org, or visit the website at www.cpancapa.org.

I. SPONSORSHIP OF CPAN®/CAPA® CERTIFICATION PROGRAMS
   A. ABPANC, a not-for-profit corporation established in 1985, is responsible for providing the CPAN® and CAPA® certification programs for registered nurses caring for perianesthesia patients.
   B. ABPANC's vision: "Recognizing and respecting the unequaled excellence in the mark of the CPAN® and CAPA® credential perianesthesia nurses will seek it, managers will require it, employers will support it and the public will demand it."
   C. ABPANC's activities are focused on achieving its mission: "To assure a certification process for perianesthesia nurses that validates knowledge gained through professional education and experience, ultimately promoting quality patient care."
   D. ABPANC's mission is driven by its commitment to:
      1. Professional practice
      2. Advocating the value of certification to health care decision-makers and the public
      3. Administration of valid, reliable, and fair certification programs
      4. Ongoing collaboration with
         a. The American Society of PeriAnesthesia Nurses (ASPAN)
         b. Other specialty organizations
         c. Key stakeholder groups
      5. Evolving psychometric and technological advances in testing
   E. ABPANC contracts with a nationally recognized testing company, Professional Examination Service, (PES) to assist in the development of each examination.
      1. In April 2009, ABPANC launched computer-based testing (CBT) at Prometric test centers.
      2. Candidates have access and the ability to test at testing centers nationwide (including Army Post Office [APO sites]) within the Prometric network of test sites.
II. NATIONAL ACCREDITATION OF THE CPAN® AND CAPA® CERTIFICATION PROGRAMS
   A. Both the CPAN® and CAPA® certification programs are accredited by the American Board of Nursing Specialties (ABNS)
      1. Accreditation status is granted for a period of 5 years.
      2. Accreditation status must be renewed at the end of the 5-year term.

    B. ABNS
      1. The standard setting body for specialty nursing certification programs
      2. Offers a very stringent and comprehensive accreditation process
      3. ABPANC has demonstrated compliance with the 18 ABNS standards of quality.
    C. ABNS accreditation means that:
      1. CPAN® and CAPA® credentials are based on a valid and reliable testing process.
      2. Structures are in place to administer the examinations meet and even exceed the standards of the certification industry from a legal, regulatory, and association management perspective.
    D. More and more employers recognize and reward specialty nursing certification if the certification programs are accredited.

  III. CERTIFICATION OF PERIANESTHESIA NURSES
    A. ABPANC offered the CPAN® certification examination for the first time in 1986.
      1. Given the changing health care environment and the emerging trend of outpatient surgery, ABPANC began to investigate the need for a separate certification examination related to ambulatory nursing in 1991.
      2. The first CAPA® examination related to this emerging specialty area was given in 1994.
    B. Achieving and maintaining CPAN® and/or CAPA® certification:
      1. Reflects a commitment to patients and their loved ones, colleagues, and the profession of nursing
      2. Strengthens one's sense of personal and professional pride
      3. Validates specialized knowledge and experience, promoting quality patient care
      4. Demonstrates a commitment to life-long learning
      5. Keeps one up to date on the latest developments in the specialty
      6. Gives a competitive edge in an unstable job market
      7. Provides flexibility and recognition when moving anywhere in the United States
      8. Viewed as a leader, mentor, and role model in perianesthesia nursing
      9. May result in a higher salary

  IV. DEFINITION OF CERTIFICATION
    A. As defined by ABNS: "Certification is the formal recognition of the specialized knowledge, skills, and experience demonstrated by the achievement of standards identified by a nursing specialty to promote optimal health outcomes."
    B. State licensure provides the legal authority for an individual to practice professional nursing.
    C. Private voluntary certification, as sponsored by ABPANC, reflects achievement of a standard beyond licensure for specialty nursing practice.
    D. Achievement of CPAN® and/or CAPA® certification status is indicative of the knowledge and experience necessary to practice in perianesthesia nursing.

  V. CPAN® AND CAPA® CERTIFICATION CREDENTIALS
    A. Granted to qualified registered nurses by ABPANC, are federally registered certification marks.
    B. Registered nurses who have not achieved certification status, or whose certification status has lapsed, are not legally authorized to use these credentials.

  VI. ELIGIBILITY REQUIREMENTS
    A. The National Council Licensure Examination is the basis for determining RN licensure.
      1. An unrestricted license means that an RN license, issued by a state board of nursing, must not have any provisions or conditions that would limit the nurse's practice in any way.

B. Candidates applying for *initial* CPAN® or CAPA® certification must have a minimum of 1800 hours of *direct* perianesthesia clinical experience as a registered nurse during the past 2 years before application.

1. When seeking initial certification, candidates must:
   a. Have direct experience caring for perianesthesia patients.
   b. Participate actively in the individual patient experience.
2. One does not need to be technically employed in a direct care position.
   a. If one's role (e.g., educator, manager, clinical nurse specialist) involves bedside interaction with the patient and/or family in some capacity, those hours would count toward meeting the experience requirement.
3. The ABPANC Board of Directors believes that nursing is both an art and a science, and in order to translate nursing knowledge and judgment into practice, one needs to have practiced direct, hands-on care before being CPAN® and/or CAPA® certified.
4. The CPAN® and CAPA® credentials are an affirmation of ABPANC's commitment to quality nursing care and patient safety.
   a. ABPANC is committed to ensuring that patients receive care from CPAN® and CAPA® certified nurses.
   b. Certification reflects current and the most up-to-date knowledge and experience.
   c. For those seeking certification for the first time, requiring that they have direct experience adds credibility to the certification process.
5. Candidates who are unsure whether their role would meet the clinical practice experience requirement should contact ABPANC for clarification at abpanc@proexam.org.
6. CPAN® and CAPA® certified nurses applying to sit for an examination for *recertification* purposes must have a minimum of 1200 clinical practice hours within the past 3 years
   a. Hours may be earned in the roles of staff nurse, manager, educator, or researcher in the perianesthesia specialty.
   b. Hours are not required to be *direct* care hours.
7. Determining which certification examination is most relevant to a candidate's practice.
   a. Candidate decides which examination is most relevant to his or her practice, based on
      (1) Patient needs
      (2) The amount of time patients spend in the specific phases described by the Perianesthesia continuum of care, as defined in ASPAN's Scope of Practice (ASPAN, 2008–2010).
   b. Regardless of the setting in which practice occurs, if most of a candidate's time is spent caring for patients
      (1) In phase I, the CPAN® examination is most relevant.
      (2) In preanesthesia phase, phase II, and/or extended observation, the CAPA® examination is most relevant.
   c. It is possible that candidates have sufficient hours caring for patients in all phases of the perianesthesia experience and qualify for sitting for *both* the CPAN® and CAPA® examinations.
C. Submission of an application, all required documentation of eligibility, and payment of fees
D. Successful completion of either the CPAN or CAPA certification examination
E. Additional eligibility requirements may be adopted by ABPANC at its sole discretion, from time to time.
1. For the purposes of CPAN®/CAPA® certification, requirements will be designed to establish
   a. The adequacy of a candidate's knowledge and experience in caring for the perianesthesia patient

VII. BASIS FOR EXAMINATIONS: A ROLE DELINEATION STUDY (STUDY OF PRACTICE)

    A. Examinations are based on the results of a role delineation study (RDS), or study of practice, conducted every 5 years to ensure that examination content remains relevant and current to the specialty.

    B. Various methods may be used to gather data, the findings of which are reflected in newly designed or revised test blueprints.

    C. The most recent RDS was conducted in 2005–2006, as required by ABNS standards.

    D. Examination blueprints

        1. The RDS conducted during 1999–2000 resulted in a major revision of the CPAN® and CAPA® conceptual framework underlying the examination blueprints.

        2. Based on the RDS findings, both the CPAN® and CAPA® examination blueprints are organized according to four domains (or categories) of perianesthesia patients' needs:

            a. Physiological needs

            b. Behavioral and cognitive needs

            c. Safety needs

            d. Advocacy needs

        3. Perianesthesia nurses are tested on the knowledge required to meet specific patient needs listed under each domain. Examples of the four domains are:

            a. Physiological need—stability of the respiratory system; patency of airway

                (1) Related knowledge required to meet that need includes physical assessment techniques and airway management.

            b. Behavioral and cognitive need—patient/family/significant other education: Identifying, describing, and communicating pain perception/experience

                (1) Related knowledge required to meet that need includes pain assessment and management (psychological, physiological, medical).

            c. Safety need—delivery of care based on accepted standards of practice (e.g., ASPAN *Standards*):

                (1) Related knowledge required to meet that need includes scope and standards of nursing practice (e.g., ASPAN, American Nurses' Association).

            d. Advocacy need—access to an environment that accommodates physical, mental, and/or emotional abilities/limitations

                (1) Related knowledge required to meet that need includes special needs patient issues (e.g., sign language, autism, and/or visual limitations).

        4. Given the differences in the time spent meeting patient needs in the four domains, the percentage of examination content for each domain differs depending on whether the candidate takes the CPAN® or CAPA® examination.

        5. The RDS conducted during 2005–2006 resulted in minor updates to the listing of patient needs and nursing knowledge, as well as a revision to the percentage of examination questions asked in each of the four domains of patient needs.

            a. For the most current examination blueprints that list specific patient needs and the knowledge required to meet those needs, please contact ABPANC directly or refer to its website at www.cpancapa.org.

    E. Fair, valid, and reliable examinations

        1. ABPANC is committed to offering nonbiased or against any groups of nurses because of ethnic background, geographic location, or any other demographic criterion.

        2. A valid examination accurately reflects the knowledge and skills required for competent practice.

            a. All questions appearing on the examinations have been validated using accepted psychometric rating scales.

            b. The RDS extends each examination's validity.

        3. Reliability means the examination is consistent in its measurements of the knowledge and skills of competency practice.

        a. Each scored examination question is reviewed annually for reliability, fairness, and validity.

    4. Each scored examination question has been verified for accuracy and referenced to a published source that is not more than 5 years old.

VIII. DEVELOPMENT OF EXAMINATIONS

  A. Examination questions are written by members of the examination construction committees who are practicing CPAN and/or CAPA certified perianesthesia nurses.

    1. Members of the Item Writer/Review Committee and the Exam Review Committee have undergone extensive training in the process of writing multiple-choice questions.

    2. ABNS standards require that members are selected to also represent the demographic characteristics of the certified nurse population.

IX. DESCRIPTION OF CPAN® AND CAPA® EXAMINATIONS

  A. Each examination consists of 165 multiple questions.

    1. 140 questions are scored.

    2. 25 questions are pretest pilot.

    3. Pilot questions

        a. Do not count toward final score

        b. Used to evaluate performance statistics before they are used as scored questions

        c. Randomly distributed

        d. Not specifically identified

        e. May increase from time to time

  B. Candidates may take up to 3 hours to complete the examination.

  C. Level of difficulty of examination questions

    1. Candidates are tested on their ability to

        a. Recall facts.

        b. Understand principles.

        c. Relate two or more facts to a situation.

        d. Analyze a group of facts.

        e. Synthesize information.

        f. Evaluate situations.

        g. Choose a correct course of action.

    2. Examination questions are written at various cognitive levels based on a condensed version of *Bloom's Taxonomy*. The three cognitive levels are:

        a. Knowledge and comprehension: the ability to recall a fact or understand a principle

        b. Application and analysis: the ability to relate two or more facts to a situation or analyze a group of facts

        c. Synthesis and evaluation: the ability to evaluate a situation using facts or make recommendations based on analysis and evaluation of facts

    3. Testing at higher cognitive levels provides a better indication of a candidate's ability to identify problems and plan, implement, and evaluate nursing care.

X. STUDYING FOR THE CPAN® AND/OR CAPA® CERTIFICATION EXAMINATIONS

  A. A partial listing of publications that may be helpful study materials is found in the *Certification Candidate Handbook*, found on the ABPANC website (www.cpancapa.org).

  B. After carefully reviewing the relevant examination blueprint and identifying individual learning needs, examination candidates should identify additional references, resources, and study opportunities that will meet their individual study needs.

  C. ABPANC also offers online practice examinations for a fee.

    1. Practice examinations may be accessed through the ABPANC website at www.cpancapa.org.

  D. Other helpful test-taking strategies are also described in Appendix B of this publication.

    E. Please note that ABPANC does not endorse or sponsor any review courses for CPAN® and CAPA® examinations.

XI. COMPUTER-BASED TESTING (CBT)

    A. In April 2009, computer-based testing was implemented.

    B. There are two 6-week testing windows per year.

        1. One available in April/May

        2. One available in October/November

    C. At the beginning of the examination:

        1. Each candidate will receive a brief tutorial on how to use the computer to answer questions and review responses.

        2. The time spent in the tutorial will not count against exam testing time.

        3. A Prometric test center staff member is always available to answer any additional questions.

    D. Application process

        1. Before applying for a CPAN® or CAPA® certification examination

            a. Candidates should access an online copy of the *Certification Candidate Handbook* from the ABPANC website at www.cpancapa.org.

            b. Candidates must read the *Certification Candidate Handbook* thoroughly and note ABPANC policies as well as the dates for upcoming examination administrations and application deadlines.

            c. Candidates are instructed to monitor the website for any policy changes to the *Certification Candidate Handbook*.

        2. Candidates will apply online for an examination via a link on the ABPANC website.

            a. Must have a valid e-mail address

                (1) This address will also serve as their login identification to access their account online.

                (2) Encouraged to obtain a free e-mail address such as those that can be obtained through Internet sites such as gmail.com, yahoo.com, hotmail.com, etc

                (3) Encouraged to use a work computer, a relative's computer, or a friend's computer, or go to an Internet café or public library if they do not have their own computer

            b. Once determined eligible to sit for an examination, will receive an *Authorization To Test (ATT)* letter

            c. May schedule examinations directly with Prometric for the location, time, and date most convenient during the 6-week testing window

            d. ASPAN members are eligible to receive a member discount off the ABPANC examination fee.

            e. To receive the ASPAN member discount, must already be member of ASPAN and provide their membership number

            f. Name must exactly match the name in the ASPAN database.

    E. Examination administration and scoring

        1. Candidates can navigate back and forth through the examination questions at their own pace and will have the ability to:

            a. Review answers to all questions at any time and are permitted to go back to questions that have already been answered.

            b. Change an answer once marked.

            c. Flag a question if wish to return to it later.

            d. Have the option of leaving a question blank and returning to it later.

            e. See a review screen that summarizes the status of each question and identifies which questions have been marked for review, omitted, and answered.

        2. Scoring report

            a. A preliminary, unofficial report indicating passing or failing will be immediately available at the test site.

            b. An official score report, along with a wallet identification card, wall certificate, and information about maintaining certification, will be sent after the examination in approximately 2 weeks.

  c. Specific information regarding the scoring process is contained in the *Candidate Handbook*.

XII. CERTIFICATION PERIOD: RECERTIFICATION
 A. Certified nurses possess the most up-to-date knowledge and have recent and current experience, CPAN® and/or CAPA® certification status is granted for a period of 3 years and must be renewed.
 B. CPAN® and CAPA® certified nurses must meet
  1. RN licensure
  2. Clinical practice eligibility requirements
  3. ABPANC's Continual Learning Program contact hours or retake the exam
 C. The recertification application process will occur only online beginning in Fall 2009.
 D. Specific information about the recertification program is available on the ABPANC website.

XIII. ABPANC CONTACT INFORMATION
 A. Call 800-6ABPANC (800-622-7262)
 B. Write 475 Riverside Drive, 6th Fl, New York, NY, 10115-0089
 C. E-mail abpanc@proexam.org
 D. Website: www.cpancapa.org

BIBLIOGRAPHY

1. American Board of Nursing Specialties: Available at: www.nursingcertification.org. Accessed October 7, 2008.
2. American Board of Perianesthesia Nursing Certification, Inc: *Certification Candidate Handbook*, New York, 2009, American Board of Perianesthesia Nursing Certification, Inc.
3. American Board of Perianesthesia Nursing Certification, Inc: *Recertification Handbook: ABPANC's guide to CPAN and CAPA Recertification*, New York, 2009, ABPANC.
4. ASPAN: *Standards of perianesthesia nursing practice 2008–2010*, Cherry Hill, NJ, 2008, ASPAN.
5. Niebuhr B, Muenzen P: A study of perianesthesia nursing practice: The foundation for newly revised CPAN® and CAPA® certification examinations. *J Perianesth Nurs* 16(3):163–173, 2001.
6. Niebuhr B, Muenzen P: ABPANC's 2005–2006 Role Delineation Study: The Foundation for the CPAN® and CAPA® Certification Examinations. Available at: www.cpancapa.org, 2008.

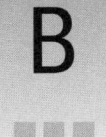

B Testing Concepts and Strategies: Certified Nurse Roles: Precepting, Coaching, and Mentoring

NANCY O'MALLEY

I. TESTING CONCEPTS
   A. Testing concepts can be applied to a variety of testing situations.
      1. Certification examinations (e.g., Certified Post Anesthesia Nurse [CPAN®] and Certified Ambulatory Perianesthesia Nurse [CAPA®] examinations)
      2. State board of nursing examinations
      3. Hospital orientation tests
      4. Continuing education tests
      5. College (academic) examinations
   B. Testing alone does not ensure competency.
      1. Written testing combined with practice of skills enhances the achievement of competency.
      2. Competency is demonstrated at the bedside when knowledge and skills are combined to provide patient care.
II. PURPOSES OF TESTING
   A. Measure knowledge of information, skills, and critical thinking skills against set standards.
   B. Validate mastery of the knowledge unique to a specific practice arena.
   C. Identify specific areas of education, critical thinking processes, and clinical practice requiring more education and development.
   D. Reduce risks for errors through increased knowledge and practice.
   E. Improve patient safety and care.
   F. Allow adapting orientation and education programs based on the participant's level of expertise.
   G. Promote continued competence in knowledge, technical skills, and critical thinking skills for meeting regulatory agencies' requirements.
III. TYPES OF QUESTIONS/ITEMS
   A. Open-ended question (not used for certification or licensure examinations)
      1. Elicits more information regarding knowledge and critical thinking skills than multiple-choice questions
      2. Allows "free thinking" of possibilities and answers
      3. Gives more insight into the thought processes of the person being tested
      4. Usually requires more time to answer
      5. May be more difficult to grade against a preset standard
   B. Multiple-choice question
      1. Composed of the following:
         a. Stem: a statement that presents a question to be answered or the problem to be solved
         b. Correct answer: usually has only one correct answer unless stated otherwise
         c. Distracter: one or more answers that are incorrect; allows a passing point to be established based on psychometric analyses and statistical criteria

C. Both open-ended and multiple-choice questions
 1. May determine knowledge of a basic fact or may present a scenario that requires applying knowledge to a situation
 2. Can be assigned a weight or value based on the question's difficulty
 3. Items may be weighted according to levels or learning domains such as those described by the Revised Bloom's Taxonomy (Table B-1).
   a. Level I: Remembering and understanding requires recalling facts or interpreting data.
   b. Level II: Applying and analyzing requires relating of two or more facts to solve the problem or analyzing the information to resolve a problem.
   c. Level III: Evaluating and creating requires evaluating and applying several concepts to identify a solution for a problem or an intervention for a situation.

IV. TESTING STRATEGIES
 A. Preparing to take an examination
  1. Six to 12 months before examination
   a. Before applying for a CPAN or CAPA certification examination, access an online copy of the *Certification Handbook* from the American Board of Perianesthesia Nursing Certification (ABPANC) website.
   b. Review the eligibility requirements carefully including experience and work environment.
   c. Apply online using the link found on the ABPANC website (www.cpancapa.org); be aware of deadlines.
   d. Investigate scholarships available through the American Society of PeriAnesthesia Nurses (ASPAN), ASPAN components, local organizations, and employers.
   e. Plan to take the examination when family/personal activities will not interfere.
   f. Obtain books or manuals on perianesthesia nursing and test-taking strategies published in the last 5 years; older reference classic reference books that have not been revised may also be acceptable.
   g. Use ASPAN's resources such as:
    (1) *Standards of Perianesthesia Nursing Practice*
    (2) *Journal of PeriAnesthesia Nursing* and other nursing journals
    (3) Education materials via digital versatile discs (DVDs), videos, and ASPAN website contact hour articles
    (4) ASPAN Certification Review courses available in various locations
   h. Obtain access to other resources such as American Heart Association literature, anesthesia, and surgery books.
  2. Six months before examination
   a. Identify your own learning preferences: alone, as part of a group, or a combination of both.
   b. Identify support resources.
    (1) Certification Coach: contact ABPANC for a list of coaches.
    (2) Support systems such as study buddy, certified colleagues, physicians, nurse educators
    (3) Consult ABPANC's *Study Tips* and website for more resources.
   c. Take practice examination available for purchase from ABPANC.
   d. Develop a general study plan.
    (1) Identify what areas you are knowledgeable about.
    (2) Identify and prioritize areas needing more study and/or practice.
  3. Three to 6 months before the examination
   a. Set aside study time in environment conducive to learning.
    (1) Remove distractions.
    (2) Ensure adequate lighting and comfortable room temperature.
    (3) Study at best time of day for learning (individual learners differ).
    (4) Study some every day and take breaks at regular intervals.
   b. Develop a personal or group study plan.

■ TABLE B-1
■ ■ **Sample of Levels of Difficulty**

	Questions	Levels Rationale
Level I	A nondepolarizing neuromuscular blocking agent is: a. Succinylcholine b. Propofol c. Pancuronium d. Ropivacaine	Requires only that candidate recalls one fact about each drug and classifies it
Level II	A healthy, 16-year-old male is admitted to PACU after an arthroscopic knee procedure. His vital signs are blood pressure180/85, heart rate 145, respiratory rate 24, and oxygen saturation is 86%. He is restless, and his breath sounds exhibit fine crackles in both bases. The most likely cause of this event is: a. Irrigation fluids used during the procedure b. Laryngospasm during extubation c. Mivacurium 0.15 mg/kg used as a neuromuscular blocking agent d. Naloxone 0.04 mg used to awaken him at the end of the case	"Most likely cause" indicates the need for applying information to a situation and analyzing it. This scenario does not say what is happening to the patient, so the nurse must analyze facts to identify the most likely cause. If the nurse had been asked to choose between various interventions, this would have been a Level III question.
Level III	After the patient's admission to PACU after a left lung resection, he suddenly becomes restless, dyspneic, and cyanotic. Initial vital signs were within normal limits. Current vital signs are blood pressure 90/64, heart rate 145, respiratory rate 32, oxygen saturation 89% and falling. During this time, the nurse observes fluid leaking from the central venous pressure line that is disconnected. The nurse's *priority* intervention is to: a. Use alcohol on end of the intravenous line tubing and immediately reconnect it to the line. b. Increase oxygen flow rate to maintain oxygen saturation above 92%. c. Position the patient in a high Fowler's position. d. Place the patient in Trendelenburg position on his left side.	This is a Level III question because it requires that the nurse evaluate facts to identify the problems, judge the implications of the situation, and then prioritize the interventions. While other answers are interventions that may be correct, the priority intervention is required to reduce adverse consequences for the patient.

Answers: Level I, **c**; Level II, **b**; Level III, **a**.
PACU, Post anesthesia care unit.

      (1) Identify areas needing more study.
      (2) Create a study schedule allowing more time for areas needing in-depth study.
      (3) Divide material into subsections and set time goals to complete each section.
   c. Develop efficient study habits such as skimming material before studying in depth.

   d. Highlight potential topics for questions and take notes.
   e. Create reference or flash cards to use in groups or individually.
   f. Review other test questions from journal articles, books, and learning modules.
   g. Translate and discuss material rather than just copying notes.
   h. Memorize material by using acronyms, acrostics, songs, or word associations.
   i. Create questions from personal clinical experiences that require critical thinking skills.
   j. Develop study groups.
      (1) Have four to eight members if possible.
      (2) Identify one or two members or a certified colleague to lead the group.
      (3) Invite physicians and other qualified resources to participate.
      (4) Have a planning session to determine the focus of each meeting.
      (5) Divide the work among the members; assign members responsibility for different chapters or topics identified during the planning session.
      (6) Meet regularly at the best time for most members.
   k. Attend educational programs provided by ASPAN, components, districts, as well as other professional organizations.
   l. Identify your personal reactions to test-taking (you may have a combination).
      (1) "Speeder"—does not read questions or answers thoroughly; misses important details; jumps to conclusions
      (2) "Slow-poke"—takes too much time on a question; gets lost in the details of a question or distracters; reads more in the question than is there; mind wanders
      (3) "Know-it-all"—assumes to know the answers based on personal experience rather than sound evidence-based practice; often does not study or use educational resources
      (4) "Crammer"—procrastinates, then relies on last-minute memorization of facts
      (5) "Overachiever"—overanalyzes questions; loses original intent of the question; feels that the questions are not phrased properly, so they cannot be answered; becomes frustrated and possibly angry if he or she does not know the answer
      (6) "Second-guesser"—not satisfied with first responses to questions; changes answers after reviewing questions even though there is not appropriate rationale for doing so; never sure he or she is right; lacks confidence in his or her own practice and may lack experience
   m. Develop strategies to improve reactions to test-taking.
      (1) Practice controlling anxiety by taking practice tests in a simulated environment.
      (2) Recognize physiological responses to test-taking and develop methods to reduce stress (e.g., deep breathing and briefly closing eyes to envision something pleasant).
      (3) Practice reading each question and all answers aloud and not skipping over possibly important words.
      (4) Practice pacing and timing each question; allot a reasonable amount of time for each question.
      (5) Ensure that responses are based on sound nursing standards and practice.
      (6) Avoid reading into a question more information than is given.
      (7) Avoid re-reading answered questions.
   n. Develop a personal study plan.
4. Day before examination
   a. Know location of test center and parking areas.
   b. Prepare materials that are listed as required for admission (e.g., driver's license or a government-issued photo identification, pencils, nursing

license) and an admission confirmation such as an "admission to test" letter from the testing vendor.

  c. Take time to relax and practice relaxation techniques.

  d. Exercise and get adequate sleep.

  e. Keep a positive attitude.

  f. Plan an after-examination reward.

5. Day of examination

  a. Eat a good breakfast.

  b. Dress in bright colors.

  c. Dress in layers; rooms may be cold or hot.

  d. Water/snacks may or may not be allowed; avoid sugary snacks.

  e. Remember to take required admission materials.

  f. Arrive at the test site at least a few minutes before your appointed testing time.

  g. Follow the proctor's directions carefully.

B. Taking the examination

1. Most professional and certification organizations strive to avoid:

  a. "Giving away" answers in the construction of the question and answers (as indicated in section IV.B.13)

  b. Creating questions to confuse test-takers

  c. Giving cues to the correct answers in the stem

  d. Asking questions that do not address nursing knowledge and skills

  e. Designing trick questions

2. Anticipate not knowing some answers; it is not expected that you know all information.

3. Read the stem carefully and completely; do not jump to an answer without fully reading the question.

4. Focus on what the question is asking; do not infer content.

5. Answer the question mentally before reading the answers if possible.

6. Read ALL of the answers before responding; two may be very similar.

7. Discard wrong or highly implausible answers first.

8. Identify prioritizing questions that ask which action to do first; all answers may be correct, but identify which takes priority.

9. Be observant for stems that are phrased negatively; look for words like *except, all except,* and *not.*

10. Remember that superlatives such as *always, never,* and *all* are usually not true.

11. If testing is by paper method, mark questions you cannot answer immediately and come back to them; be sure to skip the appropriate number on the answer sheet.

12. If testing by computer, you may not be able to return to unmarked questions or change answers; read instructions carefully.

13. For some testing situations, the following guidelines may be used for guessing the answer:

  a. If two answers are similar except for one or two words, choose one of these answers.

  b. If two answers have similar sounding or looking words, choose one of these answers.

  c. If the stem calls for sentence completion, eliminate grammatically incorrect answers.

  d. If two quantities are almost the same, choose one.

  e. If answers cover a wide numerical range, choose the middle of the range.

  f. If all else fails, choose the longest answer.

14. Candidates are usually not penalized for guessing; answer all questions (25% chance of being right if there are four possible answers; 100% of being wrong if not answered at all).

15. Change an answer if you think you have a sound reason; research has demonstrated that changing answers actually improves scores in most cases.

16. Allot time frames for completing sections of the examination, leaving time for final review; for computer testing, the computer screen will have a clock that indicates how much time is left.
17. Use relaxation techniques during the examination.
    a. Neck and shoulder rolls, tightening and relaxing muscles in different parts of the body
    b. Mental breaks (e.g., imagining being beside an ocean or in a mountain briefly)
    c. Deep breathing exercises

C. Take-home points
    1. Study areas beyond your personal experience because certification and other examinations test one's knowledge of a subject and may not cover the test-taker's personal experiences (e.g., you might be tested on your knowledge regarding caring for a patient receiving mechanical ventilation even though you may not have taken care of such a patient).
    2. Set reasonable expectations.
    3. Know that the items are designed to test your knowledge and critical thinking skills, not to confuse you.
    4. Recognize that a mild to moderate level of anxiety enhances learning.
    5. Appreciate the fact that performing well involves two components:
       a. Knowledge and understanding of information about a subject
       b. Carefully reading and comprehending the stem and all distracters
    6. Regardless of the outcome of the examination, nurses report feeling better prepared to deliver high-quality patient care by studying for it.
    7. No certification examination outcome is a measure of one's self-worth.
    8. Celebrate successes both in learning and in test-taking.

V. ROLES OF CERTIFIED NURSES: PRECEPTOR, COACH, AND MENTOR
    A. Precepting
       1. Preceptor: an expert nurse formally assigned as a teacher and guide using more structured, organizational programs to orient:
          a. Newly graduated nurse into clinical practice
          b. Novice in a clinical specialty area through the competency requirements of that unit
       2. Preceptor identifies the novice's:
          a. Learning needs—level of knowledge and skills during the course of orientation
          b. Learning preferences—visual, auditory, or kinesthetic learning preferences
          c. Cognitive style—way of gathering, processing, and evaluating information
          d. Personality style—support during integration into the unit's norms
          e. Generational influences—work ethic and perceptions of age-related care
          f. Cultural influences—perceptions of health-related issues
          g. Educational background—nursing program, previous experiences
          h. Language challenges—comprehension of English and medical terminology
          i. Gender—may influence learning preferences, communication, integration into the unit
          j. Religious preferences—observance of religious events, honoring differences in patients and other staff
       3. Preceptor education should be provided for other skills such as:
          a. Teaching styles that enhance learning
          b. Providing feedback
          c. Effective listening
          d. Conflict resolution
          e. Clinical evaluation
       4. Includes practice of technical skills and development of critical thinking skills necessary to implement the nursing process
       5. May include the use of simulation and scenarios to educate and test skills before use on a patient

6. Provides day-to-day ongoing education, resources, and evaluations
7. Develops goals with the preceptee in order to facilitate learning
8. Usually has a preset, but adaptable, time-commitment

B. Coaching
1. Coach: a knowledgeable person who assists another person master more advanced knowledge and skills through exposure to developmental experiences
   a. Involves a contractual or semicontractual relationship
   b. Provides guidance and directs toward resources
   c. May participate in or lead individual or group learning activities
   d. May provide critical thinking activities and mock testing situations
   e. Provides positive feedback focusing on what can be done better rather than what was done wrong
2. Groups may share coaching responsibilities among the members.
3. Usually involves formally established times for communication
4. Communication interactions focus more on learning a skill, knowledge acquisition, and development of critical thinking abilities.

C. Mentoring
1. Mentor: a senior person in terms of maturity and experience who provides an interactive forum for advice, emotional support, and guidance for a mentee
   a. Involves a more personal relationship built on mutual trust and commitment
   b. May occur informally as the "chemistry" of the mentor and mentee develops over time
   c. May be a longer commitment
   d. May be a more intense relationship
   e. May have informal or formalized times for communication
   f. Have less structured communication interactions that are designed to delve deeper into the thoughts and rationale behind behaviors or actions
2. Provides a strategy for recruitment and retention of nurses
3. A process that enhances confidence in the mentee's abilities

D. Roles of preceptor, coach, and mentor may be combined or separate during the course of orientation and personal growth; in some cases, a preceptor or coach may not be the best mentor for a particular novice so another person may fulfill that role.

E. Level of experience and maturity of the novice, whether the nurse is newly graduated or new to the specialty area, should determine the role of the certified nurse.
1. A medical-surgical nurse may need precepting into a specialty area such as preoperative admitting or post anesthesia care units (PACU).
2. An intensive care unit nurse or experienced PACU nurse may need coaching rather than precepting.
3. All nurses need mentors in order to enhance their professional lives.

BIBLIOGRAPHY

1. American Association of Critical-Care Nurses, AACN Certification Corporation: Safeguarding the patient and the profession: The value of critical care nurse certification. *Am J Crit Care* 12(2):154–164, 2003.
2. American Board of Perianesthesia Nursing Certification (ABPANC): *Certification handbook and application: ABPANC's guide to CPAN® and CAPA® certification*, New York, 2002, Professional Examination Service.
3. American Board of Perianesthesia Nursing Certification: *Study tips for nurses seeking perianesthesia certification*, Available at: www.cpancapa.org/studytips.htm. Accessed September 25, 2008.
4. Baghi H, Panniers TL, Smolenski M: Description of practice as an ambulatory care nurse: Psychometric properties of a practice-analysis survey. *J Nurs Meas* 15(1):62–76, 2007.

5. Byrne M, Valentine W, Carter S: The value of certification: A research journey. *AORN J* 79(4):825–828, 831–835, 2004.

6. Harton BB: Clinical staff development: Planning and teaching for desired outcomes. *J Nurses Staff Dev* 23(6):260–268, 2007.

7. Lamonte MK: Test-taking strategies for CNOR certification. *AORN J* 85(2):315–332, 2007.

8. Ludwig C: Preparing for certification: Test-taking strategies. *Medsurg Nurs* 13(2):127–128, 2004.

9. Modic MB, Harris R: Masterful precepting: Using the become method to enhance clinical teaching. *J Nurses Staff Dev* 23(1):1–9; quiz 10–11, 2007.

10. Niebuhr B, Biel M: The value of specialty nursing certification. *Nurs Outlook* 55(4):176–181, 2007.

11. Niebuhr BS, Muensen P: A study of perianesthesia nursing practice: The foundation for newly revised CPAN and CAPA certification examinations. *J Perianesth Nurs* 16(3):163–173, 2001.

12. Pethtel P: Online learning communities can provide support for nurses preparing for certification examinations. *J Contin Educ Nurs* 36(2):55–56, 2005.

13. Piazza IM, Donahue M, Dykes PC, et al: Differences in perceptions of empower-ment among nationally certified and non-certified nurses. *J Nurs Adm* 36(5):277–283, 2006.

14. Ronsten B, Anderson E, Gustafsson B: Confirming mentorship. *J Nurs Manag* 13(4):312–321, 2005.

15. Schenk S, Hartley K: Nurse coach: Healthcare resource for this millennium. *Nurs Forum* 37(3):14–20, 2002.

16. Schwarz SP, McMorris RF, DeMers LP: Reasons for changing answers: An evaluation using personal interviews. *J Educ Meas* 28(2):164–171, 1991.

17. Sechrist KR, Valentine W, Berlin LE: Perceived value of certification among certified, noncertified, and administrative perioperative nurses. *J Prof Nurs* 22(4): 242–247, 2006.

18. Smith AB, Niebuhr B: Clarification of clinical experience requirement for CPAN/ CAPA certification. *J Perianesth Nurs* 22(3):158–159, 2007.

19. Stromborg MF, Niebuhr B, Prevost S, et al: Specialty certification: More than a title. *Nurs Manage* 36(5):36–46, 2005.

20. Su WM, Osisek PJ, Starnes B: Applying the Revised Bloom's Taxonomy to a medical-surgical nursing lesson. *Nurse Educ* 29(3):116–120, 2004.

Index

---

f indicates illustrations, b indicates boxes, and t indicates tables